HEMATOPOIETIC
STEM CELL
THERAPY

HEMATOPOIETIC
STEM CELL
THERAPY

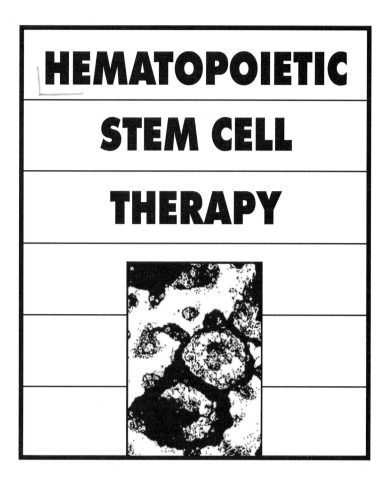

EDWARD D. BALL, M.D.
Professor of Medicine
Chief, Blood and Marrow Transplantation Division
University of California, San Diego, School of Medicine
La Jolla, California

JOHN LISTER, M.D.
Director, Blood and Marrow Transplantation Program
Western Pennsylvania Cancer Institute
The Western Pennsylvania Hospital
West Penn Allegheny Health System
Pittsburgh, Pennsylvania

PING LAW, Ph.D.
Assistant Adjunct Professor of Medicine
Director, Stem Cell Laboratory
Blood and Marrow Transplantation Division
University of California, San Diego, School of Medicine
La Jolla, California

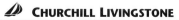 **CHURCHILL LIVINGSTONE**
A Harcourt Health Sciences Company
NEW YORK EDINBURGH LONDON PHILADELPHIA

CHURCHILL LIVINGSTONE
A Harcourt Health Sciences Company

The Curtis Center
Independence Square West
Philadelphia, Pennsylvania 19106

Library of Congress Cataloging-in-Publication Data

Hematopoietic stem cell therapy / [edited by] Edward D. Ball, John Lister,
Ping Law.—1st ed.

p.   cm.

ISBN 0–443–07622–7

1. Hematopoietic stem cells—Transplantation.   I. Ball, Edward D.
(Edward David).   II. Lister, John W.   III. Law, Ping.
[DNLM: 1. Hematopoietic Stem Cell Transplantation.   2. Neoplasms—
therapy.   WH 380 H4869 2000]

RM171.4.H46 2001   617.4′4—dc21

00-022729

Acquisitions Editor: Marc Strauss
Production Manager: Natalie Ware
Copy Editing Supervisor: Deborah Thorp
Illustration Specialist: Robert Quinn

HEMATOPOIETIC STEM CELL THERAPY   ISBN 0–443–07622–7

Printed in the United States of America.

Last digit is the print number: 9   8   7   6   5   4   3   2   1

We would like to dedicate this book to all of the patients and their loved ones who have bravely endured the considerable discomfort and emotional stress of undergoing hematopoietic stem cell transplantation (HSCT). They have contributed immensely to the improved practice of this treatment over the past two decades. We would also like to thank all of our colleagues in the medical, nursing, and allied health professions for their contributions to the life-saving treatment of HSCT. The efforts of the contributors, without whom this project would not have been possible, are deeply appreciated. We also thank Susan Shinagawa for her heroic efforts in helping us organize and manage this complex task. Finally, we are indebted to our families for their love and support and their willingness to grant us the extra time we needed to complete this task.

NOTICE

Hematology and Oncology are ever-changing fields. Standard safety precautions must be followed, but as new research and clinical experience broaden our knowledge, changes in treatment and drug therapy become necessary or appropriate. Readers are advised to check the product information currently provided by the manufacturer of each drug to be administered to verify the recommended dose, the method and duration of administration, and the contraindications. It is the responsibility of the treating physician, relying on experience and knowledge of the patient, to determine dosages and the best treatment for the patient. Neither the publisher nor the editor assumes any liability for any injury and/or damage to persons or property arising from this publication.

THE PUBLISHER

CONTRIBUTORS

ALFRED BAHNSON, Ph.D.
DIRECTOR OF CELL BIOLOGY, AUTOMATED CELL, INC., PITTS-BURGH, PENNSYLVANIA.
Gaucher Disease; Hematopoietic Stem Cells as Targets for Gene Therapy

EDWARD D. BALL, M.D.
PROFESSOR OF MEDICINE, CHIEF, BLOOD AND MARROW TRANS-PLANTATION DIVISION, UNIVERSITY OF CALIFORNIA, SAN DIEGO, SCHOOL OF MEDICINE, LA JOLLA, CALIFORNIA.
Gaucher Disease; Purging of Contaminating Tumor Cells; Hematopoietic Stem Cells as Targets for Gene Therapy; Failure of Engraftment; Late Graft Failure

BART BARLOGIE, M.D., Ph.D.
PROFESSOR OF MEDICINE AND PATHOLOGY, DIRECTOR OF AR-KANSAS CANCER RESEARCH CENTER, UNIVERSITY OF ARKAN-SAS SCHOOL OF MEDICINE, LITTLE ROCK, ARKANSAS.
Multiple Myeloma

JOHN A. BARRANGER, M.D., Ph.D.
PROFESSOR, DEPARTMENT OF HUMAN GENETICS, UNIVERSITY OF PITTSBURGH, PITTSBURGH, PENNSYLVANIA.
Gaucher Disease

ALISON A. BARTFIELD, M.D.
CLINICAL ASSISTANT PROFESSOR, DEPARTMENT OF MEDICINE, UNIVERSITY OF FLORIDA COLLEGE OF MEDICINE; CLINICAL ASSIS-TANT PROFESSOR, SHANDS HOSPITAL, GAINESVILLE, FLORIDA.
Use of Hematopoietic Growth Factors

ASAD BASHEY, M.D., Ph.D.
ASSISTANT PROFESSOR, BLOOD AND MARROW TRANSPLANTA-TION DIVISION, UNIVERSITY OF CALIFORNIA, SAN DIEGO, SCHOOL OF MEDICINE, LA JOLLA, CALIFORNIA.
Infection

MARY R. BURGUNDER, B.S.N.
BONE MARROW TRANSPLANT PROGRAM COORDINATOR, UNI-VERSITY OF PITTSBURGH MEDICAL CENTER HEALTH SYSTEM, UNI-VERSITY OF PITTSBURGH CANCER INSTITUTE, PITTSBURGH, PENN-SYLVANIA.
Coordination and Data Collection

RICHARD K. BURT, M.D.
ASSISTANT PROFESSOR OF MEDICINE, DIRECTOR OF ALLOGE-NEIC BONE MARROW TRANSPLANTATION/AUTOIMMUNE DIS-EASES, NORTHWESTERN UNIVERSITY, SCHOOL OF MEDICINE, CHICAGO, ILLINOIS.
Hematopoietic Stem Cell Transplantation for Severe Auto-immune Disease: Know Thyself

PABLO J. CAGNONI, M.D.
ASSISTANT PROFESSOR OF MEDICINE, UNIVERSITY OF COLO-RADO; ASSISTANT DIRECTOR, PHARMACOLOGY LABORATORY; UNIVERSITY OF COLORADO BONE MARROW TRANSPLANT PRO-GRAM, DENVER, COLORADO.
High-Dose Chemotherapy Conditioning Regimens for Au-tologous or Allogeneic Hematopoietic Stem Cell Trans-plantation

MATTHEW H. CARABASI, M.D.
ASSOCIATE PROFESSOR, DEPARTMENT OF MEDICINE, DIRECTOR, CLINICAL RESEARCH, BONE MARROW TRANSPLANTATION PRO-GRAM, DIVISION OF HEMATOLOGY/ONCOLOGY, UNIVERSITY OF ALABAMA AT BIRMINGHAM, BIRMINGHAM, ALABAMA.
Chronic Myelogenous Leukemia

TIMOTHY CARLOS, M.D.
ASSOCIATE PROFESSOR OF MEDICINE, UNIVERSITY OF PITTS-BURGH SCHOOL OF MEDICINE, PITTSBURGH, PENNYSLVANIA.
Hemoglobinopathies

EWA CARRIER, M.D.
ASSISTANT PROFESSOR OF MEDICINE AND PEDIATRICS, BLOOD AND MARROW TRANSPLANTATION DIVISION, UNIVERSITY OF CALIFORNIA, SAN DIEGO, SCHOOL OF MEDICINE, LA JOLLA, CALIFORNIA.
In Utero Transplantation

KELLI A. CAWLEY, M.D.
ASSISTANT PROFESSOR OF CLINICAL MEDICINE, DIVISION OF HEMATOLOGY/ONCOLOGY, OHIO STATE UNIVERSITY, COLUM-BUS, OHIO.
Acute Lymphoblastic Leukemia

RICHARD E. CHAMPLIN, M.D.
PROFESSOR OF MEDICINE, CHAIRMAN, DEPARTMENT OF BLOOD AND MARROW TRANSPLANTATION, UNIVERSITY OF TEXAS M.D. ANDERSON CANCER CENTER, HOUSTON, TEXAS.
Relapse After Hematopoietic Stem Cell Therapy: Mecha-nisms and Treatment

JIAN CHEN, M.D.
FELLOW, BLOOD AND MARROW TRANSPLANTATION DIVISION, UNIVERSITY OF CALIFORNIA, SAN DIEGO, SCHOOL OF MEDI-CINE, LA JOLLA, CALIFORNIA.
Failure of Engraftment; Late Graft Failure

IAN CHIN-YEE, M.D.

ASSOCIATE PROFESSOR OF MEDICINE, UNIVERSITY OF WESTERN ONTARIO; CONSULTANT IN HEMATOLOGY, LONDON HEALTH SCIENCES CENTRE, LONDON, ONTARIO, CANADA.

Stem Cell Quantification: The ISHAGE Guidelines for CD34+ Determination—Applications in Autologous and Allogeneic Hematopoietic Stem Cell Transplantation

MARY CLAY, M.S.

ADMINISTRATIVE SCIENTIST, DEPARTMENT OF LABORATORY MEDICINE AND PATHOLOGY, DIVISION OF TRANSFUSION MEDICINE, UNIVERSITY OF MINNESOTA, MINNEAPOLIS, MINNESOTA.

Cord Blood Stem Cells

KAREN CLEARY, M.D.

PROFESSOR OF PATHOLOGY, UNIVERSITY OF TEXAS M.D. ANDERSON CANCER CENTER, HOUSTON, TEXAS.

Therapy of Acute Graft-Versus-Host Disease

EDWARD A. COPELAN, M.D.

ASSOCIATE PROFESSOR OF INTERNAL MEDICINE, OHIO STATE UNIVERSITY COLLEGE OF MEDICINE AND PUBLIC HEALTH, BONE MARROW TRANSPLANT PROGRAM, COLUMBUS, OHIO.

Acute Lymphoblastic Leukemia

JAKE DEMETRIS, M.D.

PROFESSOR OF PATHOLOGY, UNIVERSITY OF PITTSBURGH SCHOOL OF MEDICINE; DIRECTOR, DIVISION OF TRANSPLANT PATHOLOGY, UNIVERSITY OF PITTSBURGH MEDICAL CENTER, PITTSBURGH, PENNSYLVANIA.

Liver Disease in Hematopoietic Stem Cell Transplant Recipients

ALBERT D. DONNENBERG, Ph.D.

ASSOCIATE PROFESSOR OF MEDICINE, UNIVERSITY OF PITTSBURGH; DIRECTOR, BLOOD AND MARROW PROCESSING LABORATORY, UNIVERSITY OF PITTSBURGH MEDICAL CENTER; DIRECTOR, FLOW CYTOMETRY FACILITY, UNIVERSITY OF PITTSBURGH CANCER INSTITUTE, PITTSBURGH, PENNSYLVANIA.

T-Cell Depletion and Allograft Engineering

GERALD J. ELFENBEIN, M.D.

DIRECTOR, CANCER CENTER, DIRECTOR, BLOOD AND MARROW TRANSPLANT PROGRAM, ROGER WILLIAMS MEDICAL CENTER, PROVIDENCE, RHODE ISLAND.

Breast Cancer

KAREN K. FIELDS, M.D.

PROFESSOR OF MEDICINE, UNIVERSITY OF SOUTH FLORIDA, COLLEGE OF MEDICINE, TAMPA, FLORIDA.

Breast Cancer

ALEXANDRA FILIPOVICH, M.D.

PROFESSOR OF PEDIATRICS, UNIVERSITY OF CINCINNATI SCHOOL OF MEDICINE, CHILDREN'S HOSPITAL MEDICAL CENTER, CINCINNATI, OHIO.

Hematopoietic Stem Cell Transplantation for Treatment of Congenital Immunodeficiencies

ADRIAN P. GEE, M.I. Biol., Ph.D.

PROFESSOR OF MEDICINE, DEPARTMENT OF PEDIATRICS, DIRECTOR, CLINICAL APPLICATIONS LAB, BAYLOR COLLEGE OF MEDICINE, HOUSTON, TEXAS.

Regulation of Hematopoietic Progenitor Stem Cell Therapy

ROBERT B. GELLER, M.D.

CLINICAL PROFESSOR OF MEDICINE, UNIVERSITY OF MISSOURI—KANSAS CITY; MEDICAL DIRECTOR, BLOOD AND MARROW TRANSPLANT PROGRAM, SAINT LUKE'S HOSPITAL AND ONCOLOGY-HEMATOLOGY ASSOCIATES OF KANSAS CITY, KANSAS CITY, MISSOURI.

Myelodysplasia

SERGIO A. GIRALT, M.D.

ASSOCIATE PROFESSOR OF MEDICINE, DEPARTMENT OF BLOOD AND MARROW TRANSPLANTATION, UNIVERSITY OF TEXAS M.D. ANDERSON CANCER CENTER, HOUSTON, TEXAS.

Relapse After Hematopoietic Stem Cell Therapy: Mechanisms and Treatment

WILLIAM D. HAIRE, M.D.

UNIVERSITY OF NEBRASKA MEDICAL CENTER; MEDICAL STAFF, VETERANS AFFAIRS HOSPITAL, OMAHA, NEBRASKA.

Coagulopathy During Transplantation

LISA HAMMERT, M.D.

UNIVERSITY OF PITTSBURGH MEDICAL CENTER, PITTSBURGH, PENNSYLVANIA.

Neurologic Complications

RICHARD B. HART II, M.D.

STAFF PHYSICIAN, DEPARTMENT OF INTERNAL MEDICINE, THE WASHINGTON HOSPITAL, WASHINGTON, PENNSYLVANIA.

Bacteria

JOYCE HERSCHL, M.S.W.

FIELD INSTRUCTOR, SCHOOL OF SOCIAL WORK, UNIVERSITY OF PITTSBURGH; PROGRAM COORDINATOR, UNIVERSITY OF PITTSBURGH CANCER INSTITUTE ONCOLOGY SOCIAL WORK SERVICES, UNIVERSITY OF PITTSBURGH MEDICAL CENTER, PITTSBURGH, PENNSYLVANIA.

Psychosocial Considerations: A Family Approach to Patient Care

BRUCE E. HILLNER, M.D.

PROFESSOR OF MEDICINE, VIRGINIA COMMONWEALTH UNIVERSITY, RICHMOND, VIRGINIA.

Economics

PETER R. HOLMAN, M.B., B.Ch.

ASSISTANT PROFESSOR OF MEDICINE, BLOOD AND MARROW TRANSPLANTATION DIVISION, UNIVERSITY OF CALIFORNIA, SAN DIEGO, SCHOOL OF MEDICINE, LA JOLLA, CALIFORNIA.

Myelodysplasia and Second Malignancies

SUNDAR JAGANNATH, M.D.

PROFESSOR OF MEDICINE, NEW YORK MEDICAL COLLEGE, DIRECTOR OF MULTIPLE MYELOMA PROGRAM AND BONE MARROW TRANSPLANT, ST. VINCENT'S COMPREHENSIVE CANCER CENTER, NEW YORK, NEW YORK.

Multiple Myeloma

ROY B. JONES, M.D., Ph.D.

PROFESSOR OF MEDICINE, UNIVERSITY OF COLORADO HEALTH SCIENCES CENTER; DIRECTOR, MARROW TRANSPLANTATION, UNIVERSITY OF COLORADO HOSPITAL, DENVER, COLORADO.

High-Dose Chemotherapy Conditioning Regimens for Autologous or Allogeneic Hematopoietic Stem Cell Transplantation

ARMAND KEATING, M.D.

PROFESSOR OF MEDICINE, EPSTEIN CHAIR IN CELL THERAPY AND TRANSPLANTATION, UNIVERSITY OF TORONTO; CHIEF, MEDICAL SERVICES, PRINCESS MARGARET HOSPITAL, TORONTO, ONTARIO, CANADA.

Acute Myelogenous Leukemia

MICHAEL KEENEY, A.R.T., F.I.M.L.S.

TECHNICAL SPECIALIST, FLOW CYTOMETRY/HEMATOLOGY, LONDON HEALTH SCIENCES CENTRE, LONDON, ONTARIO, CANADA.

Stem Cell Quantification: The ISHAGE Guidelines for CD34+ Determination—Applications in Autologous and Allogeneic Hematopoietic Stem Cell Transplantation

HAESOOK T. KIM, Ph.D.

DANA-FARBER CANCER INSTITUTE, BOSTON, MASSACHUSETTS.

Biostatistics

HANS-GEORG KLINGEMANN, M.D., Ph.D.

COLEMAN PROFESSOR OF MEDICINE, RUSH MEDICAL COLLEGE; DIRECTOR, BONE MARROW TRANSPLANT AND CELL THERAPY, RUSH PRESBYTERIAN-ST. LUKE'S MEDICAL CENTER, CHICAGO, ILLINOIS.

Biologic Therapy After Hematopoietic Stem Cell Transplantation

MARIA M. KOEHLER, M.D., Ph.D.

ASSOCIATE PROFESSOR, HAHNEMANN UNIVERSITY; DIRECTOR, BONE MARROW TRANSPLANTATION, ST. CHRISTOPHER'S HOSPITAL FOR CHILDREN, PHILADELPHIA, PENNSYLVANIA.

Childhood Solid Tumors

ROBERT A. KRANCE, M.D.

PROFESSOR OF PEDIATRICS/MEDICINE, BAYLOR COLLEGE OF MEDICINE; DIRECTOR, PEDIATRIC STEM CELL TRANSPLANTATION, TEXAS CHILDREN'S HOSPITAL, HOUSTON, TEXAS.

Childhood Solid Tumors

JOHN W. KREIT, M.D.

ASSISTANT PROFESSOR OF MEDICINE, DIVISION OF PULMONARY AND CRITICAL CARE MEDICINE, UNIVERSITY OF PITTSBURGH SCHOOL OF MEDICINE, PITTSBURGH, PENNSYLVANIA.

Respiratory Complications

WILLIAM KRIVIT, M.D., Ph.D.

ACTIVE PROFESSOR EMERITUS, UNIVERSITY OF MINNESOTA MEDICAL SCHOOL, FAIRVIEW-UNIVERSITY MEDICAL CENTER, DIVISION OF PEDIATRIC HEMATOLOGY-ONCOLOGY AND BLOOD AND MARROW TRANSPLANTATION, MINNEAPOLIS, MINNESOTA.

Metabolic Diseases

THOMAS A. LANE, M.D.

PROFESSOR, DEPARTMENT OF PATHOLOGY, UNIVERSITY OF CALIFORNIA, SAN DIEGO, SCHOOL OF MEDICINE, LA JOLLA, CALIFORNIA; MEDICAL DIRECTOR, WESTERN AREA COMMUNITY CORD BLOOD BANK, AMERICAN RED CROSS, PORTLAND, OREGON.

Peripheral Blood Progenitor Cell Mobilization and Collection

PING LAW, Ph.D.

ASSISTANT ADJUNCT PROFESSOR OF MEDICINE, DIRECTOR, STEM CELL LABORATORY, BLOOD AND MARROW TRANSPLANTATION DIVISION, UNIVERSITY OF CALIFORNIA, SAN DIEGO, SCHOOL OF MEDICINE, LA JOLLA, CALIFORNIA.

Graft Processing, Storage, and Infusion; Failure of Engraftment; Late Graft Failure

JOHN LISTER, M.D.

DIRECTOR, BLOOD AND MARROW TRANSPLANTATION PROGRAM, WESTERN PENNSYLVANIA CANCER INSTITUTE, THE WESTERN PENNSYLVANIA HOSPITAL, WEST PENN ALLEGHENY HEALTH SYSTEM, PITTSBURGH, PENNSYLVANIA.

Choice of Donor; Bone Marrow Harvesting

PER LJUNGMAN, M.D., Ph.D.

HEAD, SECTION OF HEMATOLOGY, DEPARTMENT OF MEDICINE, KAROLINSKA INSTITUTET; HEAD, DEPARTMENT OF HEMATOLOGY, HUDDINGE UNIVERSITY HOSPITAL, HUDDINGE, SWEDEN.

Viral Infections

ILEANA LÓPEZ-PLAZA, M.D.

ASSISTANT PROFESSOR OF PATHOLOGY, UNIVERSITY OF PITTSBURGH SCHOOL OF MEDICINE; ASSOCIATE DIRECTOR, PATIENT TRANSFUSION SERVICES; ASSOCIATE MEDICAL DIRECTOR, CENTRALIZED TRANSFUSION SERVICES, UNIVERSITY OF PITTSBURGH MEDICAL CENTER; INSTITUTE FOR TRANSFUSION MEDICINE; PITTSBURGH, PENNSYLVANIA.

Transfusion Support in Hematopoietic Stem Cell Transplantation

MARGARIDA DE MAGALHÃES-SILVERMAN, M.D.

ASSOCIATE PROFESSOR OF MEDICINE, UNIVERSITY OF IOWA COLLEGE OF MEDICINE, IOWA CITY, IOWA.

Neurologic Complications; Post-Transplant Cytotoxic Therapy

KENNETH F. MANGAN, M.D.

PROFESSOR OF MEDICINE, DIRECTOR, BONE MARROW TRANSPLANT PROGRAM, TEMPLE UNIVERSITY SCHOOL OF MEDICINE, PHILADELPHIA, PENNSYLVANIA.

Aplastic Anemia; Choice of Conditioning Regimens

DEBORAH C. MARCELLUS, M.D.

ASSISTANT PROFESSOR OF ONCOLOGY, JOHNS HOPKINS UNIVERSITY SCHOOL OF MEDICINE, BALTIMORE, MARYLAND.

Chronic Graft-Versus-Host Disease

JOAN MARTELL, C.H.S.

SUPERVISOR, HISTOCOMPATIBILITY LABORATORIES, UNIVERSITY OF PITTSBURGH MEDICAL CENTER, PITTSBURGH, PENNSYLVANIA.

Histocompatibility

AMITABHA MAZUMDER, M.D.

PROFESSOR OF MEDICINE, DIRECTOR OF BONE MARROW TRANSPLANTATION, STATE UNIVERSITY OF NEW YORK AT STONY BROOK, STONY BROOK, NEW YORK.

Immunomodulation After Transplantation

JEFFREY McCULLOUGH, M.D.

PROFESSOR, DEPARTMENT OF LABORATORY MEDICINE AND PATHOLOGY, UNIVERSITY OF MINNESOTA MEDICAL SCHOOL; VARIETY CLUB CHAIR AND DIRECTOR, CENTER FOR MOLECULAR AND CELLULAR THERAPY, UNIVERSITY OF MINNESOTA, MINNEAPOLIS, MINNESOTA.

Cord Blood Stem Cells

KENNETH R. MEEHAN, M.D.

ASSISTANT PROFESSOR OF MEDICINE, DIRECTOR, ADULT BONE MARROW TRANSPLANT RESEARCH LABORATORY, GEORGETOWN UNIVERSITY MEDICAL CENTER, VINCENT T. LOMBARDI CANCER CENTER, WASHINGTON, D.C.

Immunomodulation After Transplantation

MAURICETTE MICHALLET, M.D., Ph.D.

ASSISTANT PROFESSOR, UNIVERSITÉ CLAUDE BERNARD LYON; HEAD OF BONE MARROW TRANSPLANT UNIT, HÔPITAL EDOUARD HERRIOT, LYON, FRANCE.

Chronic Lymphocytic Leukemia

HAN MYINT, M.B.B.S., M.R.C.Path.

CONSULTANT HAEMATOLOGIST, DIRECTOR OF BONE MARROW TRANSPLANT CENTRE, CLINICAL DIRECTOR OF PATHOLOGY DIRECTORATE, ROYAL BOURNEMOUTH HOSPITAL, BOURNEMOUTH, UNITED KINGDOM.

Fungi and Other Organisms

STEVEN NEUDORF, M.D.

DIRECTOR, BLOOD AND MARROW TRANSPLANT PROGRAM, CHILDREN'S HOSPITAL OF ORANGE COUNTY, ORANGE, CALIFORNIA.

Hematopoietic Stem Cell Transplantation for Treatment of Congenital Immunodeficiencies

CRAIG R. NICHOLS, M.D.

PROFESSOR OF MEDICINE, OREGON HEALTH SCIENCES UNIVERSITY, PORTLAND, OREGON.

Germ Cell Tumors

YAGO NIETO, M.D.

INSTRUCTOR, UNIVERSITY OF COLORADO, DENVER, COLORADO.

Ex Vivo Stem Cell Expansion; High-Dose Chemotherapy Conditioning Regimens for Autologous or Allogeneic Hematopoietic Stem Cell Transplantation

DAVID J. OBLON, M.D.

CLINICAL PROFESSOR OF MEDICINE, UNIVERSITY OF CALIFORNIA, SAN DIEGO, SCHOOL OF MEDICINE, LA JOLLA; DIRECTOR, BLOOD AND BONE MARROW TRANSPLANT PROGRAM, SHARP HEALTH CARE, SAN DIEGO, CALIFORNIA.

Evaluation of Patients Before Hematopoietic Stem Cell Transplantation

ERIN O'ROURKE, M.S., O.G.C.

INSTRUCTOR, UNIVERSITY OF PITTSBURGH, PITTSBURGH, PENNSYLVANIA.

Gaucher Disease

ANDREW PECORA, M.D.

ASSOCIATE CLINICAL PROFESSOR OF MEDICINE, UNIVERSITY OF MEDICINE AND DENTISTRY, NEW JERSEY MEDICAL SCHOOL; CHIEF, ADULT BLOOD AND MARROW TRANSPLANT PROGRAM, HACKENSACK UNIVERSITY MEDICAL CENTER, HACKENSACK, NEW JERSEY.

Stem Cell Quantification: The ISHAGE Guidelines for CD34+ Determination—Applications in Autologous and Allogeneic Hematopoietic Stem Cell Transplantation

JANELLE B. PERKINS, Pharm.D.

ASSISTANT PROFESSOR, UNIVERSITY OF SOUTH FLORIDA, TAMPA, FLORIDA.

Breast Cancer

CHARLES PETERS, M.D.

ASSOCIATE PROFESSOR, UNIVERSITY OF MINNESOTA MEDICAL SCHOOL, FAIRVIEW-UNIVERSITY MEDICAL CENTER, DIVISION OF PEDIATRIC HEMATOLOGY-ONCOLOGY AND BLOOD AND MARROW TRANSPLANTATION, MINNEAPOLIS, MINNESOTA.

Metabolic Diseases

GORDON L. PHILLIPS, M.D.

PROFESSOR OF MEDICINE, DIRECTOR, BLOOD AND MARROW TRANSPLANT PROGRAM, MARKEY CANCER CENTER, UNIVERSITY OF KENTUCKY, LEXINGTON, KENTUCKY.

Hodgkin Disease

DONNA PRZEPIORKA, M.D., Ph.D.

ASSOCIATE PROFESSOR OF MEDICINE, PEDIATRICS AND IMMUNOLOGY; ASSOCIATE DIRECTOR, STEM CELL TRANSPLANT PROGRAM, BAYLOR COLLEGE OF MEDICINE, CENTER FOR CELL AND GENE THERAPY, HOUSTON, TEXAS.

Prevention of Acute Graft-Versus-Host Disease; Therapy of Acute Graft-Versus-Host Disease

JORGE RAKELA, M.D.

PROFESSOR OF MEDICINE, MAYO MEDICAL SCHOOL; CHAIR, DIVISION OF TRANSPLANTATION MEDICINE, VICE-CHAIR, DEPARTMENT OF MEDICINE, MAYO CLINIC SCOTTSDALE, SCOTTSDALE, ARIZONA.

Liver Disease in Hematopoietic Stem Cell Transplant Recipients

DONNA E. REECE, M.D.

ASSOCIATE PROFESSOR OF MEDICINE, BLOOD AND MARROW TRANSPLANT PROGRAM, MARKEY CANCER CENTER, UNIVERSITY OF KENTUCKY, LEXINGTON, KENTUCKY.

Hodgkin Disease

CHERYL L. ROCK, Ph.D., R.D.

ASSOCIATE PROFESSOR, DEPARTMENT OF FAMILY AND PREVENTIVE MEDICINE AND CANCER PREVENTION AND CONTROL PROGRAM, UNIVERSITY OF CALIFORNIA, SAN DIEGO, SCHOOL OF MEDICINE, LA JOLLA, CALIFORNIA.

Nutritional Issues and Management in Hematopoietic Stem Cell Transplantation

GAYLE ROSNER, Ph.D.

ASSISTANT PROFESSOR, DEPARTMENT OF PATHOLOGY, UNIVERSITY OF PITTSBURGH SCHOOL OF MEDICINE, PITTSBURGH, PENNSYLVANIA.

Histocompatibility

PHILLIP ROWLINGS, M.B.B.S., M.S., F.R.A.C.P., F.R.C.P.A.

HEAD, BONE MARROW TRANSPLANT SERVICE, DEPARTMENT OF HAEMATOLOGY, PRINCE OF WALES HOSPITAL, RANDWICK, SYDNEY, NSW, AUSTRALIA.

Hematopoietic Stem Cell Transplantation for Severe Autoimmune Disease: Know Thyself

JOSHUA RUBIN, M.D.

ASSOCIATE PROFESSOR OF SURGERY, UNIVERSITY OF PITTSBURGH SCHOOL OF MEDICINE, PITTSBURGH, PENNSYLVANIA.

Long-Term Venous Access During Hematopoietic Stem Cell Transplantation; Surgical Emergencies

BARBARA RUTECKI, R.N., M.S.N., M.P.H.

ADULT NURSE PRACTITIONER, DIVISION OF INFECTIOUS DISEASE, UNIVERSITY OF PITTSBURGH SCHOOL OF MEDICINE, PITTSBURGH, PENNSYLVANIA.

Bone Marrow Harvesting

ELIZABETH J. SHPALL, M.D.

PROFESSOR OF MEDICINE, ASSOCIATE DIRECTOR, BONE MARROW TRANSPLANT PROGRAM, UNIVERSITY OF COLORADO SCHOOL OF MEDICINE, DENVER, COLORADO.

Ex Vivo Stem Cell Expansion

WILLIAM B. SILVERMAN, M.D.

ASSOCIATE PROFESSOR OF MEDICINE, DIRECTOR, MEDICAL INTENSIVE CARE UNIT, PULMONARY AND CRITICAL CARE MEDICINE, UNIVERSITY OF PITTSBURGH MEDICAL CENTER, PITTSBURGH, PENNSYLVANIA.

Mucositis and Other Gastrointestinal Complications

DAVID R. SIMPSON, M.D.

ASSISTANT PROFESSOR, RUSH PRESBYTERIAN-ST. LUKE'S MEDICAL CENTER, CHICAGO, ILLINOIS.

Acute Myelogenous Leukemia

JENNIFER K. SIMPSON, M.S.N., Ph.D.

INSTRUCTOR, UNIVERSITY OF PITTSBURGH MEDICAL CENTER, PITTSBURGH, PENNSYLVANIA.

Specialized Nursing; Coordination and Data Collection

THOMAS J. SMITH M.D.

CHAIR, DIVISION OF HEMATOLOGY/ONCOLOGY, ASSOCIATE PROFESSOR OF MEDICINE AND HEALTH ADMINISTRATION, VIRGINIA COMMONWEALTH UNIVERSITY, RICHMOND, VIRGINIA.

Economics

PATRICK J. STIFF, M.D.

PROFESSOR OF MEDICINE, DIVISION OF HEMATOLOGY-ONCOLOGY, DEPARTMENT OF MEDICINE, LOYOLA UNIVERSITY MEDICAL CENTER, STRITCH SCHOOL OF MEDICINE; DIRECTOR, BONE MARROW TRANSPLANT PROGRAM, CARDINAL BERNARDI CANCER CENTER, LOYOLA UNIVERSITY MEDICAL CENTER, MAYWOOD, ILLINOIS.

Ovarian Cancer

D. ROBERT SUTHERLAND, M.Sc.

ASSOCIATE PROFESSOR, DEPARTMENT OF MEDICINE, UNIVERSITY OF TORONTO; STAFF SCIENTIST, DIVISION OF HEMATOLOGY/ONCOLOGY, SCIENTIST, AUTOLOGOUS BLOOD AND BONE MARROW TRANSPLANT PROGRAM, THE TORONTO HOSPITAL, TORONTO, ONTARIO, CANADA.

Stem Cell Quantification: The ISHAGE Guidelines for CD34+ Determination—Applications in Autologous and Allogeneic Hematopoietic Stem Cell Transplantation

MUSHTAQ SYED, M.D.

FELLOW IN ENDOCRINOLOGY AND METABOLISM, UNIVERSITY OF PITTSBURGH MEDICAL CENTER, PITTSBURGH, PENNSYLVANIA.

Endocrine and Metabolic Complications

STEFANO R. TARANTOLO, M.D.

ASSOCIATE PROFESSOR OF MEDICINE, UNIVERSITY OF NEBRASKA COLLEGE OF MEDICINE, OMAHA, NEBRASKA.

Coagulopathy During Transplantation

ANN TRAYNOR, M.D.

ASSISTANT PROFESSOR OF MEDICINE, DIVISION OF HEMATOLOGY/ONCOLOGY, NORTHWESTERN UNIVERSITY MEDICAL SCHOOL, CHICAGO, ILLINOIS.

Hematopoietic Stem Cell Transplantation for Severe Autoimmune Disease: Know Thyself

DARRELL J. TRIULTZI, M.D.

ASSOCIATE PROFESSOR OF PATHOLOGY AND MEDICINE, UNIVERSITY OF PITTSBURGH SCHOOL OF MEDICINE; DIRECTOR, DIVISION OF TRANSFUSION MEDICINE, UNIVERSITY OF PITTSBURGH MEDICAL CENTER; MEDICAL DIRECTOR, INSTITUTE FOR TRANSITION MEDICINE, PITTSBURGH, PENNSYLVANIA.

Transfusion Support in Hematopoietic Stem Cell Transplantation

MASSIMO TRUCCO, M.D.

PROFESSOR, DEPARTMENT OF PEDIATRICS, UNIVERSITY OF PITTSBURGH SCHOOL OF MEDICINE; HILLMAN PROFESSOR OF PEDIATRIC IMMUNOLOGY, HEAD, DIVISION OF IMMUNOGENETICS, DIRECTOR, CHILDREN'S HOSPITAL OF PITTSBURGH HISTOCOMPATIBILITY CENTER, CHILDREN'S HOSPITAL OF PITTSBURGH, PITTSBURGH, PENNSYLVANIA.

Histocompatibility

DAVID J. TWEARDY, M.D.

CHIEF, SECTION OF INFECTIOUS DISEASES, PROFESSOR OF MEDICINE, BAYLOR COLLEGE OF MEDICINE, HOUSTON, TEXAS.

Infection and Immunization

DAVOOD VAFAI, M.D.

ASSOCIATE PHYSICIAN, BONE MARROW TRANSPLANTATION DIVISION, UNIVERSITY OF CALIFORNIA, SAN DIEGO, SCHOOL OF MEDICINE, LA JOLLA, CALIFORNIA.

Purging of Contaminating Tumor Cells

HUGO E. VARGAS, M.D.

ASSISTANT PROFESSOR OF MEDICINE, UNIVERSITY OF PITTSBURGH SCHOOL OF MEDICINE, PITTSBURGH, PENNSYLVANIA.

Mucositis and Other Gastrointestinal Complications

UDIT N. VERMA, M.D.

INSTRUCTOR, GEORGETOWN UNIVERSITY MEDICAL CENTER, VINCENT T. LOMBARDI CANCER CENTER, WASHINGTON, D.C.

Immunomodulation After Transplantation

RAKESH VINAYEK, M.D.

MEDICAL DIRECTOR, LIVER TRANSPLANTATION, INOVA FAIRFAX HOSPITAL, FALLS CHURCH, VIRGINIA; CLINICAL ASSOCIATE PROFESSOR OF MEDICINE, UNIVERSITY OF MARYLAND SCHOOL OF MEDICINE, BALTIMORE, MARYLAND.

Liver Disease in Hematopoietic Stem Cell Transplant Recipients

GEORGIA B. VOGELSANG, M.D.

PROFESSOR OF ONCOLOGY, CLINICAL DIRECTOR, BONE MARROW TRANSPLANTATION, JOHNS HOPKINS UNIVERSITY SCHOOL OF MEDICINE, BALTIMORE, MARYLAND.

Chronic Graft-Versus-Host Disease

JULIE M. VOSE, M.D.

PROFESSOR OF MEDICINE, UNIVERSITY OF NEBRASKA MEDICAL CENTER, OMAHA, NEBRASKA.

Lymphoma

JAMES J. VREDENBURGH, M.D.

ASSOCIATE PROFESSOR OF MEDICINE, DUKE UNIVERSITY, DURHAM, NORTH CAROLINA.

Purging of Contaminating Tumor Cells

JOHN E. WAGNER, M.D.

PROFESSOR OF PEDIATRICS, UNIVERSITY OF MINNESOTA MEDICAL SCHOOL; ASSOCIATE DIRECTOR, PEDIATRIC BONE MARROW TRANSPLANTATION, ATTENDING FACULTY, FAIRVIEW-UNIVERSITY MEDICAL CENTER, MINNEAPOLIS, MINNESOTA.

Cord Blood Stem Cells

SCOTT M. WHITE, M.D.

ASSISTANT PROFESSOR OF MEDICINE, UNIVERSITY OF PITTSBURGH SCHOOL OF MEDICINE, PITTSBURGH, PENNSYLVANIA.

Infection and Immunization

JOHN W. WILSON Ph.D.

ASSISTANT PROFESSOR, DEPARTMENT OF BIOSTATISTICS, GRADUATE SCHOOL OF PUBLIC HEALTH, UNIVERSITY OF PITTSBURGH, PITTSBURGH, PENNSYLVANIA.

Biostatistics

EDWARD J. WING, M.D.

JOUKOWSKY FAMILY PROFESSOR AND CHAIRMAN, DEPARTMENT OF MEDICINE, BROWN UNIVERSITY SCHOOL OF MEDICINE; PHYSICIAN-IN-CHIEF, CHIEF OF MEDICINE, RHODE ISLAND HOSPITAL AND THE MIRIAM HOSPITAL, LIFESPAN RI ACADEMIC MEDICAL CENTER, PROVIDENCE, RHODE ISLAND.

Bacteria

JOHN R. WINGARD, M.D.

PROFESSOR OF MEDICINE AND PEDIATRICS, UNIVERSITY OF FLORIDA COLLEGE OF MEDICINE; DIRECTOR, BONE MARROW TRANSPLANT PROGRAM, SHANDS HOSPITAL, GAINESVILLE, FLORIDA.

Use of Hematopoietic Growth Factors

STEPHEN J. WINTERS, M.D.

PROFESSOR OF MEDICINE, UNIVERSITY OF LOUISVILLE SCHOOL OF MEDICINE; CHIEF, DIVISION OF ENDOCRINOLOGY AND METABOLISM, UNIVERSITY OF LOUISVILLE HEALTH SCIENCES CENTER, LOUISVILLE, KENTUCKY.

Endocrine and Metabolic Complications

SAUL A. YANOVICH, M.D.

PROFESSOR OF MEDICINE, DIRECTOR, BONE MARROW TRANSPLANT UNIT, VIRGINIA COMMONWEALTH UNIVERSITY, RICHMOND, VIRGINIA.

Economics

PREFACE

Hematopoietic stem cell (HSC) transplantation (HSCT) has emerged as a major treatment modality for a variety of malignant and nonmalignant diseases. After a turbulent period when the underlying biology of HSC, the involvement of mature leukocytes and stromal cell populations in the homing and growth of HSC, as well as the elements of supportive care were not fully understood or developed, the modern practice of HSCT has evolved dramatically. At present, more than 40,000 HSCT procedures are performed annually worldwide. Although HSCT started with allogeneic bone marrow transplantation, autologous transplantation became more frequent in the early 1990s (an equal number of autologous and allogeneic transplants were performed in 1989), especially with the replacement of bone marrow with mobilized peripheral blood progenitor cells (PBPC). Although this remains true, current trends suggest that the balance may be altered in the future. One important development is the emergence of less intense conditioning regimens, leading to the ability to treat older patients successfully with less toxicity. A second trend is the emergence of a wider array of alternative donors for allogeneic transplantation, such as mismatched related donors and use of cord blood. Use of mobilized PBPC in allogeneic transplantation has shortened neutrophil and platelet engraftment. Greater understanding of graft-versus-host disease prophylaxis and treatment has allowed an expanded donor pool to be applied to more patients who might otherwise not have been eligible to benefit from transplantation.

The explosion of knowledge of cancer biology and immunology has led to an amazing proliferation of literature. For the physician practicing HSCT, these source materials are quite diverse. In this book, we have attempted to summarize the current state of knowledge of the management of the transplant patient into a series of presentations that mirror the progress of a patient from diagnosis, through HSCT, to post-transplant complications (i.e., situations commonly encountered in the real world of the practitioner). Thus, we begin by outlining the approach to the patient with a variety of diseases treated by high-dose chemotherapy and HSCT, including the specific issues of transplantation in these subgroups. We then focus on the specifics of the preparation of the patient and donor for the transplant procedure. The third section concentrates on the specific issues of the transplant process itself, the conditioning regimen, the expected post-transplant problems, and the expected longer-term transplant problems. Possible therapies for relapse and/or treatments in addition to HSCT are discussed in the next group of chapters. Last, but not least, important issues such as psychosocial evaluation, HSCT nursing, data management, statistical methods and analyses, economics, and the regulatory environment of HSCT are addressed. We have asked that the contributors focus on practical approaches to the common and not-so-common problems encountered by the practitioner of this treatment modality. Specific recommendations are included, whenever possible.

PBPC has been used increasingly as the source of HSC. Historically, the replacement of malignant or abnormal HSC is accomplished by conditioning the patient and infusing healthy bone marrow from a matched sibling donor. When autologous transplantation gained in popularity in the 1980s, the increase in HSC in the peripheral blood following chemotherapy was recognized and was quickly adopted as a source of HSC. Rapid engraftment of PBPC, as compared with bone marrow, which has led to fewer transfusions, earlier hospital discharge, and lower costs, has made PBPC the primary source of HSC in autologous transplantation. The development and widespread use of hematopoietic growth factors coupled with the success in autologous PBPC transplantation raised the possibility of mobilizing healthy allogeneic donors. Within 2 years, the percentage of allogeneic PBPC increased from less than 10% in 1995 to more than 20% in 1997. Allogeneic PBPC transplants have been found to be safe and to have the same advantages found in autologous transplantation. The incidence of acute graft-versus-host disease appears to be increased over that of bone marrow allografts; however, chronic graft-versus-host disease may be more common. On balance, the trend appears to be that increasing numbers of transplants will utilize PBPC.

The first case of cord blood transplantation was reported in 1989. Since then, many cord blood banks have been established for public and private use. Although most cord blood HSCT were performed in pediatric patients, application in the adult setting is increasing. Clinical results for cord blood transplantation are reviewed and summarized in Chapter 26. Included in the same chapter is a description of the operation of cord blood banks. An understanding of issues, such as donation consent, processing, and storage, will facilitate interaction among transplanters and banks to select the best possible unit for a potential recipient.

In a book with so many contributors, overlap in discussion of similar topics cannot be avoided. Instead of limiting each chapter to its focus, we allowed the contributors to present a complete discourse of the subject matter, such that each chapter can be independently helpful to a reader. The different styles and approaches in addressing a common topic will also allow the readers to digest the complex and sometimes conflicting information.

To progress and communicate in the 21st century more quickly, many Web site addresses are listed herein that contain information relevant to the patient, donor, and/or physician. The International Bone Marrow Transplant Registry (IBMTR) (Web site: www.ibmtr.org) posts summary results of HSCT listed by diseases and staging, and autologous vs. allogeneic transplantation. The National Marrow Donor Program (NMDP) (Web site: www.marrow.org) lists the requirements of becoming an HSC donor and provides information for potential donors. The American Society of Hematology (ASH) (Web site: www.hematology.org) has helpful educational material. The American Association of Blood Banks (AABB) (Web site: www.aabb.org) provides information about becoming a blood component donor and about current tests performed on each unit of blood to minimize diseases associated with transfusion. The Foundation for the Accreditation of Hematopoietic Cell Therapy (FAHCT) (Web site: www.fahct.org) is an organization that produces standards for HSCT, inspects transplant centers, and accredits those programs that have met the stringent criteria. The Leukemia and Lymphoma Society (Web site: www.leukemia.org) gives material specifically related to diseases on hematologic malignancy, including HSCT information on donors and patients. Other academic societies and organizations associated with HSCT, including the International Society of Hematotherapy and Graft Engineering (ISHAGE) (Web site: www.ishage.org), the American Society of Clinical Oncology (ASCO) (Web site: www.asco.org), the International Society for Experimental Hematology (ISEH) (Web site: www.iseh.org), and the American Society for Blood and Marrow Transplantation (ASBMT) (Web site: www.asbmt.org), frequently post important and relevant information on their Web sites. Other useful Web sites include: http://cancernet.nci.nih.gov, www.bmtsupport.org, www.bmtinfo.org, www.bonemarrow.org, and www.bmtnews.org. Those listed above represent established professional organizations with direct interest or involvement in HSCT. There are many other professional and voluntary organizations, some of which may provide information directed to physicians or laymen. An exhaustive listing is not possible and is outside the scope of this book. For those organizations not mentioned here, the reader should be careful in accepting any Web site posting as fact, without independent verification, as with any information posted on the Internet.

It is difficult to capture a moving target, which may describe HSCT. The dynamic nature of this field is one of its greatest attractions to physicians. We hope that this book can aid the physician in the approach to the many patients who will benefit from the intellectual force of this very exciting field.

EDWARD D. BALL, M.D.
JOHN LISTER, M.D.
PING LAW, PH.D.

CONTENTS

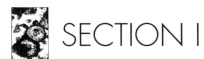 SECTION I

Issues Relevant to the Pre-transplant Period

Clinical Indications

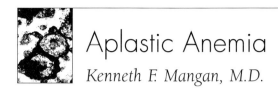

CHAPTER ONE

Aplastic Anemia

Kenneth F. Mangan, M.D.

Aplastic anemia is a bone marrow failure state characterized by insufficient production of red blood cells, white blood cells, and platelets. The bone marrow is fatty or empty. In most cases, the disorder is due to a defective or damaged multipotential stem cell leading to trilineage deficiencies of erythroid, myeloid, and megakaryocyte progenitor cells and their progeny. A diagnosis of *severe aplastic anemia* (SAA) is made if the absolute neutrophil count is less than 500/mm³, platelets are less than 20,000/mm³, and reticulocyte counts are less than 40,000/mm³ or the corrected reticulocyte count is less than 1%. Only two of the three blood criteria are required to make the diagnosis in the presence of a severely hypocellular marrow (<25%).[1] Typically, the bone marrow biopsy shows scattered residual lymphocytes and plasma cells, increased marrow fat, and only rare erythroid, myeloid, and megakaryocyte precursors. The peripheral blood smear typically shows increased proportions of lymphocytes which, when analyzed by flow cytometry, overexpress the activated IL-2 receptor–positive, HLA-DR–positive cytotoxic/suppressor CD8+ phenotype.[2] *Very severe aplastic anemia* is diagnosed when the absolute neutrophil count at presentation is less than 200/mm³ and denotes a poor prognosis.[3] In *moderately severe aplastic anemia,* bone marrow cellularity may be less than 50% but with less than 30% hematopoietic cells remaining.

CLINICAL FEATURES

DIFFERENTIAL DIAGNOSIS

Aplastic anemia is in the differential diagnosis of pancytopenia (Table 1–1). The presence or absence of a enlarged spleen on physical examination helps distinguish many causes of pancytopenia that may be confused with aplastic anemia. The spleen is never enlarged at diagnosis in SAA. In contrast, severe pancytopenia, with invasion of bone marrow by tumor, granulomatous disease, lymphoma, or leukemia, often is accompanied by an enlarged spleen. Certain viral infections, rarely autoimmune cytopenias, advanced vitamin B_{12} or folate deficiency, and paroxysmal nocturnal hemoglobinuria (PNH) may all have pancytopenia without an enlarged spleen as a presenting feature. These conditions can usually be distinguished from SAA on bone marrow biopsy by the presence of relatively cellular marrow. In PNH, however, a proportion of patients experience SAA, and some patients with SAA exhibit clinical features of PNH.[4] The vast majority of cases of aplastic anemia are acquired, but in young patients under age 20 with skeletal abnormalities on physical examination, a congenital disorder of marrow aplasia, especially Fanconi anemia, should be suspected.[5]

DIAGNOSTIC TESTS

A thorough history, physical examination, and inspection of the blood smear with complete blood count, reticulocyte count, and a generous (>2.0 cm) bone marrow biopsy should quickly establish the diagnosis of SAA in most cases. Cytogenetic studies are useful in excluding cases of hypoplastic myelodysplastic syndrome or established aplastic anemia, which may have evolved into myelodysplastic syndromes. In young patients, cytogenetic tests should be performed with clastogens such diepoxybutane or mitomycin to detect the chromosome fragility characteristic of Fanconi anemia.[5, 6] Screening tests for PNH should be performed, including acidified serum lysis (Ham test) or sucrose lysis tests. These tests, however, are less sensitive than flow cytometry of red cells, lymphocytes, and monocytes with monoclonal antibodies (CD14, CD16, CD55, CD58, CD59, and CD67) that identify glycosyl phosphatidyl inositol–linked proteins deficient in PNH.[7] Some blood tests may aid in the search for the etiology of the aplastic anemia or exclude other causes of pancytopenia, including B_{12} and folate levels (to exclude megaloblastic anemia). Serologic analysis for hepatitis A, B, and C viruses; cytomegalovirus (CMV); Epstein-Barr virus; and parvovirus is useful to exclude a viral cause for the aplastic anemia.[8]

Imaging studies are generally unproductive except in selected cases associated with altered immune states, such as systemic lupus erythematosus, rheumatoid arthritis, or eosinophilic fasciitis.[9] Computed tomography scans of the chest may help exclude a thymoma, which may be associated with aplastic anemia.[10] Magnetic resonance imaging (MRI) of the marrow space may be useful in difficult cases to help distinguish early aplastic anemia from pre-leukemia.

TABLE 1–1. DIFFERENTIAL DIAGNOSIS OF PANCYTOPENIA

Severe aplastic anemia
Autoimmune pancytopenia
Vitamin B_{12}, folate deficiency
Paroxysmal nocturnal hemoglobinuria
Fanconi anemia
Viral infections
Myelophthisic conditions*
    (tumor, granulomatous disease leukemia, lymphoma)

*Enlarged spleen may be present.

TABLE 1–2. USEFUL DIAGNOSTIC TESTS IN THE INITIAL MANAGEMENT AND EVALUATION OF THE PATIENT WITH APLASTIC ANEMIA

- Complete blood count with differential
- Platelet count
- Reticulocyte count
- Generous bone marrow biopsy and aspirate
- Marrow cytogenetics ± mitogens
- PNH tests (flow cytometry, Ham test, sucrose lysis tests)
- Viral serologic analysis for cytomegalovirus, hepatitis A, B, C, parvovirus, Epstein-Barr virus
- Serum vitamin B$_{12}$, folate levels
- Autoimmune antibody tests (Rh factor, ANA)*
- CT scan of chest for thymoma*
- Bone marrow magnetic resonance imaging*
- In vitro colony assays*
- HLA-A, -B, -D locus typing of patients, all siblings, parents

*Selected cases only.
ANA, antinuclear antigen; CT, computed tomography; HLA, human leukocyte antigen; PNH, paroxysmal nocturnal hemoglobinuria.

MRI may demonstrate increased hydrophobic fat on T1-weighted images in the vertebral bodies and may provide an overall estimate of marrow cellularity when bone marrow biopsies are inconclusive.[11]

SAA is one of the strongest indications for bone marrow transplantation. All patients who are potential allogeneic transplant candidates (<60 years of age) should undergo complete HLA-A, -B, and -D locus typing at diagnosis in preparation for a donor search. For transplant candidates, all available full siblings and parents should be tissue typed for HLA-A, -B, and -D locus antigens. HLA typing should also be performed at diagnosis to assist in future management of blood product support should a patient's condition become refractory to pooled platelets. A summary of useful clinical tests in the initial work-up of patients with SAA is shown in Table 1–2.

PATHOGENESIS

STEM CELL DEFECTS

For many years, the severe trilineage impairment of the hematopoietic compartment in SAA was thought to be due to either an acquired defect in multipotential stem cells or a defect in microenvironmental stromal cells that support stem cells. Both the WW^v mouse, with defective stem cells due to lack of stem cell factor receptor encoded by the c-kit gene, and the S^{l}S^L mouse, with defective stromal cells that fail to make stem cell factor, may experience aplastic anemia, which supports the concept that aplastic anemia may occur from damage to either the stem cell or the stromal cell tissues.[12, 13] In fact, infusion of normal stem cells from S^{l}S^L mice may cure the aplastic anemia in WW^v mice, and infusion of stromal cells from WW^v mice could cure the aplastic anemia in S^{l}S^L mice, lending support to the concept that aplastic anemia could occur from damage to stem cells, supporting tissue, or both.

In humans with aplastic anemia, measurement of stem cells by virtually any assay has shown them to be severely deficient. Short-term colony assays of erythroid (BFU-E), myeloid (CFU-GM), and megakaryocyte progenitors (CFU-Meg) all show deficiency.[8] Long-term colony assays (LT-C1C) that measure multipotential stem cells suggest that, in most patients, absolute numbers of stem cells are less than 1% of normal.[8] Direct measurement of the stem cell numbers using flow cytometry and antibodies to CD34 has also confirmed the profound deficiency of stem cells in patients with aplastic anemia.[2, 14, 15] Hematopoiesis in patients with newly diagnosed or partially recovered SAA may be sustained by only a few functioning or damaged stem cells (oligoclonal hematopoiesis). These defects may persist for months to years.[16]

STROMAL CELL DEFECTS AND HEMATOPOIETIC GROWTH FACTOR PRODUCTION

Holmberg et al. have shown that stromal cell growth in patients with aplastic anemia is normal in approximately 50% of patients and only modestly deficient in another 40%.[17] Hematopoietic growth factor levels in serum such as granulocyte-macrophage colony–stimulating factor (GM-CSF), granulocyte colony–stimulating factor (G-CSF), erythropoietin, megakaryocyte-derived growth factor, stem cell factor, and Flt-3 ligand are all preserved or elevated, suggesting that absolute defects in supporting stromal tissue that produce these growth factors are rare.[8, 18] Overproduction of negative hematopoietic growth regulatory factors such as interferon-γ and tumor necrosis factor has occasionally been shown. These factors may contribute to marrow failure by depressing hematopoietic stem cell production.[19, 20]

LYMPHOCYTE-MEDIATED SUPPRESSION OF HEMATOPOIESIS

In contrast with the relative paucity of data implicating stromal cell dysfunction in aplastic anemia, a large body of evidence has accumulated in the last couple of decades implicating immune lymphocytes in the pathogenesis of stem cell destruction in patients with aplastic anemia. Several lines of evidence suggest an immunologically mediated pathogenesis for SAA. First, patients with SAA who underwent transplantation with syngeneic (identical twin) marrow without receiving conditioning regimens showed a high rate of graft rejection.[21, 22] Graft rejection was largely avoided by conditioning the patient with immunosuppressive doses of cyclophosphamide, which would then allow engraftment in aplastic patients. Furthermore, it was observed that autologous (self) marrow recovery occurred in a small number of patients undergoing allogeneic (sex-mismatched) marrow transplants after graft rejection.[23, 24] These clinical data strongly suggested that engraftment was a result of removal of immune lymphocytes from the microenvironment by immunosuppressive doses of cyclophosphamide used to condition patients for transplantation. In animal models, infusions of mismatched lymphocytes could induce SAA as part of a graft-versus-host disease (GVHD) reaction.[25, 26] Early in vitro co-culture experiments in humans demonstrate that unfractionated or CD8-positive activated lymphocyte fractions from patients with aplastic anemia could suppress in vitro progenitor cell growth[27–29] and that these effects were not due to nonspecific immunologic effects of transfusion-induced sensitization.[30-32] Young et al. extended these data by showing that aplastic patients' T cells (in culture or cloned) overproduced negative hematopoietic growth factors, such as tumor necrosis factor or interferon-γ, which could inhibit progenitor cell growth and that this suppression was maximal when these cytokines were secreted into the marrow microenvironment.[20, 33, 34] Furthermore, interferon-γ and tumor necrosis factor could induce expression of the fas receptor on aplastic anemia CD34+ stem cells, leading to programmed cell death (apoptosis).[35, 36] In contrast with data implicating T lymphocytes in suppression of hematopoiesis in SAA, there are very few data to suggest that serum IgG antibodies mediate this disorder; only a rare case of trilineage suppression of hematopoiesis due to a serum IgG antibody is reported.[37-39]

UNIFYING HYPOTHESIS FOR PATHOGENESIS OF SEVERE APLASTIC ANEMIA

Young and Maciejewski have argued that an acquired aplastic anemia in most patients results from immunologically mediated destruction of bone marrow.[8] Viruses including hepatitis viruses, CMV, Epstein-Barr virus, and parvovirus have been implicated in the pathogenesis of aplastic anemia in selected cases. In addition, a variety of medications such as chloramphenicol, sulfonamides, anti-thyroid, antiseizure drugs, and others have also been implicated in triggering aplastic anemia. Aplastic anemia is associated with a wide range of clinical conditions characterized by altered immunity (Table 1–3). Young et al. have hypothesized that viruses may infect or bind to hematopoietic stem cells or that reactive drug metabolites may be taken up by antigen presenting cells and ultimately trigger cytotoxic lymphocytes, which may lead to the autoimmune destruction of progenitor or stem cells. Direct toxicity to stem cells by certain toxins such as benzene or insecticides may lead to genetically altered cellular peptides, which may also initiate a cytotoxic T-cell response leading to marrow destruction. Thus, the seemingly diverse inciting events (virus, drug, toxins) may all eventually lead to a common pathway for activation of immune lymphocytes, which may then ultimately destroy the marrow stem cell compartment, resulting in aplastic anemia.[8]

TABLE 1–3. CLINICAL CONDITIONS OF ALTERED IMMUNITY ASSOCIATED WITH SEVERE APLASTIC ANEMIA

- Collagen-vascular disease (systemic lupus erythematosus, rheumatoid arthritis)[38]
- Eosinophilic fasciitis[9]
- Post-transfusion graft-vs.-host disease[106]
- Thymoma[10]
- Pregnancy[107]
- Chronic α-interferon administration[108]
- Graft rejection[111]
- Chronic viral infection (hepatitis, Epstein-Barr virus, cytomegalovirus, parvovirus)[8, 94–97, 110]
- Post liver transplantation[96]

NONTRANSPLANT IMMUNOSUPPRESSIVE THERAPY

MONOTHERAPY

Before 1970, the mainstay of treatment of SAA was supportive care with red blood cell and platelet transfusions and aggressive use of antibiotics to treat infection. Eighty to 90% of patients expired within 1 year.[40] Although androgens proved useful in patients with SAA,[41] randomized controlled studies indicated that androgen therapy was no better than supportive care.[40] The clinical, laboratory, and animal model studies carried out in the 1970s that implicated immune-mediated suppression of hematopoiesis in the pathogenesis of SAA led to the rational application of immunosuppressive agents for the treatment of aplastic anemia in the late 1970s and 1980s. Early studies carried out by Mathe et al. in Europe were the first to suggest that anti-lymphocyte globulin (ALG) could induce remission in patients with SAA.[42] These studies were subsequently confirmed in a randomized study carried out by Champlin et al.[43] and a multicenter trial by Young et al.[44] providing convincing clinical evidence for the first time that immunosuppressive therapy with ALG or anti-thymocyte globulin (ATG) improved overall survival over supportive care alone.[43] Subsequently it was shown that cyclosporine alone was as effective as ALG given as a single agent.[45, 46] Massive doses of corticosteroids could induce remissions in patients with SAA as single agents, but moderate doses of corticosteroids were not beneficial or possibly detrimental.[47] In a more recent study, high-dose cyclophosphamide (45 mg/kg/day × 4 doses) also induced remissions in patients with SAA, and none of the responders experienced late clonal disorders.[48]

COMBINATION THERAPY

In an attempt to improve on the positive results of immunosuppressive monotherapy, ALG and cyclosporine were combined and tested in SAA. Methylprednisolone was administered with ALG or ATG only to prevent serum sickness side effects of these medications.

Frickhoven et al. showed that combination therapy with cyclosporine and ALG resulted in significantly better responses at 3 and 6 months versus ALG and methylprednisolone alone.[49] Sixty-five to 70% of patients were able to achieve complete response. Speed of response and response rates may be improved further by addition of G-CSF to ATG plus cyclosporine. Although responses are high and early survival 2–3 years after treatment is excellent, long-term follow-up studies have shown that up to 20% of patients may experience relapse. Hematologic recovery may be incomplete, and up to 50% of patients may experience clonal disorders or other malignancies 10–15 years after treatment.[50] The evolution to PNH and myelodysplasia is particularly disturbing and has important implications for management of SAA, particularly in younger patients (see later discussion of immunosuppressive vs. allogeneic transplantation).

In a large National Institutes of Health aplastic anemia

TABLE 1–4. USEFUL NONTRANSPLANT IMMUNOSUPPRESSIVE THERAPY FOR SEVERE APLASTIC ANEMIA

German Regimen[49]
- Anti-lymphocyte globulin (ALG, Institut Mérièux) 0.75 mL/kg/d IV days 1–8
- Methylprednisolone 5 mg/kg/d IV days 1–8, then taper and D/C on day 29
- Cyclosporine 6 mg/kg p.o. b.i.d. × 3 mo minimum

NIH Regimen[51]
- Anti-thymocyte globulin (Atgam, Upjohn) 40 mg/kg/d IV days 1–4
- Methylprednisolone 1 mg/kg/d (max 40 mg/kg/d IV), then 40 mg p.o. QD × 10 d, then taper and D/C on day 24
- Cyclosporine 6.0 mg/kg p.o. b.i.d. days 1–180, then D/C
- G-CSF 5–10 µg/kg/d for neutropenic fevers

Johns Hopkins Regimen[48]
- Cyclophosphamide 45 mg/kg/d IV days 1–4 alone or with cyclosporine 5 mg/kg IV. Taper to 1.5 mg/kg IV by day 32, then 7.5–10 mg/kg/d p.o. days 33–100, then D/C.

D/C, discontinue.

study reported by Rosenfeld et al., ATG was administered at 40 mg/kg/day for 4 days IV with cyclosporine at 12 mg/kg/day orally for 180 days in 51 patients without previous immunosuppressive therapy.[51] Methylprednisolone was administered with the ATG to prevent serum sickness. At 12 months, 78% responded, 28% had relapsed, and 10% had died. Eight percent were subsequently shown to have a PNH clone. Actuarial survival at 12 months was 86% but only 62% at 36 months, and event-free survival had dropped from 78% to 50% at 36 months. Patients with an absolute neutrophil count less than 200/mm³ (i.e., very severe aplastic anemia), and those who delayed treatment several months after initial diagnosis, and patients with pre-therapy marrow cellularity less than 10% were all likely to do more poorly with immunosuppressive therapy. Useful immunosuppressive regimens for treatment of SAA are shown in Table 1–4.

MANAGEMENT WITH ANTI-THYMOCYTE GLOBULIN AND CYCLOSPORINE

ATG and cyclosporine are toxic. Several precautions should be taken when managing SAA with these medications (Table 1–5). First, ATG is a foreign protein raised in either horse, rabbit, or mouse. All patients should undergo skin

TABLE 1–5. PRACTICAL TIPS FOR USE OF ANTI-THYMOCYTE GLOBULIN (ATG) IN SEVERE APLASTIC ANEMIA

- Skin-test all recipients—be prepared for possible anaphylactic reaction.
- Use large-bore catheter with filter and infuse slowly over 4–6 hours in normal saline.
- Premedicate patient with acetaminophen (650 mg), diphenhydramine (50 mg), and methylprednisolone (1 mg/kg) and add meperidine (50 mg) for rigors.
- Keep platelet count ≥30,000/mm³ before daily infusion.
- Cover for serum sickness 7–14 days after infusion with tapering doses of corticosteroids.
- For repeat course of ATG, use preparation raised in another animal (rabbit).

testing prior to administration. Although ATG is administered to lyse T lymphocytes, most preparations are not T-cell specific and ATG may react with B lymphocytes, platelets, red blood cells, and other tissues. ATG may work in SAA to release growth factors or directly enhance response of stem cells to growth factors.[52] ATG should be administered through a large-bore catheter to prevent phlebitis, and patients should be premedicated with antihistamines (diphenhydramine [Benadryl]), antipyretics (acetaminophen [Tylenol]), and corticosteroids to prevent hypersensitivity reactions or serum sickness. Fever and chills are common and may require intravenous meperidine (Demerol) to control chills. Skin rashes, particularly a serpiginous rash, and serositis may occur 7–10 days after discontinuance of ATG. Third, platelet counts should be maintained over 30,000/mm³ before infusion of ATG because ATG may cause a precipitous drop of the platelet count in patients who are already thrombocytopenic. Cyclosporine dosing should be adjusted to maintain therapeutic levels between 200 and 400 ng/mL, and liver and kidney functions should be monitored frequently to avoid organ toxicity.

RESULTS OF SYNGENEIC BONE MARROW TRANSPLANTS

As noted earlier, the clinical results of identical-twin transplants provided important clues to the pathogenesis of SAA.[21, 22] Because patients with aplastic anemia already exhibited an aplastic marrow, it was initially thought that infusion of fully syngeneic marrow with normal stem cells without conditioning could correct the hematopoietic defect. If aplastic anemia was due to an abnormality of the microenvironment, an infusion of normal stem cells that were fully genotypically identical may not cure the defect. Alternatively, if aplastic anemia was immunologically mediated, an immunosuppressive regimen might be required.

The International Bone Marrow Transplant Registry (IBMTR) reported on the results of 40 patients with aplastic anemia who received marrow transplants from genotypically identical twins between 1964 and 1992.[53] Of the 17 patients who underwent transplantation with an immunosuppressive conditioning regimen, 13, or 76%, sustained engraftment and 4 suffered an early death. Twenty-three underwent transplantation with no conditioning regimen; only 7 of 23, or 30%, recovered. Sixteen of 23, or 70%, experienced rejection of their grafts, and 3 subsequently died before receiving a second transplant. Thirteen of the 16 rejections were salvaged by a second transplant employing an immunosuppressive conditioning regimen. As noted earlier, these data strongly suggest that immune lymphocytes contribute to the pathogenesis of aplastic anemia and that these suppressor cells can be eliminated by an immunosuppressive conditioning regimen. Therefore, the likelihood of hematologic recovery was greater in patients who underwent conditioning before the first transplantation. The overall actuarial 10-year survival rate for the 40 patients was 78%. Interestingly, because the salvage rate with a second transplant with preparative conditioning was so good, the overall survival rate was higher in patients who did not undergo conditioning before the first transplantation compared with patients who were conditioned. The authors therefore concluded that pretransplant conditioning may increase the chance of bone marrow recovery but does not seem to improve overall survival.

Although these data may appear to argue for withholding a conditioning regimen in identical twins with SAA, the results should be interpreted cautiously. Physicians managing these cases should be prepared to perform a second transplantation with an immunosuppressive conditioning regimen as soon as it becomes apparent that graft rejection has occurred. Cyclophosphamide at 200 mg/kg with or without ATG at a total dose of 90 mg/kg should provide enough immunosuppression to overcome immune-mediated graft rejection mechanisms in this setting.

RESULTS OF ALLOGENEIC-MATCHED RELATED DONOR TRANSPLANTS

The curative potential of HLA-identical related marrow donor transplantation in SAA was first demonstrated in the early 1970s.[54, 55] These early allogeneic transplant studies provided the first real hope that SAA could be cured in a substantial number of patients using an HLA-identical matched bone marrow donor. Transplantations performed in the 1970s using HLA-identical marrow grafts cured approximately 50% of patients with SAA.[56] Since then, improvements in selection, management, and treatment have gradually improved long-term survival rates from 50% to 60% in the large 1970s series at the Fred Hutchinson Cancer Research Center to as high as 80–90% in the 1990s.[57] In the IBMTR series 5-year survival rate increased from 48% ± 7% for 1976 to 1980 to 60 ± 6% for 1982 to 1992.[58] The IBMTR attributed improvements in survival primarily to the institution of cyclosporine to prevent GVHD. Other notable improvements since the 1970s include earlier referral of SAA patients to transplant centers and reduction of exposure to CMV-positive blood products. These factors may also have affected survival and cure rates in patients with aplastic anemia.

Since the 1960s, clinical studies in allografting have identified five major problems that affect the curative potential of HLA-identical transplants for SAA: (1) graft rejection, (2) acute GVHD, (3) interstitial pneumonia, (4) chronic GVHD, and (5) development of late side effects including retarded growth, infertility, and late malignant tumors. These problems are discussed in detail.

DEFINITIONS AND RISK FACTORS FOR GRAFT REJECTION

Primary graft failure occurs if there is no evidence of engraftment within the first 3–4 weeks post transplant. *Delayed engraftment* occurs if there are declining counts after transient evidence of engraftment. *Late secondary graft failure* may occur in up to 5% of patients after withdrawal of post-transplant immunosuppression.[59] *Primary graft failure* is treated by a second transplant using the same donor and carries with it a high fatality rate (70–80%).[60, 61] Management of late graft failure is more favorable, with 25–75% of patients surviving a second transplant. For threatened or

delayed graft failure, the use of hematopoietic growth factors such as GM-CSF and re-institution of aggressive immunosuppression may rescue patients before irreversible graft failure occurs.[62]

Recipient T lymphocytes that survive the conditioning regimen may recognize minor antigens on donor stem cells and mediate graft rejection. Five major factors that increase risk of graft rejection include (1) sensitization of the recipient to blood cells through multiple blood or platelet transfusions prior to transplantation, (2) any degree of HLA mismatching between donor and recipient, (3) infusion of low numbers by donor cells, (4) reduction in the strength of the immunosuppressive conditioning regimen employed, and (5) use of T-cell depletion of donor marrow to prevent GVHD and/or reduction in post-transplant immunosuppression of the recipient. A summary of risk factors and possible solutions to prevent graft rejection in SAA allografts is shown in Table 1–6.

Effect of Transfusion-Induced Allosensitization on Graft Rejection

Transfusion of blood products prior to transplantation dramatically increases the risk of graft rejection because of potential sensitization of recipient to antigens on donor stem cells.[63] Blood products from family members should never be administered to potential transplant recipients, and blood products from non–family members should be kept to an absolute minimum to reduce risk of graft rejection after HLA-identical transplantation.

Studies from the Fred Hutchinson Cancer Research Center have shown that the incidence of graft rejection increases after any transfusion and is greatly increased after 20 donor exposures.[64] For a patient who will be undergoing allogeneic transplant, red cell transfusions should be leukodepleted to reduce risks of allosensitization and are indicated only for physiologic purposes. Many young aplastic patients can tolerate hemoglobin transfusions of

TABLE 1–6. ALLOGRAFT REJECTION IN SEVERE APLASTIC ANEMIA: RISK FACTORS AND SOLUTIONS

RISK FACTORS	SOLUTIONS
Transfusion-induced sensitization	Limit transfusion to minimum
	Use leukodepleted products
	Use irradiated products
HLA disparity between donor/ recipient	Use best match available
	Confirm with molecular typing
	Avoid mismatched transplants
Low donor marrow cells	Infuse greater than 3.5 × 10⁸ nucleated marrow donor cells/kg recipient
	Prime donor with G-CSF
	Use post-transplant growth factors
	Increase strength of preparation regimen
Low strength of preparative regimen	Add ATG or low-dose TBI or TLI
	Increase marrow cell dose
T-cell depletion of donor marrow	Increase strength of preparative regimen
	Increase dose of donor cells

ATG, anti-thymocyte globulin; G-CSF, granulocyte colony-stimulating factor; HLA, human leukocyte antigen; TBI, total body irradiation; TLI, total lymphoid irradiation.

TABLE 1–7. TRANSFUSION PRINCIPLES FOR MANAGING APLASTIC ANEMIA

Transfuse RBCs for symptoms only or for hemoglobin <8.0 g/dL.
Transfuse platelets for bleeding only or if platelets ≤10,000/mm³.
Employ prophylactic epsilon-aminocaproic acid (Amicar) to reduce mucosal bleeding.
Use leukopoor filtered and irradiated blood products to minimize allosensitization.
Use leukopoor and/or cytomegalovirus-negative selected products to maintain cytomegalovirus negativity.
Avoid use of family members as donors of blood products.

6–7 g/dL without physiologic compromise. Transfusion of older patients should never exceed 8 g/dL unless serious cardiovascular symptoms intervene.

To reduce donor exposures, single-donor platelets prior to transplantation that are leukodepleted are the most appropriate. All blood and platelet products should be irradiated to further minimize the risk of sensitization to minor histocompatibility antigens.[65] The transfusion management goals for supporting aplastic anemia patients with blood products prior to transplantation are summarized in Table 1–7. The use of leukodepleted products also reduces the acquisition of CMV. Maintaining CMV negativity in recipients reduces the incidence of post-transplant CMV interstitial pneumonia and other CMV complications, particularly in patients receiving marrow from CMV-negative donors. The application of these effective transfusion practices has probably accounted for the reduced incidence of graft rejection in the 1990s.[66]

Effect of Mismatching on Graft Rejection

As noted earlier, graft rejection can occur with syngeneic transplants when there are no histocompatible differences between donor and recipient. Graft rejection rates increase as the degree of major or minor histocompatibility differences increases. Patients with any degree of HLA-A, -B, or -D locus disparity have an increased risk for graft rejection, and these patients probably require more intense pre-transplant conditioning to prevent graft rejection.[67, 68] Removal of T lymphocytes from donor marrow or CD34 selection (which reduces T lymphocytes significantly) in donor marrow may reduce the risk of GVHD but at the expense of an increased risk of graft rejection.[69] Graft rejection rates tend to be higher in alternative-donor transplants, wherein differences in major and minor histocompatibility antigens

are greater. Overcoming these tendencies dictates that patients undergoing alternative-donor transplants should receive greater numbers of donor cells, preferably close to 4 × 10⁸/kg nucleated marrow cells, and/or more intense immunosuppressive conditioning regimens.

Effect of Donor Marrow Dose on Graft Rejection

The influence of donor cell dose on graft rejection has been noted. Marrow cell doses of less than 2 × 10⁸ nucleated marrow cells per kilogram body weight of the recipient have been associated with increased risk of graft rejection.[56, 70, 71] Supplementing marrow cells with donor buffy coat cells greatly reduces the incidence of graft rejection in SAA but at the expense of an increased incidence and severity of chronic GVHD.[72] This observation led to the abandonment of donor buffy coat cells to overcome transfusion-induced sensitization and low donor cell dose. Recent studies suggest that primed bone marrow harvests may provide increased numbers of donor stem cells with rapid engrafting potential equivalent to the engrafting potential of peripheral blood progenitor cells.[73] Unfortunately, although large numbers of peripheral blood progenitor cells can be procured with G-CSF–stimulated donors, increasing evidence suggests that allogeneic peripheral blood progenitor cell transplants are accompanied by increased severity of chronic GVHD.[74] Therefore, at present, until randomized controlled data become available, every attempt should be made to obtain greater than 3 × 10⁸ nucleated marrow cells/kilogram body weight from an HLA-identical donor. Whether priming the bone marrow with G-CSF will improve on engraftment potential in aplastic anemia is still unknown.

Effect of Conditioning Regimen on Graft Rejection

The primary purpose of the conditioning regimen for patients with SAA is to provide enough immunosuppression to allow engraftment without exposing the patient to excess toxicity. Since the mid-1970s, four major conditioning regimens have been developed. These regimens employ cyclophosphamide alone or add total body irradiation (TBI) (300–1200 cGy) or limited field irradiation (total lymphoid irradiation or thoracoabdominal irradiation) or ATG (Table 1–8).

Early series that employed cyclophosphamide alone at a dose of 200 mg/kg to prepare patients with SAA showed

TABLE 1–8. FOUR COMMON CONDITIONING REGIMENS FOR TRANSPLANTATION IN SEVERE APLASTIC ANEMIA

CYCLOPHOSPHAMIDE				
Total Dose	**Schedule**	**ATG**	**RADIATION**	**REFERENCES**
200 mg/kg	50 mg/kg IV × 4 d	None	None	Storb et al.[55]
200 mg/kg	50 mg/kg IV × 4 d	None	TBI 300 cGy × 1 d	Feig et al.[75]
200 mg/kg	50 mg/kg IV × 4 d	None	TLI 750 cGy × 1 d	McGlave et al.[77]
200 mg/kg	50 mg/kg IV × 4 d	30 mg/kg IV × 3 d	None	Storb et al.[60, 80]

ATG, antithymocyte globulin; TBI, total body irradiation; TLI, total lymphoid irradiation.

graft rejection rates of 10–25%.[63, 64, 71] The addition of TBI, total lymphoid irradiation, or thoraco-abdominal irradiation reduced graft rejection rates to under 10% by increasing the intensity of the conditioning regimen.[75–77] Irradiation may increase the risk of acute and chronic GVHD, interstitial pneumonia, and secondary malignant tumors.[75–78] In the younger patient, irradiation may result in significant suppression of growth and development and infertility.[79] These risks, however, may be offset by greater risk of graft rejection and subsequent mortality in patients undergoing unrelated-donor transplantation. The addition of ATG to cyclophosphamide may reduce graft rejection rates while avoiding the risk of irradiation altogether.[80]

For patients with aplastic anemia whose disease may have evolved to hypoplastic myelodysplastic syndrome with cytogenetic abnormalities, a myeloablative regimen is also preferred.[81] For these patients, TBI or busulfan (16 mg/kg) plus cyclophosphamide (120–200 mg/kg) is recommended to eradicate the malignant clone.

Impact of GVHD Prophylaxis on Graft Rejection

With HLA-identical donor transplants, the development of acute GVHD presents the most serious threat to long-term disease-free survival in patients who engraft. Post-transplant immunosuppression with cyclosporine, methotrexate, and other immunosuppressive agents designed to prevent donor lymphocytes from attacking host tissues may also modulate the ability of host T lymphocytes from rejecting donor marrow. Early withdrawal of cyclosporine after 6 months has resulted in delayed graft rejection in up to 5% of patients and therefore prolonged administration of cyclosporine for at least 1 year after transplantation is recommended to reduce risk of delayed graft failure.[59] During this interval, cyclosporine level should be closely monitored to keep levels between 200 and 300 ng/mL. Liver and kidney functions should also be monitored closely to avoid long-term toxicity of cyclosporine.

T-cell depletion of donor marrow or enrichment of CD34+ cells by positive selection may reduce the risks of acute GVHD but at the expense of increased risk of graft rejection. If this strategy is pursued, modest T-cell depletion (1–2 logs) and infusion of larger numbers of stem cells may counterbalance the tendency to graft rejection.

ACUTE GVHD

Studies of HLA-identical transplantations in patients with aplastic anemia from the Fred Hutchinson Cancer Research Center and from the IBMTR clearly demonstrate the negative impact of advanced GVHD on overall long-term survival.[82] Greater than 80% of patients will achieve long-term disease-free survival with grade 0–I GVHD, but this result drops to about 40% in patients in whom advanced grade II–IV GVHD develops. As noted earlier, the improvement of survival in recent years has been largely attributed to the addition of cyclosporine to methotrexate therapy for the prevention of GVHD. Patients given methotrexate alone had a 50% long-term survival rate, but those treated with methotrexate and cyclosporine had an 80% long-term survival rate.[76]

In the modern era, with the use of methotrexate and cyclosporine, most centers are reporting advanced grade II–IV GVHD in less than 15–20% of patients with SAA.[83] Cyclosporine and prednisone may also be useful in reducing the incidence of acute GVHD and may accelerate engraftment, but there are no randomized controlled studies to determine whether it is any better than methotrexate and cyclosporine in the management of SAA transplants.

The risk of acute GVHD may be increased by use of multiparous female donors into male recipients or in older patients over the age of 40.[76] Laminar air flow isolation may also reduce the incidence of acute GVHD in patients undergoing HLA-identical transplantation for SAA.[82]

INTERSTITIAL PNEUMONIA

The development of interstitial pneumonia in the first 150 days may present an obstacle to success with transplantation for SAA. In a retrospective study, Weiner et al. reviewed 547 patients undergoing HLA-identical transplants with SAA from the IBMTR to determine the incidence of interstitial pneumonia.[84] Seventeen percent of patients experienced interstitial pneumonia, and in 37% of patients it was due to CMV infection, in 41% no organism could be identified, and in 22% an organism other than CMV was identified. The overall mortality rate was 11%. Risk factors for interstitial pneumonia included use of methotrexate after bone marrow transplantation (BMT), grade II–IV GVHD, use of TBI, and increased patient age.

Similar data were observed in a large series of 329 patients from the Fred Hutchinson Cancer Research Center except that in this series methotrexate was not a risk factor.[57] These data emphasized the importance of management of patients with SAA with leukodepleted blood products. For patients whose CMV titers are negative prior to transplantation, CMV-negative selected products should be employed. After the transplantation, aggressive surveillance for CMV should prompt the institution of early prophylactic or pre-emptive use of ganciclovir during the first 120 days after the transplantation. Evidence suggests that these aggressive measures may already be reducing mortality from interstitial pneumonia in SAA.[57]

CHRONIC GVHD

Both the Fred Hutchinson Cancer Research Center series and IBMTR data document only a modest improvement in reduction of chronic GVHD after HLA-identical transplantation for SAA despite the clear reduction in incidence of acute GVHD.[57, 76] Approximately one-third of patients may suffer from significant chronic GVHD. Patients who have antecedent acute GVHD, older patients, patients who receive TBI, patients who have undergone buffy coat infusions, or patients with large numbers of allogeneic peripheral blood progenitor cells are at increased risk for development of chronic GVHD.[74, 85] Deaths from chronic GVHD are frequently due to gram-positive sinopulmonary infection. The use of prophylactic trimethoprim-sulfamethoxazole and IV immunoglobulin was strongly associated with improved survival in the IBMTR series.[58] Prolonged administration of cyclosporine may not only prevent delayed graft rejection but may also have a positive benefit by reducing the severity of chronic GVHD in the first year.

Chronic GVHD is usually managed with alternate-day therapy with corticosteroids and cyclosporine. Whether newer approaches for management of chronic GVHD, which include FK506, thalidomide, mycophenolate, or psoralen with UVA therapy, will affect morbidity and mortality in patients undergoing transplantation for SAA is still unknown.

LATE SIDE EFFECTS

Late side effects of BMT in patients with SAA are particularly important because many patients undergoing transplantation for aplastic anemia are relatively young (<40 years of age). Patients undergoing cyclophosphamide-only conditioning regimens have well-preserved growth and development, thyroid function, and fertility compared with patients receiving a conditioning regimen including TBI.[79] For younger patients, TBI should be avoided unless there is evidence for clonal evolution or concern about engraftment as noted earlier.

A large study reported by Socie et al. compared the incidence of malignant tumors in 748 patients undergoing allogeneic BMT with HLA-identical donors with the incidence in 860 patients receiving immunosuppressive therapies without transplantation.[86] Nine patients experienced malignancies in the BMT group for an incidence of 3.1%; 7% of them were solid tumors. In contrast, 42 patients receiving immunosuppressive therapy experienced secondary malignancies—34 of them were either myelodysplastic syndrome or acute myelogenous leukemia, for a 10-year incidence of 18.8%, and 7 experienced solid tumors. In the Seattle series of 330 patients with aplastic anemia followed for up to 20 years and conditioned with cyclophosphamide alone, the cumulative cancer incidence was only 3.8% at 15 years with a preponderance of cancer in the head and neck area.[87] Socie et al. reported a 22% incidence of cancer in aplastic anemia patients conditioned with cyclophosphamide and thoracoabdominal irradiation.[78] Collectively these data suggest that the incidence of solid tumor cancer risk is minimal in patients undergoing allogeneic transplantation and conditioned with cyclophosphamide alone and increases significantly with the addition of a radiation-based regimen and in Fanconi anemia. In a large survey from Seattle and Paris of 700 patients with aplastic anemia, only 23 patients experienced malignancies 1–221 months post transplant. Multivariate analysis identified Fanconi anemia, azathioprine therapy, and irradiation as risk factors.[88]

RESULTS OF ALTERNATIVE-DONOR TRANSPLANTATION

Only 25–30% of patients with SAA will find an HLA-identical sibling donor suitable for transplantation. In contrast with the donor pool in the National Marrow Donor Program and other registries now exceeding 3 million persons, non-minority patients may have up to a 75% chance of finding an HLA-identical donor from these registries.

The chance of finding an HLA-identical donor from the National Marrow Donor Program is considerably less for minority populations (African Americans, Asian Americans, Hispanic Americans).

Recent results from the National Marrow Donor Program in 141 patients undergoing matched unrelated donor transplantation for treatment of SAA who had no HLA-identical siblings are encouraging[84]: 85% of these patients were conditioned with a TBI-based regimen. A minority received cyclophosphamide and ATG alone: 76% underwent transplantation with a complete HLA-A, -B, and -DR serologically identical unrelated donor; 24% had at least one class I or class II mismatched antigen; 78% experienced engraftment and 22% experienced graft failure; and 84% developed acute grade II–IV GVHD. The overall survival rate was 36%, with the longer survivors now 9 years from transplantation.[89] This study suggested that TBI may be reduced (to 300 cGy) in patients receiving cyclophosphamide and ATG and still allow engraftment.[89] Further follow-up is needed with this cohort of patients to determine whether TBI can be avoided completely in the unrelated donor transplant setting. Although these results are encouraging, because of the high incidence of advanced GVHD, it is difficult to recommend an unrelated donor transplant in patients who have not first been given a trial of immunosuppressive therapy. A randomized controlled study is needed to determine whether unrelated donor transplants should be recommended before immunosuppressive therapy.

Only a small number of patients with aplastic anemia have received allogeneic marrow transplants from haploidentical related donors who are less than perfect matches. Patients who are haploidentical with their marrow donors and who are phenotypically identical on the nonshared haplotype appear to do as well as patients with SAA who receive fully genotypically HLA-matched marrow, and these patients can be conditioned with cyclophosphamide alone with no additional immunosuppression.[68] In contrast, small numbers of aplastic patients receiving HLA locus *mismatched marrow (at one, two, or more loci) from related donors* have sustained high rates of graft rejection and infection. These patients require aggressive immunosuppressive conditioning regimens, and only 10–20% can be expected to achieve long-term survival.[68] Results are considerably better in patients under age 20 years.[90] At present, given the results with matched unrelated donor transplants, mismatched related donor transplants cannot be recommended if there is a fully matched unrelated donor available, especially in the adult patient.

IMMUNOSUPPRESSIVE THERAPY VS. ALLOGENEIC TRANSPLANTS—WHICH IS BETTER?

The European Group for Blood and Marrow Transplantation (EBMT) could find no differences in 6-year outcome between 218 patients treated with BMT and 291 treated with ALG, although BMT gave superior results in younger (<20 years) patients.[91] Paquette et al. compared survival rates for patients treated with ATG and those given BMT in the decade 1977–1988 at University of California, Los

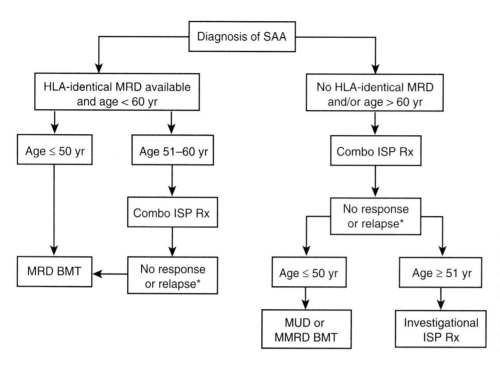

FIGURE 1–1. Suggested algorithm for transplantation decisions in severe aplastic anemia (SAA). MRD, matched related donor; MUD, matched unrelated donor; BMT, bone marrow transplant; Combo ISP Rx, combination immunosuppressive therapy with anti-thymocyte globulin and cyclosporine; MMRD, mismatched related donor. * = Retreatment with second course of ISP Rx may be useful for relapses.

Angeles.[92] Six-year survival rates remained at 46% in the ATG group but improved from 43% to 72% in the BMT group. These investigators concluded that BMT yielded a superior long-term outcome in adults with SAA.[92]

Doney et al. compared 168 BMT recipients with 227 patients who received immunosuppressive therapy for treatment of SAA.[93] Actuarial survival rates at 15 years were 69% for BMT recipients and 38% for patients receiving immunosuppressive therapy. In their series, almost 15% of patients experienced a malignant clonal disorder or PNH. These authors concluded that BMT is preferable in younger patients with aplastic anemia who have matched related donors.

As noted earlier, patients with aplastic anemia who are treated with immunosuppressive regimens alone are at high risk for clonal evolution to myelodysplasia and acute leukemia as well as PNH. Persistence of a defective or damaged clone that sustains hematopoiesis but is inherently unstable may contribute to the alarming incidence of late leukemia and PNH in patients initially responding to immunosuppressive therapies. These concerns are avoided by use of an allogeneic transplant and therefore favor the use of an HLA-identical matched related donor transplant in the younger patient whenever possible. A suggested algorithm for transplant decisions in SAA is shown in Figure 1–1.

SPECIAL SITUATIONS

Patients with aplastic anemia associated with hepatitis, PNH, or Fanconi anemia present special problems that require a different approach than the average aplastic anemia patient. These conditions are considered separately.

HEPATITIS-ASSOCIATED SEVERE APLASTIC ANEMIA

The association between acute hepatitis and aplastic anemia has been known for 50 years, and over 200 cases have been reported in the literature.[94] Aplastic anemia may occur after hepatitis A, B, or C, but a 1997 report from Brown et al. did not identify any of the known hepatitis viruses in 10 well-studied cases with hepatitis-associated aplastic anemia.[95] Aplastic anemia may also occur after liver transplantation performed for non A, non B hepatitis.[96] Immunologic studies implicate the presence of activated CD8+ T lymphocytes in the pathogenesis of this disorder.[95] For patients with HLA-identical donors, early transplantation results suggested a particularly poor prognosis,[97] but more recent studies from single centers and registry data indicate that the hepatitis did not affect rates of graft failure, acute or chronic GVHD, or long-term survival.[98–100] Cyclophosphamide may be safely administered to these patients despite abnormal liver function test results, and surprisingly there was no excess incidence of hepatic veno-occlusive disease in these patients. For patients with persistent hepatitis B antigenemia or hepatitis C in whom engraftment is successful, withdrawal of cyclosporine and immune reconstitution may lead to reactivation of cytotoxic lymphocytes, which can potentially cause fulminant viral hepatitis.[100, 101] These patients may require prolonged tapering of cyclosporine to prevent liver failure. Patients without HLA-identical donors may also be successfully treated with cyclosporine and ATG,[95] and young patients in whom immunosuppressive therapy fails are candidates for unrelated donor transplantation.

MANAGEMENT OF FANCONI ANEMIA

Fanconi anemia (FA) is a rare autosomal recessive disease characterized by multiple congenital abnormalities associated with bone marrow failure and increased susceptibility to cancer. The average age at presentation is 8 years, and patients may present with growth retardation, abnormalities of the skin, and defects in the upper extremities, particularly the thumb and forearms, gastrointestinal system, and kidneys.[5] Not all patients present with physical abnormalities, however, and the diagnosis of FA relies on demonstration of increased spontaneous chromosomal breakage in standard cytogenetic testing using clastogens such as diepoxybutane or mitomycin-C.[6] At least two of five known FA genes have been cloned.[5]

The only known curative therapy for FA is allogeneic bone marrow transplantation with an HLA-identical sibling or a volunteer donor. In 1995, Gluckman et al. summarized the international experience from the IBMTR[102]; 151 patients with FA underwent transplantation with HLA-identical sibling donors, and 48 underwent transplantation with volunteer alternative related or unrelated donors, between 1978 and 1994. Approximately two-thirds of patients survived after HLA-identical sibling transplantation, and 30% survived after alternative-donor transplants. Younger patient age, higher pre-transplant platelet counts, and use of ATG and low-dose cyclophosphamide plus limited field irradiation in the pre-transplant conditioning regimen and use of cyclosporine for GVHD prophylaxis were all associated with increased survival.

Because of the increased chromosome fragility, conditioning of these patients requires modification of the regimen to reduce the dose of cyclophosphamide and TBI.[102] Limited field irradiation (500 cGy) plus low dose (15–25 mg/kg) cyclophosphamide with or without ATG is commonly used. TBI is usually reduced to 600 cGy. When no irradiation is used, high-dose cyclophosphamide (100 mg/kg) with or without ATG has been used; however, this approach was clearly associated with a poorer outcome. Use of low-dose cyclophosphamide with limited field irradiation with or without ATG provides adequate immune suppression for stable engraftment in patients with FA without excess cancer risk. Based on the IBMTR experience, all patients with FA should be conditioned with lower doses of cyclophosphamide (15–25 mg/kg) and reduced dosages of limited field or TBI in the range of 500–600 cGy. Because of a poorer outcome associated with increasing age and lower pre-transplant platelet count, patients with FA should undergo transplantation earlier, before their clinical condition deteriorates.

PAROXYSMAL NOCTURNAL HEMOGLOBINURIA

Paroxysmal nocturnal hemoglobinemia (PNH) is an acquired clonal stem cell disorder that is characterized by intravascular hemolysis and evolution to bone marrow failure or aplastic anemia and an increased tendency to venous thrombosis in unusual locations (hepatic vein or cerebral vessels). In PNH, a somatic mutation that involves a primitive hematopoietic stem cell occurs because of a mutation of the X-linked Pig-A gene.[7] The Pig-A gene encodes a protein that is essential for the normal biosynthesis of glycosylphosphatidyl inositol, which serves as a membrane anchor for a large number of cellular proteins. The deficiency of these cellular proteins explains the heightened sensitivity of red blood cells to complement, resulting in a chronic hemolytic state. Patients with life-threatening thrombotic complications and/or marrow failure are candidates for early transplantation.[103] Allogeneic marrow trans-

plantation with an HLA-identical sibling donor is curative; however, elimination of the abnormal clone requires the use of a myeloablative conditioning regimen such as busulfan (16 mg/kg) plus cyclophosphamide (120–200 mg/kg). Cyclophosphamide with TBI is an acceptable alternative to busulfan-cyclophosphamide in this setting.

The IBMTR has reported the largest series of patients undergoing allogeneic or syngeneic bone marrow transplantation for PNH.[104] Most patients received myeloablative preparative regimens (busulfan-cyclophosphamide or cyclophosphamide TBI). There was a high incidence of graft failure (24%) and deaths related to graft failure. The 2-year probability of survival was 47%. A patient with PNH who received a syngeneic marrow transplant without a myeloablative conditioning regimen relapsed with PNH.[105] This case further suggested that without myeloablation, PNH clones could persist and have a survival advantage over normal stem cells.

REFERENCES

1. Camitta BM, Thomas ED, Nathan DG, et al: Severe aplastic anemia: a prospective study of the effect of early marrow transplantation on mortality. Blood 48:63–69, 1976.
2. Maciejewski JP, Hibbs TR, Anderson S, et al: Bone marrow and peripheral blood lymphocyte phenotype in patients with bone marrow failure. Exp Hematol 22:1102–1110, 1994.
3. Marsh JCW, How JM, Bryett KA, et al: Survival after anti-lymphocyte globulin therapy for aplastic anemia depends on disease severity. Blood 70:1046–1051, 1987.
4. Griscelli-Bennaceur A, Gluckman, E, Scrobohaci MC, et al: Aplastic anemia and paroxysmal nocturnal hemoglobinuria: search for a pathogenic link. Blood 85:1354–1363, 1995.
5. D'Andrea AD, Grompe M: Molecular biology of Fanconi anemia: implications for diagnosis and therapy. Blood 90:1725–1736, 1997.
6. Kuffel D, Lindow N, Litzow M, et al: Mitomycin C chromosome stress test to identify hypersensitivity to bi-functional alkylating agents in patients with Fanconi anemia or aplastic anemia. Mayo Clin Proc 72:579–580, 1997.
7. Rosse WF, Ware RE: The molecular basis of paroxysmal nocturnal hemoglobinuria. Blood 86:3277–3286, 1995.
8. Young NS, Maciejewski J: The pathophysiology of acquired aplastic anemia. N Engl J Med 336:1365–1372, 1997.
9. Hoffman R, Young N, Ershler W, et al: Diffuse fasciitis and aplastic anemia: a report of four cases revealing an unusual association between rheumatologic and hematologic disorders. Medicine 61:373–381, 1982.
10. Josse JW, Zacks SI: Thymoma and pancytopenia. N Engl J Med 259:113–117, 1958.
11. Moulopoulos LA, Dimopoulos MA: Magnetic residence imaging of the bone marrow in hematologic malignancies. Blood 90:2127–2147, 1997.
12. Harrison DE: Use of genetic anemias in mice as tools for hematologic research. Clinic Haematol 8:239–262, 1979.
13. Russell ES: Hereditary anemias of the mouse: a review for geneticists. Adv Genet 200:357, 1979.
14. Maciejewski JP, Selleri C, Sato T, et al: Severe and consistent deficit in marrow and circulating primitive hematopoietic cells (long term culture initiating cells) in acquired aplastic anemia. Blood 88:1983–1991, 1996.
15. Scopes J, Daly S, Atkinson R, et al: Aplastic anemia: evidence for dysfunctional bone marrow progenitor cells and the corrective effect of granulocyte colony-stimulating factor in vitro. Blood 87:3179–3185, 1996.
16. Betticher DC, Huxal H, Muller R, et al: Colony growth in cultures from bone marrow and peripheral blood after curative treatment for leukemia and severe aplastic anemia. Exp Hematol 21:1517–1521, 1993.
17. Holmberg LA, Seidel K, Leisenring W, Torok-Storb B: Aplastic anemia: analysis of stromal cell function in long term marrow cultures. Blood 84:3685–3690, 1994.

18. Lyman SD, Seaberg M, Hanna R, et al: Plasma serum levels of flt-3 ligand are low in normal individuals and highly elevated in patients with Fanconi anemia and acquired aplastic anemia. Blood 86:4091–4096, 1995.

19. Selleri C, Maciejewski JP, Sato T, Young NS: Interferon gamma constitutively expressed in the stromal microenvironment of human marrow cultures mediates potent hematopoietic inhibition. Blood 87:4149–4159, 1996.

20. Selleri C, Sato T, Anderson S, et al: Interferon gamma and tumor necrosis factor alpha suppress both early and late stages of hematopoiesis and induce programmed cell death. J Cell Physiol 165:538–546, 1992.

21. Appelbaum F, Fefer A, Cheever M, et al: Treatment of aplastic anemia by bone marrow transplantation in identical twins. Blood 55:1033–1039, 1980.

22. Champlin R, Feig S, Sparks R, Gale RP: Bone marrow transplantation from identical twins in the treatment of aplastic anemia: implication for the pathogenesis of the disease. Br J Haematol 56:455–463, 1984.

23. Baran DT, Griner PF, Klemperer MR: Recovery from aplastic anemia after treatment with cyclophosphamide. N Engl J Med 295:1522–1523, 1976.

24. Thomas ED, Storb R, Giblett ER, et al: Recovery from aplastic anemia following attempted marrow transplantation. Exp Hematol 4:97–102, 1976.

25. Barnes D, Mole RH: Aplastic anemia in sublethally irradiated mice given allogeneic lymph node cells. Br J Haematol 13:482–491, 1967.

26. Knospe WH, Steinberg D, Speck B: Experimental immunologically mediated aplastic anemia in H-2^k identical M/S(M) locus different mice. Exp Hematol 11:542–552, 1983.

27. Ascensao J, Kagan W, Moore M, et al: Aplastic anemia: evidence for an immunological mechanism. Lancet 1:669–671, 1976.

28. Hoffman R, Zanjani ED, Lutton JD, et al: Suppression of erythroid colony formation by lymphocytes from patients with aplastic anemia. N Engl J Med 296:10–13, 1977.

29. Zoumbos N, Gascon P, Trost S, et al: Circulating activated suppressor T lymphocytes in aplastic anemia. N Engl J Med 312:257–265, 1985.

30. Singer JW, Doney KC, Thomas ED: Coculture studies of 16 untransfused patients with aplastic anemia. Blood 54:180–185, 1979.

31. Torok-Storb BJ, Sieff C, Storb R, et al: In vitro tests for distinguishing possible immune-mediated aplastic anemia from transfusion induced sensitization. Blood 55:211–215, 1980.

32. Mangan KF, Mullaney MT, Rosenfeld CS, Shadduck RK: In vitro evidence for disappearance of erythroid progenitor T suppressor cells following allogeneic bone marrow transplantation for severe aplastic anemia. Blood 71:144–150, 1988.

33. Zoumbos NC, Gascon P, Djeu J, Young NS: Interferon is a mediator of hematopoietic suppression in aplastic anemia in vitro and possibly in vivo. Proc Natl Acad Sci U S A 82:188–192, 1985.

34. Tong J, Bacigalupo A, Piaggio G, et al: In vitro response of T-cells from aplastic anemia patients to anti-lymphocyte globulin and phytohemagglutinin: colony stimulating activity and lymphokine production. Exp Hematol 19:312–316, 1991.

35. Maciejewski JP, Selleri C, Sato T, et al: Increased expression of Fas antigen on bone marrow CD34+ cells of patients with aplastic anemia. Br J Haematol 91:245–252, 1995.

36. Philpott NJ, Scopes J, Marsh JC, et al: Increased apoptosis in aplastic anemia bone marrow progenitor cells: possible pathophysiologic significance. Exp Hematol 23:1642–1648, 1995.

37. Freedman MH, Gilfand EW, Sanders EH: Acquired aplastic anemia: antibody mediated hematopoietic failure. Am J Hematol 6:131–141, 1979.

38. Fitchen JJ, Cline MJ, Saxon A, Golde DW: Serum inhibition of hematopoiesis in a patients with aplastic anemia and systemic lupus erythematosus: recovery after exchange plasma pheresis. Am J Med 66:537–542, 1979.

39. Cline MJ, Opelz G, Saxon A, et al: Autoimmune panleukopenia. N Engl J Med 295:1480–1493, 1976.

40. Camitta BM, Thomas ED: Severe aplastic anemia: a prospective study of the affect of androgens or transplantation on hematologic recovery and survival. Clin Hematol 7:587–595, 1978.

41. Najean Y: Androgen therapy in aplastic anemia: a comparative study of high and low doses and four different androgens. Scand J Haematol 36:346–352, 1986.

42. Mathe G, Amiel JL, Schwarzenberg L: Bone marrow graft in man after conditioning by antilymphocyte serum. Br Med J 2:131–136, 1970.

43. Champlin RE, Ho W, Gale RP: Antithymocyte globulin treatment in patients with aplastic anemia: a prospective randomized trial. N Engl J Med 308:113–120, 1983.

44. Young M, Griffith P, Brittain E, et al: A multi center trial of antithymocyte globulin in aplastic anemia and related diseases. Blood 72:1861–1866, 1988.

45. Finlay JC, Toretsky J, Hoffman L, et al: Cyclosporin A in refractory severe aplastic anemia. Blood 64:104a, 1984.

46. Esperou A, Devergie A, Lehor P, et al: A randomized study comparing cyclosporin A and antithymocyte globulin for treatment of severe aplastic anemia. Nouv Rev Fr Hematol 31:65–68, 1989.

47. Bacigalupo A, Van Lint MT, Cervi R: Treatment of severe aplastic anemia with bolus 6-methylprednisolone and antilymphocyte globulin. Blood 41:168–171, 1980.

48. Brodsky RA, Sensebrenner LL, Jones RJ: Complete remission of severe aplastic anemia after high dose cyclophosphamide without bone marrow transplantation. Blood 87:491–494, 1996.

49. Frickhofen N, Kaltwasser JP, Schezenmeier H, et al: Treatment of aplastic anemia with antilymphocyte globulin and methylprednisolone with or without cyclosporine. N Engl J Med 324:1297–1304, 1991.

50. Najean Y, Haguenauer O: Longterm (5 to 20 years) evolution of nongrafted aplastic anemia. Blood 76:2222–2228, 1990.

51. Rosenfeld SJ, Kimball J, Vining D, Young NS: Intensive immunosuppression with antithymocyte globulin and cyclosporine as treatment for severe acquired aplastic anemia. Blood 85:3058–3065, 1995.

52. Mangan KF, D'Alessandro L, Mullaney M: Action of horse antihuman thymocyte globulin on normal human erythroid progenitor cell proliferation in vitro: erythropoietic growth enhancing factors are released by marrow accessory cells. J Lab Clin Med 107:353–364, 1986.

53. Hinterberger W, Rowlings PA, Hinterberger-Fischer M, et al: Results of transplanting bone marrow from genetically identical twins into patients with aplastic anemia. Ann Intern Med 126:116–122, 1977.

54. Thomas ED, Buckner CD, Storb R, et al: Aplastic anemia treated by marrow transplantation. Lancet 1:284–289, 1972.

55. Storb R, Thomas ED, Buckner CD, et al: Allogeneic marrow grafting for treatment of aplastic anemia. Blood 43:157–180, 1974.

56. Storb R, Prentice RL, Thomas ED: Marrow transplantation for aplastic anemia. N Engl J Med 296:61–66, 1977.

57. Storb R, Longton G, Anasetti C, et al: Changing trends in marrow transplantation for severe aplastic anemia. Bone Marrow Transplant 10:45–52, 1992.

58. Passweg JR, Socie G, Hinterberger W, et al: Bone marrow transplantation for severe aplastic anemia: has outcome improved? Blood 90:858–864, 1997.

59. Hows J, Palmer S, Gordon Smith EC: Cyclosporine and graft failure following bone marrow transplantation for severe aplastic anemia. Br J Haematol 60:611–617, 1985.

60. Storb R, Weiden PL, Sullivan KM, et al: Second marrow transplants in patients with aplastic anemia rejecting their first graft: use of conditioning regimen including cyclophosphamide and antithymocyte globulin. Blood 70:116–122, 1987.

61. McCann SR, Bacigalupo A, Gluckman E, et al: Graft rejection and second bone marrow transplants for aplastic anemia: a report from the Aplastic Anemia Working Group of the European Bone Marrow Transplant Group. Bone Marrow Transplant 13:233, 1994.

62. Nemunitis J, Singer JW, Buckner CD: Use of recombinant human granulocyte macrophage colony stimulating factor in graft failure after bone marrow transplantation. Blood 76:245–253, 1990.

63. Storb R, Thomas ED, Buckner CD: Marrow transplantation in 30 untransfused patients with severe aplastic anemia. Ann Intern Med 92:30–36, 1980.

64. Anasetti C, Doney KC, Storb R, et al: Marrow transplantation for severe aplastic anemia: long term outcome in fifty untransfused patients. Ann Intern Med 104:461–466, 1986.

65. Bean MA, Storb R, Graham T, et al: Prevention of transfusion induced sensitization to minor histocompatibility antigens in DLA-identical canine marrow grafts by gamma irradiation of marrow donor blood. Transplantation 52:956–960, 1991.

66. Deeg HJ, Self S, Storb R, et al: Decreased incidence of marrow graft rejection in patients with severe aplastic anemia changing impact of risk factors. Blood 68:1363–1368, 1986.

67. Gordon Smith EC, Hows J, Bacigalupo A, et al: Bone marrow transplantation for severe aplastic anemia from donors other than HLA identical siblings: a report of the EBMT working party. Semin Hematol 21:100–108, 1994.
68. Beatty PG, DiBartolomeo P, Storb R, et al: The treatment of aplastic anemia with marrow grafts from related donors other than HLA genotypically match siblings. Clin Transplant 1:117–124, 1987.
69. Patterson J, Prentice HG, Brennor M: Graft rejection following HLA matched T lymphocyte depleted bone marrow transplantation. Br J Haematol 64:225–230, 1986.
70. Storb R, Prentice R, Thomas ED: Factors associated with graft rejection after HLA identical marrow transplantation for aplastic anemia. Br J Haematol 55:573–585, 1983.
71. Niederweiser D, Pepe M, Storb R, et al: Improvement in rejection, engraftment rate and survival with increase in graft versus host disease by high marrow cell dose in patients transplanted for aplastic anemia. Br J Haematol 69:23–28, 1988.
72. Storb R, Doney KC, Thomas ED, et al: Marrow transplantation with or without donor buffy coat cells for 65 transfused aplastic anemia patients. Blood 59:236–246, 1982.
73. Damiane D, Fanin R, Silvestri F, et al: A randomized trial of autologous filgrastim primed bone marrow transplantation versus filgrastim mobilized peripheral blood stem cell transplantation in lymphoma patients. Blood 90:36–42, 1997.
74. Storek G, Gooby T, Siadel M, et al: Allogeneic peripheral blood stem cell transplantation maybe associated with a high risk of chronic graft versus host disease. Blood 90:4705–4709, 1997.
75. Feig SA, Champlin R, Arenson E, et al: Improved survival following bone marrow transplantation for severe aplastic anemia. Br J Haematol 54:509–517, 1983.
76. Gluckman E, Horowitz M, Champlin RE, et al: Bone marrow transplantation for severe aplastic anemia: influence of conditioning and graft versus host disease prophylaxis regimens on outcome. Blood 79:269–275, 1992.
77. McGlave PB, Haake R, Miller W, et al: Therapy of severe aplastic anemia in young adults and children with allogeneic bone marrow transplantation. Blood 70:1325–1330, 1987.
78. Socie G, Henry-Amar M, Cosset JM, et al: Increased incidence of solid malignant tumors after bone marrow transplantation for severe aplastic anemia. Blood 78:277–279, 1991.
79. Sanders JE: The impact of marrow transplant preparative regimens on subsequent growth and development. Semin Hematol 28:244–249, 1991.
80. Storb R, Etzioni R, Anasetti C, et al: Cyclophosphamide combined with antithymocyte globulin in preparation for allogeneic marrow transplants in aplastic anemia. Blood 84:941–947, 1994.
81. Appelbaum F, Storb R, Ramberg K, et al: Allogeneic bone marrow transplantation in the treatment of preleukemia. Ann Intern Med 100:689–693, 1984.
82. Storb R, Prentice R, Buckner D, et al: Graft versus host disease and survival in patients with aplastic anemia treated by marrow grafts from HLA identical siblings. N Engl J Med 308:302–307, 1983.
83. Storb R, Deeg HJ, Farewell K, et al: Marrow transplantation for severe aplastic anemia: methotrexate alone compared with the combination of methotrexate and cyclosporine for prevention of acute graft-versus-host disease. Blood 68:119–125, 1986.
84. Weiner RS, Horowitz M, Gale RP, et al: Risk factors for interstitial pneumonia following bone marrow transplantation for severe aplastic anemia. Br J Haematol 71:535–543, 1989.
85. Storb R, Prentice R, Sullivan K, et al: Predictive factors in chronic graft versus host disease in patients with aplastic anemia treated by marrow transplantation from HLA identical siblings. Ann Intern Med 98:461–466, 1983.
86. Socie G, Henry Amar M, Bacigalupo A, et al: Malignant tumors occurring after treatment of aplastic anemia. N Engl J Med 329:1152–1157, 1993.
87. Witherspoon RP, Storb R, Pepe M, et al: Cumulative incidence of secondary solid malignant tumors in aplastic anemia patients given marrow grafts after conditioning with chemotherapy alone. Blood 79:289–290, 1992.
88. Deeg HJ, Socie G, Schoch G, et al: Malignancies after marrow transplantation for aplastic anemia and Fanconi anemia: a joint Seattle Paris analysis of results in 700 patients. Blood 87:386–392, 1996.
89. Deeg HJ, Schoch G, Ramsey N, et al: Marrow transplantation from unrelated donors for patients with aplastic anemia who failed immunosuppressive therapy. Blood 90(Suppl 1):397a, 1997.
90. Camitta B, Ash R, Menitove J, et al: Bone marrow transplantation for children with severe aplastic anemia: use of donors other than HLA identical siblings. Blood 74:1852–1857, 1989.
91. Bacigalupo A, Hows J, Gluckman E: Bone marrow transplantation versus immunosuppression for treatment of severe aplastic anemia: a report of the EBMT SAA Working Party. Br J Haematol 70:171–182, 1988.
92. Paquette PL, Tabjani N, Franc M, et al: Long term outcome of aplastic anemia in adults treated with antithymocyte globulin: comparison with bone marrow transplantation. Blood 85:283–290, 1995.
93. Doney K, Leisenring W, Storb A, Appelbaum F: Primary treatment of acquired aplastic anemia: outcomes with bone marrow transplantation and immunosuppressive therapy. Ann Intern Med 126:107–115, 1997.
94. Hagler L, Pastore R, Bergin J, Wrensch N: Aplastic anemia following viral hepatitis: report of two fatal cases and literature review. Medicine 54:139–164, 1975.
95. Brown KE, Tisdale J, Barrett AJ, et al: Hepatitis-associated aplastic anemia. N Engl J Med 336:1049–1064, 1997.
96. Tzakis AG, Arditi M, Whitingon PF, et al: Aplastic anemia complicating orthotopic liver transplantation for non-A, non-B hepatitis. N Engl J Med 319:393–396, 1988.
97. Camitta B, Nathan DG, Forman EN, et al: Post hepatitis severe aplastic anemia: an indication for early bone marrow transplantation. Blood 43:473–483, 1974.
98. Witherspoon RP, Storb R, Schulman H, et al: Marrow transplantation in hepatitis associated aplastic anemia. Am J Hematol 17:269–278, 1984.
99. Kojima S, Matsuyami M, Kodin Y: Bone marrow transplantation for hepatitis associated aplastic anemia. Acta Haematol 79:7–11, 1988.
100. Parienti EA, Gordeau A, Dubois F, et al: Fulminant hepatitis due to reactivation of chronic hepatitis B infection after allogeneic bone marrow transplantation. Dig Dis Sci 33:1185–1191, 1988.
101. Kanamori H, Fukawa H, Maruton A: Case report: fulminant hepatitis C viral infection after allogeneic bone marrow transplant. Am J Med Sci 303:109–111, 1992.
102. Gluckman E, Auerbach A, Horowitz M, et al: Bone marrow transplantation for Fanconi anemia. Blood 86:2856–2862, 1995.
103. Ware R, Hall SE, Rosse WH: Paroxysmal nocturnal hemoglobinuria with onset in childhood and adolescence. N Engl J Med 325:991–996, 1991.
104. Saso R, Marsh J, Ceverska L, et al: Bone marrow transplants for paroxysmal nocturnal hemoglobinuria. Br J Haematol 104:392–396, 1999.
105. Endo M, Beatty PG, Vrecke TM, et al: Syngeneic bone marrow transplantation without conditioning in a patient with PNH: in vivo evidence that the mutant stem cells have a survival advantage. Blood 88:742–750, 1996.
106. Leitman SF: Use of blood cell irradiation in the prevention of post transfusion graft-versus-host disease. Transfus Sci 10:219–232, 1989.
107. Aitchison R, Marsh JC, Hows J, et al: Pregnancy associated aplastic anemia: a report of five cases and review of current management. Br J Haematol 73:541–545, 1989.
108. Mangan KF, Zidar B, Shadduck RK, et al: Interferon-induced aplasia: evidence for T cell mediated suppression of hematopoiesis and recovery after treatment with house antihuman thymocyte globulin. Am J Hematol 19:401–413, 1985.
109. Mangan KF: Immunologic control of hematopoiesis: implication for quality of the graft after allogeneic bone marrow transplantation. Transplant Proc 19:23–28, 1987.
110. Shadduck RK, Winkelstein A, Zeigler Z, et al: Aplastic anemia following infectious mononucleosis: possible immune etiology. Exp Hematol 7:265–271, 1979.

CHAPTER TWO

Acute Myelogenous Leukemia

David R. Simpson, M.D., and Armand Keating, M.D.

Transplant options for acute myelogenous leukemia (AML), also called acute myeloid or myeloblastic leukemia, have increased in recent years. Initially, bone marrow transplants (BMT) were designed to exploit the steep dose-response curve of leukemic cells to increased doses of specific drugs. Immune mechanisms however—especially after allogeneic bone marrow transplantation (alloBMT)—are important in preventing relapse and are emphasized by results of twin studies,[1] donor lymphocyte infusions,[2] and the correlation between graft-versus-host disease (GVHD) and relapse.[3]

Current induction protocols can achieve complete remission in up to 80% of patients with de novo AML, depending on the selection criteria.[4–6] Postremission chemotherapy cures only 25–40%,[6] however, and most patients experience relapse and die. Remission consolidation with high-dose therapy and BMT has reduced the relapse rate and achieves long-term disease-free survival (DFS) in about 60% of patients undergoing the procedure.[7, 8]

Hemotopoietic stem cell transplantation (HSCT) was initially performed with marrow from a matched sibling donor. Now transplantation may also be performed from autologous, syngeneic, mismatched sibling or unrelated donors and, in addition to bone marrow, the stem cell source may be peripheral blood progenitor cells or cord blood. The origin of the graft determines the extent of GVHD. More GVHD, greater treatment-related mortality, and fewer relapses occur in transplants from donors with greater degrees of human leukocyte antigen (HLA) disparity.

Prospective studies and registry databases have provided the means to quantify the overall relapse probability and regimen-related mortality according to the type of transplant and stage of disease. Individualization of treatment is important, however. Patient factors such as age and coexistent disease affect the risk of regimen-related death, whereas disease factors influence the risk of relapse. Factors predicting for relapse after transplantation are similar to those after chemotherapy and include the white cell count at diagnosis,[8] chromosomal abnormalities,[9, 10] and French-American-British (FAB) morphologic classification subtype.[11] Clonal chromosomal and molecular lesions are especially important because many are associated with distinct clinical patterns and predict response to specific therapy. Detection of minimal residual disease after induction therapy is also useful in predicting outcome[12, 13] and likely to become more important in the future.

Controversy remains, but a matched sibling is still the preferred donor source for young patients with AML. In those with a matched sibling donor there are few indications for other forms of HSCT. The majority of patients presenting with AML, however, do not have a suitable sibling donor or are too old for an allogeneic transplant. Other types of transplant may offer these patients greater hope for cure than the use of chemotherapy alone.

ALLOGENEIC SIBLING TRANSPLANTATION

Bone marrow transplantation (BMT) was first performed in humans in 1957. The initial work arose from studies of radiation toxicity. As early as 1922, it was observed that shielding the legs of lethally irradiated guinea pigs could prevent hematologic toxicity.[14] It was not until after the bombing of Hiroshima, however, when much research was directed at overcoming the problems of radiation toxicity, that transplantation technology progressed. Subsequent studies showed that lethally irradiated mice survived when their spleens were removed prior to irradiation and later reinfused into the peritoneum.[15] Initially, BMT was reserved for patients with a poor prognosis who had no other therapeutic option, because mortality from infection and GVHD was high. Better management of these complications has broadened the indications for alloBMT. Although GVHD remains a major cause of morbidity, immune-mediated mechanisms against leukemia or the graft-versus-leukemia (GVL) effect are probably responsible for most of the success of allogeneic transplantation.[3] Unfortunately, the reduction of GVHD by T-cell depletion[16] or increased immunosuppression[17] results in increased relapse, and as yet GVL and GVH effects have not been separated.

The main decision regarding transplants for patients with AML who have a matched sibling donor is the timing of transplantation. Many centers routinely transplant during the first remission, although this policy results in treating some patients already cured by chemotherapy alone. The reliable selection of patients in whom transplantation can be safely delayed until relapse or second remission remains a challenge.

FIRST COMPLETE REMISSION (CR1)

Thomas et al. from the Fred Hutchinson Cancer Research Center in Seattle demonstrated that matched-sibling alloBMT was effective therapy for patients with relapsed AML, especially those with high-performance status. In 1976, they began the first study of alloBMT for AML in first remission.[18] They reasoned that patients with a low burden of leukemic cells would be more readily cured and their better clinical condition would result in less transplant-related morbidity. The results of the first 19 patients receiving an HLA-matched sibling BMT after cyclophosphamide and total-body irradiation (TBI) conditioning experienced a 5-year survival rate of 50%. Two deaths were due to relapse, and seven were due to treatment-related causes. Many series published since show similar results (Table 2–1).

The International Bone Marrow Transplant Registry (IBMTR) reported the results of 647 patients receiving an unmanipulated BMT from a matched-sibling donor between January 1989 and December 1993.[7] The conditioning regimen was cyclophosphamide and TBI–based in 50% and busulfan and cyclophosphamide–based in the remainder; all patients received GVHD prophylaxis that included cyclosporine. Treatment-related mortality was 23% (95% confidence index [CI] = 19–27%), the probability of relapse was 23% (95% CI = 18–26%), and DFS was 60% (95% CI = 56–64%) at 3 years. These results are similar to data from the European Group for Blood and Marrow Transplantation (EBMT) on 516 patients, 69% of whom received TBI. Four-year treatment-related mortality was 27 ± 2%, the relapse rate was 25 ± 3%, and DFS was 55 ± 3%.[11]

To avoid overtreating patients already cured by chemotherapy, an alternative strategy is to delay alloHSCT until relapse. This is best justified in patients whose relapse probability is low. Data from the UK MRC (United Kingdom Medical Research Council) AML 10 study show that chemotherapy alone can achieve 5-year DFS of 61% in patients with t(8;21) translocation (n = 129), 54% in patients with inversion (16) (n = 48), and 53% in patients with chromosomal translocation t(15;17) (n = 194).[19] Another study has shown that patients with promyelocytic leukemia (AML M3 subtype), who experience complete remission after all-trans-retinoic acid (ATRA) and chemotherapy, experience a 90% DFS at 1 year.[20] Many centers do not routinely perform transplantation in patients with t(15;17) translocations who achieve molecular remission—defined as lack of the reverse transcriptase-polymerase chain reaction (RT-PCR) signal for the promyelocytic/retinoic acid receptor (PML/RARα) transcript—because of their excellent prognosis.[5, 21] Most patients with persistent molecular evidence of disease, however, suffer relapse within 6 months.[12, 13, 22] Therefore, failure to achieve molecular complete remission after induction therapy may warrant alloHSCT for patients in morphologic complete remission.

It is a tantalizing prospect to predict relapse by detection of minimal residual disease and then target the positive group for early transplantation. Caution must be used in extrapolating the findings from studies of molecular detection of PML-RARα to patients with other translocations, however. Molecular techniques are available for the detection of t(8;21), t(6;9), t(9;11), t(9;22), and inv(16), which together account for about 40% of de novo AML cases.[19] The 8;21 translocation has been detected by PCR in patients with stable long-term remission after chemotherapy[23–25] and alloHSCT.[26] The prognostic implication of the presence of other molecular markers is unclear.

The role of intensive chemotherapy prior to transplantation is also unclear. High-dose cytarabine prolongs remission duration but has not been shown to affect the induction rate.[27, 28] Standard or intermediate-dose cytarabine

induction regimens may be preferable because their lower toxicity may result in lower transplant-related mortality. The ideal number of cycles of consolidation chemotherapy (if any) prior to alloHSCT has not been determined. An IBMTR study is currently in progress to address this issue.

RELAPSE

Patients who do not undergo transplantation during remission may proceed to HSCT at the first sign of relapse. The rationale for this approach is that the toxicity of reinduction regimens is avoided and some patients not responsive to reinduction may be salvaged by transplantation. A report from Seattle describes patients who received alloBMT either in untreated (n = 54) or chemotherapy-resistant (n = 29) first relapse.[29] In the untreated cohort, relapse at 5 years was 36% (95% CI = 16–45%) with an overall survival rate of 28% (95% CI = 12–43%). Patients with chemotherapy-resistant relapse experienced a 5-year relapse rate of 56% (95% CI = 32–81%) and an overall survival rate of 24% (95% CI = 9–40%). In this study most patients in untreated relapse had relapse detected at the time of BMT planned for first remission (34 of 54 patients). Most of these patients (20 of 34) were in early relapse with less than 30% blasts on bone marrow biopsy. In contrast, for those whose transplantation was electively delayed until relapse, early relapse occurred in only 4 of 20 cases. Thus, care should be taken in extrapolating these results when planning clinical strategies. HSCT at the time of molecular detection of relapse, when the disease burden is low, may improve the outcome of patients with untreated relapse, although data to support this are lacking.

SECOND REMISSION

Delaying HSCT until second remission has the advantage of selecting patients who do poorly with conventional treatment and excludes those with chemotherapy-resistant disease. The disadvantage of this approach is that the reinduction chemotherapy may render some patients ineligible for HSCT because of infection or organ toxicity. Overall, approximately 60% of patients experience a second remission with salvage chemotherapy.[32] Success of induction of second remission depends on the duration of the first remission, the salvage regimen used, and cytogenetic abnormalities. Patients with inv(16) or t(8;21) are more likely to have responsive disease at relapse.[9, 30, 31]

In a series from the Fred Hutchinson Cancer Research Center, 49 patients received transplant in second remission after cyclophosphamide-TBI conditioning and methotrexate GVHD prophylaxis.[29] Treatment-related mortality (55%) and 100-day mortality (39%) were high. At 5 years, the probability of relapse was 37 ± 20% and overall survival was 28% (95% CI = 12–43%). Treatment-related mortality rates have fallen since this study was performed.[33] The EMBT reported the outcome of 98 patients receiving an HLA-identical sibling transplant in second remission between 1987 and 1993 using a variety of conditioning and GVHD regimens. At 4 years, the regimen-related mortality rate was 32 ± 5%, the relapse rate was 42 ± 8%, and

TABLE 2–1. TRIALS OF ALLOGENEIC BONE MARROW TRANSPLANTATION FOR ACUTE MYELOGENOUS LEUKEMIA

DISEASE STAGE	NUMBER OF PATIENTS	CONDITIONING REGIMEN	STUDY GROUP/AUTHOR	Dx TO BMT (MONTHS)	CR TO BMT (MONTHS)	RELAPSE RATE	REGIMEN-RELATED MORTALITY	DFS	STUDY PERIOD	REFERENCE NO.
CR1	71	BuCy	Copelan et al	4.5		14%	23%	63%	1984–1989	108
	50	CyTBI	Blaise et al	4		14%	8%	72%	1987–1990	110
	51	BuCy	Blaise et al	4		34%	27%	47%	1987–1990	110
	647	Various	IBMTR, Keating et al			22 ± 4%	23 ± 4%	60 ± 4%	1989–1993	7
	516	Various	EBMT, Gorin et al	4.75		25 ± 3%	27 ± 2%	55 ± 3%	1987–1993	11
	129 (Children)	Various	EBMTR, Gorin et al			25 ± 5%	9 ± 3%	68 ± 5%	1987–1993	11
	144/168*	Various	EORTC/GIMEMA, Zittoun et al			24.4%	17%	58%	1986–1993	5
CR2	113	BuCy	Cassileth et al	4.5	1–11	29%	20%	43 ± 10%	1990–1995	59
	704	CyTBI	IBMTR, Gale et al	4.5	3	20 ± 4%	NA	48 ± 5%	1978–1986	8
	98	Various	EBMTR, Gorin et al		2	42 ± 8%	32 ± 5%	29 ± 7%	1987–1993	11
	17 (Children)	Various	EBMTR, Gorin et al			52 ± 16%	18 ± 9%	39 ± 13%	1987–1993	11
	129	Various	IBMTR, Keating et al					53 ± 5%	1989–1993	34

*Denotes patients in randomized trial completing assigned treatment/patients assigned treatment.

BMT, bone marrow transplantation; CR, complete remission; Dx, diagnosis; Bu, busulfan; Cy, cyclophosphamide; TBI, total body irradiation; DFS, disease-free survival; IBMTR, International Bone Marrow Transplant Registry; EBMTR, European Blood and Marrow Transplant Registry; GIMEMA, Gruppo Italiana Malattie Ematologiche Maligne dell'Adulto; CR1, first complete remission; CR2, second complete remission.

DFS was 39 ± 7%.[11] Similar results were reported by the IBMTR.[34] For 129 patients receiving an HLA-identical sibling transplant in second remission between 1989 and 1993, the 2-year DFS was 50% (95% CI = 38–58%).

As stated earlier, patients with a good prognosis should be considered for allogeneic sibling transplantation at relapse, whereas patients with a poorer prognosis should receive HSCT in the first remission. The debate about what constitutes a low risk of relapse has led to different practices among transplantation centers.

INDUCTION FAILURE

Although 70–80% of patients who present with de novo AML enter remission with one or two cycles of standard induction chemotherapy,[4–6] those in whom induction fails do poorly with salvage chemotherapy.[35] A study reported in 1985 suggested that such patients should be considered for alloBMT.[36] All patients (9 of 9) with disease resistant to 2–4 cycles of induction chemotherapy entered remission after a TBI-based conditioning regimen and an HLA-identical sibling BMT. Three patients were alive with no evidence of disease at 3–60 months post transplant. Supporting this approach, the City of Hope Cancer Center treated 16 patients in whom two cycles of induction failed. Eight patients, including seven who had received high-dose cytarabine, were alive and disease-free 18 months to 11 years after BMT.[37] The results from a Vancouver study were less encouraging. Of 19 patients with AML resistant to high-dose cytarabine induction and who received a sibling or unrelated BMT after TBI- or busulfan-based conditioning, only one was a long-term survivor.[38] Most studies, however, show little difference in induction rates with the use of high-dose cytarabine[27, 28] or the addition of etoposide[39] compared with standard-dose cytarabine and an anthracycline. Patients in whom induction chemotherapy fails are therefore likely to experience resistance to standard-dose chemotherapy and may reasonably proceed directly to HSCT rather than attempt remission induction with further chemotherapy. The poor outcome in some studies suggests that a conservative approach should be adopted in patients who are borderline transplant candidates.

SECOND TRANSPLANTS FOR RELAPSED AML AFTER BMT

Despite the success of alloBMT, relapse still occurs in 20–70% of patients, with most relapses occuring within 2 years.[10, 11, 34] Twenty-six patients from Fred Hutchinson Cancer Research Center, including 11 with AML, received a second transplant 5–78 months after initial BMT.[40] Regimen-related toxicity was high, with 23% dying of veno-occlusive disease and 23% dying of interstitial pneumonia. The relapse rate was 60%, and DFS was 17% at a median follow-up of 32 months. No patient undergoing transplantation within 1 year of initial BMT survived more than 100 days. One of 15 patients undergoing transplantation within 2 years of initial BMT was alive with relapsed disease; however, 6 of 11 patients who underwent transplantation more than 2 years after BMT were alive and

disease-free. Similar results were reported from Johns Hopkins Oncology Center in patients who experienced relapse more than 6 months after BMT and who had no major complications with the initial transplant.[41] The median time to second BMT was 23 months. Regimen-related mortality was high, with a 100-day mortality rate of 35%. Although 9 of 23 patients survived, this included only one of seven patients with AML. These results indicate that patients who experience relapse less than 1 year after HSCT should not receive a second transplant. Moreover, a transplant should be offered to patients who experience relapse within 2 years of HSCT only if there was no major toxicity with the first transplant. As noted earlier, this excludes the majority of patients who experience relapse after the initial HSCT because most relapses occur early. For patients who experience late relapse however, a second HSCT may offer a reasonable chance of long-term survival. These patients may also benefit from donor leukocyte transfusions, as discussed later.

PERIPHERAL BLOOD PROGENITOR CELL (PBPC) TRANSPLANTS

Mobilized PBPC for autotransplantation result in more-rapid neutrophil and platelet engraftment[42, 43] and faster immune reconstitution[44] than do marrow cells. Acceptance of their use for allogeneic transplantation has been slower because of concerns about the incidence and severity of GVHD, because PBPC grafts typically contain 10 times more T cells than marrow grafts.[45–47] A major difference between autoHSCT and alloHSCT is that in the former most of the toxicity is related to the duration of neutropenia; in the latter, toxicity is related to GVHD. Despite this concern, no dramatic increase in the incidence of acute GVHD has been seen with PBPC allotransplants. In the first 119 transplants reported, 46 patients (39%) experienced grade II–IV acute GVHD,[48–52] similar to the outcome after BMT; however, there is a suggestion of increased chronic GVHD.[48] In a series of 47 patients from the M.D. Anderson Cancer Center receiving T-replete PBPC transplants, the 1-year probability of extensive chronic GVHD was 48%.[52] This was higher than with a control arm of patients receiving marrow (35%), although GVHD prophylaxis was different in each group. Patients receiving PBPC transplants were given steroids and either tacrolimus or cyclosporine, whereas BMT patients received cyclosporine and methotrexate.

It is possible that an increase in GVHD after alloPBPC transplantation, if confirmed, may result in a lower rate of relapse with improved survival in patients who are likely to relapse, and inferior survival and poorer quality of life in those with a low relapse risk, compared with BMT. If this is the case marrow- or T-depleted PBPC may be better for patients with good-risk disease and unmanipulated PBPC grafts may be preferred for poor-risk patients. Prospective randomized studies in Canada and Europe comparing BMT and PBPC transplant for severity of GVHD and rate of engraftment are underway. Theoretically, the use of marrow primed with granulocyte colony-stimulating factor (G-CSF) may result in rapid engraftment without the problems associated with an increased T-cell dose, but this issue is largely unexplored. T cell–depleted PBPC grafts given alone or with marrow have also been used, but the results have not been reported. Given the concerns regarding GVHD, PBPC transplant should not be considered standard therapy until additional studies address this important issue.

HAPLOIDENTICAL DONOR TRANSPLANTATION

Although the majority of patients with AML lack an HLA-identical sibling donor, most have a haploidentical donor mismatched at one or more loci. In a retrospective study, 105 consecutive haploidentical transplants were compared with 728 patients who received HLA genotypically identical transplants.[53] The degree of mismatch was genotypic but not phenotypic in 12 patients, one locus in 63 patients, two loci in 24 patients, and three loci in 6 patients. All patients received unmanipulated marrow, cyclophosphamide-TBI conditioning, and methotrexate alone for GVHD prophylaxis. There was a greater risk of graft failure (5% vs. 0.1%), engraftment delayed beyond day 40 (19% vs 9%, $P \leq .005$), and acute GVHD grade 2 or higher (70% vs. 42%, $P \leq .001$) in the haploidentical versus identical cohorts, respectively. Survival was not affected by mismatch at one locus. There were too few patients with a greater mismatch for statistical testing. The majority of patients in this series were young, with median ages of 18 and 20 years in the haploidentical and control arms, respectively; older age was associated with increased GVHD.

In an update to assess risk factors for graft failure, 269 patients receiving haploidentical transplants were compared with 930 controls.[54] The degree of mismatch was genotypic but not phenotypic in 43, one locus in 121, two loci in 86, and three loci in 19 patients. Patients received unmanipulated marrow, cyclophosphamide-TBI conditioning, and one of three GVHD prophylactic regimens (methotrexate alone (n = 174), cyclosporine alone (n = 17), or cyclosporine and methotrexate (n = 80)). Failure to engraft (8.5 vs. 1.6%, $P \leq .0001$), late graft failure (4.1% vs. 0.4%, $P \leq .0001$), and total graft failures (12% vs. 2%, $P \leq .0001$) were increased in recipients of mismatched donor transplants. Indeed, mismatch was the only significant factor associated with failure to engraft in multivariate analysis. There was also a correlation between the degree of mismatch and the risk of graft failure. In patients mismatched at one locus, mismatch at class I (HLA-A or -B) or class II (HLA-DR) conferred the same risk of engraftment failure (7% vs. 11%, P = NS). In patients with two loci mismatches, however, graft failure was significantly more frequent in patients with HLA-B and -DR (28%) mismatches than in patients with other combinations (HLA-A and -B [13%], HLA-A and -DR [6%]). The direction of mismatch in patient/donor pairs homozygous at one locus did not affect graft failure. TBI was given either as 1000 cGy in one fraction, 1575 cGy in seven fractions, or 1200 cGy in six fractions. There was a trend toward more graft failures with each of these regimens, respectively. A radiation dose of 1200 cGy in six fractions was associated with a relative risk of graft failure of 3.6 (P = .05) by multivariate analysis.

Increasing the dose of infused stem cells reduces early graft failure in mice.[55] The effect of increasing the stem cell dose in humans was studied in 17 patients (median age 23 years), who received a combination of PBPC and bone marrow from haploidentical donors mismatched at three loci.[56] All patients were conditioned with 800 cGy single-fraction TBI, anti-thymocyte globulin, cyclophosphamide, and thiotepa. GVHD prophylaxis consisted of T-cell depletion of the graft using soybean agglutination and E-rosetting. Despite the T-cell depletion, only one patient experienced failure to engraft. One patient died of grade IV GVHD, but no other patient experienced more than grade II acute GVHD. Six patients died of interstitial pneumonitis, mainly due to cytomegalovirus (CMV) (four patients) and two patients, both with acute lymphoblastic leukemia (ALL), experienced relapse. Six patients were alive and well at a median of 230 days post transplant.

These studies support the feasibility of haploidentical transplantation in young patients. Graft failure and GVHD remain barriers to the more widespread use of this approach, however. The immunosuppression needed to prevent these complications results in a high incidence of opportunistic infections, especially CMV. Increasing the stem cell dose may help decrease the rate of graft failure and improve the outcome with this type of transplant.

AUTOLOGOUS TRANSPLANTATION

In patients with AML for whom alloHSCT is not an option, high-dose therapy and autoHSCT reinfusion may improve outcome.[57] The success of autoHCST depends on the collection of sufficient viable cells, reinfusion of minimal numbers of clonogenic leukemic cells, and the effectiveness of intensive therapy to eradicate leukemic cells within the body. The interpretation of autoHSCT studies in the medical literature is confounded by several factors. The time from remission to autoHSCT is critical. Patients who receive autoHSCT after prolonged remissions have lower relapse rates because poor-risk patients will have already experienced relapse and do not proceed to transplantation. Duration of first remission, timing of marrow or PBPC collection, age, intensive therapy regimen, and the use of purged versus unpurged grafts all make comparisons of single-arm studies difficult. Several large prospective randomized studies have been reported[4–6, 58, 59] but the number of patients reaching transplantation has been low, raising concerns about patient selection and the ability to generalize from the results. Patients with AML who lack a sibling donor may be consolidated with chemotherapy, undergo autoHSCT, or receive alternative-donor HSCT. If an autograft is chosen, the optimal timing of transplantation, choice of intensive therapy regimen, and type of graft are still debatable. For example, the use of autoHSCT in first relapse is likely to increase the regimen-related toxicity of a subsequent unrelated-donor HSCT should the patient experience relapse. However, the regimen-related mortality of unrelated donor transplantation precludes its use in first relapse, except in patients with a very high probability of relapse. In older patients with AML, autoHSCT or consolidation chemotherapy alone is the main therapeutic option.

FIRST COMPLETE REMISSION (CR1)

Several randomized studies have compared remission consolidation with autoHSCT or chemotherapy (Table 2–2). In a study by the European Organization for Research and Treatment of Cancer (EORTC) and Gruppo Italiana Malattie Ematologiche Maligne dell'Adulto (GIMEMA), patients with AML in first remission received an HLA-matched sibling BMT or, if no sibling donor was available, were randomized to receive an unpurged autograft or high-dose cytarabine and daunorubicin.[5] Induction chemotherapy consisted of daunorubicin and conventional-dose ara-C, followed by consolidation with intermediate-dose cytarabine and amsacrine. Of 941 patients who entered the study, 623 patients (66%) entered CR, 230 patients had a sibling donor, and of the remaining 393 eligible patients, 254 were randomized to autoBMT or chemotherapy. The main reasons for nonrandomization were toxic effects from the chemotherapy or patient refusal. Assigned therapy was completed in 95 of 128 patients randomized to autoBMT and 104 of 126 patients randomized to chemotherapy. The 4-year DFS for the autoBMT cohort was 48% versus 30% for the chemotherapy group ($P = .05$). Overall survival was not significantly different ($56 \pm 5\%$ and $46 \pm 5\%$; $P = .43$) because patients assigned to the chemotherapy arm were salvaged by autoBMT at relapse.

In a study of patients with pediatric AML randomized in first remission to receive a 4-hydroperoxycyclophosphamide (4-HC)–purged autoBMT or 6 cycles of chemotherapy as consolidation, there was no significant survival advantage in the autoBMT arm (3-year survival 38% vs. 36%, respectively).[4] Despite 666 patients entering the study and 85% entering CR, only 71 patients actually received autoBMT. The intention to treat analysis reflects the outcome of the entire treatment protocol, but it could be argued that a strategy that allowed more patients to undergo autoBMT may have shown a different outcome.

In the MRC AML 10 study, patients were randomized to receive either ADE (cytarabine, daunorubicin, and etoposide) or DAT (daunorubicin, cytarabine, and thioguanine) for two cycles followed by one cycle each of MACE (m-amsacrine, cytarabine, etoposide) and MiDAC (mitozantrone, cytarabine).[6] After this, patients without a sibling donor were randomized to autoBMT or observation. Of the 1820 patients entered into the trial, only 38% underwent the randomization to autoBMT and only 66% actually received autoBMT. The outcome of this trial was that both disease-free and overall survival were superior for both BMT arms.[58] Cassileth and coworkers reported a somewhat different outcome in a trial conducted by several cooperative groups in North America.[59] In this trial, there was no benefit in disease-free survival or overall survival associated with either autoBMT or alloBMT compared with a single course of high-dose cytarabine. These trials illustrate the importance of salvage therapy with autoBMT after relapse and question the notion that all patients should receive transplants in first remission.

In a study of modifiable prognostic factors, 74 consecutive patients underwent unpurged autoBMT for AML in first remission after melphalan and TBI.[60] The regimen-related mortality rate was 19%, the relapse rate was 53%, and the 5-year DFS was 34%. The number of courses of consolidation therapy, use of anthracycline-based induction therapy, CR–autoBMT interval, FAB subtype, and year of transplantation all significantly influenced the risk of relapse and DFS in univariate analysis. The 5-year DFS for patients receiving two or more cycles of consolidation chemotherapy was $56 \pm 14\%$ compared with $15 \pm 12\%$ in patients who received less ($P = .0008$). In multivariate analysis, administration of two or more cycles of consolidation chemotherapy emerged as the strongest predictor of decreased relapse and increased leukemia-free survival. Although concern about time to transplantation bias is raised by the correlation of receiving two or more cycles of consolidation chemotherapy and a longer CR–BMT time, subgroup analysis suggested that the effect of consolidation therapy was still beneficial.

Despite the difficulties of randomized studies, autoHSCT appears to result in lower relapse rates compared with chemotherapy when given as consolidation therapy for patients in first remission.

FIRST RELAPSE

Approximately 50–60% of patients in first relapse achieve a second remission and become eligible for autoHSCT as consolidation.[61] Patients who fail to enter second remission may be offered an alternative-donor transplant, although outcome is poor. After their success in performing allogeneic sibling transplantation during early first relapse, the group at Fred Hutchinson Cancer Research Center elected to harvest marrow from all patients without a suitable sibling donor in first remission and proceed to autoBMT at the first sign of relapse.[62] Of 98 patients for whom marrow was harvested, 65 subsequently experienced relapse and 38 proceeded to autoBMT using the cyclophosphamide-TBI, busulfan-cyclophosphamide, or busulfan-cyclophosphamide-TBI regimens. The main reason for not proceeding to autoBMT was election by the physician or patient to undergo second-remission induction with conventional-dose chemotherapy. At 4 years, the nonrelapse mortality rate was 54%, the relapse probability was 72%, and the DFS was 13%. Surviving patients had a lower peripheral blood blast count at the time of transplant ($100/\text{mm}^3$ vs $1,500/\text{mm}^3$; $P = .02$) and a trend for a longer first remission duration (25 months vs. 11 months; $P = .08$). Analyzing the 17 most recently treated patients, the treatment-related mortality was 39%, the probability of relapse was 32%, and the DFS was 41%. The main differences in this latter group are that five patients, including four survivors, received interleukin-2 (IL-2) or IL-2 plus lymphokine-activated killer (LAK) cells after transplantation and all received busulfan-containing regimens. In an earlier study by Chopra et al., nine patients received autoBMT at first relapse after the busulfan-cyclophosphamide regimen. At a median follow-up of 20 months, the relapse rate was 70% and the DFS was 33%.[63]

These studies show that the results of autoBMT in first relapse are inferior to those in second remission (see later). Although the latter population is more selected, it is likely that long-term survivors after BMT at relapse are also those

TABLE 2–2. TRIALS OF AUTOLOGOUS BONE MARROW TRANSPLANTATION FOR ACUTE MYELOGENOUS LEUKEMIA

DISEASE STAGE	NUMBER OF PATIENTS	STUDY GROUP/AUTHOR	CONDITIONING REGIMEN	PURGED MARROWS	CR TO BMT (MONTHS)	RELAPSE RATE	TREATMENT-RELATED MORTALITY	DFS	YEARS OF STUDY	REFERENCE NO.
CR1	285	ABMTR, Keating et al	Various		NA	47±8%*	12±4%*	45±6%*	1989–1993	7
	598	EBMTR, Gorin et al	Various			52±3%†	12±2%†	42±3%†	1987–1993	11
	113 (Children)	EBMTR, Gorin et al	Various			48±6%†	8±4%†	47±6%†	1987–1993	11
	95/128	EORTC/GIMEMA, Zittoun et al	Various	6%		41%†	9%†	64%†	1986–1993	5
	116	Cassileth et al	Bu/Cy	100%	4.5	48%†	14%†	35±9%†	1990–1995	59
	190	Burnett et al	Cy/TRI	0%		37%	12%	53%		58
	74	Mehta et al	Mel/TBI		NA	53±13%‡	19%‡	34±12%‡	1986–1994	60
CR2	94	ABMTR, Keating et al	Various		NA			28±10%*	1989–1993	34
	190	EBMTR, Gorin et al	Various			63±5%†	20±3%†	30±4%†	1987–1993	11
	35 (Children)	EBMTR Gorin et al	Various			54±9%†	12±7%†	40±9%†	1987–1993	11

*At 3 years
†At 4 years
‡At 5 years
BMT, bone marrow transplantation; CR, complete remission; CR1, first complete remission; CR2, second complete remission; DFS, disease free survival; ABMTR, American Bone Marrow Transplant Registry—North America; EBMTR, European Group for Blood and Marrow Transplant Registry; GIMEMA, Gruppo Italiana Malattie Ematologiche Maligne dell'Adulto.

with chemosensitive disease and therefore those likely to enter second remission. Re-induction at relapse seems a reasonable strategy to select those who should receive autoHSCT.

SECOND REMISSION

To avoid the toxicity of HSCT, some centers prefer to treat patients lacking a matched sibling donor with chemotherapy alone, reserving autoHSCT until relapse or PBPC. If this course of treatment is anticipated, the marrow or PBPC may be harvested in first remission and cryopreserved. Alternatively, marrow or PBPC can be harvested in second remission. The treatment of patients in second remission provides insight into the relative merits of chemotherapy and autoHSCT. Because each remission tends to be shorter than the preceding one, if autoHSCT is better at preventing relapse than chemotherapy, the duration of second remission may be longer than the first. A longer duration of second remission is called *remission inversion*. There are several studies in which patients who received an autoHSCT in a CR beyond CR2 were compared with historical controls. The largest reported series is from the EBMT[11] study of 190 patients. A variety of conditioning regimens were used, 40% of which contained TBI. The regimen-related mortality rate was 20 ± 3%, the relapse rate was 42 ± 8%, and the 5-year DFS was 30 ± 4%. The median time from remission to HSCT was 2 months. These results are similar to data from the Autologous Blood and Marrow Transplant Registry—North America (ABMTR) of 94 patients who experienced a 2-year leukemia-free survival of 28 ± 10%[34] and from other single-arm studies.[64, 65]

In a United Kingdom study, 25 patients received autoBMT in second remission using busulfan-cyclophosphamide as the intensive therapy regimen.[63] Six patients underwent marrow harvesting in first remission, and 19 underwent harvesting in second remission. There was a trend for delayed platelet engraftment in the patients receiving second remission marrow but no significant increase in relapse. The times to neutrophil engraftment in patients receiving marrow harvested in first and second remission were 22 days (range 17–46) and 22 days (range 11–72), respectively, and for platelet engraftment were 51 days (range 23–29) and 75 days (range 34–1020), respectively. At a median follow-up of 25 months, overall survival was 52%, DFS was 48% and relapse rate was 43%. In patients who had a first remission exceeding 12 months, the DFS was 50% compared with 43% for those whose first remission lasted less than 12 months. Remission inversion occurred in 10 of 25 patients. These results compare favorably with those of chemotherapy-treated patients in second remission in the MRC AML 8 study, time-censored at 2 months, who experienced a DFS of 18% at 3 years.[63]

If autoHSCT is to be performed in second remission, the marrow is preferably harvested in early first remission despite the additional cost of cryopreservation. PBPC collected in second remission is likely to contain hematopoietic cells that are more damaged by the additional chemotherapy. Although salvage rates of 30% are obtainable in patients in second remission after autotransplantation, only 60% will enter second remission after conventional chemotherapy. In addition, these series are not randomized and may reflect bias in the patients selected for autoHSCT. The frequency of remission inversions suggests that autoHSCT is more effective at preventing relapse than chemotherapy and argues in favor of its use in first remission.

PURGING

A concern in autoHSCT is the re-infusion of leukemic cells in the graft. There are two lines of evidence that support the concept of in vitro purging. The first is the demonstration in the rat model that marrow purging with 4-HC eliminates tumor cells without destroying cells capable of normal hematopoietic reconstitution.[66] This effect is dose-dependent, with lower doses of 4-HC delaying the onset of leukemia and higher doses preventing it. The second is the demonstration that retrovirally marked leukemic cells contribute to relapse after autografting. Brenner et al. transferred the neomycin resistance gene into marrow harvested from children with AML in remission.[67] Two patients experienced relapse after autoBMT, and in both cases leukemic blasts containing the neomycin resistance gene were detected. Although this suggests that leukemic cells in the graft contribute to relapse, the relative importance of graft contamination compared with residual disease in the patient remains controversial. A mathematical model to predict relapse for a given burden of leukemic cells was validated in the brown Norway rat and extrapolated to humans.[68] This model suggests that most relapses are due to persistent cells in the patient. Although transplants using purged marrow are often compared with autoBMT using unpurged cryopreserved marrow, cryopreservation itself can be considered a form of purging. In a rat model, normal early progenitor cells are more resistant to cryopreservation, because only 1–2% of leukemic blasts survive the freezing/thawing process.[69]

A possible model of the ideally purged autograft is a syngeneic transplant. IBMTR data from 45 twins with AML in first remission who underwent syngeneic BMT showed a probability of relapse of 52 ± 15% and a DFS of 42 ± 15% at 3 years,[1] results similar to reports with unpurged autografts. Many single-arm studies however, show results with purged autografts that are superior to outcomes after syngeneic transplantation. This may be possible if the purging process stimulates an immune response against the leukemia by priming GVL effector cells. Laboratory data to support this concept are lacking, however.

There is a lack of large prospective trials investigating the role of purging in autoHSCT. A review of cases reported to the EBMT registry of patients with AML who received autoBMT in first remission showed a lower relapse rate and higher leukemia-free survival for patients who received mafosfamide-purged marrow.[70] Of 263 patients, 69 patients received marrow purged in vitro with mafosfamide and 194 patients received unpurged marrow. The relapse rate was significantly less in patients receiving purged marrows, 40 ± 6% versus 59 ± 4%, by univariate but not multivariate analysis. Purging resulted in delayed engraftment and significantly more veno-occlusive disease, infections, and pneumonitis. When a retrospectively identified subset of patients with good-risk disease who received a TBI-containing regimen was analyzed, the results were significant. At a median follow-up of 28 months, the relapse rate was 23% in 30 patients who received purged marrow compared with 55% in 77 recipients of unpurged marrow (P = .005). DFS was 63% and 34% (P = .05), respectively. The greatest benefit of purging was seen in patients who underwent autograft within 6 months of achieving remission, with relapse rates of 20% versus 60% (P = .01). Although these results are encouraging (they are better than those reported after twin transplants and this was a retrospective study), selection bias cannot be excluded.

Data from the ABMTR also showed a benefit to purging. The outcome of 212 patients receiving 4-HC–purged autografts was compared with that of 83 recipients of unpurged marrow.[71] For patients receiving a purged autograft in first remission, the 3-year DFS was 48% (95% CI = 39–57%) compared with 29% (95% CI = 9–49%) with unpurged marrow. Patients in second remission experienced a 3-year DFS of 39% (95% CI = 25–53%) and 24% (95% CI = 3–45%) for purged and unpurged marrow, respectively. The better results were due to similar regimen-related mortality but fewer relapses in the purged transplant recipients.

Purging delays engraftment to a degree predictable by the colony forming unit–granulocyte macrophage (CFU-GM) content of the graft.[72] Individualizing the mafosfamide dose may optimize the purge while avoiding delayed engraftment. Aliquots of the marrow graft are incubated with different concentrations of drug, and the dose predicted to allow 5% CFU-GM survival is used to treat the whole marrow.[73] The use of individualized dosages is associated with very low relapse rates, but again these data are better than data from twin studies.[70] The cyclophosphamide derivatives, 4-HC (in North America) and mafosfamide (in Europe), are the most commonly used pharmacologic purging agents, but other antineoplastic drugs, such as etoposide[74, 75] and adriamycin,[76] show promise in preclinical models. Clinical use of these agents has been limited.

Another approach is immunologic purging using monoclonal antibodies directed at myeloid-specific antigens, such as CD14, CD15, and CD33. These antigens are absent or expressed at low levels on normal hematopoietic progenitors. In most studies, one or two antibodies and complement are incubated with the marrow. After encouraging results in high-risk patients,[77] a multicenter study using CD14, CD15 and complement for purging was initiated.[78] Fifty-five patients (7 in first remission, 44 in second or third remission, and 5 in first relapse) received a purged autoBMT after high-dose therapy with cyclophosphamide-TBI or busulfan-cyclophosphamide. The relapse rates for patients in first and second or later relapse were 49 ± 20% and 39 ± 8%, with DFS of 51 ± 10% and 30 ± 9%, respectively. In the patients treated in first relapse, three of five had sustained relapse-free survival. Remission inversions were documented in 11 of the 15 patients undergoing transplantation during second relapse who are alive and whose disease is in remission. One criticism of this study is that transplantations were carried out in late first remission (median 10 months, range 6–14 months), suggesting possible time-censoring. A randomized study is planned. Robertson et al., at the Dana-Farber Cancer Institute, used anti-CD33 purging for 12 patients with AML, mainly in second relapse.[79] Five patients were in remission at a median follow-up of 12 months (range 1–33 months) for a DFS of 29%. Both these studies also demonstrated that immunologic purging causes loss of myeloid progenitors, delayed engraftment, and an increased complication rate.

In single-arm studies, marrow purging seems to reduce the relapse rate after autoBMT with no obvious advantage to particular method. The lack of controlled studies makes quantifying the benefit difficult. Moreover, purging is associated with increased toxicity due to delayed engraftment. Peripheral blood progenitor cell collections may offset the delay in engraftment but could be associated with the infusion of a greater clonogenic leukemic cell burden (see later).

AUTOLOGOUS PERIPHERAL BLOOD PROGENITOR CELL (PBPC) TRANSPLANTS

Autologous transplantations performed using PBPC result in faster neutrophil and platelet engraftment and more-rapid immune reconstitution.[43, 44] This is particularly important for patients with AML who often experience delayed engraftment after HSCT; however, there were concerns about increased relapse after a study by Korbling et al. of 43 patients receiving PBPC or purged marrow. Despite faster engraftment, a trend toward lower DFS (35% vs. 51%; P = NS) was detected in the PBPC arm.[80] Unfortunately, the study was closed prematurely. The Seattle group showed that the times to neutrophil and platelet engraftment after PBPC transplant in first or second relapse were shorter than with historical controls.[81] Although there was a decrease in treatment-related mortality at day 100 (14% vs. 32%), the relapse rate at 2 years was higher (65% compared with 37%). A retrospective study by the EBMT compared 84 PBPC transplants with 168 BMT for patients with AML in first relapse matched for FAB subtype and the intervals from diagnosis to first remission and from first remission to autoHSCT.[82] There was no difference in relapse or survival between the two cohorts. In another study, preliminary results from 135 patients randomized to PBPC transplant or autoBMT noted more-rapid neutrophil engraftment but no difference in the 3-year DFS (41% vs. 48%).[83]

UNRELATED DONOR TRANSPLANTS

Unrelated donor transplant is an option for patients without an HLA-matched sibling. When registries are combined worldwide, approximately 2.5 million available donors have been typed at the HLA-A and -B loci. A third are also typed at the HLA-DR locus.[84] Growth in the number of listed donors has increased the success of donor searches, but the majority of registered donors are Caucasian and the chance of a successful match in ethnic minorities is lower. Recent figures show the overall probability of finding a donor serologically matched at HLA-A, -B, and -DR is 64%.[84] The probabilities by ethnic group are: white, 71%; Hispanic, 62%; Asian-Pacific, 45%; and black, 24%. The use of unrelated donors has increased over recent years. The National Marrow Donor Program (NMDP) of the United States provided donors for 177 patients in 1989, 551 in 1992, and up to 80 per month for a total of 3380 transplants through June 1995.[84] Currently, GVHD is the major factor limiting the more widespread use of unrelated donor transplants, and much effort has been directed at maneuvers to circumvent this problem using both ex vivo and in vivo techniques. The World Marrow Donor Association has issued guidelines for standardized practice in the use of unrelated marrow transplantation.[85] Indications are divided into two categories: (1) in accordance with a clinical research program, and (2) a generally accepted indication. Patients with AML in remission but with high-risk features are accepted in either category. Patients in relapse may be treated only in category 1. Patients in refractory relapse are generally not accepted.

FIRST COMPLETE REMISSION (CR1)

High regimen-related mortality prevents the routine use of unrelated donor transplantation for patients in first remission and outweighs any reduction in relapse from a GVL effect. Exceptions might include cases with a very high probability of relapse, i.e., those with unfavorable cytogenetics, such as del(5), del(5q), del(7), or t(9;22). In these patients, the relapse rate after chemotherapy alone is 80–90%[19, 30] and 58% after matched sibling BMT.[10] The advantage to performing transplantation in such patients early is to avoid the additional conventional therapy that may increase the risk of a subsequent transplant.

BEYOND FIRST REMISSION

The largest analysis of outcome after unrelated-donor BMT is an NMDP review of 462 transplants, including 70 in patients with AML.[86] A variety of conditioning regimens were used, and 21% received T cell–depleted marrow grafts. Engraftment was successful in 94% of patients, although 8% experienced late graft failure. Grade II–IV acute GVHD occurred in 64 ± 5%, and grade III–IV disease occurred in 47 ± 6% of patients. Chronic GVHD occurred in 55 ± 7% of patients and was extensive in 35 ± 7%. Patients with leukemia in CR1 or CR2 experienced a 2-year DFS of 45 ± 13% compared with 18 ± 8% for those with more advanced disease. Survival was best in patients under age 18, 53 ± 15% (n = 41). Although more patients in this group had ALL, most deaths were due to nonrelapse mortality. The 2-year probability of relapse was 19 ± 6% for all leukemias, including chronic myelogenous leukemia (CML). Patients receiving T cell–depleted marrow grafts had less GVHD but no increase in relapse and experienced improved overall survival (P = .01).

The results of another series of 55 patients, 27 with AML and 28 with ALL, who received an unrelated BMT beyond first remission were similar.[87] The majority underwent TBI-based conditioning regimens (n = 40) and received cyclosporine, methotrexate, and methylprednisolone for GVHD prophylaxis (n = 32). Four patients received T cell–depleted marrow. The incidence of grade II or higher acute GVHD was 57%. Outcomes were not affected by leukemia subtype, and the actuarial risk of relapse at 1 year was 24 ± 16%. The DFS at 3 years was 23 ± 12%. Thirty-four patients died from transplant-related causes, including GVHD (n = 14), infection (n = 9), organ failure (n = 6), graft failure (n = 3), or other cause (n = 2). Survival was higher in younger patients. In patients 21 years old or younger, the 3-year DFS was 44 ± 23% compared with 12 ± 11% in older patients (P = .05). Survival was also better for patients in remission at the time of BMT, who had a 3-year DFS of 33 ± 19% compared with 15 ± 14% for patients undergoing transplantation at relapse (P = .02). Chromosomal abnormalities were a predictor of poor leukemia-free survival.

In a study of T cell–depleted unrelated-donor BMT, 42 patients with a myeloid malignancy (AML n = 23; myelodysplasia n = 8; secondary AML n = 11) received αβT-cell receptor antibody–depleted marrow after cyclophosphamide, cytarabine, methylprednisolone, and TBI conditioning.[88] Cyclosporine was also given for GVHD prophylaxis. Twenty patients had one or more HLA locus mismatches. One patient experienced failure to engraft. Acute GVHD grade II or higher occurred in 31%, and grade III or higher occurred in 8%. Extensive GVHD was present in 9%. Thirteen died of regimen-related causes; the relapse probability was 40 ± 19%, and DFS was 38 ± 16% at 4 years.

Despite the morbidity and mortality from GVHD associated with unrelated-donor BMT, reported relapse rates are consistently low. Unrelated transplants are therefore of most benefit in patients with poor-risk disease, especially those who are young and likely to have less GVHD. T-cell depletion appears to decrease GVHD mortality, with only a modest increase in relapse in this setting.

MISMATCHED UNRELATED TRANSPLANTS

Despite the severity of GVHD after matched unrelated transplants, donors with minor or major mismatches have been used in patients without a matched donor. The definition of a minor mismatch is a difference in class I antigens wherein the different HLA-A or -B antigen is within the same cross-reactive group. Class II minor mismatches are matches by serologic but not molecular typing. A review from Fred Hutchinson Cancer Research Center compared the outcome of 42 patients younger than 36 years, including 21 with acute leukemia, who received a minor-mismatched unrelated-donor BMT with an age-matched control group of 70 patients, including 27 with acute leukemia, receiving marrow from a matched unrelated donor.[89] All patients received T cell–replete marrow, cyclophosphamide-TBI conditioning, and cyclosporine and methotrexate GVHD prophylaxis. The time to engraftment was the same in both groups, with no increase in graft failure in mismatched and matched donor recipients (4.9% vs. 3.1%).

There was in increase in grade II or higher GVHD (94% [85–99%] vs. 78% [67–88%]) (P = .001) and grade III or higher acute GVHD (51% [37–66%] vs. 36% [26–48%] [NS]) in mismatched donor recipients. Chronic GVHD in the mismatched recipients was also higher at 74% (59–89%) compared with 61% (45–76%) for those receiving a matched allograft. Although death from chronic GVHD was more common in mismatched transplants (55% vs. 32%), there was a trend for less relapse, 12% versus 23% (P = .19). The 1.5-year DFS for mismatched and matched recipients, respectively, was 46% (27–64%) versus 51% (34–64%) in good-risk patients, and 44% (20–66%) versus 30% (15–47%) in patients with poor-risk disease.

These results show an increased incidence and severity of GVHD for patients receiving marrow from donors who have minor mismatches on HLA typing. A lower relapse rate may result in similar rates of survival, especially in young patients with poor-risk disease. Given the higher incidence of GVHD, the upper age limit for mismatched unrelated-donor BMT should be lower than is accepted for matched unrelated-donor BMT.

PLACENTAL BLOOD TRANSPLANTS

Human cord blood contains a higher proportion of primitive hematopoietic stem cells than marrow or PBPC. This was initially used as a source of stem cells in matched sibling transplants in children because collecting cord blood was simpler than harvesting marrow from a newborn infant. The first cord blood transplantation was performed in 1988 in a patient with Fanconi anemia. This patient was alive and well 7 years after transplantation.[90] The analysis of the first 50 patients[91] included 44 sibling transplants (34 matched, 10 haploidentical) and 6 unrelated donor transplants, only 1 of whom was fully matched. Engraftment was successful in 85% of patients. The median time to neutrophil engraftment was 22 days (range 12–46 days) and to platelet engraftment was 49 days (range 15–117 days). This is slower than would be expected after BMT. Growth factors (G-CSF or granulocyte macrophage-colony stimulating factor [GM-CSF]) did not hasten neutrophil engraftment. The incidence of GVHD was very low. Of 30 patients receiving a matched or single antigen mismatched transplant, only one (3%) experienced grade II acute GVHD and two experienced limited chronic GVHD. All four evaluable patients with two or three antigen disparate donors experienced GVHD. An interesting observation was that the GVHD was only grade I in the two patients disparate at the non-inherited maternal allele, supporting earlier observations that partial tolerance to the non-inherited maternal allele may develop during gestation. Possible reasons for the low incidence of GVHD include the young age of the recipient and donor, less-developed immune cells in the cord blood at birth, tolerance due to contaminating maternal cells, and more-naive donor lymphocytes.

Encouraged by the low incidence of GVHD, several groups have established cord blood banks for use in unrelated transplants. In a study of 25 patients (including 5 with AML) lacking a suitable sibling or unrelated donor who received an unrelated placental blood transplant, 23 patients experienced successful engraftment.[92] HLA were discordant in 24 donors. Nine of 21 evaluable patients experienced acute GVHD. This was grade II in seven and grade III in two, but no patient experienced grade IV disease. The median time to neutrophil engraftment was 22 days (range 14–37 days) and to platelet engraftment was 56 days (range 35–89 days). There was a correlation between nucleated cell dose infused and myeloid engraftment, but the largest patient, who weighed 79 kg, experienced engraftment after receiving only 1.1×10^7 nucleated cells/kg.

Although these results are encouraging, the majority of cord blood transplants to date have been in children, and the incidence of GVHD in adults is unknown. Cord blood grafts also have limited cell numbers, and this may be inadequate to reconstitute long-term hematopoiesis in larger patients without ex vivo expansion. Although mononuclear cell numbers are lower than in marrow, the primitive stem-cell dose assayed by long-term culture assay appears to be comparable.[93] Despite these limitations, in small young patients, cord blood transplants may offer an alternative stem cell source for those who lack a suitable sibling or unrelated donor.

CONDITIONING REGIMENS

The conditioning regimen in alloHSCT has two roles: to eliminate the leukemic clone and to immunosuppress the recipient in order to avoid graft rejection. The initial regimen used in Fred Hutchinson Cancer Research Center was TBI alone.[94] Cyclophosphamide was added for its dose-dependent antineoplastic activity and lack of overlapping toxicity with TBI. Also, when given prior to TBI, cyclophosphamide reduced the risk of tumor lysis in patients with relapsed leukemia.[95] Cyclophosphamide (60 mg/kg IV daily for 2 days) followed by TBI (920–1000 cGy administered as a single fraction) became the standard myeloablative conditioning regimen.[96] In an attempt to decrease relapse after transplantation, the group at Fred Hutchinson Cancer Research Center added other chemotherapeutic agents, including busulfan, carmustine, and daunorubicin, to the basic cyclophosphamide-TBI regimen.[97] These agents did not decrease relapse or prolong survival, however, and the approach was abandoned. Modification of the radiation dose was explored. Dose-escalation studies found that the maximal tolerated doses of TBI, in combination with cyclophosphamide (60 mg/kg daily for 2 days), was 1000 cGy in a single fraction, 1440 cGy in 120-cGy fractions t.i.d., 1600 cGy in 200-cGy fractions b.i.d., and 1575 cGy in daily 225-cGy fractions.[98–100] In matched sibling transplants, 1200 cGy in six fractions was better tolerated than 1000 cGy in a single fraction, did not increase relapse, and was associated with greater DFS.[100] In a randomized study, 1575 cGy in seven fractions compared with 1200 cGy in six fractions led to less relapse but more GVHD and greater regimen-related toxicity with no improvement in overall survival.[101] Because of increased mucositis, fewer patients given the higher dose of radiation received full-dose methotrexate. This may explain the higher incidence of GVHD that in turn contributed to lower relapse.

TBI is associated with long-term complications, including second malignancies, premature cataract formation, impaired growth, and endocrine dysfunction.[102–105] Non–TBI-containing regimens were studied in an attempt to avoid these late complications. The use of busulfan (16 mg/kg over 4 days) and cyclophosphamide (200 mg/kg) was associated with a very low relapse rate but high morbidity.[106] By reducing the dose of cyclophosphamide to 120 mg/kg, the regimen remained effective but was better tolerated.[107] Several studies show a similar outcome for patients with early disease treated with busulfan-cyclophosphamide with compared cyclophosphamide-TBI.[108, 109] Patients with more-advanced disease fared better with TBI,[109, 110] although these results are confounded by the inclusion of patients with advanced-stage CML who poorly tolerate high-dose therapy.[109] Substitution of cyclophosphamide in the cyclophosphamide-TBI regimen with an alternative cytotoxic agent has also been studied. Melphalan,[111, 112] etoposide,[113] and cytarabine[114] have all been used with outcomes comparable to those of standard cyclophosphamide-TBI. In another approach, radiolabeled antibodies are targeted to marrow to deliver greater doses of radiation without increased organ toxicity. A phase I/II study of ^{131}I-labeled anti-CD45 combined with busulfan-cyclophosphamide at standard doses caused increased mucositis but resulted in disease-free status in 14 of 15 patients receiving matched-sibling BMT for AML in first remission.[115]

In the autologous setting, the objectives of the conditioning regimen are different. Because immunosuppression is not required, the sole purpose of the regimen is to eradicate disease by high-dose therapy. There have been two approaches in the design of new regimens—one is dose escalation of multiagent chemotherapy, the other is replacement of components or introduction of new drugs to the standard cyclophosphamide-TBI regimen used in allogeneic transplantation. Substitution for cyclophosphamide (a drug rarely used in AML chemotherapy but shown to be effective with dose escalation) by melphalan, etoposide, and cytarabine has been studied in phase I trials. Phase II/III studies are limited, but although the toxicity profile is different, there is little change in overall toxicity or DFS compared with standard regimens.[112] Dose-escalation studies of busulfan or etoposide as a third agent to cyclophosphamide-TBI were systematically explored by the group at Fred Hutchinson Cancer Research Center using a fixed dose of 1200 cGy of fractionated TBI. The maximum tolerated doses were 7 mg/kg of busulfan in combination with 50 mg/kg cyclophosphamide[116] and 44 mg/kg of etoposide with 103 mg/kg of cyclophosphamide.[99] The efficacy of these regimens has not been addressed.

Encouraging results have been reported with non-TBI regimens. In one study, 58 patients in first remission (n = 32), second or third remission (n = 21), or induction failure (n = 5) received busulfan (16 mg/kg) and etoposide (60 mg/kg) prior to 4-HC–purged autoBMT.[117] In patients in first remission, the relapse rate was 22 ± 9% with a 3-year leukemia-free survival of 76 ± 9%, and in patients in CR2 or later the relapse rate was 25 ± 11% with a 3-year leukemia-free survival of 56 ± 11%. Similar results were reported in another study of 30 patients (19 in first remission, 9 in second remission, 2 in relapse) treated in the same way (relapse 28%, leukemia-free survival 57%).[118] However, 20 patients (15 in first remission, 3 in second remission, 2 in relapse) treated by the same group with busulfan/etoposide but who received unpurged marrow had inferior results (relapse 62%, DFS 32%).[119] Busulfan and melphalan have also been used, but the number of patients treated is too small to determine effectiveness.[120]

The feasibility of alternative conditioning regimens has been demonstrated. The number of patients treated thus far has been small, but the results, particularly with busulfan/etoposide and purged marrow, are encouraging and warrant further study.

POST-TRANSPLANT IMMUNE MODULATION

There is now good evidence that immunologic mechanisms contribute to the low relapse rate of AML after allogeneic transplantation. Clinical data supporting this GVL effect include the higher relapse rate after syngeneic[1] and T cell–depleted allogeneic transplants,[16] the ability to induce remission by donor T-cell infusion in patients who experience relapse after transplantation,[2, 121] and lower relapse in patients with clinical GVHD.[3] The GVL effector cells include both CD4 and CD8 T cells as well as natural killer cells, but their relative importance is debated. Effector cells demonstrating leukemia-specific activity exist,[122] but down-regulation of all host hematopoiesis, presumably including any malignant hematopoiesis, has also been demonstrated[123] and is supported by the prominence of aplasia in transfusion-related GVHD.[124] The relative importance of specific antileukemic and the more general antihost hematopoiesis mechanisms has not yet been determined.

Kolb et al. demonstrated that patients who experience relapse after alloBMT for CML could experience remission induced by infusion of donor buffy coat.[118] Despite its success, this procedure resulted in significant GVHD, aplasia, and a 10% mortality rate. Earlier relapses have been successfully treated with lower T-cell doses and are associated with less morbidity. Best results are in patients with only molecular evidence of relapse.[123] Donor lymphocyte infusion has been extended to the treatment of patients experiencing relapse with AML. A review of patients receiving donor lymphocyte at relapse reported to EBMT included 23 patients with AML.[2] Four were treated as remission consolidation after chemotherapy, with two durable responses. In the other 19 patients, including 15 untreated patients and 4 in whom reinduction chemotherapy failed, there were two early deaths and five entered remission, but all subsequently relapsed within 2 years. Results from a North American survey were similar.[125] Six of 36 patients (15%) receiving donor lymphocyte infusion at relapse achieved CR. The median time to remission was 34 days (range 16–99 days). The median remission duration for complete responders was 17.9 months, with two remissions ongoing at 4.5 and 40 months. Seven additional patients underwent donor lymphocyte infusion after CR was reinduced with chemotherapy; three had experienced relapse at a median follow-up of 12 months. The disappointing results in relapsed AML may reflect the different kinetics of relapse between CML and AML. Treatment of patients with low leukemic burden, such as after reinduction chemotherapy or at molecular relapse, may be more successful.

The optimal timing and dose of donor lymphocyte infusions in patients with relapsing AML after allogeneic transplantations are still being defined.

There are some encouraging preclinical and clinical reports of IL-2 in the treatment of AML. IL-2 is thought to induce lymphokine-activated killer (LAK) cells and increase leukemic cell kill. Its use is largely limited to recipients of autoHSCT because it exacerbates GVHD in allograft recipients. In the rat syngeneic transplant model, low doses of IL-2 caused a decrease in relapse.[126] In the rat allograft model, although low levels of IL-2 did not prevent relapse and high levels caused lethal GVHD, intermediate doses caused a significant decrease in relapse without induction of fatal GVHD.[123] In a pilot study, 14 patients with chemotherapy-resistant AML and 5–30% blasts in the marrow received four 5-day cycles of IL-2 followed by monthly maintenance courses.[127] CR was induced in eight patients, with five patients in sustained remission (four in third remission, one in fourth remission) at a median follow-up of 32 months. These results with overt disease suggest that an even greater effect may occur in patients with minimal disease. In a study of seven patients treated with a 5-day course of IL-2 commencing at engraftment after autoBMT (n = 6) or syngeneic BMT (n = 1), only one patient (who received syngeneic BMT) had experienced relapse at a median follow-up of 32 months.[128] Because IL-2 is associated with significant side effects, including fever, rash, hypotension, and capillary leak, one strategy has been to incubate the marrow with high-dose IL-2 and give lower doses to the patient after reinfusion.[128] Of 10 poor-risk patients receiving this regimen, five have experienced prolonged relapse-free survival. In another study, a small number of patients receiving autografts followed by IL-2 ± LAK cells experienced relapse rates that were lower than expected.[62]

A GVHD-like syndrome sometimes occuring after autoHSCT presents with fever, pulmonary infiltrates, and a rash with pathologic skin changes identical to GVHD. This syndrome is usually not followed by signs of chronic GVHD or suppressed hematopoiesis and is similar to a condition observed with lymphocyte recovery after chemotherapy.[130] In the rat model, GVHD after syngeneic BMT appears to be mediated by autoreactive lymphocytes directed against HLA-DR (anti-Ia),[131] and in vitro and in vivo antitumor activity has been demonstrated in cell lines expressing HLA-DR.[132, 133] Interferon-γ upregulates the expression of HLA-DR and can increase the antitumor effect in vitro.[132] Human studies show that HLA-DR reactive lymphocytes can be induced in about 80% of patients after autoBMT by the use of cyclosporine.[134] A randomized study of the

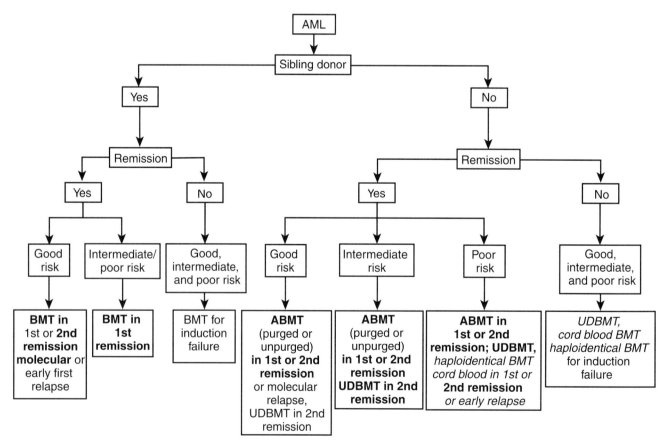

FIGURE 2–1. Recommendations are in boldface, generally accepted treatments are in regular text, and controversial treatments are in italics. The options listed are for young patients. In older patients or those with coexistent disease, some options may not apply or may be less acceptable. Treatment decisions should be based on the expected relapse rate and regimen related mortality in an individual. ABMT, autologous bone marrow transplant; UDBMT, unrelated donor BMT; AML, acute myelogenous leukemia.

efficacy of this approach in preventing relapse in patients with lymphoma is underway. There are no data on its efficacy in AML.

CONCLUSION

AlloHSCT has improved the outcome of patients with AML, largely because of a GVL effect. Best results are in CR1 with a matched sibling donor transplant. For patients with a suitable donor, the key issue is the timing of transplantation. Subjects whose disease has favorable prognostic factors perhaps are best delayed until CR2 in order to avoid overtreating those cured by remission induction chemotherapy alone. Patients without a matched sibling donor have other, albeit less satisfactory options. Autotransplants, although less toxic, yield higher relapse rates. Alternative-donor transplants, in contrast, yield more complications and higher transplant-related mortality but lower relapse risk. Transplant options for patients with AML are schematically outlined in Figure 2–1. In order to choose the best transplant option for a given patient, numerous subject- and disease-related factors need to be considered. For example, in alternative-donor transplants, treatment related mortality is primarily due to GVHD and largely influenced by age. Given the inverse relationship between GVHD and relapse, such toxic therapy is best justified in young patients with high-risk disease.

Attention is increasingly directed at augmenting or inducing GVL effects. Results of donor leukocyte infusions in patients experiencing relapse after allotransplantation are preliminary but appear promising. Immune modulation after autotransplantation is conceptually attractive but is at an early developmental stage. Important tasks include better harnessing the GVL effect, especially for autotransplants, and reducing treatment related mortality, particularly for unrelated or mismatched related donor transplants. A critical goal is the development of the most effective and least toxic treatment option for each of the genetic lesions encompassed by the diagnosis of AML.

HSCT has been used as consolidation or salvage therapy for AML for several decades. In many instances, such as primary induction failure or after first relapse, HSCT is possibly the only curative therapy. Significant questions remain regarding the role of HSCT as consolidation therapy in first remission. Several randomized trials have shown that HSCT performed in first remission does not improve overall survival compared with chemotherapy alone. These trials have not adequately accounted for the influence of prognostic indicators in patient subgroups. The application of HSCT as consolidation therapy in first remission should probably be restricted to patients with high- to intermediate-risk profiles based on leukemia cell karyotype. Continued clinical investigation is necessary to define the optimal application and timing of HSCT in this disease.

REFERENCES

1. Gale RP, et al: Identical twin transplants for leukemia. Ann Intern Med 120:646, 1994.
2. Kolb H-J, et al: Graft-versus-leukemia effect of donor lymphocyte transfusions in marrow grafted patients. Blood 86:2041, 1995.
3. Sullivan KM, et al: Influence of acute and chronic graft-versus-host disease on relapse and survival after bone marrow transplantation from HLA-identical siblings as treatment of acute and chronic leukemia. Blood 73:1720, 1989.
4. Ravindranath Y, et al: Autologous bone marrow transplantation versus intensive consolidation chemotherapy for acute myeloid leukemia in childhood. N Engl J Med 334:1428, 1996.
5. Zittoun RA, et al: Autologous or allogeneic bone marrow transplantation compared with intensive chemotherapy in acute myelogenous leukemia. N Engl J Med 332:217, 1995.
6. Burnett AK, et al: Progress report on MRC AML 10. *In* Autologous Marrow and Blood Transplantation: Proceedings of the Seventh International Symposium, Arlington, TX, 7:9, 1994.
7. Imrie K, Dicke K, Keating A: Autologous bone marrow transplantation for acute myelogenous leukemia. Stem Cells 14:69–78, 1996.
8. Gale RP, Buchner T, Zhang MJ, et al: HLA identical sibling bone marrow transplants vs chemotherapy for acute myelogenous leukemia in first remission. Leukemia 10:1687–1691; 1996.
9. Arthur DC, et al: The clinical significance of karyotype in acute myelogenous leukemia. Cancer Genet Cytogenet 40:203, 1989.
10. Gale RP, et al: Impact of cytogenetic abnormalities on outcome of bone marrow transplants in acute myelogenous leukaemia in first remission. Bone Marrow Transplant 16:203, 1995.
11. Gorin NC, et al: Retrospective evaluation of autologous bone marrow transplantation vs allogeneic bone marrow transplantation from an HLA identical related donor in acute myelocytic leukemia: A study of the European Cooperative Group for Blood and Marrow Transplantation (EBMT). Bone Marrow Transplant 18:111, 1996.
12. Miller WHJ, et al: Detection of minimal residual disease in acute promyelocytic leukemia by reverse transcription polymerase chain reaction assay for the PML/RAR-a fusion mRNA. Blood 82:1689, 1993.
13. Coco FL, et al: Molecular evaluation of residual disease as a predictor of relapse in acute promyelocytic leukemia. Lancet 340:1437, 1992.
14. Fabricious-Moeller, et al: Experimental Studies of the Hemorrhagic Diathesis from X-Ray Sickness. Copenhagen, Levin and Munksgaard, 1922.
15. Jacobsen, et al: Effects of spleen protection on mortality following x-irradiation. J Clin Med 34:1538, 1949.
16. Marmont AM, et al: T-cell depletion of HLA-identical transplants in leukemia. Blood 78:2120, 1991.
17. Weaver C, et al: Effect of graft-versus-host disease prophylaxis on relapse in patients transplanted for acute myeloid leukemia. Bone Marrow Transplant 14:885, 1994.
18. Thomas ED, et al: Marrow transplantation for acute nonlymphoblastic leukemia in first remission. N Engl J Med 301:597, 1979.
19. Grimwade D, et al: Impact of cytogenetics on outcome on AML: analysis of 1613 patients entered into the UK MRC AML 10 trial [Abstract]. Blood 92:2322, 1998.
20. Tallman MS, Anderson JW, Schiffer CA, et al: All trans-retinoic acid in acute promyelocytic leukemia [see comments] [published erratum appears in N Engl J Med 337:1639; 1997] N Engl J Med 337:1021–1028, 1997.
21. Miggiano MC, et al: Autologous bone marrow transplantation in late first complete remission improves outcome in acute myelogenous leukemia. Leukemia 10:402, 1996.
22. Jurcic J, et al: Prognostic significance of minimal residual disease detection and PML/RARa isoform type: long-term follow-up in acute promyelocytic leukemia (APL) [Abstract]. Blood 88:485a, 1996.
23. Nucifora G, Larson RA, Rowley JD: Persistence of the 8;21 translocation in patients with acute myeloid leukemia type M2 in long term remission. Blood 82:712, 1993.
24. Chang K-S, et al: Expression of AML1-ETO transcripts and detection of minimal residual disease in t(8;21)-positive acute myeloid leukemia. Oncogene 8:983, 1993.
25. Kusec R, et al: AML1/ETO transcripts can be detected in remission blood samples of all patients with t(8;21) acute myeloid leukemia after chemotherapy or autologous bone marrow transplantation. Leukemia 8:735, 1994.
26. Jurlander J, et al: Persistence of the AML1/ETO fusion transcript in patients treated with allogeneic bone marrow transplantation for t(8;21) leukemia. Blood 88:2183, 1996.
27. Bishop JF, Matthews JP, Young G, et al: The influence of induction chemotherapy dose and dose intensity on the duration of remission in acute myeloid leukemia. Australian Leukemia Study Group. Leukemia and Lymphoma 15:79–84, 1994

28. Weick J, Kopecky KJ, Appelbaum FR, et al: A randomized investigation of high-dose versus standard dose cytosine arabinoside with daunorubicin in patients with previously untreated acute myelogenous leukemia. A Southwest Oncology Group Study. Blood 88:841–851, 1996.

29. Clift RA, et al: The treatment of acute non-lymphoblastic leukemia by allogeneic marrow transplantation. Bone Marrow Transplant 2:243, 1987.

30. Swansbury GJ, et al: Long-term survival in acute myelogenous leukemia: a second follow-up of the Fourth International Workshop on Chromosomes in Leukemia. Cancer Genet Cytogenet 73:1, 1994.

31. Fenaux, et al: Cytogenetics and their prognostic value in de novo acute myeloid leukemia: a report on 283 cases. Br J Haematol 73:61, 1989.

32. Gale R, Foon KA: Therapy of acute myelogenous leukemia. Semin Hematol 24:40, 1987.

33. Frassoni F, et al: Results of allogeneic bone marrow transplantation for acute leukemia have improved in Europe with time—a report of the acute leukemia working party of the European group for blood and marrow transplantation. Bone Marrow Transplant 17:13, 1996.

34. Gale RP, Horowitz MM, Rees JK, et al: Chemotherapy versus transplants for acute myelogenous leukemia in second remission. Leukemia 10:13–19, 1996.

35. Liso V, et al: Outcome of patients with acute myeloid leukemia who failed to respond to a single course of first-line induction therapy: a GIMEMA study of 218 unselected consecutive patients. Leukemia 10:1443, 1996.

36. Zander AR, et al: Allogeneic bone marrow transplantation for acute leukemia refractory to induction chemotherapy. Cancer 56:1374, 1985.

37. Forman SJ, et al: Allogeneic bone marrow transplantation as therapy for primary induction failure for patients with acute leukemia. J Clin Oncol 9:1570, 1991.

38. Fung HC, et al: Allogeneic bone marrow transplantation for patients with acute leukemia and refractory anaemia with excess blasts in transformation for whom primary therapy failed to bring about complete remission [Abstract]. Clin Invest Med Suppl 18:433a, 1995.

39. Bishop JF, et al: Etoposide in acute nonlymphoblastic leukemia. Blood 75:27, 1990.

40. Sanders JE, et al: Second marrow transplants in patients with leukemia who relapse after allogeneic marrow transplantation. Bone Marrow Transplant 3:11, 1988.

41. Wagner JE, et al: Relapse of leukaemia after bone marrow transplantation: effect of second myeloablative therapy. Bone Marrow Transplant 9:205, 1992.

42. Schmitz N, et al: Randomized trial of filgrastim-mobilized peripheral blood progenitor cell transplantation in lymphoma patients. Lancet 347:353, 1996.

43. To LB, et al: Comparison of haematological recovery times and supportive care requirements of autologous recovery phase peripheral blood stem cell transplants and allogeneic bone marrow transplants. Bone Marrow Transplant 9:277, 1992.

44. Roberts MM, et al: Immune reconstitution following peripheral blood stem cell transplantation and allogeneic bone marrow transplantation. Bone Marrow Transplant 12:469, 1993.

45. Dreger P, et al: Timing of harvesting and composition of the leukapheresis product. Br J Cancer 68:950, 1993.

46. Weaver CH, et al: Lymphocyte content in peripheral blood mononuclear cells collected after administration of granulocyte colony-stimulating factor. Bone Marrow Transplant 13:411, 1994.

47. Dreger P, et al: Harvesting of G-CSF mobilized peripheral blood progenitor cells for allogeneic transplantation: safety kinetics of mobilization and composition of the graft. Br J Haematol 87:609, 1994.

48. Majolino I, et al: High incidence of chronic GVHD after primary allogeneic peripheral blood stem cell transplantation in patients with hematologic malignancies. Bone Marrow Transplant 17:555–560, 1996.

49. Brown RA, Adkins D, Khoury H, et al: Long term follow-up of high risk allogeneic peripheral blood stem cell transplant recipients: graft versus host disease and transplant related mortality. J Clin Oncol 17:806–812; 1999.

50. Tarantolo S, et al: Incidence of acute graft versus host disease in allogeneic blood stem cell transplantation. Blood Suppl 86:394a, 1995.

51. Urbano-Isizua A, et al: Allogeneic peripheral blood progenitor cell transplantation (alloBCT): analysis of short-term engraftment and acute GVHD in 33 cases. Blood Suppl 86:394a, 1995.

52. Anderlini P, et al: Chronic graft-vs-host disease (GVHD) after allogeneic marrow or blood stem cell transplantation, Blood 86:109a, 1995.

53. Beatty G, et al: Marrow transplantation from related donors other than HLA-identical siblings. N Engl J Med 313:765, 1985.

54. Anasetti C, et al: Effect of HLA compatibility on engraftment of bone marrow transplants in patients with leukemia or lymphoma. N Engl J Med 320:197, 1989.

55. Reisner Y, et al: Hematopoietic stem cell transplantation using mouse bone marrow and stem cells fractionated by lectins. Proc Natl Acad Sci USA 75:2933, 1978.

56. Aversa F, et al: Successful engraftment of T-cell-deleted haploidentical "three-loci" incompatible transplants in leukemia patients by addition of recombinant human granulocyte colony-stimulating factor-mobilized peripheral blood progenitor cells to bone marrow inoculum. Blood 84:3948, 1994.

57. Gorin NC: Autologous stem cell transplantation in acute myelocytic leukemia. Blood 92:1074, 1998.

58. Burnett AK, Goldstone AH, Stevens RM, et al: Randomised comparison of addition of autologous bone-marrow transplantation to intensive chemotherapy for acute myeloid leukaemia in first remission: results of MRC AML 10 trial. UK Medical Research Council Adult and Children's Leukaemia Working Parties. Lancet 351:700, 1998.

59. Cassileth PA, Harrinton DP, Appelbaum FR, et al: Chemotherapy compared with autologous or allogeneic bone marrow transplantation in the management of acute myeloid leukemia in first remission. N Engl J Med 339:1649, 1998.

60. Mehta J, et al: Autologous bone marrow transplantation for acute myeloid leukaemia in first remission: identification of modifiable prognostic factors. Bone Marrow Transplant 16:499, 1995.

61. Hiddeman W, et al: High-dose versus intermediate dose cytosine arabinoside combined with mitoxantrone for the treatment of relapsed and refractory acute myeloid leukemia: results of an age adjusted randomized comparison. Leuk Lymph 10:133, 1993.

62. Schiffman K, et al: Consequences of cryopreserving first remission autologous marrow for use after relapse in patients with acute myeloid leukaemia. Bone Marrow Transplant 11:227, 1993.

63. Chopra R, et al: Successful treatment of acute myeloid leukemia beyond first remission with autologous bone marrow transplantation using busulphan/cyclophosphamide and unpurged marrow: the British Autograft Group experience. J Clin Oncol 9:1840, 1991.

64. Spinolo JA, et al: High-dose chemotherapy and unpurged autologous bone marrow transplantation for acute leukemia in second or subsequent remission. Cancer 66:619, 1990.

65. Meloni G, et al: BAVC regimen and autologous bone marrow transplantation in patients with acute myelogenous leukemia in second remission. Blood 75:2882, 1990.

66. Sharkis SJ, Santos GW, Colvin M: Elimination of acute myelogenous leukemic cells from marrow and tumor suspension in the rat with 4-hydroxycyclophosphamide. Blood 61:521, 1980.

67. Brenner MK, et al: Gene-marking to trace origin of relapse after autologous bone marrow transplantation. Lancet 341:85, 1993.

68. Schultz FW, Martens ACM, Hagenbeek A: The contribution of residual leukemic cells in the graft to leukemia relapse after autologous bone marrow transplantation: mathematical considerations. Leukemia 3:530, 1989.

69. Hagenbeek A, Martens ACM: Cryopreservation of autologous marrow grafts in acute leukemia: survival of in vivo clonogenic leukemic cells and normal hematopoietic stem cells. Leukemia 3:535, 1989.

70. Gorin NC, et al: Autologous bone marrow transplantation for acute myelocytic leukemia in first remission: a European survey of the role of marrow urging. Blood 75:1606, 1990.

71. Miller CB, et al: Autotransplants for acute myeloid leukemia (AML): effect of purging with 4-hydroxycyclophosphamide (4HC). Proc Am Soc Clin Oncol 15:338, 1996.

72. Rowley SD, et al: CFU-GM content of bone marrow graft correlates with time to hematologic reconstitution following autologous bone marrow transplantation with 4-hydroxycyclophosphamide-purged bone marrow. Blood 70:271, 1987.

73. Gorin NC, et al: Autologous bone marrow transplantation using marrow incubated with Asta Z 7557 in adult acute leukemia. Blood 67:1367, 1986.

74. Stiff J, Koester AR: In vitro chemoseparation of leukemic cells from murine bone marrow using V16-213: importance of stem cell assays. Exp Hematol 15:263, 1987.

75. Kushner BH, et al: Preclinical assessment of urging with V-16-213: key role of long term marrow cultures. Blood 69:65, 1987.

76. Chang TT, et al: Comparative cytotoxicity of various drug combinations for human leukemic cells and normal hematopoietic precursors. Cancer Res 47:119, 1987.

77. Ball ED, et al: Autologous bone marrow transplantation in acute myelogenous leukemia: in vitro treatment with myeloid cell-specific monoclonal antibodies. Blood 68:1311, 1986.

78. Ball ED, et al: Autologous bone marrow transplantation of acute myeloid leukemia using monoclonal antibody-urged bone marrow progress. Clin Biol Res 377:97, 1992.

79. Robertson MJ, et al: Human bone marrow deleted of CD33-positive cells mediates delayed but durable reconstitution of hematopoiesis: clinical trial of MY9 monoclonal antibody-urged autografts for the treatment of acute myeloid leukemia. Blood 79:2229, 1992.

80. Korbling M, et al: Autologous blood stem cell (ABSCT) versus urged bone marrow transplantation (ABMT) in standard risk AML: influence of source and cell composition of the autograft on haematopoietic reconstitution and disease free survival. Bone Marrow Transplant 7:343, 1991.

81. Demirer T, et al: Autologous transplantation with peripheral blood stem cells collected after granulocyte colony-stimulating factor in patients with acute myelogenous leukaemia. Bone Marrow Transplant 18:29, 1996.

82. Reiffers J, et al: The source of stem cells does not affect the outcome of patients undergoing autologous stem cell transplantation for acute myeloid leukemia in first remission [Abstract]. Blood 88:684a, 1996.

83. Reiffers J, et al: Is there a place for blood stem-cell transplantation for the younger adult with acute myelogenous leukemia? J Clin Oncol 12:1100, 1994.

84. Sierra J, Anasetti C: Marrow transplantation from unrelated donors. Curr Opin Hematol 2:444, 1995.

85. Goldman JM: A special report: bone marrow transplants using volunteer donors—recommendations and requirements for a standardized practice throughout the world—1994 update. Blood 84:2833, 1994.

86. Kernan NA, et al: Analysis of 462 transplantation from unrelated donors facilitated by the National Marrow Donor Program. N Engl J Med 328:593, 1993.

87. Schiller G, et al: Treatment of advanced acute leukemia with allogeneic bone marrow transplantation from unrelated donors. Br J Haematol 88:72, 1994.

88. Drobyski W, et al: Unrelated donor transplantation for acute myelogenous leukemia myelodysplasia and secondary AML [Abstract]. Blood 88:269a, 1996.

89. Beatty PG, et al: Marrow transplantation from unrelated donors for treatment of hematological malignancies: effect of mismatching for one HLA locus. Blood 81:249, 1993.

90. Gluckman E: Umbilical cord blood biology and transplantation. Curr Opin Hematol 2:413, 1995.

91. Wagner JE, et al: Allogeneic sibling umbilical-cord blood transplantation in children with malignant and non-malignant disease. Lancet 346:214, 1995.

92. Kurtzberg J, et al: Placental blood as a source of hematopoietic stem cells for transplantation into unrelated recipients. N Engl J Med 335:157, 1996.

93. Pettengell R, et al: Direct comparison by limiting dilution analysis of long-term culture-initiating cells in human bone marrow umbilical cord blood and blood stem cells. Blood 84:3653, 1994.

94. Thomas ED, Storb R, Buckner CD: Total-body irradiation in preparation for marrow engraftment. Transplant Proc 8:591, 1976.

95. Buckner CD, et al: High-dose cyclophosphamide therapy for malignant disease. Cancer 29:357, 1972.

96. Thomas ED, et al: One hundred patients with acute leukemia treated by chemotherapy total body irradiation and allogeneic bone marrow transplantation. Blood 49:511, 1977.

97. Badger C, et al: Allogeneic marrow transplantation for acute leukemia in relapse. Leuk Res 6:383, 1982.

98. Petersen FB, et al: Marrow transplantation following escalating doses of fractionated total body irradiation and cyclophosphamide—a phase I trial. Int J Radiat Oncol Biol Phys 23:1027, 1992.

99. Petersen FB, et al: Etoposide cyclophosphamide and fractionated total body irradiation as a preparatory regimen for marrow transplantation in patients with advanced haematological malignancies: a phase I study. Bone Marrow Transplant 10:83, 1992.

100. Clift RA, et al: Allogeneic marrow transplantation using fractionated total body irradiation in patients with acute lymphoblastic leukemia in relapse. Leuk Res 6:401, 1982.

101. Clift R, et al: Allogeneic marrow transplantation in patients with acute myeloid leukemia in first remission: a randomized trial of two irradiation regimens. Blood 76:1867, 1990.

102. Weiner RS, et al: Interstitial pneumonitis after bone marrow transplantation: assessment of risk factors. Ann Intern Med 104:168, 1986.

103. Deeg HJ, et al: Cataracts after total body irradiation and marrow transplantation: a sparing effect of dose fractionation. Int J Radiat Oncol Biol Phys 10:957, 1984.

104. Witherspoon R, et al: Secondary cancers after bone marrow transplantation for leukemia or aplastic anemia. N Engl J Med 321:784, 1989.

105. Sanders JE: The impact of the marrow transplant preparative regimens on subsequent growth and development: Seattle Marrow Transplant Team. Semin Hematol 28:244, 1991.

106. Santos GW, et al: Marrow transplantation for acute nonlymphocytic leukemia after treatment with busulphan and cyclophosphamide. N Engl J Med 309:1347, 1983.

107. Tutschka JE, Coelan A, Klein J: Bone marrow transplantation for leukemia following a new busulfan and cyclophosphamide regimen. Blood 70:1382, 1987.

108. Copelan EA, et al: Treatment for acute myelocytic leukemia with allogeneic bone marrow transplantation following preparation with BuCy2. Blood 78:838, 1991.

109. Ringden O, et al: A randomized trial comparing busulfan with total body irradiation as conditioning in allogeneic marrow transplant recipients with leukemia: a report from the Nordic Bone Marrow Transplantation Group. Blood 83:2723, 1994.

110. Blaise D, et al: Allogeneic bone marrow transplantation for acute myeloid leukemia in first remission: a randomized trial of a busulfan-cytoxan versus a cytoxan-total body irradiation as preparative regimen: a report from the Group d'Etude de la Greffe de Moelle Osseuse. Blood 79:2578, 1992.

111. Powles RL, Milliken S, Helenglass G: The use of melphalan in conjunction with total body irradiation as treatment for leukemia. Transplant Proc 21:2955, 1989.

112. Mehta J, et al: Melphalan-total body irradiation and autologous bone marrow transplantation for acute leukaemia beyond first remission. Bone Marrow Transplant 18:119, 1996.

113. Blume KG, et al: Total body irradiation and high-dose etoposide: a new preparative regimen for bone marrow transplantation in patients with advanced hematologic malignancies. Blood 69:1015, 1987.

114. Ridell S, et al: High-dose cytarabine and total body irradiation with or without cyclophosphamide as a preparative regimen for marrow transplantation for acute leukemia. J Clin Oncol 6:576, 1988.

115. Matthews D, et al: ^{131}I-anti-CD45 antibody plus busulfan/cyclophosphamide in matched related transplants for AML in first remission [Abstract]. Blood 10:142a, 1996.

116. Petersen FB, et al: Busulfan cyclophosphamide and fractionated total body irradiation as a preparatory regimen for marrow transplantation in patients with advanced haematological malignancies: a phase I trial. Bone Marrow Transplant 4:617, 1989.

117. Linker CA, Ries CA, Damon LE: Autologous bone marrow transplantation for acute myeloid leukemia using busulfan plus etoposide as a preparative regimen. Blood 81:311, 1993.

118. Kolb HJ, et al: Donor leukocyte transfusions for treatment of recurrent chronic myelogenous leukemia in marrow transplant patients. Blood 76:2462, 1993.

119. Chao NJ, et al: Busulfan/etoposide—initial experience with a new preparatory regimen for autologous bone marrow transplantation in patients with acute nonlymphoblastic leukemia. Blood 81:319, 1993.

120. Martino R, et al: High-dose busulfan and melphalan before bone marrow transplantation for acute nonlymphoblastic leukaemia. Bone Marrow Transplant 16:209, 1995.

121. Buzyn-Veil A, et al: Sustained complete cytologic and molecular remission induced by donor leukocyte infusions alone in an acute myeloblastic leukaemia in relapse after bone marrow transplantation. Br J Haematol 92:423, 1996.

122. Lowdell MW, Craston R, Prentice HG: Specific anti-leukemic activity after autologous bone marrow transplantation. *In* Proceedings of the Sixth Biennial Sandoz-Keystone Symposium on Bone Marrow Transplantation, Keystone, CO, 1996.

123. Mackinnon S, et al: Adoptive immunotherapy evaluating escalating doses of donor leukocytes for relapse of chronic myeloid leukemia after bone marrow transplantation. Blood 86:1261, 1995.

124. van der Mast B, et al: Transfusion-associated graft-versus-host disease in immunocompetent patients: a self protective mechanism. Lancet 343:753, 1994.

125. Collins RHJ, et al: Donor leukocyte infusions in 140 patients with relapsed malignancy after allogeneic bone marrow transplantation. J Clin Oncol 15:433, 1997.

126. Kloosterman TC, et al: Interleukin-2 therapy after allogeneic bone marrow transplantation for acute myelocytic leukaemia: studies in a relevant rat model for AML. Bone Marrow Transplant 14:965, 1994.

127. Meloni G, et al: Interleukin-2 may induce prolonged remissions in advanced acute myelogenous leukemia. Blood 84:2158, 1994.

128. Hamon MD, et al: Immunotherapy with interleukin 2 after ABMT in AML. Bone Marrow Transplant 11:399, 1993.

129. Klingemann H-G, et al: Transplantation of patients with high risk acute myeloid leukaemia in first remission with autologous marrow cultured in interleukin-2 followed by interleukin-2 administration. Bone Marrow Transplant 14:389, 1994.

130. Horn TD: Acute cutaneous eruptions after marrow ablation: roses by other names? J Cutan Pathol 21:385, 1994.

131. Hess AD, et al: Development of graft-versus-host disease like syndrome in cyclosporine-treated rats after syngeneic bone marrow transplantation. J Exp Med 161:718, 1985.

132. Geller RB, et al: Successful in vitro graft-versus-tumor effect against an Ia-bearing tumor using cyclosporine-induced syngeneic graft-versus-host disease in the rat. Blood 74:1165, 1989.

133. Noga S, Horwitz L, Hess A: Gamma-interferon (INF) augments the graft-vs-host-disease (SGVHD) in the rat. J Leukocyte Biol Suppl 1:36, 1990.

134. Jones RJ, Santos GW: New conditioning regimens for high risk marrow transplants. Bone Marrow Transplant 4:15, 1989.

CHAPTER THREE

Acute Lymphoblastic Leukemia

Edward A. Copelan, M.D., and Kelli A. Cawley, M.D.

Acute lymphoblastic leukemia (ALL) is a disseminated hematologic malignancy characterized by clonal proliferation of immature lymphoblasts descended from a single transformed progenitor cell. At diagnosis, the marrow has usually been replaced by immature lymphoblasts that interrupt normal hematopoiesis. As reported in 1948, ALL was the first disseminated malignancy to respond to chemotherapy.[1] Today, with systemic chemotherapy, ALL is a curable malignancy.

EPIDEMIOLOGY

Long-term survival and cure after conventional chemotherapy is far more common in children with ALL than in adults. The incidence of ALL is also higher in children. It is the most common malignancy before age 15 years, accounting for 25% of all childhood malignancy. ALL has a weak bimodal incidence. The greatest number of cases occur in children less than 10 years old. A modest second peak occurs in adults over age 50 years. It occurs less commonly in African American children[2] and more commonly among upper social classes.[3] More than 75% of children but only approximately 20% of adults are cured of ALL.

Acute leukemias occur with an increased incidence in children and adults with congenital chromosomal abnormalities. ALL occurs with increased incidence in persons with Down syndrome, Kleinfelter syndrome, Fanconi anemia, Bloom syndrome, ataxia-telangiectasia, and neurofibromatosis.

Atomic bomb survivors in Japan exposed to 1 Gy of radiation showed a peak incidence of acute myelogenous and lymphoid leukemias approximately 6–7 years following exposure.[5] Radiation has also been implicated in cases of ALL in children living near nuclear power plants; one study showed that the incidence of ALL was directly related to emissions from a nuclear power plant.[6] An increased incidence of ALL has been demonstrated in children whose fathers had preconceptual radiation exposure.[7] Other significant toxic exposures include chemical substances such as benzene, alkylating agents, anthracyclines, and epipodophyllotoxins.[8]

CLASSIFICATION

Advances in the treatment of ALL have evolved in part as a result of subclassification of the disease based on morphology, cytogenetics, and immunophenotyping. ALL cells exhibit significant heterogeneity. The French-American-British (FAB) morphologic classification is based on cytoplasmic and nuclear morphology and describes three types of lymphoblasts: L1, L2, and L3. An overwhelming proportion of children have L1 morphology; most adults have L2 morphologic features.[9]

ALL is a heterogeneous disease. The lymphoblasts are derived from a single B- or T-cell progenitor arrested at a specific level of maturation. Immunophenotyping using monoclonal antibodies to surface proteins on normal lymphoid cells is important in categorizing leukemias as lymphoid versus myeloid, in the delineation of T- or B-cell origin, and in defining the stage of maturation.

ALL of B-cell lineage occurs at an incidence of approximately 75% in affected adults and in an even higher percentage of children. Over 20 differentiation antigens have been determined on B cells. CD19, an antigen in B-cell development recognized by the antibodies B4 and Leu-12, is expressed early and is present in more than 95% of cases of B-cell ALL. Three levels of maturation of B-cell ALL are widely recognized: (1) early pre-B ALL, (2) pre-B ALL, and (3) B ALL. These distinctions are used both therapeutically and prognostically. Early pre-B-cell is the most common immunophenotype in children but is less frequent in adults.[10–12]

CD7 is the most commonly expressed T-cell antigen in T-cell ALL, distinguishing it from B-cell or myeloid malignancy. The characterization of T-cell ALL is also based on the level of maturation. Early T-cell-precursor ALL occurs in 7% of adult ALL cases and 1% of childhood ALL cases. The more mature T-cell ALL makes up 17% of adult cases and 11% of childhood cases.[13–15] Myeloid antigens, most commonly CD13 or CD33, are detected in approximately 20% of adult ALL cases.

The most important prognostic test in ALL is cytogenetic analysis.[16] Clonal chromosomal aberrations are detectable in 50–70% of patients with ALL.[17, 18] Higher percentages are found in studies using better methods for bone marrow cell collection.[19] Translocations are the most widely studied chromosomal abnormality in ALL. Chromosomal translocations create aberrant expression of a normal gene product or the formation of a hybrid gene. Hybrid genes result in the formation of abnormal mRNA, which are translated into abnormal proteins such as transcription factors. Inappropriate expression of transcription factors may be associated with leukemogenesis.[20, 21]

The most common translocation in ALL is that of the Philadelphia chromosome, t(9;22), which is detected in approximately 30% of affected adults and 5% of children.[22] The translocation of 9;22 is similar to the translocation

TABLE 3–1. FREQUENCY, PROGNOSIS, AND CYTOGENETIC ABNORMALITIES OF ACUTE LYMPHOBLASTIC LEUKEMIA IMMUNOPHENOTYPES

SUBTYPE	DEFINITION	APPROXIMATE FREQUENCY (%)	EFFECT ON PROGNOSIS	ASSOCIATED STRUCTURAL CYTOGENETIC ABNORMALITIES
Early pre-B	CD19, SIg−, CIg−	50	Favorable	t(4;11)*, t(9;22)*
Pre-B	CD19, SIg−, CIg+	20	Moderately unfavorable	t(4;11)*, t(1;19), t(9;22)*
B	CD19, CD22, SIg+, CIg−	4	Unfavorable	t(8;14), t(8;22), t(2;8)
Pre-T	CD7, CD3	6	Unfavorable	
T	CD1, CD3, CD4, CD7, CD8	20	Favorable	Translocations involving TCR αδ(14q11) or TCR β(7q34)

S, surface; C, cytoplasmic; Ig, immunoglobulin; −, negative; +, positive.
*Abnormalities associated with a poorer prognosis compared with leukemias of similar phenotype lacking the translocation.
Modified from Copelan EA, McGuire EA: The biology and treatment of ALL in adults. Blood 85(5):1151–1168, 1995.

in chronic myelogenous leukemia (CML), although the breakpoint on chromosome 22 may differ and the product associated with ALL may be of different molecular size. The second most common translocation is t(4;11)(q21;q23) involving 11q23.[23, 24] This translocation is most common in patients less than 1 year old. It also occurs in 3–6% of adults with ALL.[16, 25, 26] This translocation in both age groups is associated with hyperleukocytosis. The third most common translocation in ALL is t(1;19)(q23;q13), found in pre-B ALL.[27] Specific cytogenetic abnormalities are commonly associated with specific immunophenotypes (Table 3–1).

DIAGNOSIS

Clinical features leading to the diagnosis of ALL are similar for both children and adults. The most common symptoms are nonspecific and are associated with anemia. The most common problems result from complications of thrombocytopenia. Two consecutive German trials analyzed 938 patients of ages 15–65 years. Approximately 33% of patients presented with infection, 33% with hemorrhage, 50% with lymph node enlargement and hepatosplenomegaly, 14% with mediastinal mass, 7% with central nervous system (CNS) involvement, and 4% with CNS symptoms.

The complete blood count is variable at the time of diagnosis. An increased white blood cell count (WBC) is found in 59% of patients a normal count in 14%, and a low WBC in 27%.[28] In more than 90% of cases, circulating lymphoblasts can be seen on the peripheral blood smear. The bone marrow is most commonly hypercellular and usually contains more than 50% blasts. Patients may have increased uric acid, calcium, lactate dehydrogenase, and occasionally decreased immunoglobulin levels.

PROGNOSTIC FEATURES

Once the diagnosis is established, treatment strategies can be tailored to the subclassification of disease. Age has the greatest impact on duration of remission and survival.[12, 29–31] Children younger than 1 year have a very poor prognosis.[32] In children older than 1 year, complete remission (CR) rates approach 95%. In adults more than 50 years old, however, CR rates are only approximately 40–60%.[33] These differing prognoses result primarily from differences

in disease biology. For example, a higher number of poor prognostic translocations are found in adult ALL. In addition, children tolerate aggressive treatment better, with a lower incidence of delays due to marrow toxicity and a lower incidence of injury to extramedullary organs (Table 3–2).

A variety of other factors influence prognosis. A WBC count in excess of 25,000/mm³ is associated with a poor prognosis. If CR is achieved in less than 5 weeks, sustained disease-free survival (DFS) occurs at twice the frequency associated with longer durations to achieve remission. CNS involvement is a predictor of poor prognosis.

The Philadelphia chromosome (characterized by the translocation t[9;22]) is associated with a dismal prognosis in children and adults. Adults with t(9;22) have a CR rate of 60% with a median duration of 5–10 months. The survival rate at 3 years is under 20%.[35, 36] Allogeneic hematopoietic stem cell transplantation (alloHSCT) is the most promising approach at present for treatment of Philadelphia

TABLE 3–2. FEATURES OF ADULT ALL THAT CONTRIBUTE TO POOR PROGNOSIS COMPARED WITH THOSE IN CHILDREN

DISEASE BIOLOGY

Cytogenetics
  Higher incidence of poor prognostic changes (e.g., t[9;22], t[8;14])
Immunophenotype
  Increased incidence of expression of myeloid antigens
  Less frequent early pre-B immunophenotype
Drug metabolism
  Decreased formation of methotrexate polyglutamates
  Increased incidence of expression of MDR-1 at relapse
Other
  Higher incidence of high leukocyte count at presentation
  Slow response to therapy
  Increased frequency of mediastinal masses

TREATMENT TOLERANCE

Marrow
  Decreased tolerance-treatment delays, increased life-threatening infections
Extramedullary organs
  Increased toxicity (hepatic, cardiotoxicity)
Poor tolerance of specific agents (e.g., high doses of L-asparaginase)
Poor compliance with intensive protocols

Modified from Copelan EA, McGuire EA: The biology and treatment of ALL in adults. Blood 85(5):1151–1168, 1995.

chromosome–positive ALL.[37] Translocations t(4;11) and t(8;14) are also associated with a poor prognosis.

TREATMENT

The precise role of HSCT in the therapy of ALL has not been firmly established. Standard induction therapy regimens have been established in children and used in adult ALL. Induction with vincristine, prednisone, asparaginase, and an anthracycline is standard. Induction therapy has also recently been tailored to biologic subsets of ALL. CR rates in T-cell malignancies are higher with higher doses of cyclophosphamide and cytarabine.[38] Improved survival has also been demonstrated with the addition of radiation to mediastinal masses associated with T-cell malignancies.[39] B-cell neoplasms in both children and adults have responded to high doses of cyclophosphamide, methotrexate, and cytarabine.[40–42]

HEMATOPOIETIC STEM CELL TRANSPLANTATION FOR ACUTE LYMPHOBLASTIC LEUKEMIA

Myeloablative therapy with radiation and chemotherapy or chemotherapy alone followed by alloHSCT is the most effective method to achieve eradication of leukemic cells. The elimination of malignant cells occurs by two mechanisms, the direct lethal effect of chemo-radiotherapy and the antileukemic activity of the allograft.[43–47] The antileukemic effectiveness of alloHSCT must be balanced against the high risk of the procedure. The heterogeneous nature of ALL precludes a singular approach to HSCT in persons with this disorder. Still, a general approach to HSCT in patients with ALL can be formulated. First, blood should be drawn for histocompatibility typing prior to initiation of treatment. Not only does this permit subsequent identification of sibling or unrelated donors, but it permits procurement of human leukocyte antigen (HLA)-matched platelet products in patients who subsequently become refractory to platelet transfusions during chemotherapy. Second, marrow specimens should undergo immunophenotypic, cytogenetic, and, where pertinent, molecular analysis. Only with adequate categorization of the patient's leukemia by these tests can an appropriate therapeutic strategy be devised.

AGE

The age range for which patients should be considered for alloHSCT is not well defined. Increased age is associated with greater risk of transplant-related mortality after alloHSCT,[48–50] especially that due to graft-versus-host disease (GVHD).[51] In recent years, however, the safety of alloHSCT has improved. Several studies have illustrated the usefulness of alloHSCT in selected older patients.[52–54] AlloHSCT from sibling donors has been safely performed in persons up to 65 years of age at several centers, although the bulk of data is from patients with CML,[54] in whom prior treatment is generally less extensive. Patients up to 65 years of age should be considered in appropriate circumstances for alloHSCT from HLA-matched sibling donors. Because of the higher transplant-related mortality associated with matched unrelated donor transplants, especially in older persons, it appears that an upper age limit of 50–55 years is most appropriate among these patients. Decisions must always be based on the characteristics of each patient as well as the potential for other therapies to result in sustained DFS.

STAGE OF DISEASE

CR can be attained in 90–95% of children and 70–80% of adults with ALL.[12] Patients who achieve CR and are not treated with alloHSCT while in first complete remission (CR1) and patients who experience relapse are candidates for alloHSCT. In general, because the majority of patients with ALL can be induced into a second complete remission (CR2), induction of CR2 should be attempted. Patients with HLA-identical sibling or unrelated donors should then be evaluated for transplantation. There is little justification for delaying transplantation beyond CR2 in eligible persons. Results of numerous studies demonstrate that few patients are cured by conventional chemotherapeutic regimens once they experience relapse. Furthermore, delay of transplantation beyond CR2 compromises the safety and effectiveness of transplantation.

Two large studies in children with ALL in CR2 demonstrated that when compared with chemotherapy, HSCT from HLA-identical siblings results in fewer relapses and superior DFS.[55, 56] Five-year DFS was achieved in approximately 40% of children who underwent transplantation compared with less than 20% of those treated with chemotherapy. In adults with ALL in CR2, most studies indicate a DFS rate of approximately 30%,[57–59] comparing favorably with the dismal rates for sustained DFS achieved with chemotherapy. Thus, the risk of transplantation is generally outweighed by the poor outcome of patients who do not undergo transplantation.

At present, a substantial number of patients with ALL undergo transplantation beyond CR2. Transplantation is often the best strategy in patients in more advanced stages of disease because results are superior to those obtained with chemotherapy alone. For most patients, however, earlier transplantation offers the best chance for cure with minimal risk.

Over the last several years, results have improved substantially with alloHSCT. The European Group for Blood and Marrow Transplantation (EBMT) noted lowering of transplant-related mortality from 39% to 25% for patients with ALL between 1979 and 1991.[60] Furthermore, in patients who have experienced relapse, long-term outcome of alloHSCT using matched unrelated donors is similar to those achieved with sibling donors.[61, 62] The increased incidence of transplant-related mortality using unrelated donors is offset by a lower relapse rate.

In patients who do not achieve a first remission with standard induction therapy, the prognosis is poor. Attempts to induce remission with alternative chemotherapeutic agents rarely result in long-term DFS, and aggressive attempts with second-line therapy may compromise the safety and effectiveness of transplantation. Patients who fail to enter CR should undergo alloHSCT if appropriate related or unrelated donors are available. Large studies suggest that approximately 20% of patients in whom primary induction therapy fails achieve sustained DFS after alloHSCT.[63, 64] The fewer cycles of induction chemotherapy patients receive, the more likely a successful outcome becomes. Thus, transplantation should be considered early for patients in whom induction therapy fails.

TRANSPLANTATION IN FIRST COMPLETE REMISSION (CR1)

Far more controversial, despite extensive data, is transplantation of patients with ALL in CR1. The majority of children who achieve a first remission will be cured and should not be considered for transplantation. Nevertheless, subgroups of children with very high-risk features—such as a WBC of 100,000/mm^3 or greater—might benefit from alloHSCT in CR1.[65] This issue has not been definitively answered, however.

Although the risk of relapse in adults is substantially higher than in children, it is clear that some adults who are at low risk for relapse can be identified, whereas others face far more dismal prospects with conventional approaches. The latter should be considered for transplantation. The Ph chromosome is the most frequently identifiable translocation in adults with ALL and is present in approximately 30% of these patients. It confers a dismal prognosis on patients who undergo treatment with conventional chemotherapy.[35, 66] The International Bone Marrow Transplant Registry (IBMTR) reported sustained DFS in 38% of 33 ALL patients who had the Ph chromosome and underwent alloHSCT beyond first remission—a substantially better result than that reported with chemotherapy regimens.[67] The Ph chromosome identifies a group of patients who should be considered for transplantation in CR1. Translocations such as t(4;11) are known to confer a similarly poor prognosis on patients treated with conventional chemotherapy. Patients with this disorder have been cured with alloHSCT,[68] but insufficient data limit conclusions as to the proportion of patients who could be cured with this approach.

Many investigators and clinicians have used other prognostic factors to identify patients in CR1 who are at high risk for relapse, and these workers have used alloHSCT during CR1 in these patients. Many factors that place patients at high risk for relapse with chemotherapy treatment however, such as high presenting WBC, older age, and slow response to chemotherapy, also adversely affect outcome after transplantation.[69–71] For the majority of adults with ALL, it is not clear whether transplantation in CR1 offers the best results. IBMTR studies compared adults with ALL in CR1 who underwent alloHSCT (reported to the Registry) with two cooperative group trials in West Germany in which patients received intensive postremission chemotherapy. Similar probabilities for 5-year DFS were achieved.[69, 70] This was not a randomized study, however, and the group of patients undergoing transplantation had an unusually high mortality rate of nearly 40%. A

study by the French Group for Therapy of Adult ALL used alloHSCT for patients who had HLA-matched sibling donors and either autologous bone marrow transplantation (autoBMT) or chemotherapy in those who did not. The group undergoing alloHSCT had a 3-year DFS of 47 ± 5%, whereas the chemotherapy group had a 3-year DFS of 32 ± 5%.[72] Additional relapses continued to occur beyond 36 months in the chemotherapy arm.

It can be reasonably concluded that patients with certain high-risk factors, including specific cytogenetic abnormalities such as the Philadelphia chromosome, should be treated with alloHSCT while in CR1 if a suitable donor is available. Children and adults with no high-risk factors are probably best treated with chemotherapy; alloHSCT may be reserved for those in whom disease recurs.

In patients in CR, the ability to detect, quantify, and monitor malignant cells using techniques such as flow cytometry, immunophenotyping, or polymerase chain reaction (PCR) for amplification of leukemia-specific sequences of RNA or DNA promises to permit early identification of patients destined to experience relapse on conventional treatment. These patients could be considered for alloHSCT while still in hematologic CR1. For patients with specific high-risk factors such as other cytogenetic abnormalities, a high presenting WBC, or slow but complete response to initial therapy, data are insufficient at this time to clearly define whether alloHSCT in CR1 will improve outcome. Ongoing clinical studies are designed to address these questions.

A problem that has complicated analysis of outcome in patients who achieve CR1 is the role of transplantation at a later time. It is clear that a large proportion of patients who would be eligible for alloHSCT at a later time fail to undergo this procedure once they experience relapse for a variety of reasons, including failure to achieve CR2, early relapse after induction of a second remission, or extramedullary toxicity of chemotherapy.[73]

CONDITIONING REGIMENS

There have been many attempts to improve on the traditional cyclophosphamide and total body irradiation (TBI) regimen developed and modified by Thomas et al. at the Fred Hutchinson Cancer Research Center. Numerous regimens have been investigated, many of which appear to have results similar to those with cyclophosphamide-TBI therapy. A collaborative study by Snyder et al. from the City of Hope Cancer Center and Stanford University achieved favorable results using etoposide and TBI.[74] No regimen has clearly demonstrated superiority to cyclophosphamide-TBI, however.

TBI remains a critical component of most effective regimens. Radiation-free regimens are useful in patients who have undergone extensive prior irradiation to the CNS or mediastinum.[75, 76] Interestingly, Uckun et al. have demonstrated an association between immunophenotype and radiation sensitivity of leukemic cells.[78] T-cell ALL blasts that express CD3[77] and B-cell ALL blasts that lack CD24[78] demonstrate radiation resistance. Radiation-free conditioning regimens might offer increased effectiveness in this situation; this has not been adequately addressed clinically.

Similarly, no substantial data exist as to whether patients whose blasts demonstrate multi-drug-resistant-1 (MDR-1) gene–mediated resistance fare better with radiation than with chemotherapy-only regimens, but this is clearly an area worthy of study.

In an attempt to decrease leukemic relapse without increasing toxicity to nontarget organs, radiolabeled antibodies reactive with hematopoietic antigens have been developed. Matthews et al. at the Fred Hutchinson Cancer Research Center have developed an ^{131}I-anti-CD45 antibody.[79] CD45 is present in all myeloid and lymphoid precursors and most blasts in patients with acute leukemia. Phase I dose-escalation studies in patients with acute myeloid leukemia (AML) and ALL have demonstrated the ability to deliver sizable radiation doses to target tissues without excessive regimen-related toxicity. Preliminary data have been favorable, but it is too early to determine the effectiveness of this approach.

GVHD PROPHYLAXIS

Some studies have suggested that the use of corticosteroids[43, 80] for prevention of GVHD is associated with a decreased rate of relapse and improved DFS in ALL. It is unclear whether this effect is a direct cytolytic effect of steroids or an indirect effect through an increased incidence of chronic GVHD.[80] At present, most centers employ a combination of methotrexate and cyclosporine to prevent GVHD after alloHSCT.

GROWTH FACTORS

The substantial duration of pancytopenia after alloHSCT is associated with life-threatening infections and bleeding. In addition, the numerous antibiotics used during this period themselves contribute to organ toxicity. Initial attempts to shorten the duration of neutropenia utilized hematopoietic growth factors such as granulocyte (G) or granulocyte-macrophage colony–stimulating factor (GM-CSF) after matched sibling transplantation. Randomized studies demonstrated substantial shortening of the duration of neutropenia.[81, 82] Not only was the time to achieve neutrophils of 500/mm³ significantly less in patients receiving growth factor, but the incidences of life-threatening mucositis and infection were also substantially reduced. Duration of hospitalization was shortened modestly. In general, no differences in platelet recovery, red blood cell recovery, incidence of hepatic veno-occlusive disease, GVHD, or relapse were seen. Higher doses of growth factors have led to more-rapid myeloid recovery after alloHSCT.

MOBILIZED PERIPHERAL BLOOD PROGENITOR CELLS

To further speed hematopoietic recovery, numerous investigators have performed pilot studies using mobilized peripheral blood progenitor cells (PBPC) after myeloablative therapy.[83–85] Neutrophil and platelet engraftment occurred more rapidly than with marrow. Generally, normal donors have been given G-CSF at doses ranging from 5 to 16 μg/kg/day for 2–5 days in order to mobilize PBPC. There is no evidence that brief G-CSF administration to normal donors is responsible for any significant risk. In most cases more than 5×10^6 CD34+ cells/kg were collected. Neutrophil counts of greater than 500/mm³ and platelet counts exceeding 20,000/mm³ were achieved by 2 weeks post transplantation. Patients undergoing transplantation using PBPC received fewer units of red blood cells and platelets than did recipients of bone marrow. Interestingly, despite the infusion of much higher doses of T-cells, the incidence of acute GVHD does not appear to be higher in PBPC recipients, compared with the incidence in patients receiving bone marrow. Conclusive studies have not been performed, however, and patients have not been followed for sufficient durations to determine the incidence of chronic GVHD. There is some evidence that immunologic recovery of recipients of allogeneic peripheral blood progenitor cells (alloPBPC) occurs more rapidly than with marrow. Studies designed to investigate depletion of T-cell subsets and CD34+-selected PBPC are under way.

AUTOLOGOUS BONE MARROW TRANSPLANTATION

The BGMT G-group compared allogeneic bone marrow transplant (alloBMT) in CR1 with autoBMT in 135 previously untreated adult patients under age 55.[86] The 3-year probability of DFS was 68% in the group undergoing alloBMT and 26% in the group undergoing autoBMT. The investigators concluded that early alloBMT was effective but that no conclusive data exist that autoBMT improves outcome for the majority of adults with ALL. This study is illustrative of a vast majority of studies in which results reported with autoBMT in ALL have been disappointing.[87, 88] Furthermore, patients undergoing autoBMT in the BGMT study were randomized to receive interleukin-2 (IL-2) or not after transplant. No benefit for IL-2 could be demonstrated. The limited effectiveness of autoBMT in ALL in this setting might be due to the presence of malignant cells in cryopreserved marrow or PBPC[89] and the lack of an effective mechanism for eradicating minimal residual disease after transplantation such as that conferred by GVHD in allogeneic transplants. Despite extensive experience with attempts to use antibodies or chemotherapy to purge malignant cells in vitro, clinical studies have failed to demonstrate a benefit for purging.[90, 91] At this point, no clear benefit for autoBMT over conventional chemotherapeutic approaches has been demonstrated. An ongoing international study involving the Eastern Cooperative Oncology Group from the United States and the Medical Research Council of the United Kingdom is designed to determine the relative benefits of allogeneic and autologous HSCT.

RELAPSE AFTER MARROW TRANSPLANTATION

Second allogeneic transplants for relapsed leukemia after alloHSCT have relatively low chances for success— approximately 10%—if performed soon after initial transplantation. For those patients whose transplants are performed much later than the first transplantation, survival is substantially better.[92–94] The EBMT Leukemia Working Party reported substantially improved survival in patients undergoing transplantation more than 18 months from the first transplantation.[53] Interestingly, long-term survival has been achieved in some patients with ALL who experience relapse after transplantation with relatively conservative chemotherapy.[92]

Donor lymphocyte infusions are increasingly used for the treatment of leukemia relapsing after alloBMT. The first patient ever to receive donor lymphocytes experienced relapse after alloHSCT for ALL. This patient was reported by Slavin et al.[95] to have been treated in November 1986 and was reported to be alive and well 8 years after transplantation. Their team also reported successful reversal of relapse in four of six patients with ALL and in three after the addition of recombinant human IL-2 in addition to infusion of donor peripheral blood lymphocytes.[96] In contrast, Kolb et al., upon reviewing extensive data, concluded that infusion of peripheral blood lymphocytes is relatively ineffective in ALL.[97] This issue remains controversial. In general, in patients who experience relapse within 1 year of HSCT, success rates are relatively poor with any of these treatments, whereas patients who experience further out have a better chance for long-term survival.

CONCLUSION

Allogeneic transplantation is an effective treatment in persons who cannot be induced into a first remission or who experience relapse. Allogeneic transplantation in CR1 is the best approach in certain individuals at high risk for relapse (e.g., those with the Ph chromosome). Current and future clinical studies may elucidate the role of allogeneic transplantation in other persons in first remission and the role, if any, autotransplants might have in the treatment of ALL.

REFERENCES

1. Farber S, Diamond LK, Mercer RD: Temporary remission in acute leukemia in children produced by folic acid antagonist 4-aminopteroyl-glutamic acid caminopoterin. N Engl J Med 238:787, 1948.
2. Young JI, Miller RW: Incidence of malignant tumors in the U.S. children. J Pediatr 86:254, 1975.
3. McWhirter WR: The relationship of incidence of childhood lymphoblastic leukaemia to social class. Br J Cancer 46:640, 1982.
4. Chaganti RSK, Miller DR, Meyers PA, German J: Cytogenetic evidence of the intrauterine origin of acute leukemia in monozygotic twins. N Engl J Med 300:1032, 1979.
5. Health CW: Leukomogenesis and low-dose exposure to radiation and chemical agents. In Yohn DE, Blakeslee JR (eds): Advances in Comparative Leukemia Research. Amsterdam, North-Holland/Elsevier, 1982, p 23.
6. Haerman MA, Kemp JW, MacLaren A-M: Incidence of leukaemia in young persons in west of Scotland. Lancet 1:1188, 1984.
7. Gardner MJ, Snee MP, Hall AJ: Results of case-controlled study of leukaemia and lymphoma among young people near Sellafield nuclear plant in West Cambria. Br Med J 300:423, 1990.
8. Aksoy M, Erdem S, Dineol G: Types of leukemia in chronic benzene poisoning: A study in 34 patients. Acta Haematol 55:65, 1976.
9. Loeffler H, Kayser W, Schmitz N, et al: Morphological and cytochemical classification of adult acute leukaemias in two multicenter studies in the Federal Republic of Germany. Haematol Blood Transfus 30:21, 1987.
10. Pui C-H, Behm FG, Crist WM: Clinical and biological relevance of immunologic marker studies in childhood acute lymphoblastic leukemia. Blood 82:343, 1993.
11. Crist W, Pullen J, Boyett J, et al: Acute lymphoid leukemia in adolescents: clinical and biologic features predict a poor prognosis—a Pediatric Oncology Group Study. J Clin Oncol 6:34, 1988.
12. Copelan EA, McGuire EA: The biology and treatment of acute lymphoblastic leukemia in adults. Blood 85:1151, 1995.
13. Kersey J, Nesbit M, Hallgren H, et al: Evidence of origin of certain childhood acute lymphoblastic leukemia and lymphoma in thymus-derived lymphocytes. Cancer 36:1348, 1975.
14. Reinherz EL, Kung PC, Goldstein G, et al: Discrete stages of human intrathymic differentiation: Analysis of normal thymocytes and leukemic lymphoblasts of T-cell lineage. Proc Natl Acad Sci U S A 77:1588, 1980.
15. Theil E, Kranz BK, Raghavachar A, et al: Prethymic phenotype and genotype of pre-T (CD7+/ER−) cell leukemia and its clinical significance within acute lymphoblastic leukemia. Blood 73:1247, 1989.
16. Bloomfield CD, Secker-Walker LM, Goldman AI, et al: Six year follow up of the clinical significance of karyotype in acute lymphoblastic leukemia. Cancer Genet Cytogenet 40:171, 1989.
17. Bloomfield CD, Lindquist LL, Arthur D, et al: Chromosome abnormalities and their clinical significance in acute lymphoblastic leukemia (for the Third International Workshop on Chromosomes in Leukemia). Cancer Res 43:868, 1986.
18. Bloomfield CD, Goldman AI, Alimena G, et al: Chromosome abnormalities identify high-risk and low-risk patients with acute lymphoblastic leukemia. Blood 67:415, 1986.
19. Williams PL, Ramondi SC, Rivera G, et al: Presence of clonal abnormalities in virtually all cases of acute lymphoblastic leukemia. N Engl J Med 313:640, 1985.
20. Rabbitts TH: Translocations, master genes and difference between origins of acute and chronic leukemias. Cell 67:641, 1991.
21. Nichols J, Nimer SD: Transcription factors, translocations, and leukemia. Blood 80:2953, 1992.
22. Bloomfield CD, Lindquist LL, Brunning RD, et al: The Philadelphia chromosome in acute leukemia. Virchows Arch 29:81, 1978.
23. Arthur DC, Bloomfield CD, Lindquist LL, Nesbit ME Jr: Translocation 4;11 in acute lymphoblastic leukemia: clinical characteristics and prognostic significance. Blood 59:96, 1982.
24. Levin MD, Michael PM, Garson OM, et al: Clinical pathological characteristics of acute lymphoblastic leukemia with the 4;11 chromosome translocation. Pathology 16:63, 1984.
25. Rieder H, Ludwig WD, Gassmann W, et al: Chromosomal abnormalities in adult acute lymphoblastic leukemia: results of the German ALL/AUL Study Group. Recent Results Cancer Res 131:133, 1993.
26. Pui C-H: Acute leukemias with the t(4;11)(q21;q23). Leuk Lymphoma 7:173, 1992.
27. Michael PM, Levin MD, Garson OM: Translocation 1:19—a new cytogenetic abnormality in acute lymphoblastic leukemia. Cancer Genet Cytogenet 12:333, 1984.
28. Hoffman R: Hematology: Basic Principles and Practice. New York, Churchill Livingstone, 1995, p 1087.
29. Hammond D, Sather H, Nesbit M, et al: Analysis of prognostic factors in acute lymphoblastic leukemia. Med Pediatr Oncol 14:124, 1986.
30. Sather HN: Age at diagnosis in childhood acute lymphoblastic leukemia. Med Pediatr Oncol 14:166, 1986.
31. Leumert JT, Burns CP, Wiltse CG, et al: Prognostic information of pretreatment characteristics in adult acute lymphoblastic leukemia. Blood 56:510, 1980.
32. Forman SJ, Blume KG, Thomas ED, et al: Bone Marrow Transplantation. Boston, Blackwell Scientific Publications, 1994, p 619.
33. Hoelzer D: Change in treatment strategies for adult acute lymphoblastic leukaemia (ALL) according to prognostic factors and minimal residual disease. Bone Marrow Transplant. Suppl 6:66, 1990.
34. Michael PM, Garson OM, Ekert H, et al: A prospective study of childhood acute lymphoblastic leukemia: hematology and cytogenetic correlation. Med Pediatr Oncol 14:153, 1988.
35. Secker-Walker LM, Craig JM, Hawkins JM, Hoffbrand AV: Philadelphia positive acute lymphoblastic leukemia in adults: age distribution, BCR break-point, and prognostic significance. Leukemia 5:196, 1991.
36. Lestingi TM, Hooberman AL: Philadelphia positive acute lymphoblastic leukemia. Hematol Oncol Clin North Am 7:161, 1993.
37. Blume KG, Schmidt GM, Chao NJ: Bone marrow transplant for acute lymphoblastic leukemia. In Gale KP, Hoelzzer D (eds): Acute Lymphoblastic Leukemia. New York, Wiley-Liss, 1990, p 279.
38. Hoelzer D: Therapy of the newly diagnosed adult with acute lymphoblastic leukemia. In Bloomfield CD, Herzig GP (eds): Hematology/

Oncology Clinics of North America. WB Saunders, Philadelphia, 1993, pp 139–160.

39. Hoelzer D, Thiel E, Löffler H, et al: Intensified chemotherapy and mediastinal irradiation in adult T-cell acute lymphoblastic leukemia. *In* Gale RP, Hoelzer D (eds): Acute Lymphoblastic Leukemia. Liss, New York, 1990, pp 221–229.

40. Schwenn MR, Blattner SR, Lynch E, Weinstein HJ: HiC-COM: a 2-month intensive chemotherapy regimen for children with stage III and IV Burkitt's lymphoma and B-cell acute lymphoblastic leukemia. J Clin Oncol 9:133, 1991.

41. Reiter A, Schrappe M, Ludwig W-D, et al: Favorable outcome of B-cell acute lymphoblastic leukemia in childhood: a report of three consecutive studies of the BFM group. Blood 80:2471, 1992.

42. Pees HW, Radtke H, Schwamborn J, Graf N: The BFM protocol for HIV-negative Burkitt's lymphomas and L₃ ALL in adult patients: a high chance for cure. Ann Hematol 65:201, 1992.

43. Barrett AJ, Horowitz MM, Gale RP, et al: Marrow transplantation for acute lymphoblastic leukemia: factors affecting relapse and survival. Blood 74:862, 1989.

44. Bortin MM, Truitt RL, Rimm AA, Bach FH: Graft-versus-leukaemia reactivity induced by alloimmunisation without augmentation of graft-versus-host reactivity. Nature 281:490, 1979.

45. Weisdorf DJ, Nesbit ME, Ramsay NCK, et al: Allogeneic bone marrow transplantation for acute lymphoblastic leukemia in remission: prolonged survival associated with acute graft-versus-host disease. J Clin Oncol 5:1348, 1987.

46. Doney K, Fisher LD, Appelbaum FR, et al: Treatment of adult acute lymphoblastic leukaemia with allogeneic bone marrow transplantation: multivariate analysis of factors affecting acute graft-versus-host disease, relapse, and relapse-free survival. Bone Marrow Transplant 7:453, 1991.

47. Horowitz MM, Gale RP, Sondel PM, et al: Graft-versus-leukemia reactions after bone marrow transplantation. Blood 75:555, 1990.

48. Bortin MM, Gale RP, Rim AA: Allogeneic bone marrow transplantation for 144 patients with severe aplastic anemia. JAMA 245:1132, 1981.

49. Forman SJ, Spruce WE, Farbstein MJ, et al: Bone marrow ablation followed by allogeneic marrow grafting during first complete remission of acute nonlymphocytic leukemia. Blood 61:439, 1983.

50. Thomas ED, Clift RA, Fefer A, et al: Marrow transplantation for the treatment of chronic myelogenous leukemia. Ann Intern Med 104:155, 1986.

51. Bross DS, Tutschka PJ, Farmer ER, et al: Predictive factors for acute graft-vs-host disease in patients transplanted with HLA-identical bone marrow. Blood 63:1265, 1984.

52. Klingemann HG, Storb R, Fefer A, et al: Bone marrow transplantation in patients aged 45 years and older. Blood 67:770, 1986.

53. Copelan EA, Kapoor N, Berliner M, Tutschka PJ: Bone marrow transplantation without total-body irradiation in patients aged 40 and older. Transplantation 48:65, 1989.

54. Appelbaum FR, Clift R, Radich J, et al: Bone marrow transplantation for chronic myelogenous leukemia. Semin Oncol 22:405, 1995.

55. Uderzo C, Valsecchi MG, Bacigalupo A, et al: Treatment of childhood acute lymphoblastic leukemia in second remission with allogeneic bone marrow transplantation and chemotherapy: ten-year experience of the Italian Bone Marrow Transplantation Group and the Italian Pediatric Hematology Oncology Association. J Clin Oncol 13:352, 1995.

56. Barrett AJ, Horowitz MM, Pollock BH, et al: Bone marrow transplants from HLA-identical siblings as compared with chemotherapy for children with acute lymphoblastic leukemia in a second remission. N Engl J Med 331:1253, 1994.

57. Gratwhol A, Hermans J, Zwaan F for the EBMT: Bone marrow transplantation for ALL in Europe. *In* Gale RP, Hoelzer D (eds): Acute Lymphoblastic Leukemia. Liss, New York, 1990, p 271.

58. Herzig RH, Barrett AJ, Gluckman E, et al: Bone marrow transplantation in high-risk acute lymphoblastic leukaemia in first and second remission. Lancet 1:786, 1987.

59. Butturini A, Gale RP: Chemotherapy versus transplantation in acute leukaemia. Br J Haematol 72:1, 1989.

60. Frassoni F, Lobopin M, Gluckman E, et al: Results of allogeneic bone marrow transplantation for acute leukaemia have improved in Europe with time—a report of the Acute Leukaemia Working Party of the European Group for Blood and Marrow Transplantation (EBMT). Bone Marrow Transplant 17:13, 1996.

61. Kernan MA, Bartsch G, Ash RC, et al: Retrospective analysis of 462 unrelated marrow transplants facilitated by the National Marrow Donor Program for treatment of acquired and congenital disorders of the lymphohematopoietic system and congenital metabolic disorders. N Engl J Med 328:592, 1993.

62. Beatty PG, Hansen JA, Longton GM, et al: Marrow transplantation from HLA-matched unrelated donors for treatment of hematologic malignancies. Transplantation 51:443, 1991.

63. Forman S, Schmidt G, Nademanee A, et al: Allogeneic bone marrow transplantation as therapy for primary induction failure for patients with acute leukemia. J Clin Oncol 9:1570, 1991.

64. Biggs JC, Horowitz MM, Gale RP, et al: Bone marrow transplants may cure patients with acute leukemia never achieving remission with chemotherapy. Blood 80:1090, 1992.

65. Chessells JM, Bailey C, Wheeler K, Richards SM: Bone marrow transplantation for high-risk childhood lymphoblastic leukaemia in first remission: experience in MRC UKALL X. Lancet 340:565, 1992.

66. Champlin R, Gale RP: Acute lymphoblastic leukemia: recent advances in biology and therapy. Blood 73:2051, 1989.

67. Barrett AJ, Horowitz MM, Ash RC, et al: Bone marrow transplantation for Philadelphia chromosome–positive acute lymphoblastic leukemia. Blood 79:3067, 1992.

68. Copelan EA, Kapoor N, Murcek M, et al: Marrow transplantation following busulfan and cyclophosphamide as treatment for transloca-tion (4;11) acute leukaemia. Br J Haematol 70:127, 1988.

69. Horowitz MM, Messerer D, Hoelzer D, et al: Chemotherapy compared with bone marrow transplantation for adults with acute lymphoblastic leukemia in first remission. Ann Intern Med 115:13, 1991.

70. Zhang MJ, Hoelzer D, Horowitz MM, et al: Long-term follow-up of adults with acute lymphoblastic leukemia in first remission treated with chemotherapy or bone marrow transplantation: the Acute Lymphoblastic Leukemia Working Committee. Ann Intern Med 123:428, 1995.

71. Slovak ML, Kopecky KJ, Wolman SR, et al: Cytogenetic correlation with disease status and treatment outcome in advanced stage leukemia post bone marrow transplantation: a Southwest Oncology Group study (SWOG-8612). Leuk Res 19:381, 1995.

72. Fiere D, Lepage E, Sebban C, et al: for the French Group on Therapy for Adult Acute Lymphoblastic Leukemia: Adult acute lymphoblastic leukemia: a multicenter randomized trial testing bone marrow transplantation as postremission therapy. J Clin Oncol 11:1990, 1993.

73. Berman E, Little C, Gee T, et al: Reasons that patients with acute myelogenous leukemia do not undergo allogeneic bone marrow transplantation. N Engl J Med 326:156, 1992.

74. Snyder DS, Chao NJ, Amylon MD, et al: Fractionated total body irradiation and high-dose etoposide as a preparatory regimen for bone marrow transplantation for 99 patients with acute leukemia in first complete remission. Blood 82:2920, 1993.

75. Van der Jagt RHC, Appelbaum FR, Petersen FB, et al: Busulfan and cyclophosphamide as a preparative regimen for bone marrow transplantation in patients with prior chest radiotherapy. Bone Marrow Transplant 8:211, 1991.

76. Copelan EA, Deeg HJ: Conditioning for allogeneic marrow transplantation in patients with lymphohematopoietic malignancies without the use of total body irradiation. Blood 80:1648, 1992.

77. Uckun FM, Ramsay NKC, Waddick KG, et al: In vitro and in vivo radiation resistance associated with CD3 surface antigen expression in T-lineage acute lymphoblastic leukemia. Blood 78:2945, 1991.

78. Uckun FM, Song CW: Lack of CD24 antigen expression in B-lineage acute lymphoblastic leukemia is associated with intrinsic radiation resistance of primary clonogenic blasts. Blood 81:1323, 1993.

79. Matthews DC, Appelbaum FR, Eary JF, et al: Development of a marrow transplant regimen for acute leukemia using targeted hemato-poietic irradiation delivered by ¹³¹I-labeled anti-CD45 antibody, combined with cyclophosphamide and total body irradiation. Blood 85:1122, 1995.

80. Copelan EA, Biggs JC, Avalos BR, et al: Radiation-free preparation for allogeneic bone marrow transplantation in adults with acute lymphoblastic leukemia. J Clin Oncol 10:237, 1992.

81. Neumanitis J, Rosenfeld CS, Ash R, et al: Phase III randomized, double-blind placebo-controlled trial of rhGM-CSF following allogeneic bone marrow transplantation. Bone Marrow Transplant 15:949, 1995.

82. Schriber JR, Chao NJ, Long GD, et al: Granulocyte colony-stimulating factor after allogeneic bone marrow transplantation. Blood 84:1680, 1994.

83. Korbling M, Przepiorka YO, Huh H, et al: Allogeneic blood stem cell transplantation for refractory leukemia and lymphoma: potential advantage of blood over marrow allografts. Blood 85:1659, 1995.

84. Schmitz N, Dreger P, Suttorp M, et al: Primary transplantation of allogeneic peripheral blood progenitor cells mobilized by filgrastim (granulocyte colony-stimulating factor). Blood 85:1666, 1995.

85. Bensinger WI, Weaver CH, Appelbaum FR, et al: Transplantation of allogeneic peripheral blood stem cells mobilized by recombinant human granulocyte colony-stimulating factor. Blood 85:1655, 1995.

86. Attal M, Blaise D, Marit G, et al: Consolidation treatment of adult acute lymphoblastic leukemia: a prospective, randomized trial comparing allogeneic versus autologous bone marrow transplantation and testing the impact of recombinant interleukin-2 after autologous bone marrow transplantation. Blood 86:1619, 1995.

87. Kersey J, Weisdorf D, Uckun F, et al: Allogeneic and autologous bone marrow transplantation for high risk acute lymphoblastic leukemia. Leukemia 6:191, 1992.

88. Doney K, Buckner CD, Fisher L, et al: Autologous bone marrow transplantation for acute lymphoblastic leukaemia. Bone Marrow Transplant 12:315, 1993.

89. Brenner MK, Rill DR, Moen RC, et al: Gene-marking to trace origin or relapse after autologous bone marrow transplantation. Lancet 341:85, 1993.

90. Uckun FM, Kersey JH, Haake R, et al: Autologous bone marrow transplantation in high-risk remission B-lineage acute lymphoblastic leukemia using a cocktail of three monoclonal antibodies (BA-1/CD24, BA-2/CD9, and BA-3/CD10) plus complement and 4-hydrox-yperoxycyclophosphamide for ex vivo bone marrow purging. Blood 79:1094, 1992.

91. Gilmore MJML, Hamon MD, Prentice HG, et al: Failure of purged autologous bone marrow transplantation in high risk acute lymphoblastic leukemia in first complete remission. Bone Marrow Transplant 8:19, 1991.

92. Barrett AJ, Joshi R, Tew CJ: Which treatment for patients relapsing after bone marrow transplantation for acute lymphoblastic leukaemia? Lancet 1:1188, 1985.

93. Sanders JE, Buckner CD, Clift RA, et al: Second marrow transplants in patients with leukaemia who relapse after allogeneic bone marrow transplantation. Bone Marrow Transplant 3:11, 1988.

94. Barrett AJ, Locatelli F, Treleaven JG, et al: Second marrow transplants for leukaemic relapse after bone marrow transplantation: high early mortality but favourable effect of chronic GVHD on continued remission: a report by the EBMT Leukaemia Working Party. Br J Haematol 79:567, 1991.

95. Slavin S, Naparstek E, Nagler A, et al: Allogeneic cell therapy: the treatment of choice for all hematopoietic malignancies relapsing post BMT [Letter]. Blood 87:4010, 1996.

96. Slavin S, Naparstek E, Nagler A, et al: Allogeneic cell therapy with donor peripheral blood cells and recombinant human interleukin-2 to treat leukemia relapse post allogeneic bone marrow transplantation. Blood 87:2195, 1996.

97. Kolb HJ, Schattenberg A, Goldman JM, et al: Graft-versus-host effect of donor lymphocyte transfusions in marrow grafted patients. Blood 86:2041, 1995.

CHAPTER FOUR

Chronic Myelogenous Leukemia

Matthew H. Carabasi, M.D.

First described by three investigators in 1845,[1–3] chronic myelogenous leukemia (CML) is a disease process characterized by specific hematologic and cytogenic abnormalities resulting from the malignant transformation of a single pluripotent stem cell. CML is of historical interest because it was the first malignant process associated with a specific genetic marker: the Philadelphia chromosome (Ph). This abnormality was first described in 1960[4] and later identified as a shortened chromosome 22.[5] In more than 90% of patients with CML, this shortening is the result of a translocation between the breakpoint cluster region (bcr) on the long arm of chromosome 22 and the c-abl proto-oncogene on the long arm of chromosome 9.[6] This leads to rearrangement of both genes and the production of an abnormal 8.5-kb bcr-abl mRNA[7] whose translation product is the 210-kd protein $p210^{bcr-abl}$, or bcr-abl.[8, 9] In situ hybridization and polymerase chain reaction (PCR) techniques have shown that a bcr rearrangement similar to that in Ph^+ CML is present in most cases of Ph^- CML.[10–15] Thus, the BCR gene rearrangement and production of $p210^{bcr-abl}$ uniquely define this disease whether Ph^+ cells are detected or not.

We now know that bcr-abl plays a crucial role in the pathogenesis of CML. This was first suggested by the observation that irradiated mice rescued with syngeneic bone marrow infected with a retrovirus encoding $p210^{bcr-abl}$ develop a myeloproliferative disorder resembling chronic-phase CML.[16] The specific changes caused by the presence of bcr-abl are now coming into focus. For example, although an excess of hematopoietic cells characterizes this disease state, CML progenitors have less proliferative potential than their normal counterparts.[17–22] In addition, CML and normal progenitors respond similarly to some, but not all, growth and inhibition signals.[23] What has become clear in more recent investigations is that bcr-abl works instead by inhibiting the process of apoptosis, or programmed cell death, that occurs in response to certain signals.[23–25] Interestingly, bcr-abl specifically inhibits apoptosis in response to cellular damage by cytotoxic agents[24] but not by immune-mediated mechanisms.[25, 26] This is consistent with the observation (described later) that allogeneic transplants often cure CML through immune effects mediated by donor T cells rather than the cytotoxic effects of the conditioning regimens.

Unlike acute leukemia, which can sometimes be cured with less than marrow-ablative doses of chemotherapy, CML was uniformly fatal until the development of syngeneic, and later, allogeneic hematopoietic stem cell transplant (HSCT) techniques. Despite this, physicians have been reluctant to refer patients with CML for HSCT because good disease control associated with prolonged survival can usually be achieved with less aggressive treatment approaches. In contrast, patients undergoing allogeneic HSCT may experience considerable morbidity or shortened survival due to either regimen-related toxicity or post-transplant complications such as infection or graft-versus-host disease (GVHD). These problems are even more severe when an alternative donor (either a family member who is not human leukocyte antigen [HLA]-identical or a volunteer unrelated donor) is used.

Fortunately, transplant outcomes using either HLA-identical sibling or alternative-donor grafts have steadily improved. However, results with newer nontransplant strategies are also improving. This makes an understanding of the risks and benefits associated with both transplant and nontransplant treatment options an absolute requirement for providing effective guidance to patients. Specific areas to be considered include (1) accurate assessment of survival based on proper staging at diagnosis as well as recognition of signs of disease progression, (2) results with allogeneic transplants from all potential donor sources, (3) results with nontransplant treatment strategies, and (4) alternative strategies such as allogeneic HSCT using non-myeloablative conditioning regimens or autologous transplants. This chapter surveys each of these areas.

NATURAL HISTORY

The current incidence of adult CML in Western countries is about 1 case per 100,000,[27] accounting for 20–25% of all cases of leukemia. Although the interval from diagnosis to death in patients with CML is variable, the disease usually runs a "triphasic" course through chronic, accelerated, and blast phases.[28] Most patients are in the chronic phase at the time of diagnosis, easily achieving normalization of hematologic parameters with relatively benign therapy. Patients show tremendous variability in the duration of their chronic phase. Prior to the introduction of interferon, the median survival from diagnosis was about 40 months.[29] Because of this variability, prognostic models have been developed based on the presence of certain features at the time of diagnosis, summarized in Table 4–1, that identify patients who may progress quickly to blast crisis.[30–32]

Multivariate regression analysis of the characteristics just described was performed on patients with chronic-phase CML evaluated either at a single center[29] or in a large cooperative study.[31] Both models identified patients that could be grouped in low-, intermediate-, and high-risk categories. Although these models were initially derived

TABLE 4–1. FEATURES ASSOCIATED WITH SHORTER SURVIVAL IN CML (AT TIME OF DIAGNOSIS)

Increasing patient age
Physical examination
    Large spleen (>5–6 cm below left costal margin)
Peripheral blood
    Elevated platelet count (>700,000/mm³)
    Increased
        Blasts (>1%)
        Basophils + eosinophils (>15%)
        Nucleated red blood cells
Bone marrow
    Increased blasts (>5%)
    Chromosome abnormalities in addition to Ph

from patients receiving either busulfan or hydroxyurea, they also have prognostic value regarding response and survival for patients treated with interferon-α.[33] Patients may remain in the chronic phase for up to 20 years before progressing to the second or accelerated phase. This classification is the least clearly characterized because patients may show a variety of signs, symptoms, or hematologic findings indicating increasing resistance to therapy. Specific cytogenetic abnormalities are associated with disease progression. Eighty percent of patients have additional abnormalities at the time of blast transformation,[34–37] with a second Philadelphia chromosome (+Ph); trisomy 8 (+8), 19 (+19), or 21 (+21); isochrome 17; or gain or loss of the Y chromosome (+Y or −Y) being most common.[34, 35, 38, 39] Characteristics associated with accelerated phase disease are listed in Table 4–2.

The terminal or blastic phase of CML classically presents with blood and marrow findings indistinguishable from acute leukemia, although rarely it develops initially at an extramedullary site. The criteria of the international CML Prognosis Study Group commonly used to define blast phase CML are (a) blasts 20% or greater in blood or bone marrow; (b) blasts plus promyelocytes 30% or greater in peripheral blood or 50% or greater in bone marrow; or (c) extramedullary disease defined as the presence of leukemic tumor masses or tissue infiltration with blasts.[31] Patients progressing to blast crisis have a median survival of 4–6 months.[32, 40–42]

As will be discussed later in more detail, results with allogeneic HSCT are best when patients undergo transplantation within a year of diagnosis while still in chronic

TABLE 4–2. SIGNS OF ACCELERATED DISEASE

Blasts >5% in blood or marrow
Basophils >20%
Frequent Pelger-Huët–like neutrophils, nucleated red blood cells, or
    megakaryocytic nuclear fragments
Collagen fibrosis of marrow
Appearance of new karyotypic abnormalities
Development of anemia or thrombocytopenia, not otherwise explained,
    after hemoglobin and platelet count had been normal
Development of marked thrombocytosis (10⁶/mm³) on therapy after the
    platelet count had been controlled
Progressive splenic enlargement after splenomegaly had been reversed
Leukocyte doubling time <5 days
Fever of unknown origin

phase. The foregoing criteria can be used to guide patients in a number of ways. Patients with HLA-identical siblings who are unsure about transplantation can be given a more realistic assessment of the potential benefit of nontransplant strategies. Alternatively, patients unlikely to respond to interferon or patients in accelerated or blast phase can be encouraged to pursue riskier transplant options. Again, the importance of proper staging and risk assessment in evaluating a patient with CML for transplant cannot be overstated.

ALLOGENEIC TRANSPLANT FOR PATIENTS WITH CML

TRANSPLANTS USING HLA-IDENTICAL FAMILY MEMBERS

Although this may change in the future, allogeneic HSCT is the only treatment with the demonstrable ability to consistently cure patients with CML. Encouraging results with bone marrow from identical twins[43] were followed by trials using HLA-identical family members.[44, 45] In addition, the routine use of cyclosporine and methotrexate for GVHD prophylaxis reduced the incidence and severity of this complication.[46]

The long-term survival with such transplants between 1990 and 1995 based on disease state at the time of transplantation, as reported by the International Bone Marrow Transplant Registry (IBMTR), is shown in Figure 4–1. As can be seen, survival is significantly better when patients undergo transplantation in chronic phase as opposed to more advanced stages of the disease, primarily because of a lower relapse rate. The impact of the timing of the transplantation on survival is shown in Figure 4–2. These data clearly show the advantage of performing transplantation in the first year after diagnosis, primarily due to a decrease in transplant-related mortality.[47, 48] As discussed later, this has important implications for patients wishing to try interferon before proceeding to transplantation.

Although disease status and interval from diagnosis to transplantation are clearly important, they are not the only risk factors shown to influence outcome after allogeneic transplantation using HLA-identical siblings. Analysis of 450 patients undergoing transplantation at different centers between 1985 and 1990 confirmed the importance of early transplantation in reducing the risk of transplant-related mortality. Pretransplant treatment with busulfan was also associated with increased toxicity compared with hydroxyurea.[48] The European Group for Blood and Marrow Transplantation (EBMT) performed a retrospective analysis of 373 consecutive patients who underwent transplantation between 1980 and 1988. They noted an association between male donors and late relapse and confirmed the positive effect of early treatment on transplant-related mortality.[47] Multivariate analysis of 177 recipients of related-donor transplants at the University of Minnesota[49] demonstrated that bone marrow eosinophilia was associated with an increased risk of relapse. In contrast to other studies, prolonged interval between diagnosis and transplantation was also associated with an increased risk of relapse.

More recently, several investigators have examined the

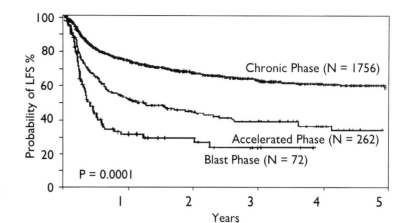

FIGURE 4–1. Probability of disease-free survival after HLA-identical sibling bone marrow transplant for chronic myelogenous leukemia in first chronic phase, 1990–1995 (methotrexate and cyclosporine given for prophylaxis of graft-vs.-host disease), based on state of disease at time of transplant.

value of the pretransplant evaluation in predicting early nonrelapse mortality. A review of 383 patients undergoing autologous or allogeneic transplantation for either hematologic malignancies or solid tumors identified several patient characteristics that were predictive for early nonrelapse mortality.[50] These included diminished forced expiratory volume in 1 second (FEV_1), diminished diffusion capacity, serum creatinine greater than 1.1 mg/dL, Eastern Cooperative Oncology Group performance status greater than 0, and modest elevation of either serum ALT or bilirubin. Goldberg et al. commented that the multivariate model was more predictive than any of the factors identified in the univariate analysis, and they emphasized the importance of global assessment of risk rather than focusing on individual factors.

A more pertinent analysis of 3142 patients undergoing transplantation for CML was conducted by the EBMT.[51] Gratwoni et al. used retrospective data to generate a risk score based on pretransplant characteristics considered to be predictive of survival. Patients were assigned a score based on the sum of the risk factors: donor type (0 for HLA-identical donor, 1 for an unrelated donor); disease state (0 for chronic phase, 1 for accelerated phase, 2 for blast crisis); age (0 for <20 years, 1 for 20–40 years, and 2 for >40 years); sex combination (0 for all except 1 for male recipient/female donor); and time from diagnosis to transplantation (0 for <12 months, 1 for >12 months). The final scoring system was highly predictive for disease-free survival, which ranged from 72% at 5 years for patients

with a score of 0 to only 22% for patients with a score of 6. Although this analysis may be helpful, there are some obvious problems. For example, a patient whose only risk factor is blast-phase disease would have a score of 2 and a predicted survival rate of 62% at 5 years rather than the known survival of less than 20% actually seen with these patients. Regardless, these results demonstrate that careful assessment of patients can be useful in evaluating the potential risk associated with allogeneic transplantation.

Currently, transplants for patients in chronic phase using HLA-identical family members as donors are most commonly performed after cytoreduction with cyclophosphamide combined with either total-body irradiation (TBI) or busulfan. Clift et al. at the Fred Hutchinson Cancer Research Center[52] performed a randomized comparison of these regimens: 142 consecutive patients in chronic phase were conditioned with either cyclophosphamide (60 mg/kg/day × 2 days) followed by TBI (2.0 Gy for 6 consecutive days) (cyclophosphamide-TBI) or oral busulfan (4 mg/kg/day × 4 days) followed by cyclophosphamide (60 mg/kg/day × 2 days) (busulfan-cyclophosphamide). Patients received CSA starting day −1 combined with short-course methotrexate. When these two regimens were compared, there was no difference in event-free survival or probability of relapse. Specifically, the probability of 3-year survival for both arms was 0.80 and the probability of relapse was 0.13. The probability of event-free survival was also identical: 0.68 for the cyclophosphamide-TBI group versus 0.71 for the busulfan-cyclophosphamide group. The probabili-

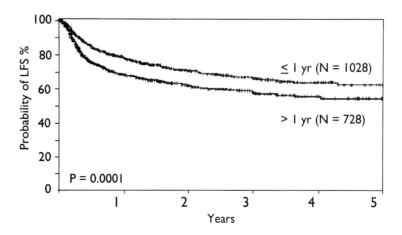

FIGURE 4–2. Probability of disease-free survival after HLA-identical sibling bone marrow transplant for chronic myelogenous leukemia in first chronic phase, 1990–1995 (methotrexate and cyclosporine given for prophylaxis of graft-vs.-host disease), based on interval from diagnosis to transplant.

ties of survival and event-free survival for 101 patients who underwent transplantation within 1 year of diagnosis were 0.86 and 0.72, respectively, for both groups. One difference seen was that the radiation-containing regimen was associated with a higher rate of acute GVHD. The probabilities of serious (grade 2, 3, or 4) acute GVHD were 0.48 and 0.35 for recipients of cyclophosphamide-TBI and busulfan-cyclophosphamide (P = .049). Extensive chronic GVHD developed in 59 patients. This study, along with the IBMTR data (see Fig. 4–1), clearly demonstrates the ability of allogeneic transplant to cure CML. Transplantation, however, caries with it a significant risk of either GVHD, especially in patients older than 30 years, or death.

TREATMENT OF RELAPSE AFTER ALLOGENEIC TRANSPLANTATION

Until 1990, relapse after allogeneic transplantation carried a poor prognosis because second transplants were associated with mortality rates approaching 100% in adults. This changed dramatically with the first published report[53] describing the use of donor lymphocyte infusion (DLI), typically at doses of 10^8 T cells/kg, to successfully reverse this complication. The EBMT has expanded on this initial experience, reporting on 75 evaluable patients with CML treated between 1992 and 1994.[54] Fifty-four patients achieved complete hematologic and cytogenetic remission, which was durable in 80% of the cases. Thirty-six patients experienced at least grade 2 GVHD, and 27 experienced myelosuppression, although this was rarely fatal.

An alternative approach was described by Mackinnon et al. at Memorial Sloan-Kettering Cancer Center,[55] who performed a dose-escalation trial in 22 relapsed recipients of T cell–depleted transplants for CML. Patients were treated with an initial dose of 10^5 donor T lymphocytes per kilogram of body weight, followed by increasing doses in nonresponders over eight levels to a maximum of 5 × 10^8 cells/kg. Nineteen patients achieved complete remission using this strategy, including 15 who became bcr-abl negative by PCR assay. A response occurred in eight patients after treatment with 10^7 T lymphocytes per kilogram, with GVHD occurring in only one responder at this dose level. This clearly demonstrates that the graft-versus-leukemia effect can be separated from GVHD, and established the minimum dose needed to induce a remission. Both groups noted that these infusions are best performed on patients while at least still in chronic phase because such infusions are seldom effective once patients progress beyond this stage.

Because of the negative impact of GVHD on survival with allogeneic transplants, strategies have been developed to remove the T lymphocytes responsible for this complication from the graft. Although T-cell depletion (TCD) is often effective in decreasing serious (grade 2 or higher) acute and chronic GVHD, its use in patients with CML has been limited by the associated increased rate of relapse.[56, 57] DLI is now routinely used to treat relapse, and two groups have published results combining TCD transplants with DLI in patients with CML.

Sehn et al. from Dana-Farber Cancer Institute compared results in patients undergoing transplantation using this approach with patients who received non-TCD trans-

plants.[58] All patients were conditioned with a combination of TBI and cyclophosphamide. Forty-six patients received TCD grafts with an anti-CD6 monoclonal antibody as their only GVHD prophylaxis. This group was compared with 40 recipients of non-TCD grafts combined with standard GVHD prophylaxis. As expected, the TCD group had a lower incidence of both grade 2–4 acute GVHD immediately after transplantation (15% vs. 37%, P = .026) and chronic GVHD (18% vs. 42%, P = .024). A trend suggesting decreased mortality at 1 year was also detected (13% vs. 29%, P = .07). Twenty-three patients required DLI for relapse, including three in the non-TCD group. After response to DLI was assessed, the fractions of patients in each group alive and disease-free 3 years after transplantation were similar: 65% (TCD group) compared with 67% (non-TCD group). In addition, there was no difference in the overall prevalence of GVHD or the proportion of patients requiring immunosuppressive agents between groups.

Papadopoulos et al. from Memorial Sloan-Kettering Cancer Center have performed a similar analysis (with no control group) in 60 consecutive patients with CML in first chronic phase who received TCD transplants followed by DLI as needed.[59] Thirty-three patients received DLI 11–116 months after transplantation using the dose escalation approach described earlier. Consistent with the low doses of T cells given at relapse, the overall incidence of serious acute or chronic GVHD was only 16% for the whole group, and the probability of disease-free survival at 39 months was 64%. Together these studies suggest that TCD transplants combined with DLI are a reasonable alternative to standard transplant approaches, although the combination has not significantly improved overall survival. This approach may decrease the risk of early mortality, however, and it restricts the risk of GVHD primarily to those patients who need it to cure their disease.

UNRELATED DONOR TRANSPLANTS

Because only 30% of patients have an HLA-compatible family member donor, patients with CML are now more often undergoing transplantation using unrelated donors. As with other transplant strategies, initial results were not encouraging. Four centers reported their combined experience with 102 patients with CML (54 in first chronic phase) who received grafts from unrelated donors.[60] The results included patients receiving either TCD or unmanipulated marrow after a number of different conditioning regimens. Estimated disease-free survival for the group was only 29% at 2½ years, with GVHD and failure to engraft accounting for much of the mortality. Fortunately, results with this type of transplant have rapidly improved, making it a more reasonable treatment option.

Hansen et al. at the Fred Hutchinson Cancer Research Center have published considerably better results in 196 patients with chronic-phase CML who underwent transplantation using unrelated donors between 1985 and 1994.[61] All patients were conditioned with a combination of cyclophosphamide-TBI, and GVHD prophylaxis consisted of cyclosporine and methotrexate. The Kaplan-Meier estimate of survival at 5 years for the entire group was 57%, approaching the results seen with HLA-identical family members. Multivariate analysis identified six factors associated with increased mortality. These include extent of HLA matching, time from diagnosis to transplantation, body-weight index, cytomegalovirus prophylaxis, fungal prophylaxis, and age greater than 50 years. The probability of 5-year survival in 51 patients aged 50 years or less who underwent transplantation within 1 year of diagnosis and who received grafts from donors matched at HLA-A, -B, and -DRB1 was 74%; this probability was 87% at 3 years in 30 patients in this group who received routine prophylaxis with fluconazole and ganciclovir.

Enthusiasm over these results must be tempered by other observations made in this group of patients. First, the incidence of serious acute (grade 2–4) GVHD was 75% in patients receiving grafts perfectly matched at HLA-A, -B, and -DRB1, rising to 95% in patients with even a minor mismatch at one locus (DRB1). The incidence of clinically extensive chronic GVHD in 161 patients surviving at least 80 days was 67%, and patients often required lengthy courses of immunosuppressive therapy. In addition, transplants from unrelated donors remain a high-risk procedure for patients older than 50 years, who account for a significant portion of patients with CML. Nevertheless, these results clearly demonstrate that transplants from unrelated donors are a viable treatment option for younger patients with CML and raise the possibility that further advances will improve outcomes in other subsets of patients.

NONTRANSPLANT TREATMENT OPTIONS

Chemotherapy

Nontransplant treatment options for CML patients include treatment with chemotherapy, interferon-α, or both. Chemotherapy used outside the transplant setting is a noncurative modality that temporarily normalizes hematologic parameters and corrects the physical abnormalities (i.e., splenomegaly) associated with CML. This results in symptomatic relief, but patients almost always remain Ph-positive. Patients typically receive one of two available oral agents, busulfan (also used in the transplant setting) or hydroxyurea. Busulfan is an alkylating agent that exerts its antileukemic effect[62, 63] by suppressing early leukemic progenitor cell populations.[64] Hydroxyurea is a ribonucleotide reductase inhibitor that inhibits DNA synthesis in late progenitor cell populations.[65–67] Hydroxyurea does not usually cause any of the serious side effects associated with busulfan, although blood counts must be checked more frequently.

Median survival with either drug is equivalent,[68, 69] although one study demonstrated superior survival with hydroxyurea.[70] In addition, busulfan should be used with caution in patients who may undergo bone marrow transplantation because IBMTR data suggest its use in this setting is associated with poor outcome.[71] More-intensive chemotherapy regimens given to patients in chronic phase may result in partial or complete suppression of Ph+ metaphases.[72–76] This effect is transient and does not improve median survival in most patients, although subgroups may benefit from this approach.[29] There are no consistently effective treatment options once the disease progresses to the blastic phase.

Interferon-α

Without a doubt, the improved survival reported for patients with CML who are receiving interferon-based regimens represents a major advance in the treatment of this disease. Interferons are biologic agents with antiproliferative as well as antiviral and differentiating activity,[77] and interferon-α has been used to treat chronic-phase CML since 1981.[78] In two studies, daily doses of either 3–9 million IU/m^2 of partially purified[78] or 5 million IU/m^2 recombinant human[79] interferon-α yielded hematologic response rates of 80–90%. A surprisingly high number (20%) of patients demonstrate significant (>35%) suppression of Ph1-positive cells, especially patients starting treatment less than 12 months after diagnosis. The median survival for the earlier study[78] was 64 months, suggesting that patients treated with interferon-α survived longer than patients treated with either busulfan or hydroxyurea.

These initial reports generated important follow-up studies that made a number of important observations, well summarized recently by Faderl et al. at M. D. Anderson Cancer Center.[80] Single-arm studies involving larger numbers of patients showed median survival times of 60–89 months,[81–84] and most randomized studies have shown both higher responses rates and prolonged survival with interferon-α compared with either hydroxyurea or busulfan.[85–88] More-recent studies have shown that the combination of low-dose cytarabine given 7–10 days/month plus interferon can further improve both survival and response rates.[89, 90]

Although this represents an impressive improvement in survival, several problems are associated with the use of interferon-α. This is illustrated by a recent update on 322 consecutive patients with CML treated by the Italian Cooperative Study Group on CML.[33] First, the benefit of interferon-α is greatest in low-risk patients, with a median survival of 104 months versus a median survival of 69 months in patients not at low risk. Unfortunately, less than half of all patients with CML are classified as low risk at diagnosis. Second, interferon-α does not improve survival in patients failing to achieve at least a hematologic response. Third, the use of interferon-α is associated with a number of side effects that can preclude continued use in up to 25% of patients.

One final problem with assessing interferon-α as a treatment alternative to allogeneic transplantation is the time needed to respond to this agent. Patients usually require 12–14 months of therapy before being considered a treatment failure. Because a delay of this magnitude can negatively affect outcome after allogeneic HSCT, patients wishing to try interferon-α faced a difficult decision if a suitable donor was available. Further analysis by Sacchi et al. at M. D. Anderson may help with this dilemma.[91] They analyzed data on 274 patients treated with interferon-α from 1982 through 1990 as well as an additional 137 patients treated with interferon-α plus cytarabine between 1990 and 1994. By careful analysis of pretreatment characteristics and response status after 6 months of therapy, they identified a group of patients unlikely to have a meaningful cytogenetic response. Briefly, patients with either a partial hematologic response or resistant disease after 6 months of therapy had a less than 10% probability of a major cytogenetic response. Patients with either splenomegaly of 5 cm or more below the costal margin or platelet count of 700,000/mm³ or higher prior to starting treatment were also unlikely to benefit. The availability of a model to predict response at 6 months may allow patients for whom transplant is a less-desirable treatment option to try interferon-α without adversely affecting outcome after transplantation.

COMPARISON OF TRANSPLANT AND NONTRANSPLANT TREATMENT OPTIONS

As discussed earlier, several good treatment options are available to patients with CML depending on the availability of either an acceptable family member or an unrelated donor. Although there may be an obvious factor suggesting the most appropriate strategy for individual patients, most fall into intermediate-risk categories for both transplant or nontransplant treatment options, especially if an HLA-identical family member is identified. At present, there is no randomized trial comparing transplantation with therapy based on interferon-α, but studies have compared transplant recipients with matched controls from large published studies in an attempt to quantitate the risk/benefit ratio associated with transplantation when compared with potentially "safer" treatments.

Gale et al. compared results reported to the IBMTR for 548 recipients of transplants from HLA-identical siblings with data collected on 196 patients treated with either hydroxyurea (n = 121) or interferon-α (n = 75) in a randomized trial conducted by the German CML group.[92] The transplant group included only recipients of unmanipulated bone marrow grafts who received cyclosporine and methotrexate as GVHD prophylaxis. Statistical adjustments were made to compensate for patient differences between the two groups and changing risks over time, since the relative risk associated with each approach changed over time.

For the first 18 months after diagnosis, mortality was higher in the transplant group, survival between 18 and 56 months was equivalent, and after 56 months, mortality was lower in the transplant group. The probability of survival at 7 years was 58% in the transplant group and only 32% in the nontransplant group. The survival advantage associated with transplant was seen earlier in patients who underwent transplantation less than 1 year after diagnosis and in patients with intermediate- or high-risk characteristics at diagnosis. One problem with this analysis is the relatively low number of patients treated with interferon-α in the nontransplant cohort. Although the inclusion of more patients treated with interferon-α might change how long it takes for the survival advantage to switch to the transplant cohort, it is not likely to effect the overall results of the study.

A similar analysis of the impact of transplant from an unrelated donor on survival at various intervals from diagnosis compared with no transplant has also been performed.[93] Lee et al. considered the impact of various treatment strategies on a hypothetical patient with CML, looking at the impact of risk assessment as well as age (25, 35, and 45 years old) on survival. The nontransplant survival curves were estimated from six published studies, including interferon trials as well as determinants of prognosis. The predicted outcome after unrelated donor transplant was calculated from data obtained from the IBMTR and the National Marrow Donor Program (NMDP): 778 patients with chronic-phase CML undergoing transplantation between 1987 and 1994 were analyzed; the median age at transplant was 36 years, and the median interval from diagnosis to transplant was 20 months.

In virtually all scenarios, patients undergoing transplantation showed superior survival, although this could take up to 12 years to become apparent. The only exception was in older (age 45 years) low-risk patients, in whom survival was equivalent with or without transplant. It is important to note that the control group did not include patients treated with interferon-α combined with cytarabine, which might have affected the analysis. It is equally likely, however, that improvements in the transplant arm would be seen with the incorporation of routine prophylaxis against cytomegalovirus and fungal infections, as described by the investigators at the Fred Hutchinson Cancer Research Center cited earlier. The cost-effectiveness of transplants using unrelated donors has also been analyzed[94] using data from 157 patients who underwent transplantation at Brigham and Women's Hospital and the Fred Hutchinson Cancer Research Center. Lee et al. concluded that unrelated donor transplants, although costly, have a cost-effectiveness ratio comparable to that of other accepted treatments for both malignant and nonmalignant conditions.

Finally, data have been published that investigate the impact of interferon treatment on outcome after transplants from unrelated donors.[95] Morton et al. at the Fred Hutchinson Cancer Research Center compared 114 recipients of transplants from unrelated donors who had not been treated with interferon-α with 70 patients treated with interferon-α for varying intervals prior to transplantation. Patients treated with interferon-α for 6 months or more before transplantation had an increased risk of grade 3 or 4 acute GVHD and decreased survival compared with patients treated with interferon-α for less than 6 months or other treatments. Potential problems with this study include the relatively low number of patients in some of the subsets as well as the presence of other factors that could also affect outcome. The study, however, does suggest that interferon should be used with caution in patients committed to transplantation using unrelated donors until this question has been definitively answered. It also suggests that patients 50 years of age or younger with an appropriate unrelated donor should consider proceeding to transplantation in lieu of a trial of interferon-α because such patients had a 5-year survival rate of 87% if they also received prophylaxis against cytomegalovirus and fungal infections after transplantation.

FUTURE DIRECTIONS

As can be seen from the preceding discussion, transplant offers the potential for cure but can actually shorten survival in some patients. Two strategies to lower transplant-related mortality are currently under investigation. The first involves the use of autologous HSCT. Autologous transplants have been used in the past to treat patients after blast transformation, utilizing cryopreserved chronic-phase marrow or peripheral blood progenitor cells (PBPC) infused after myeloablative therapy. Although occasional long-term survivors were reported, this approach often failed because of rapid return to blast crisis.[96, 97] Patients have also undergone autologous transplantation in chronic phase after aggressive cytoreduction in an attempt to prolong survival. In a review of 200 patients with CML who underwent autologous HSCT between 1984 and 1992, the median survival of 142 patients undergoing transplantation in chronic phase had not been reached at 42 months post transplant, and the median survival of patients who underwent transplantation in accelerated phase was 35.9 months.[98] Only disease status was predictive for survival. An extensive review of this topic is available elsewhere[99] that also discusses potential strategies to improve our ability to purge leukemic cells from the graft.

A second strategy involves the use of nonablative conditioning regimens to reduce transplant-related mortality. This approach involves the use of low-dose chemotherapy followed by an infusion of unmanipulated PBPC from an HLA-identical donor. The chemotherapy, usually fludarabine combined with other agents, is given to stabilize disease and is immunosuppressive enough to allow engraftment of donor cells, although GVHD prophylaxis is required early after transplant. Patients who fail to achieve full donor chimerism or who experience relapse can often be salvaged with withdrawal of immunosuppressive agents or DLI.

Results from a group of 26 patients treated with this approach in Israel have been reported.[100] This group included six patients with CML in chronic phase and one patient with CML in accelerated phase. At the time of last observation, 21 patients were alive and disease-free, including four patients treated for CML. Twenty-two of 26 patients survived, and the probability of disease-free survival was 77.5% at 14 months. Twelve patients experienced grade 2–4 acute GVHD, which was fatal in four. Khouri et al. at M. D. Anderson have also described their experience with 15 patients treated for advanced lymphoid malignancies.[101] Eleven patients experienced engraftment, with seven patients surviving 90–767 days (median follow-up of 180 days). Grade 1 skin GVHD occurred in four patients after initial treatment, and one patient experienced grade 2 acute GVHD of the liver. Three patients experienced acute GVHD after DLI, which was fatal in one case. Both studies show that this approach is capable of completely eradicating disease, even in patients refractory to chemotherapy prior to transplantation. This approach does not completely eliminate the risk of fatal GVHD, however, in part because it relies on graft-versus-recipient reactions to eliminate malignant cells and ensure durable engraftment. In addition, patients often experience infectious complications similar to those seen in recipients of standard transplant regimens, especially if GVHD occurs. Nevertheless, this approach appears to be extremely promising in patients with CML, in whom immune-mediated effects are central to cure.

A new Abl tyrosine kinase inhibitor, STI571, has been recently developed. Preliminary clinical data showed that the drug can induce remission in CML patients in chronic and accelerated phases.[104] Its implications for HSCT remain to be studied.

CONCLUSION

Patients with CML have a number of available treatment options, each associated with a unique set of risks and benefits. Despite this, there is some consensus among transplant physicians[102] and advocates of nontransplant strategies such as interferon-α on certain issues.[103] First, patients with an HLA-identical family member should not be discouraged from pursuing transplantation unless other medical or social issues preclude a successful outcome. The impact of age on outcome in this setting is not clear, with such transplantation routinely being performed on patients at least up to age 60 years. Similarly, a subset of patients younger than 50 years who undergo transplantation early in their disease have a high likelihood of cure when the transplant is from HLA-identical unrelated donors.

For other patients, risks and benefits are less clear. Patients who are unsure about undergoing transplantation must often balance the potential short-term survival advantage associated with interferon-α treatment against the risk of increased mortality associated with either delaying transplantation or treatment with interferon-α prior to unrelated donor transplantation. If it is possible to assess the likelihood of a major response after only 6 months of therapy, as suggested by investigators at M. D. Anderson Cancer Center, a trial of interferon-α may be a reasonable option for such patients. In addition, newer approaches using less intensive conditioning regimens may eliminate some of the early survival advantage associated with interferon-α when compared with transplant, especially if they are successfully applied to transplants from unrelated donors. In the future, comparisons using patient populations treated with the latest approaches may more clearly define the appropriate use of both transplant and nontransplant treatment options in patients with CML.

ACKNOWLEDGEMENT

Data presented in this chapter were obtained from the Statistical Center of the IBMTR. The analysis has not been reviewed or approved by the Advisory Committee of the IBMTR.

REFERENCES

1. Craigie D: Case of disease of the spleen, in which death took place in consequence of the presence of purulent matter in the blood. Edinburgh Med Surg J 64:400–413, 1954.
2. Bennett JH: Case of hypertrophy of the spleen and liver, in which death took place from suppuration of the blood. Edinburgh Med Surg J 64:413–423, 1845.
3. Virchow R: Weisses blut. Froiep Notizen 36:151–156, 1845.
4. Nowell PC, Hungerford DA: Chromosome studies on normal and leukemic human leukocytes. J Natl Cancer Inst 25:85–109, 1960.
5. Caspersson T, Gahrton G, Lindsten J, et al: Identification of the Philadelphia chromosome on a number 22 by quinacrine mustard fluorescence analysis. Exp Cell Res 63:238–240, 1970.
6. Rowley JD: A new consistent chromosomal abnormality in chronic myelogenous leukemia identified by quinacrine fluorescence and giemsa staining. Nature 243:290–293, 1973.
7. Shtivelman E, Lifshitz B, Gale RP, et al: Fused transcript of abl and bcr genes in chronic myelogenous leukemia. Nature 315:550–554, 1985.
8. Konopka JB, Watanabe SM, Witte ON: An alteration of the human

c-abl protein in K562 leukemia cells unmasks associated tyrosine kinase activity. Cell 37:1035–1042, 1984.

9. Kloetzer W, Kurzrock R, Smith L, et al: The human cellular abl gene product in the chronic myelogenous leukemia cell line K562 has an associated tyrosine protein kinase activity. Virology 140:230–238, 1985.

10. Kurzrock R, Blick MB, Talpaz M, et al: Rearrangement in the breakpoint cluster region and the clinical course in Philadelphia negative chronic myelogenous leukemia. Ann Intern Med 105:673–679, 1986.

11. Bartram CR, Kleihauer E, de Klein A, et al: C-abl and bcr are rearranged in a Ph¹-negative CML patient. EMBO J 4:683–686, 1985.

12. Morris CM, Reeve AE, Fitzgerald PH, et al: Genomic diversity correlates with clinical variation in Ph¹-negative chronic myeloid leukaemia. Nature 320:281–283, 1986.

13. Bartran CR: bcr rearrangement without juxtaposition of c-abl in chronic myeloid leukemia. J Exp Med 162:2175–2179, 1985.

14. Dreazen O, Klisak I, Rassool F, et al: Do oncogenes determine clinical features in chronic myeloid leukaemia? Lancet 1:1402–1405, 1987.

15. Wiederman LM, Karhi KK, Shivji MK, et al: The correlation of breakpoint cluster region rearrangement and p210 phl/abl expression with morphological analysis of Ph-negative chronic myeloid leukemia and other myeloproliferative diseases. Blood 71:349–355, 1988.

16. Daley GQ, Van Etten RA, Baltimore D: Induction of chronic myelogenous leukemia in mice by the P210$^{bcr/abl}$ gene of the Philadelphia chromosome. Science 247:824–830, 1990.

17. Goto T, Nishikori M, Arlin Z, et al: Growth characteristics of leukemic and normal hematopoietic cells in Ph¹+ chronic myelogenous leukemia and effects of intensive treatment. Blood 59:793–808, 1982.

18. Strife A, Clarkson B: Biology of chronic myelogenous leukemia: is discordant maturation the primary defect? Semin Hematol 25:1–19, 1988.

19. Strife A, Lambek C, Wisniewski D, et al: Proliferative potential of subpopulations of granulocyte-macrophage progenitor cells in normal subjects and chronic myelogenous leukemia patients. Blood 62:389–397, 1983.

20. Strife A, Lambek C, Wisniewski D, et al: Discordant maturation as the primary biological defect in chronic myelogenous leukemia. Cancer Res 48:1035–1041, 1988.

21. Wisniewski D, Strife A, Atzpodien J, et al: Effects of recombinant human tumor necrosis factor on highly enriched hematopoietic progenitor cell populations from normal human bone marrow and peripheral blood and bone marrow from patients with chronic myeloid leukemia. Cancer Res 47:4788–4794, 1987.

22. Clarkson B, Strife A: Discordant maturation in chronic myelogenous leukemia. In Deisseroth AB, Arlinghaus RB (eds): Chronic Myelogenous Leukemia, New York, Marcel Dekker, 1991, pp 3–90.

23. Eaves C, Cashman J, Eaves A: Defective regulation of leukemic hematopoiesis in chronic myeloid leukemia. Leuk Res 22:1085–1096, 1998.

24. Bedi A, Barber JP, Bedi GC, et al: BCR-ABL-mediated inhibition of apoptosis with delay of G2/M transition following DNA damage: a mechanism of resistance to multiple anticancer agents. Blood 86:1148–1168, 1995.

25. Fuchs EJ, Bedi A, Jones RJ, et al: Cytotoxic T cells overcome BCR-ABL-mediated resistance to apoptosis. Cancer Res 55:463–466, 1995.

26. Roger R, Issaad C, Pallardy M, et al: BCR-ABL does not prevent apoptotic death induced by human natural killer or lymphokine-activated killer cells. Blood 87:1113–1122, 1996.

27. Surveillance Epidemiology End Results Incidence and Mortality Data: 1973–1977. NCI Monograph 57. Bethesda, MD, National Cancer Institute, 1981, p 10.

28. Sokal JE, Baccarani M, Russo D, et al: Staging and Prognosis in Chronic Myelogenous Leukemia. Semin Hematol 25:49–61, 1988.

29. Kantarjian HM, Smith TL, McCredie KG, et al: Chronic myelogenous leukemia: a multivariate analysis of the associations of patient characteristics and therapy with survival. Blood 66:1326–1355, 1985.

30. Gomez GA, Herrmann R, Sokal JE: Prognostic value of serial measurements of leukocyte thymidine uptake in well controlled chronic myelocytic leukemia. Leuk Res 5:497–503, 1981.

31. Sokal JE, Cox EB, Baccarani M, et al: Prognostic discrimination in

32. Marianni G, Annino L, Solinas S, et al: Blastic transformation in chronic myelogenous leukemia: experience with 50 patients. Med Pediatr Oncol 4:159–167, 1978.

33. The Italian Cooperative Study Group on Chronic Myeloid Leukemia: Long-term follow-up of the Italian trial of interferon-α versus conventional chemotherapy in chronic myeloid leukemia. Blood 92:1541–1548, 1998.

34. Sandberg AA: The Chromosomes in Human Cancer and Leukemia. New York, Elsevier North Holland, 1980, p 185.

35. Whang-Peng J, Knutsen T: Chromosomal abnormalities in chronic granulocytic leukaemia. In Shaw MT (ed): Chronic Granulocytic Leukemia. Eastbourne, U.K., Praeger, 1982, p 49.

36. Swolin B, Weinfeld A, Westin J, et al: Karyotypic evolution in Ph-positive chronic myeloid leukemia in relation to management and disease progression. Cancer Genet Cytogenet 18:65–79, 1985.

37. Singh S, Wass J, Vincent PC, et al: Significance of secondary cytogenetic changes in patients with Ph-positive chronic granulocytic leukemia in the acute phase. Cancer Genet Cytogenet 21:209–220, 1986.

38. Sokal JE, Gomez GA, Baccarani M, et al: Prognostic significance of additional cytogenetic abnormalities at diagnosis of Philadelphia chromosome–positive granulocytic leukemia. Blood 72:294–298, 1988.

39. Bernstein R: Cytogenetics of chronic myelogenous leukemia. Semin Hematol 25:20–34, 1988.

40. Alimena G, Dallapiccola B, Gastaldi R, et al: Chromosomal, morphological and clinical correlations in blastic crisis of chronic myeloid leukaemia: a study of 69 cases. Scand J Haematol 28:103–117, 1982.

41. Bertanzzoni U, Brusamolino E, Isernia P, et al: Prognostic significance of terminal transferase and adenosine deaminase in acute and chronic myeloid leukemia. Blood 60:685–692, 1982.

42. Cervantes F, Ballesta F, Mila M, et al: Cytogenetic studies in blast crisis of Ph-positive chronic granulocytic leukemia: results and prognostic evaluation in 52 patients. Cancer Genet Cytogenet 21:239–246, 1986.

43. Fefer A, Cheever MA, Greenberg PD, et al: Treatment of chronic granulocytic leukemia with chemoradiotherapy and transplantation of marrow from identical twins. N Engl J Med 306:63–68, 1982.

44. Thomas ED, Clift RA, Fefer A, et al: Marrow transplantation for the treatment of chronic myelogenous leukemia. Ann Intern Med 104:155–163, 1986.

45. Goldman JM, Apperley JF, Jones L, et al: Bone marrow transplantation for patients with chronic myeloid leukemia. N Engl J Med 314:202, 1986.

46. Storb R, Deeg HJ, Whitehead J, et al: Methotrexate and cyclosporine compared with cyclosporine alone for prophylaxis of acute graft verus host disease after marrow transplantation for leukemia. N Engl J Med 314:729, 1986.

47. Van Rhee F, Szydlo RM, Hermans J, et al: Long-term results after allogeneic bone marrow transplantation for chronic myelogenous leukemia in chronic phase: a report from the Chronic Leukemia Working Party of the European Group for Blood and Marrow Transplantation. Bone Marrow Transplant 20:553–560, 1997.

48. Goldman JM, Szydlo R, Horowitz MM, et al: Choice of pretransplant treatment and timing of transplants for chronic myelogenous leukemia in chronic phase. Blood 82(7):2235–2238, 1993.

49. Enright H, Davies SM, DeFor T, et al: Relapse after non-T-cell-depleted allogeneic bone marrow transplantation for chronic myelogenous leukemia: early transplantation, use of an unrelated donor, and chronic graft-versus-host disease are protective. Blood 88 (2):714–720, 1996.

50. Goldberg SL, Klumpp TR, Magdalinski AJ, et al: Value of the pretransplant evaluation in predicting toxic day-100 mortality among blood stem-cell and bone marrow transplant recipients. J Clin Oncol 16 (12):3796–3802, 1998.

51. Gratwoni A, Hermans J, Goldman JM: Risk assessment for patients with chronic myeloid leukemia before allogeneic blood or marrow transplantation. Lancet 352:1087–1092, 1998.

52. Clift RA, Buckner CD, Thomas ED, et al: Marrow transplantation for chronic myeloid leukemia: a randomized study comparing cyclophosphamide and total body irradiation with busulfan and cyclophosphamide. Blood 84(6):2036–2043, 1994.

53. Kolb HJ, Mittermueller J, Clemm C, et al: Donor leukocyte transfu-

sions for treatment of recurrent chronic myelogenous leukemia in marrow transplant patients. Blood 76:2462, 1990.

54. Kolb H-J, Schattenberg A, Goldman JM, et al: Graft-versus-leukemia effect of donor lymphocyte transfusions in marrow grafted patients. Blood 86(5):2041–2050, 1995.

55. Mackinnon S, Papadopoulos EB, Carabasi MH, et al: Adoptive immunotherapy evaluating escalating doses of donor leukocytes for relapse of chronic cyeloid leukemia after bone marrow transplantation: separation of graft-versus-leukemia responses from graft-versus-host disease. Blood 86(4):1261–1268, 1995.

56. Cunningham I, Castro-Malaspina H, Flomenberg N, et al: T-cell depleted bone marrow transplant for chronic myelogenous leukemia. Blood 72:384a, 1988.

57. Goldman JM, Gale RP, Horowitz MM, et al: Bone marrow transplantation for chronic myelogenous leukemia in chronic phase: increased risk for relapse associated with T cell depletion. Ann Intern Med 108:806–184, 1988.

58. Sehn LH, Alyea EP, Weller E, et al: Comparative outcomes of T-cell-depleted and non-T-cell-depleted allogeneic bone marrow transplantation for chronic myelogenous leukemia: impact of donor lymphocyte infusion. J Clin Oncol 17(2):561–568, 1999.

59. Papadopoulos EB, Young JW, Barnett L, et al: Combined use of T-cell depleted bone marrow transplants (TCDBMT) with donor leukocyte infusions (DLI) for treatment of patients with chronic myelogenous leukemia (CML). Blood 92(Suppl 1):322a, 1998.

60. McGlave PB, Beatty P, Ash R, et al: Therapy for chronic myelogenous leukemia with unrelated donor bone marrow transplantation: results in 102 cases. Blood 75:1728–1732, 1990.

61. Hansen JA, Gooley TA, Martin PJ, et al: Bone marrow transplants from unrelated donors for patients with chronic myeloid leukemia. N Engl J Med 338:962–968, 1998.

62. Galton DAG: Myleran in chronic myeloid leukaemia. Lancet 1:208, 1953.

63. Haut A, Abbot WS, Wintrobe MM, et al: Busulfan in the treatment of chronic myelocytic leukemia: the effect of long term intermittent therapy. Blood 17:1, 1961.

64. Haddow A, Timmis GM: Myleran in chronic myeloid leukaemia: chemical constitution and biological action. Lancet 1:207, 1953.

65. Fishbein WN, Carbone PP, Freireich EJ: Clinical trials of hydroxyurea in patients with cancer and leukemia. Clin Pharmacol Ther 5:574, 1964.

66. Kennedy BJ: Hydroxyurea therapy in chronic myelogenous leukemia. Cancer 29:1052, 1971.

67. Schwartz JH, Canellos GP: Hydroxyurea in the management of the hematologic complications of chronic granulocytic leukemia. Blood 46:11, 1975.

68. Bolin RW, Robinson WA, Sutherland J, et al: Busulfan vs hydroxyurea in long-term therapy of chronic myelogenous leukemia. Cancer 50:1683–1686, 1982.

69. Rushing D, Goldman JM, Gibbs G, et al: Hydroxyurea versus busulfan in the treatment of chronic myelogenous leukemia. Am J Clin Oncol 5:307–313, 1982.

70. Talpaz M, Kantarjian HM, McCredie K, et al: Clinical investigation of human alpha interferon in chronic myelogenous leukemia. Blood 69:1280, 1987.

71. Goldman J, Szydlo R, Horowitz M, et al: Choice of pretransplant treatment and timing of transplants for chronic myelogenous leukemia in chronic phase. Blood 82:2235, 1993.

72. Brodsky I, Fuscaldo KE, Kahn SB, et al: Chronic myelogenous leukemia: a clinical and experimental evaluation of splenectomy and intensive chemotherapy. Ser Haematol 6:143, 1975.

73. Clarkson B: Chronic myelogenous leukemia: is aggressive treatment indicated? J Clin Oncol 3:135, 1985.

74. Denz H, Lechleitner M, Marth CH, et al: Effects of human recombinant alpha-2 and gamma interferon on the growth of human cell lines from solid tumors and hematologic malignancies. J Interferon Res 5:147, 1985.

75. Sharp JC, Wayne AW, Crofts M, et al: Karyotypic conversion in Ph[1]-positive chronic myeloid leukaemia with combination chemotherapy. Lancet 1:1370, 1979.

76. Smalley RV, Vogel J, Huguley CM, et al: Chronic granulocytic leukemia: cytogenetic conversion of the bone marrow with cycle-specific chemotherapy. Blood 50:107, 1977.

77. Borden EC, Fall LA: Interferons: biochemical, cell growth, inhibitory and immunological effects. Prog Hematol 350:1, 1981.

78. Talpaz M, Kantarjian HM, McCredie KG, et al: Clinical investigation of human alpha interferon in chronic myelogenous leukemia. Blood 69:1280–1288, 1987.

79. Talpaz M, Kantarjian HM, McCredie K, et al: Hematologic remission and cytogenetic improvement induced by recombinant human interferon alpha A in chronic myelogenous leukemia. N Engl J Med 314:1065–1069, 1986.

80. Faderl S, Kantarjian HM, Talpaz M: Chronic myelogenous leukemia: update on biology and treatment. Oncology 13:169–180, 1999.

81. Kantarjian HM, Smith TL, O'Brien SM, et al: Prolonged survival in chronic myelogenous leukemia after cytogenetic response to interferon-α therapy. Ann Intern Med 122:254–261, 1995.

82. Alimena G, Morra E, Lazzarino M, et al: Interferon alpha-2b as therapy for Ph-positive chronic myelogenous leukemia: a study of 82 patients treated with intermittent or daily administration. Blood 72:642–647, 1988.

83. Ozer H, George SL, Schiffer CA, et al: Prolonged subcutaneous administration of recombinant α2b interferon in patients with previously untreated Philadelphia chromosome–positive chronic-phase chronic myelogenous leukemia: effect on remission duration and survival: Cancer and Leukemia Group B study 8583. Blood 82:2975–2984, 1993.

84. Mahon F, Montastruc M, Faberes C, et al: Predicting complete cytogenetic response in chronic myelogenous leukemia patients treated with recombinant interferon-α. Blood 84:3592–3594, 1994.

85. Ohnishi K, Ohno R, Tomonaga M, et al: A randomized trial comparing interferon-α with busulfan for newly diagnosed chronic myelogenous leukemia in chronic phase. Blood 86:906–916, 1995.

86. Allan NC, Richards SM, Shepherd PCA on behalf of the UK Medical Research Council's Working Parties for Therapeutic Trials in Adult Leukaemia: UK medical research council randomized, multicentre trial of interferon-α n1 for chronic myeloid leukemia: improved survival irrespective of cytogenetic response. Lancet 345:1392–1397, 1995.

87. The Italian Cooperative Study Group on Chronic Myeloid Leukemia: Interferon-alpha-2a as compared with conventional chemotherapy for the treatment of chronic myeloid leukemia. N Engl J Med 330:820–825, 1994.

88. Hehlmann R, Heimpel H, Hasford J: Randomized comparison of interferon-α with busulfan and hydroxyurea in chronic myelogenous leukemia: the German CML Study Group. Blood 84:4064–4077, 1994.

89. Kantarjian HM, O'Brien S, Smith TL, et al: Treatment of Philadelphia chromosome–positive early chronic phase chronic myelogenous leukemia with daily doses of interferon alpha and low-dose cytosine arabinoside. J Clin Oncol 17:284–292, 1999.

90. Guillhot F, Chastang C, Michallet M, et al: Interferon alpha-2b combined with cytarabine versus interferon alone in chronic myelogenous leukemia. N Engl J Med 337:223–229, 1997.

91. Sacchi S, Kantarjian HM, Smith T, et al: Early treatment decisions with interferon-alfa therapy in early chronic-phase chronic myelogenous leukemia. J Clin Oncol 16:882–889, 1998.

92. Gale RP, Hehlmann R, Zhang M-J, et al: Survival with bone marrow transplantation versus hydroxyurea or interferon for chronic myelogenous leukemia. Blood 91:1810–1819, 1998.

93. Lee S, Kuntz K, Horowitz M, et al: Unrelated donor bone marrow transplantation for chronic myelogenous leukemia: a decision analysis. Ann Intern Med 127:1080–1088, 1997.

94. Lee S, Anasetti C, Kuntz K, et al: The cost and cost-effectiveness of unrelated donor bone marrow transplantation for chronic myelogenous leukemia. Blood 92:4047–4052, 1998.

95. Morton AJ, Gooley T, Hansen JA, et al: Association between pretransplant interferon-α and outcome after unrelated donor marrow transplantation for chronic myelogenous leukemia in chronic phase. Blood 92:394–401, 1998.

96. Haines ME, Goldman JM, Worsley AM, et al: Chemotherapy and autografting for patients with chronic granulocytic leukaemia in transformation: probable prolongation of life for some patients. Br J Haematol 58:711–722, 1984.

97. Buckner CD, Clift RA, Fefer A, et al: Treatment of blastic transformation of chronic granulocytic leukemia by high dose cyclophosphamide, total-body irradiation and infusion of cryopreserved autologous marrow. Exp Hematol 6:96–109, 1978.

98. McGlave PB, De Fabritis P, Deisseroth A, et al: Autologous transplants for chronic myelogenous leukemia: results from eight transplant groups. Lancet 343:1486, 1994.
99. Bhatia R, Verfaillie C, Miller J, et al: Autologous transplantation therapy for chronic myelogenous leukemia. Blood 88:2623–2634, 1997.
100. Slavin S, Nagler A, Naparstek, et al: Nonmyeloblative stem cell transplantation and cell therapy as an alternative to conventional bone marrow transplantation with lethal cytoreduction for the treatment of malignant and nonmalignant hematologic diseases. Blood 91:756–763, 1998.
101. Khouri IF, Keating M, Korbling M, et al: Transplant-lite: induction of graft-versus-malignancy using fludarabine-based nonablative chemotherapy and allogeneic blood progenitor-cell transplantation as treatment for lymphoid malignancies. J Clin Oncol 16:2817–2824, 1998.
102. Lee S, Anasetti C, Horowitz M, et al: Initial therapy for chronic myelogenous leukemia: playing the odds. J Clin Oncol 16:2897–2903, 1998.
103. Kantarjian HM, O'Brien S, Anderlini P, et al: Treatment of chronic myelogenous leukemia: current status and investigational options. Blood 87:3069–3081, 1996.
104. Druker BJ, Lydon NB: Lessons learned from the development of an Abl tyrosine kinase inhibitor for chronic myelogenous leukemia. J Clin Invest 105:3–7, 2000.

CHAPTER FIVE

Myelodysplasia

Robert B. Geller, M.D.

The role of hematopoietic stem cell transplantation (HSCT) to treat myelodysplastic syndromes (MDS) is an evolving and controversial topic.[1] Several factors contribute to the perplexity of this issue, most notably the difficulty in distinguishing MDS from other hematopoietic diseases, such as polycythemia vera,[2, 3] chronic myelogenous leukemia (CML) and other chronic myeloproliferative diseases,[4–6] acute myelogenous leukemia (AML), and aplastic anemia.[7] MDS represents a diverse group of malignant disorders of the hematopoietic stem cell with varied clinical and laboratory features. Indeed, studies that include conditions that do not meet the French-American-British (FAB) Cooperative Group diagnostic criteria of MDS, such as aplastic anemia with cytogenetic abnormalities, acute malignant myelosclerosis, or myelofibrosis, make the evaluation of the role of BMT even more difficult.[8–10]

A second factor complicating the assessment of BMT in MDS has been the lack of prognostic factors predictive of poor clinical outcome for an individual patient. This is in part due to the clinical heterogeneity that exists within each FAB subtype.[11] The clinical course may vary from an indolent disease with a survival of greater than 10 years without significant intervention to a rapidly progressive and fatal disease.[12] Despite the ability to determine molecular, genetic, and immunophenotype characteristics and chromosome status, no uniform method exists to predict patient outcome[13–18]; however, the International Prognostic Scoring System (IPSS) has been developed to evaluate prognostics in MDS using clinical characteristics.[19] This chapter focuses on the evaluation of patients with MDS for HSCT using the FAB classification and the IPSS as a clinical guide. In addition, the role of allogeneic HSCT (alloHSCT), including the use of alternative donors, and the potential role of autologous HSCT (autoHSCT) are addressed.

CLASSIFICATION OF MYELODYSPLASIA

MDS represents a group of clonal hematopoietic disorders characterized by impaired maturation of hematopoietic stem cells, progressive peripheral cytopenias, and a tendency to progress to AML. In 1982, the FAB group referred to the "myelodysplastic syndromes" as a group of bone marrow disorders that share common features of ineffective hematopoiesis and dyspoiesis.[8] This classification listed the qualitative changes that can be seen in the erythroid, granulocytic, and megakaryocytic series. Using these morphologic abnormalities, the percentage of blasts in the peripheral blood and bone marrow, the percentage of ring sideroblasts in the bone marrow, the presence of Auer rods,

and the number of monocytes in the peripheral blood, the FAB classification defined five subtypes of MDS[8, 11] (Table 5–1): refractory anemia (RA), refractory anemia with ringed sideroblasts (RARS), refractory anemia with excess of blasts (RAEB), chronic myelomonocytic leukemia (CMML), and refractory anemia with excess of blasts in transformation (RAEB-t). This classification has been widely accepted, although it has been found to have limited prognostic significance.[20–22] Results from the third meeting of the Morphologic, Immunologic and Cytogenetic Cooperative Study Group in 1988 showed a relatively good prognosis for RA and RARS, a worse prognosis for RAEB and CMML, and a poor prognosis for RAEB-t.[23]

Although the FAB classification has provided useful morphologic guidelines and has defined diagnostic groups, it has been noted to be deficient in several ways. For example, FAB requires that all cases of MDS show evidence of "ineffective hematopoiesis" (peripheral cytopenias with either normocellular or hypercellular bone marrow). Other authors have shown that some patients can have a hypocellular bone marrow and have all the morphologic and clinical features of an MDS.[24–26] This has been called *hypocellular MDS* and is not recognized in the FAB classification. Other disease categories not recognized by the FAB classification include MDS with myelofibrosis, refractory cytopenias with trilineage dysplasia, and treatment-related MDS.[9, 10, 27] Another common criticism has been either the addition of CMML as a myelodysplastic syndrome or, with its inclusion, the inability of this classification schema to appropriately distinguish CMML from other chronic myeloproliferative syndromes.[4]

In addition, it is not uncommon for a patient's disease to progress from one subtype to another. Of primary concern is a percentage of blast cells between 25% and 30%, which requires a pathologic diagnosis of RAEB-t, but clinically this may be more characteristic of "de novo" AML; these patients may simply have presented relatively early in the course of AML or their blast percentages may have been underestimated, resulting in a diagnosis of RAEB-t instead of AML. In these cases, other clinical characteristics and/or another bone marrow examination may be required to accurately distinguish MDS from de novo AML, especially because optimal treatment depends on an accurate diagnosis.

Common to all subtypes of MDS and less frequently seen in de novo AML are dysplastic features of the bone marrow, which may occur in one, two, or all three lineages of the myeloid precursors.[28] Within the FAB classification, these features include dyserythropoiesis with or without ringed sideroblasts; dysgranulopoiesis with hypogranula-

TABLE 5–1. MYELODYSPLASTIC SYNDROMES AS CLASSIFIED BY THE FRENCH-AMERICAN-BRITISH COOPERATIVE GROUP

TYPE	BLASTS, PERIPHERAL BLOOD (%)	FEATURES OF MARROW ASPIRATE BLASTS, MARROW	PERIPHERAL BLOOD/ABSOLUTE MONOCYTOSIS ($>1 \times 10^9$/L)	RINGED SIDEROBLASTS MARROW	TYPICAL MORPHOLOGIC FEATURES, PERIPHERAL BLOOD	TYPICAL MORPHOLOGIC FEATURES, BONE MARROW BIOPSY
Refractory anemia (RA)	≤1% (usually not seen)	Dyserythropoiesis Granulocytic and megakaryotic series appear normal <5% blasts	No	Ringed sideroblasts may be seen	Reticulocytopenia Variable dyserythropoiesis Infrequent dysgranulopoiesis	Normocellular or hypercellular marrow Erythroid hyperplasia
Refractory anemia with ringed sideroblasts (RARS)	≤1%	Similar to RA but with >15% of all nucleated cells in marrow representing ringed sideroblasts	No	>15% of all nucleated cells	Similar to RA Often dimorphic population of red blood cells	Similar to RA but with >15% ringed sideroblasts
Refractory anemia with excess of blasts (RAEB)	<5%	Always dysgranulopoiesis, dyserythropoiesis, and/or dysmegakaryocytopoiesis 5–20% blasts	No	Ringed sideroblasts may be seen	Cytopenias in two or more cell lines Conspicuous abnormalities in all three cell lines	Hypercellular marrow Granulocytic or erythroid hyperplasia
Refractory anemia in excess of blasts in transformation (RAEB-t)	≥5%	Similar to RAEB >20–30% blasts	No	Ringed sideroblasts may be seen	May see Auer rods in granulocytic precursors	Similar to RAEB May see Auer rods
Chronic myelomonocytic leukemia (CMML)	<5%	Resembles RAEB ≤20% blasts	Yes	Ringed sideroblasts may be seen	Absolute monocytosis often associated with increase in mature granulocytes with or without dysgranulopoiesis	Resembles RAEB but with significant increase in monocyte precursors

tion, hyposegmentation, and megaloblastic changes; and dysmegakaryocytopoiesis with micromegakaryocytes.

EPIDEMIOLOGY AND CLINICAL AND LABORATORY FEATURES

The incidence of MDS has been reported to be 1–2 per 100,000,[29, 30] although as many as 16% of patients admitted to a general hospital setting for evaluation of pancytopenia have been reported to have MDS.[31] The majority of patients with MDS are elderly males (modestly more often than females), with a median age of 60–75 years, although MDS does occur in younger patients and children.[32, 33] The degree of bone marrow failure significantly correlates with the clinical signs and symptoms of the patient. Many patients are symptom free, and the condition is detected by routine clinical tests. Other patients present with fatigue and exertional dyspnea or, less commonly, signs of bleeding, including petechiae, gingival bleeding, or the presence of a hematoma.[32] The most common infections in patients with MDS are lower respiratory tract bacterial infections and skin abscesses.[34] Less than 20% of patients have splenomegaly; however, in patients in whom CMML is diagnosed, the incidence is between 30% and 50%.[32] Hepatosplenomegaly is found in up to 25% of patients with MDS[32]; Sanz et al. found lymphadenopathy to be present in only 13% of 370 patients with MDS.[16]

The etiology of MDS is unknown in the majority of cases. In an increasing number of patients in whom MDS is diagnosed, however, the disease follows a previous exposure to chemotherapy and/or ionizing radiation.[27] Alkylating therapy used for Hodgkin disease and non-Hodgkin lymphoma has been most associated with the development of therapy-related MDS.[35–37] The addition of ionizing radiation to prolonged alkylating exposure, as used to treat patients with lymphoma receiving combined-modality therapy, has significantly increased this risk.[38] Therapy-related MDS has also been reported in patients with multiple myeloma receiving alkylating therapy,[39] children receiving prolonged therapy with etoposide for acute lymphoblastic leukemia,[40] and female patients receiving adjuvant therapy for breast cancer.[41, 42]

Several subtypes of treatment-related or secondary MDS have been described, depending on the toxin exposure and the clinical features. For patients exposed to alkylating therapy, therapy-related MDS generally occurs 3–4 years after use of the inciting agent and is associated with chromosomal abnormalities, specifically chromosomes 5 and/or 7.[43] In addition, these patients generally present with periods of prolonged cytopenia. Therapy-related MDS following exposure to topoisomerase II inhibitors, such as the epipodophyllotoxins, is generally characterized by relatively short progression to MDS after exposure (1–2 years), short evolution of MDS to AML, and a characteristic chromosomal abnormality involving chromosome 11q23.[44] In addition, there appears to be an increased incidence of therapy-related MDS in patients with a diagnosis of breast cancer, lymphoma, or multiple myeloma receiving high-dose chemotherapy followed by autologous stem cell transplant.[45] It is, however, difficult to ascertain whether the previous induction or salvage chemotherapy regimens or the intensity of the high-dose chemotherapy regimen prior to the autologous reinfusion is the precipitating event for the development of therapy-related MDS.

The original descriptions of the laboratory features of each type of MDS are from the FAB classification[8] (see Table 5–1). Patients with RA uniformly have anemia associated with reticulocytopenia. Although the peripheral blood granulocyte and platelet counts are generally normal, the rare patient without anemia but with thrombocytopenia or neutropenia or both can also be considered in this group. By definition, leukemic blasts are less than 1% of the total white blood cell count in the peripheral blood. Blasts account for less than 5% of the total marrow cells. The laboratory findings in patients with RARS are similar to those in patients with RA except that more than 15% of all nucleated marrow cells are ringed sideroblasts. The presence of a double or dimorphic red blood cell population can also be observed on peripheral blood smear preparations from patients with RARS.[46]

In RAEB, the degree of cytopenia is more severe than in RA and RARS, affecting at least two or more of the bone marrow cell lines. Blasts may be seen in the peripheral blood but account for less than 5% of the total white blood cell count. In the bone marrow, blasts must account for 5–20% of the total marrow cells. RAEB-t differs from RAEB primarily by numeric criteria. The laboratory findings for RAEB-t include a peripheral blast count of 5% or more, a bone marrow blast count of more than 20% but no greater than 30%, or the presence of Auer rods in the granulocyte series. If more than 30% blasts are counted in the bone marrow, a diagnosis of AML is rendered. CMML is characterized by an absolute monocytosis of greater than 1×10^9/L that is often associated with elevated numbers of granulocytes. Numbers of monocytic precursors may be increased in the bone marrow. The blasts in the bone marrow may be as high as 20%. In the peripheral blood, blasts are less than 5%.

Since the original laboratory descriptions of the five subtypes of MDS, specific chromosomal abnormalities have been described in patients with MDS that are associated with unique syndromes characterized by distinctive clinical and laboratory findings.[47] One such syndrome found in MDS is the 5q− syndrome, for which females are more often affected than males, and the laboratory values show macrocytic anemia, thrombocytosis, and erythroid hypoplasia in at least 50% of patients. The megakaryocytes frequently have unilobed nuclei and bizarre atypical morphologic features. Monosomy 7 has also been associated with MDS and has a distinct group of clincial and laboratory findings. Patients are usually in their fifth or sixth decade of life and are more commonly men. Laboratory findings include anemia and thrombocytopenia. Clinically, patients have splenomegaly. Pronounced dysgranulopoiesis is often present on peripheral blood smears.

Other chromosomal abnormalities have also been reported in 40–60% of patients with MDS. Chromosomal abnormalities in patients with MDS may be complex, with multiple abnormalities. The most common abnormalities include, singly or in combination, loss of part or all of chromosome 7 and/or 5, trisomy +8, del(20q), and the loss of chromosome Y (−Y).[19, 48–51] Those chromosomal abnormalities primarily found in patients with de novo

AML, such as t(8;21), inv(16), or t(15;17), which generally carry a good prognosis, are rarely encountered in patients with MDS.

NATURAL HISTORY AND PROGNOSTIC FACTORS

Since the acceptance of the FAB classification, researchers have shown that MDS is indeed a clonal proliferation of multipotent bone marrow stem cells.[33] Although neoplastic, the stem cells in MDS retain their capacity to differentiate but do so inefficiently. Mature blood elements are variably reduced, and eventually bone marrow failure ensues because of the progressive impairment of the stem cells to differentiate. Compounding the problems of ineffective hematopoiesis is the increased propensity for leukemic transformation.[19, 52–54] Because the neoplastic stem cells of MDS progress so variably, the clinical course for patients with MDS is extremely variable. Whereas some patients remain symptom free for many years, others die from complications of cytopenia or from defects in neutrophil function within weeks to months of diagnosis. For some patients, death results from disease progression to acute leukemia. Because the treatment modalities are so diverse and range from supportive care to HSCT, clinicians need objective criteria to stratify patients into reliable prognostic groups and to select patients who should be treated immediately and aggressively.

The prognostic value of the FAB classification has been demonstrated in several studies.[20–22] Most of these analyses suggest that the subtypes of MDS can be divided into two general groups to predict overall survival. In a large meta-analysis of 1914 patients from several studies, Sanz and Sanz demonstrated that median survival is longer for patients with RA and RARS (37 and 49 months, respectively) compared with patients with RAEB and RAEB-t (9 and 6 months, respectively).[55] CMML was found to have an intermediate prognosis. In addition, this analysis found that the likelihood of leukemia transformation also depended on disease subtype. Patients with RA and RARS had an average percentage of leukemia transformation of 11% and 5%, respectively, whereas the average percentage of leukemia transformation was 23% for RAEB and 48% for RAEB-t.

Even though the FAB classification of MDS is of some prognostic value, clinicians have attempted to identify risk factors for individual patients that more accurately predict survival. A number of prognostic scoring systems have been developed in an attempt to determine oucome, particularly survival, in patients with MDS.[13–19] This is particularly important given the heterogeneous nature of this malignancy.

The most recent prognostic scoring system combined cytogenetic, morphologic, and clinical data from several large, previously reported risk-based studies on a total of 816 patients.[19] In this prognostic scoring system, IPSS (Table 5–2), significant variables for scoring included the number of cytopenias, the marrow blast percentage, and the karyotype. Three cytogenetic subgroups were identified: (1) a good risk including del(20q) only, del(5q) only, −Y, or normal karyotypes; (2) an intermediate group including

+8, single miscellaneous or double abnormalities; and (3) a poor-risk subgroup including complex (three or more abnormalities) or chromosome 7 abnormalities. By combining the risk scores for these three major variables, patients were stratified into four distinct risk groups in terms of overall survival and the risk of AML evolution. These four risk groups are (1) low, (2) intermediate-1 (INT-1), (3) intermediate-2 (INT-2), and (4) high. Median overall survival in the low-risk group was 5.7 years; for INT-1 and INT-2 it was 3.5 and 1.2 years, respectively; and for the high-risk group it was only 0.4 years.

Age at diagnosis was also shown to be an important variable for overall survival.[19] For patients under 60 years of age, the median survival for low, INT-1, INT-2, and high was 11.8 years, 5.2 years, 1.2 years, and 0.4 years, respectively. For patients 60 years of age or older, median survival was 4.8 years, 2.7 years, 1.1 years, and 0.5 years for low, INT-1, INT-2, and high-risk groups, respectively. Patients with therapy-related MDS were not included in this prognostic analysis; overall, patients with secondary MDS have a worse prognosis than patients with primary MDS.[27]

HEMATOPOIETIC STEM CELL TRANSPLANTATION FOR MDS

Despite the wide range of therapy available for managing MDS, including differentiating agents (13-*cis*-retinoic acid, all-*trans* retinoic acid, vitamin D_3 analogs),[56–61] myeloid growth factors (granulocyte colony-stimulating factor; granulocyte macrophage–colony-stimulating factor), either alone or in combination with erythropoietin,[62–64] or single-agent and combination chemotherapy with cytarabine,[65–69] HSCT offers the only treatment approach that may prolong survival and potentially cure the patient. AlloHSCT has been the treatment of choice in the majority of young patients with histocompatible siblings.[70] More recent alternatives include volunteer matched unrelated donors and placental cord or umbilical cord blood transplants.[71, 72] In addition, autologous transplants have also been evaluated in appropriate patients when a compatible donor has not been found.[73]

Table 5–3 summarizes results obtained in patients with MDS undergoing alloHSCT.[1, 74–81] The majority of patients undergoing transplantation in these trials were less than 55 years old and received bone marrow from phenotypically identical siblings or family members with a single antigen mismatch. Preparative regimens differed widely but usually included either busulfan or total body irradiation.

ROLE OF PROGNOSTIC INDICATORS IN EVALUATING RESULTS WITH HSCT

Results from these series generally suggest that certain clinical features convey a favorable prognosis: younger age, less-advanced disease status, compatible sibling donor, and short duration of disease. Other prognostic factors, such as chromosomal abnormalities, the use of pretransplantation induction therapy, and the presence of marrow fibrosis, may be of importance, although data are conflicting.

TABLE 5-2. SUMMARY OF STUDIES OF ALLOGENEIC BLOOD AND MARROW TRANSPLANTATION IN MYELODYSPLASTIC SYNDROMES

AUTHOR	NO. OF PATIENTS	DISEASE SUBTYPE (n)	PREPARATIVE REGIMEN (n)	NON-RELAPSE-RELATED DEATHS	DISEASE-FREE SURVIVAL (%)	FAVORABLE PROGNOSTIC FACTORS	UNFAVORABLE PROGNOSTIC FACTORS
Leblond et al.[74]	84	RA (20) RAEB (25) RAEB-t (17) SAML (17) Other (5)	Not discussed	Not discussed	38	RA, RAEB with stable disease	Not discussed
DeWitte et al.[75]	78	RA (9) RAEB (16) RAEB-t (20) SAML (32) CMML (1)	TBI and chemotherapy (69) Chemotherapy (9)	25	45	RA, RAEB, RAEB-t Untreated myelodysplasia	Not discussed
Longmore et al.[76]	23	RA (6) RAEB (6) RAEB-t (5) SAML (6)	Ara-C, Cy, TBI (1) Ara-C, Cy, FTBI (13) Cy and FTBI (5) CAR, Cy, ETOP (3) Bu and Cy (1)	9	43	Treatment early in course of disease	Use of T cell–depleted marrow in patients with marrow fibrosis
O'Donnell et al.[77]	20	RAEB (4) RAEB-t (8) SAML (1) CMML (2) Other (5)	Ara-C, Cy, TBI (4) FTBI and Cy (3) FTBI and VP16 (6) TBI and VP16 (1) TBI, Bu, VP16 (1) Bu and Cy (5)	9	35	Not discussed	Increase in marrow blasts >10%
Anderson et al.[78]	93	RA (RARS) (29) RAEB (31) RAEB-t (14) CMML (2) Other (17)	Cy and Bu (5) Cy and TBI (88)	44	43	Age < 40 yr Less-advanced disease	Excess blasts Older age
Marmont & Horowitz[79]	123	RA (16) RAEB (51) RAEB-t (35) CMML (6) Other (15)	Cy and TBI (92) Cy, Bu, Cy (31)	Not discussed	10–42	Not discussed	Splenomegaly before conditioning Chromosomal abnormalities
Nevill et al.[80]	19	RA (2) RAEB (2) REAB-t (10) CMML (1) Other (4)	Cy and Bu	6	37	Age < 40 yr Shorter disease duration of <1 yr Normal cytogenetics	Not discussed
Sutton et al.[81]	86	RA (20) RAEB (26) RAEB-t (18) SAML (17) Other (5)	TBI (23) Cy and TBI (30) Bu and Cy (27) Chemotherapy only (3)	33	38	RA or RAEB with stable disease No previous treatment	Delay to transplantation allowing for progression SAML RA or RAEB with progressive disease

TBI, total body irradiation; SAML, secondary AML; Bu, busulfan; Cy, cyclophosphamide; FTBI, fractionated TBI; VP16, etoposide; Ara-C, cytarabine; ETOP, etoposide; CAR, carmustine; RA, refractory anemia; RARS, refractory anemia with ring sideroblasts; RAEB, refractory anemia with excess of blasts; RAEB-t, RAEB in transformation; CMML, chronic myelomonocytic leukemia.

From Schultz AB, Geller RB, Hillyer CD: The role of bone marrow transplantation in the treatment of myelodysplastic syndromes. J Hematother 4:323, 1995.

TABLE 5–3. INTERNATIONAL PROGNOSTIC SCORING SYSTEM (IPSS) FOR MYELODYEPLASTIC SYNDROMES

PROGNOSTIC VARIABLE	SURVIVAL AND AML EVOLUTION— SCORE VALUE				
	0	0.5	1.0	1.5	2.0
Marrow blasts (%)	<5	5–10	—	11–20	21–30
Karyotype*	Good	Intermediate		Poor	
Cytopenias†	0/1	2/3			

RISK CATEGORY	COMBINED SCORE
Low	0
INT-1	0.5–1.0
INT-2	1.5–2.0
High	≥2.5

*Cytogenetics: good = normal, -Y, del(5q), del(20q); poor = complex (> three abnormalities) or chromosome 7 anomalies; intermediate = other abnormalities.
†Cytopenias: neutrophil count <1800/μL, platelets < 100,000/μL, hemoglobin <10 g/dL.
INT-1, intermediate-1; INT-2, intermediate-2.
From Greenberg P, Cox C, LeBeau MM, et al: International scoring system for evaluating prognosis in myelodysplastic syndromes. Blood 89:2079, 1997.

In 1998, Appelbaum and Anderson published an analysis wherein post-transplant outcome was evaluated according to the IPSS risk categorization.[82] In this review, 251 patients with MDS (median age, 38 years; range, 1–66) who underwent transplantation from 1981 through 1996 at the Fred Hutchinson Cancer Research Center were evaluated. Median time from diagnosis to transplantation was 8 months (1–192 months), and 14% of the patients had therapy-related MDS; 43% of the patients had less-advanced MDS (RA, RARS, and hypoplastic anemia with a clonal cytogenetic abnormality). Fifty-seven percent of these patients had advanced MDS (RAEB, RAEB-t, and CMML). According to the IPSS cytogenetics subgrouping, 44% had good-risk cytogenetics, 21% had intermediate-risk cytogenetics, and 31% had poor-risk cytogenetics. Cytogenetic analysis was not available for 4% of patients. In addition, 59% of the transplants were from human leukocyte antigen (HLA)-matched related donors, 13% from HLA partially matched related donors, and 28% of the transplants were from unrelated donors.[82]

Overall, the disease-free survival (DFS) was 40% with a

relapse rate of 18%.[82] From the multivariate analysis, older age, increasing disease duration, mismatched donors, male sex, and therapy-related MDS were factors that predicted for increased nonrelapse mortality (Table 5–4). Patients over the age of 50 years had approximately a 50% chance of dying from transplant-related complications; patients under 20 years of age had a 20% risk. Prolonged disease duration, disease subtype, and cytogenetics were significant in predicting the risk of relapse. Patients with less-advanced MDS rarely experienced relapse, whereas the risk of relapse was significantly higher (≈25%) in advanced MDS. Patients with low- or intermediate-risk cytogenetics had a significantly lower risk of relapse than did patients with high-risk cytogenetics. This difference was found to be independent of disease subtype.[82]

Increasing age, disease subtype, and cytogenetics predicted for DFS as shown in Figure 5–1.[82] In addition, patients with less-advanced MDS had a 55% DFS rate at 6 years compared with a 30% DFS rate for patients with advanced MDS. Patients with low- or intermediate-risk cytogenetics experienced significantly higher DFS than did patients with high-risk cytogenetics.

Figure 5–2 demonstrates the impact of IPSS on nonrelapse mortality, risk of relapse, and DFS.[82] At 5 years, DFS was 60% for the low and INT-1 risk groups, 36% for the INT-2 risk groups, and 20% for the high-risk patients.

USE OF ALTERNATIVE DONORS

With the increasing size of the national and worldwide donor registries of HLA-typed volunteers, the potential use of unrelated donors is expanding. Castro-Malaspina et al. reported on 320 patients with MDS treated with allografts from unrelated donors recruited through the National Marrow Donor Program from 1988 through 1997.[83] Median age was 37 years, and median disease duration prior to transplantation was 9 months. Donors were serologically identical in 267 patients and mismatched in 53 cases. The probability of DFS at 2 years was 30%, with a 24% probability of relapse. Of the 320 patients, 210 have expired because of treatment-related complications, including acute and chronic graft-versus-host disease (GVHD) (17%), graft failure (3%), and infections (30%). The relapse mortality rate was 12%.

TABLE 5–4. MULTIVARIATE ANALYSIS OF PROGNOSTIC FACTORS IN PATIENTS WITH MYELODYSPLASTIC SYNDROMES UNDERGOING ALLOGENEIC BLOOD AND MARROW TRANSPLANTATION

VARIABLE	DISEASE-FREE SURVIVAL (P)	RELAPSE (P)	NONRELAPSE MORTALITY (P)
Increasing age	.003	NS	.0003
Increasing disease duration	NS	.002	.0002
FAB subtype	.011	.0002	NS
Cytogenetics (poor vs. good)	.003	.0001	NS
Donor	NS	NS	.007
Gender	NS	NS	.007
Therapy-related disease	NS	NS	.011

NS, not significant.
From Appelbaum FR, Anderson J: Allogeneic bone marrow transplantation for myelodysplastic syndrome: outcome analysis according to IPSS score. Leukemia 12(Suppl 1):525, 1998.

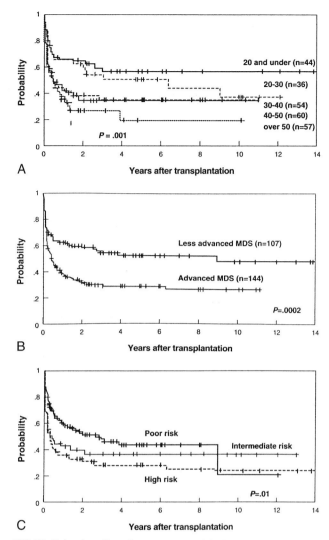

FIGURE 5–1. The effect of increasing age (A), disease subtype (B), and cytogenetics (C) on disease-free survival for 251 patients with myelodysplastic syndromes undergoing alloBMT. (From Appelbaum FR, Anderson J: Allogeneic bone marrow transplantation for myelodysplastic syndrome: outcome analysis according to IPSS score. Leukemia 12 [Suppl 1]: 525, 1998.)

A 1998 retrospective analysis of the effect of T-cell depletion included evaluation of patients with MDS receiving bone marrows from unrelated donors.[84] A total of 420 patients were evaluated, with 111 patients undergoing T-cell depletion and 309 patients receiving conventional immunosuppressive therapy; 311 patients were HLA-compatible and 109 were mismatched. There was no significant difference in survival or relapse risk with the use of T-cell depletion, regardless of patient-donor compatibility.

Anderson et al. reported on 52 patients with MDS or MDS-related AML treated between 1987 and 1993 with unmanipulated unrelated donor marrow transplantation.[71] Median age was 33 years (range, 1–53); donors were phenotypically identical at HLA-A -B and -DRB1 loci in 34 cases and mismatched in 18 cases. The 2-year DFS relapse mortality, and nonrelapse mortality rates were 38%, 28%, and 48%, respectively. Relapse rates were significantly higher for RAEB-t and MDS-related AML compared with

RA, RAEB, or CMML. The risk of treatment-related mortality was significantly higher in older patients and patients with longer disease duration.

It has been shown that transplantation of hematopoietic stem cells from unrelated placental blood or umbilical-cord blood can restore the function of bone marrow and sustain hematopoietic recovery in patients.[85] For patients with MDS who do not have a suitable related donor, umbilical-cord blood transplants may offer certain advantages over unrelated bone marrow transplants, including a decreased risk of GVHD and the ease and rapid availability of the cord blood to the transplant center.[86–89] The decreased risk of GVHD is desirable because the median age of patients in whom MDS is diagnosed tends to be older; therefore, these patients are not only at greater risk for GVHD but are more likely to die from complications.

In 1998, Rubinstein et al.[72] reported on 562 recipients of umbilical-cord transplants from unrelated donors, of

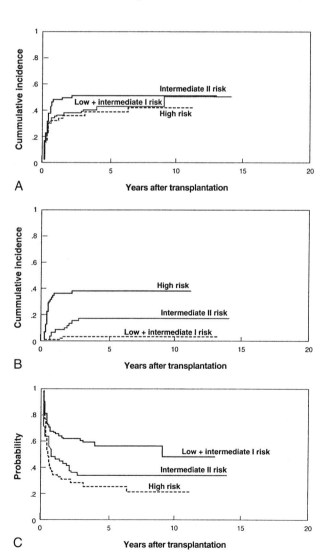

FIGURE 5–2. The impact of the International Prognostic Scoring System (IPSS) on nonrelapse mortality (A), risk of relapse (B), and disease-free survival (C) for 251 patients with myelodysplastic syndromes undergoing allogeneic blood and marrow transplantation. (From Appelbaum FR, Anderson J: Allogeneic bone marrow transplantation for myelodysplastic syndrome: outcome analysis according to IPSS score. Leukemia 12 [Suppl 1]: 525, 1998.)

whom 21 patients had MDS. Their results confirmed earlier studies that demonstrated that umbilical-cord transplants result in trilineage engraftment, cause GVHD less often than unrelated bone marrow transplants, and result in survival rates similar to those of unrelated bone marrow transplants. Only 18% of these recipients were older than 18 years, however, with the oldest patient being 58 years; in addition, 17% of these patients weighed more than 60 kg, with the heaviest patient weighing 116 kg. Successful myeloid recovery was associated with younger age, a higher number of nucleated cells in the umbilical-cord blood product per kilogram of patient body weight, and the absence of HLA mismatching. Event-free survival correlated with the recipient's age and diagnosis, the number of nucleated cells in the blood product, the extent of HLA disparity, and the transplant center.

Even though umbilical-cord transplants offer an alternative source of stem cells, experience with this technique in older patients is currently limited. Its more general use in older patients will probably be restricted until successful techniques of umbilical-cord stem cell expansion are developed.

ROLE OF AUTOLOGOUS HSCT

The majority of patients with MDS may be ineligible for allografting because of older age and lack of a histocompatible donor. Several trials evaluating the role of allogeneic hematopoietic stem cell transplant (alloHSCT) have clearly shown the effect of increasing age on treatment-related mortality after alloHSCT, with patients over the age of 50 years experiencing a worse survival than younger patients. Induction chemotherapy may produce complete remission (CR), but remission is generally short.[68, 69] In particular, patients with complex cytogenetic abnormalities have a significantly worse prognosis.[19] Until recently, autografting in patients with MDS was limited to small numbers of patients.[90–92] More recently, however, studies in larger numbers of selected patients suggest that autografting may be a potential treatment option.[73, 93] Obstacles to expanding its use in patients with MDS continue to be the ability to procure autografts of normal progenitor cells, which are relatively free of malignant cells, and minimizing the treatment-related mortality in an older population.

DeWitte et al. published the results of the European Group for Blood and Marrow Transplantation (EBMT) for 79 patients with MDS or secondary AML.[73] Two-year survival, DFS, and risk-of-relapse rates were 39%, 34%, and 64%, respectively. Interestingly, within this group of 79 patients, 55 patients for whom the duration of first CR was known were compared with a matched control group of 110 patients with de novo AML. DFS at 2 years for patients with MDS or secondary AML was lower than in the de novo AML group (28% vs. 51%, $P = .025$), primarily because of an increased risk of relapse (69% vs. 40%, $P = .007$). This higher relapse risk may suggest more residual malignant cells or residual disease more resistant to therapy. In addition, a substantial number of patients in this series were not eligible for autoHSCT because of delayed hematopoietic recovery after induction chemotherapy and/or poor marrow harvests.

In addition, the role of chemotherapy-purged autoHSCT has also been evaluated in a small series of patients.[93] In seven patients with MDS (3 with RAEB, 1 with RAEB-t, 1 with CMML, and 2 with secondary MDS) who achieved CR, consolidation was with myeloablative therapy followed by reinfusion of autologous bone marrow purged with mafosfamide. Six patients were evaluated for myeloid engraftment; median recovery was 41 days (range, 27–60 days). Five patients were evaluable for platelet recovery; recovery occurred at a median of 120 days (range, 60–140 days). Two patients are alive and disease free at 10 and 28 months post transplant; four patients experienced relapse at a median of 9 months after autografting. When compared with recovery from de novo AML in patients undergoing a similar procedure, recovery for both neutrophils and platelets was slower even though the number of colony forming units-granulocyte macrophages collected per kilogram was similar.

Recent studies have suggested the feasibility of peripheral blood stem cell (PBSC) harvests.[94, 95] A major advantage is the possibility of collecting large numbers of progenitor cells to aid in accelerated hematopoietic recovery compared with conventional autoHSCT. Hastened myeloid recovery may reduce the need for prolonged supportive care and reduce the overall toxicity and mortality.

Demuynck et al. investigated the feasibility of PBSC collection in 11 patients with high-risk MDS.[94] PBSC harvest was undertaken only after CR was achieved. Six patients underwent mobilization with granulocyte colony-stimulating factor (G-CSF) for 7 days after completion of induction and consolidation therapy; the remaining five patients underwent harvesting during the recovery phase following chemotherapy. In 7 of the 11 patients, 5 patients after G-CSF mobilization alone, sufficient cell numbers ($> 1 \times 10^6$ CD34+ cells/kg) were obtained in a median of five collections. Cytogenetic analysis at the time of collection revealed normal karyotype in all patients. Five patients subsequently underwent transplantation; the median time to absolute neutrophil count of greater than 1000/μL was 16 days (range, 11–25 days). Untransfused platelet counts greater than 20,000/μL occurred at a median of 41 days (range, 8–144 days) in four patients.

Carella et al. reported the results of nine patients with RAEB-t, secondary AML from a precedent MDS, or therapy-related AML who underwent apheresis after intensive chemotherapy with idarubicin, cytosine arabinoside, and etoposide and G-CSF.[95] All patients had double or complex cytogenetic abnormalities in marrow cells prior to mobilization. In six patients, the leukapheresis product was entirely karyotypically normal and contained a sufficient number of CD34+ progenitor cells.

These small trials demonstrate the feasibility of PBSC collections in selected patients with high-risk MDS or secondary AML. A major concern remains the possible contamination of the HSC by clonal malignant cells. In the cases discussed earlier, all patients were found to have normal karyotypes in the harvested samples.[94, 95] In addition, other techniques, including X-chromosome inactivation, have demonstrated polyclonal remission in several of these patients.[96] Therefore, even though MDS is a clonal disorder of the malignant stem cell, it may be possible to collect and cryopreserve a sufficient number of normal progenitor cells. In doing so, autoHSCT may be an alternative for those patients who lack an allogeneic donor or who may not be able to tolerate the complications associated with the allograft procedure.

THE TRANSPLANTATION PROCEDURE

EVALUATION OF A PATIENT FOR TRANSPLANTATION

Patients with MDS who are referred for transplant present specific problems for the transplant center related to confirmation of the diagnosis and appropriate classification of the patient's disease. It is particularly important to distinguish primary MDS from AML as well as to accurately classify the subtype of MDS, because this may affect the timing of the transplantation and decisions related to a recommendation of induction chemotherapy prior to transplantation. It is necessary not only to classify the patient according to the FAB classification schema but to accurately determine the clinical score according to the IPSS. Therefore, the clinical history should include an accurate assessment of the disease course, including the timing and severity of cytopenias and the documentation of any infections or bleeding problems. Recent bone marrow aspirates and biopsies are required to describe the marrow cellularity, the degree of dysplasia, the percentage of marrow blasts, and the presence or absence of ringed sideroblasts and fibrosis. Marrow cytogenetics are critical for prognosis.

If there is any question regarding the diagnosis of MDS, other useful screening tests include serum erythropoietin, vitamin B_{12}, ferritin, and red blood cell folate levels. In addition, for all patients considered potential condidates for an allograft, HLA typing of the patient and siblings and other appropriate family members is required.

Because most patients in whom either MDS or acute leukemia is diagnosed present with cytopenias, it is extremely important to distinquish primary MDS from rapidly evolving de novo AML because the treatment approaches and overall prognosis may differ significantly. This is particularly important in those patients who present with less than 30% blasts in the bone marrow and are initially classified as having RAEB-t. The patient's history is particularly important because patients with primary MDS tend to have a history of cytopenia and may have presented to a physician previously for complications of their disease. For those patients without any previous history who are found to have advanced MDS at diagnosis, a repeat bone marrow aspirate and biopsy may be required to adequately determine the progression of the disease and to distinguish MDS from AML. In addition, the history is particularly important in determining whether the patient has any known exposure to radiation, chemotherapy, or other known toxins to differentiate secondary MDS from primary MDS.

The patient's age and performance status are also critical determinants of HSCT eligibility. Transplant centers vary regarding their age requirements for either alloHSCT or autoHSCT. Generally, patients under the age of 60–65 years are considered for more intensive or aggressive therapies. With the use of peripheral blood as a source for either allogeneic or autologous stem cells, the upper age limits

may become less important, and physiologic rather than chronologic age might be used to establish patient eligibility.

Performance status is often a measurement of the patient's ability to tolerate more intensive therapy. In 1998, Goldberg et al. published a retrospective review of 383 patients undergoing HSCT to determine the value of pretransplant variables in predicting day-100 treatment related mortality.[97] Performance status (Eastern Cooperative Oncology Group [ECOG] > 0) was found to be highly predictive in both univariate and multivariate analysis. The authors' analysis was unable to correlate toxicity with age. The impact of age on transplant-related morbidity and mortality has been controversial, with several trials noting higher risks but other trials not demonstrating this increased risk.

TIMING FOR HSCT

The most appropriate timing for transplantation continues to be controversial. Most transplant trials, either allogeneic or autologous, have demonstrated that DFS is improved in patients with short disease duration, in patients with fewer blasts compared with patients with advanced MDS, and in patients with IPSS low-risk or INT-1 risk.[73–82] These are the same variables, however, that predict for increased survival with conventional therapy and/or supportive care. Even though HSCT can potentially provide long-term DFS and cure, it continues to be associated with relatively high risk; therefore, there may be subgroups of patients in whom transplantation can be delayed and considered later.

A short period of observation, generally several months, may be required to determine the clinical stability of patients with MDS. This may be particularly important in patients with IPSS low-risk or INT-1 disease. In addition, during this time the patient's performance status can be adequately assessed, and for those patients considered for alloHSCT, HLA typing can be performed. For patients with stable low-risk disease (IPSS low-risk or INT-1) the timing of HSCT needs to be addressed individually. Clearly, the age of the patient, performance status, availability of a donor, and willingness of the patient to pursue aggressive therapy needs to be considered. Patients electing to delay HSCT should be closely monitored and referred for transplantation as the disease begins to show signs of progression.

It is important, however, to emphasize the negative impact that disease progression may have on transplant outcome. Sutton et al. found that patients with stable RA at the time of alloHSCT experienced a significantly higher DFS than did patients with other MDS subtypes;[81] however, patients whose disease progressed between diagnosis and HSCT did poorly after transplantation. Patients with more-advanced disease at presentation (IPSS INT-2 or high-risk disease) should be considered for HSCT early in their treatment plan to avoid further progression of disease.

DETERMINING THE BEST TRANSPLANT OPTION

As discussed earlier, different transplant options may be considered depending on the patient's age, performance status, disease subtype and stage, and even weight. All patients with a good performance status should be considered for HSCT. As discussed previously, the chronologic age alone may no longer be an eligibility criterion; rather, the biologic or physiologic age may be the determinant. For those "younger" patients with an HLA-compatible family member, alloHSCT should be considered (Fig. 5–3). If no family member is HLA compatible, either an unrelated donor or an autologous transplant may be pursued. Clearly, many factors determine the appropriate role for an unrelated donor transplant given the significant early mortality rate associated with this procedure, especially in older patients. For "smaller" adult patients (<60 kg), an unrelated umbilical-cord transplant may be considered as an option.

In 1998, Arnold et al. compared the results of 130 patients with MDS or secondary AML who received an unrelated bone marrow transplant with the results of 177 patients with similar diagnoses receiving an autograft.[98] The two cohorts were equally matched for age, disease subtype, stage of disease, interval from diagnosis to transplantation, and year of transplantation. At 3 years, the overall survival and DFS were identical; however the treatment-related mortality was significantly higher in the unrelated transplant group (55% vs. 22%) and the relapse rate was significantly lower compared with the patients undergoing autologous transplantation (36% vs. 60%). The multivariate analysis revealed that type of transplant and age of the patient were independent prognostic indicators for survival. Using this analysis, the investigators recommend that remission induction therapy be administered to patients with advanced MDS (RAEB or RAEB-t). If the patient enters CR; autoHSCT should be considered. If the patient does not enter remission and is less than 40 years old, the search for an unrelated donor should proceed. For patients older than 40 years, an unrelated donor transplant should not be considered because of the significant early mortality associated with the procedure.

For those patients who do not wish to pursue alloHSCT or for "older" patients, autoHSCT may now be considered as an option (see Fig. 5–3). To be a candidate for autografting, however, the patient should be in CR after intensive induction chemotherapy, and a bone marrow or PBSC product should be harvested or collected during CR. In addition, the karyotype of the stem cell product clearly needs to be normal.

PREPARATIVE REGIMENS

A variety of preparative regimens have been used to treat patients prior to either autoHSCT or alloHSCT (see Table 5–3). These regimens primarily consist of cyclophosphamide/total body irradiation (TBI), busulfan and cyclophosphamide, and intensive chemotherapy and TBI. Attempts to intensify the preparative regimen for patients with advanced MDS to reduce the risk of relapse have demonstrated increased treatment-related toxicity and mortality; improvement in DFS has not occurred. At present, it does not appear that any single regimen is superior to another.

Alternatives to conventional radiation-containing regimens are required in treating patients with therapy-related MDS because many of these patients have already been exposed to radiation and may not be candidates for TBI. In addition, chemotherapy-based regimens may offer more flexibility and do not require the radiation support. O'Donnell et al.[99] reported on 38 patients with MDS receiving busulfan and cyclophosphamide as a preparative regimen; compared with patients receiving TBI-containing regimens, gastrointestinal toxicity appeared to be less severe in patients receiving busulfan, with less than half of patients requiring parenteral nutrition.[99] In 72% of patients, however, hepatic dysfunction developed, with 16% experiencing hepatic veno-occlusive disease. Because of the wide variability of busulfan absorption, monitoring busulfan levels in patients may reduce hepatic toxicity and should be considered in patients at risk for hepatic toxicity.[100]

Thus far, conditioning regimens for patients with MDS and other hematologic malignancies undergoing alloHSCT have been intensified to the point at which dose-limiting toxicity is frequently encountered. Because of toxicity, allografts have been limited primarily to younger patients.

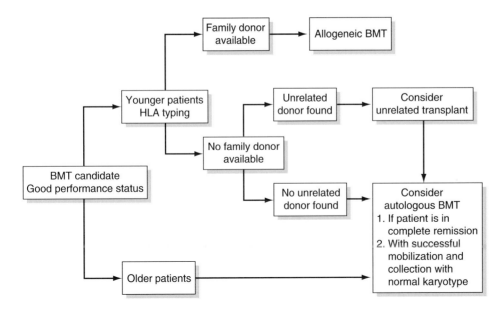

FIGURE 5–3. Blood and marrow transplantation (BMT) options for appropriate patients with myelodysplastic syndromes. HLA, human leukocyte antigen.

Because MDS is a disease diagnosed more frequently in patients in their fifth, sixth, and seventh decades of life than in younger patients, less-intensified regimens will be required if more patients with MDS are to benefit from allografting. Because of this, nonmyeloablative preparative regimens are being developed in which intensive cytoreductive conditioning regimens are being replaced by much less-intense therapy followed by nonmyelotoxic immunosuppression and the possible use of donor lymphocyte infusions to stabilize the donor graft and to use the graft-versus-host reaction to control the malignancy.[101–103]

Giralt et al. have incorporated fludarabine or 2-chlorodeoxyadenosine–containing regimens in patients with myeloid or lymphoid malignancies.[101] Twelve of 15 patients with myeloid malignancies were evaluable; in 8, donor cell engraftment was documented in the bone marrow within 30 days after transplantation. Overall survival was poor, and only one patient achieved a sustained CR. Slavin et al. reported on a strategy in 26 patients receiving fludarabine, lower doses of busulfan, and antithymocyte globulin followed by PBSC transplantation.[102] Initial results were promising with good overall survival and the development of full donor chimerism after transient mixed chimerism in a significant number of patients.

In 1998, Storb reported on a strategy in which four patients, aged 53–60 years (one each with chronic lymphocytic leukemia, multiple myeloma, MDS, and AML in first remission), were conditioned with only 200 cGy TBI and were reinfused with PBSC from their HLA-identical siblings.[103] Patients received post-transplant immunosuppression with cyclosporine and mycophenolate mofetil, which blocks the "de novo" purine synthesis pathway by binding to inosine monophate dehydrogenase, thereby interfering with lymphocyte replication. All patients experienced mixed chimerism, and three were given donor lymphocyte infusions on post-transplant day 65. All transplant and post-transplant care was delivered in the outpatient setting and, except for one patient who received a red blood cell transfusion, no transfusions were required. In addition, with one exception, granulocyte counts did not fall below 1000/μL and platelet counts did not fall below 100,000/μL. Even though follow-up is short, these preliminary results are encouraging.

USE OF INDUCTION CHEMOTHERAPY PRIOR TO ALLOGENEIC HSCT

The use of induction chemotherapy prior to alloHSCT is controversial. Results from multiple transplant trials have demonstrated that MDS subtype and/or marrow blast percentage at the time of transplantation may significantly affect transplant outcome.[74–83] Several recent trials have suggested successful remission induction rates for patients in whom MDS has been newly diagnosed using standard AML regimens.[104, 105] Bernstein et al. reported on 33 patients in whom the original diagnosis was AML but was reclassified as MDS (1 with RA, 7 with RAEB, and 25 with RAEB-t) on central pathology review.[104] Treatment outcomes for patients with MDS and AML were similar, with CR rates of 79% and 68%, respectively. This study clearly represented a subgroup of patients who presented without prior history of cytopenia and in whom the original diagnosis was based on FAB classification for blast cell percentages.

Estey et al.[105] reported on 52 patients with RAEB and 106 patients with RAEB-t, as defined by the FAB criteria, who were treated with the same regimens used for patients with AML. Patients with RAEB underwent treatment because of thrombocytopenia, red blood cell transfusion requirements, or an abnormal karyotype. The CR rate was essentially identical in all three groups (62% for RAEB, 66% for RAEB-t, and 66% for AML). As expected, patients with either RAEB or RAEB-t were more likely to have poor prognostic characteristics, in particular complex cytogenetic abnormalities including chromosomes 5 and/or 7. The results of this analysis suggest that treatment results for patients with RAEB or RAEB-t are essentially identical to those of patients with de novo AML, who have similar prognostic characteristics.

Sutton et al. reported on 71 patients with MDS (16 with RA, 27 with RAEB, and 28 with RAEB-t) who received allografts from HLA-compatible sibling donors; 17 of these patients received induction chemotherapy prior to HSCT.[81] The use of cytoreductive chemotherapy prior to transplantation did not show any clear benefit in this small series of patients. For those patients who entered CR, the survival rate was 43% but the relapse rate was not significantly lower when compared with the other patients. Of the six patients who entered remission prior to HSCT, four experienced relapse. All patients in whom induction chemotherapy failed prior to transplantation died from relapse (six patients) or treatment-related complications (five patients). Therefore, in this series, chemotherapy prior to HSCT yielded a low rate of remission and did not appear to affect the relapse rate, even in those patients who achieved remission prior to transplantation. In fact, Cox regression analysis demonstrated that prior chemotherapy had a negative impact on HSCT outcome.

De Witte et al., however, published results on 78 patients with MDS or secondary AML who received alloHSCT with a different conclusion than the previous study.[75] Thirty-four of these patients received intensive chemotherapy prior to transplantation, of whom 16 (1 with RAEB, 6 with RAEB-t, and 9 with secondary AML) entered CR. Of those patients in whom induction therapy failed or who experienced relapse prior to transplantation, none survived beyond 2 years. Of the 16 patients who achieved remission, DFS at 2 years was 60% ± 13%. In addition, 10 patients underwent transplantation during hypoplasia after induction chemotherapy or during a partial remission. Transplant-related mortality was high, with six patients dying soon after allografting and two patients experiencing relapse early in the post-transplant course.

The results evaluating the role of induction chemotherapy prior to allogeneic transplantation are conflicting. For patients with advanced MDS, primarily RAEB or RAEB-t, recent chemotherapy trials suggest CR rates comparable to those of patients with AML, especially in patients with MDS who present without cytopenias and/or with good- or intermediate-risk cytogenetic subgroups.[104, 105] If remission is achieved, overall survival after allografting may be improved. For those patients with resistant disease, however, the role of alloHSCT may be more limited. For patients with high-risk RA, prior induction chemotherapy appears to offer no significant improvement in post-transplant outcome.

CONCLUSIONS

MDS is a heterogeneous group of clonal hematopoietic diseases characterized by progressive cytopenia. Not only can patients with MDS present the clinician with a diagnostic dilemma but they can also present treatment challenges. In the past, treatment strategies for patients with MDS varied from supportive care only to intensive induction therapy followed by HSCT. Results were often conflicting because of the variability of disease subgroups and disease duration, age, and performance status of the patients as well as the interests and expertise of the treatment centers. More recently, however, MDS classification by morphology and prognostic variables has become more standardized. Even though treatment strategies continue to vary, interpretation of results has improved because of these classification schemas.

The role of HSCT as a viable treatment option for patients with MDS has continued to expand. Initially, these procedures were limited to younger patients with HLA-compatible sibling donors. With the use of unrelated donors, allografting is now available for a larger number of patients. In addition, with the use of more innovative procedures, including PBSC transplants, T cell–depletion techniques, and donor lymphocyte infusions as well as less-toxic nonmyeloablative preparative regimens, treatment-related toxicity and mortality may significantly decrease. This will allow allografting to become more attractive to an older population. For those patients who are in CR, autografting may also be an option. More innovative procedures for mobilization and stem-cell collection will allow for further expansion of this procedure.

REFERENCES

1. Schultz AB, Geller RB, Hillyer CD: The role of bone marrow transplantation in the treatment of myelodysplastic syndromes. J Hematother 4:323, 1995.
2. Najean Y, Deschamps A, Dresch C, et al: Acute leukemia and myelodysplasia in polcythemia vera: a clinical study with long-term follow-up. Cancer 61:89, 1988.
3. Shamdas GJ, Spier CM, List AF: Myelodysplastic transformation of polycythemia vera: case report and review of the literature. Am J Hematol 37:45, 1991.
4. Tefferi A, Hoagland HC, Therneau TM, et al: Chronic myelomonocytic leukemia: natural history and prognostic determinants. Mayo Clin Proc 64:1264, 1989.
5. Galton DAG: The myelodysplastic syndromes. Scand J Haematol 36(Suppl 45):16, 1986.
6. Bennett JM, Catovsky D, Daniet MT, et al: The chronic myeloid leukemias: guidelines for distinguishing chronic granulocytic, atypical chronic myeloid, and chronic myelomonocytic leukemia. Proposals by the French-American-British Cooperative Leukemia Group. Br J Haematol 87:746, 1994.
7. Kouides PA, Bennett JM: Morphology and classification of the myelodysplastic syndromes and their pathologic variants. Semin Hematol 33:95, 1996.
8. Bennett JM, Catovsky D, Daniel MT, et al: Proposals for the classification of the myelodysplastic syndromes. Br J Haematol 51:189, 1982.
9. Rosati S, Anastasi J, Vardiman J: Recurring diagnostic problems in the pathology of the myelodysplastic syndromes. Semin Hematol 33:111, 1996.
10. Maschek H, Georgii A, Kaloutsi V, et al: Myelofibrosis in primary myelodysplastic syndromes: a retrospective study of 352 patients. Eur J Haematol 48:208, 1992.
11. Ho PJ, Gibson J, Vincent P, et al: The myelodysplastic syndromes: diagnostic criteria and laboratory evaluation. Pathology 25:297, 1993.
12. Mufti G: A guide to risk assessment in the primary myelodysplastic syndrome. Hematol Oncol Clin North Am 6:587, 1992.
13. Taylor KM, Rodwell RL, Taylor DL, et al: Myelodysplasia. Curr Opin Oncol 6:32, 1994.
14. Mufti GJ, Stevens JR, Oscier DG, et al: Myelodysplastic syndromes: a scoring system with prognostic significance. Br J Haematol 59:425, 1985.
15. Worsley A, Oscier DG, Stevens J, et al: Prognostic features of chronic myelomonocytic leukemia: a modified Bournemouth score gives the best prediction of survival. Br J Haematol 68:17, 1988.
16. Sanz GF, Sanz MA, Vallespi T, et al: Two regression models and a scoring system for predicting survival and planning treatment in myelodysplastic syndromes: a multivariate analysis of prognostic factors in 370 patients. Blood 74:395, 1989.
17. Goasguen JE, Garand R, Bizet M, et al: Prognostic factors of myelodysplastic syndromes—a simplified 3-D scoring system. Leuk Res 14:255, 1990.
18. Aul C, Gattermann N, Heyll A, et al: Primary myelodysplastic syndromes: analysis of prognostic factors in 235 patients and proposals for an improved scoring system. Leukemia 6:52, 1992.
19. Greenberg P, Cox C, LeBeau MM, et al: International scoring system for evaluating prognosis in myelodysplastic syndromes. Blood 89:2079, 1997.
20. Foucar K, Langdon RM, Armitage JO, et al: Myelodysplastic syndromes: a clinical and pathologic analysis of 109 cases. Cancer 56:553, 1984.
21. Tricot G, Vlietinck R, Boogaerts MA, et al: Prognostic factors in myelodysplastic syndrome: importance of initial data on peripheral blood counts, bone marrow cytology, trephine biopsy and chromosomal analysis. Br J Haematol 60:19, 1985.
22. Varela BL, Chuang C, Woll JE, et al: Modifications in the classification of primary myelodysplastic syndromes: the addition of a scoring system. Hematol Oncol 3:55, 1985.
23. Third MIC Cooperative Study Group: Recommendations for a morphologic, immunologic, and cytogenetic (MIC) working classification of the primary and therapy-related myelodysplastic disorders: report of the workshop held in Scottsdale, AZ Feb. 23–25, 1987. Cancer Genet Cytogenet 32:1, 1988.
24. Yoshida Y, Oguma S, Uchino H, et al: Refractory myelodysplastic anaemias with hypocellular bone marrow. J Clin Pathol 41:703, 1988.
25. Hand S, Goodwin JE: Hypoplastic myelodysplastic syndrome. Cancer 62:958, 1988.
26. Fohlmeister I, Fisher R, Modder B, et al: Aplastic anemia and the hypocellular myelodysplastic syndrome: histomorphological, diagnostic and prognostic features. J Clin Pathol 38:1218, 1985.
27. Thirman MJ, Larson RA: Therapy-related myeloid leukemia [Review]. Hematol Oncol Clin North Am 10:293, 1996.
28. Kampmeier P, Anastasi J, Vardiman JW: Issues in the pathology of the myelodysplastic syndromes. Hematol Oncol Clin North Am 6:501, 1992.
29. Aul C, Gattermann N, Schneider W: Age-related incidence and other epidemiological aspects of myelodysplastic syndromes. Br J Haematol 82:358, 1992.
30. Williamson PJ, Kruger AR, Reynolds PJ, et al: Establishing the incidence of myelodysplastic syndrome. Br J Haematol 87:743, 1994.
31. Imbert M, Scoazec J-Y, Mary J-Y, et al: Adult patients presenting with pancytopenia: a reappraisal of underlying pathology and diagnostic procedures in 213 cases. Hematol Pathol 3:159, 1987.
32. Ganser A, Hoelzer D: Clinical course of myelodysplastic syndromes. Hematol Oncol Clin North Am 6:607, 1992.
33. Noel P, Solberg LA: Myelodysplastic syndromes: pathogenesis, diagnosis and treatment. Crit Rev Oncol Hematol 12:193, 1992.
34. Pomeroy C, Oken MM, Rydell RE, et al: Infection in the myelodysplastic syndromes. Am J Med 90:338, 1991.
35. Kaldor JM, Day NE, Clarke EA, et al: Leukemia following Hodgkin's disease. N Engl J Med 322:7, 1990.

36. Pedersen-Bjergaard J, Larsen SO: Incidence of acute nonlymphocytic leukemia, preleukemia, and acute myeloproliferative syndrome up to 10 years after treatment of Hodgkin's disease. N Engl J Med 307:965, 1982.

37. Pedersen-Bjergaard J, Ersboll J, Mygind H, et al: Risk of acute nonlymphocytic leukemia and preleukemia in patients treated with cyclophosphamide for non-Hodgkin's lymphoma. Ann Intern Med 103:195, 1985.

38. Andrieu, J-M, Ifrah N, Payen C, et al: Increased risk of secondary acute nonlymphocytic leukemia after extended-field radiation therapy combined with MOPP chemotherapy for Hodgkin's disease. J Clin Oncol 8:1148, 1990.

39. De Gramont A, Louvet C, Krulik M, et al: Preleukemic changes in cases of nonlymphocytic leukemia secondary to cytoxic therapy. Cancer 58:630, 1986.

40. Pui C-H, Behm FG, Raimondi SC, et al: Secondary acute myeloid leukemia in children treated for acute lymphoid leukemia. N Engl J Med 321:136, 1989.

41. Curtis RE, Boice JD, Jr, Stovall M, et al: Risk of leukemia after chemotherapy and radiation treatment for breast cancer. N Engl J Med 326:1745, 1992.

42. Daimandidou E, Buzdar AU, Smith TL, et al: Treatment-related leukemia in breast cancer patients treated with fluorouracil-doxorubicin-cyclophosphamide combination adjuvant chemotherapy: the University of Texas M.D. Anderson Cancer Center experience. J Clin Oncol 14:2722, 1996.

43. Pedersen-Bjergaard J, Pedersen M, Roulston D, Philip P: Different genetic pathways in leukemogenesis for patients presenting with therapy-related myelodysplasia and therapy-related acute myeloid leukemia. Blood 86:3542, 1995.

44. Pedersen-Bjergaard J, Philip P: Balanced translocations involving chromosome bands 11q23 and 21q22 are highly characteristic of myelodysplasia and leukemia following therapy with cytostatic agents targeting at DNA-topoisomerase II. Blood 78:1147, 1991.

45. Stone RM: Myelodysplastic syndrome after autologous transplantation for lymphoma: the price of progress? Blood 83:3437, 1994.

46. Dacie JV, Smith MD, White JC, et al: Refractory normoblastic anemia: a clinical and hematological study of seven cases. Br J Haematol 5:56, 1959.

47. Bick RL, Laughlin WR: Myelodysplastic syndromes. Lab Med 24:712, 1993.

48. Michels SD, McKenna RW, Arthur DC, et al: Therapy-related acute myeloid leukemia and myelodysplastic syndrome: a clinical and morphologic study of 65 cases. Blood 65:1364, 1985.

49. Morel P, Hebbar M, Lai J-L, et al: Cytogenetic analysis has strong independent prognostic value in de novo myelodysplastic syndromes and can be incorporated in a new scoring system: a report on 408 cases. Leukemia 7:1315, 1993.

50. Ohyashiki K, Sasao I, Ohyashiki JH, et al: Cytogenetic and clinical findings of myelodysplastic syndromes with a poor prognosis. Cancer 70:94, 1992.

51. Gonzales Manso AI, Garcia Marcilla AG, Barreiro E, et al: Cytohematologic and cytogenetic prognostic factors at diagnosis and in the evaluation in 46 primary myelodysplastic syndromes. Cancer Genet Cytogenet 61:174, 1992.

52. Cazzola M, Ponchio L, Rosti V, et al: Diagnostic approach to the myelodysplastic syndromes. Leukemia 6(Suppl 4):19, 1992.

53. Weisdorf DJ, Oken MM, Johnson GJ, et al: Chronic myelodysplastic syndrome: short survival with or without evolution to acute leukemia. Br J Haematol 55:691, 1983.

54. Vallespi T, Torrabadella M, Julia A, et al: Myelodysplastic syndromes: a study of 101 cases according to the FAB classification. Br J Haematol 61:83, 1985.

55. Sanz GF, Sanz MA: Prognostic factors in myelodysplastic syndromes. Leuk Res 16:77, 1992.

56. Yoshida Y, Yamagishi M, Oguma S, et al: Conservative treatment for refractory myelodysplastic anemias: a Japanese cooperative study. Acta Haematol Jpn 51:1448, 1988.

57. Stadtmauer E, Cassileth PA, Edelstein M, et al: Danazol treatment of myelodysplastic syndromes. Br J Haematol 77:502, 1991.

58. Douer D, Koeffler HP: Retinoic acid: inhibition of the clonal growth of human myeloid leukemia cells. J Clin Invest 69:277, 1982.

59. Castaigne S, Chomienne C, Daniel MT, et al: All-*trans*-retinoic acid as a differentiation therapy for acute promyelocytic leukemia: I. Clinical results. Blood 76:1704, 1990.

60. Richard C, Mazo E, Cuadrado M, et al: Treatment of myelodysplastic syndrome with 1.25-dihydroxyvitamin D$_3$. Am J Hematol 23:175, 1986.

61. Koeffler HP, Hirji K, Intri L, and the Southern California Leukemia Group: 1.25-Dihydroxyvitamin D$_3$: in vivo and in vitro effects on human preleukemic and leukemic cells. Cancer Treat Rep 69:1399, 1985.

62. Ganser A, Hoelzer D: Treatment of myelodysplastic syndromes with hematopoietic growth factors. Hematol Oncol Clin North Am 6:633, 1992.

63. Greenberg PL, Negrin R, Nagler A: The use of hemopoietic growth factors in the treatment of myelodysplastic syndromes. Cancer Surv 9:199, 1990.

64. Negrin RS, Stein R, Doherty K, et al: Maintenance treatment of the anemia of myelodysplastic syndromes with recombinant human granulocyte colony-stimulating factor and erythropoietin: evidence for in vivo synergy. Blood 87:4076, 1996.

65. Miller KB, Kyungmann K, Morrison FS, et al: The evaluation of low-dose cytarabine in the treatment of myelodysplastic syndromes: a phase-III intergroup study. Ann Hematol 65:162, 1992.

66. Omoto E, Deguchi S, Takaba S, et al: Low-dose melphalan for treatment of high-risk myelodysplastic syndromes. Leukemia 10:609, 1996.

67. Beran M, Kantarjian H, O'Brien S, et al: Topotecan, a topoisomerase I inhibitor, is active in the treatment of myelodysplastic syndrome and chronic myelomonocytic leukemia. Blood 88:2473, 1996.

68. DeWitte T, Suciu S, Peetermans M, et al: Intensive chemotherapy for poor prognosis myelodysplasia (MDS) and secondary acute myeloid leukemia (sAML) following MDS of more than 6 months duration: a pilot study by the Leukemia Cooperative Group of the European Organization for Research and Treatment in Cancer (EORTC-LCG). Leukemia 9:1805, 1995.

69. Ruutu T, Hanninen A, Jarventie G, et al: Intensive chemotherapy of poor prognosis myelodysplastic syndromes (MDS) and acute myeloid leukemia following MDS with idarubicin and cytarabine. Leuk Res 21:133, 1997.

70. Appelbaum FR, Storb R, Ramberg RE, et al: Allogeneic marrow transplantation in the treatment of preleukemia. Ann Intern Med 100:689, 1984.

71. Anderson JE, Anasetti C, Appelbaum FR, et al: Unrelated donor marrow transplantation for myelodysplasia (MDS) and MDS-related acute myeloid leukemia. Br J Haematol 93:59, 1996.

72. Rubinstein P, Carrier C, Scaradavou A, et al: Outcomes among 562 recipients of placental-blood transplants from unrelated donors. N Engl J Med 339:1565, 1998.

73. DeWitte T, VanBiezen A, Hermans J, et al: Autologous bone marrow transplantation for patients with myelodysplastic syndrome (MDS) or acute myeloid leukemia following MDS. Blood 90:3853, 1997.

74. Leblond V, Jouet JP, Ribaud P, et al: Bone marrow transplantation for myelodysplastic syndrome and secondary leukemias (AML): outcome of 84 patients. Leukemia 5:179, 1991.

75. DeWitte TD, Zwann F, Hermans J, et al: Allogeneic bone marrow transplantation for secondary leukemia and myelodysplastic syndrome: a survey by the Leukemia Working Party of the European Bone Marrow Transplantation Group (EBMTG). Br J Haematol 74:151, 1990.

76. Longmore G, Guinan EC, Weintein HJ, et al: Bone marrow transplantation for myelodysplasia and secondary acute nonlymphoblastic leukemia. J Clin Oncol 8:1707, 1990.

77. O'Donnell MR, Nademanee AP, Snyder DS, et al: Bone marrow transplantation for myelodysplastic and myeloproliferative syndromes. J Clin Oncol 5:1822, 1987.

78. Anderson JE, Appelbaum FR, Fisher LD, et al: Allogeneic bone marrow transplantation for 93 patients with myelodysplastic syndrome. Blood 82:677, 1993.

79. Marmont AM, Horowitz MM: Outcome of allogeneic bone marrow transplantation for myelodysplastic syndromes. Bone Marrow Transplant 5(Suppl 2):71, 1990.

80. Nevill TJ, Shepherd JD, Reece DE, et al: Treatment of myelodysplastic syndromes (MDS) with busulfan-cyclophosphamide (BUCY) conditioning and allogeneic bone marrow transplantation (BMT). Blood 76(Suppl 1):557a, 1990.

81. Sutton L, Leblond V, LeMaignan C, et al: Bone marrow transplantation for myelodysplastic syndrome and secondary leukemia: outcome of 86 patients. Bone Marrow Transplant 7(Suppl 2):39, 1991.

82. Appelbaum FR, Anderson J: Allogeneic bone marrow transplantation for myelodysplastic syndrome: outcome analysis according to IPSS score. Leukemia 12(Suppl 1):525, 1998.

83. Castro-Malaspina H, Collins JER, Gajewski J, et al: Unrelated donor marrow transplantation for myelodysplastic syndromes [Abstract]. Blood 92:106a, 1998.

84. Wagner JE, King R, Kollman C, et al: Unrelated donor bone marrow transplantation in 5075 patients with malignant and non-malignant disorders: impact of marrow T-cell depletion [Abstract] Blood 92:686a, 1998.

85. Gluckman E, Broxmeyer HE, Auerbach AD, et al: Hematopoietic reconstitution in a patient with Fanconi's anemia by means of umbilical-cord blood from an HLA-identical sibling. N Engl J Med 321:1174, 1989.

86. Wagner JE, Kernan NA, Steinbuch M, et al: Allogeneic sibling umbilical-cord blood transplantation in children with malignant and non-malignant disease. Lancet 346:214, 1995.

87. Kurtzberg J, Laughlin M, Graham ML, et al: Placental blood as a source of hematopoietic stem cells for transplantation into unrelated recipients. N Engl J Med 335:157, 1996.

88. Gluckman E, Rocha V, Boyer-Chammard A, et al: Outcome of cord-blood transplantation from related and unrelated donors. N Engl J Med 337:373, 1997.

89. Wagner JE, Rosenthal J, Sweetman R, et al: Successful transplantation of HLA-matched and HLA-mismatched umbilical cord blood from unrelated donors: analysis of engraftment and acute graft-versus-host disease. Blood 88:795, 1996.

90. Geller RB, Vogelsang GB, Wingard JR, et al: Successful marrow transplantation for acute myelocytic leukemia following therapy for Hodgkin's disease. J Clin Oncol 6:1558, 1988.

91. McMillan AK, Goldstone AH, Linch DC, et al: High dose chemotherapy and autologous bone marrow transplantation in acute myeloid leukemia. Blood 76:480, 1990.

92. Öberg G, Simonsson B, Smedmyr B, et al: Is haematological reconstitution seen after ABMT in MDS patients? Bone Marrow Transplant 4(Suppl 2):52, 1989.

93. Laporte JP, Isnard F, Lesage S, et al: Autologous bone marrow transplantation with marrow purged by Mafosfamide in seven patients with myelodysplastic syndromes in transformation (AML-MDS): a pilot study. Leukemia 7:2030, 1993.

94. Demuynck H, Delforge G, Verhoef P, et al: Feasibility of peripheral blood progenitor cell harvest and transplantation in patients with poor-risk myelodysplastic syndromes. Br J Haematol 92:351, 1996.

95. Carella AM, Delana A, Lerma E, et al: In vivo mobilization of karyotypically normal peripheral blood progenitor cells in high-risk MDS, secondary or therapy-related acute myelogenous leukemia. Br J Haematol 95:127, 1996.

96. Delforge M, Demuynck H, Vandenberghe P, et al: Polyclonal primitive hematopoietic progenitors can be detected in mobilized peripheral blood from patients with high-risk myelodysplastic syndromes. Blood 86:3660, 1995.

97. Goldberg SK, Klumpp TR, Magdalinski AJ, Mangan KF: Value of the pretransplant evaluation in predicting toxic day-100 mortality among blood stem-cell and bone marrow transplant recipients. J Clin Oncol 16:3796, 1988.

98. Arnold R, Hermans J, De Witte TH, et al: Unrelated bone marrow transplantation compared with autologous transplantation in patients with myelodysplastic syndrome and secondary acute myeloid leukemia: an EBMT survey [Abstract]. Blood 92:142a, 1998.

99. O'Donnell MR, Long GD, Parker PM, et al: Busulfan/cyclophosphamide as conditioning regimen for allogeneic bone marrow transplantation for myelodysplasia. J Clin Oncol 13:2973, 1995.

100. Dix SP, Wingard JR, Mullins RE, et al: Association of busulfan area under the curve with veno-occlusive disease following BMT. Bone Marrow Transplant 17:225, 1996.

101. Giralt S, Estey E, Albitar M, et al: Engraftment of allogeneic hematopoietic progenitor cells with purine analog-containing chemotherapy: harnessing graft-versus-leukemia without myeloablative therapy. Blood 89:4531, 1997.

102. Slavin S, Nagler A, Naparstek E, et al: Nonmyeloablative stem cell transplantation and cell therapy as an alternative to conventional bone marrow transplantation with lethal cytoreduction for the treatment of malignant and nonmalignant hematologic disease. Blood 91:756, 1998.

103. Storb R: Nonmyeloablative preparative regimens: theory and practice. Hematology, 1998, pp 342–353.

104. Bernstein SH, Brunetto VL, Davey FR, et al: Acute myeloid leukemia-type chemotherapy for newly diagnosed patients without antecedent cytopenias having myelodysplastic syndrome as defined by French-American-British criteria: a cancer and leukemia. Group B study. J Clin Oncol 14:2486, 1996.

105. Estey E, Thall P, Beran M, et al: Effect of diagnosis (refractory anemia with excess blasts, refractory anemia with excess blasts in transformation, or acute myeloid leukemia) on the outcome of AML-type chemotherapy. Blood 90:2969, 1997.

Hodgkin Disease

Donna E. Reece, M.D., and Gordon L. Phillips, M.D.

Hodgkin disease is the most common malignancy in persons in the age range of 10–30 years. This malignancy develops in approximately 14,000 persons in the United States and Canada each year. A number of distinctive biologic features characterize this disease, and recent studies have contributed to a better understanding of its pathogenesis. In addition, the results of conventional chemotherapy and radiotherapy in this disease represent a relative success story for modern oncology in that most patients can be cured with conventional first-line therapy.[1]

Since the 1970s, intensive therapy and hematopoietic stem cell (HSC) transplantation (HSCT) have been evaluated in patients who have a low likelihood of cure with conventional therapy. Although there is only one small published randomized trial in patients with relapsed or refractory disease that shows an advantage of autologous HSCT over nontransplant therapy, considerable data from other studies demonstrate the efficacy of this modality.[2] Allogeneic HSCT has been performed much less commonly in Hodgkin disease because a number of problems have limited its use, particularly the higher nonrelapse mortality that occurs with this HSC source. This chapter briefly discusses issues related to the biology of Hodgkin disease and results of conventional therapy. It then focuses on the optimal role of autologous HSCT in this disease.

BIOLOGY

Hodgkin disease is notable in that the malignant cell, the Hodgkin–Reed-Sternberg (H-RS) cell, constitutes less than 5% of the tumor mass. Rather, the majority of cells in tumor masses are composed of T and B cells, macrophages, histiocytes, fibroblasts, neutrophils, stromal cells, eosinophils, and plasma cells.[3] The histologic subtype depends on the reactive cellular environment in which the H-RS cells are found, and classic Hodgkin disease can be categorized as nodular sclerosis, mixed cellularity, lymphocyte depletion, and a provisional subtype called lymphocyte-rich (formerly, diffuse lymphocyte predominance).[4]

The nodular lymphocyte predominance form of Hodgkin disease is now considered an immunophenotypically distinct B-cell entity that clinically resembles a low-grade lymphoma.[3–5] The clonality and lineage derivation of the H-RS cells have long been debated. Cytogenetic studies have identified clonal karyotypic changes in lymph nodes from some patients, although no specific aberration has been found; most karyotypes are complex with hyperdiploidy.[3, 6] Previous work from numerous investigators has demonstrated the expression of markers associated with T-cell or B-cell lineage in many cases. Nevertheless, a uniform immunophenotype of cells in classic Hodgkin disease has not been defined.[3] Recent studies have used single-cell polymerase chain reaction in H-RS cells to evaluate lineage origin and clonality in classic Hodgkin disease. Kuppers et al. identified rearranged immunoglobulin genes, consistent with B-cell lineage origin, in most patients evaluated, although other investigators, using different techniques, have described either polyclonal or mixed populations of H-RS cells.[7–9] Roth et al. reported the absence of rearrangements in the majority of patients.[10] A common B-cell precursor, however, has been identified for two patients with both non-Hodgkin lymphoma and classic Hodgkin disease; this finding provides convincing evidence of the B-cell derivation of H-RS cells.[11]

The role of Epstein-Barr virus (EBV) infection in the pathogenesis of Hodgkin disease remains speculative. The EBV genome can be found in at least 50% of cases, often associated with expression of the latent membrane protein (LMP1).[12] Possible transforming potential and/or protection from apoptosis has been proposed as a consequence of LMP1 expression in Hodgkin disease.[13–15]

The role of cytokines and cytokine receptors in Hodgkin disease is being increasingly recognized because H-RS cells are thought to actively interact with adjacent lymphocytes.[16] H-RS cells express a number of adhesion and co-stimulatory molecules as well as members of the tumor necrosis factor (TNF)-receptor family, such as CD30, CD40, and Fas/CD95 receptors.[3, 16–20] With the exception of the nodular lymphocyte predominance subtype, approximately 85–90% of cells in classic Hodgkin disease express CD30, an antigen found on certain lymphomas and lymphoma cell lines, virally infected B cells, and activated T cells. The CD30 ligand exerts a number of biologic activities ranging from stimulation of proliferation to induction of apoptosis.[16–18]

H-RS cells may secrete a multitude of cytokines, including interleukin (IL)-1, IL-3, IL-5, IL-6, IL-9, macrophage colony-stimulating factor (M-CSF), TNF, lymphotoxin, and receptors for IL-2, IL-6, IL-9, M-CSF, stem cell factor (SCF) (c-kit), and IL-12. These may be involved in the attraction to or activation of immune cells at the tumor site and in their aberrant immune response as well as in the constitutional symptoms observed in this disease.[3, 16–20] In one series, a majority of patients with Hodgkin disease had elevated serum levels of TNF, which correlated with disease stage and the presence of "B" (constitutional) symptoms.[21]

Other clinical correlates have been observed. CD30 expression of H-RS cells has been described as a favorable prognostic factor, whereas high levels of soluble CD30 in the serum correlate with a poor prognosis.[17, 22, 23] It has been hypothesized that the CD30 ligand inhibits the growth of tumors expressing CD30 and that soluble CD30 may block this effect.[16] Immunotherapy that exploits surface molecules such as CD30 is under investigation, as is discussed later.

RESULTS OF CONVENTIONAL THERAPY

Fortunately, a majority of patients can be cured with conventional chemotherapy and/or radiotherapy, and efforts have focused on designing treatment that produces the greatest efficacy with the lowest toxicity. Cure rates exceed 75–80% in patients with early-stage disease confirmed by staging laparotomy and treated with radiation therapy.[24, 25] Results from two centers have shown that cure rates approach 100% in patients with stage IA or IIA nonbulky disease who receive brief chemotherapy with ABVD (doxorubicin, bleomycin, vinblastine, and dacarbazine) followed by radiation therapy; such an approach obviates the need for laparotomy because subclinical disease outside the radiotherapy port is addressed by systemic therapy.[26, 27]

Almost two thirds of patients with more advanced Hodgkin disease can be cured with chemotherapy with or without radiation therapy. Data from randomized clinical trials have established the superiority of ABVD over other regimens such as MOPP (nitrogen mustard, vincristine, procarbazine, prednisone), or combinations of MOPP and ABVD, in terms of both antitumor effect and toxicity.[28, 29] Newer protocols such as the 12-week Stanford V program and the dose-escalated BEACOPP regimen (bleomycin, etoposide, doxorubicin, cyclophosphamide, vincristine, procarbazine, and prednisone) from Germany are under evaluation.[30, 31]

Despite these advances, about 10% of patients with advanced disease do not enter a remission with conventional chemotherapy, and approximately 20–30% may suffer a relapse of disease.[28] Radiation therapy can be curative in some patients.[32–34] Most patients, however, require further systemic therapy after chemotherapy fails. Results of salvage chemotherapy or radiotherapy in patients in whom disease progresses after an initial chemotherapy-induced complete remission (CR) depend on the presence or absence of adverse prognostic features, such as failure to enter CR, an initial CR duration of 1 year or less, presence of B symptoms, advanced stage at diagnosis, and extranodal disease.[32–39] Fortunately, in a significant proportion of these patients, autologous HSCT offers the chance of long-term disease-free survival in Hodgkin disease.

INTENSIVE THERAPY AND AUTOLOGOUS HSCT

The various time points during the course of Hodgkin disease at which intensive therapy and autologous transplantation can be performed are listed in Table 6–1. The following discussions consider patient selection based on these time points as well as other issues related to the relevance of chemosensitivity status, selection of conditioning regimen, and choice of HSC to be used for transplantation.

TABLE 6–1. TIMING OF AUTOLOGOUS TRANSPLANTATION IN HODGKIN DISEASE

WHEN	DETAILS
As part of initial therapy	Early PR1, CR1
Failure of induction chemotherapy	Late PR, other, untested
First relapse after chemotherapy-induced CR1	Chemosensitive Chemoresistant
Second remission	
Second relapse	
Subsequent remission/relapse	

CR, complete remission; PR, partial remission.

OVERVIEW OF RESULTS OF AUTOLOGOUS TRANSPLANTATION

For most malignant disease, disease status is an important criterion for patient selection for transplantation. Many studies of autologous HSCT in Hodgkin disease have combined the results in patients with relapsed and refractory disease. In addition to heterogeneity in terms of timing of autologous HSCT, factors such as the extent of prior therapy, chemosensitivity status, conditioning regimen, HSC source, and use of peritransplantation conventional chemotherapy or radiotherapy have often varied. In such studies, the long-term progression-free survival rates have ranged from 35–50%. Although early transplant-related mortality rates, described as deaths due to causes other than relapse within the first 100 days after autologous HSCT, were as high as 20% in some of the initial studies,[47] other more recent studies report rates of 5–10%[42, 44, 45] or even lower.[40, 41, 43, 46]

Many series have identified adverse prognostic factors for overall or progression-free survival. These have usually included parameters associated with more advanced disease, such as failure of more than two or three prior regimens, bulky disease, tumor size greater than or equal to 2 cm, poor performance status, chemoresistance, extranodal disease, B symptoms, and lack of CR at autologous HSCT.[42–58] Female sex, elevated lactate dehydrogenase level, and relapse in a previously irradiated field have also been reported as unfavorable features, whereas the use of posttransplantation radiotherapy has been reported to improve survival.[40, 50, 51, 59] Of note, the histologic subtype of Hodgkin disease has not been identified as a significant prognostic determinant in autologous transplant recipients. Table 6–2 shows the most commonly reported factors, in decreasing order of frequency, in published series.

Examination of the results of autologous transplantation specifically by disease status is also helpful. As shown in Figure 6–1, the results of autologous HSCT were strongly correlated with the time point in the disease course at which transplantation was performed in our initial 100 patients treated in Vancouver Hospital.[60] In the absence of randomized clinical trials, the use of such information may allow comparison of results of autologous HSCT with those anticipated from conventional therapy in a similar setting. One must keep in mind, however, that such comparisons are, by nature, subject to the selection bias inherent in all

TABLE 6-2. ADVERSE RISK FACTORS
IN PATIENTS UNDERGOING AUTOLOGOUS
TRANSPLANTATION FOR HODGKIN DISEASE

FACTOR	NUMBER OF REFERENCES IN TEXT
Failure of $\geq$ 2–3 regimens	7
Abnormal performance status	6
Chemoresistance	6
Extranodal disease	6
B symptoms	4
Bulky disease	3
Initial CR duration $\leq$ 1 year	2
Disease $\geq$ 2 cm at autologous HSCT	2
Lack of CR at autologous HSCT	2

CR, complete remission; HSCT, hematopoietic stem cell transplantation.

transplant studies in terms of age, performance status, and other features.

RESULTS BY DISEASE STATUS

Autologous Transplantation as Part of Initial Therapy

The rationale for the use of intensive therapy as part of primary therapy depends on the identification of reliable prognostic factors early in the disease course that can define a group of patients at high risk for relapse. Using clinical and laboratory features present at diagnosis, a number of prognostic systems for newly diagnosed advanced-stage Hodgkin disease have been described.[61–65] Findings of three of the larger series are summarized in Table 6–3. Each of these can identify groups of patients with a very good outcome and relatively small groups with unfavorable prognosis with chemotherapy.[61–65] Even the worst prognostic

groups still experience 5-year freedom-from-progression rates on the order of 50%. A large project, similar to the International Prognostic Index for Non-Hodgkin's Lymphoma, has now been completed for Hodgkin disease and has identified seven prognostic factors: hemoglobin less than or equal to 10.5 g/dL, albumin less than 4 g/dL, stage IV disease, male sex, white blood cell count greater than or equal to 15,000, absolute lymphocyte count less than 600/mm³, and age greater than or equal to 45 years.[63] The presence of any one of these factors decreases tumor control rates by 7–8% at 5 years. This system can discriminate patients with 5-year tumor control rates ranging from 42% in patients with five factors to 80% in those with none of the factors. The proportion of patients in the poor prognostic groups is small, less than 10%.[63]

These efforts are noteworthy and can define a small group of patients at high risk for treatment failure. It remains controversial, however, whether a progression-free survival rate of 42–50% warrants HSCT in responding patients, particularly because autologous HSCT can salvage a proportion of patients if disease recurs.

New efforts to use more specific biologic markers to define prognosis are under evaluation. For example, preliminary observations from the M.D. Anderson Cancer Center and the Mayo Clinic have identified serum IL-10 levels as a prognostic factor in patients with stage III or IV disease, although the most unfavorable risk group still experienced a relatively high failure-free survival rate of 57%.[66] Another preliminary report from the M.D. Anderson Cancer Center has noted that patients with low serum albumin, high lactate dehydrogenase, and high β_2-microglobulin levels experience a failure-free survival rate of 43%.[67] Other studies have described a relationship between levels of soluble IL-2 receptor, levels of TNF and its receptor, or level of expression of several gene products and clinical outcome in Hodgkin disease.[68–70]

Nevertheless, several series have reported the result of

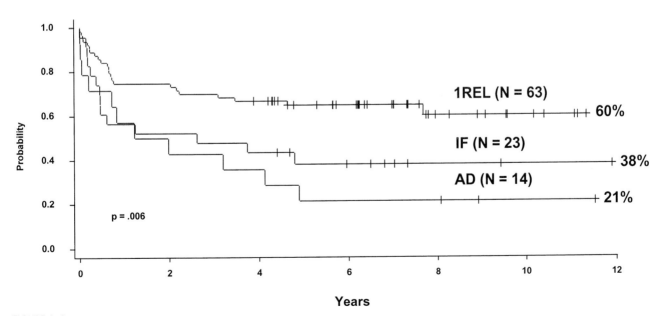

FIGURE 6–1. Progression-free survival by disease status in 100 patients with Hodgkin disease treated in Vancouver Hospital with high-dose cyclophosphamide, carmustine, and etoposide ± cisplatin (CBV ± P) and autologous HSCT. 1REL, first relapse; IF, induction failure; AD, advanced disease (second relapse or beyond).

TABLE 6-3. PROGNOSTIC SYSTEMS IN HODGKIN DISEASE

INSTITUTION AUTHOR (YEAR)	N	FACTORS	WORST PROGNOSTIC GROUP	
			% of Patients	FFP (%)
Straus et al.[61] (1990)	185	Hct Age LDH Inguinal nodes Med mass > 0.45 cm Positive marrow	20	52
Lee et al.[62] (1997)	453	Stage Bulk/B symptoms ALC/positive marrow	12	57
Hasenclever and Diehl[63] (1998)	5141	Hb Age Sex WBC ALC Albumin Stage	7	42

N, number; Hct, hematocrit; LDH, lactate dehydrogenase; med, mediastinal; ALC, absolute lymphocyte count; FFP, freedom from progression.

variably defined high-risk patients who underwent autologous transplantation in an initial CR or partial remission (PR) (Table 6–4). In general, treatment-related mortality rates have been very low and long-term progression-free survival rates have been 70–100%.[71-76] Despite the use of HSCT very early in the disease course, secondary malignancy has been described in this population of patients.[74-76]

More information regarding the potential use of intensive therapy and autologous transplantation as part of primary therapy will become available in the next few years. First, the European Bone Marrow Transplant (EBMT) group has an ongoing randomized study for high-risk patients defined by a modification of the Straus criteria.[61, 77] In this study, patients receive initial therapy with regimens containing ABVD. After four cycles, responding patients are randomized to continue chemotherapy or to undergo autologous HSCT. Even if this study shows superior results in the autologous transplant arm, it is likely that autologous HSCT will be applicable in only a small proportion of patients as part of initial therapy.

Induction Failure

As mentioned previously, approximately 10% of patients with Hodgkin disease treated with multidrug chemotherapy regimens fail to enter a CR. Moreover, others already may be cured without further therapy because the residual radiographic lesions may represent fibrosis alone.[32, 78] Observation of such patients, rather than proceeding with more therapy, is the generally accepted approach.[28, 78] A few of these patients with minimal tumor volume can achieve durable remission using radiation therapy in this setting, but most patients in whom induction chemotherapy fails have an extremely poor prognosis and ultimately succumb to their disease. For the purpose of this discussion, the term *induction failure* refers to those patients with disease progression during chemotherapy, those who have unequivocal radiologic disease progression after attainment of a PR, or those who have biopsy-documented residual Hodgkin disease after primary chemotherapy.[79]

A number of centers have described the results of the use of intensive therapy and autologous HSCT for induction failure in Hodgkin disease (Table 6–5). Patients experiencing induction failure conditioned with any of a number of regimens have a 25–40% probability of prolonged progression-free survival.[53, 55, 79-83] The Autologous Bone Marrow Transplant Registry (ABMTR) analysis found that the presence of B symptoms at diagnosis and an abnormal performance status prior to transplantation correlated with a poorer survival.[53] In the latter study, patients with neither risk factor experienced an overall survival rate of 88%, those with both factors experienced a survival rate of 36%,

TABLE 6-4. RESULTS OF AUTOLOGOUS HSCT AS PART OF INITIAL THERAPY

AUTHOR/YEAR	NUMBER	STATUS*	EARLY TRM (%)	PFS
Bradley et al., 1995[71]	23	CR	4	70% at 4 years
Carella et al., 1996[73]	22	CR	4	77% at 6 years
Sureda et al., 1997[74]	27	CR	0	78% at 2 years
Nademanee et al., 1999[75]	20	CR (14); PR (6)	0	100% at 4 years
Moreau et al., 1998[72]	130	CR (45); PR (85)	3	74% at 5 years

*Numbers in parentheses. TRM, transplant-related mortality; CR, complete remission; PR, partial remission; PFS, progression-free survival.

TABLE 6–5. RESULTS OF AUTOLOGOUS HSCT IN PATIENTS IN WHOM INDUCTION CHEMOTHERAPY FAILS

AUTHOR/YEAR	N	SELECTION CRITERIA*	CONDITIONING	STEM CELL SOURCE	EARLY TRM	SURVIVAL
Gianni et al., 1993[80]	16	PR→progression (9) Progression on MOPP/ABVD (7)	Sequential program with melphalan + TBI or IFRT	BM + PB	0%	31% PFS at 6 years
Chopra et al., 1993[50]	46	No CR with MOPP + "poor features" No CR with MOPP/ABVD or LOPP/EVAP Failure of ≥2 chemotherapy regimens	BEAM	BM	N/A	33% PFS at 5 years
Reece et al., 1995[79]	30	PR→progression (21) Progression on chemotherapy (8) PR with + biopsy (1)	CBV ± P	BM (19) PB (8) Both (3)	17%	42% PFS at 4 years
Prince et al., 1996[81]	30	Persistent disease after initial chemotherapy (23) Progression on chemotherapy (7) Tumor sensitivity preautologous HSCT (30)	Etoposide + melphalan	BM PB Both	10%	34% PFS at 3 years
Sweetenham et al., 1999[82]	175	NR Progression after one or two chemotherapy regimens	BEAM (47%) CBV (22%) Other chemotherapy (23%) TBI-based (8%)	BM (79%) PB (18%) Both (3%)	14%	32% PFS at 6 years
Horning et al., 1997[44]	29	Progression on chemotherapy (14) Progression <4 weeks of best response (9) PR→progression (6)	fTBI/VP/Cy BCNU/VP/Cy CCNU/VP/Cy	BM PB Both	N/A	~50% OS at 4 years
Lazarus et al., 1999[53]	122	No CR with progression or + biopsy	Chemotherapy-based (107) TBI-based (15)	BM (86) PB (25) Both (11)	12%	40% PFS at 3 years
André et al., 1999[55]	86	Progression on first chemotherapy No CR + progression within 3 months of stopping first chemotherapy	BEAM (51%) CBV (25%) TBI-based (2%) Others (22%)	BM (52) PB (34)	8.1%	25% EFS and 35% OS at 5 years

TRM, transplant-related mortality; IFRT, involved field radiation therapy; BEAM, carmustine, etoposide, cytosine arabinoside, melphalan; CBV ± P, cyclophosphamide, carmustine, etoposide ± cisplatin; fTBI/VP/Cy, fractionated TBI, etoposide, cyclophosphamide; BCNU, carmustine; CCNU, lomustine; MOPP/ABVD, nitrogen mustard, vincristine, procarbazine, prednisone/doxorubicin, bleomycin, vinblastine, dacarbazine; LOPP/EVAP, lomustine, vincristine, prednisone, procarbazine/etoposide, vinblastine, doxorubicin, prednisone.
*Numbers or percentages of patients are in parentheses.

and those with only one factor experienced an intermediate survival rate. The 1999 French registry report found that patients experiencing induction failure who were responsive to second-line chemotherapy before autologous HSCT fared much better than those who remained resistant to chemotherapy.[55]

In view of the disappointing results of conventional therapy and the established effectiveness of autologous HSCT in patients experiencing induction failure, a randomized study to confirm the superiority of transplantation is highly unlikely. A comparative study of autologous HSCT versus conventional therapy has been performed at the Stanford University Medical Center, however, and patients who underwent transplantation had a significantly better outcome, with a 4-year progression-free survival rate of 52% versus 19%.[83] Also, the French group performed a matched comparison between further conventional therapy and autologous HSCT after failure of induction chemotherapy; the 5-year survival was superior in the patients who underwent transplantation.[55] Given these findings, one might conclude that autologous transplantation is the treat-

ment of choice in patients in whom conventional induction chemotherapy fails.

First Relapse After Complete Remission

The preferred therapy for patients who experience relapse after a CR achieved by primary radiotherapy alone is usually combination chemotherapy.[48] These patients are not routinely considered for transplantation unless they subsequently experience relapse after salvage chemotherapy.

On the other hand, most patients who experience recurrence after achieving a CR with combination chemotherapy are potential candidates for intensive therapy and autologous transplantation. As discussed earlier, a few selected patients may be cured by radiotherapy alone.[34] The outcome of patients treated with salvage chemotherapy particularly depends on the duration of initial CR.[35–39] Those patients who experience relapse within 1 year after achieving a CR have a low long-term disease-free survival rate. Patients with a longer initial CR fare somewhat better.

Second CR rates are high in this instance, and overall survival rates have ranged from 24%–55% or even higher.[35–39] Death in remission from other causes, particularly secondary myelodysplastic syndrome or acute myelogenous leukemia, adversely affects the survival rate in patients in second CR.[36, 38]

Table 6–6 summarizes the results of larger series evaluating intensive therapy and autologous transplantation in patients in first relapse after chemotherapy. Some series have excluded patients considered to have a high probability of cure with radiotherapy or conventional chemotherapy.[42, 44, 57] Progression-free survival rates have ranged from 40%–60%.[42, 48, 50, 56, 57, 83, 86] Reported early transplant-related mortality rates have ranged from 3%–5%.[48, 86, 87]

As with conventional salvage chemotherapy, biologic features of the disease influence the outcome after autologous HSCT. Several studies in first-relapse patients have reported that a length of initial CR of less than 1 year, presence of extranodal disease at relapse, and B symptoms at relapse are adverse risk factors for outcome after autologous transplantation.[56, 57] These factors overlap both with those risk factors defined for first-relapse patients receiving nontransplant salvage therapy and with ones identified in larger, more heterogeneous series combining patients undergoing transplantation at different time points.

Tumor response to conventional salvage chemotherapy administered before autologous HSCT has also correlated with outcome in several series of first-relapse patients. In a series from the University of Nebraska Medical Center,

patients who underwent transplantation without pretransplantation conventional chemotherapy ("untested" relapse) had the best outcome.[48] A 1997 EBMT registry analysis found that progression-free survival was better for those in a second CR compared with those in an untested, partially sensitive, or resistant first relapse, in that order. A confusing finding in this series was that patients with 5–10 cm of residual disease prior to autologous HSCT experienced a progression-free survival rate comparable to that in patients in second CR and better than that in patients with masses measuring either less than 5 cm or greater than 10 cm.[87] Other factors that temper these observations include the selection bias inherent in registry data and the difficulty in accurately assessing responses in Hodgkin disease, as noted earlier. In a French registry analysis, all first-relapse patients received conventional salvage chemotherapy before autologous HSCT; patients with chemosensitivity experienced better survival than those whose disease was resistant, with no difference between those in a CR or a PR.[56]

The experience from Vancouver Hospital with autologous transplantation for patients in first relapse has been instructive.[57, 86] In Vancouver, all patients with Hodgkin disease were managed through a centralized provincial cancer center, which helped assess the influence of both disease status and selection bias on autologous HSCT results. Beginning in 1985, autologous HSCT was offered to the majority of patients with Hodgkin disease in a first relapse after chemotherapy. A small number of patients were excluded from autologous HSCT because of the presence of very

TABLE 6–6. RESULTS OF AUTOLOGOUS HSCT IN PATIENTS IN FIRST RELAPSE AFTER CHEMOTHERAPY

AUTHOR/YEAR	N	SELECTION CRITERIA*	CONDITIONING*	STEM CELL SOURCE	EARLY TRM	SURVIVAL
Chopra et al., 1993[50]	52	Relapse < 1 year after MOPP/ABVD-like therapy (22) Failure of ≥2 chemotherapy regimens (30)	BEAM	BM	N/A	47% PFS at 5 years
Nadamanee et al., 1995[42]	43†	Relapse < 1 year after chemotherapy No CR with salvage therapy Extranodal relapse	BCNU/VP-16/CTX fTBI/VP-16/CTX	BM PB Both	N/A	~40% PFS at 3 years
Bierman et al., 1996[48]	85	Relapse after CR with MOPP, ABVD, or MOPP/ABV-like therapy	CBV	BM PB	4%	40% PFS at 5 years
Reece et al., 1996[86]	58	Relapse after CR	CBV ± P	BM	3%	61% PFS at 5 years
Yuen et al., 1997[83]	47	Relapse after CR ≤ 1 year (25) > 1 year (22)	BCNU/VP-16/Cy fTBI/VP-16/Cy	BM PB Both	N/A	56% PFS ≤ 1 year ~50% PFS > 1 year at 4 years
Wheeler et al., 1997[52]	42	Relapse after CR	CBV	BM PB Both	N/A	44% PFS at 4 years
Brice et al., 1997[56]	220†	Relapse after CR Pretransplantation salvage chemotherapy	BEAC, CBV, BEAM, and other	BM PB Both	N/A	71% OS at 4 years
Sweetenham et al., 1997[87]	139†	Relapse after CR	BEAM (81) CBV (28) Other chemotherapy (19) TBI-containing (11)	BM (94) PB (35) Both (10)	6.5%	44.7% PFS at 5 years

TRM, transplant-related mortality; BEAM, carmustine, etoposide, cytosine arabinoside, melphalan; BCNU/VP-16/CTX, carmustine, etoposide, cyclophosphamide; fTBI, fractionated TBI; CBV ± P, cyclophosphamide, carmustine, etoposide ± cisplatin; BCNU/VP-16/Cy, carmustine, etoposide, cyclophosphamide; BEAC, carmustine, etoposide, cytosine arabinoside, cyclophosphamide; BM, bone marrow; PB, peripheral blood; MOPP/ABVD, nitrogen mustard, vincristine, procarbazine, prednisone/doxorubicin, bleomycin, vinblastine, dacarbazine.
*Numbers of patients are in parentheses.
†Also includes patients in second CR.

good prognostic factors for cure with further conventional therapy or refusal of any further treatment; only one patient was excluded for other reasons. Therefore, autologous HSCT in our population was not skewed toward good-risk patients. Our study design also differed from that of other centers in that a majority of patients received standardized brief conventional chemotherapy with two cycles of a MOPP variant, MVPP (mechlorethamine, vinblastine, procarbazine, and prednisone), local radiation therapy, or both. Autologous bone marrow was the HSC source in all but two patients. Patients were not restaged for chemosensitivity after conventional cytoreductive therapy, and all subsequently underwent autologous HSCT. Patients were conditioned with either CBV (cyclophosphamide, carmustine, etoposide) or CBV plus conventional dose cisplatin (CBVP). The agents in CBV were administered in doses higher than those originally described because we hoped that patients would tolerate an augmented conditioning regimen well if treated early in the disease course.[45]

Fifty-eight patients in first relapse from CR underwent transplantation using CBVP over a 7-year period between 1985 and 1992. The early nonrelapse mortality rate was low, less than 5% one year post transplantation. The current progression-free survival rate is 63% (95% CI, 48–75%), with a median follow-up of 8 (range, 4–14) years. There have been several late nonrelapse deaths due primarily to pulmonary fibrosis or secondary solid malignancy; no cases of secondary acute myelogenous leukemia have been observed in this population.[86]

As previously reported, multivariate analysis of progression-free survival in this group of patients identified three adverse risk factors: initial complete remission duration less than 1 year, extranodal disease at relapse, and B symptoms at relapse. The number of adverse risk factors has continued to correlate well with the progression-free survival. The updated progression-free survival is 77% in those with no risk factors compared with 75% for those with one, 47% for those with two, and 25% for those with all three risk factors, respectively. Sixty-five percent of those with an initial CR duration of less than 1 year survive without progression versus 76% of those with a longer CR duration. Because the main reason for failure was disease recurrence, these risk factors, not surprisingly, also correlate with the probability of recurrent disease.

A 1997 historical comparison study from Stanford University Medical Center compared the outcome of autologous HSCT versus conventional salvage therapy in first-relapse patients. Patients with an initial CR duration of less than 1 year had significantly improved progression-free survival with autologous HSCT. Those with a longer duration of CR did not have a significantly better outcome with autologous HSCT at 4 years, although longer follow-up would be of interest.[83] Obviously, randomized clinical trials comparing chemotherapy salvage regimens with autologous HSCT in first-relapse patients would be optimal. Such studies, however, are hindered not only by logistic considerations such as requirements for sample size but also by the documented efficacy, relatively low risk, and general acceptance of autologous HSCT as a therapeutic option in this setting.

Experience to date shows that autologous HSCT is indicated at the time of first relapse for those patients with an initial CR duration of less than 1 year as well as for patients with any length of first CR who have other poor prognostic features such as B symptoms or extranodal disease. For the group of patients in whom the initial CR duration exceeds 1 year, particularly those who are asymptomatic and have limited nodal relapse, cure rates are relatively high with conventional therapy. The excellent results with autologous HSCT in this favorable subset, however, support autologous HSCT as an alternative strategy. It will be critical to assess the impact of late nonrelapse mortality in these patients to determine the best strategy.

Second Complete Remission

Patients who achieve a second CR with conventional therapy are expected to be in a favorable position to proceed with autologous HSCT. As mentioned earlier, patients who achieve a second CR after salvage chemotherapy have been reported to have a better outcome than those with a lesser degree of response in some, but not all, autologous HSCT series.[56, 87] This finding may reflect the intrinsically better prognosis of those with highly chemosensitive disease rather than support the need to use repetitive cycles of pretransplantation conventional chemotherapy to attempt to achieve a full response. There is also concern that the use of extensive salvage chemotherapy before autologous HSCT could be deleterious to the transplantation procedure, as discussed later.

Second Relapse or Later in the Disease Course

When autologous HSCT has been deferred until later in the disease course—that is, second relapse or beyond after chemotherapy—progression-free survival rates have varied. Chopra et al. reported that the outcome of patients who underwent transplantation in second or greater CR was better than that in first-CR patients.[50] They pointed out, however, that some patients who undergo transplantation in advanced relapse may have a "chronic relapsing" form of Hodgkin disease and may need prolonged follow-up to accurately assess the effect of autologous HSCT.[50, 88] Wheeler et al. reported 3-year progression-free survival rates of 40% and 44% for patients undergoing autologous transplantation in second and more advanced relapse, respectively. These results were comparable to those in first-relapse patients.[52] Brice et al., however, reported that the 4-year overall survival rate was significantly worse in patients in second or greater relapse (51%) compared with those in first relapse (71%).[56] The findings from Vancouver Hospital also demonstrate an inferior outcome for patients who undergo transplantation in a second or greater relapse, primarily because of an increased risk of transplant-related mortality as demonstrated in Figure 6–1.[60]

No information is available regarding the proportion of patients in second or greater relapse who are actually able to undergo autologous HSCT. Also, issues related to the extent of prior cytotoxic agent exposure become increasingly important in more heavily pretreated patients. For example, cumulative HSC damage may be encountered, leading to difficulty in mobilizing adequate numbers of PBPC for transplantation or even to cytogenetic changes suggestive of myelodysplasia precluding autologous transplantation.[89–92] Moreover, there is evidence to suggest that transplant-related mortality increases with the extent of prior cytotoxic therapy.[60, 93] Given the considerations of both antitumor effect and toxicity, the use of autologous HSCT earlier in the disease course, rather than waiting until second relapse or later, is preferable.

A decision analysis study reported in 1992 by Desch et al. defined second relapse as the optimal time for use of autologous HSCT, at least in a patient experiencing relapse within 1 year of completing standard four-drug chemotherapy.[94] This analysis raises a number of interesting points but is based on assumptions that may not be valid given the current results of autologous HSCT in Hodgkin disease, particularly the now-routine low early transplant-related mortality.

CHEMOSENSITIVITY STATUS

It has become acceptable practice in non-Hodgkin lymphoma to base patient selection for autologous HSCT on the demonstration of chemosensitivity to conventional agents; patients without significant cytoreduction may be excluded from transplantation.[95] Similar chemosensitivity "testing" has occasionally been used in Hodgkin disease, but more commonly chemotherapy has been given for several cycles to initiate tumor shrinkage while financial and logistic arrangements are underway for autologous HSCT without denying transplantation to those with a suboptimal response.[40] Available data also suggest that some patients can proceed directly to transplantation in an "untested relapse," particularly if the tumor volume is small and the transplantation can be performed promptly.[46, 48, 87]

The persuasive study by Chopra et al. established the efficacy of autologous HSCT in patients with Hodgkin disease in whom salvage chemotherapy fails.[96] In this study, the outcome of high-dose therapy with BEAM (BCNU [carmustine], etoposide, cytarabine, melphalan) and autologous HSCT was compared in patients who had either responded to or had not responded to several cycles of salvage chemotherapy with mini-BEAM, a moderately myelosuppressive regimen not requiring HSC support. The results of autologous HSCT in these two groups were similar. Other series have demonstrated that up to 30% of patients who do not respond to chemotherapy may benefit from autologous transplantation.[50]

The use of pretransplantation conventional salvage chemotherapy is likely best individualized according to factors such as tumor burden, estimated HSC reserve, and anticipated time to the transplantation. Usually, one to three cycles should be sufficient, and additional treatment to try to achieve full remission may not be necessary. Although the outcome of autologous HSCT is better in patients responsive to chemotherapy, patients who are not responsive should not routinely be excluded from transplantation.

SELECTION OF HEMATOPOIETIC STEM CELLS FOR TRANSPLANTATION

Although bone marrow is involved in approximately 30% of new diagnoses, only about 10% of patients at the time

of first relapse after chemotherapy have marrow disease (J. Connors, personal communication). Patients with a history of bone marrow involvement, but whose marrow is histologically in remission at the time of HSC procurement, can undergo autologous HSCT using either bone marrow or PBPC. In the retrospective analyses of Bierman et al., recipients of PBPC transplants with a history of but no active histologic marrow involvement at the time of PBPC collection experienced a failure-free survival rate of 46%; the failure-free survival rate was 27% in those patients who had never had bone marrow involvement and who received PBPC grafts. On the other hand, PBPC recipients with active marrow involvement at the time of apheresis experienced a failure-free survival rate of only 11%.[97] Two other groups have identified active marrow involvement as an adverse prognostic factor in patients undergoing PBPC transplantation.[44, 98] Whether the inferior outcome in patients with active marrow disease is due to the absolute tumor burden, biologic features of the disease, or infusion of occult tumor cells is uncertain. Gene marking studies in patients with acute myelogenous leukemia and neuroblastoma undergoing autologous HSCT have demonstrated that tumor cells in the graft can contribute to relapse; studies of this nature in Hodgkin disease are not available.[99]

For selected patients with Hodgkin disease and poor-risk features, and/or bone marrow involvement, allogeneic HSCT may be considered. Age restrictions, donor unavailability, and the high transplant-related mortality rate have hindered this approach. In addition, a case-control analysis of autologous versus allogeneic transplantation performed by the EBMT group showed no advantage for the allogeneic group.[100] Long-term survival, however, can be achieved in some patients undergoing allogeneic transplantation, and further studies using new, less toxic allogeneic grafting techniques such as the nonmyeloablative conditioning regimens are appropriate.[49, 101–103]

Currently, most centers preferentially use autologous mobilized PBPC because of the ability to perform transplantation in patients with active marrow disease, the more rapid engraftment, the potential economic advantage, and the comparable short-term antitumor results when compared with the use of bone marrow. Issues relating to long-term results need to be monitored, however. A 1997 matched pair analysis from the EBMT group unexpectedly found that the 4-year progression-free survival (52.1% vs. 37.9%) and overall survival rates (65.3% vs. 52.7%) were superior in patients receiving bone marrow rather than PBPC transplants.[104] In addition, three retrospective studies have found that the risk of secondary myelodysplastic syndrome/acute myelogenous leukemia was higher in patients receiving PBPC rather than marrow transplants, although this finding reached statistical significance in only one analysis.[76, 105, 106] This worrisome finding is not readily explained and will be further evaluated in a large ongoing study by the ABMTR and U.S. National Cancer Institute.

INTENSIVE CONDITIONING REGIMEN

Numerous intensive conditioning regimens have been used in patients with Hodgkin disease undergoing autologous

HSCT and have been summarized previously.[107] This discussion highlights the more common regimens and discusses new strategies rather than providing a complete listing of all regimens.

Total body irradiation (TBI)-based regimens are effective in patients with Hodgkin disease previously unexposed to radiotherapy.[42, 44] Given the frequency of prior mediastinal radiotherapy in Hodgkin disease, however, most centers have used chemotherapy-only regimens to avoid the excessive pulmonary toxicity seen when TBI is given to such patients.[84, 107] Two commonly used regimens are BEAM (BCNU, etoposide, cytarabine, and melphalan) and variations of CBV, in which cyclophosphamide, BCNU, and etoposide are given in one of several dose schedules.[42, 44–46, 50, 57, 58, 108] Although the toxicity profiles differ with these regimens, there is currently no evidence to support the superiority of any particular intensive therapy regimen in Hodgkin disease. When BCNU-containing regimens are used, attentiveness to delayed lung toxicity requiring steroid therapy is important, particularly when the doses exceed 450 mg/m^2.[108–110] In patients receiving high-dose melphalan-based regimens such as BEAM, mucositis and enterocolitis constitute the most significant nonhematologic toxicity.[50]

The results of conditioning with high-dose melphalan as a single agent were reported in 1997 by Stewart et al.[111] Among 23 relapsed or refractory Hodgkin disease cases, no autologous HSCT transplant-related deaths occurred and the progression-free survival rate at 5 years was 50%. Notably, there was a significant reduction in expense when compared with multidrug conditioning regimens.[111]

On the other hand, a strategy involving two cycles of multiagent intensive therapy, each followed by autologous HSCT, in patients with Hodgkin disease resistant to chemotherapy, was reported in 1997. Toxicity was considerable, and only 57% of patients were able to receive a second transplant. Both CR and progression-free survival rates, however, were improved in patients receiving the second transplant, and further investigation of such double transplants, especially with measures to decrease toxicity, would be of interest.[112]

PERITRANSPLANTATION RADIOTHERAPY

Most relapses after autologous transplantation occur in sites of previous disease, and adjunctive involved-field radiotherapy has been given either before or after transplantation to attempt to reduce this risk.[40, 47, 50, 51, 57, 79] Peritransplantation radiotherapy has most often been used in patients receiving intensive therapy without TBI, largely because of concerns about pulmonary toxicity.[84, 113] Criteria for involved-field radiotherapy have varied but often have included the presence of bulky disease or disease encompassable by a standard field as measured before transplantation or persistent disease after transplantation, taking into account prior radiation exposure and normal tissue tolerance. Radiotherapy techniques have also varied, but total doses in the range of 2000–3000 cGy have generally been used.[47, 51, 114, 118] Such radiotherapy can be given without excessive toxicity in most patients. Serious pulmonary complications can occur, however, particularly when

involved-field radiotherapy to the chest is given before or after autologous HSCT in patients receiving an intensive therapy regimen containing TBI or high doses of nitrosourea or to those with a history of mantle irradiation.[47, 84, 108, 116] In addition, hepatic veno-occlusive disease and radiation-induced gastrointestinal toxicity have been observed after autologous HSCT when involved-field radiotherapy has immediately preceded the transplant procedure.[116] When radiotherapy is administered after autologous HSCT, blood counts should be followed carefully because diminished marrow reserve may lead to cytopenia in some patients.[119]

The available data indicate that pre- or post-transplantation involved-field radiotherapy can decrease recurrence in sites of previous disease and that post-transplantation radiotherapy can convert incomplete responses to CR in some patients.[114, 118] In addition, a beneficial effect on freedom from relapse and overall survival has been described.[51, 118] Judicious use of radiotherapy, particularly in patients previously unexposed to radiation who have nodal disease, is reasonable to try to optimize the curative potential of autologous HSCT, although many issues regarding the best treatment volume, dose, and sequencing of such therapy with autologous transplantation, as well as the risk of late complications, are unresolved.

LATE COMPLICATIONS

Late fatal complications after autologous transplantation are primarily due to chronic lung damage, infection, and second malignancy—particularly "treatment-related" myelodysplastic syndrome/acute myelogenous leukemia (MDS/AML).[120] The raw incidence of late fatal pulmonary fibrosis ranges from 0%–6% and appears to be related to the use of high doses of BCNU or TBI in the conditioning regimen.[44, 56, 76, 90, 120] Late fatal infection has been described in approximately 1%–2% of autologous transplant recipients; bacterial, viral, and fungal infections have all been implicated.[42–44, 50, 54–56, 90, 98, 120] The cumulative incidence of MDS/AML in patients undergoing autologous transplantation for Hodgkin disease has ranged from 5%–24%, although it must be kept in mind that the use of actuarial methods to calculate the incidence may magnify the risk because many patients may be censored at intervals shorter than those at which MDS/AML may occur.[76, 105, 106, 121, 124]

The relative contributions of HSC damage from prior therapy and of the intensive regimen to the development of MDS/AML are uncertain, although the former problem is thought to play the dominant role. First, the large matched comparison by André et al. found that the incidence of secondary MDS/AML was similar in patients with Hodgkin disease whether they received conventional therapy or autologous HSCT.[76] Second, chromosomal abnormalities typical of therapy-related MDS/AML have been detected via sensitive techniques such as fluorescence in situ hybridization (FISH) in morphologically normal marrow specimens and PBPC products obtained before transplantation. These abnormalities were the same as those detectable by conventional cytogenetic techniques at the time that clinical MDS/AML was later diagnosed after autologous HSCT.[125]

Non-Hodgkin lymphoma and a variety of solid tumors have also been described after autologous HSCT for Hodgkin's disease.[40, 43, 44, 46, 48, 51, 52, 76, 86] Similar tumor types also occur after conventional therapy in this disease.[76, 126–128] In the analyses by André et al., the risk of secondary solid tumors after autologous HSCT was 4%, significantly higher than that in a matched group of patients treated with conventional therapy.[76]

FUTURE DIRECTIONS

Further efforts to define the incidence of and risk factors for late transplant-related toxicity, particularly secondary malignancy, and to develop a strategy to try to minimize such complications are needed to optimize the results in Hodgkin disease. The identification of subgroups with relatively good outcomes post transplantation may allow the use of less intensive but still potentially curative conditioning regimens. Measures to collect HSC that are minimally damaged by prior cytotoxic therapy may also be appropriate. Despite concerns about transplant-related mortality, however, disease recurrence after autologous HSCT remains the major limitation of this procedure and novel approaches are required.

Given the limited enthusiasm for further simple dose intensification of existing agents, several studies have described the feasibility of using immunomodulatory techniques in conjunction with autologous HSCT. The use of agents such as interferon-α or interleukin-2 with or without lymphokine-activated killer or activated natural killer cells after autologous HSCT in Hodgkin disease has been explored.[129–131] Interferon-α may be of particular interest because a randomized study reported in 1998 that the continuous CR rate and survival rates were superior in those receiving interferon maintenance.[132] As mentioned previously, use of specific monoclonal antibody preparations directed at antigens expressed at high levels on Hodgkin–Reed-Sternberg cells have considerable appeal. Both anti-CD25 immunotoxin and anti-CD16/CD30 bispecific antibody have shown activity in patients with refractory Hodgkin disease, and such immunotherapy could potentially be combined with transplantation in the future.[133, 134] Recent studies are evaluating the generation and adoptive transfer of autologous lymphocytes for the treatment of patients with Epstein-Barr virus antigen–positive Hodgkin disease.[135] Finally, allogeneic transplantation could be re-evaluated in selected, less heavily pretreated patients to try to reduce the transplant-related mortality of previous studies. Potential candidates include those with active bone marrow involvement, those resistant to chemotherapy, or those with poor-risk features at the time of induction failure.

CONCLUSION

Current data support the use of autologous HSCT in the majority of patients with disease progression despite initial combination chemotherapy. In most instances, it should be used soon after it is apparent that initial chemotherapy has failed to cure, specifically at the time of failure of induction chemotherapy or first relapse/second CR. Adverse prognos-

tic factors reflecting both unfavorable biologic features of the disease and resistance to conventional chemotherapy have been identified; patients at high risk for disease recurrence are potential candidates for innovative treatment. Although early transplant-related mortality is low, late mortality due to causes other than relapse has been increasingly recognized and deserves evaluation.

REFERENCES

1. Aisenberg AC: Problems in Hodgkin's disease management. Blood 93:761, 1999.
2. Linch DC, Winfield D, Goldstone AH, et al: Dose intensification with autologous bone-marrow transplantation in relapsed and resistant Hodgkin's disease: results of a BNLI randomised trial. Lancet 341:1051, 1993.
3. Haluska FG, Brufsky AM, Canellos GP: The cellular biology of the Reed-Sternberg cell [see comments]. Blood 84:1005, 1994.
4. Harris NL, Jaffe ES, Stein H, et al: A revised European-American classification of lymphoid neoplasms: a proposal from the International Lymphoma Study Group [see comments]. Blood 84:1361, 1994.
5. Timens W, Visser L, Poppema S: Nodular lymphocyte predominance type of Hodgkin's disease is a germinal center lymphoma. Lab Invest 54:457, 1986.
6. Deerberg-Wittram J, Weber-Matthiesen K, Schlegelberger B: Cytogenetics and molecular cytogenetics in Hodgkin's disease. Ann Oncol 7:49, 1996.
7. Kuppers R, Rajewsky K, Zhao M, et al: Hodgkin disease: Hodgkin and Reed-Sternberg cells picked from histological sections show clonal immunoglobulin gene rearrangements and appear to be derived from B cells at various stages of development. Proc Natl Acad Sci U S A 91:10962, 1994.
8. Delabie J, Tierens A, Gavriil T, et al: Phenotype, genotype, and clonality of Reed-Sternberg cells in nodular sclerosis Hodgkin's disease: results of a single-cell study. Br J Haematol 94:198, 1996.
9. Hummel M, Ziemann K, Lammert H, et al: Hodgkin's disease with monoclonal and polyclonal populations of Reed-Sternberg cells [see comments]. N Engl J Med 333:901, 1995.
10. Roth J, Daus H, Trumper L, et al: Detection of immunoglobulin heavy-chain gene rearrangement at the single-cell level in malignant lymphomas: no rearrangement is found in Hodgkin and Reed-Sternberg cells. Int J Cancer 57:799, 1994.
11. Brauninger A, Hansmann ML, Strickler JG, et al: Identification of common germinal-center B-cell precursors in two patients with both Hodgkin's disease and non-Hodgkin's lymphoma [see comments]. N Engl J Med 340:1239, 1999.
12. Knecht H, Odermatt BF, Bachmann E, et al: Frequent detection of Epstein-Barr virus DNA by the polymerase chain reaction in lymph node biopsies from patients with Hodgkin's disease without genomic evidence of B- or T-cell clonality. Blood 78:760, 1991.
13. Hennessy K, Fennewald S, Hummel M, et al: A membrane protein encoded by Epstein-Barr virus in latent growth-transforming infection. Proc Natl Acad Sci U S A 81:7207, 1984.
14. Wang D, Liebowitz D, Kieff E: An EBV membrane protein expressed in immortalized lymphocytes transforms established rodent cells. Cell 43:831, 1985.
15. Henderson S, Rowe M, Gregory C, et al: Induction of bcl-2 expression by Epstein-Barr virus latent membrane protein 1 protects infected B cells from programmed cell death. Cell 65:1107, 1991.
16. Pinto A, Gattei V, Zagonel V, et al: Hodgkin's disease: a disorder of dysregulated cellular cross-talk. Biotherapy 10:309, 1998.
17. Clodi K, Younes A: Reed-Sternberg cells and the TNF family of receptors/ligands. Leuk Lymphoma 27:195, 1997.
18. Gruss HJ, Pinto A, Gloghini A, et al: CD30 ligand expression in nonmalignant and Hodgkin's disease-involved lymphoid tissues. Am J Pathol 149:469, 1996.
19. Gruss HJ, Hirschstein D, Wright B, et al: Expression and function of CD40 on Hodgkin and Reed-Sternberg cells and the possible relevance for Hodgkin's disease. Blood 84:2305, 1994.
20. Cossman J, Messineo C, Bagg A: Reed-Sternberg cell: survival in a hostile sea. Lab Invest 78:229, 1998.
21. Gruss HJ, Dolken G, Brach MA, et al: The significance of serum

levels of soluble 60kDa receptors for tumor necrosis factor in patients with Hodgkin's disease. Leukemia 7:1339, 1993.

22. Gause A, Pohl C, Tschiersch A, et al: Clinical significance of soluble CD30 antigen in the sera of patients with untreated Hodgkin's disease. Blood 77:1983, 1991.

23. Nadali G, Tavecchia L, Zanolin E, et al: Serum level of the soluble form of the CD30 molecule identifies patients with Hodgkin's disease at high risk of unfavorable outcome. Blood 91:3011, 1998.

24. Longo DL, Glatstein E, Duffey PL, et al: Radiation therapy versus combination chemotherapy in the treatment of early-stage Hodgkin's disease: seven-year results of a prospective randomized trial [see comments]. J Clin Oncol 9:906, 1991.

25. Biti GP, Cimino G, Cartoni C, et al: Extended-field radiotherapy is superior to MOPP chemotherapy for the treatment of pathologic stage I-IIA Hodgkin's disease: eight-year update of an Italian prospective randomized study [see comments]. J Clin Oncol 10:378, 1992.

26. Klasa RJ, Connors JM, Fairey R, et al: Treatment of early stage Hodgkin's disease: improved outcome with brief chemotherapy and radiotherapy without staging laparotomy. Ann Oncol 7:21, 1996.

27. Santoro A, Bonfante V, Viviani S, et al: Subtotal nodal (STNI) versus involved field (IFRT) irradiation after four cycles of ABVD in early stage Hodgkin's disease. Proc Am Soc Clin Oncol 15:415, 1996.

28. Canellos GP, Anderson JR, Propert KJ, et al: Chemotherapy of advanced Hodgkin's disease with MOPP, ABVD, or MOPP alternating with ABVD [see comments]. N Engl J Med 327:1478, 1992.

29. Duggan D, Petroni G, Johnson J, et al: MOPP/ABV versus ABVD for advanced Hodgkin's disease—a preliminary report of CALGB 8952 (with SWOG, ECOG, NCIC). Proc Am Soc Clin Oncol 16:12a, 1997.

30. Horning SJ, Rosenberg SA, Hoppe RT: Brief chemotherapy (Stanford V) and adjuvant radiotherapy for bulky or advanced Hodgkin's disease: an update. Ann Oncol 7:105, 1996.

31. Diehl V, Franklin J, Hasenclever D, et al: BEACOPP, a new dose-escalated and accelerated regimen, is at least as effective as COPP/ABVD in patients with advanced-stage Hodgkin's lymphoma: interim report from a trial of the German Hodgkin's Lymphoma Study Group. J Clin Oncol 16:3810, 1998.

32. Thomas F, Cosset JM, Cherel P, et al: Thoracic CT-scanning follow-up of residual mediastinal masses after treatment of Hodgkin's disease. Radiother Oncol 11:119, 1988.

33. Mauch P, Tarbell N, Skarin A, et al: Wide-field radiation therapy alone or with chemotherapy for Hodgkin's disease in relapse from combination chemotherapy. J Clin Oncol 5:544, 1987.

34. Wirth A, Corry J, Laidlaw C, et al: Salvage radiotherapy for Hodgkin's disease following chemotherapy failure [see comments]. Int J Radiat Oncol Biol Phys 39:599, 1997.

35. Bonadonna G, Santoro A, Gianni AM, et al: Primary and salvage chemotherapy in advanced Hodgkin's disease: the Milan Cancer Institute experience. Ann Oncol 2(Suppl 1):9, 1991.

36. Longo DL, Duffey PL, Young RC, et al: Conventional-dose salvage combination chemotherapy in patients relapsing with Hodgkin's disease after combination chemotherapy: the low probability for cure. J Clin Oncol 10:210, 1992.

37. Buzaid AC, Lippman SM, Miller TP: Salvage therapy of advanced Hodgkin's disease: critical appraisal of curative potential [published erratum appears in Am J Med 1987 Dec;83(6):A11]. Am J Med 83:523, 1987.

38. Bonfante V, Santoro A, Viviani S, et al: Outcome of patients with Hodgkin's disease failing after primary MOPP-ABVD [see comments]. J Clin Oncol 15:528, 1997.

39. Lohri A, Barnett M, Fairey RN, et al: Outcome of treatment of first relapse of Hodgkin's disease after primary chemotherapy: identification of risk factors from the British Columbia experience 1970 to 1988. Blood 77:2292, 1991.

40. Crump M, Smith AM, Brandwein J, et al: High-dose etoposide and melphalan, and autologous bone marrow transplantation for patients with advanced Hodgkin's disease: importance of disease status at transplant. J Clin Oncol 11:704, 1993.

41. Bierman PJ, Bagin RG, Jagannath S, et al: High dose chemotherapy followed by autologous hematopoietic rescue in Hodgkin's disease: long-term follow-up in 128 patients. Ann Oncol 4:767, 1993.

42. Nademanee A, O'Donnell MR, Snyder DS, et al: High-dose chemotherapy with or without total body irradiation followed by autologous bone marrow and/or peripheral blood stem cell transplantation for patients with relapsed and refractory Hodgkin's disease: results in 85 patients with analysis of prognostic factors. Blood 85:1381, 1995.

43. O'Brien ME, Milan S, Cunningham D, et al: High-dose chemotherapy and autologous bone marrow transplant in relapsed Hodgkin's disease—a pragmatic prognostic index. Br J Cancer 73:1272, 1996.

44. Horning SJ, Chao NJ, Negrin RS, et al: High-dose therapy and autologous hematopoietic progenitor cell transplantation for recurrent or refractory Hodgkin's disease: analysis of the Stanford University results and prognostic indices. Blood 89:801, 1997.

45. Jagannath S, Armitage JO, Dicke KA, et al: Prognostic factors for response and survival after high-dose cyclophosphamide, carmustine, and etoposide with autologous bone marrow transplantation for relapsed Hodgkin's disease. J Clin Oncol 7:179, 1989.

46. Burns LJ, Daniels KA, McGlave PB, et al: Autologous stem cell transplantation for refractory and relapsed Hodgkin's disease: factors predictive of prolonged survival. Bone Marrow Transplant 16:13, 1995.

47. Reece DE, Barnett MJ, Connors JM, et al: Intensive chemotherapy with cyclophosphamide, carmustine, and etoposide followed by autologous bone marrow transplantation for relapsed Hodgkin's disease [published erratum appears in J Clin Oncol 1992 Jan;10(1):170]. J Clin Oncol 9:1871, 1991.

48. Bierman PJ, Anderson JR, Freeman MB, et al: High-dose chemotherapy followed by autologous hematopoietic rescue for Hodgkin's disease patients following first relapse after chemotherapy. Ann Oncol 7:151, 1996.

49. Anderson JE, Litzow MR, Appelbaum FR, et al: Allogeneic, syngeneic, and autologous marrow transplantation for Hodgkin's disease: the 21-year Seattle experience. J Clin Oncol 11:2342, 1993.

50. Chopra R, McMillan AK, Linch DC, et al: The place of high-dose BEAM therapy and autologous bone marrow transplantation in poor-risk Hodgkin's disease. A single-center eight-year study of 155 patients. Blood 81:1137, 1993.

51. Lancet JE, Rapoport AP, Brasacchio R, et al: Autotransplantation for relapsed or refractory Hodgkin's disease: long-term follow-up and analysis of prognostic factors. Bone Marrow Transplant 22:265, 1998.

52. Wheeler C, Eickhoff C, Elias A, et al: High-dose cyclophosphamide, carmustine, and etoposide with autologous transplantation in Hodgkin's disease: a prognostic model for treatment outcomes. Biol Blood Marrow Transplant 3:98, 1997.

53. Lazarus HM, Rowlings PA, Zhang MJ, et al: Autotransplants for Hodgkin's disease in patients never achieving remission: a report from the Autologous Blood and Marrow Transplant Registry. J Clin Oncol 17:534, 1999.

54. Jost LM, Widmer L, Honegger HP, Stahel RA: Index of pretreatment intensity predicts outcome of high-dose chemotherapy and autologous progenitor cell transplantation in chemosensitive relapse of Hodgkin's disease. Ann Oncol 8:785, 1997.

55. André M, Henry-Amar M, Pico J-L, et al: Comparison of high-dose therapy and autologous stem-cell transplantation with conventional therapy for Hodgkin's disease induction failure: a case-control study. J Clin Oncol 17:222, 1999.

56. Brice P, Bouabdallah R, Moreau P, et al: Prognostic factors for survival after high-dose therapy and autologous stem cell transplantation for patients with relapsing Hodgkin's disease: analysis of 280 patients from the French registry. Societé Française de Greffe de Moelle. Bone Marrow Transplant 20:21, 1997.

57. Reece DE, Connors JM, Spinelli JJ, et al: Intensive therapy with cyclophosphamide, carmustine, etoposide ± cisplatin, and autologous bone marrow transplantation for Hodgkin's disease in first relapse after combination chemotherapy [see comments]. Blood 83:1193, 1994.

58. Arranz R, Tomas JF, Gil-Fernandez JJ, et al: Autologous stem cell transplantation (ASCT) for poor prognostic Hodgkin's disease (HD): comparative results with two CBV regimens and importance of disease status at transplant. Bone Marrow Transplant 21:779, 1998.

59. Lumley MA, Milligan DW, Knechtli CJ, et al: High lactate dehydrogenase level is associated with an adverse outlook in autografting for Hodgkin's disease. Bone Marrow Transplant 17:383, 1996.

60. Reece D: Should high risk patients with Hodgkin's disease be singled out for heavier therapeutic regimens while low risk patients are spared such therapies? Leuk Lymphoma 15:19, 1995.

61. Straus DJ, Gaynor JJ, Myers J, et al: Prognostic factors among 185 adults with newly diagnosed advanced Hodgkin's disease treated with alternating potentially noncross-resistant chemotherapy and intermediate-dose radiation therapy. J Clin Oncol 8:1173, 1990.

62. Lee SM, Radford JA, Ryder WD, et al: Prognostic factors for disease progression in advanced Hodgkin's disease: an analysis of patients aged under 60 years showing no progression in the first 6 months after starting primary chemotherapy. Br J Cancer 75:110, 1997.

63. Hasenclever D, Diehl V: A prognostic score for advanced Hodgkin's disease: International Prognostic Factors Project on Advanced Hodgkin's Disease [see comments]. N Engl J Med 339:1506, 1998.

64. Proctor SJ, Taylor P, Donnan P, et al: A numerical prognostic index for clinical use in identification of poor-risk patients with Hodgkin's disease at diagnosis: Scotland and Newcastle Lymphoma Group (SNLG) Therapy Working Party. Eur J Cancer 27:624, 1991.

65. Ferme C, Bastion Y, Brice P, et al: Prognosis of patients with advanced Hodgkin's disease: evaluation of four prognostic models using 344 patients included in the Group d'Etudes des Lymphomes de l'Adulte Study. Cancer 80:1124, 1997.

66. Sarris AH, Preti A, Smith T, et al: A predictive model for failure-free survival (FFS) of adults with Hodgkin's disease (HD) treated with ABVD or equivalent regimens. Blood 90:388a, 1997.

67. Sarris AH, Kliche KO, Pethambaram P, et al: Interleukin-10 levels are often elevated in serum of adults with Hodgkin's disease and are associated with inferior failure-free survival. Ann Oncol 10:433, 1999.

68. Viviani S, Camerini E, Bonfante V, et al: Soluble interleukin-2 receptors (sIL-2R) in Hodgkin's disease: outcome and clinical implications. Br J Cancer 77:992, 1998.

69. Warzocha K, Bienvenu J, Ribeiro P, et al: Plasma levels of tumour necrosis factor and its soluble receptors correlate with clinical features and outcome of Hodgkin's disease patients. Br J Cancer 77:2357, 1998.

70. Morente MM, Piris MA, Abraira V, et al: Adverse clinical outcome in Hodgkin's disease is associated with loss of retinoblastoma protein expression, high Ki67 proliferation index, and absence of Epstein-Barr virus–latent membrane protein 1 expression. Blood 90:2429, 1997.

71. Bradley SJ, Pearce R, Taghipour G, et al: First remission autologous bone marrow transplantation for Hodgkin's disease—preliminary EBMT data. Leuk Lymphoma 15:51, 1995.

72. Moreau P, Fleury J, Brice P, et al: Early intensive therapy with autologous stem cell transplantation in advanced Hodgkin's disease: retrospective analysis of 158 cases from the French registry. Bone Marrow Transplant 21:787, 1998.

73. Carella AM, Prencipe E, Pungolino E, et al: Twelve years experience with high-dose therapy and autologous stem cell transplantation for high-risk Hodgkin's disease patients in first remission after MOPP/ABVD chemotherapy. Leuk Lymphoma 21:63, 1996.

74. Sureda A, Mataix R, Hernandez-Navarro F, et al: Autologous stem cell transplantation for poor prognosis Hodgkin's disease in first complete remission: a retrospective study from the Spanish GEL-TAMO cooperative group. Bone Marrow Transplant 20:283, 1997.

75. Nademanee A, Molina A, Fung H, et al: High-dose chemo/radiotherapy and autologous bone marrow or stem cell transplantation for poor risk advanced-stage Hodgkin's disease during first partial or complete remission. Biol Blood Marrow Transplant 5:292–298, 1999.

76. André M, Henry-Amar M, Blaise D, et al: Treatment-related deaths and second cancer risk after autologous stem-cell transplantation for Hodgkin's disease. Blood 92:1933, 1998.

77. Federico M, Clo V, Carella AM: Preliminary analysis of clinical characteristics of patients enrolled in the HD01 protocol: a randomised trial of high dose therapy and autologous stem cell transplantation versus conventional therapy for patients with advanced Hodgkin's disease responding to first line therapy. Leuk Lymphoma 15:63, 1995.

78. Connors JM, Klimo P, Adams G, et al: Treatment of advanced Hodgkin's disease with chemotherapy—comparison of MOPP/ABV hybrid regimen with alternating courses of MOPP and ABVD: a report from the National Cancer Institute of Canada clinical trials group [published erratum appears in J Clin Oncol 1997 Jul;15(7):2762]. J Clin Oncol 15:1638, 1997.

79. Reece DE, Barnett MJ, Shepherd JD, et al: High-dose cyclophosphamide, carmustine (BCNU), and etoposide (VP16–213) with or without cisplatin (CBV ± P) and autologous transplantation for patients with Hodgkin's disease who fail to enter a complete remission after combination chemotherapy. Blood 86:451, 1995.

80. Gianni AM, Siena S, Bregni M, et al: High-dose sequential chemo-radiotherapy with peripheral blood progenitor cell support for relapsed or refractory Hodgkin's disease—a 6-year update. Ann Oncol 4:889, 1993.

81. Prince HM, Crump M, Imrie K, et al: Intensive therapy and autotransplant for patients with an incomplete response to front-line therapy for lymphoma. Ann Oncol 7:1043, 1996.

82. Sweetenham JW, Carella AM, Taghipour G, et al: High-dose therapy and autologous stem cell transplantation for adult patients with Hodgkin's disease who do not enter remission after induction chemotherapy: results in 175 patients reported to the European Group for Blood and Marrow Transplantation. J Clin Oncol 17:3101–3109, 1999.

83. Yuen AR, Rosenberg SA, Hoppe RT, et al: Comparison between conventional salvage therapy and high-dose therapy with autografting for recurrent or refractory Hodgkin's disease. Blood 89:814, 1997.

84. Phillips GL, Wolff SN, Herzig RH, et al: Treatment of progressive Hodgkin's disease with intensive chemoradiotherapy and autologous bone marrow transplantation. Blood 73:2086, 1989.

85. Rapoport AP, Rowe JM, Kouides PA, et al: One hundred autotransplants for relapsed or refractory Hodgkin's disease and lymphoma: value of pretransplant disease status for predicting outcome. J Clin Oncol 11:2351, 1993.

86. Reece DE, Phillips GL: Intensive therapy and autologous stem cell transplantation for Hodgkin's disease in first relapse after combination chemotherapy. Leuk Lymphoma 21:245, 1996.

87. Sweetenham JW, Taghipour G, Milligan D, et al: High-dose therapy and autologous stem cell rescue for patients with Hodgkin's disease in first relapse after chemotherapy: results from the EBMT. Lymphoma Working Party of the European Group for Blood and Marrow Transplantation. Bone Marrow Transplant 20:745, 1997.

88. Goldstone AH, McMillan AK: The place of high-dose therapy with haemopoietic stem cell transplantation in relapsed and refractory Hodgkin's disease. Ann Oncol 4:21, 1993.

89. Bensinger W, Appelbaum F, Rowley S, et al: Factors that influence collection and engraftment of autologous peripheral-blood stem cells. J Clin Oncol 13:2547, 1995.

90. Weaver CH, Schwartzberg L, Li W, et al: High-dose chemotherapy and autologous peripheral blood progenitor cell transplant for the treatment of Hodgkin's disease. Bone Marrow Transplant 17:715, 1996.

91. Moskowitz CH, Glassman JR, Wuest D, et al: Factors affecting mobilization of peripheral blood progenitor cells in patients with lymphoma. Clin Cancer Res 4:311, 1998.

92. Chao NJ, Nademanee AP, Long GD, et al: Importance of bone marrow cytogenetic evaluation before autologous bone marrow transplantation for Hodgkin's disease. J Clin Oncol 9:1575, 1991.

93. Schiffman K, Buckner CD, Maziarz R, et al: High-dose busulfan, melphalan, and thiotepa followed by autologous peripheral blood stem cell transplantation in patients with aggressive lymphoma or relapsed Hodgkin's disease [published erratum appears in Biol Blood Marrow Transplant 1998;4(1):56]. Biol Blood Marrow Transplant 3:261, 1997.

94. Desch CE, Lasala MR, Smith TJ, Hillner BE: The optimal timing of autologous bone marrow transplantation in Hodgkin's disease patients after a chemotherapy relapse [see comments]. J Clin Oncol 10:200, 1992.

95. Philip T, Guglielmi C, Hagenbeek A, et al: Autologous bone marrow transplantation as compared with salvage chemotherapy in relapses of chemotherapy-sensitive non-Hodgkin's lymphoma [see comments]. N Engl J Med 333:1540, 1995.

96. Chopra R, Linch DC, McMillan AK, et al: Mini-BEAM followed by BEAM and ABMT for very poor risk Hodgkin's disease. Br J Haematol 81:197, 1992.

97. Bierman P, Vose J, Anderson J, et al: Comparison of autologous bone marrow transplant (ABMT) with peripheral stem cell transplantation (PSCT) for patients (PTS) with Hodgkin's disease (HD). Blood 82:445a, 1993.

98. Hurd DD, Haake RJ, Lasky LC, et al: Treatment of refractory and relapsed Hodgkin's disease: intensive chemotherapy and autologous bone marrow or peripheral blood stem cell support. Med Pediatr Oncol 18:447, 1990.

99. Brenner MK, Rill DR, Moen RC, et al: Gene marking and autologous bone marrow transplantation. Ann N Y Acad Sci 716:204, 1994.

100. Milpied N, Fielding AK, Pearce RM, et al: Allogeneic bone marrow

transplant is not better than autologous transplant for patients with relapsed Hodgkin's disease. European Group for Blood and Bone Marrow Transplantation. J Clin Oncol 14:1291, 1996.

101. Jones RJ, Piantadosi S, Mann RB, et al: High-dose cytotoxic therapy and bone marrow transplantation for relapsed Hodgkin's disease. J Clin Oncol 8:527, 1990.

102. Phillips GL, Reece DE, Barnett MJ, et al: Allogeneic marrow transplantation for refractory Hodgkin's disease. J Clin Oncol 7:1039, 1989.

103. Slavin S, Nagler A, Naparstek E, et al: Nonmyeloablative stem cell transplantation and cell therapy as an alternative to conventional bone marrow transplantation with lethal cytoreduction for the treatment of malignant and nonmalignant hematologic disease. Blood 91:756, 1998.

104. Majolino I, Pearce R, Taghipour G, Goldstone AH: Peripheral-blood stem-cell transplantation versus autologous bone marrow transplantation in Hodgkin's and non-Hodgkin's lymphomas: a new matched-pair analysis of the European Group for Blood and Marrow Transplantation Registry Data. Lymphoma Working Party of the European Group for Blood and Marrow Transplantation. J Clin Oncol 15:509, 1997.

105. Traweek ST, Slovak ML, Nademanee AP, et al: Clonal karyotypic hematopoietic cell abnormalities occurring after autologous bone marrow transplantation for Hodgkin's disease and non-Hodgkin's lymphoma. Blood 84:957, 1994.

106. Bhatia S, Ramsay NK, Steinbuch M, et al: Malignant neoplasms following bone marrow transplantation. Blood 87:3633, 1996.

107. Reece DE, Phillips GL: Intensive therapy and autotransplantation in Hodgkin's disease. Stem Cells (Dayt) 12:477, 1994.

108. Wheeler C, Antin JH, Churchill WH, et al: Cyclophosphamide, carmustine, and etoposide with autologous bone marrow transplantation in refractory Hodgkin's disease and non-Hodgkin's lymphoma: a dose-finding study. J Clin Oncol 8:648, 1990.

109. Rubio C, Hill ME, Milan S, et al: Idiopathic pneumonia syndrome after high-dose chemotherapy for relapsed Hodgkin's disease. Br J Cancer 75:1044, 1997.

110. Ager S, Mahendra P, Richards EM, et al: High-dose carmustine, etoposide and melphalan ("BEM") with autologous stem cell transplantation: a dose-toxicity study. Bone Marrow Transplant 17:335, 1996.

111. Stewart DA, Guo D, Sutherland JA, et al: Single-agent high-dose melphalan salvage therapy for Hodgkin's disease: cost, safety, and long-term efficacy. Ann Oncol 8:1277, 1997.

112. Ahmed T, Lake DE, Beer M, et al: Single and double autotransplants for relapsing/refractory Hodgkin's disease: results of two consecutive trials. Bone Marrow Transplant 19:449, 1997.

113. Pecego R, Hill R, Appelbaum FR, et al: Interstitial pneumonitis following autologous bone marrow transplantation. Transplantation 42:515, 1986.

114. Mundt AJ, Sibley G, Williams S, et al: Patterns of failure following high-dose chemotherapy and autologous bone marrow transplantation with involved field radiotherapy for relapsed/refractory Hodgkin's disease [see comments]. Int J Radiat Oncol Biol Phys 33:261, 1995.

115. Tsang RW, Gospodarowicz MK, Sutcliffe SB, et al: Thoracic radiation therapy before autologous bone marrow transplantation in relapsed or refractory Hodgkin's disease: PMH Lymphoma Group, and the Toronto Autologous BMT Group. Eur J Cancer 35:73, 1999.

116. Pezner RD, Nademanee A, Niland JC, et al: Involved field radiation therapy for Hodgkin's disease autologous bone marrow transplantation regimens. Radiother Oncol 34:23, 1995.

117. Constine LS, Rapoport AP: Hodgkin's disease, bone marrow transplantation, and involved field radiation therapy: coming full circle from 1902 to 1996 [editorial; comment]. Int J Radiat Oncol Biol Phys 36:253, 1996.

118. Poen JC, Hoppe RT, Horning SJ: High-dose therapy and autologous bone marrow transplantation for relapsed/refractory Hodgkin's disease: the impact of involved field radiotherapy on patterns of failure and survival [see comments]. Int J Radiat Oncol Biol Phys 36:3, 1996.

119. Toren A, Nagler R, Nagler A: Involved field radiation post autologous stem cell transplantation in lymphoma patients is associated with major haematological toxicities. Med Oncol 15:113, 1998.

120. Reece DE, Nevill TJ, Sayegh A, et al: Regimen-related toxicity and non-relapse mortality with high-dose cyclophosphamide, carmustine (BCNU) and etoposide (VP16-213) (CBV) and CBV plus cisplatin (CBVP) followed by autologous stem cell transplantation in patients with Hodgkin's disease. Bone Marrow Transplant 23:1131, 1999.

121. Darrington DL, Vose JM, Anderson JR, et al: Incidence and characterization of secondary myelodysplastic syndrome and acute myelogenous leukemia following high-dose chemoradiotherapy and autologous stem-cell transplantation for lymphoid malignancies. J Clin Oncol 12:2527, 1994.

122. Miller JS, Arthur DC, Litz CE, et al: Myelodysplastic syndrome after autologous bone marrow transplantation: an additional late complication of curative cancer therapy [see comments]. Blood 83:3780, 1994.

123. Pedersen-Bjergaard J, Pedersen M, Myhre J, Geisler C: High risk of therapy-related leukemia after BEAM chemotherapy and autologous stem cell transplantation for previously treated lymphomas is mainly related to primary chemotherapy and not to the BEAM-transplantation procedure. Leukemia 11:1654, 1997.

124. Donaldson SS, Hancock SL: Second cancers after Hodgkin's disease in childhood [editorial; comment]. N Engl J Med 334:792, 1996.

125. Radford JE, Abruzzese EA, Pettenati MJ: Presence in pretransplant marrow of abnormal progenitor clones that give rise to post transplant myelodysplasia: implications for high-dose chemoradiotherapy with autologous hematopoietic cell transplantation. Autologous Blood and Marrow Transplantation. Proceedings of the Ninth International Symposium. Arlington, Texas, 1999, p 483.

126. van Leeuwen FE, Klokman WJ, Hagenbeek A, et al: Second cancer risk following Hodgkin's disease: a 20-year follow-up study. J Clin Oncol 12:312, 1994.

127. DeVita VT Jr: Late sequelae of treatment of Hodgkin's disease. Curr Opin Oncol 9:428, 1997.

128. Hoppe RT: Hodgkin's disease: complications of therapy and excess mortality. Ann Oncol 8:115, 1997.

129. Schenkein DP, Dixon P, Desforges JF, et al: Phase I/II study of cyclophosphamide, carboplatin, and etoposide and autologous hematopoietic stem-cell transplantation with posttransplant interferon alfa-2b for patients with lymphoma and Hodgkin's disease. J Clin Oncol 12:2423, 1994.

130. Benyunes MC, Higuchi C, York A, et al: Immunotherapy with interleukin 2 with or without lymphokine-activated killer cells after autologous bone marrow transplantation for malignant lymphoma: a feasibility trial. Bone Marrow Transplant 16:283, 1995.

131. Lister J, Rybka WB, Donnenberg AD, et al: Autologous peripheral blood stem cell transplantation and adoptive immunotherapy with activated natural killer cells in the immediate posttransplant period. Clin Cancer Res 1:607, 1995.

132. Aviles A, Diaz-Maqueo JC, Talavera A, et al: Maintenance therapy with interferon alfa 2b in Hodgkin's disease. Leuk Lymphoma 30:651, 1998.

133. Engert A, Diehl V, Schnell R, et al: A phase-I study of an anti-CD25 ricin A-chain immunotoxin (RFT5-SMPT-dgA) in patients with refractory Hodgkin's lymphoma. Blood 89:403, 1997.

134. Hartmann F, Renner C, Jung W, et al: Treatment of refractory Hodgkin's disease with an anti-CD16/CD30 bispecific antibody [published erratum appears in Blood 1998 Mar 1;91(5):1832]. Blood 89:2042, 1997.

135. Roskrow MA, Suzuki N, Gan Y, et al: Epstein-Barr virus (EBV)-specific cytotoxic T lymphocytes for the treatment of patients with EBV-positive relapsed Hodgkin's disease. Blood 91:2925, 1998.

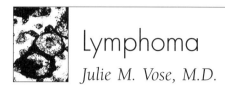

CHAPTER SEVEN

Lymphoma

Julie M. Vose, M.D.

The non-Hodgkin lymphomas (NHL) are a heterogeneous group of malignant disorders that exhibit distinct clinical behavior. The histopathologic classification of lymphoma allowed for the comparison of clinical outcome in patients grouped according to their pathologically defined entity. The first broadly applied classifications such as the Rappaport system were based on histologic and cytologic characteristics of lymphoma cells and were mainly descriptive.[1] Subsequent classifications such as the Kiel and the Lukes and Collins schemes attempted to relate the malignant cell that characterized each lymphoma to its normal counterpart within the lymphatic system.[2, 3] The Working Formulation, developed through the National Cancer Institute as a means for translating between existing lymphoma classifications, based its classification on clinical parameters, morphology, and grouping the lymphomas according to their natural history, response to therapy, and overall survival.[4] This scheme was rapidly adopted by clinicians and has been widely used as the basis for determining first therapy.

Further insight into the pathogenesis of lymphoid malignancy from genetic, molecular, and immunologic methods expanded our knowledge about the cellular origin of lymphoma. In addition, distinct phenotypic and genetic changes were identified that allowed more-precise definition of each lymphoma. In 1994, a new classification was proposed by the International Lymphoma Study Group and was designated the Revised European American Lymphoma (REAL) classification system.[5] Although the REAL classification has clarified many of the clinicopathologic entities that were lacking in the older systems of classification, it does not translate all the entities into prognostically and therapeutically relevant categories. With some further modification and clinical input, this classification system could be helpful in future study evaluations and therapeutic management decisions. Recent modifications of the REAL system are being incorporated into the revised World Health Organization (WHO) classification, whose publication should provide for further reproducibility and clinical relevance. Although a simplified scheme is not ideal, the lymphomas are divided into aggressive, highly aggressive, and indolent categories for the purposes of this discussion. This allows interpretation of data previously based on the Working Formulation.

AGGRESSIVE NON-HODGKIN LYMPHOMA

The development of combination chemotherapy for therapy of patients with newly diagnosed aggressive NHL has provided cure of approximately a third of patients. The devel-

opment of the original CHOP regimen (cyclophosphamide, doxorubicin, vincristine, and prednisone) for the treatment of patients with aggressive NHL produced a 45–60% complete response rate with a 30–35% long-term disease-free survival rate in patients with advanced-stage disease.[6] Further development led to the addition of agents to the original CHOP backbone and the use of alternating therapy with nonoverlapping toxicity in an attempt to improve the outcome without increasing toxicity. Regimens such as M-BACOD (methotrexate, bleomycin, cyclophosphamide, vincristine, and dexamethasone), MACOP-B (methotrexate, Adriamycin [doxorubicin], cyclophosphamide, vincristine, prednisone, and bleomycin), and ProMACE-CytaBOM (prednisone, Adriamycin [doxorubicin], cyclophosphamide, and etoposide, followed by cytarabine, bleomycin, vincristine, and methotrexate) initially produced improved complete response rates of 60–80%.[7–9] In a prospective randomized trial, however, the long-term disease-free survival of these patients appeared similar to those treated with the original CHOP regimen.[10] Subset analysis of the high-risk patients also failed to identify any group that benefited from specific regimens.[10] Subsequent trials have confirmed the lack of superior efficacy of any of the more-intensive regimens except in patients with an adverse International Prognostic Index score. It may well be that more-aggressive therapy benefits patients with a predicted higher relapse rate after conventional-dose chemotherapy. Reports from cooperative group trials are eagerly awaited in this area.

Despite progress in the initial therapy of patients with aggressive NHL, the treatment of relapsed NHL with conventional salvage chemotherapy has remained difficult. Many salvage regimens have been formulated since the 1970s such as DHAP (dexamethasone, high-dose cytarabine, and cisplatin), or MINE (ifosfamide, mitoxantrone, and etoposide).[11, 12] Although patients may respond transiently to these regimens, the complete response rates are typically 20–30% at best.[11, 12] In a review of 16 studies, Singer and Goldstone found that only 12 of 398 patients in relapse who were treated with a variety of different chemotherapeutic programs were in continuous complete remission at 2 years.[13] This poor result with conventional chemotherapy for relapsed or high-risk disease has prompted the investigation of high-dose chemotherapy with hematopoietic stem cell (HSC) rescue in these patient populations.

LYMPHOMA BIOLOGIC FACTORS

In relapsed aggressive NHL, the factor most predictive for success of high-dose chemotherapy and autologous HSC transplantation (HSCT) is the sensitivity of the lymphoma to chemotherapy. As demonstrated by Philip et al.[14], patients whose disease was in complete remission with initial chemotherapy and was responsive to further salvage chemotherapy were reported to have a long-term disease-free survival rate of 40%. Several other studies have also reported long-term disease-free survival rates in patients with chemotherapy-sensitive relapse of 35–50%.[15–17] This compares with patients with chemotherapy-resistant disease, in whom long-term disease-free survival rates of 14–25% have been reported.[14–17] Patients who have primary refractory aggressive lymphoma and have never experienced a complete remission have been reported to have a 0–15% chance of long-term disease-free survival.[14, 15]

Other factors that have been reported to be predictive for a poorer outcome of transplantation for aggressive NHL include the presence of a large mass at the time of transplantation, an elevated lactate dehydrogenase (LDH) level at the time of transplantation, and extensive prior treatment (≥ 3 treatment regimens).[18] It is therefore the policy of many transplant centers only to perform transplantation with patients with chemotherapy-sensitive, relapsed disease without evidence of bulky disease. When this policy is used, however, only approximately 50% of patients with relapsed disease are able to undergo high-dose therapy and autologous HSCT.[19] The utility of high-dose chemotherapy and autologous HSCT has now been demonstrated in a prospective randomized trial to be superior to conventional-dose salvage chemotherapy with the DHAP regimen for patients with chemotherapy-sensitive disease.[19] High-dose chemotherapy and autologous HSCT should be considered the standard of care for patients with chemotherapy-sensitive, recurrent NHL.

Probably the most important area of current research is in the selection of patients for HSCT in first partial or complete remission who are identified at the time of diagnosis as high-risk for relapse. Many different prognostic factors have been identified as important in predicting the outcome of patients with high-risk disease. These include bulky disease, number of extranodal sites, high LDH, stage at diagnosis, and rapidity of achieving a complete remission.[20–22] The International Prognostic Index was developed by Shipp et al. and has identified a group of patients under age 60 years who are at high-risk for relapse with doxorubicin-based therapy.[23] In this analysis, patients under age 60 years who have two or three of the following characteristics have a 25–30% chance of 5-year disease-free survival: stage 3 or 4, Eastern Cooperative Oncology Group performance status of 2 or higher, or an LDH level above the upper limits of normal.[23] Many centers are now using these prognostic factors to choose patients at the time of diagnosis who are thought to be at a very high risk for relapse and entering them into trials with the use of alternative approaches such as high-dose chemotherapy and autologous HSCT in very good first partial or complete response.

Several pilot trials have now been initiated in this high-risk patient group, with many studies reporting 60–80% of the patients to be long-term disease-free survivors.[24, 25] This concept has not been fully tested in a prospective randomized trial compared with conventional chemotherapy. The trial that comes closest to a retrospective analysis of this high-risk population, however, was published by Haioun et al.[26] In this study, all patients with aggressive NHL at the time of diagnosis were entered into a trial in which all patients received an anthracycline-containing regimen for four cycles. If their disease was in complete remission after four cycles, they were randomized to receive either an intensive consolidation protocol with an ifosfamide-based regimen or they received the CVB (cyclophosphamide, etoposide, and carmustine [BCNU]) regimen and underwent autologous bone marrow transplantation. At the time of the initial publication, the 3-year failure-free survival rate of the consolidation group was 57% and 56% for the transplant arm (P = NS). There was no difference in the low- or low-intermediate risk patients according to the International Prognostic Group; however, the high-intermediate-risk and high-risk patients had a 3-year failure-free survival rate of 60% in the HSCT arm compared with 44% in the consolidation chemotherapy arm (P = .07).[26] With additional follow-up, the difference between these two arms in the high-intermediate-risk and high-risk groups became statistically significant, with the 5-year failure-free survival rate in the transplant group at 57% and 36% in the consolidation group (P = .01)[27]

For patients who did not experience complete remission with induction therapy but did experience a partial response, the utility of high-dose chemotherapy and autologous HSCT has also been evaluated in the LNH-87 trial. Of 96 patients in this trial who experienced an initial partial response with induction therapy, 32 patients went on to receive high-dose chemotherapy and undergo autologous HSCT. The 4-year event-free survival rate of the transplant patients was 58% compared with 20% for the conventionally treated patients (P < .0001).[27] For those patients who experience a good partial remission from their initial induction therapy and are still responding to chemotherapy, high-dose chemo/radiotherapy and autologous HSCT should be strongly considered.

A vast majority of patients with intermediate-grade NHL who undergo high-dose therapy and autologous HSCT have been diagnosed with diffuse large-cell or immunoblastic NHL. Several other histologic subtypes are also included in the intermediate-grade category, however, such as follicular large cell, diffuse small cleaved cell, diffuse mixed small and large cell, and diffuse intermediate cell lymphoma (mantle cell lymphoma). Most series demonstrate consistent results in the chemotherapy-sensitive diffuse large cell and immunoblastic histologic subtypes, with approximately 40% of patients failure-free at 3–5 years post transplantation. The effect of the other histologies on the outcome for transplantation, however, is controversial, with some studies demonstrating an improved outcome for patients with a follicular large cell pattern as opposed to a diffuse growth pattern.[28] The role of transplantation for mantle cell NHL has not yet been well established; however, early studies of patients undergoing autologous HSCT for relapsed mantle cell lymphoma has demonstrated a 40% 2-year failure-free survival rate with no obvious plateau on the curve at an early time point.[29] A 1997 abstract from Dana-Farber Cancer Institute evaluated 26 patients undergoing transplantation for mantle cell lymphoma. At 4 years post transplantation, the disease-free survival rate was 21% and the overall survival rate 53%.[30]

PATIENT FACTORS

Patient selection for HSCT must include factors related to overall health status in addition to those related to the risk factors associated with the status of the patient's lymphoma. Factors routinely assessed and found to be adequate prior to HSCT should include the patient's overall Karnofsky performance status, renal status, cardiac status, pulmonary function, and liver function. An adequate pretransplantation evaluation of renal function should demonstrate a serum creatinine of 1.5–2.0 mg/dL or less and/or a creatinine clearance of at least 50 mL/hour. With the use of potentially nephrotoxic agents such as aminoglycoside antibiotics or amphotericin during the transplant procedure and large volume shifts, renal impairment can occur in some patients. Therefore, an adequate baseline function is mandatory. The cardiac function should also be adequate to allow for a potential drop in the ejection fraction during the procedure from cardiotoxic agents or problems with volume overload. In young patients with no clinical history of cardiac disfunction and limited anthracycline exposure, a formal measurement of the ejection fraction may not necessarily be of additional benefit in predicting cardiac dysfunction during transplantation.[31] For patients with any clinical history of cardiac dysfunction, older patients, or those with extensive prior anthracycline exposure, a baseline ejection fraction or further cardiac evaluation is warranted.

The pulmonary toxicity associated with high-dose therapy and HSCT is occasionally clinically significant. A baseline pulmonary function with pulmonary mechanics and diffusion capacity (DLCO) can be helpful in assessing the pulmonary status of the candidate. In addition, if any question remains, a pulmonary exercise stress test may be helpful in the evaluation. Concerns of pulmonary functional status deterioration during or after the transplantation related to volume overload, infectious agents, or pulmonary parenchymal damage causing a deterioration of the pulmonary status. Although there is no set standard for the pulmonary status prior to transplantation, a general guideline in many transplant centers is that the mechanics and DLCO should be greater than 50% of the patient's predicted normal values. A poor pretransplantation pulmonary function and/or a history of radiation to the thorax is sometimes associated with an increase in the risk of pulmonary complications.[32]

Pretransplantation liver functional and synthetic status are also important. In some studies, the presence of elevated liver transaminases and/or bilirubin can be associated with an increased risk of veno-occlusive disease (VOD).[33] McDonald et al. also reported that patients who start conditioning therapy while being treated for bacterial and/or viral infections appear to be at increased risk for fatal VOD.[33] In addition, VOD has been reported to be more common in patients with liver metastases or in patients who have received prior irradiation to the liver field.[34] Detailed description of pretransplant patient evaluation is found in Chapter 20.

HIGHLY AGGRESSIVE NON-HODGKIN LYMPHOMA

Lymphoblastic lymphoma typically is diagnosed in children or young adolescent patients with a high incidence of a mediastinal mass at diagnosis. It has now become standard practice to use an acute lymphoblastic leukemia (ALL)-type regimen with this histologic picture, including central nervous system (CNS) prophylaxis because of the high risk of CNS disease. With the use of such a regimen, CNS prophylaxis, and maintenance therapy, most young patients have an excellent chance of long-term disease-free survival.[35, 36] Patients who experience relapse after receiving a conventional ALL-type regime, however, have a poor salvage rate with conventional chemotherapy. Patients with relapsed lymphoblastic NHL should receive conventional salvage therapy such as a high-dose cytarabine regimen to establish chemotherapy sensitivity and reduce the tumor burden. If they are found to still be chemotherapy-sensitive, high-dose chemotherapy and HSCT should be strongly considered at that time. Autologous HSCT for relapsed lymphoblastic lymphoma has been reported to produce a long-term disease-free survival rate of 30–40% in most series.[37, 38] Some studies have advocated an allogeneic source of HSC as possibly being superior to an autologous source because of the high incidence of marrow and blood involvement with this histologic subtype. Although no prospective randomized studies have been performed to address this issue, a case-matched study from the European Group for Blood and Marrow Transplantation (EBMT) by Chopra et al. evaluated this issue.[39] In this analysis, only patients who received transplants after the first complete remission benefited from an allogeneic HSCT, with a progression-free survival rate of 19% for those undergoing autologous HSCT and 40% for those with an allogeneic HSCT ($P = .029$).

Because of the aggressiveness of lymphoblastic lymphoma, particularly in adult patients, some physicians have advocated the use of high-dose chemotherapy and HSCT during first complete remission. Clinical characteristics that have been associated with a poorer prognosis at the time of initial diagnosis have included a positive bone marrow and/or CNS involvement associated with elevated LDH.[36, 40] Several studies evaluated the results of HSCT for patients with lymphoblastic lymphoma using autologous transplants during first complete remission, demonstrating a 57–85% survival rate for patients at high risk.[37–39] We currently recommend high-dose chemotherapy and HSCT for patients with these high-risk characteristics and a human leukocyte antigen (HLA)-identical sibling as the source of HSC in cases of relapsed lymphoblastic lymphoma.

Burkitt lymphoma is also a very aggressive lymphoma that is difficult to manage in adults. Autologous or allogeneic HSCT used as therapy during first complete remission for patients with high-risk features, such as elevated LDH and CNS and/or bone marrow involvement, has been reported to produce long-term disease-free survival in a high percentage of adult patients.[41] The case-control study by Chopra et al.[39] failed to demonstrate an advantage for the use of allogeneic HSC over an autologous HSC in this type of lymphoma.

The choice of a transplant candidate with NHL depends on lymphoma factors such as histologic subtype, LDH, stage, number of extranodal sites, and remission status as well as patient factors such as age, organ function, and performance status. Each clinical situation must be individualized with respect to the choice of therapy for the patient.

INDOLENT NON-HODGKIN LYMPHOMA

The use of high-dose chemo/radiotherapy and HSCT for indolent NHL is more controversial than its use for the aggressive lymphomas. With conservative therapy, patients receiving conventional radiation or chemotherapy who have indolent lymphoma can look forward to a relatively long life expectancy, with a median of 6–9 years in many series.[42–44] Because of the relatively long natural history of this illness, physicians have been hesitant to perform HSCT in these patients. Despite the prolonged survival, however patients with indolent NHL have continuous pattern of relapse, with only 10–20% of all patients alive at 10–20 years after the original diagnosis.

Because of the incurability of this illness in most advanced cases, the use of high-dose chemotherapy and HSCT has been applied to patients with relapsed disease. Several trials have now been published evaluating the outcome of high-dose chemo/radiotherapy and autologous HSCT for patients with recurrent indolent NHL.[45–47] Rohatiner et al.[45] evaluated 64 patients with recurrent follicular lymphoma who received cyclophosphamide with total body irradiation (TBI) and a purged autologous bone marrow transplant. With a median follow-up of 3.5 years, 35 patients continued in remission between 1 and 8 years posttransplantation. Another study by Bastion et al.[46] evaluated 60 patients with poor-prognosis follicular lymphoma who received either BEAM (BCNU [carmustine], etoposide, cytarabine, and melphalan) or cyclophosphamide and TBI and unpurged autologous peripheral blood progenitor cells (PBPC). With a median follow-up of 21 months, 48 patients were alive and 18 patients were in relapse.

The largest series of HSCT for recurrent indolent NHL has been published by Bierman et al.[47] In this series, 141 patients with recurrent follicular NHL received high-dose chemo/radiotherapy and autologous unpurged PBPC or bone marrow transplantation. The patients had received one to four or more prior chemotherapy regimens prior to HSCT. The 4-year overall survival rate was 65%, and the failure-free survival rate was 44%. In a multivariate analysis, the number of prior regimens the patients had undergone and a follicular large cell histology were significantly associated with a poorer outcome. The patients who had undergone only one prior regimen had a 5-year failure-free survival rate of 70% compared with 15% for those who had undergone four or more prior regimens ($P > .001$).

Because patients with indolent NHL often have bone marrow involvement with lymphoma at some point in their disease, the consideration for purging of the HSC, whether derived from the bone marrow or from PBPC, by chemotherapy, monoclonal antibodies with complement, or positive selection is an issue in transplantation for this histologic subtype. Gribben et al.[48] evaluated 114 patients who received cyclophosphamide and TBI followed by a monoclonal antibody–purged autologous bone marrow graft for indolent NHL. In this analysis, 57 (50%) of patient's bone marrow was able to be purged successfully to bcl-2 negativity by polymerase chain reaction. Of the 57 cases in which it was possible to purge to negativity 3 of 57 (5%) had relapsed compared with 26 of 57 (46%) that could not be purged to negativity ($P \leq .0001$). Other studies, however, have not always confirmed this analysis, with a smaller

percentage of cases able to be purged to negativity and less of a correlation with the eventual outcome.[49] A case-matching study of transplants with purged marrow for indolent lymphoma and analyzed in the European Bone Marrow Transplant Registry did not demonstrate any difference in the outcome compared with a matched set of patients who received an unpurged marrow transplant.[50] In addition, the short- and long-term effects of using a purged or selected product on immunologic reconstitution is unknown. A prospective, randomized trial would be the best confirmation of the outcome of patients receiving a purged autologous transplant; however, no such trial has been reported to date. Discussion on purging can be found in Chapter 29.

Some centers have also performed pilot trials using high-dose chemo/radiotherapy and autologous HSCT in first complete remission as part of the patient's initial management after routine induction chemotherapy. One such study from the Dana Farber Cancer Institute evaluated 77 patients with bulky stage 3 or 4 follicular NHL who received six cycles of CHOP induction therapy to first complete remission followed by cyclophosphamide/TBI and autologous purged bone marrow transplantation. This study demonstrated a 3-year disease-free survival rate of 63% and a 3-year survival rate of 89%.[51] A pilot study of autologous HSCT in 34 patients with follicular lymphoma and one of the established high-risk features (involvement of three or more lymph nodes measuring >3 cm, tumor size >7 cm, massive pleural or peritoneal effusion, massive splenomegaly, B symptoms or a platelet count of <100,000/mm³) was reported by Morel et al.[52] The patients were in complete remission or very good partial remission with 75% tumor volume reduction and then received high-dose BEAM followed by mafosfamide-purged autologous HSCT. The estimated treatment failure rate and overall survival were 43% and 80%, respectively at 48 months with a median follow-up of 36 months.[52] In comparison with a historical control group treated with chemotherapy alone, the treatment failure rate was 26%. A prospective randomized comparison is needed to accurately reflect the effect of early transplantation in high-risk follicular lymphoma.

The use of an HLA-matched sibling donor has also been recommended for patients with indolent NHL. Van Besien et al. reported 10 patients with chemotherapy-refractory indolent lymphoma who received myeloablative therapy and allogeneic HSCT. In this study, both the actuarial and failure-free survival rates were the same at 80% ± 13%, with a median follow-up of 816 days.[53] For the surviving patients, the duration of the current remission exceeds that of any prior remission achieved. In information from the International Bone Marrow Transplant Registry, 81 patients who received an allogeneic HLA-matched HSCT for multiply recurrent and resistant indolent NHL experienced an estimated 3-year survival rate of 46% and disease-free survival rate of 43%.[54] Because of the questionable curability of indolent lymphoma with an autologous transplant, some centers are now recommending an HLA-matched sibling donor for young patients if that is possible. In addition, if a patient has a chemotherapy-resistant indolent lymphoma or evidence of extensive blood and bone marrow involvement, an HLA-matched related allogeneic HSCT would be preferred. Because of the wide variation in the natural

TABLE 7–1. INDICATIONS FOR HSCT IN NON-HODGKIN LYMPHOMA (NHL)

NHL HISTOLOGY	INDICATION FOR TRANSPLANT
Diffuse/aggressive	Relapsed, chemotherapy-sensitive
	First partial remission after induction
	First complete remission—high/intermediate-risk or high risk according to international index
Highly aggressive	Relapsed chemotherapy-sensitive
	First partial or complete remission in high-risk disease—high lactate dehydrogenase, central nervous system–positive and/or bone marrow–positive
Indolent	Consider: relapsed after conventional therapy—autologous vs. allogeneic

history of patients with indolent lymphoma, choosing the correct form of management for certain patients should be based on prognostic factor analysis. An outline of clinical indications for HSCT according to NHL histology is presented in Table 7–1.

CONCLUSION AND FUTURE DIRECTIONS

Despite all of the progress in HSCT techniques, the major cause of failure for lymphoma is relapse of disease. Unfortunately, different combinations of chemotherapeutic agents with or without radiation have not improved the outcome of patients undergoing HSCT for NHL. Current areas of active investigation in the autologous setting include the use of various purging or positive-selection techniques, the addition of monoclonal antibodies to the transplant regimen, or the addition of cytokines or other immunomodulating agents after transplantation. Research trends in the allogeneic setting include the use of selection devices for T-cell depletion with specific cell subpopulation add-back or the use of less intensive transplant chemotherapy regimens with the use of planned delayed donor-leukocyte infusions. Clinical trials over the next few years should greatly add to our knowledge base in this area.

REFERENCES

1. Rappaport H: Tumors of the hematopoietic system. *In* Atlas of Tumor Pathology, Series I, Section III, Fascicle 8. Washington, DC, Armed Forces Institute of Pathology, 1966.
2. Lennert K, Mohri N, Stein H, et al: The histopathology of malignant lymphoma. Br J Haematol 31(Suppl):193–203, 1975.
3. Lukes R, Collins R: Immunologic characterization of human malignant lymphomas. Cancer 34:1488–1503, 1974.
4. Non-Hodgkin's lymphoma pathologic classification project: National Cancer Institute sponsored study of classifications of non-Hodgkin's lymphomas: summary and description of a Working Formulation for clinical usage. Cancer 49:2112–2135, 1982.
5. Harris NL, Jaffe ES, Stein H, et al: A revised European-American classification of lymphoid neoplasms: a proposal from the International Lymphoma Study Group. Blood 84:1361–1392, 1994.
6. DeVita VT Jr, Canellos GP, Chabner B, et al: Advanced diffuse histiocytic lymphoma, a potentially curable disease. Lancet 1:248 250, 1975.
7. Shipp MA, Harrington DP, Klatt MM, et al: Identification of major prognostic subgroups of patients with large-cell lymphoma treated with m-BACOD or M-BACOD. Ann Intern Med 104:757–756, 1986.
8. Klimo P, Connors JM: MACOP-B chemotherapy for the treatment of diffuse large-cell lymphoma. Ann Intern Med 102:596–602, 1985.
9. Fisher RI, DeVita VT, Hubbard SM, et al: Randomized trial of Pro-MACE-MOPP vs. ProMACE-CytaBOM in previously untreated, advanced stage, diffuse aggressive lymphomas. Proc Am Soc Clin Oncol 3:242, 1984.
10. Fisher RI, Gaynor ER, Dahlberg S, et al: Comparison of a standard regimen (CHOP) with three intensive chemotherapy regimens for advanced non-Hodgkin's lymphoma. N Engl J Med 328:1002–1006, 1993.
11. Velasquez WS, Cabanillas F, Salvador P, et al: Effective salvage therapy for lymphoma with cisplatin in combination with high-dose Ara C and dexamethasone (DHAP). Blood 71:117–122, 1988.
12. Rodriguez MA, Cabanillas FC, Hagemeister FB, et al: A phase II trial of mesna/ifosfamide, mitoxantrone, and etoposide for refractory lymphomas. Ann Oncol 6:609–611, 1995.
13. Singer CRJ, Goldstone AH: Clinical studies of ABMT in non-Hodgkin's lymphoma. Clin Hematol 15:105–150, 1986.
14. Philip T, Armitage JO, Spitzer G, et al: High-dose therapy and autologous bone marrow transplantation after failure of conventional chemotherapy in adults with intermediate-grade or high-grade non-Hodgkin's lymphoma. N Engl J Med 316:1493–1498, 1987.
15. Lazarus HM, Crilley P, Ciobanu N, et al: High-dose carmustine, etoposide, and cisplatin and autologous bone marrow transplantation for relapsed and refractory lymphoma. J Clin Oncol 10:1682–1689, 1992.
16. Vose JM, Armitage JO, Bierman PJ, et al: Salvage therapy for relapsed or refractory non-Hodgkin's lymphoma utilizing autologous bone marrow transplantation. Am J Med 87:285–288, 1989.
17. Gribben JG, Goldstone AH, Linch DC, et al: Effectiveness of high-dose combination chemotherapy and autologous bone marrow transplantation for patients with non-Hodgkin's lymphomas who are still responsive to conventional-dose therapy. J Clin Oncol 7:1621–1629, 1989.
18. Vose JM, Anderson JR, Kessinger A, et al: High-dose chemotherapy and autologous hematopoietic stem-cell transplantation for aggressive non-Hodgkin's lymphoma. J Clin Oncol 11:1846–1851, 1993.
19. Philip T, Guglielmi C, Hagenbeek A, et al: Autologous bone marrow transplantation as compared with salvage chemotherapy in relapses of chemotherapy-sensitive non-Hodgkin's lymphoma. N Engl J Med 333:1540–1545, 1995.
20. Fisher RI, Hubbard SM, DeVita VT, et al: Factors predicting long-term survival in diffuse mixed, histiocytic, or undifferentiated lymphoma. Blood 58:45–51, 1981.
21. Shipp MA, Harrington DP, Klatt MM, et al: Identification of major prognostic subgroups of patients with large-cell lymphoma treated with m-BACOD or M-BACOD. Ann Intern Med 104:757–756, 1986.
22. Coiffier B, Gisselbrecht C, Vose JM, et al: Prognostic factors in aggressive malignant lymphomas: description and validation of a prognostic index that could identify patients requiring a more intensive therapy. J Clin Oncol 74:558–564, 1991.
23. Shipp MA, Harrington DP, Anderson JR, et al: A predictive model for aggressive non-Hodgkin's lymphoma, the international non-Hodgkin's lymphoma prognostic factor project. N Engl J Med 329:987–994, 1993.
24. Gulati SC, Shank B, Black P, et al: Autologous bone marrow transplantation for patients with poor-prognosis lymphomas. J Clin Oncol 6:1303–1313, 1988.
25. Philip T, Hartmann O, Biron P, et al: High-dose therapy and autologous bone marrow transplantation in partial remission after first-line induction therapy for diffuse non-Hodgkin's lymphoma. J Clin Oncol 6:1118–1124, 1988.
26. Haioun C, Lepage E, Gisselbrecht C, et al: Comparison of autologous bone marrow transplantation with sequential chemotherapy for intermediate-grade and high-grade non-Hodgkin's lymphoma in first complete remission: a study of 464 patients. J Clin Oncol 12:2543–2551, 1994.
27. Haioun C, Lepage E, Gisselbrecht C, et al: High-dose therapy followed by stem cell transplantation in partial response after first-line induction therapy for aggressive non-Hodgkin's lymphoma. Ann Oncol 9:55 60, 1990.
28. Vose JM, Bierman PJ, Lynch JC, et al: Effect of follicularity on autologous transplantation for large-cell non-Hodgkin's lymphoma. J Clin Oncol 16:844–849, 1998.
29. Stewart DA, Vose JM, Weisenburger DD, et al: The role of high-dose

therapy and autologous hematopoietic stem cell transplantation for mantle cell lymphoma. Ann Oncol 6:263–266, 1995.

30. Freedman A, Neuberg D, Aster J, et al: High-dose chemoradiotherapy and anti-B cell monoclonal antibody purged autologous bone marrow transplantation in mantle cell lymphoma: no evidence for long-term remission. Proc Am Soc Clin Oncol 16:316a, 1997.

31. Hertenstein B, Stefanic M, Schmeiser T, et al: Cardiac toxicity of bone marrow transplantation: predictive value of cardiologic evaluation before transplantation. J Clin Oncol 12: 998–1004, 1994.

32. Clark JG, Schwartz DA, Flournoy N, et al: Risk factors for airflow obstruction in recipients of bone marrow transplants. Ann Intern Med 107:648–656, 1987.

33. McDonald GB, Hinds MS, Fisher LD, et al: Venooclusive disease of the liver after bone marrow transplantation: diagnosis, incidence, and predisposing factors. Hepatology 4:16–20, 1984.

34. Ayash LJ, Hunt M, Antman K, et al: Hepatic venooclusive disease in autologous bone marrow transplantation of solid tumors and lymphomas. J Clin Oncol 8:1699–1703, 1990.

35. Anderson JR, Derek R, Jenkin T, et al: Long-term follow-up of patients treated with COMP or LSA2-L2 therapy for childhood non-Hodgkin's lymphoma: a report of CCG-551 from the childrens cancer group. J Clin Oncol 11:1024–1032, 1993.

36. Morel P, Lepage E, Brice P, et al: Prognosis and treatment of lymphoblastic lymphoma in adults: a report on 80 patients. J Clin Oncol 10:1078–1085, 1992.

37. Sweetenham JW, Liberti G, Pearce R, et al: High-dose therapy and autologous bone marrow transplantation for adult patients with lymphoblastic lymphoma: results of the European group for bone marrow transplantation. J Clin Oncol 12:1358–1365, 1994.

38. Baro J, Richard C, Sierra J, et al: Autologous bone marrow transplantation in 22 adults patients with lymphoblastic lymphoma responsive to conventional dose chemotherapy. Bone Marrow Transplant 10:33–38, 1992.

39. Chopra R, Goldstone AH, Pearce R, et al: Autologous versus allogeneic bone marrow transplantation for non-Hodgkin's lymphoma: a case-controlled analysis of the European Bone Marrow transplant Group Registry data. J Clin Oncol 10:1690–1695, 1992.

40. Coleman CN, Piccozi VJ, Cox RS, et al: Treatment of lymphoblastic lymphoma in adults. J Clin Oncol 4:1628–1637, 1986.

41. Troussard X, Leblond V, Kuentz, et al: Allogeneic bone marrow transplantation in adults with Burkitt's lymphoma or acute lymphoblastic leukemia in first complete remission. J Clin Oncol 8:809–812, 1990.

42. Young RC, Longo DL, Glatstein E, et al: The treatment of indolent lymphomas: watchful waiting vs. aggressive combined modality treatment. Semin Hematol 25:11–16, 1988.

43. Portlock CS: Management of the low-grade non-Hodgkin's lymphomas. Semin Oncol 17:51–59, 1990.

44. Morrison VA, Peterson BA: Combination chemotherapy in the treatment of follicular low-grade lymphoma. Leukemia Lymphoma 10:29–33, 1993.

45. Rohatiner AZS, Johnson PAWM, Price CGA, et al: Myeloablative therapy with autologous bone marrow transplantation as consolidation therapy for recurrent follicular lymphoma. J Clin Oncol 12:1177–1184, 1994.

46. Bastion Y, Brice P, Haioun C, et al: Intensive therapy with peripheral blood progenitor cell transplantation in 60 patients with poor-prognosis follicular lymphoma. Blood 86:3257–3262, 1995.

47. Bierman PJ, Vose JM, Anderson JR, et al: High-dose therapy with autologous hematopoietic rescue for follicular low-grade non-Hodgkin's lymphoma. J Clin Oncol 15:445–450, 1997.

48. Gribben JG, Freedman AS, Neuberg D, et al: Immunologic purging of marrow assessed by PCR before autologous bone marrow transplantation for B-cell lymphoma. N Engl J Med 325:1525–1533, 1991.

49. Johnson PWM, Price CGA, Smith T, et al: Detection of cells bearing the t(14;18) translocation following myeloablative treatment and autologous bone marrow transplantation for follicular lymphoma. J Clin Oncol 12:798–805, 1994.

50. Williams CD, Goldstone AH, Pearce RM, et al: Purging of bone marrow in autologous bone marrow transplantation for non-Hodgkin's lymphoma: a case-matched comparison with unpurged cases by the European blood and marrow transplant lymphoma registry. J Clin Oncol 14:2454–2464, 1996.

51. Freedman A, Gribben J, Neuberg D, et al: High-dose therapy and autologous bone marrow transplantation in patients with follicular lymphoma during first remission. Blood 88:2780–2786, 1996.

52. Morel P, Laporte JP, Noel MP, et al: Autologous bone marrow transplantation as consolidation therapy may prolong remission in newly diagnosed high-risk follicular lymphoma: a pilot study of 34 cases. Leukemia 9:576–582, 1995.

53. Van Besien KW, Khouri IF, Giralt SA, et al: Allogeneic bone marrow transplantation for refractory and recurrent low-grade lymphoma: the case for aggressive management. J Clin Oncol 13:1096–1102, 1995.

54. van Besien K, Sobocinski KA, Rowlings PA, et al: Allogeneic bone marrow transplantation for low-grade lymphoma. Blood 92:1832–1836, 1998.

CHAPTER EIGHT

Multiple Myeloma

Sundar Jagannath, M.D., and Bart Barlogie, M.D., Ph.D.

Multiple myeloma (MM) is a hematologic malignancy characterized by monoclonal proliferation of plasma cells, accounting for 1% of all cancers and 10% of hematologic tumors nationwide with an average annual age-adjusted incidence rate of 5 per 100,000.[1] The incidence of MM is twice the national rate for African Americans (10 of 10^5) and lower in Asians (2 of 10^5). MM is rare in patients under 40 years (<2%), with a progressive rise in incidence with increasing age.[2] Median age of onset is 65 years. Ten thousand deaths each year in the United States are attributable to this disease. The etiology of MM remains elusive, although association with prior radiation exposure (e.g., atomic bomb survivors, radiologists, and radium dial workers), occupational exposure (e.g., agriculture, metal, rubber, paper, leather, and textile industries), and chemical exposure (e.g., to paint sprays and silicone breast implants) have been reported.[1, 3]

DIAGNOSIS AND STAGING

The most common clinical manifestations of MM include bone pain from osteolytic bone lesions and fractures, anemia, hypercalcemia, renal failure, and recurrent infections. Less frequently, hyperviscosity, bleeding diathesis, or organ dysfunction from light chain deposition are noted at presentation. Diagnosis of MM is established by the presence of marked marrow plasmacytosis (>30%), plasmacytoma in tissue biopsy, multiple lytic bone lesions, and monoclonal immunoglobulins spike on serum (IgG >3.5 g/dL; IgA >2.0 g/dL) or urine electrophoresis (>1 g/day). It is important to distinguish MM from monoclonal gammopathy of undetermined significance (MGUS), solitary plasmacytoma, and indolent myeloma.

MGUS is characterized by lower levels of serum monoclonal protein (<3 g/dL), minimal or absent light chain excretion, marrow plasmacytosis (<5%), the absence of lytic bone lesions, anemia, hypercalcemia, renal insufficiency, and, most importantly, stability of the monoclonal protein during follow-up.[4] Indolent or smoldering myeloma defines an asymptomatic stage of the disease, with minimal tumor burden reflected by minimal marrow plasmacytosis (<30%), mild anemia (Hgb >10 g/dL), no renal insufficiency, and absent or asymptomatic small lytic bone lesions (fewer than three lesions).[5, 6] Such patients can be recognized only retrospectively. The indolent nature of the disease is reflected by a low plasma cell labeling index of less than 1%.[7]

Occasionally, plasma cell tumors present as an isolated lesion in the bone (solitary plasmacytoma of bone) or as an extraosseous soft tissue mass (extramedullary plasmacytoma). These patients are typically male and are generally younger than patients presenting with MM by a decade.[8] Solitary plasmacytoma of the bone often involves the spine (40%) and is frequently accompanied by paraprotein (<60%) but with preserved, uninvolved immunoglobulins (>90%). The cure rate of solitary bone lesions is only 30% with local radiotherapy (RT),[9–11] reflecting frequent subclinical dissemination, now often appreciated by the use of magnetic resonance imaging (MRI) of the axial bone marrow.[12] Disappearance of paraprotein postlocal RT portends good prognosis. Extramedullary plasmacytoma often presents in the upper respiratory tract (>70%), and local radiation therapy is often curative.[10, 11]

When a diagnosis of plasma cell dyscrasia is suspected, the standard work-up should include serum and urine protein electrophoresis, immunofixation of serum and urine to identify the nature of the monoclonal protein, and quantitation of immunoglobulin levels. A complete blood count, sedimentation rate, and blood chemistries, including total protein, albumin, electrolytes, blood urea nitrogen (BUN), creatinine, calcium, uric acid, and lactate dehydrogenase, should be obtained. Urinalysis and 24-hour urine collection for determination of total protein and light chain excretion as well as creatinine clearance should be performed. A skeletal survey is necessary to delineate the extent of lytic bone lesions. MRI with T1-weighted and inversion recovery sequences of the skull, entire spine, and pelvis is recommended to image the extent of marrow involvement, along with extraosseous soft tissue mass to rule out impending spinal cord or nerve root compression. Bone scans are of limited value because the osteoblastic activity is suppressed in this disease unless there is associated fracture or osteosclerotic myeloma.[13]

The Durie-Salmon staging system, which correlates presenting clinical features of MM with measured myeloma tumor mass, is widely used.[14] This system divides MM into three tumor burden groups: stage I (low, 0.6×10^{12} cells/m^2), II (intermediate, $0.6–1.2 \times 10^{12}$), and III (high, $>1.2 \times 10^{12}$). Subclassifications A and B refer to normal or abnormal renal function (creatinine, 2.0 mg/dL). For better delineation of prognosis and choice of therapy, determination of serum β_2-microglobulin and C-reactive protein, serum lactate dehydrogenase, plasma cell labeling index, and cytogenetics are highly recommended (see later). The combined use of serum β_2-microglobulin and C-reactive protein is probably the easiest approach to assess prognosis.[15]

STANDARD TREATMENT

WATCH AND WAIT FOR EARLY ASYMPTOMATIC DISEASE

Patients presenting with asymptomatic Durie-Salmon stage IA disease with low β_2-microglobulin and normal C-reactive protein should not be treated but carefully monitored at 3-month intervals ("wait and watch") for possible indolent or smoldering myeloma. A normal MRI pattern of spine and pelvis provides additional clinically important information to defer therapy.[16] Should these patients experience symptoms, show doubling of their M-component values in less than 1 year, or show progression of bone disease, therapy should be initiated immediately. Although early detection and prompt initiation of therapy is the dictum for most malignancies, a wait-and-watch policy for MM allows for better quality of life with no compromise of the ultimate outcome. For example, among patients with MGUS, the interval from the recognition of the monoclonal gammopathy to diagnosis of MM ranged from 2–29 years (median, 10 years) and median survival after diagnosis was 34 months.[17] Patients with indolent myeloma did not require therapy for 3 years, and their survival time from the initiation of therapy was also 3 years, similar to that for newly diagnosed symptomatic myeloma.[17]

PALLIATIVE RADIATION THERAPY

Symptomatic myeloma requires prompt initiation of systemic chemotherapy. Palliative radiotherapy should be restricted to patients with disabling pain who have a well-defined focal process that has not responded to chemotherapy. Even in the case of an extraosseous soft tissue plasmacytoma impinging on the spinal cord or a nerve root, prompt initiation of chemotherapy with a high-dose glucocorticoid-based regimen such as VAD (vincristine, doxorubicin, and dexamethasone) would be as effective as local radiotherapy. Should local radiotherapy need to be administered to the spine, the total dose should not preclude the future use of total body irradiation (TBI; total dose < 3000 cGy) in the management of the systemic disease. Also, the radiation port should be restricted to the focal site of disease so as not to compromise the bone marrow reserve.

STANDARD CHEMOTHERAPY

Before the advent of chemotherapy, the median life expectancy of patients with myeloma was about 1 year.[18, 19] Introduction of oral melphalan and prednisone in the 1960s produced substantial improvement in the palliation of these patients, with objective responses (>50% tumor mass reduction) in over half of the patients lasting a median of 18 months and prolongation of life expectancy to a median of 3 years.[20, 21] Unfortunately, these results could not be improved by the introduction of multiagent combination chemotherapy as shown by large randomized clinical trials (Table 8–1).[22] VAD administration induced rapid tumor cytoreduction, but the median duration of response and overall survival remained unchanged.[23–25] Combination chemotherapy generally induces a rapid and slightly higher response rate, and as such patients presenting with high-tumor-mass myeloma should be treated with multiagent combination chemotherapy. Chemotherapy should be administered until the patient reaches a plateau phase and subsequently should be discontinued.

MAINTENANCE THERAPY

There is no role for maintenance chemotherapy with alkylating agents in MM. Although continuation of alkylating agents may result in longer duration of remission, there is no survival benefit.[26] Furthermore, chronic exposure to alkylating agents for 2 or more years reduces hematopoietic

TABLE 8–1. RANDOMIZED TRIALS COMPARING MELPHALAN AND PREDNISONE WITH COMBINATION CHEMOTHERAPY

TRIAL	CHEMOTHERAPY	NO. OF PATIENTS	RESPONSE %	MEDIAN SURVIVAL IN MONTHS
Bergsagel et al., 1979[27]	MP	125	40	28
	MP/CP/BP	123	31	31
Salmon et al., 1994[25]	MP	77	32	23
	VMCP/VCAP VMCP × 3/VBAP	160	54	43
Pavlovsky et al., 1988[91]	MP	145	33	42
	VMCCP	115	44	44
Cooper et al., 1986[92]	MP	146	47	34
	MCBP	156	56	29
	sequential MCBP	156	47	22
	MCBAP	157	44	26
Peest et al., 1988[93]	MP	170	33	>40
	VMCP	150	33	40
Boccadoro et al., 1991[94]	MP	146	64	37
	VMCP/VBAP	138	77	52

VMCP, vincristine, melphalan, cyclophosphamide, prednisone; VBAP, vincristine, carmustine, doxorubicin, prednisone; MP, melphalan, prednisone; CP, cyclophosphamide, prednisone; BP, carmustine, prednisone; VMCCP, vincristine, melphalan, cyclophosphamide, semustine, prednisone; MCBP, melphalan, cyclophosphamide, carmustine, prednisone; MCBAP, melphalan, cyclophosphamide, carmustine, doxorubicin, prednisone.

stem cell (HSC) reserve and increases the chance for development of myelodysplasia and acute myelogenous leukemia.[26, 27] Although glucocorticoids have significant antimyeloma effect, their role in maintenance therapy has not been studied. Interferon-α (IFN-α) has been used as maintenance treatment for responding patients in the plateau phase of their disease. A 1995 meta-analysis of randomized clinical trials with or without IFN-α by Ludwig et al. indicates that more studies show a beneficial rather than indifferent or harmful effect from IFN-α.[28] There is some concern, however, that IFN-α maintenance could also lead to an increased risk of a second neoplasm as has been reported for hairy cell leukemia.[29] In addition, IFN-α may not be effective in patients with myeloma overexpressing bcl-2 in their tumors, a common finding in this disease.[30]

HIGH-DOSE CHEMOTHERAPY—DOSE INTENSITY

Application of dose-intensive chemotherapy has been a challenge in this disease. First, unlike Hodgkin disease or lymphoma, MM is not a chemotherapy-sensitive disease as noted by infrequent complete remissions (CR) and no cures with standard therapy. Second, this disease predominantly afflicts elderly patients, with a median age of onset of 65 years.[2] Third, renal impairment (serum creatinine >2 mg/dL) is encountered frequently as a part of the disease manifestation, either at diagnosis or during the course of the disease.[31] And finally, prolonged alkylating agent exposure, IFN-α maintenance, and radiation to the spine and pelvis often compromise the HSC and predispose these elderly patients to myelodysplasia.

Because of these reasons, systematic evaluation of dose-intensive therapy was not performed until McElwain and Powles from Royal Marsden reported on the marked antitumor activity of high-dose melphalan at 140 mg/m² in nine patients with high-risk, newly diagnosed (n = 5) or refractory myeloma.[32] Several investigators have subsequently shown that melphalan induced CR even in alkylating agent-resistant disease and established for the first time that relative drug resistance to alkylating agents could be overcome by dose escalation in myeloma.[33–40] A dose relationship has been observed for overall and CR rates as the IV dose of melphalan was increased from 100–200 mg/m² to

TABLE 8–2. DOSE INTENSITY IN REFRACTORY MYELOMA

	N	% ED	% CR	MEDIAN OS (MONTHS)
Melphalan 200 × 2	198	4	19	29
Melphalan 140 + TBI	18	28	11	14
Melphalan 100 × 1	47	19	6	7
		0.0001	0.09	0.0006

CR, complete remission; OS, overall survival; TBI, total body irradiation; ED, early death.

400 mg/m² (the latter administered in two cycles) or to 140 mg/m² with TBI (Table 8–2).

NEWLY DIAGNOSED DISEASE

TOTAL THERAPY

Investigators at the University of Arkansas designed a "total therapy" protocol for all newly diagnosed symptomatic MM in patients 70 years or younger.[41] The study was an intensive remission induction followed by tandem transplants and subsequent IFN-α maintenance (treatment schema in Fig. 8–1). The primary objective of the study was to increase the CR rate and thereby improve disease-free survival (DFS) and overall survival (OS). VAD chemotherapy induces rapid tumor cytoreduction, requires no dose alteration for renal impairment, and has no HSC toxicity. High-dose cyclophosphamide followed by sargramostim (granulocyte macrophage colony-stimulating factor, or GM-CSF) was employed for its antitumor effect as well as for HSC mobilization. Adequate HSC to support at least two transplants were collected. EDAP (etoposide, dexamethasone, cytosine arabinoside, cisplatin) is an effective treatment for patients presenting with elevated lactate dehydrogenase or plasmablastic features.[42] This was followed by first high-dose chemotherapy (HDCT) with melphalan at 200 mg/m² and HSC rescue. Between 3 and 6 months later, responding patients received a second autotransplant with the same regimen. Patients who did not achieve a partial remission received a second autotransplant with melphalan at 140 mg/m² and TBI.

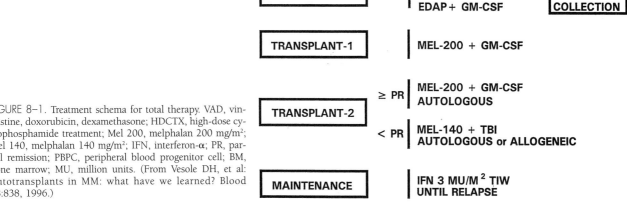

FIGURE 8–1. Treatment schema for total therapy. VAD, vincristine, doxorubicin, dexamethasone; HDCTX, high-dose cyclophosphamide treatment; Mel 200, melphalan 200 mg/m²; Mel 140, melphalan 140 mg/m²; IFN, interferon-α; PR, partial remission; PBPC, peripheral blood progenitor cell; BM, bone marrow; MU, million units. (From Vesole DH, et al: Autotransplants in MM: what have we learned? Blood 88:838, 1996.)

IFN-α maintenance was offered to all patients. Patients younger than 56 years in whom the first autotransplant failed (less than partial remission [PR]) and had matched sibling donors received allogeneic transplants.

Total therapy was administered to 231 patients with newly diagnosed symptomatic MM. Median age was 51 years (range, 26–71 years), and 50 patients were 60 years or older. Over half the patients had Durie-Salmon stage III disease, 30% had β_2-microglobulin levels exceeding 3 mg/L, and 9% had impaired renal function (creatinine >2 mg/dL). Ninety percent of patients participating in the study completed induction chemotherapy, 84% received one and 71% received two transplants. The CR rate progressively increased from 5% after VAD, to 17% at the end of induction chemotherapy, to 30% after completion of first transplantation, and to 41% at the end of two transplantations. Using an intent-to-treat approach to account for all 231 patients, the actuarial 5-year median event-free survival (EFS) and OS times were 42 and 58 months, respectively. The transplant-related mortality rate was 1% with the first autotransplant and 4% after the second transplant.[43] Actuarial survival curves are shown in Figure 8–2.

PAIR-MATE ANALYSIS

The results of total therapy were compared with the outcome of untreated patients receiving standard therapy according to Southwest Oncology Group (SWOG) trials (Fig. 8–3): 124 pair mates were selected from both total therapy and among 1123 SWOG patients to match for the three major prognostic features recognized on SWOG trials (age, β_2-microglobulin, and creatinine). With the intent-to-treat approach, total therapy was superior to standard treatment with a higher PR rate of 85% versus 52% ($P = .0001$) and longer median duration of EFS (49 vs. 20 months, $P = .0001$) and OS (62+ vs. 46 months, $P = .003$), with projected 5-year rates of EFS of 36% versus 20% and OS of 59% versus 42%.[44]

RANDOMIZED TRIALS

The French Intergroup for Myeloma (the Intergroupe Francais du Myelome) were the first to report a prospective, randomized clinical trial comparing autologous bone marrow transplantation as a part of initial therapy to standard chemotherapy alone.[45] Schema of this trial is shown in Figure 8–4. Two hundred previously untreated patients with MM who were less than 65 years of age and who had Durie-Salmon stage II or III disease were randomly assigned at the time of diagnosis to receive either conventional chemotherapy with VMCP (vincristine, melphalan, cyclophosphamide, prednisone)/VBAP (vincristine, carmustine, doxorubicin, prednisone) or HDCT with melphalan, 140 mg/m², and TBI, 800 cGy. Autologous marrow was collected after four cycles of induction with VMCP/VBAP. Plasma cell infiltration of marrow up to 30% was allowed at the time of harvest. Only 74% of patients randomized to the HDCT arm received a transplant because of inadequate response to the first four cycles of VMCP/VBAP. Analysis of the data by an intent-to-treat approach accounting for all 200 patients showed that the HDCT arm resulted in a significantly higher CR rate (22% vs. 5%), EFS rate (28% vs. 10% at 5 years), and OS rate (52% vs. 12% at 5 years) compared with the standard therapy arm.[45]

Fermand et al. examined the question of whether high-dose therapy at the time of progression was as effective as when used early in the disease process.[46] They found that overall survival was similar between those undergoing transplantation early and later at the time of progression. Patients treated early with high-dose therapy, however, experienced significantly longer periods of time symptom-free and off chemotherapy compared with those receiving transplants later.

SUMMARY OF MULTIPLE TRIALS

Table 8–3 summarizes seven large studies conducted predominantly among patients with recently diagnosed dis-

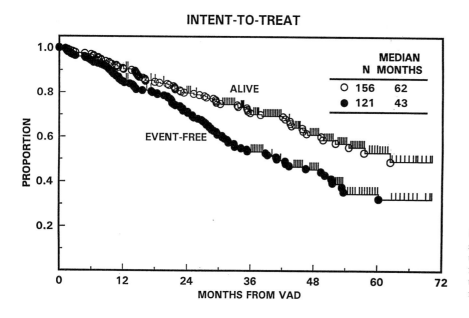

FIGURE 8–2. Overall survival and event-free survival curves for all 231 patients on an intent-to-treat basis; 156 patients are alive for a median survival of 62 months, and 121 patients are alive and free of progression for a median event-free survival of 43 months.

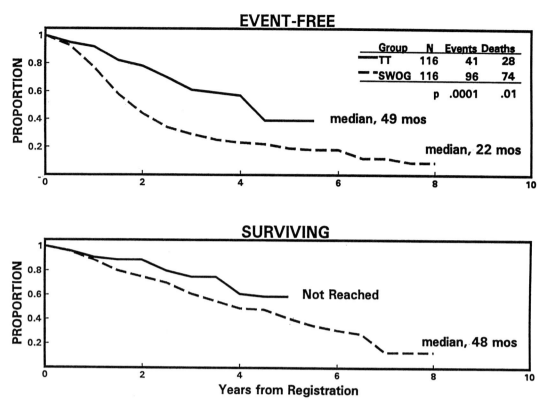

FIGURE 8–3. Survival curves for the 116 pair-mates treated either on standard Southwest Oncology Group trials (*dashed lines*) or total therapy (*solid lines*). (From Barlogie B, et al: Superiority of tandem autologous transplantation over standard therapy for previously untreated MM. Blood 89:789, 1997.)

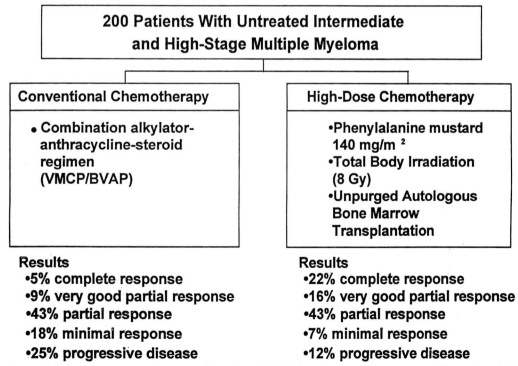

FIGURE 8–4. Schema of the French Intergroup Phase III randomized trial of high-dose therapy versus conventional therapy (1995). (From Attal M, et al: A prospective, randomized trial of autologous bone marrow transplantation and chemotherapy in MM. N Engl J Med 335:91, 1996.)

TABLE 8-3. SUMMARY OF AUTOTRANSPLANTATION IN MULTIPLE MYELOMA

AUTHORS	CHEMOSENSITIVE	NO. OF PATIENTS	REGIMEN	% ED	% CR	MEDIAN SURVIVAL
Cunningham et al., 1994[47]	Yes	53	Mel 200	2%	75%	63% at 5 yr
Anderson et al., 1993[48]	Yes	52	Mel + TBI	2%	40%	4.2 yr
Schiller et al., 1995[49]	Yes	51	Bu-Cy			4.8 yr
Attal et al., 1992[50]	Yes	35	Mel ± TBI	3%	43%	81% at 3.5 yr
Bensinger et al., 1996[51]	Resistant 65%	64	Bu-Cy TBI + Bu-Cy Bu Mel TBI	24%	30%	3 yr
Fermand et al., 1993[52]	Resistant 70%	63	BEMC + TBI	11%	20%	5 yr
Harousseau et al., 1995[53]	Resistant 23%	133	Mel ± TBI	4%	37%	4 yr
EBMTR, 1995[54]		207	Mel ± TBI	4%	46%	2.7 yr

CR, complete remission; Mel, melphalan; TBI, total body irradiation; Bu-Cy, busulfan/cyclophosphamide; BEMC, carmustine, etoposide, melphalan, cyclophosphamide; ED, early death.

ease.[47–54] Collectively, these trials demonstrate that the treatment-related mortality (TRM) rate can drop to below 5%, CR rates increase from about 5% with standard therapy to about 40% with myeloablative therapy, and median duration of EFS and OS exceed 3 and 5 years, respectively, depending on patient selection and treatment regimens employed.

HEMATOPOIETIC STEM CELL PROCUREMENT

Peripheral blood progenitor cells (PBPC) supplanted marrow as the source of HSC in the nineties. Chemotherapy and/or cytokine-mobilized PBPC provided significantly faster granulocyte and platelet recoveries to critical levels than did bone marrow autografts (Fig. 8–5). As a result, the TRM rate has declined from a range of 10–15% to less than 2%.[55, 56] PBPC collection lends itself easily to collection of a preset goal of CD34+ cells. There is a highly significant correlation between the number of CD34+ cells/kg body weight infused and prompt recovery of both granulocytes and platelets. The threshold dose for CD34+ cells necessary for prompt engraftment is greater than or equal to 2×10^6/kg; however, patients with more-extensive prior therapy required more ($\geq 5 \times 10^6$/kg CD34+ cells).[57, 58] Such quantities of HSC were easily collected in the large majority of patients with limited prior therapy (85%) compared with only 52% of patients with more than 24 months of prior chemotherapy (Fig. 8–6). Therefore, it is important to harvest PBPC early in the course of the treatment. Mobilization of progenitor cells with filgrastim (granulocyte

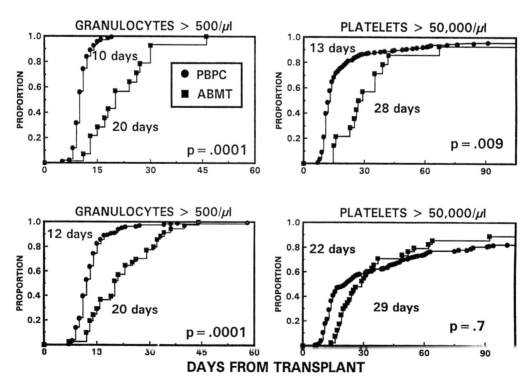

FIGURE 8–5. Hematologic recovery after bone marrow transplant (■) or peripheral blood progenitor cell transplant (●). *Top panels,* Patients with ≤12 months of prior therapy are shown; *Bottom panels,* patients who had received >12 months of prior therapy are shown.

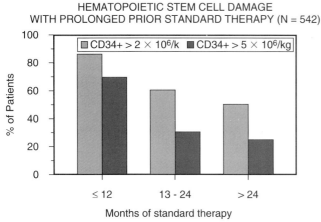

HEMATOPOIETIC STEM CELL DAMAGE
WITH PROLONGED PRIOR STANDARD THERAPY (N = 542)

FIGURE 8–6. Stem cell damage as measured by ability to collect adequate CD34+ cells by leukapheresis in 542 patients. Adequate stem cells to support at least one transplant (CD34+ > 2 × 10⁶/kg body weight) could be obtained in 50% of patients with >12 months of prior therapy, but enough stem cells to support two transplants (CD34+ > 5 × 10⁶/kg body weight) could be obtained in only 20% of patients.

colony-stimulating factor, or G-CSF) alone is easily accomplished with fewer side effects and discomfort to the patient and is cost effective. Minimally treated patients with extensive marrow disease, however, may benefit from tumor cytoreduction along with stem cell mobilization with cyclophosphamide.[59]

CD34+ SELECTION/TUMOR CELL CONTAMINATION

Tumor cell contamination of marrow harvest is expected even when marrow is harvested in remission. Marrow contamination of up to 30% of plasma cells has been allowed at the time of the harvest, especially with relapsed or refractory disease. No adverse clinical outcome in either remission duration or OS could be attributed to reinfusion of visibly contaminated marrow cells.[45, 55] Gene marking studies of autologous bone marrow by Brenner et al., however, have clearly indicated that reinfused tumor cells can contribute to relapse.[60]

PBPC harvests have fewer clonal B cells (using CDRIII-PCR technology) than marrow harvests.[61] Several groups have shown that the process of PBPC mobilization with chemotherapy and growth factor also results in tumor cell mobilization.[62, 63] It is conceivable that circulating clonal B cells represent the immature proliferative compartment of myeloma tumor cells as opposed to the predominantly mature plasma cell noted in the bone marrow.[64, 65] Gazitt et al. showed that there was differential mobilization of HSC and tumor cells after high-dose cyclophosphamide.[62] CD34+ cells were detected in higher frequency during the early phase of recovery from cytosine arabinoside when the white blood cell (WBC) count had reached 500/mm³, whereas plasma cells were mobilized in greater numbers later when the WBC count had already reached 5000/mm³.[62] Thus, even without purging techniques, tumor cell contamination of the PBPC product can be minimized if PBPC collection can be completed within the first 2 days, which is facilitated by large-volume leukapheresis.

It is possible to remove tumor cells from the transplant either by enrichment of CD34+ HSC or by depletion of tumor cells. Because a substantial number of patients do not achieve CR after an autotransplant, it is unlikely that in vitro manipulation of the HSC product alone would result in long-term disease control in MM. Preliminary results to date indicate that there is no substantial difference in the relapse pattern of the disease after tumor cell purging, indicating that the major reason for failure is the inadequacy of HDCT to eradicate MM in the patient.[48, 49, 63]

RENAL FAILURE

Renal failure occurs in half of patients with MM at some time during the course of their illness,[31] adversely affecting their life expectancy and quality of life.[66–69] These patients are excluded from intensive therapy trials. In 1996, Tricot et al. demonstrated comparable pharmacokinetics of high-dose IV melphalan regardless of renal function, thus justifying the administration of this key agent to patients with impaired renal failure.[70] Indeed, dialysis-dependent patients have been successfully treated with high-dose melphalan and HSC rescue without undue morbidity or mortality.[71]

PREVIOUSLY TREATED PATIENTS

Standard chemotherapy induces objective response in 40%, partial response in 20%, stable disease in 30%, and progressive disease in 10% of patients.[25] Thus, approximately 60% of patients respond to initial standard chemotherapy. Responding patients have a median life expectancy of 4 years from the start of chemotherapy. Those who do not respond to initial chemotherapy survive approximately 1 year with subsequent salvage chemotherapy and palliative radiation.[72] Salvage therapy with VAD or glucocorticoids induces responses in one third of these patients, seldom complete, resulting in a response duration of 1 year and OS time of 14 months. Patients in whom both alkylating agents and VAD fail have a short median survival time of less than 1 year.[73]

AUTOTRANSPLANTATION FOR RECURRENT OR REFRACTORY MYELOMA

HDCT was first explored among previously treated myeloma patients. Barlogie et al. performed a series of dose-escalation studies of melphalan in previously treated patients with myeloma over a period of 15 years.[33, 35, 37, 55] A summary of their experience in 135 patients with refractory myeloma was reviewed by Vesole et al. (see Table 8–2).[74] Melphalan at doses of 90–100 mg/m² without HSC rescue was given to 47 patients; 21 patients received TBI (850 cGy) with either melphalan or thiotepa and autologous bone marrow transplantation. More recently, 67 patients with refractory disease were offered a tandem (double) transplant approach with marrow and/or PBPC rescue and growth factor support (G-CSF or GM-CSF): 42 of 67 patients received the intended two transplants. There was a progressive increase in the CR, EFS, and OS with increasing dose intensity (see Table 8–2). Patients achieving CR experience improved quality of life with absence of bone pain and improvement in the performance status. Therefore, HDCT can and should be made available for patients with recurrent myeloma.

Patients with refractory myeloma benefit from early intervention with myeloablative therapy.[74, 75] In a group of patients with MM refractory to standard therapy, 109 patients with primary unresponsive disease experienced superior EFS (23 vs. 14 months, $P = .002$) and OS (39 vs. 25 months, $P = .008$) compared with 69 patients with resistant relapse.[76] Intensive treatment, however, has only limited value in the control of disease when it has become refractory to prolonged exposure to chemotherapy beyond a year.[77]

PROGNOSTIC FACTORS

In order to determine who benefits most from HDCT, over a dozen pretransplantation variables pertinent to disease and host parameters were examined in 550 patients entered on tandem transplant trials at the University of Arkansas.[76] The risk factors that predict for survival outcome after standard therapy also predict for outcome after transplantation (Fig. 8–7). These include serum values of β_2-microglobulin level, C-reactive protein, creatinine, albumin, and lactate dehydrogenase, as well as chemotherapy responsiveness, duration of prior therapy, disease stage, immuno-

globulin isotype, and marrow plasmacytosis. In addition, similar to the case with leukemia and lymphoma, tumor cytogenetics plays a pivotal role in defining the prognosis. The karyotypic abnormality in myeloma is often complex; however, presence of a translocation, a deletion of chromosome 13 or 13q, or an abnormality involving the long arm of chromosome 11 portend a very poor outcome and are considered to be unfavorable karyotypes. On a multivariate Cox regression analysis, favorable karyotype, β_2-microglobulin as a reflector of tumor burden, C-reactive protein reflecting interleukin-6 cytokine activity, and duration of prior chemotherapy reflecting drug resistance were the four critical and independent prognostic variables determining the duration of EFS and OS (Table 8–4). Using β_2-microglobulin, duration of prior chemotherapy, and cytogenetics, three risk categories could be clearly discerned with markedly different remission duration and survival outcome. Surprisingly, age and renal function were unimportant. Further analysis of carefully matched patients according to the aforementioned critical variables revealed no significant difference, especially in OS among patients under 65 years of age versus those 65 years and older.[78]

MYELODYSPLASIA/SECONDARY LEUKEMIA

An increased risk of acute leukemia and myelodysplasia has been reported in patients with myeloma.[27, 79] Treatment with leukemogenic agents (alkylating agents and radiation)

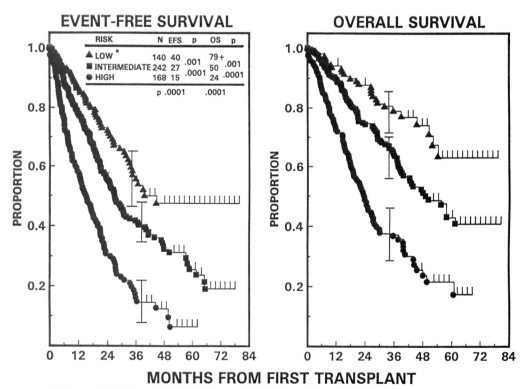

FIGURE 8–7. The overall and event-free survival curves for 550 patients receiving tandem transplants are presented on an intent-to-treat basis by risk categories; 78% of the patients actually received the intended second transplant. All three favorable risk factors, namely β_2-microglobulin <2.5 mg/L, less than 12 months of prior therapy before first transplantation and favorable cytogenetics (see text) constituted low risk; any one unfavorable risk factor resulted in intermediate risk; two or all three unfavorable risk factors was categorized as high risk. (From Vesole DH, et al: Autotransplants in MM: what have we learned? Blood 88:838, 1996.)

TABLE 8-4. TANDEM TRANSPLANTATION FOR MYELOMA (N = 550): MULTIVARIATE ANALYSIS

EVENT-FREE SURVIVAL	P	OVERALL SURVIVAL	P
Favorable cytogenetics	.0001	Favorable cytogenetics	.0001
≤12 months of prior therapy	.0001	β_2-microglobulin ≤2.5 mg/L	.0001
β_2-microglobulin ≤2.5 mg/L	.0001	Sensitive disease	.0001
C-reactive protein ≤4.0 mg/L	.0009	C-reactive protein ≤4.0 mg/L	.0004
Sensitive disease	.01	≤12 months of prior therapy	.005
Non-IgA isotype	.03	Non-IgA isotype	.04

perhaps contributes to the high actuarial risk of leukemia—17% at 4 years.[27] The occurrence of acute leukemia even before the start of therapy would indicate that this is perhaps a part of the natural history of this disease.[80] Similarly, myelodysplasia has been reported after high-dose melphalan and autotransplantation.[81] These data suggest that avoidance of HSC-damaging chemotherapy prior to transplantation is the key to preventing secondary hematologic malignancies after autotransplantation.

ALLOGENEIC TRANSPLANTATION

Allogeneic transplants offer the advantage of lack of tumor cell contamination as well as a graft-versus-myeloma effect.[82] The report from the European Blood and Marrow Transplant Registry summarizing the allotransplant experience in Europe over a decade indicates a long-term survival rate of 30% at 8 years.[83] Patients who achieved CR after allotransplantation had the best outcome, with a 32% EFS rate at 7 years. Even so, the first-year mortality rate of greater than 40% and late relapses beyond 5 years have limited the role of allotransplantation in this patient population with a median age well over 40 years. Single-center results have not been any better, as noted by the recent results from Fred Hutchinson Cancer Research Center in 80 patients conditioned with busulfan and cyclophosphamide (n = 57) or modified TBI (n = 23); TRM occurred in 35 patients within 100 days, and the EFS rate was only 20% at 4 years.[84] Pair-mate analysis of allotransplants and autotransplants showed a superior EFS and OS for patients undergoing autotransplantation, mainly due to a considerably higher mortality rate with allotransplants within the first 100 days (25% compared with 2%).[85, 86] Matched sibling transplants should be the treatment of choice for patients younger than 60 years presenting with unfavorable karyotypes.

CONCLUSION AND FUTURE DIRECTIONS

Progress in myeloma therapy has been achieved at last through pursuit of the "more is better" concept aiming at more-marked tumor cytoreduction in order to increase the incidence of CR, including molecular CR, as a first step

toward cure.[87] The demonstration of certain cytogenetic abnormalities conferring poor outcome along with standard variables such as β_2-microglobulin and C-reactive protein affords a risk-oriented treatment. It is conceivable that autograft decontamination of tumor cells through either positive selection or removal of tumor cells by monoclonal antibodies and/or cytotoxic agents will only benefit the group in whom marked and sustained reduction in tumor burden can be achieved through HDCT alone and in whom tumor cell reinfusion may become clinically relevant. Posttransplantation immune modulation may be important for both good-risk and poor-risk patients. This can be accomplished with the help of idiotype vaccination or, more recently, the dendritic cell vaccination program.[88, 89] A 1990 report of the significant antimyeloma activity of thalidomide in patients with residual or relapsed disease after high-dose therapy is of interest.[90] It is likely that this observation will lead to adjuvant use of thalidomide after high-dose therapy.

The safety of allogeneic transplantation needs to be improved so that patients with MM can benefit from a graft-versus-myeloma effect. This may be accomplished by T-cell depletion to reduce the incidence and severity of graft-versus-host disease (GVHD); in order to elicit a graft-versus-myeloma effect, a fixed dose of thymidine kinase gene-transduced donor T cells can be administered upon completion of hematopoietic engraftment. These cells can be eliminated by administration of ganciclovir in cases of severe GVHD.

With the increasing incidence of myeloma, patients and physicians alike can be expected to look toward a treatment approach with curative intent rather than a palliative approach. The management of myeloma has improved enough in recent years, incorporating safe and effective intensive therapy approaches, that it is conceivable that 20–30% of patients with MM can be expected to be alive at 10 years.

REFERENCES

1. Riedel DA, Pottern LM: The epidemiology of multiple myeloma. Hematol Oncol Clin North Am 6:225, 1992.
2. Kyle RA: Multiple myeloma: review of 869 cases. Mayo Clin Proc 50:29, 1975.
3. Rabkin CS, Silverman S, Tricot G, et al: The National Cancer Institute Silicone Implant/Multiple Myeloma Registry. Curr Top Microbiol Immunol 210:385, 1996.
4. Kyle RA: Monoclonal gammopathy of undetermined significance. Am J Med 64:814, 1978.
5. Alexanian R: Localized and indolent myeloma. Blood 56:521, 1980.
6. Kyle RA, Greipp PR: Smoldering multiple myeloma. N Engl J Med 302:1347, 1980.
7. Witzig TE, Gonchoroff NH, Katzmann JA, et al: Peripheral blood B cell labeling indices are a measure of disease activity in patients with monoclonal gammopathies. J Clin Oncol 6:1041, 1988.
8. Dimopoulos MA, Moulopoulos A, Delasalle K, Alexanian R: Solitary plasmacytoma of bone and asymptomatic MM. Hematol Oncol Clin North Am 6:359, 1992.
9. Dimopoulos MA, Goldstein J, Fuller L, et al: Curability of solitary bone plasmacytoma. J Clin Oncol 10:587, 1992.
10. Galieni P, Cavo M, Avvisati G, et al: Solitary plasmacytoma of bone and extramedullary plasmacytoma: two different entities? Ann Oncol 6:687, 1995.
11. Bolek TW, Marcus RB, Mendenhall NP: Solitary plasmacytoma of bone and soft tissue. Int J Radiat Oncol Biol Phys 36:329, 1996.
12. Moulopoulos LA, Dimopoulos MA, Weber D, et al: Magnetic reso-

nance imaging in the staging of solitary plasmacytoma of bone. J Clin Oncol 11:1311, 1993.

13. Woolfenden JM, Pitto MJ, Durie BGM, et al: Comparison of bone scintigraphy and radiography in MM. Radiology 134:723, 1980.

14. Durie BGM, Salmon SE: A clinical staging system for MM. Cancer 36:842, 1975.

15. Bataille R, Boccadoro M, Klein B, et al: C-Reactive protein and beta-2 microglobulin produce a simple and powerful myeloma staging system. Blood 80:733, 1992.

16. Moulopoulos LA, Dimopoulos MA, Smith TL, et al: Prognostic significance of magnetic resonance imaging in patients with asymptomatic MM. J Clin Oncol 13:251, 1995.

17. Kyle RA: "Benign" monoclonal gammapathy: after 20 to 35 years of follow-up. Mayo Clin Proc 68:26, 1993.

18. Feinleib M, MacMahon B: Duration of survival in MM. J Natl Cancer Inst 24:1259, 1960.

19. Holland JR, Hosley H, Scharlau C, et al: A controlled trial of urethane treatment in MM. Blood 27(3):328–342, 1966.

20. Bergsagel DE, Sprague CC, Austin C, Griffith KM: Evaluation of new chemotherapeutic agents in the treatment of MM. Cancer Chemother Rep 21:87, 1962.

21. Alexanian R, Haut A, Khan AU, et al: Treatment for MM: combination chemotherapy with different melphalan dose regimens. JAMA 208:1680, 1969.

22. Alexanian R, Dimopoulos M: The treatment of MM. N Engl J Med 330:484, 1994.

23. Samson D, Newland A, Kearney J, et al: Infusion of vincristine and doxorubicin with oral dexamethasone as first-line therapy for MM. Lancet 2:882, 1989.

24. Alexanian R, Barlogie B, Tucker S: VAD-based regimens as primary treatment for MM. Am J Hematol 33:86, 1990.

25. Salmon SE, Crowley JJ, Grogan TM, et al: Combination chemotherapy, glucocorticoids, and interferon alfa in the treatment of multiple myeloma: a Southwest Oncology Group study [see comments]. J Clin Oncol 12:2405, 1994.

26. Belch A, Shelley W, Bergsagel D, et al: A randomized trial of maintenance versus no maintenance melphalan and prednisone in responding MM patients. Br J Cancer 57:94, 1988.

27. Bergsagel DE, Bailey AJ, Langley R, et al: The chemotherapy of plasma-cell myeloma and the incidence of acute leukemia. N Engl J Med 301:743, 1979.

28. Ludwig H, Cohen AM, Polliack A, et al: Interferon-alpha for induction and maintenance in MM: results of two multicenter randomized trials and summary of other studies. Ann Oncol 6:467, 1995.

29. Kampmeier P, Spielberger R, Dickstein J, et al: Increased incidence of second neoplasms in patients treated with interferon alpha 2b for hairy cell leukemia: a clinicopathologic assessment [see comments]. Blood 83:2931, 1994.

30. Sangfelt O, Osterborg A, Grander D, et al: Response to interferon therapy in patients with MM correlates with expression of the Bcl-2 oncoprotein. Int J Cancer 63:190, 1995.

31. Kyle RA: Monoclonal proteins and renal disease. Annu Rev Med 45:71, 1994.

32. McElwain TJ, Powles RL: High-dose intravenous melphalan for plasma-cell leukemia and myeloma. Lancet 1:822, 1983.

33. Barlogie B, Hall R, Zander A, et al: High-dose melphalan with autologous bone marrow transplantation for multiple myeloma. Blood 67:1298, 1986.

34. Selby P, McElwain TJ, Nandi AC, et al: MM treated with high dose intravenous melphalan. Br J Haematol 66:55, 1987.

35. Barlogie B, Alexanian R, Dicke KA, et al: High-dose chemoradiotherapy and autologous bone marrow transplantation for resistant MM. Blood 70:869, 1987.

36. Harousseau JL, Milpied N, Garand R, Bourhis JH: High dose melphalan and autologous bone marrow transplantation in high-risk myeloma [Letter]. Br J Haematol 67:493, 1987.

37. Barlogie B, Alexanian R, Smallwood L, et al: Prognostic factors with high-dose melphalan for refractory multiple myeloma. Blood 72:2015, 1988.

38. Fermand JP, Levy Y, Gerota J, et al: Treatment of aggressive MM by high-dose chemotherapy and total body irradiation followed by blood stem cells autologous graft. Blood 73:20, 1989.

39. Gore ME, Selby PJ, Viner C, et al: Intensive treatment of MM and criteria for complete remission [see comments]. Lancet 2:879, 1989.

40. Reiffers J, Marit G, Boiron JM: Autologous blood stem cell transplanta-

tion in high-risk multiple myeloma [Letter]. Br J Haematol 72:296, 1989.

41. Jagannath S, Vesole DH, Tricot G, et al: Hemopoietic stem cell transplants for MM. Oncology 8:89, 1994.

42. Barlogie B, Velasquez WS, Alexanian R, Cabanillas F: Etoposide, dexamethasone, cytarabine, cisplatin in vincristine, doxorubicin, and dexamethasone–refractory myeloma. J Clin Oncol 7:1514, 1989.

43. Barlogie B, Jagannath S, Desikan KR, et al: Total therapy with tandem transplants for newly diagnosed multiple myeloma. Blood 93(1):55–65, 1999.

44. Barlogie B, Jagannath S, Vesole DH, et al: Superiority of tandem autologous transplantation over standard therapy for previously untreated MM. Blood 89:789, 1997.

45. Attal M, Harousseau JL, Stoppa AM, et al: A prospective, randomized trial of autologous bone marrow transplantation and chemotherapy in MM. Intergroupe Francais du Myelome. N Engl J Med 335:91, 1996.

46. Fermand JP, Ravaud P, Chevret S, et al: High-dose therapy and autologous peripheral blood stem cell transplantation in multiple myeloma: up-front or rescue treatment? Results of a multicenter sequential randomized clinical trial. Blood 92(9):3131–3136, 1998.

47. Cunningham D, Paz-Ares L, Milan S, et al: High-dose melphalan and autologous bone marrow transplantation as consolidation in previously untreated myeloma. J Clin Oncol 12:759, 1994.

48. Anderson KC, Andersen J, Soiffer R, et al: Monoclonal antibody-purged bone marrow transplantation therapy for MM. Blood 82:2568, 1993.

49. Schiller G, Vescio R, Freytes C, et al: Transplantation of CD34$^+$ peripheral blood progenitor cells after high-dose chemotherapy for patients with advanced MM. Blood 86:390, 1995.

50. Attal M, Huguet F, Schlaifer D, et al: Intensive combined therapy for previously untreated aggressive myeloma. Blood 79:1130, 1992.

51. Bensinger WI, Rowley SD, Demirer T, et al: High-dose therapy followed by autologous hematopoietic stem-cell infusion for patients with MM. J Clin Oncol 14:1447, 1996.

52. Fermand JP, Chevret S, Ravaud P, et al: High-dose chemoradiotherapy and autologous blood stem cell transplantation in MM: results of a phase III trial involving 63 patients. Blood 82:2005, 1993.

53. Harousseau JL, Attal M, Divine M, et al: Autologous stem cell transplantation after first remission induction treatment in MM: a report of the French Registry on Autologous Transplantation in MM. Blood 85:3077, 1995.

54. Bjorkstrand B, Ljungman P, Bird JM, et al: Autologous stem cell transplantation in multiple myeloma: results of the European Group for Bone Marrow Transplantation. Stem Cells 13:140, 1995.

55. Jagannath S, Barlogie B, Dicke K, et al: Autologous bone marrow transplantation in MM: identification of prognostic factors. Blood 76:1860, 1990.

56. Jagannath S, Vesole DH, Glenn L, et al: Low-risk intensive therapy for MM with combined autologous bone marrow and blood stem cell support. Blood 80:1666, 1992.

57. Tricot G, Jagannath S, Vesole D, et al: Peripheral blood stem cell transplants for MM: identification of favorable variables for rapid engraftment in 225 patients. Blood 85:588, 1995.

58. Prince HM, Imrie K, Sutherland DR, et al: Peripheral blood progenitor cell collections in multiple myeloma: predictors and management of inadequate collections. Br J Haematol 93:142, 1996.

59. Desikan KR, Jagannath S, Siegel D, et al: Post-transplant engraftment kinetics and toxicities in MM patients are comparable following mobilization of PBSC with G-CSF with or without high-dose cyclophosphamide. Blood 88:679a, 1996.

60. Brenner MK, Rill DR, Moen RC, et al: Gene-marking to trace origin of relapse after autologous bone-marrow transplantation. Lancet 341:85, 1993.

61. Henry JM, Sykes PJ, Brisco MJ, et al: Comparison of myeloma cell contamination of bone marrow and peripheral blood stem cell harvests. Br J Haematol 92:614, 1996.

62. Gazitt Y, Tian E, Barlogie B, et al: Differential mobilization of myeloma cells and normal hematopoietic stem cells in MM after treatment with cyclophosphamide and granulocyte-macrophage colony-stimulating factor. Blood 87:805, 1996.

63. Lemoli RM, Fortuna A, Motta MR, et al: Concomitant mobilization of plasma cells and hematopoietic progenitors into peripheral blood of MM patients: positive selection and transplantation of enriched CD34 + cells to remove circulating tumor cells. Blood 87:1625, 1996.

64. Billadeau D, Quam L, Thomas W, et al: Detection and quantitation

of malignant cells in the peripheral blood of MM patients. Blood 80:1818, 1992.

65. Bergsagel PL, Smith AM, Szczepek A, et al: In multiple myeloma, clonotypic B lymphocytes are detectable among CD19+ peripheral blood cells expressing CD38, CD56, and monotypic Ig light chain [published erratum appears in Blood 1995 Jun 1; 85(11):3365]. Blood 85(2):436–447, 1995.

66. Bataille R, Durie BGM, Grenier J, Sany J: Prognostic factors and staging in multiple myeloma: a reappraisal. J Clin Oncol 4(1):80–87, 1986.

67. Durie BGM, Stock-Novack D, Salmon SE, et al: Prognostic value of pretreatment serum 02 microglobulin in myeloma: a Southwest Oncology Group Study. Blood 75:823, 1990.

68. Blade J, Lopez-Guillermo A, Bosch F, et al: Impact of response to treatment on survival in MM: results in a series of 243 patients. Br J Haematol 88:117, 1994.

69. Torra R, Blade J, Cases A, et al: Patients with MM requiring long-term dialysis: presenting features, response to therapy, and outcome in a series of 20 cases. Br J Haematol 91:854, 1995.

70. Tricot G, Alberts DS, Johnson C, et al: Safety of autotransplants with high-dose melphalan in renal failure: a pharmacokinetic and toxicity study. Clin Cancer Res 2:947, 1996.

71. Jagannath S, Barlogie B, Vesole D: Autotransplants can be performed safely in MM patients with renal insufficiency. Blood 86:809a, 1995.

72. Dalton WS, Salmon SE: Drug resistance in myeloma: mechanisms and approaches to circumvention. Hematol Oncol Clin North Am 6:383, 1992.

73. Barlogie B, Smith L, Alexanian R: Effective treatment of advanced MM refractory to alkylating agents. N Engl J Med 310:1353, 1984.

74. Vesole DH, Barlogie B, Jagannath S, et al: High-dose therapy for refractory MM: improved prognosis with better supportive care and double transplants. Blood 84:950, 1994.

75. Alexanian R, Dimopoulos MA, Hester J, et al: Early myeloablative therapy for MM. Blood 84:4278, 1994.

76. Vesole DH, Tricot G, Jagannath S, et al: Autotransplants in MM: what have we learned? Blood 88:838, 1996.

77. Alexanian R, Dimopoulos M, Smith T, et al: Limited value of myeloablative therapy for late MM. Blood 83:512, 1994.

78. Siegel DS, Desikan KR, Mehta J, et al: Age is not a prognostic variable with autotransplants for multiple myeloma. Blood 93(1):51–54, 1999.

79. Rosner F, Grunwald H: MM terminating in acute leukemia: report of 12 cases and review of the literature. Am J Med 57:927, 1974.

80. Cleary B, Binder RA, Kales AN, et al: Simultaneous presentation of acute myelomonocytic leukemia and MM. Cancer 41:1381, 1978.

81. Govindarajan R, Jagannath S, Flick JT, et al: Preceding standard therapy is the likely cause of NMS after autotransplants for MM. Br J Haematol 95:349, 1996.

82. Tricot G, Vesole DH, Jagannath S, et al: Graft-versus-myeloma effect: proof of principle. Blood 87:1196, 1996.

83. Gahrton G, Tura S, Ljungman P, et al: Prognostic factors in allogeneic bone marrow transplantation for MM [see comments]. J Clin Oncol 13:1312, 1995.

84. Bensinger W, Buckner C, Anasetti C, et al: Allogeneic marrow transplantation for MM: an analysis of risk factors on outcome. Blood 88:2787, 1996.

85. Mehta J, Tricot G, Jagannath S, et al: A single-center matched-pair comparison of auto- and allografting in MM. Blood 88:618a, 1996.

86. Bjorkstrand B, Ljungman P, Svensson H, et al: Allogeneic bone marrow transplantation versus autologous stem cell transplantation in multiple myeloma: a retrospective case-matched study from the European group for blood and marrow transplantation. Blood 88:4711, 1996.

87. Bjorkstrand B, Ljungman P, Bird JM, et al: Double high-dose chemoradiotherapy with autologous stem cell transplantation can induce molecular remissions in MM. Bone Marrow Transplant 15:367, 1995.

88. Kwak LW, Taub DD, Duffey PL, et al: Transfer of myeloma idiotype-specific immunity from an actively immunized marrow donor. Lancet 345:1016, 1995.

89. Hsu FJ, Benike C, Fagnoni F, et al: Vaccination of patients with B-cell lymphoma using autologous antigen-pulsed dendritic cells. Nature Med 2:52, 1996.

90. Singhal S, Mehta J, Desikan R, et al: Antitumor activity of thalidomide in refractory multiple myeloma. N Engl J Med 341(21):1565–1571, 1999.

91. Pavlovsky S, Corrado C, Santarelli MT, et al: An update of two randomized trials in previously untreated multiple myeloma comparing melphalan and prednisone versus three- and five-drug combinations: an Argentine Group for the Treatment of Acute Leukemia Study. J Clin Oncol 6:769–775, 1988.

92. Cooper MR, McIntyre OR, Propert KJ, et al: Single, sequential, and multiple alkylating agent therapy for multiple myeloma: a CALGB study. J Clin Oncol 4:1331–1339, 1986.

93. Peest D, Deicher H, Coldewey R, et al: Induction and maintenance therapy in multiple myeloma: a multicenter trial of MP versus VCMP. Eur J Cancer Clin Oncol 24:1061–1067, 1988.

94. Boccadoro M, Marmont F, Tribalto M, et al: Multiple myeloma: VMCP/VBAP alternating combination chemotherapy is not superior to melphalan and prednisone even in high-risk patients. J Clin Oncol 9:444–448, 1991.

CHAPTER NINE

Chronic Lymphocytic Leukemia

Mauricette Michallet, M.D., Ph.D.

Chronic lymphocytic leukemia (CLL) is the most prevalent adult leukemia in North America and Europe. Although CLL is usually a disease of the elderly, it is being diagnosed with increasing frequency in younger people. A recent report indicates that about 10% of patients are less than 50 years of age.[1] Current conventional chemotherapy is not curative and hence can be considered inappropriate as sole therapy for younger patients who request a curative therapeutic attempt. Clinical stage, bone marrow histology, blood lymphocyte count, lymphocyte doubling time, and cytogenetics are reliable predictors of patient outcome.[2–6] CLL in younger adults has no major distinctive features, and prognostic factors are not altered by patient age. The median survival is less than 3 years in younger patients with advanced CLL and hence, in such cases, innovative dose-intensive therapy can be justified.[1]

The choice of therapy for advanced-stage CLL remains problematic. Considerable interest and clinical experience has demonstrated the effectiveness of the purine analogues fludarabine, deoxycoformycin, and 2-chlorodeoxyadenosine.[7, 8] Initial treatment with alkylating agents has been standard therapy, although fludarabine can also be considered for first-line treatment.[6] The addition of an anthracycline may improve the response rate, but the median survival time remains less than 4 and 6 years for Binet stages C and B, respectively.[9, 10] Despite a high response rate, there is little evidence that fludarabine alone or in combination with other agents results in cure of a significant proportion of patients so treated. The prognosis of patients failing therapy with fludarabine depends on the extent of prior therapy and other clinical variables.[11] The combination of fludarabine with cyclophosphamide and an anthracycline or the use of 2-chlorodeoxyadenosine may be effective salvage treatment for a patient previously treated with fludarabine.[7] The dismal prognosis in relapsed and refractory patients allows consideration of autologous and allogeneic hematopoietic stem cell therapy (HSCT).

Newer agents alone or in combination with fludarabine may improve the efficacy of conventional-dose chemotherapy but may also provide for an increased therapeutic effect with HSCT. Monoclonal antibodies, such as rituximab (anti-CD20), directed against B-cell antigens, may provide ways of enhancing the therapeutic effect of chemotherapy and also offer attractive ex-vivo purging possibilities.

ALLOGENEIC AND AUTOLOGOUS TRANSPLANTATION IN CLL

The choice of conditioning regimen, type of transplant, and source of hematopoietic stem cells (HSC) are not well defined for patients with CLL who wish to undergo transplantation. However, the feasibility of both autologous and allogeneic HSCT has been convincingly demonstrated in patients with advanced-stage CLL. As in low-grade lymphoma, autologous transplantation for CLL raises the question of the degree to which leukemia cells contaminating the autologous graft contribute to relapse. Allogeneic transplantation may be associated with a graft-versus-leukemia (GVL) effect that is responsible for a reduced relapse rate when compared with autologous transplantation. The relative contribution of leukemia graft contamination to relapse in autologous transplantation and the magnitude of the GVL effect to prevent it in allogeneic HSCT are unknown.

As CLL is a relatively indolent disease, clinical trial design based purely on clinical relapse requires very-long-term follow-up of patients before definitive conclusions can be reached regarding the efficacy of transplantation. For this reason, investigators have looked for surrogate markers of relapse. The immunoglobulin heavy chain locus (IgH) is rearranged in a clonal fashion and can be detected by polymerase chain reaction (PCR) of the CDRIII region. Several investigators have shown that detection of a clonal rearrangement of the IgH locus or detection of clonal B cells by flow cytometry correlates with minimal residual disease (MRD) and subsequent relapse.[12–15] Furthermore, contamination of autologous grafts can be detected in this fashion.

Dreger et al. reported autologous HSCT using chemoradiotherapy and Dexa-BEAM (dexamethasone, BCNU, etoposide, ara-C, melphalan) for HSC mobilization in 18 patients with early- and late-stage CLL.[16] Post-transplant molecular MRD monitoring by PCR amplification of CDRIII rearrangements was performed. The median age was 49 (range 29–61 years), and adverse prognostic factors were present in 16 of 18 patients. HSC harvesting was successful in 14 patients (3 bone marrow and 11 peripheral blood progenitor cells), and all grafts were purged using immunomagnetic procedures (see Chapter 29). No transplant-related mortality (TRM) was reported. MRD monitoring detected three cases of persistent or recurrent disease with one clinical relapse.

Esteve et al. reported on autologous (n = 5) and allogeneic (n = 7) HSCT in 12 patients with high-risk CLL.[17] MRD was assessed by flow cytometry and PCR. In the patients undergoing allogeneic HSCT, two of seven died from TRM, three of seven experienced graft-vs.-host disease (GVHD), and engraftment occurred in all patients. In the patients undergoing autologous HSCT, engraftment occurred in all, and none died of transplant-related causes. After transplantation, the complete remission (CR) rate was 10/11 clinically and 9/11 molecularly. The patient in clinical CR but molecular relapse experienced relapse 9 months after transplant and died. Seven patients remained in molecular CR for a median of 16 months (range 1–58 months). Relapse risk at 2 years was 13%.

Khouri et al. reported 22 patients with advanced CLL who received anti-CD19 monoclonal antibody–purged autologous bone marrow transplantation (BMT) (n = 11) and allogeneic or syngeneic BMT (n = 11).[18] Six of 11 autologous transplant patients survived in remission 2–29 months after BMT. Ten of 11 allogeneic and syngeneic transplant recipients survived 2–36 months after BMT. TRM was minimal (<10%). More recently, the same authors reported 24 allogeneic transplants and 14 autologous transplants in CLL patients.[19] They showed better results after allogeneic transplant than after autologous transplant, with a 3-year survival of 57% and 24%, respectively. Case matching showed superiority of allogeneic and autologous transplant over a variety of conventional therapies.[19] The same group also has shown the feasibility of allogeneic transplant after a nonmyeloablative regimen in this disease.[20]

Michallet et al. reported the outcome of human leukocyte antigen (HLA)-identical sibling BMT for CLL in patients younger than 60 years.[21] Retrospective data from 30 transplant centers worldwide was collected from the European Group for Blood and Marrow Transplantation (EBMTR) and the International Bone Marrow Transplant Registry (IBMTR). Fifty-four patients undergoing transplantation between 1984 and 1992 with a median interval from diagnosis to transplantation of 37 months (range 5–130 months) were included. At the time of transplantation, 3 patients were Rai stage 0, 10 were stage 1, 10 were stage 2, 7 were stage 3, and 22 were stage 4. Thirty-eight patients (70%) achieved hematologic remission post transplantation. Twenty-four (44%) remained alive for a median of 27 months (range 5–80 months) after transplantation. The three patients who received transplants at Rai stage 0 remained alive 21, 32, and 45 months after transplantation. The 3-year stage-specific survival probabilities with confidence intervals were 68% (38–98%), 30% (2–58%), 57% (21–93%), and 34% (12–56%) in Rai stages 1 to 4, respectively. Five patients (9%) died of progressive leukemia and 25 (46%) of treatment-related complications. The authors concluded that allogeneic HSCT can provide extended hematologic remission but that superiority over other forms of therapy is not established.

Pavletic et al. reported on 16 previously treated patients with CLL who were undergoing transplantation using autologous peripheral blood progenitor cell (PBPC) (n = 13) or bone marrow (n = 3) HSC.[22] The median age of the patients was 49 years (range 44–60 years), the median number of prior chemotherapy regimens was two, and disease was responsive to chemotherapy at the time of transplantation. Engraftment occurred in all patients and all achieved CR post transplant. Ten of 16 patients were alive at a median of 41 months (range 22–125 months) and five were disease-free. Eight patients had relapsed, and six had died. The projected 3-year overall survival, failure-free survival, and relapse rates were 68%, 37%, and 56%, respectively. The authors concluded that there was no evidence that autologous transplantation was curative.

Rabinowe et al. reported on 20 patients with poor-prognosis B-cell CLL who underwent high-dose chemoradiotherapy followed by rescue with multiple monoclonal

antibody–purged autologous bone marrow (n = 12) or T cell–depleted allogeneic bone marrow from HLA-identical siblings (n = 8).[23] All had poor-prognosis disease as determined by staging, bone marrow pattern, tumor doubling time criteria, or cytogenetics. All patients responded to treatment before BMT and engrafted fully after transplantation. The toxicity profile was not significantly different between autologous and allogeneic transplant recipients. Two treatment-related deaths were observed. Clinical CR was documented in 17 of 19 patients and confirmed by flow cytometry in 15 of 15 and by IgH gene rearrangement study in 11 of 14. The same authors have recently updated the results of 81 purged autologous transplants and 23 HLA-identical T-depleted allogeneic transplants.[24] In this study, the median overall survival has not been reached and the 4-year overall survival and disease-free survival were 85% and 63% after autologous transplant and 50% and 44% after allogeneic transplant, respectively.

Sutton et al. reported their experience with 20 patients treated with ESHAP (etoposide, Solu-Medrol, high-dose ara-C, Platinol).[25] Only 13 patients responded to ESHAP, and only 8 of 12 patients in whom PBPC collection was attempted had adequate numbers of HSC for autologous HSCT. Six of eight patients who underwent transplantation were alive in CR at a median of 30 months after transplantation. The authors noted that, using their criteria, they were only able to perform transplantation in 40% of the patients entered in their study and argued for collection of HSC in first remission for later use.

Table 9–1 summarizes the autologous and allogeneic transplant experience in CLL. No series of patients undergoing transplantation from unrelated donors has been reported.

We recently updated data on the outcome of allogeneic transplants (n = 88) and autologous transplants (n = 225) from the EBMTR. Among the 188 allogeneic transplants reported to the EBMTR between 1983 and 1998, 157 patients were transplanted from HLA-identical sibling donors, 5 from syngeneic donors, 7 from matched related donors, 5 from mismatched related donors, and 7 from unrelated donors (3 matched, 4 mismatched). The median age was 44 years (range 21–58 years) and there were 143 males and 45 females. The median interval from diagnosis to transplant was 35 months (range 4–171 months). Of 141 evaluable patients, 113 (80%) were considered to have responsive disease at transplant including 40 in CR (28%). Patients were selected for transplant according to separate criteria at individual transplant centers. One hundred fifty-three (81%) received bone marrow as the HSC source, 33 (17%) received allogeneic PBPC recruited by granulocyte colony–stimulating factor (G-CSF), and 2 (23%) received bone marrow and PBPC. Twenty-three patients (12%) received a T-depleted transplant.

Two hundred twenty-five patients receiving autologous transplant for CLL were reported to the EBMTR between 1988 and 1998. There were 179 males and 46 females with a median age of 50 years (range 22–66 years). All patients had received pretransplant therapy and the median interval between diagnosis and transplant was 30 months (range 2–216 months). Of 159 evaluable patients, 111 (70%) were considered to have responsive disease at trans-

TABLE 9–1. RESULTS OF AUTOLOGOUS (AUTO) AND ALLOGENEIC (ALLO) TRANSPLANTATION FOR CHRONIC LYMPHOCYTIC LEUKEMIA

FIRST AUTHOR	NUMBER OF PATIENTS	TYPE OF TRANSPLANT	CONDITIONING REGIMEN	CR	FOLLOW-UP
Dreger[16]	18 (14 E)	AUTO	Cy + TBI	11	13 A
Esteve[17]	12	ALLO AUTO		10	7 CR
Khouri[18]	11	ALLO	Cy + TBI	6	10 A
	11	AUTO	Cy + TBI	2	6 A
Michallet[21]	54	ALLO	Variable	38	24 A
Pavletic[22]	16	AUTO	Cy + TBI ± Ara-C BEAC	16	10 A
Rabinowe[23]	8	ALLO	Cy + TBI	7	7 CR
	12	AUTO	Cy + TBI	11	10 CR
Sutton[25]	20 (8 E)	AUTO			6 A

A, alive; Ara-C, cytosine arabinoside; BEAC, BCNU, etoposide, Ara-C, cyclophosphamide; CR, complete remission; Cy, cyclophosphamide; E, evaluable; TBI, total body irradiation.

plant including 81 in CR (51%). One hundred sixty-four patients received PBPC (73%), 50 BM (22%), and 11 BM and PBPC (5%). Seventy-four patients (33%) received a purged graft, either by negative selection (n = 51) or positive selection of CD-34 positive cells (n = 23).

One hundred six of 153 patients at risk (69%) developed acute GVHD, 71 greater than grade 2 (39%), and 48 of 101 (48%) patients at risk developed chronic GVHD, which was extensive in 20 (20%). Seventy-one (86%) in the allogeneic group and 106 (85%) in the autologous group achieved a hematologic remission post-transplant. In the allogeneic group, 94 patients are alive post-transplant, and in the autologous group, 190 patients are alive post-transplant. As demonstrated in Figure 9–1, the 3-year survival probability for the allogeneic transplant group is 46% with a median follow-up of 20 months and 78% for the autologous transplant group with a median follow-up of 10 months (P<.001). The 3-year risk of relapse and TRM after allogeneic transplant is 15% and 49%, respectively and after autologous transplant 48% and 14%, respectively (Fig. 9–2). We did not find any difference in survival by compar-

ing the HSC source for allogeneic and autologous transplant (BM or PBPC), and in the autologous group there is no difference with purging. In addition, we found a significant difference in survival between patients receiving autologous transplants early after CLL diagnosis (≤36 months) and receiving later transplants, and we also demonstrated, as in myeloma, a difference of survival after allogeneic transplant between male and female recipients (Figs. 9–3 and 9–4).

This analysis clearly demonstrates the feasibility of performing autologous and allogeneic HSCT in patients with CLL. No randomized clinical trial has performed a comparison of transplant and standard therapy. For this reason, the efficacy of transplant as compared with other therapy is uncertain. Hence, the selection of patients for transplantation should take into account the age of the patient, existence of an HLA-identical sibling donor, CLL prognostic factors, and evolution of the disease on conventional therapy. For allogeneic transplantation, high morbidity and TRM may still exist, although this may be improving with the advent of more effective supportive care. Allogeneic transplantation may cure some patients with CLL as evi-

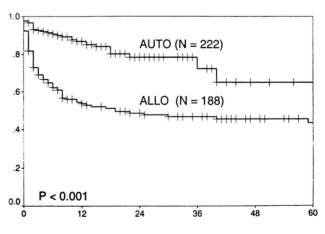

FIGURE 9–1. Survival of CLL patients undergoing autologous (AUTO) and allogeneic (ALLO) transplantation. AUTO, 13 patients at risk >36 months; median follow-up, 10 months; overall survival, 78%. ALLO, 41 patients at risk >36 months; median follow-up, 20 months; overall survival, 46%.

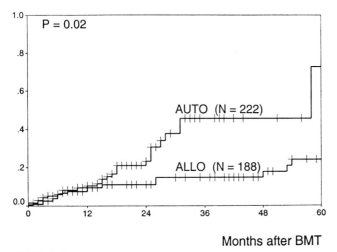

FIGURE 9–2. Incidence of relapse in CLL patients undergoing autologous (AUTO) and allogeneic (ALLO) transplantation. AUTO, 10 patients at risk >36 months; relapse, 48%. ALLO, 39 patients at risk >36 months; relapse, 15%.

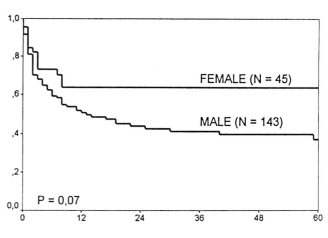

FIGURE 9–4. Survival for male and female patients after allogeneic transplantation. FEMALE, 14 patients at risk >36 months; survival, 63%. MALE, 27 patients at risk >36 months; survival, 41%.

denced by persisting molecular remission after a very long follow-up period after transplantation. GVL has been demonstrated with withdrawal of immunosuppression and donor leukocyte infusion—couple this with the fact that there appears to be little potential cure associated with autologous transplantation and one is forced to conclude that cure may be immunologically mediated.[26, 27] In an effort to provide a GVL effect and to decrease the toxicity of the conditioning regimen, investigators have used a fludarabine-based nonablative preparative regimen and donor lymphocyte infusion after transplantation in patients with hematologic malignancy.[28, 29] This and other less toxic approaches may provide a feasible means for extending allogeneic transplantation to older patients with CLL.

CONCLUSION

Autologous transplantation in CLL results in a very high percentage of hematologic CR after transplant. In a propor-

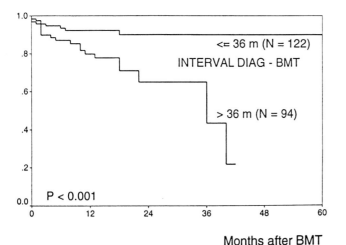

FIGURE 9–3. Survival for CLL patients after autologous HSCT according to the interval between diagnosis and transplant (i.e., ≤36 months or >36 months). Transplant within 36 months of diagnosis, 10 patients at risk >36 months after HSCT; overall survival, 89%. Transplant >36 months from diagnosis, 3 patients at risk >36 months after HSCT; overall survival, 64%.

tion of "complete remitters," molecular techniques and flow cytometry confirm remission status. As in allogeneic transplantation, these more sensitive techniques appear to be predictive of eventual clinical relapse. The design of clinical trials aimed at proving efficacy will need to use such surrogate markers to provide timely data for analysis. Autologous HSCT has lower TRM than allogeneic HSCT. From this standpoint, autologous HSCT presents an attractive therapeutic option for otherwise healthy patients.

REFERENCES

1. Montserrat E, Gomis F, Vallespi T, et al: Presenting features and prognosis of chronic lymphocytic leukemia in younger adults [see Comments]. Blood 78:1545, 1991.
2. Rai KR, Sawitsky A, Cronkite EP, et al: Clinical staging of chronic lymphocytic leukemia. Blood 46:219, 1975.
3. Binet JL, Auquier A, Dighiero G, et al: A new prognostic classification of chronic lymphocytic leukemia derived from a multivariate survival analysis. Cancer 48:198, 1981.
4. Rozman C, Montserrat E, Rodriguez-Fernandez JM, et al: Bone marrow histologic pattern—the best single prognostic parameter in chronic lymphocytic leukemia: a multivariate survival analysis of 329 cases. Blood 64:642, 1984.
5. Pangalis GA, Roussou PA, Kittas C, et al: B-chronic lymphocytic leukemia: prognostic implication of bone marrow histology in 120 patients experience from a single hematology unit. Cancer 59:767, 1987.
6. Cheson BD, Bennett JM, Grever M, et al: National Cancer Institute–sponsored Working Group guidelines for chronic lymphocytic leukemia: revised guidelines for diagnosis and treatment. Blood 87:4990, 1996.
7. Juliusson G, Elmhorn-Rosenborg A, Liliemark J: Response to 2-chlorodeoxyadenosine in patients with B-cell chronic lymphocytic leukemia resistant to fludarabine [see comments]. N Engl J Med 327:1056, 1992.
8. Keating MJ, O'Brien S, Lerner S, et al: Long-term follow-up of patients with chronic lymphocytic leukemia (CLL) receiving fludarabine regimens as initial therapy. Blood 92:1165, 1998.
9. Effectiveness of "CHOP" regimen in advanced untreated chronic lymphocytic leukaemia: French Cooperative Group on Chronic Lymphocytic Leukaemia. Lancet 1:1346, 1986.
10. Long-term results of the CHOP regimen in stage C chronic lymphocytic leukaemia: French Cooperative Group on Chronic Lymphocytic Leukaemia [see comments]. Br J Haematol 73:334, 1989.
11. Seymour JF, Robertson LE, O'Brien S, et al: Survival of young patients with chronic lymphocytic leukemia failing fludarabine therapy: a basis for the use of myeloablative therapies. Leuk Lymphoma 18:493, 1995.

12. Cabezudo E, Matutes E, Ramrattan M, et al: Analysis of residual disease in chronic lymphocytic leukemia by flow cytometry. Leukemia 11:1909, 1997.
13. Kipps TJ: Chronic lymphocytic leukemia. Curr Opin Hematol 5:244, 1998.
14. Provan D, Bartlett-Pandite L, Zwicky C, et al: Eradication of polymerase chain reaction–detectable chronic lymphocytic leukemia cells is associated with improved outcome after bone marrow transplantation. Blood 88:2228, 1996.
15. Schultze JL, Donovan JW, Gribben JG: Minimal residual disease detection after myeloablative chemotherapy in chronic lymphatic leukemia. J Mol Med 77:259, 1999.
16. Dreger P, von Neuhoff N, Kuse R, et al: Early stem cell transplantation for chronic lymphocytic leukaemia: a chance for cure? Br J Cancer 77:2291, 1998.
17. Esteve J, Villamor N, Colomer D, et al: Hematopoietic stem cell transplantation in chronic lymphocytic leukemia: a report of 12 patients from a single institution [see comments]. Ann Oncol 9:167, 1998.
18. Khouri IF, Keating MJ, Vriesendorp HM, et al: Autologous and allogeneic bone marrow transplantation for chronic lymphocytic leukemia: preliminary results. J Clin Oncol 12:748, 1994.
19. Khouri I, Keating M, Lerner S, et al: Improved survival with allogeneic and autologous stem cell transplantation for chronic lymphocytic leukemia (CLL): a case-matched analysis with conventional chemotherapy. Blood 92:287a, 1998.
20. Khouri IF, Keating M, Korbling M, et al: Transplant-lite: induction of graft-versus-malignancy using fludarabine-based nonablative chemotherapy and allogeneic blood progenitor-cell transplantation as treatment for lymphoid malignancies. J Clin Oncol 16:2817, 1998.
21. Michallet M, Archimbaud E, Bandini G, et al: HLA-identical sibling bone marrow transplantation in younger patients with chronic lymphocytic leukemia: European Group for Blood and Marrow Transplantation and the International Bone Marrow Transplant Registry [see comments]. Ann Intern Med 124:311, 1996.
22. Pavletic ZS, Bierman PJ, Vose JM, et al: High incidence of relapse after autologous stem-cell transplantation for B-cell chronic lymphocytic leukemia or small lymphocytic lymphoma. Ann Oncol 9:1023, 1998.
23. Rabinowe SN, Soiffer RJ, Gribben JG, et al: Autologous and allogeneic bone marrow transplantation for poor prognosis patients with B-cell chronic lymphocytic leukemia. Blood 82:1366, 1993.
24. Gribben J, Neuberg D, Soiffier R, et al: Autologous versus allogeneic bone marrow transplantation for patients with poor prognosis CLL. Blood 92:322a, 1998.
25. Sutton L, Maloum K, Gonzalez H, et al: Autologous hematopoietic stem cell transplantation as salvage treatment for advanced B cell chronic lymphocytic leukemia. Leukemia 12:1699, 1998.
26. deMagalhaes-Silverman M, Donnenberg A, Hammert L, et al: Induction of graft-versus-leukemia effect in a patient with chronic lymphocytic leukemia. Bone Marrow Transplant 20:175, 1997.
27. Rondon G, Giralt S, Huh Y, et al: Graft-versus-leukemia effect after allogeneic bone marrow transplantation for chronic lymphocytic leukemia. Bone Marrow Transplant 18:669, 1996.
28. Khouri IF, Przepiorka D, van Besien K, et al: Allogeneic blood or marrow transplantation for chronic lymphocytic leukaemia: timing of transplantation and potential effect of fludarabine on acute graft-versus-host disease. Br J Haematol 97:466, 1997.
29. Giralt S, Estey E, Albitar M, et al: Engraftment of allogeneic hematopoietic progenitor cells with purine analog-containing chemotherapy: harnessing graft-versus-leukemia without myeloablative therapy. Blood 89:4531, 1997.

CHAPTER TEN

Breast Cancer

Gerald J. Elfenbein, M.D., Janelle B. Perkins, Pharm. D., and Karen K. Fields, M.D.

The strategy of high-dose chemotherapy (HDCT) is relatively simple: eradication of the malignancy using supralethal doses of cytotoxic therapy that also produces fatal myeloablation and, therefore, necessitates hematopoietic stem cell transplantation (HSCT). The intent is curative, not palliative. Two fundamental properties of disease necessary for success of HDCT are (1) the malignancy must be therapy-sensitive at conventional doses and (2) an adequate source of "good" stem cells must be available. A third requirement for a successful outcome is also necessary—the patient must be able to tolerate nonhematopoietic toxicity. Breast cancer met the two principal criteria predictive of success. First, adjuvant chemotherapy has been documented to improve event-free survival (EFS) of patients with locoregional disease.[1, 2] Further, combination chemotherapy (including doxorubicin) has produced a high rate of complete response (20–25%) and complete and partial response (60–70%) for patients with metastatic disease.[3] Second, an adequate source of "good" stem cells could be derived from bone marrow because many patients had no marrow metastases by the criterion of histologic evaluation of several bone marrow biopsies or the cells could be derived from the peripheral blood in patients with marrow metastases.[4, 5]

Performance of autologous HSCT for breast cancer began in the 1980s.[6, 7] HDCT for breast cancer was worthy of exploration at that time because there were essentially no cures (<2%) produced for patients with metastatic disease by conventional chemotherapeutic doses[8] and because there were frequent relapses for patients with advanced locoregional disease despite the use of the best available, conventional, multimodal adjuvant therapy (surgery, radiation therapy, and chemotherapy). Furthermore, breast cancer was often sensitive to the alkylating drugs that were used in HDCT protocols. In addition, although increased dose intensity of conventional therapy has not been demonstrated to produce an increased cure rate for metastatic disease,[9] it has been shown to improve the EFS for patients in the adjuvant setting.[10] According to the Autologous Blood and Marrow Transplant Registry—North America (ABMTR), since 1989 breast cancer has become the number-one diagnosis for which autologous transplants (autotransplants) have been used in North America.[11]

INDICATIONS

At present, the sole indication for transplantation for breast cancer is "high-risk" disease. One reasonable definition of high-risk breast cancer is, at the time of presentation to the medical oncologist, the patient has a probability of relapse that exceeds 30% during the next 5 years despite the use of best available, conventional, multimodal therapy. High-risk breast cancer, then, includes metastatic disease, inflammatory disease, and locally advanced disease. By this criterion, patients with stage II breast cancer with four or more positive lymph nodes fit into this category.[12]

To predict how many patients nationwide will meet this criterion of high risk, a 10-year retrospective analysis of data collected by the H. Lee Moffitt Cancer Center (HLMCC) and Research Institute (when patients with breast masses came to our surgical team under the same set of conditions as they would to any primary care breast surgeon) was conducted. Of 1836 analytic cases (new patients), 1241 (67.6%) were under the age of 65 years and 595 (32.4%) were 65 years of age or older. As shown in Table 10–1, 358 women under the age of 65 years presented with stage II (≥4 positive lymph nodes) or higher-stage disease (19.5%). Only 65 patients (3.5%) under the age of 65 presented with stage II disease with four to nine positive lymph nodes.

Nationwide, in 1999, if all patients in these high-risk categories underwent transplantation at presentation (Table 10–2), approximately 34,848 (178,700 × 19.5%) patients would do so as part of primary management.[13] Estimating how many patients with less than stage II disease (≥4 positive nodes) who will experience relapse in the next 5 years and would ultimately be candidates for transplantation in the future as salvage therapy is not easy; however, sensible estimates are that 2% of stage 0 patients, 5% of stage I patients, and 10% of stage II patients (≤3 positive nodes) will experience relapse in the next 5 years. Then, an additional 56 patients under the age of 65 (or 3.05% of all 1836 patients) will be candidates for transplantation because of relapse. Applying these proportions to national incidence data, this will bring an additional 5450 (178,700 × 3.05%) patients to transplantation for a grand total of 40,297 patients nationwide (or 22.55% of all 178,700 patients) in 1996.

The strategy of waiting to use transplants as salvage therapy for those who have experienced metastatic disease is not as sound as using transplants as part of the primary management (see later). At HLMCC, transplanting in the adjuvant setting would mean that only about 130 patients (56 + 74; 7.1%) would need transplants for metastatic disease and 284 patients (65 + 64 + 115 + 40; 15.5%) would need transplants in the adjuvant setting. Thus, under

TABLE 10–1. INCIDENCE OF STAGE AND SUBSTAGE OF BREAST CANCER AT PRESENTATION BETWEEN 1986 AND 1995 (N = 1836)*

DISEASE STAGE	DISEASE SUBSTAGE	NO. (%) OF PATIENTS <65 YR	NO. (%) OF PATIENTS ≥65 YR
0	All	147 (11.8)	77 (12.9)
I	All	414 (33.4)	280 (47.1)
II	All		184 (30.9)
II	0–3 + nodes	317 (25.5)	
II	4–9 + nodes	65 (5.2)	
II	>9 + nodes	64 (5.2)	
III	All		21 (3.5)
III	Noninflammatory	115 (9.3)	
III	Inflammatory	40 (3.2)	
IV	All	74 (6.0)	23 (3.8)
Unstaged	All	5 (0.4)	10 (1.7)
Total	All	1241 (100)	595 (99.9)

*As recorded by the Tumor Registry of the H. Lee Moffitt Cancer Center, University of South Florida.

ideal circumstances, nationwide, two patients in the adjuvant setting would undergo transplantation for each patient with metastatic disease. This is not yet the case. Too many patients with locally advanced disease are being followed after conventional therapy until relapse before HDCT is offered as a therapeutic option.

CONTRAINDICATIONS

There are two basic contraindications to performing transplantation with high-risk breast cancer. First, the patient has an expected reduced survivability from the procedure because of vital organ dysfunction due to pre-existing conditions or as a consequence of prior cytotoxic therapy for breast cancer. Vital organs that must have sufficient functional reserve to tolerate nonhematopoietic toxicities without failing (and being responsible for death) are the heart, lungs, kidneys, and liver. Various cutoff levels have been established for functional performance for each of these organs. Excess mortality is anticipated with functional performance below these levels. The HLMCC uses a left ventricular ejection fraction of 50% (as measured by radiolabled blood pool studies), a pulmonary diffusion capacity of 60% of predicted (as measured by carbon monoxide inhalation), a creatinine clearance of 60 mL/min (as measured from a 24-hour urine collection), and a bilirubin in the normal range with hepatic enzymes no higher than

twice the upper limits of normal.[14, 15] Patients deficient in one vital organ functional reserve may still be candidates for HDCT provided (1) the specific high-dose regimen does not ordinarily cause major problems with the organ system in question, (2) the cure rate of the stage of breast cancer is sufficiently high to warrant the extra risk of mortality as well as increased morbidity, and (3) the patient and her family are fully aware of the anticipated problems and accept the risks.

Second, there are disease-specific circumstances that suggest the procedure cannot be applied with curative intent. In breast cancer, the principal disease-related contraindication for transplant is central nervous system (CNS) metastases, whether it be space-occupying lesions in the CNS or carcinomatous meningitis (meningeal carcinomatosis). Only radiotherapy and a limited number of chemotherapeutic agents penetrate the CNS with sufficient ease to be therapeutic for these disease processes. There has been precious little success with HDCT in this setting.[16]

A third relative contraindication to HDCT is a psychosocial circumstance that impairs patient compliance and therefore exposes the patient to excess morbidity and mortality. The issue of an age level to determine ineligibility is discussed later.

OUTCOMES

The major outcomes for transplantation for breast cancer that deserve attention are divided into two types: (1) those

TABLE 10–2. ESTIMATED NUMBER OF PATIENTS NATIONWIDE ELIGIBLE FOR HIGH-DOSE CHEMOTHERAPY FOR HIGH-RISK BREAST CANCER AT PRESENTATION*

DISEASE STAGE	DISEASE SUBSTAGE	NO. (%) OF HLMCC PATIENTS	NO. OF PATIENTS NATIONWIDE
II	4–9 + nodes	65 (3.54)	6,326
II	>9 + nodes	64 (3.49)	6,237
III	Noninflammatory	115 (6.26)	11,187
III	Inflammatory	40 (2.18)	3,896
IV	At presentation	74 (4.03)	7,202
Total	High-risk cases	358 (19.5)	34,848

*Using American Cancer Society estimate of 178,700 new invasive cases of breast cancer for 1998 and H. Lee Moffitt Cancer Center (University of South Florida) Tumor Registry distribution of 1836 analytic cases (as shown in Table 10–1).

outcomes for which data are *immediately available* to be evaluated, of which toxic death is the most prominent example, but also including chronic organ system damage leading to functional impairment that disables the patient, and (2) those outcomes which require a considerable period of time before data may be evaluated (i.e., they have *delayed availability*), of which the most prominent examples are EFS and overall survival (OS), but also including quality-of-life measures at a time remote from the procedure.

Intrinsic to a successful therapeutic strategy delivered with curative intent are an adequate study population and a sufficient follow-up period to analyze the effectiveness of the strategy (i.e., determining the cure rate). What are discreetly measurable are relapse and death—evidence of failure. Cure can be achieved only among patients for whom neither of these events has occurred over a prolonged period of time. Just how long (what minimum duration) patients in EFS must be followed and just what median duration of follow-up should be for these patients are unclear. Should the minimum or median follow-up be 3 years, 5 years, 7 years, 10 years, or more? Evidence of failure may appear quickly, but proving success takes a lot more time.

For procedures delivered with curative intent, the most important outcome is EFS at a biologically significant period of time (based on the natural history of the patient's disease) after the procedure and not the median duration of EFS. The only candidates for cure are event-free survivors. It is altogether possible that only a brief median EFS would become infinite. Although the improvement in median EFS so observed may be mathematically significant, it would be difficult to prove that the improvement in cure rate was mathematically significant (even though it may be biologically significant) without a large cohort of patients being followed for a considerable period of time.

It is altogether possible that, for a therapeutic strategy delivered with curative intent, the OS for patients could be less during the first or second year after the procedure even though the cure rate is superior as measured at the 5-year mark. Choosing between two different treatment strategies, then, becomes a difficult decision for the patient and should be based on the utility of different segments of time to the patient (i.e., what risk of early mortality is the patient willing to accept for a higher probability of being cured?).

Table 10–3 shows toxic deaths in the immediate post-transplantation period, OS, and EFS at 1, 3, and 5 years

posttransplantation by disease stage at the HLMCC between 1989 and 1997. With these concepts and available data, comments about major outcomes are limited at this time.

As seen in Table 10–3, stage of disease at time of transplantation is a major factor in determining outcome. This parallels the experience observed for allogeneic HSCT (alloHSCT) for leukemias and autologous HSCT (autoHSCT) for lymphomas in which patients with early-stage disease (first complete remission [CR1]) do better than patients with intermediate-stage disease (once relapsed but chemosensitive), who do better than patients with advanced-stage (chemorefractory) disease.[17] Locally advanced but noninflammatory breast cancer may be considered early-stage disease, inflammatory breast cancer may be considered intermediate-stage disease, and metastatic breast cancer may be considered advanced-stage disease.

HLMCC data show plateaus appearing in EFS curves (Fig. 10–1), indicative of "stability" in the long-term EFS patient population, which is suggestive of "cure." Similar results have been reported by the ABMTR.[18] It will, however, be necessary to have long-term follow-up of a large cohort of patients before cure rates can be definitively established. Five years is a sensible minimum follow-up for the cohort of event-free survivors before cure rates can be established. Although this conservative stance is reasonable, it has two drawbacks. First, cure rates will be established but only for patients treated during the time period ending 5 years in the past. Second, although changes in HDCT and supportive care in the most recent 5-year time period may improve cure rates as compared with the preceding 5-year time period, it will take an additional 5 years to demonstrate the improvement. As an example of how changes in supportive care strategies can produce unanticipated and often paradoxical results, consider T-cell depletion, which successfully prevented acute graft-versus-host disease (GVHD) in patients with chronic myelogenous leukemia (CML) in first chronic phase but deleteriously affected EFS.[19, 20]

There are now sufficient data to address the strategy question: Should transplantation for locally advanced breast cancer (≥stage II with 10 or more positive nodes) be performed in the adjuvant setting or at time of relapse with metastatic disease? To answer this question, estimates of the cure rates for locally advanced breast cancer and metastatic disease are required. HLMCC transplant data (Fig. 10–2) make the following assumptions for locally advanced breast

TABLE 10–3. MAJOR CLINICAL OUTCOMES AFTER HIGH-DOSE CHEMOTHERAPY AND AUTOLOGOUS TRANSPLANTATION FOR HIGH-RISK BREAST CANCER*

DISEASE STAGE	TOXIC DEATHS (%)	OVERALL SURVIVAL (%)			EVENT-FREE SURVIVAL (%)		
		1 Year	3 Years	5 Years	1 Year	3 Years	5 Years
II (N > 7)	8	90	71	64	78	47	47
III (any N)	6	88	61	48	75	45	45
III (inflammatory)	7	56	35	23†	33	27	27†
IV (nonrefractory)	13	58	28	22	30	15	0
IV (refractory)	17	44	12	7	18	15	2

*Data from the H. Lee Moffitt Cancer Center for the first 400 patients with breast cancer treated, 1989–1997.
†Values from 4 years after transplantation.

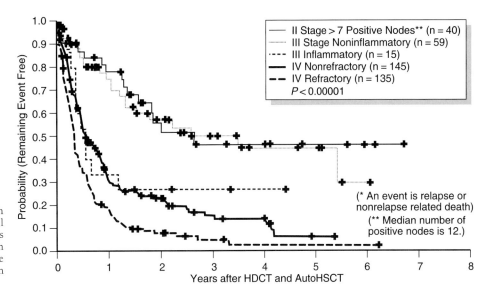

FIGURE 10–1. Event-free survival with autologous hematopoietic stem cell transplantation (auto-SCT) for patients with high-risk breast cancer treated with high-dose chemotherapy (HDCT) at the H. Lee Moffitt Cancer Center between 1989 and 1996, by disease stage.

cancer in the adjuvant setting reasonable: (1) the toxic death rate is 5%, (2) the cure rate is 50%, and (3) the relapse rate is 45%. Further, it is reasonable to assume that none of the patients who experience relapse after transplantation is curable. The strategy of transplanting in the adjuvant setting, then, would cure 50 women of 100 so treated. Next, reasonable (and ambitious) assumptions for the same category of patients treated with conventional

multimodal therapy are (1) the cure rate is 30% and (2) the relapse rate is 70% within the first 5 years after treatment. Again, extrapolating data from the HLMCC, it is reasonable to assume that 15% (or 10) of the patients who experience relapse with metastatic disease are curable with transplantation. The strategy of waiting to offer transplantation until metastatic disease is present would cure only 40 (30 + 10) women of 100 so treated. The difference in

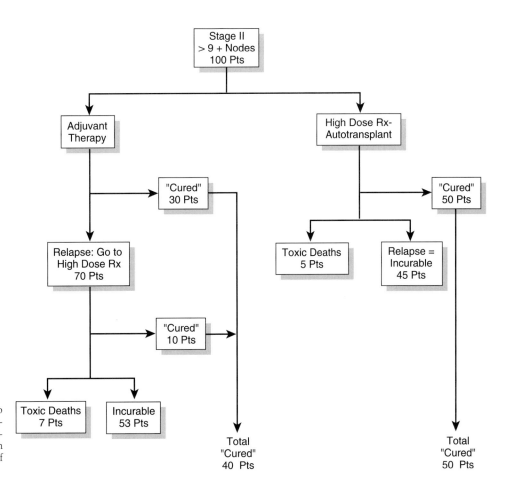

FIGURE 10–2. Comparison of two treatment strategies. High-dose chemotherapy (Rx) in the adjuvant setting produces more "cures" than when administered at the time of metastatic disease development.

total cured patients between the two strategies is 10 using these assumptions (see Fig. 10–2).

It would appear, then, that the strategy of transplantation in the adjuvant setting is superior even if it means over-treating 30% of patients who would have been cured with conventional treatment alone. Delaying transplantation would result in the undertreatment of at least 10% of patients (those who might have been cured if transplantation had been offered in the adjuvant setting but couldn't be salvaged with transplantation in the metastatic setting). It takes but a simple mathematical calculation to determine what the cure rate for transplants for metastatic disease must be for the two strategies to result in the same cure rate ultimately—that is, 29% ($\times = 100* [50-30]/70$). This number exceeds the current estimated cure rate for transplantation in the metastatic setting by a factor of 2. Thus, if the objective of treatment of high-risk breast cancer is to cure the most women, the strategy of transplantation in the adjuvant setting is the strategy of choice until the salvage rate for metastatic disease (by transplantation) is vastly improved or the cure rate with conventional multimodal therapy is vastly improved in the adjuvant setting.

COMPARATIVE STUDIES

The reason why so many women with locally advanced breast cancer do not receive transplants is stated to be that there are no published, comparative trials in peer-reviewed journals "proving" that transplantation is superior to conventional treatment. Further, it is asserted that what might appear to be superior results in phase II studies of HDCT for locally advanced breast cancer is really the consequence of bias introduced by the manner and the time of patient selection. These are both valid criticisms. The issue of which treatment strategy produces the best EFS at 5 years can only be answered definitively by a phase III, stratified, randomized trial comparing the two strategies. Fortunately (at the time of writing), at least two such trials are ongoing in the United States and at least six are in progress in Europe (G. Rosti, personal communication). Unfortunately, even if these studies completed accrual today, it would take 5 or more years before measurable outcomes could be established.

In the meantime, two existing bodies of data may shed some light on this question: Which is better—conventional therapy or HDCT for locally advanced breast cancer? The first body of data comes from a theoretical approach using the mathematical model of decision analysis. Using outcome data extant at the time of analysis, HDCT for locally advanced breast cancer would be superior to conventional adjuvant therapy alone if the following criteria were met: (1) less than 15% toxic death rate for HDCT; (2) greater than 45% EFS rate for HDCT at 5 years; and (3) at least 20 years' life for all patients treated by either therapy if none had breast cancer. Because the median age of women undergoing transplantation for locally advanced breast cancer at the HLMCC and in North America is 40–45 years and the first two criteria appear to be met, it is easy to see why a Monte Carlo analysis selects HDCT over conventional treatment.[21]

A separate type of analysis comparing conventional therapy with HDCT has been performed using historical and simultaneous data. Duke University Medical Center compared their EFS results for locally advanced breast cancer with historical data from two previous Cancer and Leukemia Group B (CALGB, an NCI-sponsored multi-institutional clinical trials cooperative group) adjuvant chemotherapy trials and one ongoing trial.[12] Case matching for risk factors was attempted. In the first two comparisons, HDCT was superior at year 3 post transplantation. In the latter comparison, in which more-intensive therapy was delivered to the conventionally treated patients, it was projected that HDCT would yield a superior EFS (but not until 5 years after treatment).

Although neither of these approaches proves the superiority of HDCT over conventional therapy for locally advanced breast cancer, they support using HDCT for locally advanced breast cancer in patients who would be eligible for, but are not enrolled in, randomized trials because of accessibility and other valid reasons, especially because the HDCT toxic death rate is now less than 5% and because many of these patients can receive their treatment in the outpatient setting.

With respect to metastatic disease, there is one randomized phase III trial comparing transplantation to conventional treatment ongoing in the United States, at least one trial in progress in Europe (G. Rosti, personal communication), and one trial, published in peer-reviewed literature, from South Africa.[22] The latter trial has shown the superiority of transplantation to conventional therapy to be statistically significant. Neither treatment arm fared particularly well, however, rendering the biologic significance of this study questionable at best.

Two additional bodies of data have shed some light on the question: For metastatic breast cancer, which is better, transplantation or conventional therapy? The EFS for HLMCC patients with metastatic breast cancer treated with HDCT has been compared with that of patients on the best chemotherapy arm of two different, randomized, large cooperative group, peer-reviewed published trials.[23] Approximately 25% of our patients had metastatic disease sensitive to doxorubicin-based CT. The other 75% had failed at least one chemotherapy regimen, of which one included doxorubicin. In the first trial selected for comparison,[24] patients received no chemotherapy prior to enrollment in the trial using a doxorubicin-based regimen. They were considered chemotherapy-naive. In the second,[25] all patients experienced failure of one prior chemotherapy regimen without doxorubicin prior to enrollment in the trial comparing doxorubicin against two other agents (doxorubicin was found to be superior). These two trials can be seen to have patient populations with risk factors (disease chemosensitivity) that bracket our patients treated with HDCT.

As seen in Figure 10–3, the two trials used for comparison have different EFS rates under 2 years post treatment with the chemotherapy-naive patients faring better than those in whom prior chemotherapy (without doxorubicin) had failed. At 1½ years post treatment, EFS was the same for HDCT patients and chemotherapy-naive patients; 3 years after treatment, EFS was superior for HDCT patients. One might have anticipated this result because HDCT may

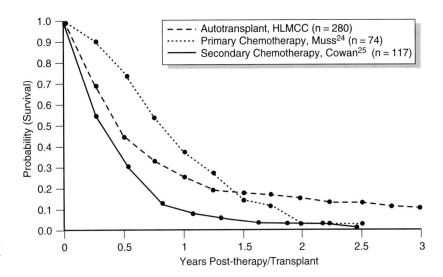

FIGURE 10–3. Progression-free survival with metastatic breast cancer. HLMCC, H. Lee Moffitt Cancer Center.

have the potential to cure metastatic breast cancer whereas conventional CT does not. (Statistical analysis could not be performed because raw data from the two reference studies[24, 25] were unavailable.)

A 1996 report of a study performed at Duke University Medical Center[26] evaluated the 5-year EFS and OS rates for chemotherapy-naive patients with metastatic breast cancer consolidated with HDCT and for those who received HDCT only at progression after CR with AFM (doxorubicin, 5-fluorouracil [5FU], and methotrexate [MTX]). In other words, after highly successful induction therapy, patients were randomized to receive transplants early or at relapse (later). The results are interesting. EFS was clearly better for patients receiving HDCT as consolidation, but OS was better for patients who received HDCT at relapse. Complete responders experiencing relapse after receiving AFM were not prevented from achieving success with a (late) transplant. Long-term follow-up is necessary to determine which HDCT strategy results in better OS. Furthermore, conclusions drawn from this study are restricted to the limited population of chemotherapy-naive patients with metastatic breast cancer who achieve CR after AFM treatment. Finally, if the transplant-at-relapse strategy were to be pursued, all patients would have to be treated (pretransplantation) in a manner identical to that used with those in the study.

Again, these data are insufficient to prove that HDCT is superior to conventional therapy for patients with metastatic disease. They do support the use of HDCT, especially for patients with chemosensitive metastatic breast cancer for whom randomized clinical trials remain inaccessible. Although any hint of "cure" (e.g., ≥15%) from phase II trials would, biologically speaking, be significantly better than conventional chemotherapy, the present lack of sufficient long-term data prevents us from making definitive conclusions.

Five randomized studies[26–31] comparing high-dose therapy for breast cancer with "control" therapy were presented in abstract form at the 35th Annual Meeting of the American Society of Clinical Oncology (ASCO) in Atlanta, May 15–19 1999. One of these studies has been found to be potentially fraudulent and will not be discussed further in this chapter.[29] There was considerable interest in this opportunity to see new data from randomized trials that had been ongoing for many years. A concise summary of the available data is provided in Table 10–4. The analysis follows.

Of the four studies presented, two trials were in the adjuvant setting and two concerned patients with metastatic disease. These two different disease state trials must be interpreted separately. Three of the studies were large (in terms of numbers of patients accrued) cooperative group trials (one metastatic, two adjuvant), and one was a small trial (a cooperative group trial). Three trials compared "control" arms with high-dose therapy that could not be considered "conventional" because they were augmented in intensity or duration of therapy, and two had control arms that could be deemed reasonable for comparison. Using more aggressive therapy in control arms is not intrinsically bad, but it changes the nature of the question being asked such that the question no longer can be phrased "Is high-dose therapy an improvement over *conventional* therapy?" Finally, and most disappointingly, of the four studies presented, three reported patients for whom the median duration of follow-up was insufficient to draw conclusions and only one had long enough follow-up to permit scientifically meaningful conclusions to be drawn.

Taking all the issues into consideration, only one of the four studies could be deemed completed and interpretable. This was a small study, appropriately controlled, and had sufficient follow-up, and was in the metastatic setting. These data underscore the need for continued study in this area by centers well established for conducting trials and tracking patients. Continued referral of patients for the procedure (to centers conducting trials to improve the results over what has already been achieved) is essential. The studies did not support any change in public policy with respect to funding the procedure for eligible patients.

TABLE 10-4. HIGH-DOSE THERAPY FOR HIGH-RISK BREAST CANCER—FOUR RECENTLY PRESENTED STUDIES

AUTHOR/ GROUP/START OF STUDY	DISEASE STATUS	NO. OF PATIENTS	HIGH-DOSE REGIMEN	"CONTROL" ARM	CLINICAL OUTCOME PARAMETER — High-Dose	Control	COMMENTS ABOUT STUDY (Based on ASCO Meeting, 5/99)
Peters et al.[27]/CALGB, 1/91	Adjuvant >9+ LNs	884 enrolled 785 randomized	**Induction: Cyclophosphamide, doxorubicin, and fluorouracil (CAF) × 4 cycles** BCNU (600 mg/m²) Cyclophosphamide (5625 mg/m²) Cisplatin (165 mg/m²) (N = 394)	BCNU (90 mg/m²) Cyclophosphamide (900 mg/m²) Cisplatin (90 mg/m²) with G-CSF (N = 391)	Treatment-related mortality 7.4% / **Relapse rate** 25% / Progression-free survival at 3 yr 68% / Overall survival at 3 yr 78%	0.0% / 37% / 64% / 80%	1. "Control" arm (lower-dose BCP) is more intense than standard therapy (ordinarily, nothing after CAF × 4 cycles) 2. Median follow-up is 37 mo 3. Difference is not expected until 5 yr after high-dose therapy 4. Next analysis in 5/01 5. Too early to draw conclusions
Bergh et al,[28] (Scandinavia 3/94)	Adjuvant >9+ LNs	525 randomized	Fluorouracil, epirubicin, and cyclophosphamide, (FEC) × 3 cycles Cyclophosphamide, thiotepa, and carboplatin (CTCb)	"Tailored" (augmented-dose) FEC × 9 cycles with G-CSF and ciprofloxacin	Number of relapses 50 / Number of deaths 78 / Myelodysplasia and secondary AMLs 2	50 / 40 / 8	1. "Control" arm (9 courses of aggressive FEC) is much more intense than standard therapy and is compared to standard dose FEC × 3 cycles and 1 course of CTCb 2. Median follow-up is 42 mo 3. Myelopathies appear independent of treatment arm 4. Difficult to draw conclusions when "control" arm is 6 courses of aggressive FEC
Stadtmauer et al.[30] ECOG/1/90	Metastatic responders	545 enrolled 199 randomized	**Induction: Cyclophosphamide, methotrexate, and fluorouracil (CMF) or CAF × 4-6 cycles** CTCb (N = 110)	CMF × 2 yr (N = 89)	Overall survival at 3 yr for CRs 42% / Overall survival at 3 yr for PRs 27% / Progression-free survival at 3 yr 6% / ($P = 0.03$)	49% / 36% / 12%	1. Median follow-up is 37 mo 2. Only half of anticipated CRs and PRs were randomized to participate in trial 3. Continuation of CMF for 2 years in "control" arm is not standard care for stage IV patients 4. Remarkably poor results for high-dose arm and unexpectedly good results for "control" arm 5. No comment about quality of life relative to time "off therapy" after high-dose regimen
Lotz et al.[31] (France, PEGASE/9/92)	Metastatic responders	61 randomized	**Induction: Anthracycline-based therapy × 4-6 cycles** Mobilization with intermediate dose cyclophosphamide, mitoxantrone, and melphalan (CNL) (N = 32)	Continued intermediate-dose cyclophosphamide × 2-4 total cycles (N = 29)	Median progression-free survival 35 mo ($P = 0.01$ at 3 yr) / **Median overall survival** 43 mo ($P = 0.03$ at 3 yr) / **Overall survival at 5 yr** 30% ($P = 0.12$ at 5 yr)	20 mo / 20 mo / 18%	1. Median follow-up is 53 mo 2. Delay in time to relapse noted 3. Longer "off therapy" period noted 4. Trend toward better overall survival noted 5. Beta error for survival is large because sample size is small 6. Positive outcome for high-dose CNL therapy

AML, acute myelogenous leukemia; ASCO, American Society of Clinical Oncologists; CR, complete responder; ECOG, European Clinical Oncology Group; LN, lymph node; PR, partial responder.

As discussed earlier in this chapter under Outcomes, premature presentation and interpretation of data from trials such as the studies presented at the 1999 ASCO meeting may lead to erroneous conclusions about clinical value (or lack thereof) and, subsequently, to inappropriate alterations in policy. At the time of this writing, plans for additional randomized clinical trials for both high-risk and metastatic disease are in development by many institutions. It is anticipated that continued follow-up analysis of the CALGB trial and results of other ongoing trials will continue to help define the role of high-dose therapy with HSCT in the management of breast cancer.

REGIMENS

With over 5500 women receiving HDCT for high-risk breast cancer between 1989 and 1995, it is not difficult to imagine that a wide variety of regimens have been used. The philosophy and data behind the development of these regimens are relatively simple. (1) Agents explored for activity should be dose-escalatable because of primarily hematopoietic toxicity and should have manageable, non-hematopoietic dose-limiting toxicities. (2) Drug selection should be based on its individual efficacy or synergy in combination with other efficacious drugs. (3) Combinations of drugs with non–cross-resistant mechanisms of action and nonoverlapping toxicities are preferred. According to our available data and the extent to which analyses have been completed, there appears to be no significant difference among transplant regimens in terms of EFS in the adjuvant[32] or metastatic[11] settings. This suggests that EFS for patients receiving HDCT for high-risk breast cancer is less dependent on specific drug combinations than on dose intensity. Intuitively, the first part of this hypothesis is difficult to accept. Even so, in light of the outcome of the large, multicenter, prospective randomized trial comparing four different regimens for intermediate-grade and selected high-grade non-Hodgkin lymphoma, which showed no differences in disease-free survival, it may very well be true.

Over 800 patients have undergone transplantation at HLMCC since 1989, of whom more than 400 have been treated for breast cancer. One of the goals of our program was to develop novel regimens for breast cancer and to determine the impact of dose intensity on EFS for patients with high-risk breast cancer. Table 10–5 lists the six different regimens used at our institution between 1989 and

1996. Maximum tolerated doses (MTD) of the drugs in combinations for the four unique regimens, ICE (ifosfamide, carboplatin, etoposide), MITT (mitoxantrone, thiotepa), TNT (paclitaxel, mitoxantrone, thiotepa), and TIME (topotecan, ifosfamide, etoposide), developed in our institution are also shown. Two interesting observations are noted. First, for patients with noninflammatory locally advanced stage III breast cancer, no differences have been observed among the four regimens used nor has there been any evidence of a dose-intensity effect for one specific regimen (i.e., ICE) (Fig. 10–4).[33, 34] Consequently, it is our belief that outpatient transplants with regimens that have but modest nonhematologic toxicities (such as CTC [cyclophosphamide, thiotepa, carboplatin] and BUCY2 [busulfan, cyclophosphamide]) and for which the duration of aplasia can be minimized (with mobilized peripheral blood stem cells) are safe, less expensive, and efficacious for these patients with locally advanced breast cancer.

Our second observation is that, for patients with inflammatory and metastatic breast cancer, there appears to be a dose-intensity effect with the ICE regimen[23, 34, 35] but no regimen effect[33] when all regimens are studied at the MTD. Figure 10–5 shows the comparison of EFS for the ICE, MITT, TNT, and CTC regimens for doxorubicin-responsive stage IV disease. Figure 10–6 shows the comparison of EFS for the ICE, MITT, TNT, and TIME regimens for stage IV disease refractory to doxorubicin, mini-ICE,[14, 36] or paclitaxel. Consequently, we think that patients with chemosensitive metastatic or inflammatory disease should be treated at the MTD of the regimen with the least morbidity and mortality (such as CTC in the case of doxorubicin complete responders). Conversely, patients with chemoresistant metastatic disease should be enrolled in dose escalation, phase I/II trials exploring new drugs in high-dose or new drug combinations (such as TIME for doxorubicin- and paclitaxel-resistant disease. At the HLMCC, the number and severity of side effects and the duration of aplasia even with mobilized peripheral blood progenitor cells (PBPC)[37] usually requires that these patients be hospitalized. Further improvement in supportive care and home health care capabilities may reverse this trend, at least for a subgroup of these patients.

Many centers, including our own, are now performing outpatient transplantation for selected patients with high-risk breast cancer. The factors driving this shift are economy and preference. The latter factor reflects the well-

TABLE 10–5. HIGH-DOSE CHEMOTHERAPY REGIMENS (PHASE II) USED FOR HIGH-RISK BREAST CANCER BY THE H. LEE MOFFITT CANCER CENTER, UNIVERSITY OF SOUTH FLORIDA

REGIMEN	DRUG 1	DRUG 2	DRUG 3
ICE	Ifosfamide* (20.1 g/m^2)	Carboplatin (1.8 g/m^2)	Etoposide (3.0 g/m^2)
MITT	Mitoxantrone (90 mg/m^2)	Thiotepa (1.2 g/m^2)	
TNT	Paclitaxel (360 mg/m^2)	Mitoxantrone (48 mg/m^2)	Thiotepa (0.72 g/m^2)
BUCY2	Busulfan (16 mg/kg)	Cyclophosphamide (120 mg/kg)	—
CTC	Cyclophosphamide (6.0 g/m^2)	Thiotepa (500 mg/m^2)	Carboplatin (0.8 g/m^2)
TIME	Topotecan (escalating)	Ifosfamide* (10.0 g/m^2)	Etoposide (1.5 g/m^2)

*With equivalent doses of mesna as a uroprotectant.

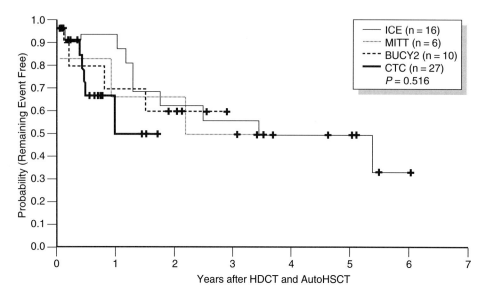

FIGURE 10–4. Comparison of four high-dose chemotherapeutic regimens (HDCT) given to sequential cohorts of patients with noninflammatory stage III breast cancer. No differences occurred in event-free survival. BUCY2, busulfan, cyclophosphamide; CTC, cyclophosphamide, thiotepa, carboplatin; ICE, ifosfamide, carboplatin, etoposide; MITT, mitoxantrone, thiotepa.

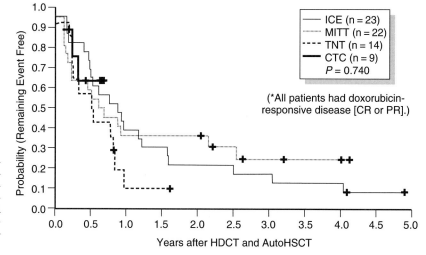

FIGURE 10–5. Comparison of four high-dose chemotherapeutic regimens (HDCT) given to sequential cohorts of patients with stage IV breast cancer responsive to doxorubicin. No differences occurred in event-free survival. CTC, cyclophosphamide, thiotepa, and carboplatin; ICE, ifosfamide, carboplatin, and etoposide; MITT, mitoxantrone and thiotepa; TNT, paclitaxel, mitoxantrone, and thiotepa.

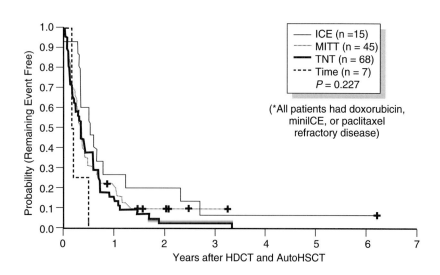

FIGURE 10–6. Comparison of four high-dose chemotherapeutic regimens (HDCT) given to sequential cohorts of patients with stage IV diseases refractory to conventional chemotherapy at the time of transplantation. No differences occurred in event-free survival. ICE, ifosfamide, carboplatin, etoposide; MITT, mitoxantrone, thiotepa; TIME, topotecan, ifosfamide, etoposide; TNT, paclitaxel, mitoxantrone, thiotepa.

known desire of patients to receive as much of their care as possible as outpatients, principally for psychologic and support reasons. Outpatient transplants have been made feasible by (1) home health care delivery, (2) a short period of aplasia, thereby minimizing the risk of acquiring *Aspergillus* pneumonia, (3) primary care providers (family member or friend) staying with patients 24 hours a day, and (4) a well-thought-out care plan by the outpatient clinic and evening and weekend coverage team to efficiently handle daily anticipated problems as well as providing rapid responses to urgent and emergent problems. The last two appear to be the limiting factors for more widespread application of outpatient HSCT. Although it is our belief that outpatient transplants will and should increase in frequency for appropriately selected patients, ultimately the selected treatment regimen should produce the greatest potential for EFS despite the toxicity or cost.

For locally advanced and for limited-extent metastatic disease (e.g., one metastatic site), it is our practice to surgically extirpate all known disease when feasible and reasonable. For locoregional disease, it is our practice to irradiate the disease area including the surgical field. Whether radiotherapy should precede or follow HDCT is unresolved. We and others have observed marked radiation recall skin toxicity when paclitaxel (or docetaxel) is given after radiotherapy.[38, 39] As a result, because we currently use paclitaxel for PBPC mobilization, our patients with locoregional disease received radiation post transplantation. For limited-extent metastatic disease, when extirpation is not feasible or reasonable, our practice is to irradiate the site with an involved-field approach. For the special circumstance of chest wall recurrence, considered a harbinger of metastatic disease, we perform excisional biopsy(ies) and irradiate if the involved area has not previously been irradiated.

No comparative trials have established these practice preferences as being of proven value in this high-risk breast cancer population receiving HDCT. These preferences, however, have been chosen because of the philosophy that HDCT is likely to be most effective when given in the setting of the lowest tumor burden possible and based on systematic evaluation of relapses.

Finally, post-transplantation hormonal therapy is worthy of discussion. For patients with locally advanced breast cancer whose primary lesion is estrogen receptor–positive and/or progesterone receptor–positive (ER/PR+), we prescribe ER antagonist therapy for 2 or more years post-

transplantation. Some investigators recommend this for 5 years. For patients with metastatic disease, we base our decision concerning hormonal therapy on the results of the metastatic disease biopsy; otherwise, we base our decision on the hormone receptor studies of the primary lesion. For patients with metastatic disease considered to be ER/PR+, we recommend ER antagonist therapy for 2 or more years after transplantation only for those patients with no prior hormonal therapy. Again, the utility of this practice preference has not been established by comparative trials in this patient population receiving HDCT. Because the transplant is offered with curative intent and because toxicity is relatively mild, however, ER antagonist therapy is prescribed for its potential contribution to the curative effect.

TOXICITY

A full discussion of generic toxicity attributable to HDCT is discussed in Chapters 34 and 35. Some of the novel regimens developed at the HLMCC for breast cancer, however, have relatively novel dose-limiting toxicities (DLT) worthy of mention. They include ifosfamide-related nephrotoxicity, ototoxicity, neuropathy, and encephalopathy,[40, 41] mitoxantrone-related cardiotoxicity and delayed engraftment,[42] busulfan-related pulmonary toxicity and delayed thrombopoiesis,[43] and paclitaxel-related severe myalgias, arthralgias, and neuropathy.[44] Some DLT, such as mitoxantrone-related cardiotoxicity, might have been anticipated, but others, such as busulfan-related delayed thrombopoiesis, came as a surprise. The important message from these observations is that when new drugs are used in high doses (e.g., mitoxantrone) or old drugs are applied in new circumstances (e.g., busulfan in the autologous setting), vigilant surveillance is required until the full spectrum of DLT is identified and recorded for each new drug, dose, and setting.

Age has long been thought to be a risk factor for poor outcome (EFS) principally because of a reduced capacity to tolerate toxicity from HDCT due to progressive loss of vital-organ functional reserve. Toxic death rates were also thought to be higher. The effect of age in the ability of our patients to tolerate regimen-related toxicity has been evaluated. As can be seen in Table 10–6, for patients treated with ICE,[45] there was no consistent or convincing evidence that older (>54 years) patients with breast cancer fared any less well than younger patients (<55 years). Although

TABLE 10–6. EFFECTS OF AGE ON TOLERANCE OF HIGH-DOSE CHEMOTHERAPY WITH THE ICE REGIMEN FOLLOWED BY AUTOLOGOUS TRANSPLANTATION AT THE H. LEE MOFFITT CANCER CENTER, UNIVERSITY OF SOUTH FLORIDA

	19–34 YEARS	35–43 YEARS	44–54 YEARS	55–59 YEARS	TWO-TAILED *P* VALUE
Number of patients	51	55	51	11	n/a
Mucositis*	75%	55%	75%	82%	0.055
Peripheral neuropathy*	0%	2%	0%	9%	0.064
Hemorrhagic cystitis*	0%	10%	4%	18%	0.042
Discharge day post transplantation	24	24	27	30	0.142
Toxic deaths	6%	9%	12%	0%	0.526

*Percentage of patients with grade 3 or 4 toxicity on the World Health Organization scale.
ICE, ifosfamide + carboplatin + etoposide.

we believe that patient selection on our part is not responsible for failure to observe an age effect for morbidity or mortality from HDCT (all patients 55–64 years of age were included in the analysis with the exception of those patients excluded from HDCT because of vital-organ system dysfunction), it is possible that referring physician preference introduced a selection bias.

HEMATOPOIETIC STEM CELLS

Discussions of hematopoietic stem cell (HSC) sources, mobilization, and function can be found in Chapter 5. Three issues relevant to HSC are worthy of discussion here, however. First, retrospective analyses of patients with large cell non-Hodgkin lymphoma[46, 47] revealed that, for one subpopulation of patients, those who received PBPC experienced an EFS superior to that of those who received bone marrow HSC. The reason for selecting PBPC over marrow was that marrow HSC was not harvestable because of histologic evidence of (1) tumor contamination, (2) hypocellularity, or (3) myelofibrosis. This same reason for choosing PBPC over marrow HSC was applied to the treatment of our patients with metastatic breast cancer. From a retrospective analysis of both the chemosensitive and the chemoresistant disease subpopulations,[5] we found identical EFS curves for patients who received marrow HSC and PBPC. Thus, we did not confirm in breast cancer what was observed in NHL.

Second, subsequent to the retrospective study already described for NHL, a prospective, randomized trial was performed for patients with harvestable bone marrow according to the reason cited. Patients received granulocyte colony-stimulating factor (G-CSF) for 9 days, underwent bone marrow harvest on day 6, and underwent four PBPC harvests on days 7–10. Prior to randomization, patients were stratified according to disease (breast cancer vs. other [principally lymphoma] and HDCT regimen [ICE vs. MITT or its successor, TNT]). On the day of transplantation, patients received either primed marrow HSC or mobilized PBPC. The majority of patients (65%) in this study had breast cancer. We found no difference in recovery of granulocytes or platelets that depended on HSC source,[48, 49] leading us to conclude that the reason that prior literature claimed that PBPC allowed faster engraftment than marrow HSC was that the PBPC were collected under stimulating conditions and the marrow HSC were not. Interestingly, in this prospective, stratified, randomized trial, no differences in relapse rates dependent on stem-cell source were found (Fig. 10–7).

Third, the clinical significance of tumor cell contamination of marrow that is histologically free of tumor cells was evaluated. A reverse transcriptase–polymerase chain reaction (RT-PCR) assay was developed using a unique primer for cytokeratin 19 that could detect one breast cancer cell among 10^7 normal marrow cells.[50] With this assay, marrow specimens collected and frozen after chemotherapy in responding patients were examined. Of patients with locally advanced disease, over 50% were found to have marrow micrometastases by this molecular test. In over 80% of patients with chemoresponsive metastatic disease to which at least a partial remission had occurred, marrow micrometastases were still present after chemotherapy. Furthermore, for patients with locoregional disease, the relapse rate in the first 2 years was 33% for marrow micrometastatic disease–positive patients but only 9% for marrow micrometastatic disease–negative patients according to this molecular test. This difference is not statistically significant but may very well be biologically significant. Moreover, 67% of patients with micrometastatic disease in their marrow, collected after conventional adjuvant therapy but before marrow collection and HDCT, did not experience relapse after HDCT. Finally, for patients with metastatic disease, the relapse rate was 85% for marrow micrometastatic disease–positive patients but only 11% for marrow micrometastatic disease–negative patients. This difference was statistically significant and clearly is biologically significant. All patients were treated with the same high-dose regimen (ICE), and all patients received marrow HSC. Median follow-up for EFS was over 2 years, and no other risk factor could be implicated in these findings.[51]

These data lead us to conclude that minimal residual disease in the marrow detectable by PCR assay prior to HDCT is predictive of a poorer outcome (higher relapse rate) after HDCT. Furthermore, these data may be used to support the hypothesis that purging harvested marrow of tumor cells prior to cryopreservation will reduce the possibility of systemic relapse after transplantation. These data,

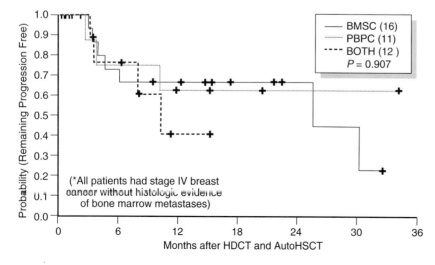

FIGURE 10–7. Comparison of progression-free survival in patients with stage IV breast cancer receiving bone marrow stem cells (BMSC), peripheral blood progenitor cells (PBPC), or both. No differences occurred in progression-free survival.

however, may also be used to support the hypothesis that the detection of minimal residual disease in the marrow is a measure of tumor burden in the body prior to transplantation and that post-transplantation antitumor therapy will be required to reduce the probability of relapse. These two hypotheses are not mutually exclusive. Both may be true, and further research is necessary to move from speculation to formal proof (see later).

RELAPSE

Although HDCT is delivered with curative intent, the principal reason for failure is relapse. In our series, for patients with locally advanced disease the relapse rate in the first 3 years is 42% and, for patients with inflammatory or metastatic breast cancer, the relapse rate is 84% (Fig. 10–8). Although these outcomes are better than for patients treated with conventional therapy, there is much room for improvement. It is noteworthy that the time to relapse curves is similar in shape for patients with locally advanced and metastatic disease and that few relapses occur in the third year after transplantation, with only rare relapses after year 3 (see Fig. 10–8). This forms the basis for our conservative recommendation that cure rates cannot be established until all patients in a study group pass 5 years from transplantation.

The distribution of sites of relapse is worthy of discussion. For patients with locoregional disease who experience relapse post transplantation, in our series there seems to be an excess of relapses in the CNS with either space-occupying lesions or meningeal carcinomatosis as the first site of relapse. This is likely due to (1) seeding of the CNS prior to any systemic chemotherapy and (2) the poor penetrability of the blood-brain barrier for many drugs used in HDCT. Notable exceptions in this "rule" are thiotepa, carmustine (BCNU), busulfan, and cytosine arabinoside, all of which are used in high doses but rarely together. For patients in our series with metastatic disease who experienced relapse after transplantation, there is no discernible pattern of preferential relapse sites. Furthermore, we cannot establish a different pattern of relapse for patients who received marrow HSC and for those who received PBPC.

What happens to patients after they relapse is an important issue to address. This is in part because relapse is common. More importantly, survival following relapse after transplantation is a measure of the palliative value of this treatment strategy even though the primary objective (cure) cannot be attained. Relapsed disease is usually treated conservatively with hormonal therapy (based on ER/PR status and prior use of hormonal therapy), single-agent chemotherapy (most recently with paclitaxel, navelbine, and lately docetaxel), combination CT (such as mitoxantrone, leucovorin, and fluorouracil if feasible, depending on prior chemotherapy) and radiotherapy (for locoregional disease control). Several observations about this salvage therapy are noteworthy. First, a surprising number of patients responded. Second, these patients tolerated myelosuppressive cytotoxic therapy poorly with significantly more frequent, severe, and prolonged myelodepression. Third, at the HLMCC, for the handful of second transplants at relapse for still-chemosensitive disease there have been objective responses but no long-term event-free survivors. This observation has been confirmed by a recently reported series from Duke University.[52] Until new regimens are developed, second transplants are not recommended unless the relapse was very late (>3 years) after the first transplant.

As shown in Figure 10–9, from a retrospective analysis of our data, the median duration of survival after relapse for all 228 (of the first 400) patients who experienced relapse was approximately 7 months.[53] From a multivariate analysis of risk factors that may determine the duration of survival after relapse following autoHSCT, the only significant factor to emerge was time between transplantation and relapse.[54] Longer time to relapse was associated with longer survival after relapse. A significant fraction of patients (~12%) were alive 2 years after relapse. Figure 10–10 shows survival following relapse after transplantation plotted on the same graph as OS from the time study treatment was begun for the two large, multicenter, conventional chemotherapy trials described earlier.[24, 25] The survival curve for transplant-failure patients was similar to that of patients in whom one chemotherapy regimen (lacking doxorubicin) had already failed. In other words, death following relapse after transplantation was no more rapid than death after second-line conventional treatment. Be-

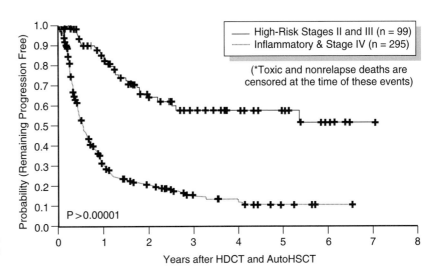

FIGURE 10–8. Progression-free survival as a function of disease stage for patients with high-risk breast cancer.

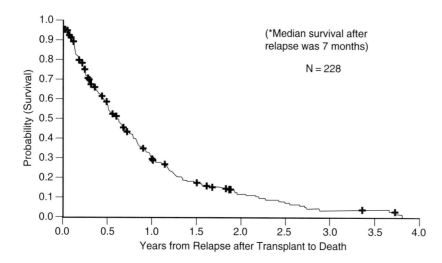

FIGURE 10-9. Survival after relapse following high-dose therapy and autologous transplantation.

cause transplant recipients experienced failure of at least two chemotherapy regimens (one containing doxorubicin and the other HDCT), it appears that HDCT provides significant palliative benefit even for patients destined to experience relapse after transplantation. (Statistical analyses could not be performed because raw data from the two reference studies[24, 25] were not available.)

PROGNOSTIC FACTORS

When a large number of patients receive the same treatment with different outcomes (i.e., EFS or OS are not uniformly obtained), it presents an opportunity to evaluate the patients and their individual clinical presentations to determine whether characteristics of their disease (or general medical circumstances) accounted for better or poorer outcomes. Such an analysis identifies prognostic factors. Subsequently, these factors may be used prospectively to select a group of patients with poor prognosis for EFS or OS for whom experimental therapy is appropriate.

Without question, the most important prognostic factor predicting an adverse outcome after transplantation for breast cancer is stage of disease (see Fig. 10–1). Patients

with metastatic disease do worse than patients with high-risk, locally advanced disease. With locally advanced breast cancer, stage still appears to play a major prognostic role. Patients with inflammatory breast cancer experience poorer EFS and OS than do other stage III patients. Finally, patients with noninflammatory stage III disease do worse than stage II patients.

The ABMTR has performed preliminary multivariate analyses[15] for more than 1000 women with metastatic breast cancer to determine prognostic factors for EFS. They have shown that for patients older than 46 years, with less than a CR to induction chemotherapy, with ER-negative disease, and with metastases to soft tissues, viscera, and/or especially the CNS, the risk of progression or death is significantly higher than for their respective counterparts (i.e., patients ≤46 years of age, in CR, with ER-positive disease, and with only bone and/or marrow metastases). In our studies of patients with metastatic disease receiving ICE, we identified a number of prognostic factors for poor EFS from univariate analyses. They are (1) presence of microscopic metastatic disease after induction therapy in the marrow as detected by PCR assay,[51] (2) anthracycline responsiveness (CR or PR),[33] and (3) dose intensity of the ICE regimen.[34] ICE was given only to patients with

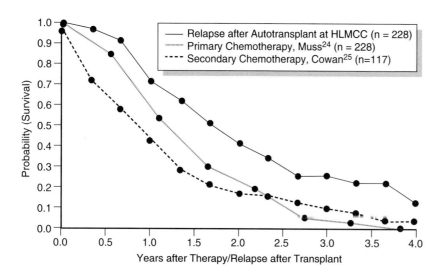

FIGURE 10–10. Overall survival with metastatic breast cancer in a comparison of three independent studies. HLMCC, H. Lee Moffitt Cancer Center.

chemosensitive disease to an anthracycline-based regimen or, failing that, to mini-ICE.[14, 36] Finally, the ABMTR presented an analysis of 758 patients with locally advanced breast cancer who received HDCT and autologous transplants. From univariate analyses, the risk factors ascertained for reduced EFS were (1) inflammatory disease and (2) ER-negative status of the primary tumor.[32]

CONTROVERSIES

Although many areas of controversy have been described in this chapter, this section has been reserved for discussion of controversial issues addressing improvement of the cure rate after transplantation presented from the point of view of (1) the current therapeutic rationale and/or interpretation of preliminary data and (2) the major pitfalls and obstacles to success. Other controversies such as economic concerns are addressed in Chapter 64.

INTERMEDIATE-DOSE THERAPY

It has been suggested that especially for locally advanced breast cancer, multiple courses of intermediate-dose, single-agent chemotherapy (given with brief interdose intervals [for improved dose intensity over conventional adjuvant therapy] with hematopoietic growth factor support with or without PBPC support) may be superior to single-event combination HDCT.[55] The preliminary results from the phase I/II trials applying this rationale are exciting, but long-term follow-up is lacking. Additionally, patient selection bias may explain the results (e.g., the average number of nodes positive for microscopic metastatic disease was 9, whereas transplants for locally advanced disease have been traditionally performed for ≥10 positive nodes). Fortunately, a large national intergroup trial comparing "standard" HDCT with multiple courses of intermediate-dose therapy has been launched. If the two treatment regimens have different results, the regimen producing the better outcome will become the strategy of choice. If the two have similar results, the least toxic and/or least expensive strategy will become the treatment of choice.

TANDEM TRANSPLANTS

Another concept being pursued by a number of centers is that of tandem transplants for metastatic disease.[56–58] The rationale for this strategy is that residual malignant cells after the first transplant, which would be the *forme fruste* for relapse, may still be chemosensitive. Because two transplants are planned, each high-dose regimen can be delivered at less than the MTD. One regimen may be repeated, or two different regimens may be employed. Conceptually, this is an attractive hypothesis. Only preliminary phase I/II data, with a potential selection bias, are available, however. Not until a phase III trial comparing a single-transplant regimen at MTD with tandem transplants is performed will we be able to determine whether one strategy is superior. Multiple courses of intermediate-dose therapy may be considered a variant of tandem transplants.

PURGING HEMATOPOIETIC STEM CELL COLLECTIONS

There is no doubt that malignant cells contaminate some, if not all, of the stem cell collections (from marrow or blood) from patients with metastatic disease.[51, 59–63] There is evidence to suggest, at least in some pediatric cancers, that tumor cells contaminating HSC product may participate in relapse of the disease after transplantation.[64] The participation of transfused tumor cells in relapse has not yet been confirmed for patients with breast cancer, however. There is no doubt that we have the technology to select positively for CD34 + cells (and achieve engraftment) and by so doing obtain an increase in reduction of tumor cell content of the stem cell product of at least 1 log[65, 66] and, alternatively, to remove tumor cells from HSC products by negative selection and thus achieve a log or more reduction of tumor contamination.[67] Preliminary phase I/II studies have shown EFS benefit in patients whose stem cell product was subjected to positive selection for CD34 + cells, eliminating tumor cells as detected by immunohistochemistry.[68] What is unclear from these studies and can only be clarified by a randomized phase III sham procedure controlled trial (such as that being performed for multiple myeloma) is whether purging HSC products to tumor-negative status is directly responsible for reducing relapse after transplantation or a surrogate marker for the low tumor cell mass remaining in the patient that must be killed in order to produce cure. In this light, those patients for whom purging to tumor-negative status cannot be achieved have a higher tumor cell mass to be destroyed by HDCT, a much more formidable task. Purging procedures and clinical efficacy are discussed in Chapter 29.

GRAFT-VERSUS-TUMOR EFFECT

The graft-versus-leukemia effect after alloHSCT has been amply demonstrated in animals and man.[69–71] The magnitude of clinical benefit derived from this phenomenon is variable, however, with chronic myelogenous leukemia benefiting most, acute lymphoblastic leukemia benefiting least, and acute myelogenous leukemia deriving intermediate benefit.[20, 72] Does an analogous allogeneic graft-versus-tumor effect exist for solid tumors?[73] This remains an unanswered clinical question. To answer it directly, alloHSCT must be compared with autologous ones in a prospective, probably allocated (by the existence of an HLA-identical sibling donor) phase III trial using a single high-dose regimen. Although allogeneic HSC should be free of tumor-cell contamination and may produce a graft-versus-tumor effect, the current study-limiting factors are the problem of GVHD and TRM associated with alloHSCT. Until these two problems (which introduce morbidity and mortality above that experienced by patients [median age, 40–45 years] receiving autologous transplants) are resolved, it will be difficult to justify this study. Further, will the best autologous transplantation regimen for EFS in patients with breast cancer be sufficiently immunosuppressive to obviate allogeneic graft rejection? Finally, even if a salutary graft-versus-tumor effect were demonstrated, only a minority of patients would have genotypically HLA-identical siblings to serve as donors, thus limiting the breadth of applicability of alloHSCT for breast cancer.

The alternative to the allogeneic graft-versus-tumor effect is the autologous graft-versus-tumor effect.[74, 75] Autologous GVHD has been induced in a significant number of patients with breast cancer receiving HDCT.[76] Even so, the last analysis performed by the Johns Hopkins Oncology Center that pioneered this field demonstrated no autologous graft-versus-tumor effect for breast cancer.[77] Further, to date, we have no evidence that transplants utilizing PBPC produce an EFS superior to those with marrow HSC,[5, 49] as has been shown for the subpopulation of patients with NHL discussed earlier.[46] One of the hypotheses generated from the retrospective study of patients with NHL was that PBPC products contain significantly more immune cells than do marrow HSC and that tumor immune destruction could be superior because of better effector-to-target-cell ratios for immune system–mediated tumor cytolysis. This hypothesis is attractive and is currently being tested in selected patients with NHL in a randomized trial,[78] the preliminary results of which do not confirm the previous report.[46] As described earlier,[48, 49] at last analysis in the stratified, randomized HSC trial that we performed comparing G-CSF–primed marrow HSC to G-CSF-mobilized PBPC (see Fig. 10–7), we did not find a significant difference in relapse-free survival between the two arms for patients with stage IV breast cancer (the single largest group of patients, accounting for 56% of total enrollment). Because the hypothesis being tested in this study dealt with the pace of hematopoietic reconstitution after transplantation, for which the required sample size was relatively small, and because the patient population enrolled was not restricted to patients with breast cancer (let alone stage IV breast cancer), we cannot exclude a small difference in relapse-free survival between the two arms of the study. Nor can we exclude the difference between the two study arms for those patients enrolled in the trial but who were not eligible for randomization because of limitations in the HSC content of the PBPC product who consequently received both HSC products at the time of transplantation. To prove that a small difference might exist and would be significant would require a significantly larger study in a homogeneous patient population.

Even if PBPC products alone do not produce an autologous graft-versus-tumor effect merely because of mass action of cells immune to tumor antigens transferred with the transplant, they are (by virtue of the higher content of immune system cells than in marrow HSC products) a perfect target for augmentation of immune function by one method or another. On the one hand it would be preferable to test any biotherapy hypothesis in patients with chemo-sensitive metastatic disease yet with a high probability of relapse after HDCT, such as our patients with metastatic disease in their marrow after induction chemotherapy detected by PCR analysis for cytokeratin-19 messenger RNA.[50] Unfortunately, these patients may still have too high a tumor-cell burden to be eradicated by the immune system in order to improve EFS. On the other hand, the least tumor cell burden is in patients treated in the adjuvant setting, in which the immune system has a better chance of eradicating MRD. Unfortunately, because of the relatively low relapse rate after transplantation for locally advanced disease, the study design would necessitate a very large sample size before a randomized controlled trial could be expected to demonstrate a positive effect from biotherapy. Furthermore, there are two few data from preclinical and phase I/II studies to choose which candidate biotherapy should be studied first.

CONCLUSION

High-dose chemotherapy supported by HSCT as a treatment for patients with "high-risk" breast cancer evolved in one decade from infancy to an advanced stage of development. Moreover, breast cancer became the most common indication for HSCT in North America. Although numerous phase II studies and some phase III studies have shown convincing improvement in survival for patients with breast cancer, there has always been controversy in the oncology community regarding the increasingly common practice of HSCT for this disease outside of clinical trials. The recent presentation of data at the annual meeting of the American Society of Clinical Oncology has further added to the confusion and controversy surrounding this field. There are many criticisms of the studies, but it is generally agreed that further research is necessary to establish the role of HSCT for patients with advanced breast cancer. There are already several ongoing randomized studies in Europe and North America and many more in the planning stages. While awaiting the results of additional trials as well as continued follow-up on already-closed trials, the patient and physician will be guided in their decision-making process by somewhat conflicting and confusing data. Enrollment in clinical trials—either phase II trials testing novel biologic, immunologic, or pharmacologic approaches or randomized phase III studies that build on the recent knowledge—should be encouraged.

REFERENCES

1. Early Breast Cancer Trialists' Collaborative Group: Systemic treatment of early breast cancer by hormonal, cytotoxic, or immune therapy: 133 randomised trials involving 31,000 recurrences and 24,000 deaths among 75,000 women. Lancet 339:1, 71, 1992.
2. Olivotto IV, Bajdik CD, Math M, et al: Adjuvant systemic therapy and survival after breast cancer. N Engl J Med 330:805, 1994.
3. Henderson IC: Chemotherapy for metastatic disease. In Harris JR, Hellman S, Henderson IC, Kinne DW (eds): Breast Diseases, 2nd ed. Philadelphia, Lippincott-Raven, 1991, p 604.
4. Elias AD, Ayash L, Anderson KC, et al: Mobilization of peripheral blood progenitor cells by chemotherapy and granulocyte-macrophage colony-stimulating factor for hematologic support after high-dose intensification for breast cancer. Blood 79:3036, 1992.
5. Fields KK, Agaliotis DP, Janssen WE, et al: High dose chemotherapy and the treatment of metastatic breast cancer: selecting the regimen and the source of stem cells. Cancer Control 1:213, 1994.
6. Cheson BD, Lacerna L, Leyland-Jones B, et al: Autologous bone marrow transplantation: current status and future directions. Ann Intern Med 110:51, 1989.
7. Antman K, Corringham R, de Vries E, et al: Dose intensive therapy in breast cancer. Bone Marrow Transplant Suppl 10:67, 1992.
8. Greenberg PA, Hortobagyi GN, Smith TL, et al: Long-term follow-up of patients with complete remission following combination chemotherapy for metastatic breast cancer. J Clin Oncol 14.2197, 1996.
9. Hortobagyi GN, Bodey SP, Buzdar AU, et al: Evaluation of high-dose versus standard FAC chemotherapy for advanced breast cancer in protected environment units: a prospective randomized study. J Clin Oncol 5:354, 1987.

10. Wood WC, Budman DR, Korzun AH, et al: Dose and dose intensity of adjuvant chemotherapy for stage II, node-positive breast carcinoma. N Engl J Med 330:1253, 1994.

11. Passweg JR, Rowlings PA, Armitage JO, et al: Report from the International Bone Marrow Transplant Registry and Autologous Blood and Marrow Transplant Registry—North America. In Cecka JM, Terasaki PI (eds): Clinical Transplants 1995. The Regents of the University of California, Los Angeles, 1996, p 117.

12. Peters WP, Ross M, Vredenburgh JJ, et al: High-dose chemotherapy and autologous bone marrow support as consolidation after standard-dose adjuvant therapy for high-risk primary breast cancer. J Clin Oncol 11:1132, 1993.

13. American Cancer Society: Cancer Facts and Figures—1999. Atlanta, American Cancer Society, 1999.

14. Fields K, Elfenbein G, Saleh R, et al: Ifosfamide, carboplatin, and etoposide in combination for induction and high-dose chemotherapy: focus on breast cancer and lymphoma. Hematol Oncol 10:61, 1992.

15. Fields KK, Perkins JP, Hiemenz JW, et al: Intensive dose ifosfamide, carboplatin, and etoposide followed by autologous stem cell rescue: results of a phase I/II study in breast cancer patients. Surg Oncol 2:87, 1993.

16. Rowlings PA, Antman KS, Horowitz MM, et al: Prognostic factors in autotransplants for metastatic breast cancer [abstract]. Blood Suppl 86:618a, 1995.

17. Sobocinski KA, Horowitz MM, Rowlings PA, et al: Bone marrow transplantation—1994: a report form the International Bone Marrow Transplant Registry and the North American Autologous Bone Marrow Transplant Registry. J Hematother 3:95, 1994.

18. Antman KH, Rowlings PA, Vaughan WP, et al: High-dose chemotherapy with autologous hematopoietic stem-cell support for breast cancer in North America. J Clin Oncol 15:1870, 1997.

19. Martin PJ, Hansen JA, Buckner CD, et al: Effects of in vitro depletion of T cells in HLA-identical allogeneic marrow grafts. Blood 66:664, 1985.

20. Goldman JM, Gale RP, Horowitz MM, et al: Bone marrow transplantation for chronic myelogenous leukemia in chronic phase: increased risk for relapse associated with T-cell depletion. Ann Intern Med 108:806, 1988.

21. Elfenbein G, Fields K, Saleh R, et al: High dose chemotherapy with autologous bone marrow rescue (HDCBMR) as adjuvant treatment of poor risk stage II breast cancer: a decision analysis [abstract]. Blood Suppl 76:536a, 1990.

22. Bezwoda WR, Seymour L, Dansey RD: High-dose chemotherapy with hematopoietic rescue as primary treatment for metastatic breast cancer: a randomized trial. J Clin Oncol 13:2483, 1995.

23. Fields KK, Elfenbein GJ, Perkins JB, Moscinski L: High dose versus standard dose chemotherapy for the treatment of breast cancer: a review of current concepts. In Sackstein R, Janssen WE, Elfenbein GJ (eds): Bone Marrow Transplantation: Foundations for the 21st Century; Annals of the New York Academy of Sciences. New York, The New York Academy of Sciences, 770:1995, p 288.

24. Muss HB, Case LD, Richards F, et al: Interrupted versus continuous chemotherapy in patients with metastatic breast cancer. N Engl J Med 325:1342, 1991.

25. Cowan JD, Neidhart J, McClure S, et al: Randomized trial of doxorubicin, bisantrene, and mitoxantrone in advanced breast cancer: a Southwest Oncology Group study. J Natl Cancer Inst 83:1077, 1991.

26. Peters WP, Jones RB, Vredenburgh J, et al: A large, prospective, randomized trial of high-dose combination alkylating agents (CPB) with autologous cellular support (ABMS) as consolidation for patients with metastatic breast cancer achieving complete remission after intensive doxorubicin-based induction therapy (AFM) [Abstract]. Proc Am Soc Clin Oncol 15:149a, 1996.

27. Peters W, Rosner G, Vredenburgh J, et al: A prospective, randomized comparison of two doses of combination alkylating agents (AA) after CAF in high-risk primary breast cancer involving 10 or more axillary lymph nodes (LN): preliminary results of CALGB 9082/SWOG 9114/NCIC MA-13 [abstract]. Proc Am Soc Clin Oncol 18:1a, 1999.

28. The Scandinavian Breast Cancer Study Group 9401: Results from a randomized adjuvant breast cancer study with high dose chemotherapy with CTCb supported by autologous bone marrow stem cells versus dose escalated and tailored FEC therapy [abstract]. Proc Am Soc Clin Oncol 18:2a, 1999.

29. Bezwoda WR: Randomized, controlled trial of high dose chemother-apy (HD-CNVp) versus standard dose (CAF) chemotherapy for high risk, surgically treated, primary breast cancer [abstract]. Proc Am Soc Clin Oncol 18:2a, 1999.

30. Stadtmauer EA, O'Neill A, Goldstein LJ, et al: Conventional-dose chemotherapy compared with high-dose chemotherapy plus autologous hematopoietic stem-cell transplantation for metastatic breast cancer. Philadelphia Bone Marrow Transplant Group. New Engl J Med 342:1069–1076, 2000.

31. Lotz J-P, Cure H, Janvier M, et al: High-dose chemotherapy (HD-CT) with hematopoietic stem cells (sic) transplantation (HSCT) for metastatic breast cancer (MBC): results of the French Protocol PEGASE 04 [abstract]. Proc Am Soc Clin Oncol 18:43a, 1999.

32. Rowlings PA, Antman KH, Fay JW, et al: Prognostic factors for outcome of autotransplants in women with high-risk primary breast cancer [Abstract]. Proc Am Soc Clin Oncol 16:117a, 1997.

33. Perkins JB, Fields KK, Partyka JS, Elfenbein GJ: Novel high dose regimens for the treatment of breast cancer. In Dicke KA, Keating A (eds): Autologous Blood and Marrow Transplantation, Proceedings of the 8th International Symposium. Arlington, TX, 1997, p 387.

34. Perkins JP, Elfenbein GJ, Fields KK: Analysis of dose response relationships in the setting of high dose ifosfamide, carboplatin, and etoposide and autologous hematopoietic stem cell transplantation: implications for the treatment of patients with advanced breast cancer. Semin Oncol Suppl 23:42, 1996.

35. Fields KK, Perkins JB, Elfenbein GJ: Reply to letter-to-the-editor. J Clin Oncol 13:1826, 1995.

36. Fields KK, Zorsky PE, Hiemenz JW, et al: Ifosfamide, carboplatin, and etoposide: a new regimen with a broad spectrum of activity. J Clin Oncol 12:544, 1994.

37. Elfenbein GJ, Perkins JB, Janssen WE, et al: Recovery of hematopoiesis after high dose therapy and autologous peripheral blood stem cell transplantation is clearly dependent upon the mobilizing regimen and the transplant regimen [abstract]. Blood Suppl 88:407a, 1996.

38. Schwietzer VG, Juillard GJ, Bajada CL, Parker RG: Radiation recall dermatitis and pneumonitis in a patient treated with paclitaxel. Cancer 76:1069, 1995.

39. Zulian GB, Aapro MS: Docetaxel and radiation-recall severe mucositis [Letter]. Ann Oncol 5:964, 1994.

40. Fields KK, Elfenbein GJ, Lazarus HM, et al: Maximum tolerated doses of ifosfamide, carboplatin, and etoposide given over six days followed by autologous stem cell rescue: toxicity profile. J Clin Oncol 13:323, 1995.

41. Agaliotis DP, Ballester OF, Mattox T, et al: Ifosfamide related nephrotoxicity in adults undergoing autologous stem cell transplantation. Am J Med Sci 1997.

42. Fields KK, Elfenbein GJ, Perkins JB, et al: Two novel high dose treatment regimens for metastatic breast cancer: ifosfamide, carboplatin plus etoposide (ICE) and mitoxantrone plus thioTEPA (MITT): outcomes and toxicities. Semin Oncol Suppl 20:59, 1993.

43. Ballester OF, Agaliotis DP, Hiemenz JW, et al: Phase I-II study of high dose busulfan and cyclophosphamide followed by autologous peripheral blood stem cell transplantation for haematological malignancies: toxicities and haematopoietic recovery. Bone Marrow Transplant 18:9, 1996.

44. Fields K, Perkins J, Elfenbein G, et al: A phase I dose escalation trial of high dose Taxol, Novantrone, and thioTEPA (TNT) followed by autologous stem cell rescue (ASCR): toxicity [abstract]. Proc Am Soc Clin Oncol 14:322, 1995.

45. Partyka JB, Fields KK, Perkins JB, et al: The effects of age on tolerance of high dose ifosfamide, carboplatin, and etoposide and autologous stem cell rescue: morbidity and mortality [Abstract]. Proc Am Soc Clin Oncol 15:506, 1996.

46. Vose J, Anderson JR, Kessinger A, et al: High-dose chemotherapy and autologous hematopoietic stem-cell transplantation for aggressive non-Hodgkin's lymphoma. J Clin Oncol 11:1846, 1993.

47. Liberti G, Pearce R, Taghipour G, et al: Comparison of peripheral blood stem-cell and autologous bone marrow transplantation for lymphoma patients: a case-controlled analysis of the EBMT Registry data. Lymphoma Working Party for the EBMT. Ann Oncol Suppl 5:151, 1994.

48. Janssen WE, Hiemenz JW, Fields KK, et al: Stem cells from bone marrow and blood for transplant: a comparative review. Cancer Control 1:225, 1994.

49. Janssen WE, Smilee RC, Elfenbein GJ: A prospective randomized trial

comparing blood vs. marrow derived stem cells for hematopoietic replacement following high dose chemotherapy. J Hematother 4:139, 1995.

50. Moscinski LC, Trudeau W, Fields KK, Elfenbein GJ: High sensitivity detection of minimal residual breast carcinoma using the polymerase chain reaction and primers for cytokeratin 19. Diagn Mol Pathol 5:173, 1996.

51. Fields KK, Elfenbein GJ, Trudeau WL, et al: The clinical significance of bone marrow metastases as detected using polymerase chain reaction methods in patients with breast cancer undergoing high dose chemotherapy and autologous bone marrow transplantation. J Clin Oncol 14:1868, 1996.

52. Bearman SI, Vredenburgh JJ, Cagnoni PJ, et al: High-dose therapy with autologous hematopoietic progenitor cell support for patients with breast cancer who failed previous stem cell-supported therapy [Abstract]. Proc Am Soc Clin Oncol 16:177a, 1997.

53. Singh B, Elfenbein GJ, Kronish LE, et al: Survival duration after relapse following high dose therapy and autologous hematopoietic stem cell transplantation for high risk breast cancer patients [abstract]. Proc Am Soc Clin Oncol 16:117a, 1997.

54. Elfenbein GJ, Singh B, Kronish LE, et al: High dose chemotherapy and autologous stem cell transplantation provides palliation for women with high risk breast cancer who are not cured by transplant [abstract]. Exp Hematol 25:821, 1997.

55. Fennelly D, Vahdat L, Schneider J, et al: High-intensity chemotherapy with peripheral blood progenitor cell support. Semin Oncol Suppl 21:21, 1994.

56. Ayash LJ, Elias A, Schwartz G, et al: Double dose intensive chemotherapy with autologous stem-cell support for metastatic breast cancer: no improvement in progression-free survival by the sequence of high-dose melphalan followed by cyclophosphamide, thioTEPA, and carboplatin. J Clin Oncol 14:2984, 1996.

57. Spitzer G, Dunphy FR, Petruska PJ, et al: Tandem transplants in solid tumors: marrow versus peripheral stem cell transplant: peripheral blood cells as now practiced are not the answer. J Hematother 2:363, 1993.

58. Bitran JD, Samuels B, Klein L, et al: Tandem high-dose chemotherapy supported by haematopoietic progenitor cells yields prolonged survival in stage IV breast cancer. Bone Marrow Transplant 17:157, 1996.

59. Datta YH, Adams PT, Drobyski WR, et al: Sensitive detection of occult breast cancer by the reverse-transcriptase polymerase chain reaction. J Clin Oncol 12:475, 1994.

60. Sharp JG, Kessinger A, Vaughan WP, et al: Detection and clinical significance of minimal tumor cell contamination of peripheral stem cell harvests. Int J Cell Cloning Suppl 10:92, 1992.

61. Ross AA, Cooper BW, Lazarus HM, et al: Detection and viability of tumor cells in peripheral blood stem cell collections from breast cancer patients using immunocytochemical and clonogenic assay techniques. Blood 82:2605, 1993.

62. Kessinger A, Reed E, Vaughan W, Sharp J: Clinical outcome of patients (pts) with breast cancer and gynecological epithelial tumors undergoing high-dose therapy and peripheral stem cell transplantation with or without minimally contaminated apheresis harvests [Abstract]. Proc Am Soc Clin Oncol 12:97a, 1993.

63. Vredenburgh J, Silva O, de Sombre K, et al: The significance of bone marrow micrometastases for patients (pts) with breast cancer and ≥10+ lymph nodes treated with high-dose chemotherapy and hematopoietic support [Abstract]. Proc Am Soc Clin Oncol 14:317a, 1995.

64. Brenner MK, Rill DR, Moen RC, et al: Gene-marking to trace origin of relapse after autologous bone-marrow transplantation. Lancet 341:85, 1993.

65. Shpall EJ, Jones RB, Bearman SI, et al: Transplantation of CD34+ hematopoietic progenitor cells. J Hematother 3:145, 1994.

66. Shpall EJ, Jones RB, Bearman SI, et al: Transplantation of enriched CD34-positive autologous marrow into breast cancer patients following high-dose chemotherapy: influence of CD34-positive peripheral-blood progenitors and growth factors on engraftment. J Clin Oncol 12:28, 1994.

67. Graham-Pole J, Casper J, Elfenbein G, et al: High-dose chemoradiotherapy supported by marrow infusions for advanced neuroblastoma: a Pediatric Oncology Group pilot study. J Clin Oncol 9:152, 1991.

68. Shpall EJ, Franklin WA, Jones RB, et al: Transplantation of CD34 positive (+) marrow and/or peripheral blood progenitor cells (PBPCS) into breast cancer patients following high-dose chemotherapy [abstract]. Blood Suppl 84:396a, 1994.

69. Sinkovics JG, Shullenberger CC, Howe CD: Immunological functions of homologous spleen cells in viral mouse leukemia. Tex Rep Biol Med 23:94, 1965.

70. Sinkovics JG, Ahern MJ, Shirato E, Shullenberger CC: Viral leukemogenesis in immunologically and hematologically altered mice. J Reticuloendothelial Soc 8:474, 1970.

71. Weiden P, Flournoy N, Thomas ED, et al: Antileukemic effect of graft-versus-host disease in human recipients of allogeneic-marrow grafts. N Engl J Med 300:1068, 1979.

72. Horowitz MM, Gale RP, Sondel PM, et al: Graft-versus-leukemia reactions after bone marrow transplantation. Blood 75:555, 1990.

73. Ueno NT, Rondon G, Mizra NQ, et al: Allogeneic versus autologous transplantation for poor risk patients with metastatic breast cancer [Abstract]. Proc Am Soc Clin Oncol 16:116a, 1997.

74. Elfenbein GJ, Green I, Paul WE: The allogeneic effect: increased affinity of serum antibody produced during a secondary response. Eur J Immunol 3:640, 1973.

75. Elfenbein GJ, Green I, Paul WE: The allogeneic effect: increased cellular immune and inflammatory responses. J Immunol 112:2166, 1974.

76. Hess AD, Kennedy MJ, Ruvolo PP, et al: Antitumor activity of syngeneic/autologous graft-versus-host disease. In Sackstein R, Janssen WE, Elfenbein GJ (eds): Bone marrow transplantation: foundations for the 21st century. Ann NY Acad Sci 770:189, 1995.

77. Kennedy MJ, Hess AD, Passos Coelho JL, et al: Autologous graft vs. host disease (AGVHD) as immune therapy after high-dose chemotherapy (HDC) for metastatic breast cancer (MBC): medium-term follow-up and comparison with historical controls [Abstract]. Proc Am Soc Clin Oncol 15:335a, 1996.

78. Vose JM, Sharp JG, Chan W, et al: High-dose chemotherapy (HDC) and autotransplant for non-Hodgkin's lymphoma (NHL): randomized trial of peripheral blood (PBST) versus bone marrow (ABMT) and evaluation of minimal residual disease (MRD) [Abstract]. Proc Am Soc Clin Oncol 16:90a, 1997.

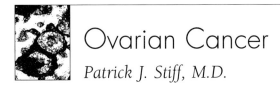

Ovarian Cancer

Patrick J. Stiff, M.D.

In 2000, ovarian cancer will be diagnosed in an estimated 23,100 women.[1] During this same year, 14,000 will die of this disease, making ovarian cancer the most lethal gynecologic malignancy and the fourth most common cause of cancer deaths in women. The incidence and mortality rates mirror those for all forms of leukemia combined.[1] Although our understanding of this disease has improved in recent years, the resources designed to improve early detection and therapy of this lethal illness are only now increasing.

Unfortunately, the death rate for this disease is unlikely to improve in the near term. Compared with the mid-1970s, the prognosis for patients with ovarian cancer has improved[2]; however, much of the improvement can be linked to the effective management of germ cell or stromal cell tumors in young women and the aggressive initial surgical management that is now undertaken for patients with the epithelial form of the disease.[3] For epithelial ovarian cancer, the most common form, newer conventional therapies that include agents such as paclitaxel are indeed improving the median survival, but this is unlikely to translate into a significantly higher cure rate, at least for those with bulky disease at diagnosis. In addition, screening for this disease, except in those with a genetic predisposition, has thus far been unsuccessful in effectively diagnosing early-stage ovarian cancer. Thus, any improvements in the prognosis of women with this disease will have to come from the treatment side of the equation.

Ovarian carcinoma is a heterogeneous group of tumors of which epithelial ovarian cancer composes the largest group (85%) and is the focus of this review. Because of their rarity and curability with conventional therapy, the other two major forms of ovarian cancer, germ cell tumors and sex/stromal cell tumors, are only occasionally seen at transplant centers. If high-dose therapy is used for these tumors, patients are most often treated with regimens similar to those used for male germ cell tumors. Their clinical outcome with high-dose therapy would be expected to mirror the results for male tumors (i.e., based on the bulk of disease and sensitivity to conventional platinum-based regimens). On the other hand, epithelial ovarian cancers are rarely cured with conventional therapy[4, 5] and have been the subject of numerous high-dose therapy approaches in recent years.[6, 7]

STAGING AND PROGNOSTIC FACTORS

The median age of onset for epithelial ovarian cancer is 63 years. The staging and the respective incidence of each stage as per the International Federation of Gynecology and Obstetrics (FIGO) classification is shown in Table 11–1.[8] As indicated, the vast majority of patients present with stage III/IV disease, largely because of the vague nature of symptoms that precede the diagnosis, which include mild bloating, constipation, vague nausea, and weight gain. These symptoms are all associated with the normal aging process; a high-fat, high-calorie, and low-bulk diet; and a sedentary lifestyle. Unfortunately, even in the younger woman, the symptoms are often ignored, largely because of the rarity of the disease.

At diagnosis, all patients undergo thorough surgical staging, including tumor debulking, total abdominal hysterectomy, bilateral salpingo-oophorectomy, omentectomy and, especially for early-stage disease, pelvic and retroperitoneal lymph node dissection to detect occult disease. The most important prognostic factor for patients with epithelial tumors remains the amount of bulk disease at the completion of the initial surgical procedure; thus, a complete surgical procedure, best accomplished by a trained gynecologic oncologist, is critical. The amount of residual disease for patients with the most common stage of disease (stage III) correlates strongly with prognosis: The median survival for patients with bulk of less than 1 cm is 45–50 months; for bulk of 1 cm or more, it is 25–30 months.[4, 5] For patients who undergo inadequate surgery at the time of diagnosis, the possibility of early re-exploration after a chemotherapy-induced remission may also be of value in improving prognosis,[9] although this is still the subject of confirmatory ongoing trials.

Other prognostic variables that have been shown to affect survival in multivariate analyses include age, performance status, grade of the tumor, and histology.[10] Of the histologic subtypes, the worst is clear cell carcinoma. It rarely re-

TABLE 11–1. FIGO (INTERNATIONAL FEDERATION OF GYNECOLOGY AND OBSTETRICS) STAGING AND SURVIVAL OF EPITHELIAL OVARIAN CANCER

STAGE	EXTENT	INCIDENCE	SURVIVAL*
I	Ovary (one or both) ± malignant ascities	25%	90%
II	Local pelvic extension	15%	75%
III	Microscopic or gross extension to peritoneum or retroperitoneal lymph nodes	45%	20%
IV	Distant spread including hematogenous	15%	5%

*Survival estimated at 5 years.

sponds completely to chemotherapy, relapses quickly in those who do respond, and typically does not respond to salvage chemotherapy. With the other subtypes, survival is best with endometrioid and mucinous carcinomas.[11] Tumor grade appears to be an important prognostic factor: The 5-year survival rate with grade III tumors is 5–25%; with grade I tumors, it is 70–80%.

Age is one of the more controversial prognostic factors, especially at both ends of the spectrum. It is well known that elderly patients receive less therapy, which includes both surgery and chemotherapy, and thus is it not surprising that they do more poorly. In fact, limited data indicate that elderly patients do as well as younger women when treated with the same aggressiveness.[12] For the young, premenopausal group, age has been shown to be a favorable prognostic variable. In a 1998 analysis by Duska et al., however, this improvement was due to a larger proportion of borderline malignant tumors; with the exclusion of such tumors from this younger age group, the 5-year survival for advanced disease is identical to that of older women.[13] Thus, all indications are that, with the same aggressive therapy for advanced disease with the most common grade of disease (grade III), age is not as important as it once was thought to be. This has obvious implications for high-dose therapy studies, especially dispelling the fact that young patients do well with conventional therapy; thus, any improvement associated with high-dose therapy must consider age.

INITIAL MANAGEMENT

The optimal initial conventional therapy of patients with ovarian cancer has been reviewed.[4, 5] Patients with stage I, low-grade tumors without malignant ascites are treated with surgery alone and have a 5-year survival rate that approaches 90%. Patients with stage I disease with ascites or grade II tumors or with stage II disease postoperatively receive some form of therapy designed to reduce their risk of relapse, which is approximately 35%. Ongoing trials are determining what that therapy should be, with most studies now testing the value of platinum-based chemotherapy. As expected, neither of these groups are being investigated with high-dose therapies.

As has been indicated, patients with stage III and IV disease have a dismal prognosis, even with newer regimens: Initial management still fails 75% of the time. In fact, patients with stage IV disease have a 5-year survival rate that approaches only 5–7%.[14] Nevertheless, newer conventional regimens do appear to have made a modest impact on median survival rates for patients with advanced disease. More importantly, these regimens appear to more effectively cytoreduce the residual disease left after initial surgery.[15–17] This should have important implications for the potential use of high-dose therapy as consolidation treatment of initial remissions.

Patients treated with platinum-based chemotherapy have response rates of roughly 70%, with the major discriminant for long-term survival based on the amount of residual disease after initial surgery.[18, 19] Optimal disease is defined as a maximal diameter of 1 cm at initial surgery, with suboptimal disease denoting larger bulk residual. Most recently reported clinical trials separate and treat these two groups separately, with platinum/cyclophosphamide regimens yielding the following results: For suboptimal stage III and IV disease, median progression-free survival (PFS) is 12 months and median 24-month overall survival (OS) is 24 months; for optimal stage III disease, median PFS is 20 months and OS is 40 months.[4, 5] The choice of platinum compound (i.e., cisplatin vs. carboplatin) has no impact on outcome, but carboplatin appears to be less neurotoxic in a randomized trial of the two agents.[20]

The current optimal chemotherapy regimen for patients with stage III/IV disease is paclitaxel with either cisplatin or carboplatin, although cisplatin has been the more extensively studied of the two (Table 11–2).[15–17] Because paclitaxel led to favorable results when used with relapsed/refractory disease, it was incorporated into front-line therapy with cisplatin and compared with cyclophosphamide and cisplatin in a phase III trial reported in 1996 by the Gynecologic Oncology Group, who studied patients with suboptimal stage III/IV disease. The paclitaxel group showed significant improvement in responses (73% vs. 60%), PFS (13 vs. 18 months), and OS (26 vs. 38 months), although the pathologic complete remission (CR) rate was no higher for the new therapy.[15]

A second study, performed internationally, explored the same combination of cisplatin and paclitaxel, although the platinum was administered as a 3-hour infusion rather than a 24-hour infusion as was used in the first study.[16, 17] Unlike the first study, this trial also included patients with optimal stage III disease (35%). Again there was a significant improvement in response rate (77% vs. 66%), PFS (16 vs. 12 months), and OS (35 vs. 25 months), a degree of survival benefit similar to that reported by the Gynecologic Oncology Group. A follow-up Gynecologic Oncology Group trial, however, compared the paclitaxel/cisplatin combination to either agent alone and showed no difference in the PFS or OS for a similar group of patients treated with cisplatin alone versus the new combination—apparently contradicting the results of the original trial.[21] Unlike the case with the initial trial, patients in the second trial were eligible to receive paclitaxel at the time of relapse if they did not receive it initially.

Taken together, these studies suggest a modest benefit to paclitaxel-based regimens, although the timing of the use

TABLE 11–2. RECENT PACLITAXEL-BASED TRIALS IN ADVANCED OVARIAN CARCINOMA

TRIAL	REGIMEN	PFS (MONTHS)	OS (MONTHS)
Suboptimal Stage III/IV Disease			
GOG 111[15]	Pac 135 mg/m² + Cisplatin 75 mg/m²	18	38
GOG 132[21]	Pac 135 mg/m² + Cisplatin 75 mg/m²	16	35
International[17]*	Pac 175 mg/m² + Cisplatin 75 mg/m²	16	35
Optimal Stage III Disease			
GOG 114[23]	Pac 135 mg/m² + Cisplatin 75 mg/m²	25	48

Pac, (paclitaxel); GOG, Gynecologic Oncology Group.
*Included 35% with optimal stage III disease; Pac given as 3-hour infusion.

of this agent (i.e., with platinum or sequentially following platinum) remains to be determined. Subsequent studies suggest that carboplatin can be used in lieu of cisplatin, with paclitaxel, over a 3-hour infusion.[22] Thus, in summary, paclitaxel with a platinum compound should be considered the initial treatment of choice for patients with advanced ovarian cancer; however, patients with suboptimal stage III/IV disease can optimally expect a median PFS of only 16–18 months. OS advantages appear greater, likely because of the increased cytoreduction with the combination and an associated increase in the number of responding patients who re-respond to either of the two agents at the time of relapse.

The ideal therapy for patients with optimal stage III disease is likely to be similar to that for patients with suboptimal disease. In the international study discussed earlier, use of paclitaxel benefited both the suboptimal and the optimal group.[16, 17] In a 1998 Gynecologic Oncology Group trial that explored intraperitoneal therapy, the control arm was the same regimen of paclitaxel plus cisplatin used in the initial trial for suboptimal disease.[23] The PFS and OS for patients with optimal stage III disease were 22.5 and 47.6 months, respectively, again showing a modest benefit for the new regimen as compared with results from other trials using platinum and cyclophosphamide. The percentage of patients who will be disease free at 5–8 years is yet to be determined by these studies. The majority of patients with optimal stage III disease, however, will still experience relapse and ultimately die of drug-refractory disease.

RATIONALE FOR HIGH-DOSE THERAPY

Ovarian cancer, like the leukemias, the lymphomas, and testes cancer but unlike most cases of extensive stage IV breast cancer, is initially chemosensitive. A majority of patients enter clinical CR, but ovarian cancer is frequently incurable using conventional therapies. Because of its dismal prognosis and the fact that it shares some of the features of other initially chemosensitive tumors that respond favorably to intensive high-dose chemotherapy regimens, interest in high-dose therapy has increased in recent years (Table 11–3). Both in vitro and in vivo data validate the utility of dose intensity in ovarian cancer, including regional high-dose therapy via the intraperitoneal route.[24–30] The latter data have been confirmed in a randomized phase III trial reported in 1996 that compared intravenous with intraperitoneal cisplatin, both combined with cyclophosphamide.[30] There is a favorable dose-response curve for a

TABLE 11–3. RATIONALE FOR HIGH-DOSE THERAPY IN OVARIAN CANCER

Despite large tumor burden at diagnosis, pathologic complete remissions occur in 25–40%
Cures occur with conventional-dose therapy
In vitro favorable dose-response curve
Active agents can be safely escalated with in vitro synergy
Improved survival using regional high-dose (intraperitoneal) chemotherapy

variety of clinically active agents,[26, 27] and synergy of these active agents in vitro has been demonstrated.[28, 29]

As with other tumors, the use of this therapy in ovarian cancer has evolved over time. Initially, both chemorefractory disease and, because of the high response rate, relapsing chemoresponsive disease were treated. Most recently, efforts have focused on patients who respond to initial therapy. As with other diseases, data strongly suggest the benefit of high-dose therapy, with patients with certain risk factors benefiting most. What appears unique to this disease is that the well-known phenomenon that long remissions induced by conventional chemotherapy increase the probability of responsiveness to subsequent therapy,[31] as described later, appears to also occur in patients responding to high-dose therapy. Thus, a prolonged remission after transplantation appears to increase the chances of a subsequent postrelapse response to conventional salvage therapy.

TRANSPLANTS FOR RELAPSED AND REFRACTORY DISEASE

Patients not responding to or experiencing relapse after initial chemotherapy are incurable with conventional chemotherapy. In fact, a 1995 National Cancer Institute Consensus Conference on Ovarian Cancer concluded that palliative salvage chemotherapy does not improve survival.[32] The authors suggested that these patients should be offered innovative, experimental forms of therapy. Nevertheless, a small percentage of patients do respond to conventional salvage therapy and, with the availability of several new active agents with different modes of action, it may now be possible that survival after relapse can be enhanced.

Patients experiencing relapse have been divided prognostically into two groups based on their platinum "sensitivity." Patients whose disease does not respond to platinum or who experience relapse within 6 months after completing a course of platinum chemotherapy have a median survival of approximately 8–12 months and a response rate to further platinum of 5–15%.[33] These together make up the platinum-resistant group. On the other hand, patients who do not experience relapse until more than 6 months after the completion of platinum-based therapy are considered platinum sensitive.[34, 35] They have a median survival rate of 16–20 months and a response rate to platinum of 35–50%, depending on the duration of their initial remission. The differences between these two groups are significant and need to be considered when new drug therapies, including dose-intensive options, are considered.

For the platinum-resistant group, a variety of agents may produce remissions, including paclitaxel,[36, 37] topotecan,[38, 39] liposomal doxorubicin,[40] oral low-dose etoposide,[41] and hexamethylmelamine.[42] When these agents are used as second-line treatments, remissions occur in approximately 20% of patients and last 3–4 months; survival from the onset of first relapse is 5–12 months. In contrast, when those with platinum-sensitive disease are traditionally re-treated with cisplatin or carboplatin, responses are in the 35–40% range. No conventional single-agent or combination chemotherapy is superior to the re-introduction of platinum for this patient group.[34, 35] Remissions last 4–6 months, and survival from first relapse is approximately 16 months. Thus, these figures serve for rough comparisons for any new drug therapy or novel treatment approach.

EARLY TRANSPLANT TRIALS IN REFRACTORY DISEASE

Although conventional salvage therapy produces responses in the range of 15–25% for platinum-refractory disease,[33, 36] early transplant trials reported response rates for drug-resistant disease of roughly 75%.[43–45] In a phase I trial, Shea et al. treated a large number of patients with refractory tumors with high-dose carboplatin and autologous bone marrow transplantation.[43] Of the 11 patients treated with ovarian cancer, seven (77%) responded, one of whom entered CR.

Shpall et al. used trialkylator therapy consisting of thiotepa, cyclophosphamide, and cisplatin in a group of 12 patients in whom a median of three prior regimens had failed and who all had platinum-resistant disease.[44] All were debulked surgically prior to transplantation and all received their cisplatin via the intraperitoneal route. Of eight evaluable patients, six (75%) entered a pathologic partial remission that lasted a median of 6 months.

Stiff et al. treated seven patients with refractory ovarian cancer with a combination of high-dose carboplatin, cyclophosphamide, and mitoxantrone as part of a phase I trial.[45] Mitoxantrone was chosen because of its in-vitro activity with platinum-resistant disease at high doses using the tumor cloning assay. This trial demonstrated that the mitoxantrone doses (75 mg/m^2) gave serum levels in the steepest part of the in-vitro dose response curve when tumor cells from patients with platinum-resistant disease were analyzed. Of six evaluable patients (there was one early death), all responded, with a median response duration of 7.5 months. One in whom platinum-based induction therapy had failed was progression-free at more than 2 years, and 29% were alive at 2 years.

Among several other studies, a phase II trial of the carboplatin, cyclophosphamide, and mitoxantrone regimen first began to suggest which patients are likely to benefit from high-dose therapy.[46] Of the 30 patients undergoing transplantation, two thirds had platinum-resistant disease and 73% had bulky disease as defined by maximum residual disease greater than 1 cm at the time of transplantation. The results were similar to those of other trials: Of the 27 patients with measurable or evaluable disease, 89% responded, with 7 of 8 patients with platinum-sensitive disease entering clinical CR versus 9 of 19 patients with platinum-resistant disease ($P = .06$). The median survival for the entire group was 29 months, and the median PFS was 7 months. The 10 patients with platinum-sensitive disease did not reach the median survival time, however, experiencing an 80% survival rate at 1 year. Given the short OS (10.4 months) for platinum-resistant disease, the study concluded that high-dose therapy may not be of any value to patients with platinum-resistant disease.

Studies from other centers reporting on small numbers of patients have generally drawn the same conclusions regarding platinum-resistant disease. The largest of these trials were reported by Weaver et al. and Holmberg et al. (Table 11–4).[47, 48] Weaver et al., using high-dose carboplatin, mitoxantrone, and melphalan, treated a group of 31 patients who had received a median of two prior regimens.[47] The CR rate was 70%, and of the seven patients who were in CR at the time of transplantation, five remained in CR at 9–19 months. Holmberg et al. treated 31 patients with the busulfan, melphalan, and thiotepa (BUMELTT) regimen.[48] Of 13 patients with platinum-sensitive disease, six were progression free; of 18 with platinum-resistant disease, only two remained in remission at a median follow-up time for all patients of 564 days. These studies taken together have led to the conclusion that patients with platinum-resistant disease should not be offered transplant therapy. Given the small proportion of patients with platinum-sensitive disease who remain in continuous remission for more than 2 years, however, it would appear that transplantation may be an advantage in this subgroup of patients experiencing relapse.

MULTIVARIATE ANALYSIS OF PROGNOSTIC FACTORS

These preliminary findings were further validated in a multivariate analysis of 100 consecutive patients treated at Loyola University Medical Center.[49] Similar to results with the initial 30-patient series, 66% had platinum-resistant disease and 61% had tumor bulk of greater than 1 cm at transplantation. Age, remission status, platinum sensitivity, bulk, months from diagnosis, histology, grade, number of prior regimens, response to induction therapy, transplant

TABLE 11–4. PROGRESSION-FREE AND OVERALL SURVIVAL FOR PATIENTS UNDERGOING TRANSPLANTATION FOR RELAPSED/REFRACTORY OVARIAN CANCER: SERIES WITH 30 OR MORE PATIENTS

SERIES	N	REGIMEN	PLATINUM RESISTANT	PLATINUM SENSITIVE
Stiff et al.[46]	30	Carboplatin 500 mg/m^2 Mitoxantrone 75 mg/m^2 Cyclophosphamide 120 mg/m^2	10.4 months OS 5.1 months PFS	>80% survival at 1 yr 10.1 months PFS
Weaver et al.[47]	31	Carboplatin 500 mg/m^2 Mitoxantrone 75 mg/m^2 Melphalan 1600 mg/m^2	10/16 alive; 8/16 progression free at 15 months*	7/12 alive; 4/12 progression free at 15 months
Holmberg et al.[48]	31	Busulfan 12 mg/m^2 Melphalan 100 mg/m^2 Thiotepa 500 mg/m^2	33% survival at 18 months, 2/18 progression free	100% survival at 18 months, 6/13 progression free

OS, overall survival; PFS, progression-free survival.
*Includes four patients without evaluable data at transplantation.

TABLE 11–5. PROGRESSION-FREE AND OVERALL SURVIVAL OF PATIENTS UNDERGOING TRANSPLANTATION FOR OVARIAN CANCER AT LOYOLA*

GROUP	N	SURVIVAL (MONTHS)	PFS (MONTHS)
All patients	164	17.3	7.7
Resistant	87	10.5	5.6
Sensitive	77	30.8	11.7
Sensitive, <1 cm	57	43.3	16.0
Sensitive, ≥1 cm	20	23.3	7.8
NED	17	43.8	33.2

NED, no evidence of disease; Resistant, platinum resistant; Sensitive, platinum sensitive.

*Data to July 1998 (N = 164).

regimen, stage at diagnosis, and response to initial conventional therapy were analyzed. For the multivariate analysis, bulk at the time of transplantation and platinum sensitivity were the two significant factors affecting PFS. For OS, age, bulk, and platinum sensitivity were the significant factors. Of all of the factors, bulk was the most important. Although the median survival was only 9.6 months for those with resistant disease, patients with resistant disease of minimal bulk (<1 cm) had a median survival of 28 months; those with bulky disease had a survival of only 8.6 months, suggesting that patients with platinum-resistant disease of low tumor burden may benefit from high-dose therapy. The best risk group comprised patients with platinum-sensitive disease and low tumor bulk. This group had a PFS of nearly 19 months and a projected OS of 29 months.

As of May 1998, 164 patients had been treated and followed for a median of 36 months.[50] Over time, proportionately fewer patients with resistant or bulky disease have been treated: Now, less than one-half of the entire group have had bulky disease (>1 cm) at the time of transplantation, and 47% of the group have platinum-sensitive disease. Of the 164 patients, 79 were treated with the initial regimen of carboplatin, mitoxantrone, and cyclophosphamide. Forty patients with resistant, primarily low-bulk disease received a new regimen of melphalan (180 mg/m^2), mitoxantrone (90 mg/m^2), and paclitaxel (450–650 mg/m^2 given as a 96-hour infusion), and 38 patients with platinum-sensitive disease received a regimen of dose-intensive paclitaxel (700 mg/m^2), carboplatin (area-under-the-curve [AUC] dose, 20–28), and mitoxantrone (90 mg/m^2). Seven received a variety of alternative regimens, including thiotepa, cisplatin, and cyclophosphamide in a Southwest Oncology Group multicenter phase II trial.

The results are shown in Table 11–5. The median PFS for all 164 patients is 7.7 months, and their OS is 17.3 months. Similar to the case with our initial report,[49] the OS for those below the median age of 48 years was 22.8 months versus 13.5 months for patients older than 48 years (P = .018). Those with platinum-resistant disease continue to do poorly, with a PFS and OS of only 5.6 and 10.5 months, respectively. Unlike the survival benefit reported in the analysis of first 100 patients for resistant disease of low tumor burden, the OS for this group is only 12 months versus the 28 months reported previously. The PFS and OS for those with platinum-sensitive disease were

11.7 and 30.8 months, respectively. For those with minimal-bulk, platinum-sensitive disease, the PFS is 16.0 months and the OS is 43.3 months, both significantly higher than for patients with platinum-sensitive, bulky disease (PFS = 7.8 months; OS = 23.3 months). Approximately 40% of this subgroup appeared to be disease-free at the median follow-up time of 2 years, and approximately 20% are projected to be disease-free at 4–5 years.

COMPARISONS WITH CONVENTIONAL THERAPY

Without randomized phase III comparative data to document a definite improvement in PFS or OS for patients undergoing transplantation after initial or subsequent conventional chemotherapy fails, it appears reasonable to compare transplant outcome with those of similar groups of patients treated with conventional options. The absence of randomized trials is largely due to the fact that no curative conventional therapy is available for this group. Although there may be differences in the types of patients treated by high-dose therapy, some conclusions can be drawn from these comparisons and suggestions made for randomized trials. We have performed several comparisons using matched patients from patients at Loyola University Medical Center to define trials of conventional salvage therapy (Table 11–6).[36, 51]

Considering all patients in first relapse, paclitaxel at conventional doses for platinum-resistant disease gives a 4-month PFS.[36] Of the first 100 patients undergoing transplantation, a group with the same prognostic factors had a survival time after transplantation identical to that of patients receiving paclitaxel. In contrast, those with platinum-sensitive disease had a 4.5-month PFS with paclitaxel versus 8 months with transplantation. Although the differences at the median are not dramatic, all conventionally treated patients with platinum-sensitive disease had experienced relapse by 20 months, whereas 30% of the transplants were progression free at the same point and the 3-year PFS for the group was projected to be 18%. The conclusion for this and similar analyses is that although transplants appear to be of limited value for platinum-resistant disease, they may confer the possibility of a long-term PFS in patients with platinum-sensitive disease—a possibility not seen with conventional options.

The patients who do best with conventional therapy are those with a prolonged first remission. In fact, for those who experience relapse after an initial remission that has lasted more than 12 months, expected median survival is 20–24 months.[49] To further evaluate the benefit of transplantation for this group, a similar analysis was performed for those with sensitive disease whose first remission lasted more than a year before first salvage therapy was administered. With either cyclophosphamide, doxorubicin, and cisplatin or single-agent paclitaxel, the median survival for this patient group ranges between 20 and 24 months according to a 1996 report that specifically evaluated treatment in this patient group.[51] In contrast, a similar group undergoing transplantation for platinum-sensitive disease whose initial remission lasted more than 12 months had a 93% survival rate at 22 months and a 60% survival rate at

TABLE 11–6. COMPARISON OF CONVENTIONAL SALVAGE CHEMOTHERAPY WITH TRANSPLANTATION FOR OVARIAN CANCER AT LOYOLA

COMPARISON	N	PFS	OS
• Conventional therapy			
Paclitaxel[36]	27	Platinum resistant: 4 mo	NA for subgroups
	16	Platinum sensitive: 4.5 mo	
Transplant therapy	30	Platinum resistant: 4 mo	
	17	Platinum sensitive: 8 mo	
• Conventional therapy			
Topotecan vs paclitaxel[38]	112	18.9 wk	63.0 wk
	114	14.7 wk	53.0 wk
Transplant therapy	90	50.1 wk	97.4 wk
• Conventional therapy*			
CAP vs paclitaxel[37]	38	18.9 mo	24.3 mo
	41	7.3 mo	20.3 mo
Transplant therapy	14	14.0 mo	93% @ 24 mo

CAP, cyclophosphamide, Adriamycin, cisplatin regimen; NA, not available; OS, overall survival; PFS, progression-free survival.
*Initial remission > 1 yr.

40 months, again suggesting the superiority of transplantation.

Finally, transplantation was compared with conventional-dose topotecan and paclitaxel for patients in whom a single-chemotherapy regimen failed.[38] These data were taken from a study used to support the licensing of topotecan in the United States by the FDA as second-line therapy for patients with advanced ovarian cancer.[38] The PFS was longer for the 90 patients who underwent transplantation and who met the same eligibility criteria in this 164-patient series (50.1 weeks vs. 14.7 and 18.9 weeks for those treated with paclitaxel and topotecan, respectively). The OS was also higher for those who underwent transplantation: 97.4 weeks versus 63.0 and 53.0 weeks for the topotecan and paclitaxel groups, respectively.

Taken together, these and several other recent reports indicate that for patients with recurrent platinum-sensitive disease of low tumor burden, transplantation offers an OS superior to that of conventional options, with approximately 20% achieving a long-term PFS. For those with platinum-resistant, especially bulky disease, however, transplantation appears to offer a PFS and OS similar to those of conventional therapies and, given the toxicity and costs of transplantation, should not be generally recommended. Patients meeting the criterion of platinum-sensitive disease of low tumor burden should be offered the option of transplantation at the time of first relapse.

TRANSPLANTS FOR RESPONDING DISEASE AT THE COMPLETION OF INITIAL THERAPY

Because platinum sensitivity and low tumor burden are important prognostic factors for patients undergoing transplantation for relapsed disease, it is logical to consider performing transplantation in this group of patients at the time of first response. Several pilot studies from France describe transplantation for this group of patients (i.e., performed at the time of second-look surgery).

The largest report to date is that by Legros et al.[52] Patients received chemotherapy with a platinum-based combination after debulking surgery; after their disease was demon-strated to be platinum sensitive, all were treated with high-dose chemotherapy with either melphalan at 140 mg/m^2 (23 patients) or carboplatin at 1600 mg/m^2 and cyclophosphamide at 6.4 g/m^2 (30 patients). At a median follow-up of over 6½ years, 23% are in continuous CR and 45% are alive. Of 31 patients with no or microscopic disease at second look, the disease-free survival rate at 5 years was 26.9%. For the 19 patients in this group with negative results on second look, the 5-year disease-free survival rate of 32.8% implies that the 12 patients with microscopic residual disease at second look experienced a similar disease-free survival after the single transplant procedure. For those patients with bulky disease at the initiation of second-look surgery, the 5-year disease-free survival rate was 19.2% and the 5-year survival rate was 33.8%.

These data for patients with positive results on second-look laparotomy appear superior to data for those treated with only conventional therapy after second-look surgery. Considering expected survival after second-look surgery for optimal (approximately 50 months) or suboptimal disease (approximately 20 months)—and the fact that 42% of this group had suboptimal disease at diagnosis—we would expect the median survival for this group to be approximately 45 months when treated with conventional therapy rather than the 66 months reported.

These data indicate that transplantion may be useful for this patient group and should be considered in the absence of a comparative trial. With the availability of a comparative phase III trial, however, all eligible patients should be enrolled. Under the auspices of the National Cancer Institute, the Gynecologic Oncology Group, as well as the Southwest Oncology Group, Cancer and Leukemia Group B, and Eastern Cooperative Oncology Group, initiated a randomized phase III trial several years ago. The design is shown in Figure 11–1. Enrolled patients have the following characteristics:

Stage III or IV disease
Patients respond to four to six cycles of a platinum-based regimen after debulking surgery
Patients are in clinical CR (suboptimal stage III and IV) or partial remission documented by second-look laparotomy (optimal stage III)

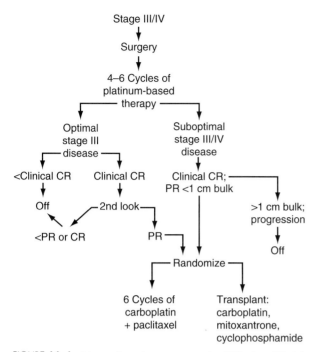

FIGURE 11–1. Advanced ovarian cancer ongoing U.S. phase-III trial.

Patients were randomized to receive either six cycles of paclitaxel (175 mg/m³ over 3 hours) combined with carboplatin at an AUC of 7.5 or a single transplant using the carboplatin, mitoxantrone, and cyclophosphamide regimen (with the carboplatin doses now at an AUC of 28). The trial was expected to take 5 years but was closed after 2 years and enrollment of only 25 patients. The reasons were the slow acceptance of this form of therapy by treating physicians, including some transplant physicians, who thought that no conventional therapy is acceptable for patients with a disease with such a poor prognosis. Several phase III trials in Europe are ongoing, and the results may assist in defining the role of this therapy in the patient group.

TRANSPLANTS AS PART OF INITIAL THERAPY

Several pilot transplant studies have used high-dose chemotherapy after induction chemotherapy for advanced ovarian cancer. The rationale for these trials comes from the fact that drug resistance develops early in this disease, and many patients reach clinical CR quickly after conventional-dose therapy is begun.

Benedetti-Panici et al. initially described 20 and more recently described 35 previously untreated patients with stage III and IV disease (bulky disease in 7, or 20%) undergoing two to four cycles of cisplatin (100–160 mg/m²) and cyclophosphamide (1500–1600 mg/m²), followed by peripheral blood progenitor cell (PBPC), with or without bone marrow harvesting.[53] Twenty patients then received high-dose cisplatin (100 mg/m²), carboplatin (1800 mg/m²), and etoposide (1800 mg/m²); 15 received carboplatin (1200 mg/m²), etoposide (900 mg/m²), and melphalan (100 mg/m²) and stem cell rescue. Four to 6 months after trans-

plantation, responders underwent second-look surgery to document response. Of the 24 completing all therapy, 10 (42%) had entered pathologic CR, including 7 who had been followed for more than 3 years. Because the results of initial surgery are not clearly defined, the pathologic CR results are uninterpretable. Because pathologic CR rates range from 25% to 40%, depending on initial bulk of disease, these results may not be better than those achieved with the best available conventional therapy at the time the study was initiated (i.e., platinum with cyclophosphamide).

Similar conclusions can be drawn from smaller trials testing early transplantation after initial chemotherapy.[54–56] Ten patients received high-dose chemotherapy with paclitaxel (700 mg/m²), carboplatin (AUC dose, 20–28), and mitoxantrone (90 mg/m²) at the conclusion of initial chemotherapy at Loyola. Five had stage IV disease and four had suboptimal stage III disease at diagnosis. At a median time from diagnosis of 26 months, 65% are disease-free. The central nervous system was the initial site of relapse in two of the patients with stage IV disease. Although patients were selected by their referral for transplantation, the PFS for this group with conventional therapy would be expected to be approximately 18 months. Overall, the results are promising but inconclusive, and again a randomized trial is required for verification.

Several trials have looked at less-intensive but multiple cycles of high-dose chemotherapy with stem cell rescue. Shinozuka et al. treated 42 patients with two cycles of modestly dose-escalated cyclophosphamide (1600–2400 mg/m²), doxorubicin (80–100 mg/m²), and cisplatin (100–150 mg/m²) with autologous bone marrow transplantation after primary surgery.[57] For the 23 patients with only microscopic residual after initial surgery, the 4-year survival rate was 70%; for those with macroscopic disease, the median survival was 3 years. These survival rates appear not to be different from those of conventional therapy with a combination of paclitaxel and platinum; this is likely because the dose intensity of this regimen is only twice that of conventional doses shown not to be effective in multiple randomized trials.[4, 5]

In the largest series to date of more-intensive, multicycle therapy, Fennelly et al. treated 16 patients (10 of whom underwent suboptimal debulking) with high-dose cyclophosphamide and paclitaxel with cytokine support and PBPC collection for two cycles, followed by four courses of carboplatin and cyclophosphamide and PBPC rescue.[58] In this small cohort, second-look surgery results were negative in five patients (38.5%), which may be higher than that achievable with paclitaxel and cisplatin conventional-dose chemotherapy.

Unpublished updates indicated that those with suboptimal stage III disease initially had a high probability of residual disease at the completion of the program, whereas those with optimal stage III did not. Because of the encouraging results for optimal stage III disease, the Gynecologic Oncology Group began a multicenter pilot trial of this therapy, but the trial was closed because of a high percentage of positive results on second-look laparotomy. The failure appears to suggest that double-dose chemotherapy, even given rapidly with stem cell support, is insufficient to eradicate this disease. This type of therapy is still being pursued, albeit with a more dose-intensive regimen, and data appear promising.[59]

CONCLUSION

It appears that high-dose chemotherapy may improve the survival of patients both when used after relapse in chemosensitive disease and when used as the conclusion of initial chemotherapy. High-dose chemotherapy appears to be the only therapy available to date that—in a fraction of these patients—provides a long-term PFS of up to 4–5 years when used for relapsed platinum-sensitive disease of low tumor burden. In addition, several sets of pilot data suggest an improvement in the PFS or OS of patients undergoing transplantation with responding first-remission disease. The benefit for this group of patients needs to be verified in a randomized phase III trial. Whether such a trial will ever take place in the United States is doubtful.

REFERENCES

1. Greenlee RT, Murray T, Bolden S, Wingo PA: Cancer statistics, 2000. CA Cancer J Clin 50:7, 2000.
2. Ries LAG, Kosary CL, Hankey BF, et al (eds): SEER cancer statistics review, 1973–1994: tables and graphs (NIH Publication 97-2789). Bethesda, MD, National Cancer Institute, 1997.
3. Williams SD, Blessing JA, Moore DH, et al: Cisplatin, vinblastine, and bleomycin in advanced and recurrent ovarian germ-cell tumors. Ann Intern Med 111:22, 1989.
4. Kristensen GB, Trope C: Epithelial ovarian cancer. Lancet 349:113, 1997.
5. McGuire WP, Ozols RF: Chemotherapy of advanced ovarian cancer. Semin Oncol 25:340, 1998.
6. Kotz KW, Schilder RJ: High-dose chemotherapy and hematopoietic progenitor cell support for patients with epithelial ovarian cancer. Semin Oncol 22:250, 1995.
7. Fennelly D: The role of high-dose chemotherapy in the management of advanced ovarian cancer. Curr Opin Oncol 8:415, 1996.
8. International Federation of Gynecology and Obstetrics: Annual report on the results of treatment in gynecological cancer. Int J Gynecol Obstet 28:189, 1989.
9. van den Burg MEL, van Lent M, Buyse M, et al: The effect of debulking surgery after induction chemotherapy on the prognosis in advanced ovarian cancer. N Engl J Med 332:629, 1995.
10. Grene MH, Clark JW, Blaney DW: The epidemiology of ovarian cancer. Semin Oncol 11:209, 1998.
11. Friedlander ML: Prognostic factors in ovarian cancer. Semin Oncol 25:305, 1998.
12. Gershenson DM, Mitchell MF, Atkinson N, et al: Age contrasts in patients with advanced ovarian cancer. Cancer 71:638S, 1993.
13. Duska I, Chang Y, Goodman A, et al: Epithelial ovarian tumors in the reproductive age group. Proc Am Soc Clin Oncol 17:355a, 1998.
14. Bonnefoi H, Macfarlane v, AHern RP, Gore ME: Stage b IV epithelial ovarian carcinoma: 20 years of experience at the Royal Marsden Hospital (RMH). Proc Am Soc Clin Oncol 15:280, 1996.
15. McGuire WP, Hoskins WJ, Brady MF, et al: Cyclophosphamide and cisplatin compared with paclitaxel and cisplatin in patients with stage III and stage IV ovarian cancer. N Engl J Med 334:1, 1996.
16. Piccart MJ, Bertelsen K, Stuart G, et al: Is cisplatin-paclitaxel (P-T) the standard in first-line treatment of advanced ovarian cancer (OvCa)? the EORTC-GCCG, NOCOVA, NCI-C and Scottish intergroup experience. Proc Am Soc Clin Oncol 16:352a, 1997.
17. Stuart G, Bertelsen K, Mangioni C, et al: Updated analysis shows a highly significant improved overall survival (OS) for cisplatin-paclitaxel as first line treatment of advanced ovarian cancer: mature results of the EORTC-GCCG, NOCOVA, NCIC CTG and Scottish intergroup trial. Proc Am Soc Clin Oncol 17:361a, 1998.
18. Hoskins WJ: Surgical staging and cytoreductive surgery of epithelial ovarian cancer. Cancer 71(Suppl 14):1534, 1993.
19. Griffiths CT: Surgical resection of tumor bulk in the primary treatment of ovarian cancer. Monogr Natl Cancer Inst 42:101, 1975.
20. Alberts DS, Green S, Hannigan EV, et al: Improved therapeutic index of carboplatin plus cyclophosphamide: final report of the Southwest Oncology Group of a phase II randomized trial in stage III and IV ovarian cancer. J Clin Oncol 10:706, 1992.
21. Muggia FM, Brally PS, Brady MF, et al: Phase III of cisplatin (P) or paclitaxel (T) versus their combination in suboptimal stage III and IV epithelial ovarian cancer (EOC): gynecologic oncology study group (GOG) study No. 132. Proc Am Soc Clin Oncol 16:352a, 1997.
22. Bookman MA, McGuire WP, Kilpatrick D, et al: Carboplatin and paclitaxel in ovarian carcinoma: a phase I trial of the gynecologic oncology group. J Clin Oncol 14:1895, 1996.
23. Markman M, Bundy B, Benda J, et al: Randomized phase 3 study of intravenous (IV) cisplatin (CIS)/paclitaxed (PAC) versus moderately high dose IV carboplatin (CARB) followed by IV PAC and intraperitoneal (IP) CIS in optimal residual ovarian cancer (OC): an intergroup trial (GOG, SWOG, ECOG). Proc Am Soc Clin Oncol 17:361a, 1998.
24. Alberts DS, Young L, Mason N, Salmon SE: In vitro evaluation of anticancer drugs against ovarian cancer at concentrations achievable by intraperitoneal administration. Semin Oncol 4(Suppl 12):38, 1985.
25. Lidor Y, Shapp EJ, Peters WP, Bast RC Jr: Alkylating agents and immunotoxins exert synergistic activity against ovarian cancer cell lines. Proc Am Assoc Cancer Res 30:401, 1989.
26. Beherns BC, Hamilton TC, Masuda H, et al: Characterization of a cis-diamine dichloro-platinum (II)–resistant human ovarian cancer cell line and its use in evaluation of platinum analogs. Cancer Res 47:414, 1987.
27. Raymond E, Hanauske A, Faivre S, et al: Effects of prolonged versus short-term exposure paclitaxel (Taxol) on human tumor colony-forming units. Anticancer Drugs 8:379, 1997.
28. Teicher B, Holden SA, Jones SM, et al: Influence of scheduling in two-day combinations of alkylating agents in vivo. Cancer Chemother Pharmacol 25:161, 1989.
29. Lidor YJ, Shpall EJ, Peters WP, Bast RC: Synergistic cytotoxicity of different alkylating agents for epithelial ovarian cancer. Int J Cancer 49:704, 1991.
30. Ablerts DS, Liu PY, Hannigan EV, et al: Phase III study of intraperitoneal cisplatin and intravenous cyclophosphamide versus intravenous cisplatin and IV cyclophosphamide in patients with optimal stage III ovarian cancer. N Engl J Med 335:1950, 1996.
31. Eisenhauer EA, Vermorken JB, van Glabbeke M: Predictors of response to subsequent chemotherapy in platinum pretreated ovarian cancer: a multivariate analysis of 704 patients. Ann Oncol 8:963, 1997.
32. NIH Consensus Conference: Ovarian cancer: screening, treatment and follow-up: NIH consensus development on ovarian cancer. JAMA 273:491, 1995.
33. Seltzer V, Vogl S, Kaplan B: Recurrent ovarian carcinoma: retreatment using combination chemotherapy including cis-diaminedichloroplatinum in patients previously responding to this agent. Gynecol Oncol 21:167, 1985.
34. Markman M, Rothman R, Hakes T, et al: Second-line platinum therapy in patients with ovarian cancer previously treated with cisplatin. J Clin Oncol 9:389, 1991.
35. Sabbatini P, Spriggs D: Salvage therapy of ovarian cancer. Oncology 12:833, 1998.
36. Thigpen JT, Blessing JA, Ball E, et al: Phase II trial of paclitaxel in patients with progressive ovarian carcinoma after platinum based chemotherapy: a gynecologic oncology group study. J Clin Oncol 12:1748, 1994.
37. Colombo N, Marzola M, Parma G, et al: Paclitaxel vs. CAP (cyclophosphamide, adriamycin, cisplatin) in recurrent platinum sensitive ovarian cancer: a randomized phase II study. Proc Am Soc Clin Oncol 15:279, 1996.
38. ten Bokkel Huinik W, Gore M, Carichael J, et al: Topotecan vs paclitaxel for the treatment of recurrent epithelial ovarian cancer. J Clin Oncol 15:2183, 1997.
39. Gordon A, Carmichael J, Malfetano J, et al: Final analysis of a phase III randomized study of topotecan (T) vs paclitaxel (p) in advanced epithelian ovarian carcinoma: International Topotecan Study Group. Proc Am Soc Clin Oncol 17:356a, 1998.
40. Muggia FM, Hainsworth JD, Jeffers S, et al: Phase II study of liposomal doxorubicin in refractory ovarian cancer: antitumor acitiviy and toxicity modification by liposomal encapsulation. J Clin Oncol 15:987, 1997.

41. Rose PG, Blessing JA, Mayer AR, Homesley HD: Prolonged oral etoposide as second-line therapy for platinum-resistant and platinum-sensitive ovarian carcinoma: a gynecologic oncology group study. J Clin Oncol 16:405, 1998.

42. Moore DH, Valea F, Crumpler LS, Fowler WC: Hexamethylmelamine/altretamine as second-line therapy for epithelial ovarian carcinoma. Gynecol Oncol 51:109, 1993.

43. Shea TC, Flaherty M, Elias A, et al: A phase I clinical and pharmacokinetic study of carboplatin and autologous bone marrow support. J Clin Oncol 7:651, 1989.

44. Shpall EJ, Clark-Pearson D, Soper JT, et al: High dose alkylating agent chemotherapy with autologous bone marrow support in patients with stage III/IV epithelial ovarian cancer. Gynecol Oncol 38:386, 1990.

45. Stiff PJ, McKenzie RS, Alberts DS, et al: Phase I clinical and pharmacokinetic study of high dose mitoxantrone combined with carboplatin, cyclophosphamide and autologous bone marrow rescue: high response rate for refractory ovarian carcinoma. J Clin Oncol 12:176, 1994.

46. Stiff P, Bayer R, Camarda M, et al: A phase II trial of high-dose mitoxantrone, carboplatin, and cyclophosphamide with autologous bone marrow rescue for recurrent epithelial ovarian carcinoma: analysis of risk factors for clinical outcome. Gynecol Oncol 57:278, 1995.

47. Weaver CH, Greco FA, Hiansworth JD, et al: A phase I-II study of high-dose melphalan, mitoxantrone and carboplatin with peripheral blood stem cell support in patients with advanced ovarian or breast carcinoma. Bone Marrow Transplant 20:84, 1991.

48. Holmberg LA, Demier T, Rowley S, et al: High-dose busulfna, melphalan and thiotepa followed by autologous peripheral blood stem cell (PBSC) rescue in patients with advanced stage III/IV ovarian cancer. Bone Marrow Transplant 22:651, 1998.

49. Stiff PJ, Bayer R, Kerger C, et al: High-dose chemotherapy with autologous transplantation for persistent/relapsed ovarian cancer: a multivariate analysis of survival for 100 consecutively treated patients. J Clin Oncol 15:1309, 1997.

50. Stiff PJ, Kerger C, Bayer RA: High dose chemotherapy and autologous stem cell transplantation for ovarian carcinoma: comparisons to conventional therapy and future directions. *In* Dicke K, Keating A (eds): Autologous Marrow and Blood Transplantation—Proceedings of the Ninth International Symposium. Arlington, TX, Cancer Treatment Research and Educational Institute, 1999, in press.

51. Colombo N, Marzola M, Parma G, et al: Paclitaxel vs. CAP (cyclophosphamide, adriamycin, cisplatin) in recurrent platinum sensitive ovarian cancer: a randomized phase II study. Proc Am Soc Clin Oncol 15:279, 1996.

52. Legros M, Dauplat J, Fluery J, et al: High-dose chemotherapy with hematopoietic rescue in patients with stage III to IV ovarian cancer: Long-term results. J Clin Oncol 15:1302, 1997.

53. Benedetti-Panici P, Pierelli L, Scambia G, et al: High dose carboplatin, etoposide and melphalan (CEM) with peripheral blood progenitor cell support as late intensificatiion for high-risk cancer: non haematological, haematological toxicities and role of growth factor administration. Br J Cancer 75:1205–1212, 1997.

54. Mencichella G, Pereli L, Foddae, et al: Autologous blood stem cell harvesting and transplantation in patients with advanced ovarian cancer. Br J Haematol 79:444, 1991.

55. Palmer PA, Schwartzberg L, Birch R, et al: High dose melphalan ± mitoxantrone with peripheral blood progenitor cell support as a component of initial treatment of patients with advanced ovarian cancer. Proc Am Soc Clin Oncol 14:991, 1995.

56. Juttner CA, Davy MLJ, To LB, et al: Autologous PBSC transplantation in stage 3 and 4 ovarian cancer. Int J Cell Cloning 10(Suppl 1):145, 1992.

57. Shinozuka T, Murakami M, Miyamoto T: High dose chemotherapy (HDC) with autologous bone marrow transplantation (ABMT) in ovarian cancer. Proc Am Soc Clin Oncol 10:193, 1991.

58. Fennelly D, Schneider J, Bengala C, et al: Escalating-dose taxol plus high-dose (HD) cyclophosphamide (C) Carboplatin (CBDCA) plus C rescued with peripheral blood progenitor cells (PBP) in patients with stace IIC-IV ovarian cancer (OC). Gynecol Oncol 56:121, 1995.

59. Schilder RJ, Shea TC: Multiple cycles of high dose chemotherapy for ovarian cancer. Semin Oncol 25:349, 1998.

CHAPTER TWELVE

Childhood Solid Tumors

Maria M. Koehler, M.D., Ph.D., and
Robert A. Krance, M.D.

The role of hematopoietic stem cell transplantation (HSCT) in the treatment of childhood malignancy has yet to be fully defined. Although childhood tumors manifest a dose-related response to chemotherapy, suggesting a potential role for high-dose therapy with stem cell rescue, the actual benefit compared with conventional dose has not been demonstrated.[24, 120, 127, 179, 183, 186, 192] Convincingly demonstrating a benefit will be difficult because malignancy is uncommon in children, clinical trials require lengthy intervals of time before the data can be interpreted, and in the end the data frequently remain inconclusive. For all of these reasons, HSCT for pediatric solid tumors must still be considered investigational therapy.

Furthermore, complications of high-dose therapy and transplantation can be appreciable in children. Growth and development, which are the essence of childhood, may be severely compromised by intensive conditioning procedures.[56, 204] After total body irradiation (TBI), children may fail to attain full adult height or may exhibit endocrine dysfunction, delayed maturation, and decreased pulmonary reserve.[178, 193] Unfortunately, these side effects are most pronounced in the youngest patients, for whom the developing brain and nervous system remain a critical concern.[56, 178] Relying on pharmacokinetic and pharmacodynamic data generated in adult subjects to improve treatment regimens is not practical in pediatric patients because the metabolism of chemotherapeutic agents is poorly characterized in children.[99, 109, 129, 132, 179, 194] As a consequence, pediatric patients are vulnerable to both under- and over-treatment. Although, in practice, most children tolerate ablative chemotherapy and radiotherapy without undue regimen-related morbidity and mortality, concerns over treatment safety and efficacy remain foremost.

Virtually every common pediatric solid tumor has been treated with intensive chemotherapy and hematopoietic stem cell rescue. The bulk of the experience has accrued in the treatment of neuroblastoma, rhabdomyosarcoma, Ewing sarcoma, high-grade glioma, and other brain tumors and will be discussed in more detail.

In making the decision to use intensive therapy to treat a child with a malignant tumor, a number of factors must be weighed. Foremost among these, the tumor must manifest a dose-response effect. Because the role of autologous transplantation is limited to rescuing hematopoietic function, success depends on how effectively the high-dose preparatory regimen destroys residual malignant cells.

Candidates for transplantation are those at highest risk for treatment failure and ultimately death. Recurrent disease almost always portends ultimate failure, but certain features present at initial diagnosis can be ominous. Thus, accurate predictors of risk are extremely useful in identifying appropriate transplantation candidates.

Consensus holds that transplantation should be reserved for the time of maximum tumor reduction.[17, 18, 52, 63, 90, 192] The method and extent of tumor reduction vary with tumor type, but a good outcome is more likely in patients treated prior to disease relapse or progression.[76, 139, 166, 192] Theoretically, allogeneic hematopoietic stem cell transplantation (alloHSCT) should be preferable for tumors in which the bone marrow is a common site of metastasis or for tumors associated with undetectable residual marrow disease. The higher rates of morbidity and mortality associated with alloHSCT, however, have limited its usefulness in most circumstances.[42, 126, 140, 169]

Autologous transplantation may be accomplished using either bone marrow or leukapheresis products. One advantage of using peripheral blood progenitor cells (PBPC) is the more rapid hematopoietic recovery compared with bone marrow (BM).[97] Shortening the interval to myeloid recovery lowers morbidity and mortality rates.[45]

For autologous transplantation, the option of purging the autograft of possible malignant cells remains under investigation.[81, 105, 149, 150, 195] Evidence that contamination of bone marrow or PBPC can contribute to relapse is scanty.[12] Data, however, do not establish whether purging effectively reduces tumor cell contamination and the risk of relapse, nor do they establish which of the various purging techniques is most effective. Because methods used to remove tumor cells from the autograft often prolong the hematopoietic recovery period, answers to these questions are actively sought.[81, 119]

Relapse often occurs at the site of disease present before transplantation. For this reason and because of the known tendency of pediatric solid tumors to recur, the origin of the relapsed disease is thought to be malignant cells surviving the conditioning regimen. Thus, the potential impact of purging may be very limited.

Finally, the conditioning regimen is of paramount importance to the transplantation strategy; eradication of residual disease depends on it. Paradoxically, this aspect remains least well defined. Until now, the design of most conditioning regimens has been largely empirical, relying on current understanding of treatment for specific tumors. Not surprisingly, no conditioning regimen has been shown to be superior to another.

NEUROBLASTOMA

BACKGROUND

Neuroblastoma is the most common malignant extracranial tumor in childhood.[13] Microscopic features characteristic of neuroblastoma are recognized, but its appearance is far too often indistinguishable from the other "small blue round cell" tumors of childhood. Findings supportive of the diagnosis include elevated urinary catecholamines. Useful adjuncts to the diagnosis include tumor cytogenetic findings (e.g., deletion 1p, homogeneously staining regions, and double minute chromatin bodies); increase in the copy number and expression of the proto-oncogene N-myc; and/or antibody detection of tumor markers (e.g., neuron-specific enolase, synaptophysin, ganglioside GD2).

Patient age at diagnosis and disease stage are recognized as important predictors of clinical behavior. Elevated serum levels of neuron-specific enolase, ganglioside GD2, and ferritin are associated with advanced stage. Diploid tumor cells, as opposed to hyperdiploid tumor cells, are associated with advanced disease. Gene amplification shown by homogeneously staining regions, double minute chromatin bodies, and increased copy number and expression of N-myc and/or deletion 1p (the presumed locus for a tumor suppressor gene p73) are highly concordant with the "diploid" tumors, advanced stage, and a poor outcome.[34]

Typically, patients more than 12 months old have diploid DNA content, N-myc amplification, advanced stage, and a poor response to treatment. Hyperdiploid DNA content and absence of both N-myc amplification and 1p deletion predict favorable treatment response regardless of the extent of disease. Neuroblastoma stage 4S (Table 12–1) is limited to infants less than 12 months of age and by definition is widely disseminated, yet it carries a good prognosis. This subset of cases is associated with hyperdiploid DNA content, low N-myc copy number, and absence of 1p deletion.

The optimal management of neuroblastoma requires a multidisciplinary team approach. Surgical attempts at complete tumor resection must be weighed against disease stage and other considerations (Table 12–1). In patients presenting with advanced disease, delayed resection may be possible after chemotherapy. Effective chemotherapy requires a combination of agents. Most active against neuroblastoma are vincristine, cyclophosphamide, doxorubicin, etoposide, carboplatin, and cisplatin.[120, 179, 200] Neuroblastoma is a radiosensitive tumor.[79, 203] The effective dose range is 15–30 Gy. Radiotherapy can serve as an effective adjunct to surgery and chemotherapy for patients with limited, as opposed to disseminated, disease.[21]

Until the mid-1980s, chemotherapy regimens for metastatic neuroblastoma produced response rates of 50% but long-term survival rates were less than 10%.[4, 24, 102, 192] In more recent chemotherapy trials, treatment has been intensified. This approach improves the response rate to 80–90% in patients with stage 4 disease, but the long-term survival rate has not shown a corresponding increase.[4, 24] Nevertheless, current protocols for treating high-risk neuroblastoma emphasize intensive chemotherapy, with or without stem cell rescue.[7, 42, 63, 76, 88, 102, 119, 127, 167, 192]

TABLE 12–1. INTERNATIONAL NEUROBLASTOMA STAGING SYSTEM

STAGE	DEFINITION
1	Localized tumor with complete gross excision, with or without microscopic residual disease; representative ipsilateral lymph nodes negative for tumor microscopically (nodes attached to and removed with the primary tumor may be positive).
2A	Localized tumor with incomplete gross excision; representative ipsilateral nonadherent lymph nodes negative for tumor microscopically.
2B	Localized tumor with or without complete gross excision, with ipsilateral nonadherent lymph node involvement; or localized unilateral tumor with contralateral regional lymph node involvement; or midline tumor with bilateral extension by infiltration (unresectable) or by lymph node involvement.
3	Unresectable unilateral tumor infiltrating across the midline;* with or without regional lymph node involvement; or localized unilateral tumor with contralateral regional lymph node involvement; or midline tumor with bilateral extension by infiltration (unresectable) or by lymph node involvement.
4	Any primary tumor with dissemination to distant lymph nodes, bone, bone marrow, liver, skin, and/or other organs (except as defined for stage 4S).
4S	Localized primary tumor (as defined for stage 1, 2A, or 2B); with dissemination limited to skin, liver, and/or bone marrow† (limited to infants <1 yr of age).

*The midline is defined as the vertebral column. Tumors originating on one side and crossing the midline must infiltrate to or beyond the opposite side of the vertebral column.

†Marrow involvement in stage 4S should be minimal, i.e., <10% of total nucleated cells identified as malignant on bone marrow biopsy or on marrow aspirate. More extensive marrow involvement would be considered to be stage 4. The MIBG (metaiodobenzylguanidine) scan (if performed) should be negative in the marrow.

PATIENT SELECTION

In identifying which patient is most likely to benefit from intensive chemotherapy and HSCT, the critical determinants are disease stage, age, and tumor biology (see Table 12–1). The overall 5-year disease-free survival (DFS) rate of patients with stage 1, 2, and 4S disease is 75–90%.[13] Advanced-stage disease, although initially responsive to chemotherapy, has a high probability of recurrence (DFS rate = 20%). It is to this cohort, accounting for more than two-thirds of patients 12 months or older, that HSCT has been extensively applied.

TIMING OF HSCT

In most current clinical trials, the appropriate time for transplantation coincides with maximum tumor reduction. Many patients with neuroblastoma can be rendered disease free by chemotherapy alone; should the response to chemotherapy be incomplete, it is common practice to perform second and even third surgical procedures to achieve complete response. Likewise, local irradiation may be used to treat sites of residual disease before proceeding to transplantation or used later to decrease toxicity. In general, results are superior if transplantation occurs prior to relapse or disease progression.[63, 76, 89, 102, 140, 143, 166, 176, 181, 192]

For patients undergoing transplantation before disease progression, while in complete remission (CR), or while in very good partial remission (defined as >90% primary tumor reduction, metastatic disease limited to bone, and >90% decrease in catecholamine excretion), the progression-free survival (PFS) rate is 25–55% after 2–4 years.[42, 63, 127, 138, 167] Approximately 10–15% of deaths result from transplant-related morbidity, and the remainder result from relapse.[63, 76, 88, 120, 138, 140, 166, 167, 182] In contrast, for patients undergoing transplantation in less than very good partial remission or after disease progression (including second CR), the PFS rate at 2 years is only 10–28%; the PFS rate is less than 5% for patients undergoing transplantation with advanced disease.[63, 76, 123, 166, 167, 170, 180–182]

New advances beyond improving chemotherapy, conventional radiation, surgery, and hematopoietic growth factor support are needed to effect an obvious increase in cure rate.

ALLOGENEIC TRANSPLANTATION

Because the patient's bone marrow is commonly involved in advanced neuroblastoma (80% of stage 4 cases), concern about residual but undetectable marrow disease suggests that the use of allogeneic bone marrow might confer a therapeutic advantage. Three reports have described the outcome of 49 patients undergoing alloHSCT (Table 12–2).[42, 126, 140] Similar to the case with autologous transplants, approximately one-fourth of patients remained disease free at 2–4 years after HSCT. The others died of procedure-related mortality or relapse. A multicenter review summarized data of 350 patients treated by autotransplantation and 124 patients treated by allografts; the authors found no difference in rates of relapse or survival but noted increased toxicity with alloHSCT (early death from veno-occlusive disease, renal failure, disseminated infections).[35, 36, 170] Toxicity of alloHSCT regimens (in part attributed to toxicity from prophylaxis for graft-versus-host disease) and relapse were the main causes of failure.[76, 77, 126, 140]

There are no reports documenting a graft-versus-tumor effect in neuroblastoma, and it has been speculated that the low rate of graft-versus-host disease reported for patients with neuroblastoma undergoing alloHSCT may explain this.[126] Because of the higher mortality rate without

improved DFS, alloHSCT has not been the preferred method of treatment in patients with neuroblastoma.

AUTOLOGOUS TRANSPLANTATION

Although autologous transplantation following high-dose chemotherapy is widely used to treat advanced-stage neuroblastoma (Table 12–3), there is no consensus as to the specific therapeutic interventions essential to improve DFS. The type of ablative chemotherapy, the role of irradiation (whether to local sites of disease or to the total body), the need for purging, and the role of post-transplantation immunomodulation are all the focus of current investigation.

Although the data are inconclusive, a number of reports claim that intensive treatment of neuroblastoma followed by stem cell rescue has resulted in 30–40% PFS rates at 2–5 years.[35, 63, 127, 138, 166, 167, 192] Preliminary data suggest that for certain groups of patients (e.g., those with N-myc amplification), chemotherapy with stem cell rescue may be better than chemotherapy alone.[192] This observation should be interpreted cautiously, however, because these results are derived from nonrandomized clinical trials. Furthermore, treatment approaches in these reports differ as to preparative regimens, use of radiation, and purging; thus, it is impossible to compare the studies directly (see Table 12–3).

As shown in Table 12–4, only four trials compare consolidation regimens that include intensive chemotherapy with similar myeloablative regimens followed by stem cell rescue.[76, 155, 184, 170, 192] Unfortunately, three of the four trials were not randomized, and the single randomized trial[170] involved a small patient cohort (24 patients in the transplant arm).

In the largest nonrandomized multicenter study (207 patients), the results of treating patients with high-risk (stage 4) neuroblastoma in remission with chemotherapy (carboplatin, etoposide, melphalan) and TBI followed by purged HSCT were compared with the results of treating similar patients with continuous postremission chemotherapy.[192] The higher risk subset (poor responders, disease positive for N-myc, older age) appeared to derive the greatest benefit from myeloablative and transplantation therapy, with an estimated overall event-free survival (EFS) rate of 40% at 4 years versus 19% in the chemotherapy arm (see Table 12–4).

Even so, in the absence of a properly randomized trial, there is no absolute evidence that myeloablative consolida-

TABLE 12–2. COMPARISON OF AutoHSCT AND AlloHSCT IN PATIENTS WITH STAGE IV OR RELAPSED NEUROBLASTOMA

	MATTHAY et al., 1994[140]		LADENSTEIN et al., 1994[126]		EVANS et al., 1994[42]	
	Auto	**Allo**	**Auto**	**Allo**	**Auto**	**Allo**
Number of patients	36	20	34	17	30	12
Early toxic deaths	3	4	4	3	5	5
Relapse	18	11	16	9	15	3
PFS or DFS in %	49	25	41	35	30	17
	At 4 years		*At 2 years*		*At 4 years*	

DFS, disease-free survival; PFS, progression-free survival.

TABLE 12–3. RESULTS OF AUTOLOGOUS HEMATOPOIETIC STEM CELL TRANSPLANTATION FOR NEUROBLASTOMA (STAGE IV OR RELAPSED)*

PREPARATIVE REGIMEN‡	NO. OF PTS	TBI	PURGE	MEDIAN FOLLOW-UP (mo)	PFS % (CR-VGPR)	TOXIC DEATH	REFERENCE
Melphalan	65	N	N	23	33	1	Pinkerton, 1991—ENSG[170]
VCR, melphalan	34	Y	N	59	29	1	Dini et al., 1991[35]
VCR, melphalan, Cis	67	Y	N	60	25	6	Dini et al., 1991[35]
BCNU, VM26, melphalan	33	N	chemo	28	48	4	Hartmann et al., 1987[88]
VAMP	17	Y	N	71	87	0	McCowage et al., 1995[143]
VAMP, DEM, CEM	67	Y	IM	40†	40	5	Stram et al., 1996[192]
VCR, melphalan	62	Y	IM	59	20	13	Philip et al., 1991[166]
VP, thiotepa	19	Y	IM	24	42	1	Kamani et al., 1996[102]
Melphalan	26	N	chemo	24	6	5	Kushner et al., 1991[119]
Cis, BCNU, melphalan, thiotepa	25	N	chemo	24	44	3	Kushner et al., 1991[118]
VAMP, PEM	101	Y	IM	39	43	21	Seeger and Reynolds[182]
Melphalan	15	N	N	31	33	0	Hartmann et al., 1986[89]
VCR, melphalan	117	Y	N	65	35	12	Garaventa et al., 1998[63]
Melphalan	74	Y	IM	24	32	7	Graham-Pole et al., 1991[76]
VCR, melphalan	35	Y	chemo	32	44	6	Philip et al., 1987[167]
Cis, BCNU, VP, melphalan	36	N	N	28	30	5	Kremens et al., 1994[117]
Cy, VCR, adria, Cis	36	Y	IM	36	66	1	Mugishma et al., 1995[151]
Thiotepa/Cy	51	Y/N		40	58	1	Kletzel et al., 1998[108]

*Restricted to studies with > 15 patients.
†Projected.
‡adria, doxorubicin (Adriamycin); BCNU, *bis*-chloroethyl-nitrosourea; CEM, cisplatin, etoposide, melphalan; chemo, chemotherapy; Cis, cisplatin; CR-VGPR, complete remission to very good partial remission; Cy, cytoxan; DEM, doxorubicin, etoposide, melphalan; IM, immunopurge with monoclonal antibodies; N, not included; PEM, cisplatin, etoposide, and melphalan; PFS, progression-free survival; TBI, total body irradiation; VAMP, teniposide, doxorubicin, melphalan, cisplatin; VCR, vincristine; VM26, teniposide; VP, etoposide; Y, included.

tion followed by stem cell rescue improves long-term disease-free rates in these patients. The current Children's Cancer Group 3891 study randomizes patients while asking just such a question. Early analysis suggests that the EFS rate at 3 years may be superior for patients undergoing transplantation versus chemotherapy: 34% versus 18%. These results are preliminary and await maturation of the study population.

Despite the lack of definitive data, several assumptions may be made regarding the indications, optimal timing, toxicity, and effectiveness of transplantation for advanced neuroblastoma. Furthermore, newer or controversial approaches to the treatment of neuroblastoma, such as the use of unconventional radiation, purging, double myeloablative regimens, and post-transplant therapy, must be discussed.

HIGH-DOSE PRETRANSPLANTATION CHEMOTHERAPY

To date, no single HSCT regimen has proven superior in the treatment of patients with neuroblastoma (see Table 12–3). The earliest intensive regimens employed single-agent chemotherapy.[5, 120, 170] The addition of other agents, such as vincristine[63, 166]; cisplatin, etoposide, and doxorubicin[181]; cisplatin and etoposide[183, 181]; and carboplatin and etoposide,[172, 192] with or without fractionated TBI (10–12 Gy), have not improved significantly upon earlier results.[35, 63, 76, 118, 155, 166, 184, 192] Comparison among preparative regimens is impossible because patient and disease status at transplantation vary among studies and the potential impact of different ancillary treatment approaches cannot be ignored (see Table 12–3).

If only the first 2 years after transplantation are considered, the overall survival of patients with advanced-stage neuroblastoma is improved by autotransplantation compared with treatment with chemotherapy alone. The few studies that report longer follow-up after transplantation, however, show that relapses continue to occur up to 7 years and that DFS at 5 years is ultimately unchanged.[42, 76, 127, 167, 192]

To explore the efficacy of added intensification to the autograft approach, Philip and colleagues performed a dou-

TABLE 12–4. PROGRESSION/DISEASE-FREE SURVIVAL RATES IN CHILDREN WITH HIGH-RISK NEUROBLASTOMA CHEMOTHERAPY VS. CHEMOTHERAPY AND HSCT

STUDY GROUP	RATE OF PFS/DFS		NO. PATIENTS	REFERENCE
	Chemotherapy (%)	Chemotherapy + HSCT (%)		
CCG	19	40	207	Stram et al., 1996[192]
POG	30	32	116	Shuster et al., 1991[184]
				Graham-Pole et al., 1991[76]
ENSG	19	33	65	Pinkerton, 1991[170]
Japan	39	50	110	Ohnuma et al., 1995[155]

Trials were not randomized, with the exception of Pinkerton's.[170]
CCG, Children's Cancer Group; ENSG, European Neuroblastoma Study Group; POG, Pediatric Oncology Group; DFS, disease-free survival; PFS, progression-free survival.

TABLE 12–5. DOUBLE TRANSPLANTS FOR NEUROBLASTOMA

STUDY	NO. PATIENTS	PREPARATORY REGIMENS	TOXIC DEATH	OUTCOME
Philip et al., 1993[164]	33	1. Teniposide, carmustine, carboplatin, and cisplatin 2. Vincristine, melphalan, total body irradiation	24%	5-year EFS 32%

Kawa-Ha et al., 1996[103]	8	1. Ifosfamide (2.5 g/m^2)
		   Melphalan (140 mg/m^2)
		2. Busulfan (5 mg/kg)
		   Thiotepa (200 mg/m^2)
			0	6/8 in complete remission 6–29 months post procedure

EFS, event-free survival.

ble harvest/double graft using two different intensive transplant preparatory regimens.[164] The intent was to test the role of increased dose intensity on tumor response, relapse pattern, and overall survival (Table 12–5). For this small group, considering that eligibility was limited to patients with delayed response or relapse, the overall survival rates of 36% at 2 years and 32% at 5 years were encouraging. As might be expected, the toxic death rate, 24%, was high.[164]

More recently, Japanese investigators reported that six of eight patients (seven patients with stage 4 disease, one patient in relapse) remained in CR or without progressive disease 6–29 months after single harvest/double intensive chemotherapy (see Table 12–5).[103]

Current Children's Cancer Group and Pediatric Oncology Group studies for patients with advanced-stage neuroblastoma examine the feasibility of performing sequential PBPC transplantation in first CR, each stage preceded by a different high-dose consolidation chemotherapy (followed by local irradiation). Although the multiple autograft approach is feasible, the question remains whether more intensive postremission chemotherapy can improve DFS in high-risk neuroblastoma.

Alternatives to conventional ablative regimens test novel antitumor agents combined with transplantation. Metaiodobenzylguanidine, an epinephrine analogue selectively accumulated by tumors of neural crest origin, is being assessed extensively in clinical trials in Europe.[66, 93, 110] Hoefnagel et al.[93] used ^{131}I-metaiodobenzylguanidine alone as a first therapeutic approach in 31 children with inoperable stage 3 or 4 neuroblastoma. Objective response—tumor size reduction between 72% and 81%—was achieved in all patients. Toxicity was mainly hematologic. Subsequently, 19 of the 27 evaluable patients underwent surgery, resulting in complete or near-complete resection.

Even so, in a German neuroblastoma trial using ^{131}I-metaiodobenzylguanidine administered over one to six courses (mean dose 8 ± 6.7 mCi/kg/course) combined with chemotherapy, no lasting clinical benefit was seen in a group of 47 patients.[111] When high-dose ^{131}I-metaiodobenzylguanidine was added to a conditioning regimen that included melphalan, carboplatin, and etoposide, followed by PBPC transplantation, rapid and complete hematopoietic recovery occurred in 19 patients.[66, 110] Experience in the United States is limited to a recently completed dose finding study that reported a 37% response rate in 30 patients.[70, 137] The clinical benefit specific to high-dose metaiodobenzylguanidine in this multiagent regimen is difficult to gauge.

RADIATION

The role of radiation in neuroblastoma is poorly defined. Both preclinical[31] and clinical studies[21, 79, 118] have differed regarding the radiosensitivity of neuroblastoma. Uncertain, too, is the role of radiation in the transplantation preparative regimen and whether local irradiation to sites of previous and/or current disease is preferable to TBI (see Table 12–3).

Some insight into this problem may be gained by studying the patterns of relapse after treatment of neuroblastoma. In a group of 99 children with high-risk neuroblastoma undergoing myeloablative chemotherapy, TBI (10 Gy), and autologous HSCT, 22 of 41 relapses included the primary site. None of 11 patients who had gross total resection of the primary tumor at diagnosis experienced relapse at the primary site. Local irradiation (10–20 Gy) administered to residual disease at the primary site or to bone metastases administered prior to transplantation did not influence the relapse rate at these sites. The relapse rate was less for patients in CR or very good partial remission (VGPR) at the time of transplantation, suggesting that disease responsiveness to induction chemotherapy was an important predictor of outcome.[139] Kushner et al.[118] and Kremens et al.[117] treated 39 patients with stage 4 neuroblastoma using intensive myeloablative chemotherapy and 21 Gy of irradiation to the primary site and adjacent lymph nodes, followed by autologous HSCT. Only five relapses occurred at the primary site.

Twenty-six patients with advanced neuroblastoma underwent consolidation/intensification with cyclophosphamide and TBI followed by transplantation.[185] Thirteen of these patients received local irradiation (8–24 Gy) to sites of primary and metastatic bone disease. Regimen-related mortality—six deaths—was significant. For the remaining patients, there were three failures among patients receiving local irradiation, but in no patient was failure limited to the sites of previous disease. In contrast, treatment failure occurred in 6 of 10 patients not receiving local irradiation, 4 in sites of previous disease. Finally, 27 patients with high-risk neuroblastoma underwent HSCT after non-TBI myeloablative therapy.[200] Local radiotherapy (15 Gy) was administered to residual tumor sites. The EFS rate at 2 years (median follow-up, 6 months) was 60% (n = 16). Only 2 of 8 patients experienced relapse in irradiated sites.

Taken together, these data suggest that for patients whose disease responds well to chemotherapy, local radiotherapy has a potential role in the context of treatment intensification and hematopoietic stem cell rescue. The local radiation does not influence cure or parameters of survival. Its use appears to be of value in patients with a single residual site or a low number of residual sites of disease. Obvious restrictions to the use of radiotherapy arise when sites of disease include the liver or multiple bones; in these circumstances, the dose of radiotherapy must be limited because of tissue tolerance and/or practicalities of administration. Should local radiotherapy prove an effective adjunct to disease control, failure at sites not previously recognized to be involved by tumor may still limit the value of this approach. Because of such considerations, the use of TBI gained interest as part of combined chemotherapy/radiotherapy consolidation.

At this time, an absolute conclusion cannot be made regarding the need for TBI in autologous HSCT conditioning regimens. Randomized studies between TBI and non-TBI regimens have not been conducted, and comparisons between studies are confounded by differences in chemotherapy regimens, status of disease at transplantation, and use of purged or unpurged stem cells. Although many investigators use TBI, the outcomes from non-TBI regimens are similar (see Table 12–3).

PURGING

Despite intensified cytotoxic therapy for neuroblastoma, relapse remains the major cause of failure. Because neuroblastoma commonly involves the bone marrow, it has been recognized that persistent, albeit clinically occult, disease in the marrow might be a source of relapse after autologous HSCT.[150] Studies using gene marking of harvested marrow cells have unequivocally demonstrated that tumor cells in autografts can contribute to post-transplantation relapse.[12] In theory, purging the marrow of neuroblastoma tumor cells may reduce or eliminate the risk of reinfusing malignant cells. To that end, clinical studies that included purging of harvested marrow began in the early 1980s.[163] The most widely adopted method for ex vivo purging combines a panel of antibodies reacting with neuroblastoma cells that adhere to magnetic microspheres.[150] Other purging regimens use chemotherapeutic agents (mafosfamide, 6-hydroxydopamine, and 4-hydroperoxycyclophosphamide) but have not been widely practiced.[6, 88, 119]

Because physical methods of purging frequently prolong the time to hematopoietic recovery, their use must be questioned until there is proof of efficacy. In addition, relapse does not occur in all patients with residual marrow disease who have undergone harvesting and transplantation. Therefore, major uncertainty exists over the significance of residual marrow disease and determining which patients, if any, will benefit from marrow purging. Although patients who receive unpurged marrow may experience recurrence of disease in patterns suggestive of tumor embolization (lung metastases),[72] the patterns of recurrence after HSCT with purged and unpurged marrow are similar—namely, at sites of the primary tumor, residual gross disease, and bone.[36, 69, 76, 139, 185, 192] The obvious inference is that inadequate cytotoxic therapy, rather than tumor contamination of harvested bone marrow, is the principal reason for relapse.

Supporting this conclusion is the fact that children un-

dergoing allografting as opposed to autografting experienced no clear benefit in PFS, other treatment being essentially the same.[42, 126, 140] Somewhat surprisingly, in some reports relapses were more frequent in allogeneic recipients (69% vs. 46%), although sites of relapse were similar. Indeed, when attempting to quantify the value of marrow tumor purging, several studies found that untreated marrow autografts produced long-term PFS rates similar to those following re-infusion of purged marrow[35, 169, 170] (see Table 12–3).

It cannot, however, be concluded that in vitro purging is of no value. The failure of purging to enhance PFS may be more a statement of the efficacy of the purging method itself than a true estimation of the value of purging. Using gene marking to distinguish purged and unpurged marrow or PBPC products, Brenner has initiated studies to examine the effectiveness of various purging methods (Brenner, personal communication, 1997). In this method, portions of the harvested product are separated and marked with different and distinguishable retroviral vectors. One portion may be purged, the other not, or each portion may undergo a distinct and different purging method. Once marker gene is returned to the patient, its presence in recurrent tumor identifies the failed purging method. The results of clinical studies are pending.

An alternative solution to the problem of marrow tumor contamination may be the selection and infusion of pure hematopoietic cells. The risk of contaminating tumor cells has been assumed to be lower when using PBPC. Sensitive detection methods, however, have identified tumor cells in PBPC in a number of patients.[81, 149, 195] It is uncertain whether removing these cells would reduce the relapse rate. What is certain is that infusion of PBPC results in a more rapid hematopoietic recovery and a lower morbidity rate.[15] Either product, marrow or blood, can be used as a source to positively select hematopoietic stem cells. A number of methods to select CD34+ cells are being used in clinical trials. Preliminary results show a rapid hematopoietic recovery after autologous grafting with enriched CD34+ progenitor cells.[26, 154, 195] With more patients and adequate follow-up, the efficacy of this approach in sustaining remission will become clear. Finally, although purging methods may produce some incremental increase in PFS, the overall data suggest that the major impediment to cure in patients undergoing transplantation continues to be residual neuroblastoma in the patient.

POST-TRANSPLANTATION THERAPY

Short of applying more chemotherapy or local radiation after transplantation, another approach to eradicate residual disease after HSCT is to promote or create an endogenous antineuroblastoma immune response. Because of the heterogeneity among patients and the diversity of therapy, the time needed to recover cellular and humoral immunity after transplantation varies widely. In general, recovery of cell-mediated immunity precedes that of humoral immunity.[10, 175]

The promotion of an adjunct immune-mediated response to eradicate residual neuroblastoma in the post-transplant setting would require that the tumor be susceptible to cell-mediated immune mechanisms (e.g., cytotoxic T cells or natural killer cells). In vitro assays indicate that neuroblastoma cells are not susceptible to cytotoxic T-cell lysis, presumably because of the low expression of human leukocyte antigens on neuroblastoma cells.[130, 152] In contrast, neuroblastoma cells demonstrate susceptibility to killing mediated by natural killer cells.[55, 130] Interleukin-2 (IL-2), a potent stimulator of natural killer cell expansion and killing, has been administered in several trials as adjuvant therapy,[47, 133, 145, 199] but results are available for only small numbers of patients with short follow-up; thus, efficacy is difficult to judge.

Ex vivo engineering and administration of antibodies directed against neuroblastoma cell surface antigens (e.g., GD2) may offer another adjunctive therapeutic approach. Reports from several pilot studies using murine antibodies 3F8,[22, 23, 25] ch14.18, and 14.G2a[61, 80] noted several objective responses in patients with relapsed, refractory, or metastatic neuroblastoma. Rare but important toxicity included human antimouse antibody formation, neurologic changes, nephrotic syndrome, and hypotension. Hank et al.[82] and Kushner et al.[121] showed that the in vitro cytotoxicity of these neuroblastoma-specific antibodies (3F8 and 14.G2a) can be enhanced by granulocyte macrophage colony-stimulating factor or IL-2. These reports have led to studies investigating the potential for cytokines to increase immune effector cell numbers and thereby increase the efficacy of anti-GD2 antibodies.[61]

Testing this approach in a severe combined immunodeficiency (SCID) mouse model of human neuroblastoma, chimeric anti-GD2 antibody (ch14.18) fused to IL-2 prolonged survival and produced a greater antitumor response than equivalent doses of IL-2 alone.[177] Likewise, retrovirus-mediated transfer of the IL-2 gene into neuroblastoma cell lines has produced IL-2 secreting clones. In vitro assays demonstrate that culture of these transduced cells with lymphocytes induced potent human leukocyte antigen unrestricted cytotoxic activity (CD16+ or CD56+, CD8−) against transduced and parental neuroblastoma cells.[128] With further refinement, both of these methods may be worthy of clinical trial.

Finally, the role of tumor-modulating agents is being examined in the treatment of neuroblastoma. After treatment with retinoic acid, neuroblastoma cell lines have exhibited a profound decrease in N-myc RNA expression and cell cycle arrest.[174] This suggests that the cellular biology of neuroblastoma may be altered via drug mediation. Several pilot and phase I trials as well as a single cooperative group trial have examined the use of 13-cis-retinoic acid after HSCT. The maximum tolerated dose has been established at 160 mg/m²/day. Toxicity, including hypercalcemia, appeared manageable, and preliminary results support further clinical trials.[151, 201]

Treatment of neuroblastoma with immunotherapy and drug modulation is still largely of unproven benefit, but these modalities may have a place in the context of intensive chemoradiotherapy with or without transplantation. The optimal time for employing these treatments would likely be the adjuvant setting at the stage of minimal residual disease. The German National Neuroblastoma Protocol exemplifies the approach of combined-modality therapy. Harvest of PBPC is followed by positive selection and cryopreservation of CD34+ hematopoietic progenitors. After myeloablative chemotherapy that may include high-dose ¹³¹I-metaiodobenzylguanidine, PBPC are reinfused and followed by adjuvant treatment with the chimeric monoclonal antibody, ch14.18. Local radiotherapy is administered to sites of "resistant" metastases. Preliminary results suggest that this multimodal approach is feasible and has no severe unanticipated side effects.[154]

At the moment, it is not clear whether transplantation can improve on the cure rate achieved by intensive induction therapy with surgery. There is no evidence that TBI, autologous double-graft protocols, or alloHSCT benefits children with neuroblastoma. Transplantation does increase the length of remission for some patients, but its effect on the cure rate requires further study. The value of purging remains to be determined. More effective chemotherapy and radiation regimens, improved purging techniques, and the use of cytokines and PBPC to hasten recovery should further increase the effectiveness of autologous transplantation. Concomitant advances in immunomodulation will undoubtedly modify the role of autologous transplantation in neuroblastoma.

BRAIN TUMORS

Although the survival rates of children with brain tumors have improved because of advances in surgery, chemotherapy, and radiotherapy, the prognosis remains dismal for most children with anaplastic astrocytoma, glioblastoma multiforme, brain stem glioma, metastatic or unresectable medulloblastoma, primitive neuroectodermal tumor (PNET), ependymoblastoma, and recurrent brain tumor.[50, 71, 188, 198] For many of these entities, the overall survival rate is less than 10%, thus demanding novel therapeutic approaches including chemotherapy/radiotherapy intensification followed by stem cell transplantation.

Ultimately, the success of transplantation will depend on the effectiveness of dose intensification. In vitro and in vivo animal models of brain tumors have defined agents with potential antitumor activity.[53, 59, 60, 187] The preclinical evidence alone is insufficient to predict in vivo activity because, to be effective, chemotherapy must penetrate the blood-brain and blood-tumor barriers in tumoricidal concentrations. A number of agents (e.g., thiotepa, cyclophosphamide, melphalan, bis-chloroethyl-nitrosourea, etoposide, and the platinum derivatives) demonstrate excellent penetration into brain parenchyma as evidenced in phase I/II trials.[1, 2, 8, 41, 57, 65, 90, 91, 190, 196] Unfortunately, in vitro studies find that many potentially useful compounds exhibit steep dose-response curves and cannot be administered safely to achieve cytotoxic concentrations at tumor sites. The potential advantage in using high-dose chemotherapy to penetrate the brain/tumor parenchyma provides a rational basis for the use of stem cell transplantation.

A number of studies using high-dose single-agent chemotherapy (e.g., bis-chloroethyl-nitrosourea or etoposide) followed by autologous transplantation have reported measurable responses and improved survival among adults with recurrent glioma.[68, 168] For children with brain tumors, there have been few clinical trials of dose-intense chemotherapy followed by autologous marrow or stem cell rescue (Table

12–6). Results of these reports are difficult to interpret and compare because of the wide diversity of variables among studies. The type of tumor, the disease status at the time of transplantation (e.g., complete response, partial or no response, or progressive disease), the number of previous relapses, and the intensity of previous therapy (radiation and/or chemotherapy) undoubtedly affect the outcome after transplantation.[48, 51, 52, 129] Confounding the interpretation

of data is the lack of a consistent benchmark to measure the response to therapy.

HIGH-GRADE ASTROCYTIC TUMORS

Ten patients with high-grade astrocytoma, which was recurrent in seven patients and secondary in two patients, under-

TABLE 12–6. HIGH-DOSE CHEMOTHERAPY STUDIES WITH AUTOLOGOUS STEM CELL RESCUE FOR BRAIN TUMORS IN CHILDREN

STUDY	NO. OF PTS/ DIAGNOSIS	TREATMENT	DISEASE STATUS	OUTCOME/TOXICITY
Primitive Neuroectodermal Tumors/Medulloblastoma/Ependymoma				
Kalifa et al., 1992[100]	8 medullo/PNET 5 ependymoma	Busulfan 600 mg/m^2 Thiotepa 1050 mg/m^2	Recurrent with measurable dis; previous chemo/radiotherapy	2 CR; 5 PR 6 SD (5–24 mo) 1 toxic death
Kalifa et al., 1993[101]	8 medullo/PNET	Busulfan 600 mg/m^2 Thiotepa 1050 mg/m^2	Recurrent; previous chemotherapy	7 CRX/PR 1 PD (8–54 mo)
Garvin et al., 1992[64]	31 brain tumors including 6 medullo/PNET	Thiotepa Etoposide Carboplatin or BCNU	29 recurrent 2 newly diagnosed	28% CR/PR (3–16 mo) 23% toxic death 32% PFS at 11.5 mo (3–36 mo)
Finlay et al., 1994[49]	24 medullo/PNET 4 pinealoblastoma	Thiotepa 900 mg/m^2 Etoposide 750 mg/m^2 Carboplatin 1500 mg/m^2	Recurrent/progressive dis; previous chemo/radiotherapy	12/28 responders (10 with MRD are PFS) 3 toxic death (11%) 41.2 ± 9.5% (EFS) at 24 mo
Finlay et al., 1996[51]	12 PNET	Thiotepa 900 mg/m^2 Etoposide 1500 mg/m^2	Recurrent 6 measurable tumor 6 previous chemo/radiotherapy	2/6 CR/PR 5 toxic death 7 dis progression No survival at 2 years
Graham et al., 1993[74]	8 medullo	Melphalan 75–120 mg/mg^2 Cytoxan 6 g/m^2	Recurrent	2/8 responded
Mahoney et al., 1996[129]	9 medullo/PNET 6 malignant glioma 5 ependy/germ	Melphalan 180 mg/m^2 Cytoxan 3–6 g/m^2	Recurrent; previous chemo/radiotherapy; 16 with measurable disease	4 CR/PR in medullo 3 CR in ependy/germ 4 toxic death PFS 1 year 17% ± 9%
Graham et al., 1987[73]	19 medullo	Melphalan 75–120 mg/m^2 Cytoxan 6 g/m^2	12 disseminated 6 localized	4 CR >24 mo in localized only
Dunkel et al., 1998[39]	21 medullo	Carboplatin 1500 mg/m^2 Thiotepa 900 mg/m^2 Etoposide 750 mg/m^2	Recurrent	34% EFS at 36 mo 3 toxic deaths
Mason et al., 1998[135]	15 ependymoma	Thiotepa 900 mg/m^2 Etoposide 900 mg/m^2 ± carboplatin 1500 mg/mg^2	Recurrent	9 PD 5 toxic deaths 1 unrelated death
Malignant Glioma/High-Grade Astrocytoma				
Finlay et al., 1990[48]	9 glioma/AA 1 brain stem glioma	Thiotepa 900–1200 mg/m^2 Etoposide 1500 mg/m^2 ± BCNU 600 mg/m^2	7 recurrent 3 primary (all measurable dis)	4 CR; 2 PR 2 CR at 15 mo 1 toxic death
Dunkel et al., 1994[38]	17 brain stem glioma	Thiotepa 900 mg/m^2 Etoposide ± carboplatin/BCNU	11 recurrent 6 new diagnosis	2 responders 2 toxic deaths No improvement
Heideman et al., 1993[90]	13 malignant glioma	Thiotepa 900 mg/m^2 Cytoxan 600 mg/m^2 Followed by XRT	2 recurrent 11 primary 10 with bulky dis	1 CR; 3 PR; 7 SD; 1 PD CR/PR 31% (1–16 mo) 3 surv with 1 CR (30 mo) and 2 recurrences 3 toxic death
Kedar et al., 1994[104]	6 brain stem glioma	Thiotepa 900 mg/m^2 Cytoxan 3000–3750 mg/m^2	Primary	1 PR 1 toxic death
Finlay et al., 1996[51]	18 high-grade glioma	Thiotepa 900 mg/m^2 Etoposide 1500 mg/m^2	Recurrent; previous chemo/radiotherapy	29% ± 10% CR/PR 5 survivors at 49 mo (39–59 mo) 2 toxic deaths
Dunkel et al., 1998[39]	16 pontine glioma	Thiotepa 900 mg/m^2 Etoposide 250–1500 mg/m^2 ± BCNU 200 mg/m^2 ± Carboplatin 1500 mg/m^2	6 primary 10 recurrent	All PD No survival >17 mo 2 toxic deaths

AA, high-grade astrocytoma; BCNU, BCNU, *bis*-chloroethyl-nitrosourea; chemo, chemotherapy; CR, complete response; dis, disease; EFS, event-free survival; ependy, ependymoma; germ, germinoma; medullo, medulloblastoma; MRD, minimal residual disease; PD, progressive disease; PFS, progression-free survival; PNET, primitive neuroectodermal tumor; PR, partial response; SD, stable disease; surv, survivors; XRT, radiation therapy.

went intensive chemotherapy followed by HSCT[48] (see Table 12–6). At the beginning of intensification, all patients had measurable disease. At day 28 post transplantation, four patients had obtained CR and two had obtained PR. Two continued in CR for more than 15 months after therapy. Regimen-related toxicity contributed to the morbidity and mortality and included mucositis, skin erythema and desquamation, systemic infection, and liver dysfunction. Given the patients' advanced disease state, the outcome justified further trial of this therapy. When essentially the same combination therapy was used to treat 17 children with brain stem tumor, however, there was no discernible improvement in survival compared with standard therapy.[38]

Receiving a combination of thiotepa with cyclophosphamide in an attempt to reduce nonhematologic toxicity, 13 patients with high-grade glioma underwent chemotherapy intensification (see Table 12–6) followed by HSCT.[90] Patients had not received prior chemotherapy or radiotherapy for their central nervous system lesion and began intensification within 4 weeks after primary resection. Post-transplantation patients received radiotherapy to appropriate fields using a variety of schedules. Ten patients manifested bulky disease at the time chemotherapy was started. The 31% response rate was considered superior when compared with that achieved with conventional therapy, but the overall survival was not improved. Three patients remained alive, one in CR, 14–30 months after transplantation. Grade 3 and 4 regimen-related toxicity, principally mucositis, skin changes, and infection, occurred in all patients. Of note, two patients died at 23 and 24 months after treatment (one of pneumonia, the other of shunt complications) but without evidence of recurrent disease. Both patients had evidence of extensive radiation necrosis. This raises the concern that intensive therapy may increase the severity of postirradiation complications. The same drugs, albeit at a lower total dose of cyclophosphamide, HSCT, and radiotherapy, resulted in two partial responses and two toxic deaths among six patients with brain stem glioma and three patients with high-grade gliomas.[104]

A 1996 summary of the results of treating recurrent high-grade brain malignancy with etoposide and thiotepa followed by autologous HSCT noted that the activity of this combination was sufficient to warrant further trial.[51] All patients (n = 45, including 18 patients with glioma) had at least one tumor recurrence, and all had received prior treatment with chemotherapy and/or radiotherapy. Among the evaluable patients, four patients with high-grade glioma (n = 14) and two with PNET/medulloblastoma (n = 6) achieved a complete or partial response. Five patients, who had high-grade glioma without measurable disease at the time of initiating therapy, remained alive beyond 3 years. In contrast, there were no survivors among those patients with radiographic evidence of bulky disease at the initiation of therapy. Treatment-related toxicity included mucositis, somnolence, hepatic veno-occlusive disease, and death (see Table 12–6). Previous therapy may exaggerate the likelihood of severe toxicity and prolong the time to neutrophil and platelet engraftment (23 and 35 days, respectively). To that end, as demonstrated in another trial, the interval to neutrophil recovery may be shortened by the administration of granulocyte colony-stimulating factor.[129]

PRIMITIVE NEUROECTODERMAL TUMORS AND MEDULLOBLASTOMA

As is true for high-grade gliomas, the treatment of locally advanced or recurrent embryonic brain tumors requires improved therapy. In evaluating reports describing the efficacy of high-dose chemotherapy and stem cell transplantation, the impact of previous and concurrent therapy must be weighed. The extent of surgical resection, whether for primary or recurrent tumor, may dramatically influence survival.

The combination of busulfan and thiotepa with stem cell rescue resulted in a partial response for four of eight patients with recurrent PNET or medulloblastoma.[100] This response rate was encouraging because disease had proved refractory to prior chemotherapy and/or radiotherapy in all patients. When essentially the same regimen was used to treat recurrent non-irradiated medulloblastoma, seven of eight patients achieved CR/PR and six were disease free 8–54 months after transplantation.[101] Furthermore, for four patients it was possible to limit the post-transplantation radiation to the posterior fossa. A recent update of these results[33] (20 patients with relapsed or progressive medulloblastoma) showed that although this treatment appeared effective for local recurrences, only a single patient with metastatic disease survived.

In a different approach to patients with recurrent medulloblastoma/PNET, all having received prior radiotherapy, high-dose etoposide was combined with thiotepa and infusion of hematopoietic stem cells.[51] Partial response was noted in two of six patients with measurable disease; however, no patient survived beyond 2 years of salvage therapy.

To increase antitumor activity, carboplatin or *bis*-chloroethyl-nitrosourea was combined with thiotepa and etoposide.[51, 64] Toxicity was appreciable, with multiorgan involvement leading to a fatality rate between 10% and 40% over several studies.[39, 49, 51, 64] In one study that included 31 children with advanced disease, 21% of patients with measurable disease achieved CR, and PFS was 32% at 11.5 months (range, 3–36 months).[64] Similarly, 12 of 28 patients with recurrent medulloblastoma had stable disease 4–34 months after chemotherapy and transplantation.[49] Patients with minimal disease prior to therapy faired best.

Finally, combining the alkylators melphalan and cyclophosphamide, Graham et al.[74] reported two responses among eight patients with either recurrent "chemosensitive" or newly diagnosed high-risk medulloblastoma. This experience has been expanded to include 37 patients (19 patients with medulloblastoma). Overall, 15 patients treated with this regimen remained free of disease. Toxicity was manageable and generally limited to mucositis.[74] Among 18 evaluable patients with recurrent or progressive brain tumors after chemotherapy/radiotherapy (including 4 patients with medulloblastoma) treated with melphalan and escalating doses of cyclophosphamide, 7 patients achieved CR (n = 4) or PR.[129]

If effective in treating pediatric brain tumors, intensive chemotherapy followed by stem cell rescue may confer the additional benefit of being able to reduce or altogether avoid brain irradiation and its consequent psychomotor toxicity in young children. This strategy was applied in 29 patients with recurrent/measurable central nervous system disease who underwent surgical resection, myeloablative consolidation chemotherapy (thiotepa, carboplatin, and etoposide), and stem cell rescue; at 11.5 months, the CR and PFS rates were 21% and 32%, respectively.[64, 136] Death from regimen-related toxicity occurred in 7 patients.[64] Of 37 of 42 patients with newly diagnosed disease who were evaluable for response, 15 were free of disease (median DFS, >44 months); 3 toxic deaths were attributed to regimen-related toxicity.[136] These important studies prove that a significant proportion of children with malignant brain tumors can avoid radiotherapy and prolonged chemotherapy yet still achieve durable remission with a brief, intensive chemotherapy regimen.

In summary, recurrent PNET and medulloblastoma appear to be responsive to alkylator-based therapy.[73, 74, 129] The combination of thiotepa and etoposide initially produced a 50% response rate among patients with medulloblastoma/PNET; with longer follow-up, however, the treatment failed.[49, 64] For most patients, the disease progressed by 6 months after transplantation. More recently, with the addition of carboplatin to the thiotepa/etoposide regimen, the 2-year EFS rate exceeded 40%.[39, 49, 51]

The use of therapy based on thiotepa and etoposide[39, 48, 51] and thiotepa/cyclophosphamide[90, 104] in high-grade glioma remains problematic: the prolonged survival rate is less than 20%. Treatment results for recurrent ependymoma and brain stem glioma are even worse.[39, 52, 90, 104, 129, 135] It appears that ablative chemotherapy regimens need to be individualized to the tumor type. In defining ablative regimens, the previous chemosensitivity of the tumor will need to be considered.

TOXICITY

Although recurrence of primary disease remains the gravest problem for those who survive, irradiation and adjuvant chemotherapy may cause significant immediate and delayed morbidity. One must be cognizant that consolidation treatment with high-dose chemotherapy and autologous stem cell rescue may add toxicity.[116]

For patients undergoing salvage therapy, the significant morbidity and mortality of myeloablative treatment are largely related to prolonged pancytopenia. Drug toxicity to other organ systems may be superimposed on sequelae of prior therapy, however. Immediate toxicity associated with high-dose chemotherapy and autologous bone marrow rescue includes mucositis, renal dysfunction, veno-occlusive disease, sepsis, hemorrhage and, in 50% of patients, various forms of acute neurologic dysfunction, including encephalopathy, coma, hallucinations, seizures, headaches, ataxia-tremor-dysarthria, anorexia, and others.[116] Patients who have received prior craniospinal radiation are more likely to encounter chronic neurologic effects.[46, 52, 129]

Patients who have received craniospinal irradiation prior to intensification/stem cell rescue require more time to recover platelet (>50 × 10⁹) and neutrophil counts (>0.5 × 10⁹) (median, day 30 vs. day 72 for platelets and day 13 vs. day 23 for neutrophils).[46] Prompt platelet recovery may be particularly important for patients considered to be at increased risk for intracranial bleeding. Although prolonged platelet and neutrophil recovery have not been

shown to affect PFS or overall survival, intervention to hasten the recovery of hematopoietic function will likely reduce morbidity. Other modifications to treatment may be important. For example, patients who receive high-dose carboplatin as a part of pre-HSCT consolidation treatment are likely to further aggravate the hearing loss frequently present after prior treatment. Although not life-threatening, hearing loss in children interferes with the acquisition of speech, a major function necessary to socialization, learning, and quality of life.[56]

SUMMARY

The improved response rate, up to 40%, is reason to continue investigation of high-dose therapy and hematopoietic stem cell transplantation in children with high-grade brain tumors. Initial efforts exploring new approaches to treatment rarely have resulted in immediate resolution of the clinical problem. These early studies provided critical observations that second-generation trials seek to improve on. The studies cited have suggested that the treatment of brain tumors needs to be oriented to the specific tumor type. Patients with minimal residual disease or those without gross residual tumor demonstrate a higher rate of response and achieve longer PFS. Patients with residual bulky disease or chemotherapy-resistant disease are unlikely to derive benefit from this approach.

Early collection of stem cells, before craniospinal radiation and substantive chemotherapy administration, provides a better yield of stem cells and more rapid hematopoietic recovery. Because the probability of durable EFS most closely correlates with the status of residual disease, the role of high-dose chemotherapy with stem cell rescue clearly must be evaluated as a consolidation approach before or after radiation therapy for patients in first remission. Logically, high-dose chemotherapy and stem cell transplantation will prove curative when administered to patients with chemoresponsive tumors and minimal residual disease. Future trials must adopt a more stringent approach in terms of eligibility and specifying tumor histology, stage, and prior therapy.

The use of myeloablative chemotherapy earlier in treatment may reduce systemic toxicity from veno-occlusive disease and multiorgan failure. Whether early high-dose chemotherapy with stem cell rescue improves DFS and increases the portion of patients cured of their disease will require proof in subsequent clinical trials. This can be accomplished only in the context of multi-institutional collaboration.

The need to identify appropriate chemotherapeutic agents remains the major goal in the treatment of brain tumors. Encouraging clinical data regarding new agents such as temozolomide, the taxanes, and the topoisomerase-I inhibitors[27, 84, 99, 156] or radiolabeled monoclonal antibodies are emerging.[9] The use of experimental agents in pilot studies must continue as a priority.

EWING SARCOMA FAMILY OF TUMORS

The Ewing sarcoma family of tumors—Ewing sarcoma, extraosseous Ewing sarcoma, small cell osteosarcoma, and (primitive) peripheral neuroectodermal (neuroepithelioma) tumor (PNET)—are characterized by one of two common chromosomal translocations: t(11;22) or t(21;22). Both fusion genes include the EWS gene on chromosome 22. For classic Ewing sarcoma, the primary site is evenly divided between the long bones of the extremities and the bones of the central axis (pelvis, chest wall, spine, or neck). The trunk is the most common primary site for extraosseous Ewing sarcoma and PNET. Despite their many similarities, it is unclear whether the various entities included in the Ewing family carry the same prognosis.

In Ewing sarcoma, tumor size and site are important prognostic factors; bulky primaries of axial skeleton generally fare worst.[43] In recent years, multimodal treatment may have diminished the prognostic importance of tumor size and site.[78, 122, 144] For patients with nonmetastatic Ewing sarcoma, the 2-year DFS rate approaches 70% after surgery, multiagent chemotherapy, and radiotherapy.[19, 78, 98, 153]

With patients who present with metastases, 3- to 5-year DFS rates are between 20% and 45%.[19, 43, 94, 148, 189] When metastases involve bone marrow or bony sites distant from the primary tumor, the DFS rate falls to less than 15%.[17–19, 147] After tumor recurrence, further treatment may salvage between 5% and 30% of patients.[18, 94]

The management of Ewing sarcoma enlists the judicious use of surgery, radiotherapy, and chemotherapy. Although treatment to achieve local control cannot be segregated from methods to eradicate or prevent metastases, it is recognized that metastatic disease is uncommon at presentation; nevertheless, most failures occur at distant sites (65% systemic, 25% local, 10% combined). Thus, all patients, regardless of the completeness of primary tumor resection, require chemotherapy (dose-intensive cyclophosphamide and doxorubicin in combination with vincristine, actinomycin D, ifosfamide, and etoposide).[48, 78, 132, 144, 148, 153] Inoperable tumors may be rendered resectable after chemotherapy. Radiotherapy (at doses between 50 and 55 cGy) is essential for incompletely resected primary tumors, but the optimal radiotherapeutic approach to localized disease control remains under investigation.[44, 148]

Ewing sarcoma presents an unmistakable dose/response relationship to both chemotherapy and radiotherapy. This observation suggests that the use of dose-intensive therapy followed by hematopoietic stem cell rescue may be effective either as salvage therapy for patients experiencing relapse or as primary therapy for patients at high risk for relapse. Both approaches have been explored in clinical trials.[3, 16, 17, 28, 75, 85, 147, 148, 157, 161, 162] Likewise, the role of TBI in the context of chemotherapy/stem cell rescue to treat poor-prognosis Ewing sarcoma has been examined in laboratory and clinical studies.[17, 18, 44, 94, 106, 107, 124, 125, 148, 191]

Table 12–7 summarizes the results of a number of clinical trials examining Ewing sarcoma that include high-dose chemotherapy/TBI followed by transplantation. It should be noted that comparison of outcomes among studies requires circumspection because of dissimilarities among patients as to tumor histology, size, and location; prior exposure to therapy; and measure of response.

Early studies in patients with the high-risk Ewing sarcoma family of tumors showed encouraging long-term results in patients with nonmetastatic disease but poor results in patients with metastatic disease.[94, 148] TBI of 5–12 Gy was administered in the majority of early studies.[17, 94, 124, 148, 191] More recent studies exclude irradiation in favor of enhanced chemotherapy; overall results are comparable.

Whether dose intensification and hematopoietic stem cell transfusion can enhance DFS ultimately rests on the effectiveness of intensified therapy to eradicate residual tumor cells. To date, melphalan, either as a single agent or in combination, has received the widest use in consolidation therapy before transplantation (see Table 12–7).

Reviewing the European experience, in which more than 80% of 63 patients with Ewing family tumors received melphalan as part of intensification and stem cell rescue, investigators judged this approach superior to conventional treatment.[125] All patients had metastatic disease, either at presentation or during recurrence, but achieved CR prior to undergoing intensification and transplantation. For patients in first CR, the 5-year EFS rate was 21%; the EFS rate was 32% for patients in second CR.

So far, no particular pre-HSCT schedule can be identified as superior. Compared with conventional therapy, consolidation with high-dose radiotherapy/chemotherapy contributed to improved EFS rates for high-risk patients. In line with this perception, the Children's Cancer Group opened a group-wide pilot study for patients with high-risk Ewing sarcoma/PNET. Eligible for this study are patients who present with disease metastatic to bone marrow or to bone distant from the primary tumor. Induction chemotherapy is followed by PBPC collection and irradiation of the primary tumor and sites of bulky metastatic disease. High-dose consolidation therapy with melphalan and etoposide are followed by TBI and stem cell rescue.

Tumor contamination in the stem cell graft may be a critical determinant of success after high-dose chemotherapy/radiotherapy and stem cell rescue. Ewing sarcoma/PNET spreads hematogenously, and it is assumed that all patients have metastatic disease at diagnosis even though clinically evident metastases are found in only 20% of patients.[94, 202] This assumption is based on two facts: (1) patients treated with local therapy alone invariably experience failure at distant sites; and (2) cure only became possible with the advent of effective systemic therapy.

Because more than 90% of Ewing sarcoma/PNET tumors are defined by the translocation t(11;22), the use of reverse transcriptase–polymerase chain reaction (RT-PCR) detection may permit screening of harvested bone marrow or blood for residual disease prior to transplantation.[197, 202] The significance of the presence of abnormal cells is uncertain, but using RT-PCR screening technology to monitor the effects of treatment may further clarify the indications for and efficacy of dose-intensive radiochemotherapy and stem cell transplantation.

In summary, high-dose chemotherapy, either single-agent (e.g., melphalan) or multiagent, possibly combined with local irradiation and/or TBI and followed by autologous stem cell transplantation, has resulted in a 20–40% EFS rate for patients with high-risk Ewing sarcoma. In other studies reporting on patients with recurrent or metastatic Ewing sarcoma, the EFS rate seldom exceeds 20%. When compared with historical data, these figures may be viewed as encouraging. Nevertheless, caution is necessary because the outcome following newer and more intensive

TABLE 12–7. AUTOLOGOUS STEM CELL RESCUE FOR EWING SARCOMA FAMILY OF TUMORS

STUDY	PATIENTS	TREATMENT	RESULTS
Mise et al., 1988[148]	Metastatic primary tumor (13) or trunk/humerus/femur primary tumor (18)	Induction: vin, adria, cyclo, actino, 50 Gy to primary site Consolidation: vin, adria, cyclo, TBI (800 cGy)	77% 3-yr EFS for nonmetastatic disease, EFS < 10% in metastatic disease
Marcus, 1989	Metastatic ES (9); primary tumor > 8 cm (11)	Similar to the above regimen	63% 3-yr EFS
Herzig, 1985	10 patients	Melphalan (120–125 mg/m^2) ± BCNU	6 PR 2 CR
Dini, 1988	Refractory ES (9)	Melphalan (140–220 mg/m^2)	2 PR 2 CR
Burdach et al. 1993[17]	Multifocal ES (7); relapsed ES (10)	Melphalan (120–180 mg/m^2) + etoposide (40–60 mg/m^2) + TBI (12 Gy)	45% 6-yr DFS
Hartmann, 1991	Metastatic disease (27)	Melphalan (140–200 mg/m^2)	CR 41% Response 81%
Horowitz et al., 1993[94]	Metastatic ES (56) or localized ES (humerus, trunk, or femur)	VADRIAC, consolidation with TBI (8 cGy) and VADRIAC	30% 6-yr EFS for entire group, 48% EFS without metastatic dis, 10% with metastatic dis
Ladenstein et al. 1995[125]	32 patients in 1 CR 31 patients in 2 CR	Melphalan-based conditioning ± TBI	21% 5-yr EFS 1st CR and 32% EFS 2nd CR
Stewart et al., 1996[191]	13 patients Relapse/refractory (4) Metastatic (2) Nonmetastatic (6)	Melphalan (140–200 mg/m^2) ± TBI (500 cGy)	3 PR (25–108 mo)
Atra et al., 1997[3]	18 patients in CR metastatic (11)	Melphalan 200 mg/m^2 Busulfan 16 mg/m^2	70% 2-yr DFS, 54% DFS with metastatic dis
Ozkaynak et al., 1998[157]	15 patients Recurrent (9)	Melphalan 200 mg/m^2 Carboplatin 1200 mg/m^2 Etoposide 800 mg/m^2 ± cytoxan 3000 mg/m^2	66 ± 19% 3-yr EFS 16% toxic deaths

actino, actinomycin D; adria, adriamycin; cyclo, cyclophosphamide; vin, vincristine; VADRIAC, vincristine, adriamycin, cyclophosphamide; BCNU, *bis*-chloroethyl-nitrosurea; CR, complete response; PR, partial response; TBI, total body irradiation; DFS, disease-free survival; EFS, event-free survival; ES, Ewing sarcoma.

multiagent primary therapy will not be comparable to that of older conventional chemotherapy and salvage regimens.

For patients whose tumors are unresponsive to chemotherapy, salvage rates rarely exceed 10%. There is a clear need for new and more effective agents. Finally, prospective trials should determine whether postgraft therapy (e.g., immunotherapy) can further increase survival.

RHABDOMYOSARCOMA AND SOFT TISSUE SARCOMAS

Rhabdomyosarcoma and the "nonrhabdo" soft tissue sarcomas are developmentally related to primitive mesenchymal cells. Rhabdomyosarcoma accounts for approximately 5% of pediatric cancers and is the most common soft tissue sarcoma in children. These tumors can arise at virtually any site and are categorized as orbit, head and neck (excluding parameningeal), parameningeal, genitourinary (excluding bladder/prostate), bladder/prostate, extremity, and other (e.g., trunk, paraspinal sites). Certainty regarding the diagnosis of rhabdomyosarcoma (as well as other sarcomas) often requires that routine histopathology be supplemented with immunohistochemistry (including the application of antibodies with specificity for muscle-specific actin, myoglobin, myosin, desmin, myogenin, and the MyoD proteins) and electron microscopy.

Pathologically, rhabdomyosarcoma is classified as embryonal (60%), alveolar (20%), or pleomorphic/undifferentiated (20%). The relevance of rhabdomyosarcoma histology relates to the observation that response to chemotherapy differs by histotype. Embryonal rhabdomyosarcoma

responds more favorably than the others. Accordingly, the relatively recent finding of specific fusion genes limited to alveolar rhabdomyosarcoma suggests that genetic factors may underlie this treatment-related observation. These fusion genes (and associated chimeric messengers) are the result of translocation, either t(2;13) (PAX3-FKHR) or t(1;13) (PAX7-FKHR). When studied using RT-PCR or FISH (fluorescent in situ hybridization), virtually every alveolar rhabdomyosarcoma is marked by one of these chimeric genes. In addition to the findings, other genetic features (e.g., tumor cell ploidy) may prove useful in characterizing rhabdomyosarcoma. Genetic characterization may help to define those patients in need of new treatments or as a method to indicate the presence of residual rhabdomyosarcoma cells.

The prognosis of patients with rhabdomyosarcoma is best characterized by tumor histology, primary tumor site, stage, and treatment (Tables 12–8 and 12–9).[32, 158, 160] Analogous to Ewing sarcoma/PNET, rhabdomyosarcoma presenting at specific unfavorable sites (e.g., extremity, parameninges, retroperitoneum, pelvis, or a paraspinal site) has been associated with high risk of treatment failure.

Sequential Intergroup Rhabdomyosarcoma Study (IRS) Group studies I, II, and III demonstrated that more aggressive chemotherapy and surgery, with or without irradiation, have significantly reduced the prognostic impact of disease site and tumor histology, except for tumors metastatic at presentation. In IRS III, the 5-year PFS rate exceeded 60% at all sites and exceeded 80% for favorable sites. Overall, the cure rate for rhabdomyosarcoma ranges between 70% and 90% for patients with localized disease and favorable histology; however, the 5-year PFS rate is less than 30%

TABLE 12–8. INTERGROUP RHABDOMYOSARCOMA STUDY CLINICAL STAGING CLASSIFICATION

GROUP	DEFINITION
I	Localized disease, completely resected tumor confined to muscle or organ of origin, infiltration beyond site of origin with regional nodes not involved
II	Gross excision but either microscopic residual disease or adjacent organ or regional nodes involved
	Grossly resected but microscopic residual disease (tumor found by pathologist at margin)
	Regional disease, completely resected, in which nodes may be involved or extension of tumor into an adjacent organ
	Regional disease with involved nodes, grossly resected, but with evidence of microscopic residual disease
III	Incomplete resection or biopsy with gross residual disease
IV	Distant metastatic disease present at onset

for patients who present with disseminated disease.[29, 30, 141, 142] Direct comparison of outcome between IRS and European studies is made somewhat problematic by differences in tumor staging; however, with metastatic disease, the outcome is similar (i.e., the 3-year DFS rate ranges between 19% and 25%).[20, 113, 114]

Likewise, the outcome is poor for patients in whom current multiagent treatment regimens fail. IRS and European data support the conclusion that salvage is poor, partly because of intolerance of further chemotherapy.[30, 94, 112, 131] The IRS reported 3-year postrelapse survival rates of 48% ± 12%, 12% ± 9%, 11% ± 5%, and 8% ± 4% in clinical groups I through IV, respectively.[30] Superior survival among group I patients alone undoubtedly reflects the fact that relapses were local and aggressive radiotherapy and chemotherapy remained a therapeutic option. Thus, patients with metastatic disease at presentation or recurrent tumor are appropriate candidates for novel therapy, including dose-intensive chemotherapy with or without radiotherapy followed by stem cell transplantation.

Experience with the use of dose intensification/stem cell transplantation in the treatment of rhabdomyosarcoma began early in the 1980s. Patients with recurrent, progressive, or refractory disease were treated with a variety of high-dose regimens, including thiotepa, melphalan, busulfan/cyclophosphamide, and cyclophosphamide/doxorubicin/dacarbazine followed by HSCT.[5, 11, 87, 96, 205] These studies demonstrated that this approach was feasible in terms of both manageable toxicity and potential for response. More recently, investigators have attempted to define the efficacy of high-dose therapy and stem cell transplantation by applying this therapy more systematically.[37, 94, 115, 123, 169] Data from these studies are presented in Table 12–10.

According to the European HSCT solid tumor registry, high-dose therapy and stem cell rescue were used as a part of primary therapy to treat more than 60 patients with rhabdomyosarcoma, the majority of whom presented with metastatic disease (see Table 12–10).[37, 123, 115, 169] Most intensification regimens included melphalan, either alone or in combination, with or without TBI. Overall, 20–25% of patients survived, but a difference in survival—28% versus 12%—favored patients undergoing transplantation as part of initial versus salvage therapy.[123] Likewise, survival for patients undergoing transplantation after achieving CR was superior to that of patients undergoing transplantation while in PR. The investigators did not claim a benefit for those patients receiving intensification with melphalan and HSCT. This strategy resulted in appreciable short-term morbidity, but it was probably no more severe than with prolonged chemotherapy. The impact of this approach, however—especially for patients presenting with metastatic disease—is unclear because the DFS and overall survival rates (20% and 25%) were little different from those achieved with conventional chemotherapy.[20, 112–114]

The German/Austrian Pediatric Bone Marrow Transplant Group recently reported on stem cell transplantation in high-risk rhabdomyosarcoma[115] (see Table 12–10). Nine patients remained alive without recurrent disease at 27 months post transplantation; however, only 5 of 27 patients with metastatic disease were disease-free survivors. Four of nine patients with recurrent disease survived disease free. Perhaps this favorable outcome is attributable to less aggressive initial therapy because relapses typically occurred at primary disease sites. No significant trends emerged to differentiate which patients or regimens merited further study. Overall, the treatment results were no better than those reported with more traditional approaches.[20, 112]

Investigators at the National Cancer Institute expanded their approach of intensification with vincristine, doxorubi-

TABLE 12–9. RHABDOMYOSARCOMA—STAGING

STAGE	SITES	T	SIZE	N	M
1	Orbit Head and neck (excluding parameningeal) GU—nonbladder/nonprostate	T_1 or T_2	A or B	N_0 or N_1 or N_x	M_0
2	Bladder/prostate Extremity Cranial parameningeal Other (includes trunk, retroperitoneum, etc.)	T_1 or T_2	A	N_0 or N_x	M_0
3	Bladder/prostate Extremity Cranial parameningeal Other (includes trunk, retroperitoneum, etc.)	T_1 or T_2	A B	N_1 N_0 or N_1 or N_x	M_0 M_0
4	All	T_1 or T_2	A or B	N_0 or N_x	M_1

GU, genitourinary.

TABLE 12–10. HIGH-DOSE CHEMOTHERAPY WITH STEM CELL RESCUE IN RHABDOMYOSARCOMA

STUDY	PATIENTS	TREATMENT	RESULTS
Pinkerton, 1991[170]	43 children with stage 4 or 3 RMS	VAC × 8 wk followed by HD melphalan with bone marrow rescue	Stage 3: 3-yr DFS 55% Stage 4: 3-yr DFS 25%
Dumontet et al., 1992[37]	11 RMS including 4 metastatic	Melphalan 140 mg/m^2 ± VCR ± TBI	1 toxic death 2-yr DFS 20% 15-month median survival
Koscielniak et al., 1997[115]	Primary metastatic (27) or relapsed RMS (9); 32 in CR; 4 in VGPR	HDC ± TBI Melphalan (4 × 30–45 mg/m^2) ± VP (40–60 mg/kg), CB (3 × 400–500 mg/m^2) 31 autologous 5 allogeneic sibling	1 toxic death 9 alive NED 57 mo (32–108 mo) (25%) including 5 of 27 with primary metastatic disease
Horowitz et al., 1993[94]	25 patients in remission Unresectable/alveolar or unresectable embryonal of extremities or trunk	TBI (8 Gy) Adriamycin 35 mg/m^2 × 2 Vincristine 2 mg/m^2 Cyclophosphamide 1.2 g/m^2 × 2	6-yr EFS 24% 6% therapy-related death

HDC, high-dose chemotherapy; VGPR, very good partial remission; VP, etoposide; NED, no evidence of disease; CB, carboplatin; VAC, vincristine, doxorubicin, cyclophosphamide; DFS, disease-free survival; EFS, event-free survival; TBI, total body irradiation; HD, high-dose; RMS, rhabdomyosarcoma.

cin, cyclophosphamide, and TBI followed by stem cell transplantation for patients with rhabdomyosarcoma.[94] Patients were eligible if they presented with unresectable alveolar disease, unresectable embryonal rhabdomyosarcoma of the extremity or trunk, or metastatic disease. Additionally, patients must have been complete responders to chemotherapy, surgery, and local radiotherapy. The 24% EFS rate at 6 years was comparable with those of other reports; the EFS rate for patients with metastatic disease was less than 20%. Most failures were at distant rather than primary tumor sites; however, the site of relapse was influenced by primary therapy. The transplantation process conferred no apparent benefit.

In the final estimation, no data establish the treatment superiority of dose-intensive chemotherapy/radiotherapy followed by stem cell transplantation for patients with advanced or recurrent rhabdomyosarcoma. Although this approach remains appealing, the direction in which to proceed to increase the cure rate is hardly obvious. Nevertheless, interest remains in developing and refining this approach. The Children's Cancer Group has developed a study in which patients with metastatic soft tissue sarcoma receive consolidation treatment with continuous-infusion carboplatin and etoposide along with melphalan and autologous stem cell transplantation. Because aggressive therapy has reduced the impact of tumor stage, histology, and primary site in other instances, the rationale underlying this approach appears to have merit.

OTHER TUMORS

Patients with advanced or recurrent/refractory germ cell tumor, retinoblastoma, Wilms tumor, and other soft tissue sarcomas may be candidates for salvage therapy with ablative chemotherapy and autologous HSCT.[14, 20, 37] Fortunately, therapy for these entities is usually effective, and relatively few patients experience treatment failure. Nevertheless, for patients with recurrent disease, investigators have employed dose-intensive therapy and stem cell rescue. For example, 10 of 25 patients with recurrent Wilms tumor, 16 with more than two recurrences, remained alive

and disease free for a median of 27 months after this approach.[62] It should be noted that the tumors of patients benefitting from treatment responded to conventional therapy prior to intensification and transplantation. Also, only one of eight patients with residual gross disease at the time of transplantation remained alive and disease free. This observation is consistent with similar findings for patients with other tumors. Elsewhere, data regarding the efficacy of intensification and transplantation in treating children with retinoblastoma, germ cell tumors, and other solid tumors are largely anecdotal.

CONCLUSION

Many issues need to be addressed in order to optimize dose escalation/stem cell transplantation. For example, what role does radiotherapy, either local or total body, play? Prior to transplantation, what is the optimal treatment, at what dose, and for what duration? Likewise, which patients are the most appropriate candidates for this approach? Will screening blood and/or bone marrow by RT-PCR or FISH for disease-specific genetic abnormalities better define patients who will benefit from transplantation? Identification of new and effective chemotherapeutic agents that can be administered in a dose-intensive schedule is critical. The advantage of purging and/or selecting for hematopoietic precursors is largely untried. Much of the work necessary to clarify this matter remains to be done.

Early toxicity is still a problem, including an unacceptable rate of death related to the transplantation regimen. With advances in supportive care and the growing experience of transplant centers, the reported death rate due to the procedure is still higher than mortality related to conventional therapy.

What seems conclusive at this moment is that the role for hematopoietic stem cell transplantation as part of an intensification/consolidation therapy for pediatric solid tumors has yet to be established. Clearly lacking is definite proof that the outcome for a definable population of patients with any pediatric tumor can be improved by this approach. Although there are encouraging reports of its efficacy in treating many childhood tumors, advances in front-line conventional therapy diminish the portion of patients for whom high-dose chemotherapy/radiotherapy and stem cell transplantation are needed. Nevertheless, as prognostic criteria are refined, it may become evident that, at least for certain patients, standard chemotherapy will always prove inadequate. For these patients, it remains to be demonstrated that therapy intensification followed by stem cell rescue will be beneficial. Regardless, new chemotherapeutic and immunologic agents will be needed to derive full benefit from this approach.

REFERENCES

1. Abrahamsen TG, Lange BJ, Packer RJ, et al: A phase I and II trial of dose-intensified cyclophosphamide and GM-CSF in pediatric malignant brain tumors. J Pediatr Hematol Oncol 17:134–139, 1995.
2. Allen JC, Bosl G, Walker R: Chemotherapy trials in recurrent primary intracranial germ cell tumors. J Neurooncol 3:147–152, 1985.
3. Atra A, Whelan JS, Calvagna V, et al: High-dose busulphan/melphalan with autologous stem cell rescue in Ewing's sarcoma. Bone Marrow Transplant 20:843–846, 1997.
4. August CS, Sarota FT, Koch PA, et al: Treatment of advanced neuroblastoma with supra-lethal chemotherapy, radiation and allogeneic or autologous marrow reconstitution. J Clin Oncol 2:609–616, 1984.
5. Bagnulo S, Perez DJ, Barrett A, et al: High dose melphalan and autologous bone marrow transplantation for solid tumours in childhood. J Paediatr Haematol Oncol 1:129, 1985.
6. Beaujean F, Hartmann O, Benhamou E, et al: Hematopoietic reconstitution after repeated autologous transplantation with mafosfamide-purged marrow. Bone Marrow Transplant 4:537–541, 1989.
7. Berthold F, Burdach S, Kremens B, et al: The role of chemotherapy in the treatment of children with neuroblastoma stage IV: the GPO (German Pediatric Oncology Society) experience. Klin Paediatr 202:262–269, 1990.
8. Bertolone SJ, Baum ES, Krivit W, Hammond GD: A phase II study of cisplatin therapy in recurrent childhood brain tumors: a report from the Children's Cancer Study Group. J Neurooncol 7:5–11, 1989.
9. Biger DD, Brown MT, Friedman AH, et al: Iodine-131-labeled anti-tenascin monoclonal antibody 81c6 treatment of patients with recurrent malignant gliomas: phase I trial results. J Clin Oncol 16:2202–2212, 1998.
10. Blaise D, Olive D, Stoppa AM, et al: Hematologic immunologic effects of the systemic administration of recombinant interleukin-2 after autologous bone marrow transplantation. Blood 76:1092–1097, 1990.
11. Blay JY, Bouhour D, Bruant-Mentigny M, et al: High-dose chemotherapy (VIC) and bone marrow support in advanced sarcomas. Bone Marrow Transplant 14(Suppl 1):S55, 1994.
12. Brenner M, Rill D, Moen R, et al: Gene-marking to trace origin of relapse after autologous bone-marrow transplantation. Lancet 341:85–86, 1993.
13. Brodeur GM, Pritchard J, Berthold F, et al: Revisions of the international criteria for neuroblastoma: diagnosis, staging, and response to treatment. J Clin Oncol 11:1466–1477, 1993.
14. Broun ER, Nichols CR, Turns M, et al: Early salvage therapy for germ cell cancer using high dose chemotherapy with autologous bone marrow support. Cancer 73:1716–1720, 1994.
15. Brunwald MW, Besinger WI, Soll E, et al: High-dose fractionated total-body irradiation, etoposide and cyclophosphamide for treatment of malignant lymphoma: comparison of autologous bone marrow and peripheral blood stem cells. Bone Marrow Transplant 18:131–141, 1996.
16. Burdach S, Peters C, Paulussen M, et al: Improved relapse free survival in patients with poor prognosis Ewing's sarcoma after consolidation with hyperfractionated total body irradiation and fractionated high dose melphalan followed by high dose etoposide and hematopoietic rescue. Bone Marrow Transplant 7(Suppl 2):95, 1991.
17. Burdach S, Jurgens H, Peters C, et al: Myeloablative radiochemotherapy and hematopoietic stem-cell rescue in poor-prognosis Ewing's sarcoma. J Clin Oncol 11:1482–1488, 1993.
18. Burdach S, Jurgens H, Pape H, et al: Myeloablative radiochemotherapy and stem cell rescue in poor prognosis Ewing Sarcoma—a 1994 update of the German-Austrian cooperative study. Bone Marrow Transplant 14(Suppl 1):S53, 1994.
19. Cangir A, Vietti TJ, Gehan EA, et al: Ewing's sarcoma metastatic at diagnosis. Cancer 66:887–893, 1990.
20. Carli M, Pinkerton P, Oberlin O, et al: Risk group analysis in metastatic soft tissue sarcomas (STS) in children: European Intergroup Study MMT 89 [Abstract 1438]. Proc Am Soc Clin Oncol 14:449, 1995.
21. Castleberry RP, Kun LE, Shuster JJ, et al: Radiotherapy improves the outlook for patients older than 1 year with Pediatric Oncology Group stage C neuroblastoma. J Clin Oncol 9:789–795, 1991.
22. Cheung NK, Yeh SDJ, Kushner BH, et al: Phase I study of radioimmunotherapy of neuroblastoma using iodine 131-labeled 3F8. Prog Clin Biol Res 385:328, 1994.
23. Cheung NK, Cheung IY, Canete A, et al: Antibody response to murine anti-GD2 monoclonal antibodies: correlation with patient survival. Cancer Res 54:2228–2233, 1994.
24. Cheung NK, Heller G: Chemotherapy dose intensity correlates strongly with response, median survival, and median progression-free survival in metastatic neuroblastoma. J Clin Oncol 9:1050–1058, 1991.
25. Cheung NK, Kushner BH, Yeh SJ, Larson SM: 3F8 monoclonal antibody treatment of patients with stage IV neuroblastoma: a phase II study. Prog Clin Biol Res 385:319–328, 1994.
26. Civin CI, Trischmann T, Kadan NS, et al: Highly purified CD34-positive cells reconstitute hematopoiesis. J Clin Oncol 14:2224–2233, 1996.
27. Coggins CA, Elion GB, Houghton PJ, et al: Enhancement of irinotecan (CPT-11) activity against central nervous system tumor xenografts by alkylating agents. Cancer Chemother Pharmacol 41:485–490, 1998.
28. Cornbleet MA, Corringham RET, Prentice HG, et al: Treatment of Ewing's sarcoma with high-dose melphalan and autologous bone marrow transplantation. Cancer Treat Rep 65:241–244, 1981.
29. Crist WM, Garnsey L, Beltangady MS, et al: Prognosis in children with rhabdomyosarcoma: a report of the Intergroup RMS Studies I and II. J Clin Oncol 8:443–452, 1990.
30. Crist W, Gehan EA, Ragab AH, et al: The Third Intergroup Rhabdomyosarcoma Study. J Clin Oncol 13:610–630, 1995.
31. Deacon JM, Wilson PA, Peckham MJ: The radiobiology of human neuroblastoma. Radiother Oncol 3:201–209, 1985.
32. De Zen L, Sommaggio A, d'Amore ESG, et al: Clinical relevance of DNA ploidy and proliferative activity in childhood rhabdomyosarcoma: a retrospective analysis of patients enrolled onto the Italian Cooperative Rhabdomyosarcoma Study 88. J Clin Oncol 15:1198–1205, 1997.
33. Dupuis-Girod S, Hartmann O, Benhamou E, et al: High dose chemotherapy in relapse of medulloblastoma in young children. Bull Cancer 84:264–272, 1997.
34. Dick S: First p53 relative may be a new tumor suppressor. Science 277:1605–1606, 1997.
35. Dini G, Lanino E, Garaventa A, et al: Myeloablative therapy and unpurged autologous bone marrow transplantation for poor-prognosis neuroblastoma: report of 34 cases. J Clin Oncol 9:962–969, 1991.
36. Dini G, Philip T, Hartmann O, et al: Bone marrow transplantation for neuroblastoma: a review of 509 cases. Bone Marrow Transplant 4(Suppl 4):42–46, 1989.
37. Dumontet C, Biron P, Bouffet E, et al: High dose chemotherapy with ABMT in soft tissue sarcomas: a report of 22 cases. Bone Marrow Transplant 10:405–408, 1992.
38. Dunkel I, Garvin J, Goldman S, et al: High-dose chemotherapy (HDCx) with autologous bone marrow rescue (ABMR) does not cure children with brainstem tumors [Abstract 83]. Pediatr Neurosurg 21:219a, 1994.
39. Dunkel IJ, Garvin JH Jr, Goldman S, et al: High dose chemotherapy with autologous bone marrow rescue for children with diffuse pontine brain stem tumors: Children's Cancer Group. J Neurooncol 37:67–73, 1998.
40. Dunkel IJ, Boyett JM, Yates A, et al: High-dose carboplatin, thiotepa, and etoposide with autologous stem-cell rescue for patients with recurrent medulloblastoma: Children's Cancer Group. J Clin Oncol 16:222–228, 1998.

41. Edwards MS, Levin VA, Seager ML, et al: Phase II evaluation of thiotepa for treatment of central nervous system tumors. Cancer Treat Rep 63:1419–1421, 1979.

42. Evans AE, August CS, Bunin N, et al: Bone marrow transplantation for high risk neuroblastoma at the Children's Hospital of Philadelphia: an update. Med Pediatr Oncol 23:232–327, 1994.

43. Evans R, Nesbit M, Askin F, et al: Local recurrence, rate and sites of metastases, and time to relapse as a function of treatment regimen, size of primary and surgical history in 62 patients presenting with non-metastatic Ewing's sarcoma of the pelvic bones. Int J Radiat Oncol Biol Phys 11:129–136, 1985.

44. Evans RG, Burgert EO, Gilchrist GS, et al: Sequential half-body irradiation (SHBI) and combination chemotherapy as salvage treatment for failed Ewing's sarcoma—a pilot study. Int J Radiat Oncol Biol Phys 10:2363–2368, 1984.

45. Faucher C, LeCorroller AG, Blaise D, et al: Comparison of G-CSF primed peripheral blood progenitor cells and bone marrow autotransplantation: clinical assessment and cost effectiveness. Bone Marrow Transplant 14:895–901, 1994.

46. Faulkner LB, Lindsley KL, Kher U, et al: High-dose chemotherapy with autologous marrow rescue for malignant brain tumors: analysis of the impact of prior chemotherapy and cranio-spinal irradiation on hematopoietic recovery. Bone Marrow Transplant 17:389–394, 1996.

47. Favrot M, Floret D, Michon J, et al: A phase-II study of adoptive immunotherapy with continuous infusion of interleukin-2 in children with advanced neuroblastoma: a report on 11 cases. Cancer Treat Rev 16(Suppl A):129–142, 1989.

48. Finlay JL, August C, Packer R, et al: High-dose multi-agent chemotherapy followed by bone marrow "rescue" for malignant astrocytomas of childhood and adolescence. J Neurooncol 9:239–248, 1990.

49. Finlay JL, Garvin J, Allen JC, et al: High-dose chemotherapy (HDCx) with autologous marrow rescue (ABMR) in patients with recurrent medulloblastoma (MB)/primitive neuroectodermal tumors (PNET) [Abstract 493]. Proc Am Soc Clin Oncol 13:176, 1994.

50. Finlay JL, Boyett JM, Yates AJ, et al: Randomized phase III trial in childhood high-grade astrocytoma comparing vincristine, lomustine and prednisone with the eight-drugs-in-1-day regimen. J Clin Oncol 13:112–123, 1995.

51. Finlay JL, Goldman S, Wong MC, et al: Pilot study of high-dose thiotepa and etoposide with autologous bone marrow rescue in children and young adults with recurrent CNS tumors. J Clin Oncol 14:2495–2503, 1996.

52. Finlay JL: The role of high-dose chemotherapy and stem cell rescue in the treatment of malignant brain tumors. Bone Marrow Transplant 18:S1–S5, 1996.

53. Finlay JL, Knipple J, Turski P, et al: Pharmaco-kinetic studies of thiotepa in dogs following delivery by various routes [Abstract 74]. J Neurooncol 4:110, 1986.

54. Finlay JL: High-dose chemotherapy with bone marrow rescue in children and young adults with malignant brain tumors [Abstract 1078]. Proc Am Assoc Cancer Res 32:181, 1991.

55. Foreman NK, Rill DR, Coustan-Smith E, et al: Mechanism of selective killing of neuroblastoma cells by natural killer cells and lymphokine adapted killer cells: potential for residual disease eradication. Br J Cancer 67:933–938, 1993.

56. Freilich RJ, Kraus DH, Budnick AS, et al: Hearing loss in children with brain tumors treated with cisplatin and carboplatin-based high-dose chemotherapy with autologous bone marrow rescue. Med Pediatr Oncol 26:95–100, 1996.

57. Friedman HS, Schold SC, Mahaley MS, et al: Phase II treatment of medulloblastoma and pineoblastoma with melphalan: clinical therapy based on experimental models of human medulloblastoma. J Clin Oncol 7:904–911, 1989.

58. Friedman HS, Colvin OM, Skapek SX, et al: Experimental chemotherapy of human medulloblastoma cell lines and transplantable xenografts with bifunctional alkylating agents. Cancer Res 48:4189–4195, 1988.

59. Friedman HS, Mahaley MS, Schold SC, et al: Efficacy of vincristine and cyclophosphamide in the therapy of recurrent medulloblastoma. Neurosurgery 18:335–340, 1986.

60. Friedman HS, Colvin OM, Ludeman SM, et al: Experimental chemotherapy of human medulloblastoma with classical alkylators. Cancer Res 46:2827–2833, 1986.

61. Frost JD, Hank JA, Reaman GH, et al: A phase I/IB trial of murine monoclonal anti-GD2 antibody 14.G2a plus interleukin-2 in children with refractory neuroblastoma: a report of the Children's Cancer Group. Cancer 80:317–333, 1997.

62. Garaventa A, Hartmann O, Bernard J-L, et al: Autologous bone marrow transplantation for pediatric Wilms' tumor: the experience of the European Bone Marrow Transplant Solid Tumor Registry. Med Pediatr Oncol 22:11–14, 1994.

63. Garaventa A, Rondelli R, Lanino E, et al: Myeloblastive therapy and bone marrow rescue in advanced neuroblastoma: report from the Italian Bone Marrow Transplant Registry. Bone Marrow Transplant 18:125–130, 1996.

64. Garvin J, Finlay J, Walker R, et al: High-dose chemotherapy and autologous bone marrow rescue for high-risk central nervous system (CNS) tumors in children under six years of age [Abstract 421]. Proc Am Soc Clin Oncol 11:150, 1992.

65. Gaynon PS, Ettinger LJ, Baum ES, et al: Carboplatin in childhood brain tumors: a Children's Cancer Study Group phase II trial. Cancer 66:2465–2469, 1990.

66. Gaze MN, Wheldon TE, O'Donoghue JA, et al: Multimodality megatherapy with ^{131}I meta-iodobenzylguanine, high dose melphalan, and total body irradiation with bone marrow rescue feasibility–study of a new strategy for advanced neuroblastoma. Eur J Cancer 31a:252–256, 1995.

67. Gazitt Y, He YJ, Rios A, et al: To purge or not to purge: the neuroblastoma experience. Prog Clin Biol Res 377:643–650, 1992.

68. Giannone L, Wolff S: Phase II treatment of central nervous system gliomas with high-dose etoposide and autologous bone marrow transplantation. Cancer Treat Rep 71:759–761, 1987.

69. Glorieux P, Bouffet E, Philip I, et al: Metastatic interstitial pneumonitis after autologous bone marrow transplantation: a consequence of reinjection of malignant cells? Cancer 58:2136–2139, 1986.

70. Goldberg SS, DeSantes K, Huberty JP, et al: Engraftment after myeloablative doses of ^{131}I-metaiodobenzylguanidine followed by autologous bone marrow transplantation for treatment of refractory neuroblastoma. Med Pediatr Oncol 30:339–346, 1998.

71. Goldwein JW, Glauser TA, Packer RJ, et al: Recurrent intracranial ependymomas in children: survival, patterns of failure, and prognostic factors. Cancer 66:557–563, 1990.

72. Graeve JL, deAlarcon PA, Sato Y, et al: Miliary pulmonary neuroblastoma: a risk of autologous bone marrow transplantation? Cancer 62:2125–2127, 1988.

73. Graham ML, Herndon JE II, Casey JR, et al: High dose chemotherapy with autologous stem-cell rescue in patients with recurrent and high risk pediatric brain tumors. J Clin Oncol 15:1814–1823, 1997.

74. Graham ML, Chaffee S, Kurtzberg J, et al: A phase I–II study of high-dose melphalan and cyclophosphamide with autologous bone marrow and/or stem cell rescue for patients with high-risk central nervous system tumors [Abstract 523]. Proc Am Soc Clin Oncol 12:182, 1993.

75. Graham-Pole J, Lazarus HM, Herzig RH, et al: High-dose melphalan therapy for the treatment of children with refractory neuroblastoma and Ewing's sarcoma. Am J Pediatr Hematol Oncol 6:1726, 1984.

76. Graham-Pole J, Casper J, Elfenbein G, et al: High-dose chemoradiotherapy supported by marrow infusions for advanced neuroblastoma: a Pediatric Oncology Group study. J Clin Oncol 9:152–158, 1991.

77. Graham-Pole J: The role of marrow autografting in neuroblastoma [Editorial]. Bone Marrow Transplant 4:3, 1989.

78. Grier H, Krailo M, Link M, et al: Improved outcome in non-metastasis Ewing's sarcoma (EWS) and PNET of bone with the addition of ifosfamide (I) and etoposide (E) to vincristine (V), Adriamycin (Ad), cyclophosphamide (C), and actinomycin (A): a Children's Cancer Group (CCG) and Pediatric Oncology Group (POG) report [Abstract 1443]. Proc Am Soc Clin Oncol 13:421, 1994.

79. Halperin EC, Cox EB: Radiation therapy in the management of neuroblastoma: the Duke University Medical Center experience 1967–1984. Int J Radiat Oncol Biol Phys 12:1829–1837, 1986.

80. Handgretinger R, Anderson K, Lank P, et al: A phase I study of human/mouse chimeric anti-ganglioside GD2 antibody ch14.18 in patients with neuroblastoma. Eur J Cancer 31A:261–267, 1995.

81. Handgretinger R, Griel J, Schurmann U, et al: Positive selection and transplantation of peripheral CD34+ progenitor cells: feasibility and purging efficacy in pediatric patients with neuroblastoma. J Hematol 6:235–242, 1997.

82. Hank JA, Surfus J, Gan J, et al: Treatment of neuroblastoma patients

with antiganglioside GD2 antibody plus interleukin-2 induces antibody dependent cellular cytotoxicity against neuroblastoma detected in vitro. J Immunother 15:29–37, 1994.

83. Hank JA, Robinson RR, Surfus J, et al: Augmentation of antibody dependent cell mediated cytotoxicity following in vivo therapy with recombinant interleukin-2. Cancer Res 50:5234–5239, 1990.

84. Hare CB, Elion GB, Houghton PJ, et al: Therapeutic efficacy of the topoisomerase I inhibitor 7-ethyl-10-(4-[1-piperidino]-carbonyloxy-camptothecin against pediatric and adult central nervous system tumor xenografts. Cancer Chemother Pharmacol 39:187–191, 1997.

85. Hartmann O, Oberlin O, Beaujean F, et al: Place de la chimiothérapie à hautes doses suivie d'autogreffe médullaire dans le traitement des sarcômes d'Ewing metastatiques de l'enfant. Bull Cancer 77:181–187, 1990.

86. Hartmann O, Vassal G, Mechinaud F, et al: High-dose busulfan and thiotepa with autologous bone marrow transplantation as a salvage therapy for non-irradiated medulloblastoma patients [Abstract 1465]. J Clin Oncol 12:425, 1993.

87. Hartmann O, Benhamou E, Beaujean F: High-dose busulfan and cyclophosphamide with autologous bone marrow transplantation support in advanced malignancies in children: a phase II study. J Clin Oncol 4:1804–1810, 1986.

88. Hartmann O, Benhamou E, Beaujean F, et al: Repeated high-dose chemotherapy followed by purged autologous bone marrow transplantation as consolidation therapy in metastatic neuroblastoma. J Clin Oncol 5:1205–1211, 1987.

89. Hartmann O, Kalifa C, Benhamou E, et al: Treatment of advanced neuroblastoma with high-dose melphalan and autologous bone marrow transplantation. Cancer Chemother Pharmacol 16:165–169, 1986.

90. Heideman RL, Douglass EC, Krance RA, et al: High-dose chemotherapy and autologous bone marrow rescue followed by interstitial and external-beam radiotherapy in newly diagnosed pediatric malignant gliomas. J Clin Oncol 11:1458–1465, 1993.

91. Heideman RL, Cole DE, Balis F, et al: Phase II and pharmacokinetic evaluation of thiotepa in the cerebrospinal fluid and plasma of pediatric patients: evidence for dose-dependent plasma clearance of thiotepa. Cancer Res 49:736–741, 1989.

92. Heideman RL, Packer RJ, Reaman GH, et al: A phase I evaluation of thiotepa in pediatric central nervous system malignancies. Cancer 72:271–275, 1993.

93. Hoefnagel CA, De Kraker H, Valdez Olmos RA, Voute PA: ^{131}I-MIBG as a first-line treatment in high-risk neuroblastoma patients. Nucl Med Commun 15:712–717, 1994.

94. Horowitz ME, Kinsella TJ, Wexler LH, et al: Total-body irradiation and autologous bone marrow transplant in the treatment of high-risk Ewing's sarcoma and rhabdomyosarcoma. J Clin Oncol 11:1911–1918, 1993.

95. Horowitz ME, Etcubanas E, Christensen ML, et al: Phase II testing of melphalan in children with newly diagnosed rhabdomyosarcoma: a model for anticancer drug development. J Clin Oncol 6:308–314, 1988.

96. Houghton JA, Cook RL, Lutz PJ, et al: Melphalan: a potential new agent in the treatment of childhood rhabdomyosarcoma. Cancer Treat Rep 69:91–96, 1985.

97. Inwards D, Kessinger A: Peripheral blood stem cell transplantation: historical perspective, current status, and prospects for the future. Transfus Med Rev 6:183–190, 1992.

98. Juergens H, Exner U, Gadner H, et al: Multidisciplinary treatment of primary Ewing's sarcoma of bone: a 6-year experience of a European Cooperative Trial. Cancer 61:23–32, 1988.

99. Kadota RP: Perspectives on investigational chemotherapy and biologic therapy for childhood brain tumors. J Pediatr Hematol Oncol 18:13–22, 1996.

100. Kalifa C, Hartmann O, Demeocq F, et al: High-dose busulfan and thiotepa with autologous bone marrow transplantation in childhood malignant brain tumors: a phase II study. Bone Marrow Transplant 9:227–233, 1992.

101. Kalifa C, Hartmann O, Vassal G, et al: High-dose busulfan (BU) and thiotepa (TT) with autologous bone marrow transplantation (ABMT) as a salvage therapy for non irradiated medulloblastoma patients (PTS) [Abstract 1465]. Proc Am Soc Clin Oncol 12:425, 1993.

102. Kamani N, August CS, Bunin N, et al: A study of thiotepa, etoposide and fractionated total body irradiation as a preparative regimen prior to bone marrow transplantation for poor prognosis patients with neuroblastoma. Bone Marrow Transplant 17:911–916, 1996.

103. Kawa-Ha K, Yumura-Yagi K, Inoue M, et al: Results of single and double autografts for high-risk neuroblastoma patients. Bone Marrow Transplant 17:957–962, 1996.

104. Kedar A, Maria BL, Graham-Pole J, et al: High-dose chemotherapy with marrow reinfusion and hyperfractionated irradiation for children with high-risk brain tumors. Med Pediatr Oncol 23:428–436, 1994.

105. Kemshed JT, Heath L, Gibson FM, et al: Magnetic microspheres and monoclonal antibodies for the depletion of neuroblastoma cells from bone marrow: experiences, improvements, and observations. Br J Cancer 54:771–778, 1986.

106. Kinsella TJ, Mitchell JB, McPherson S, et al: In vitro radiation studies on Ewing's sarcoma cell lines and human bone marrow CFU-C: application to the clinical use of total body irradiation (TBI). Int J Radiat Oncol Biol Phys 10:1005–1011, 1984.

107. Kinsella TJ, Glaubiger D, Diesseroth A, et al: Intensive combined modality therapy including low-dose TBI in high-risk Ewing's sarcoma patients. Int J Radiat Oncol Biol Phys 9:1955–1960, 1983.

108. Kletzel M, Abella EM, Sandler ES, et al: Thiotepa and cyclophosphamide with stem cell rescue for consolidation therapy for children with high-risk neuroblastoma: a phase I/II study of the Pediatric Blood and Marrow Transplant Consortium. J Pediatr Hematol Oncol 20:49–54, 1998.

109. Kletzel M, Kearns GL, Wells TG, Thompson HC: Pharmacokinetics of high dose thiotepa in children undergoing autologous bone marrow transplantation. Bone Marrow Transplant 10:171–175, 1992.

110. Klingebiel P, Handgretinger R, Herter M, et al: Peripheral stem cell transplantation in neuroblastoma stage 4 with the use of 131I MIBG. Adv Neurol Res 4:309–317, 1994.

111. Klingebiel T, Berthold F, Treuner J, et al: Metaiodobenzylguanidine (mIBG) in treatment of 47 patients with neuroblastoma: results of the German Neuroblastoma Trial. Med Pediatr Oncol 19:84–88, 1991.

112. Klingebiel TH, Bode U, Hess C, et al: Treatment of relapse in soft-tissue and Ewing's sarcoma patients—a phase II trial (CESS/CWS REZ 91) [Abstract P73]. Med Pediatr Oncol 21:573, 1993.

113. Koscielniak E, Rodary C, Flamant F, et al: Metastatic rhabdomyosarcoma and histologically similar tumors in childhood: a retrospective European multi-center analysis. Med Pediatr Oncol 20:209–214, 1992.

114. Koscielniak E, Jtrgens H, Winkler K, et al: Treatment of soft tissue sarcoma in childhood adolescence: a report of the German Cooperative Soft Tissue Sarcoma Study. Cancer 70:2557–2567, 1992.

115. Koscielniak E, Klingebiel TH, Peters C, et al: Do patients with metastatic and recurrent rhabdomyosarcoma benefit from high-dose therapy with hematopoietic rescue? Report of the German/Austrian Pediatric Bone Marrow Transplant Group. Bone Marrow Transplant 19:227–231, 1997.

116. Kramer ED, Packer RJ, Ginsberg J, et al: Acute neurologic dysfunction associated with high-dose chemotherapy and autologous bone marrow rescue for primary malignant brain tumors. Pediatr Neurosurg 24:230–237, 1997.

117. Kremens B, Klingebiel T, Herrmann F, et al: High-dose consolidation with local radiation and bone marrow rescue in patients with advanced neuroblastoma. Med Pediatr Oncol 23:470–475, 1994.

118. Kushner BH, O'Reilly RJ, Mandell LR, et al: Myeloablative combination chemotherapy without total body irradiation for neuroblastoma. J Clin Oncol 9:274–279, 1991.

119. Kushner BH, Gulati SC, Kwon JH, et al: High-dose melphalan with 6-hydroxydopamine purged autologous bone marrow transplantation for poor risk neuroblastoma. Cancer 68:242–247, 1991.

120. Kushner BH, O'Reilly RJ, LaQuaglia M, Cheung N-KV: Dose-intensive use of cyclophosphamide in ablation of neuroblastoma. Cancer 66:1095–1100, 1990.

121. Kushner BH, Cheung NKV: GM-CSF enhances 3F8 monoclonal antibody-dependent cellular cytotoxicity against human melanoma and neuroblastoma. Blood 73:1936–1941, 1989.

122. Kushner BH, Meyers PA, Gerald WL, et al: Very high dose short-term chemotherapy for poor-risk peripheral primitive neuroectodermal tumors, including Ewing's sarcoma, in children and young adults. J Clin Oncol 13:2796–2804, 1995.

123. Ladenstein R, Lasset C, Hartmann O, et al: Impact of megatherapy on survival after relapse from stage 4 neuroblastoma in patients over 1 year of age at diagnosis: a report from the European Group for Bone Marrow Transplant. J Clin Oncol 11:2330–2341, 1993.

124. Ladenstein R, Lasset C, Pinkerton R, et al: Impact of megatherapy in children with high-risk Ewing's tumors in complete remission: a report from the EBMT Solid Tumour Registry. Bone Marrow Transplant 15:697–705, 1995.

125. Ladenstein R, Gadner H, Hartmann O, et al: The European experience with megadose therapy and autologous bone marrow transplantation in solid tumors with poor prognosis Ewing sarcoma, germ cell tumors and brain tumors. Wien Med Wochenschr 145:55–57, 1995.

126. Ladenstein R, Lasset C, Hartmann O, et al: Comparison of auto versus allografting as consolidation of primary treatments in advanced neuroblastoma over one year of age at diagnosis: report from the European Group for Bone Marrow Transplant. Bone Marrow Transplant 14:37–46, 1994.

127. Ladenstein R, Philip T, Lasset C, et al: Multivariate analysis of risk factors in stage 4 neuroblastoma patients over the age of one year treated with megatherapy and stem cell transplantation: a report from the European Bone Marrow Transplant Solid Tumor Registry. J Clin Oncol 16:953–965, 1998.

128. Leimig T, Foreman N, Rill D, et al: Immunomodulatory effects of human neuroblastoma cells transduced with retroviral vector encoding interleukin-2. Cancer Gene Ther 1:253–258, 1994.

129. Mahoney DH Jr, Strother D, Camitta B, et al: High-dose melphalan and cyclophosphamide with autologous bone marrow rescue for recurrent/progressive malignant brain tumors in children: a pilot Pediatric Oncology Group study. J Clin Oncol 14:382–388, 1996.

130. Main EK, Lampson LA, Hart MK, et al: Human neuroblastoma cell lines are susceptible to lysis by natural killer cells but not by cytotoxic T lymphocytes. J Immunol 135:242–246, 1985.

131. Mameghan H, Fisher R, Tobias V, et al: Local failure in childhood rhabdomyosarcoma and undifferentiated sarcoma: prognostic factors and implications for curative therapy. Med Pediatr Oncol 21:88–95, 1993.

132. Marina NM, Rodman J, Shema S, et al: Phase I study of escalating targeted doses of carboplatin combined with ifosfamide and etoposide in children with relapsed solid tumors. J Clin Oncol 11:554–560, 1993.

133. Marti F, Pardo N, Peiro M, et al: Progression of natural immunity during one-year treatment of residual disease in neuroblastoma patients with high doses of interleukin-2 after autologous bone marrow transplantation. Exp Hematol 23:1445–1452, 1995.

134. Mason WP, Goldman S, Grovas A, Finlay JL: Intensive chemotherapy and autologous bone marrow reconstitution (ABMR) for children with new or recurrent ependymoma [Abstract 276]. J Clin Oncol 14:145, 1995.

135. Mason WP, Goldman S, Yates AJ, et al: Survival following intensive chemotherapy with bone marrow reconstitution for children with recurrent intracranial ependymoma—a report of the Children's Cancer Group. J Neurooncol 37:135–145, 1998.

136. Mason WP, Grovas A, Halpern S, et al: Intensive chemotherapy and bone marrow rescue for young children with newly diagnosed malignant brain tumors. J Clin Oncol 16:210–221, 1998.

137. Matthay KK, DeSantes K, Hasegawa B, et al: Phase I dose escalation of ^{131}I-metaiodobenzylguanidine with autologous bone marrow support in refractory neuroblastoma. J Clin Oncol 16:229–236, 1998.

138. Matthay KK, O'Leary MC, Ramsay NK, et al: Role of myeloablative therapy in improved outcome for high-risk neuroblastoma: review of recent Children's Cancer Group results. Eur J Cancer 31A:572–575, 1995.

139. Matthay KK, Atkinson JB, Stram DO, et al: Patterns of relapse after autologous purged bone marrow transplantation for neuroblastoma: a Children's Cancer Group Pilot Study. J Clin Oncol 11:2226–2233, 1993.

140. Matthay KK, Seeger RC, Reynolds CP, et al: Allogeneic versus autologous purged bone marrow transplantation for neuroblastoma: a report from the Children's Cancer Group. J Clin Oncol 12:2382–2389, 1994.

141. Mauer HM, Gehan EA, Beltangady M, et al: The Intergroup Rhabdomyosarcoma Study—II. Cancer 71:1904–1922, 1993.

142. Maurer HM, Beltangady M, Gehan EA, et al: The Intergroup Rhabdomyosarcoma Study—I: a final report. Cancer 61:209–220, 1988.

143. McCowage GB, Vowels MR, Shaw PJ, et al: Autologous bone marrow transplantation for advanced neuroblastoma using teniposide, doxorubicin, melphalan, cisplatin, and total-body irradiation. J Clin Oncol 13(11):2789–2795, 1995.

144. Meyer WH, Kun L, Marina N, et al: Ifosfamide plus etoposide in newly diagnosed Ewing's sarcoma of bone. J Clin Oncol 10:1737–1742, 1992.

145. Michon J, Hartmann O, Demeocq F, et al: Consolidation with busulfan and melphalan followed by blood progenitor cell (BPC) graft in children and young adults with high risk Ewing's sarcoma: a report of the French Society of Pediatric Oncology (SFOP). Proc Am Soc Clin Oncol 13:A1415, 1994.

146. Michon J, Negrier S, Coze C, et al: Administration of high-dose recombinant interleukin 2 after autologous bone marrow transplantation in patients with neuroblastoma: toxicity, efficacy, and survival. Prog Clin Biol Res 385:293–300, 1994.

147. Miser Js, Sanders JE: High-dose chemotherapy and systemic adjuvant irradiation in Ewing's Sarcoma. Bone Marrow Transplant 14(1):S54, 1994.

148. Miser JS, Kinsella TJ, Triche TJ, et al: Preliminary results of treatment of Ewing's sarcoma of bone in children and young adults: six months of intensive combined modality therapy without maintenance. J Clin Oncol 6:484–490, 1988.

149. Moss TJ, Sanders DG, Lasky LC, Bostrom B: Contamination of peripheral blood stem cell harvests by circulation neuroblastoma cells. Blood 76:1879–1883, 1990.

150. Moss TJ, Reynolds CP, Sather HN, et al: Prognostic value of immunocytologic detection of bone marrow metastases in neuroblastoma. N Engl J Med 324:219–226, 1991.

151. Mugishima H, Harada K, Suzuki T, et al: Comprehensive treatment of advanced neuroblastoma involving autologous bone marrow transplant. Acta Paediatr Jpn 37:493–499, 1995.

152. Negrier S, Michon J, Floret E, et al: Interleukin-2 and lymphokine-activated-killer cells in 15 children with advanced metastatic neuroblastoma. J Clin Oncol 9:1363–1370, 1991.

153. Nesbit M: Advances and management of solid tumors in children. Cancer 65:696–702, 1990.

154. Niethammer D, Handgretinger R: Clinical strategies for the treatment of neuroblastoma. Eur J Cancer 31A(4):568–571, 1995.

155. Ohnuma N, Takahashi H, Kaneko M, et al: Treatment combined with bone marrow transplantation for advanced neuroblastoma: an analysis of patients who were pretreated intensively with the protocol of the Study Group of Japan. Med Pediatr Oncol 24:181–187, 1995.

156. O'Reilly SM, Newlands ES, Glaser MG, et al: Temozolomide: a new oral cytotoxic agent with promising activity against gliomas [Abstract 499]. J Clin Oncol 12:176, 1993.

157. Ozkaynak MF, Matthay K, Cairo M, et al: Double non-total body irradiation regimen with autologous hematopoietic stem cell transplantation in pediatric solid tumors. J Clin Oncol 16:937–944, 1998.

158. Pappo AS, Crist WM, Kuttesch WM: Tumor-cell DNA content predicts outcome in children and adolescents with clinical group III embryonal rhabdomyosarcoma. J Clin Oncol 11:1901–1905, 1993.

159. Pappo AS, Etcubanas E, Santana VM, et al: A phase II trial of ifosfamide in previously untreated children and adolescents with unresectable rhabdomyosarcoma. Cancer 71:2119–2125, 1993.

160. Pappo AS, Shapiro DN, Crist WMC, Maurer HM: Biology and therapy of pediatric rhabdomyosarcoma. J Clin Oncol 13:2123–2139, 1995.

161. Paulussen M, Ansmann M, Burdach S, et al: Bone marrow transplantation in disseminated Ewing's sarcoma: the CESS experience. SIOP XXV Meeting [Abstract 40]. Med Pediatr Oncol 21:541, 1993.

162. Paulussen M, Ansmann M, Braun-Munzinger G, et al: Bone marrow transplantation in primary and secondary disseminated Ewing's sarcoma—the CESS experience. Bone Marrow Transplant 14(Suppl 1):S57, 1994.

163. Philip T, Bernard JL, Zucker JM, et al: Purged autologous bone marrow transplantation in 25 cases of very poor prognosis neuroblastoma [Letter]. Lancet 1:576–577, 1985.

164. Philip T, Ladenstein R, Zucker JM, et al: Double megatherapy and autologous bone marrow transplantation for advanced neuroblastoma: the LMCE2 study. Br J Cancer 67:119–127, 1993.

165. Philip T, Ladenstien R, Lasset C, et al: 1070 myeloablative megatherapy procedures followed by stem cell rescue for neuroblastoma: 17 years of European experience and conclusions: European Group for Blood and Marrow Transplant Registry Solid Tumor Working Party. Eur J Cancer 33:2130–2135, 1997.

166. Philip T, Zucker JM, Bernard JL, et al: Improved survival at 2 and 5 years in the LMCE1 unselected group of 72 children with stage IV neuroblastoma older than 1 year of age at diagnosis: is cure possible in a small subgroup? J Clin Oncol 9:1037–1044, 1991.

167. Philip T, Bernard JL, Zucker JM, et al: High-dose chemoradiotherapy with bone marrow transplantation as consolidation treatment in neuroblastoma: an unselected group of stage IV patients over 1 year of age. J Clin Oncol 5:266–271, 1987.

168. Phillips GL, Wolff SN, Fay JW, et al: Intensive 1,3-bis(2-chloroethyl)-1-nitrosourea (BCNU) monochemotherapy and autologous marrow transplantation for malignant glioma. J Clin Oncol 4:639–645, 1986.

169. Pinkerton CR: Megatherapy for soft tissue sarcomas: EBMT experience. Bone Marrow Transplant 7:120–122, 1991.

170. Pinkerton CR: ENSG 1—randomized study of high-dose melphalan in neuroblastoma. Bone Marrow Transplant 7:112–113, 1991.

171. Pinkerton CR: Where next with therapy in advanced neuroblastoma? Br J Cancer 61:351–353, 1990.

172. Pinkerton CR, McElwain TJ: High-dose carboplatin in combination regimens using autologous bone marrow rescue in neuroblastoma and soft tissue sarcoma. Med Pediatr Oncol 310:125, 1989.

173. Pinkerton CR, Philip T, Hartmann O, et al: High-dose chemoradiotherapy with autologous bone marrow rescue in pediatric soft tissue sarcomas. In Dicke KA, Spitzer G, Jaanath S, Evinger-Hodges MJ (eds): Autologous Bone Marrow Transplant. Houston, University of Texas MD Anderson Cancer Center, 1989, p 617.

174. Reynolds CP, Schindler P, Jones D, et al: Comparison of 13-cis-retinoic acid to trans-retinoic acid using human neuroblastoma cell lines. In Evans A, Biedler JL, Brodeur G, et al (eds): Advances in Neuroblastoma Research 4. New York, Wiley, 1994, pp 237–244.

175. Rosillo MC, Ortuno F, Moraleda JM, et al: Immune recovery after autologous or rhG-CSF primed PBS transplantation. Eur J Haematol 56:301–307, 1996.

176. Saarinen UM, Wikstrom S, Makipernaa A, et al: In vivo purging of bone marrow in children with poor-risk neuroblastoma for marrow collection and autologous bone marrow transplantation. J Clin Oncol 14:2791–2802, 1996.

177. Sabzevari H, Gilles SD, Mueller BM, et al: A recombinant antibody-IL2 fusion protein suppresses growth of hepatic human neuroblastoma metastasis in SCID mice. Proc Natl Acad Sci U S A 91:9626–9630, 1994.

178. Sanders JE: Endocrine problems in children after bone marrow transplant for hematologic malignancies. Bone Marrow Transplant 8:2–4, 1991.

179. Santana VM, Schell MJ, Williams R, et al: Escalating sequential high-dose carboplatin and etoposide with autologous marrow support in children with relapsed solid tumors. Bone Marrow Transplant 10:457–462, 1992.

180. Seeger RC, Reynolds CP, Stram D, et al: Intensive chemoradiotherapy and ABMT for high-risk neuroblastomas. Bone Marrow Transplant 14(Suppl 1):S63, 1994.

181. Seeger RC, Villablanca JG, Matthay KK, et al: Intensive chemoradiotherapy and autologous bone marrow transplantation for poor prognosis neuroblastoma. Prog Clin Biol Res 366:527–533, 1991.

182. Seeger RC, Reynolds CP: Treatment of high-risk solid tumors of childhood with intensive therapy and autologous bone marrow transplantation. Pediatr Clin North Am 38:393–424, 1991.

183. Shea TC, Storniolo AM, Mason JR, et al: A dose escalation study of carboplatin/cyclophosphamide/etoposide along with autologous bone marrow or peripheral blood stem cell rescue. Semin Oncol 19(Suppl 2):139–144, 1992.

184. Shuster JJ, Cantor AB, McWilliams N, et al: The prognostic significance of autologous bone marrow transplant in advanced neuroblastoma. J Clin Oncol 9:1045–1049, 1991.

185. Sibley GS, Mundt AJ, Goldman S, et al: Patterns of failure following total body irradiation and bone marrow transplantation with or without a radiotherapy boost for advanced neuroblastoma. Int J Radiat Oncol Biol Phys 32:1127–1135, 1995.

186. Siegert W, Beyer J, Strohscheer I, et al: High-dose treatment with carboplatin, etoposide, and ifosfamide followed by autologous stem-cell transplantation in relapsed or refractory germ cell cancer: a phase I/II study. J Clin Oncol 12:1223–1231, 1994.

187. Spigelman MK, Zappula RA, Johnson J, et al: Etoposide-induced blood-brain barrier disruption: effect of drug compared with that of solvents. J Neurosurg 61:674–678, 1984.

188. Sposto R, Ertel IJ, Jenkin RD, et al: The effectiveness of chemotherapy for treatment of high grade astrocytoma in children: results of a randomized trial: a report from the Children's Cancer Study Group. J Neurooncol 7:165–177, 1989.

189. Stea B, Kinsella TJ, Tricha TJ, et al: Treatment of pelvic sarcomas in adolescents and young adults with intensive combined modality therapy. Int J Radiat Oncol Biol Phys 13:1797–1805, 1987.

190. Stewart DJ, Richard MT, Hugenholtz H, et al: Penetration of VP-16 (etoposide) into human intracerebral and extracerebral tumors. J Neuro-Oncol 2:133–139, 1984.

191. Stewart DA, Gyonyor E, Paterson AHG, et al: High-dose melphalan ± total body irradiation and autologous hematopoietic stem cell rescue for adult patients with Ewing's sarcoma or peripheral neuroectodermal tumor. Bone Marrow Transplant 18:315–318, 1996.

192. Stram DO, Matthay KK, O'Leary M, et al: Consolidation chemoradiotherapy and autologous bone marrow transplantation versus combined chemotherapy for metastatic neuroblastoma: a report of two concurrent Children's Cancer Group studies. J Clin Oncol 14:2417–2426, 1996.

193. Sullivan KM, Mori M, Sanders J, et al: Late complications of allogeneic and autologous marrow transplantation. Bone Marrow Transplant 10:127–134, 1992.

194. Taha IAK, Ahmad RA, Rogers DW, et al: Pharmacokinetics of melphalan in children following high dose intravenous injections. Cancer Chemother Pharmacol 10:212–216, 1983.

195. Tchirkov A, Kanold J, Giollant M, et al: Molecular monitoring of tumor cell contamination in leukapheresis products from stage IV neuroblastoma patients before and after positive CD34 selection. Med Pediatr Oncol 30:288–232, 1998.

196. Tirelli U, D'Incalci M, Canetta R, et al: Etoposide (VP-16-213) in malignant brain tumors: a phase II study. J Clin Oncol 2:432–437, 1984.

197. Toretsky JA, Neckers L, Wesler LH: Detection of (11;22)(q24;q12) translocation-bearing cells in peripheral blood progenitor cells of patients with Ewing's sarcoma family of tumors. J Natl Cancer Inst 87:385–386, 1995.

198. Torres CF, Rebsamen S, Silber JH, et al: Surveillance scanning of children with medulloblastoma. N Engl J Med 330:892–895, 1994.

199. Valteau-Couanet D, Rubie H, Meresse V, et al: Phase I–II study of interleukin-2 after high-dose chemotherapy and autologous bone marrow transplantation in poorly responding neuroblastoma. Bone Marrow Transplant 16:515–520, 1995.

200. Villablanca JG, Matthay KK, Ramsay NK, et al: Carboplatin, etoposide, melphalan, and local irradiation with autologous bone marrow transplantation for high-risk neuroblastoma [Abstract 1402]. Proc Am Soc Clin Oncol 14:440, 1995.

201. Villablanca JG, Khan AA, Avramis VI, et al: Phase I trial of 13-cis-retinoic acid in children with neuroblastoma following bone marrow transplantation. J Clin Oncol 13:894–901, 1995.

202. West DC, Grier HE, Swallow MM, et al: Detection of circulating tumor cells in patients with Ewing's sarcoma and peripheral primitive neuroectodermal tumor. J Clin Oncol 15:583–588, 1997.

203. Wheldon TE, O'Donoghue JA, Gregor A: Radiobiological rationale for hyperfractionation in the radiotherapy of neuroblastoma [Letter]. Int J Radiat Oncol Biol Phys 13:1430, 1987.

204. Wingard JR, Plotnick LP, Freemer CS, et al: Growth in children after bone marrow transplantation: busulfan plus cyclophosphamide versus cyclophosphamide plus total body irradiation. Blood 79:1068–1073, 1992.

205. Wolff SN, Herzit RH, Fay JW, et al: High-dose N,N′,N″-triethylenethiophosphoramide (thiotepa) with autologous bone marrow transplantation: phase I studies. Semin Oncol 17(Suppl 3):2–6, 1990.

CHAPTER THIRTEEN

GERM CELL TUMORS

Craig R. Nichols, M.D.

Germ cell cancer is an uncommon disease, accounting for approximately 1% of all malignancies in males.[1] It is, however, an important disease in the field of oncology because it is a highly curable malignancy, occurring primarily in adolescent and young adult males. The impact of cure in this population is enormous, and a 1990 cost-benefit analysis suggests that the annual economic value of cisplatin-based chemotherapy for this disease can be estimated at $150 million.[2] In this rare and complicated, curable illness, it is important that physicians versed in the intricacies of this disease provide oversight in the decision and treatment process.

Effective therapies that can now cure the majority of patients are the product of several decades of rational drug development, well-planned clinical trials, and a small measure of serendipity. Accordingly, germ cell cancer has truly become a "model" for developing treatments for other malignancies.[3] In order to understand the role of high-dose treatment in this unique malignant disease, it is important to review the role of serum tumor markers and utility of surgical extirpation of residual cancer in the management of patients in whom germ cell tumors are diagnosed. In addition, an overview of important clinical trials using conventional-dose therapy forms a basis for understanding the value of high-dose treatment in this very chemotherapy-sensitive tumor.

TUMOR MARKERS

Management of testicular cancer has come to depend on the accurate determination of levels of serum tumor markers and the interpretation of these values in the clinical context. The most sensitive and specific markers are alpha-fetoprotein (AFP) and the beta subunit of human chorionic gonadotropin (HCG). AFP is a glycoprotein normally produced by the fetal yolk sac and is derived from yolk sac or embryonal carcinoma elements of germ cell cancers. Levels of AFP are not detectable in normal adults. The half-life of this protein in the serum is about 5 days. HCG is a smaller glycoprotein that is normally produced by trophoblastic tissues. In germ cell cancers, syncytiotrophoblastic components elaborate HCG. The protein is composed of an alpha and a beta subunit, each of which is antigenically distinct. The serum half-life of the entire protein is 18–24 hours.

Clinical decisions in patients with germ cell cancer frequently depend on precise measurement of the serum tumor markers HCG, AFP, and lactate dehydrogenase. Overall, HCG is elevated in 75% of patients with disseminated testicular and primary retroperitoneal nonseminomatous germ cell tumors; AFP is elevated in 40% of patients.

Elevated lactate dehydrogenase is a less-specific marker and is probably a correlate of disease bulk. Pure seminoma is most frequently associated with normal AFP and HCG; however, approximately 10% of all cases and up to 50% of patients with advanced disease may have low-level elevation of HCG (usually <100 mIU/mL). Any elevation of AFP in patients with seminoma must be viewed as evidence of nonseminomatous disease, and management should proceed as such.

The rate of disappearance of elevated tumor markers is very useful in determining response to treatment. HCG is most useful in this regard, and the most clinically helpful guideline is that a tenfold decrease in the HCG level over a 3-week period is consistent with disease eradication. Less-steep declines of HCG levels correlate with the emergence of drug-resistant disease in the case of chemotherapy or residual disease in the case of surgery. Likewise, reappearance of marker elevation often predates the radiographic appearance of recurrent disease and, as such, is an invaluable method of detecting early relapse.

Although the accurate determination of these markers is a luxury in the management of patients with germ cell cancer, cautious interpretation is needed to avoid errors in clinical management. First, HCG determination can be nonspecific, and there is some cross-reactivity in the radio-immunoassay with luteinizing hormone. Also, HCG can be falsely elevated in patients who use marijuana. Low-level HCG elevation is consequently difficult to interpret. A conservative approach to this dilemma is to repeat the HCG determination to ensure that the elevation is not a laboratory error. If the level is still high, the patient should be queried regarding drug use. Testosterone should be given to ensure that a hypogonadal state with resultant high levels of luteinizing hormone is not interfering with the determination of HCG. If the level remains increased, restaging procedures and investigation of sanctuary sites are in order.

False-positive elevation of AFP is rare. Differential considerations would include laboratory error, other tumor types such as hepatoma, or liver inflammation from cirrhosis or hepatitis.

MANAGEMENT OF DISSEMINATED GERM CELL CANCER

PROGNOSTIC FACTORS IN DISSEMINATED DISEASE

In recent years, a primary therapeutic strategy has diverged for the treatment of germ cell tumor patients with a low versus high risk of relapse, with corresponding emphasis on less versus more intensive treatment, respectively. As increasingly aggressive (and toxic) regimens are developed for patients with a low likelihood of achieving complete remission (CR) or a high risk of relapse, the elucidation of prognostic factors to correctly identify such patients becomes increasingly important. Different prognostic factors (and the relative importance of each) have been reported by separate groups and have evolved into a number of staging systems for advanced disease.

Such assignment of patients into "good-risk" and "poor-risk" categories has been undertaken by the National Cancer Institute,[4] European Organization for the Research and Treatment of Cancer,[5] Memorial Sloan-Kettering Cancer Center,[6] the Southeastern Cancer Study Group,[7] the Medical Research Council,[8, 9] and the Danish Testicular Carcinoma Study Group.[10] A number of characteristics are uniformly identified in poor-risk patients and include a high volume of metastatic disease, significant elevations of serum tumor markers, extragonadal primary lesions, and visceral organ involvement. New prognostic factors are being identified and include measurements of the kinetics of tumor growth, with a higher proliferative index predictive of poor outcome after therapy.[11]

Most recently, an international consortium collected clinical data on patients receiving platinum-based therapy for metastatic germ cell tumor to develop a new prognostic model for disseminated disease. Data on 5202 patients with nonseminomatous germ cell tumor and 660 patients with seminoma were analyzed and showed that independent predictors of outcome in univariate analysis included mediastinal primary site; the degree of AFP, HCG, and lactate dehydrogenase elevation; and the presence of nonpulmonary visceral metastasis. Using these factors, the consortium derived prognostic categories.[12] Good-risk nonseminomatous patients have a testis or retroperitoneal primary, favorable markers, and no nonpulmonary visceral metastases (anticipated progression-free survival [PFS] rate, 90%). Poor prognosis includes those patients with mediastinal primary nonseminoma, nonpulmonary visceral metastases, or an unfavorable elevation of tumor markers (anticipated PFS rate, 40%). An intermediate group had an anticipated PFS rate of 75%. For seminoma, only good- and intermediate-risk groups are identified, with good and intermediate risk being discriminated by the absence or presence of nonpulmonary visceral metastases.[12]

TREATMENT OF "GOOD-RISK" DISSEMINATED DISEASE

Although there is debate regarding the relative importance of a number of potential prognostic factors, in general those patients with either serum marker elevation only or small volume infradiaphragmatic or supradiaphragmatic involvement (or both) without visceral involvement have highly curable disease and are categorized as good risk. This group of patients accounts for approximately 70% of patients presenting with disseminated disease.

Stratification by selected prognostic factors in a series of randomized clinical trials has confirmed their predictive value. In the mid-1980s, several clinical trials were designed specifically for this group of patients. Because virtually all of these patients achieved CR with standard chemotherapy, these trials addressed the possibility of reducing the amount of chemotherapy administered (thus decreasing acute and chronic toxicity) while maintaining an excellent cure rate. Several approaches to this reduction in therapy have been employed, including a shortening of the duration of therapy, use of chemotherapeutic agents with less single-agent toxicity, or a reduction in the number of agents used.

A number of trials have addressed the issue of less-intensive therapy for patients with good-risk germ cell tumor.[13–16] Review of these trials suggests that good-risk germ cell cancer can be reliably cured with three courses of cisplatin, etoposide, and bleomycin or four courses of the two-drug combination, cisplatin and etoposide. The current standard of therapy in this patient population has minimal acute and probably even less long-term toxicity. Further reductions in the amount of therapy are therefore unlikely to significantly reduce toxicity but certainly have the potential to reduce the cure rate in this stage of disease.

TREATMENT OF "POOR-RISK" DISSEMINATED DISEASE

The one-third of patients with disseminated testicular cancer who present with poor prognostic features remain a therapeutic challenge. Serial clinical trials have helped to define therapy for this less-favorable clinical setting.[17–20] Most investigators use four courses of bleomycin, etoposide, and cisplatin. Such "standard treatment" results in cure for approximately 60% of patients in this risk category. The current emphasis in the initial treatment of these poor-risk patients is the exploration of dose-intensive regimens and the use of etoposide and other newer agents as initial therapy.

POSTCHEMOTHERAPY SURGERY

Depending on the stage at diagnosis, 20–50% of patients who undergo induction chemotherapy for disseminated germ cell tumor have significant residual radiographic abnormalities. In this subset of patients, postchemotherapy resection of residual disease is often performed to remove residual teratoma or viable cancer. Several points bear emphasis in this setting. First, postchemotherapy surgery should be considered only if levels of the serum markers AFP and HCG have normalized. Patients with persistently elevated serum markers should be considered for salvage chemotherapy rather than surgical "debulking." Second, postchemotherapy resection of residual abnormalities is rarely urgent, and sufficient time should be taken to allow the patient to recover from the effects of induction chemotherapy. Typically, patients undergo surgery 6 weeks after the last round of treatment. Third, repeat imaging of the areas of abnormality should be performed prior to surgery. In many patients, continued involution of residual masses occurs after the completion of therapy, making surgical resection unnecessary.

The histopathologic findings in postchemotherapy surgical specimens help define the need for further treatment.

In earlier reports, about 40% of cases revealed teratoma, 40% showed fibrous necrotic debris, and 20% showed residual viable germ cell cancer. Analysis of recent series suggests that the incidence of persistent cancer is decreasing.[13, 17]

Persistent cancer identified and totally removed at postchemotherapy surgery requires special management. If the surgical margins are free of tumor, all sites of known disease are removed; if the serum tumor markers remain normal, patients should receive two postoperative cycles of cisplatin-based therapy similar to induction therapy. Patients with unresectable disease, positive surgical margins, or elevated tumor markers should be considered for full salvage therapy using new agents and more prolonged courses of therapy. About two-thirds of patients receiving additional postoperative cisplatin-based chemotherapy after total resection of residual viable cancer remain disease free.[21]

SALVAGE CHEMOTHERAPY

To interpret the role of high-dose chemotherapy (HDC), one must understand the curative potential of conventional-dose salvage treatment. Overall, 20–30% of all patients with disseminated disease do not achieve CR with first-line therapy. These patients, as well as those who experience relapse from CR, are candidates for salvage chemotherapy. Because of the decreased efficacy and increased toxicity of second-line chemotherapy, this is an important decision point in the treatment of such patients and requires the expertise of physicians well versed in the intricacies of therapeutic options for this stage of testicular cancer.

Several clinical situations may mimic progressive or recurrent disease but are not indications for salvage chemotherapy. One such situation involves the appearance of nodular lesions on chest radiograph or chest computed tomography at the end of chemotherapy or soon thereafter. These nodules may merely represent bleomycin-induced pulmonary injury and are characteristically located in a subpleural region. This should be considered in patients who otherwise respond serologically or radiographically.

Another clinical situation frequently mistaken for progressive disease is the syndrome of "growing teratoma." For patients with elements of teratoma in their primary lesion, radiographically enlarging metastatic lesions during chemotherapy concurrent with appropriately declining serologic markers (as described earlier) are likely to represent teratomatous elements in these growing lesions. Appropriate management of such patients includes completion of induction chemotherapy with subsequent surgical resection of residual radiographic abnormalities without the administration of salvage chemotherapy.

The current standard salvage chemotherapy that serves as a basis for comparison is the regimen reported at Indiana University of VeIP (vinblastine [Velban], ifosfamide, and cisplatin [Platinol]).[22] Patients received vinblastine, 0.11 mg/kg, on days 1 and 2; ifosfamide, 1.2 g/m^2 daily, for 5 days; and cisplatin, 20 mg/m^2 daily, for 5 days. This combination was used as initial salvage chemotherapy in 124 patients who failed to improve on cisplatin. Patient characteristics reflected a poor-risk population. Advanced disease

by the Indiana classification system was present in 81 patients (65%) at initial presentation and 59 patients (48%) at the time of VeIP administration. Thirty-one patients (25%) had an extragonadal primary site. Toxicity of the regimen in this pretreated population was significant, with 73% experiencing granulocytopenic fever. Transfusions of platelets (28%) and red blood cells (48%) were common. Renal insufficiency (serum creatinine >4 mg/dL) was observed in 7% of patients. Three patients died of treatment-related causes.

Despite the formidable toxicity, the therapeutic results were gratifying. Fifty-six patients (45%) achieved disease-free status with either chemotherapy alone (34 patients, 27%) or resection of teratoma (15 patients, 12%) or viable carcinoma (7 patients, 6%). At a minimum follow-up of 27 months, 29 patients (23%) were continuously disease free and 37 (30%) were disease free. Among patients with extragonadal primaries, only 6 of 31 obtained disease-free status and only 1 remained continuously disease free. Outcome related to response to primary therapy is as follows: Of 77 patients who never obtained disease-free status with primary cisplatin, 17 (22%) became disease free with VeIP and 11 (14%) remained continuously free of disease. These results have been confirmed by other investigators.[23]

HIGH-DOSE CHEMOTHERAPY: BACKGROUND AND RATIONALE

Preliminary studies using HDC in patients with refractory germ cell cancer had mixed results. In early studies using high-dose cyclophosphamide, etoposide, or thiotepa, high rates of response were obtained but these responses were uniformly brief.[24] Subsequent studies in Europe and the United States, using principles and chemotherapy combinations more specific to germ cell cancer, had more favorable results. A review of recent and current studies of HDC in germ cell cancer using supportive autologous bone marrow transplantation (autoBMT), hematopoietic growth factors, and HDC without specific efforts to modulate myelosuppression follows. Also discussed are implications of current clinical trials and future directions.

PHASE II CLINICAL TRIALS OF INTENSIVE CHEMOTHERAPY

A variety of phase II clinical trials have been performed with the goal of intensifying the dose of available agents in patients with poor-risk germ cell cancer. Most of these protocols have used very-high-dose cisplatin with etoposide, bleomycin, and frequently the addition of agents of unknown efficacy in germ cell cancer, such as vincristine and methotrexate.[25–29] These trials have invariably reported superior outcome, and such trials have been held as validation of the concept of increased dose intensity in germ cell cancer.

These trials also illustrate some of the difficulties in drawing conclusions regarding dose intensity. The investigators used a myriad of classification systems to assign poor-risk status. Many trials include patients that by other classification systems would be good risk (particularly patients with bulky abdominal disease only). Inclusion of such patients into these poor-risk trials apparently validates the newer regimen because such patients would have excellent outcomes with standard therapy. When reclassified by other, more-stringent classification systems, response rates diminish and often are comparable to those of standard therapy. These trials are performed over a long period of time, allowing for other factors not related to treatment to influence the comparison with historical controls.[30]

AUTOLOGOUS BONE MARROW TRANSPLANTATION AND HIGH-DOSE CHEMOTHERAPY IN GERM CELL NEOPLASMS

Indiana University Studies

Investigations into the use of high-dose carboplatin and etoposide with autoBMT began at Indiana University in 1986. Initial investigations were in patients who were heavily pretreated and for whom no other curative therapeutic options existed. Subsequent studies have explored modification of the initial regimen in patients with refractory disease and the efficacy of this regimen in patients in first relapse after conventional therapy. Important insights into the need for patient selection, the particular problem of primary nonseminomatous mediastinal germ cell tumors, and the value of intervention early in the course of the disease for these toxic, expensive, yet potentially curative modes of therapy have been gained.

The initial phase I/II dose-escalation study examined the use of two courses of high-dose carboplatin and etoposide followed by autoBMT in patients with germ cell tumors refractory to cisplatin (defined as progression within 4 weeks of the last cisplatin dose) or recurring after a minimum of two prior regimens containing cisplatin.[31] Thirty-three patients were entered in this trial. The initial 13 patients were treated with escalating doses of carboplatin to establish the maximum tolerated dose in combination with etoposide at a fixed dose of 1200 mg/m². The subsequent 20 patients were treated with etoposide, 1200 mg/m², and the phase II dose of carboplatin, 1500 mg/m², given in three divided doses on days -7, -5, -3.

Toxicity in the protocol included the expected severe myelosuppression, moderate enterocolitis, and stomatitis. Grade 3 hepatic toxicity (75-fold increase in liver enzymes), usually associated with massive infections, occurred in 8 of 33 patients (24%). Of interest, significant ototoxicity, neurotoxicity, or nephrotoxicity did not occur despite extensive prior exposure to cisplatin in this patient population. Overall, 7 of 33 patients (21%) died as a consequent of treatment, 2 in the phase II portion of the study. Deaths were primarily due to infection, although one patient died of veno-occlusive disease of the liver.

Of note, this was a very heavily pretreated patient population: Over half of the patients had received three or more prior chemotherapy regimens, and 67% of patients had cisplatin-refractory disease. Eight patients obtained CR and six achieved partial remission (PR) for an overall response rate of 44% (95% confidence intervals, 27–63%). Of the eight patients obtaining CR, three were long-term disease-free survivors and a fourth died at 22 months free of germ

cell cancer from therapy-related acute nonlymphocytic leukemia. Review of responding patients reveals that CR was achieved despite advanced stage or disease refractory to cisplatin. More recently, an overview of the experience at Indiana University with the first 40 patients with multiply relapsed and refractory germ cell cancer treated with double autoBMT demonstrated a 15% long-term disease-free survival rate.[34]

After the phase I/II study, a larger multi-institutional phase II trial was carried out through the Eastern Cooperative Oncology Group using the same dose and schedule of agents as in the phase II portion of the initial study.[33] For patients to qualify, at least two prior cisplatin-based regimens (at least one of which contained ifosfamide) had to have failed or their disease had to be cisplatin-refractory. Forty patients were entered into this multi-institution cooperative group effort between July 1988 and September 1989. Two patients were deemed ineligible because of insufficient prior therapy and incorrect histologic diagnosis; 22 of 38 evaluable patients (58%) proceeded to a second course of HDC.

Toxicity was similar to that seen in the phase I trial, with 5 of 38 patients (13%) dying of treatment-related causes. Infection (one patient), hemorrhage (two patients), and hepatic toxicity (two patients) accounted for the deaths. All treatment-related deaths occurred in the first course of therapy. Other extramyeloid toxicities were comparable to those in the initial study. Nine patients (23%) achieved CR, including two patients disease-free with post-BMT surgical resection, and eight patients achieved PR for an overall response rate of 43%. Three of the CR occurred after the first BMT, and four patients entered CR with the second BMT. Five of nine were alive and free of disease with a minimum follow-up of 18 months. Of note, all PR recurred with a median duration of remission of 2.5 months. Achievement of CR was associated with a testicular rather than extragonadal primary tumor, absence of liver metastases, and embryonal cell type.

A striking finding in this study was the poor outcome in patients with nonseminomatous primary mediastinal germ cell tumors. Eleven patients with this diagnosis were enrolled in this study, and none obtained durable remission. This parallels the institutional experience at Indiana University in this patient population treated with HDC and autoBMT while in second or greater relapse.[34] Since 1987, 12 such patients were treated on serial protocols of high-dose carboplatin/etoposide with or without ifosfamide. Seven of the 12 did not receive the planned second course of therapy because of tumor progression or treatment-related toxicity. No patient achieved CR, and the median post-HDC survival time was 3.5 months. This subgroup has been identified as having poor outcome with other conventional salvage therapies and should be the focus of investigation of new approaches in treatment.[35]

The results with high-dose carboplatin/etoposide/autoBMT in patients with recurrent and refractory germ cell cancer indicated that a fraction of patients could be rendered permanently disease free. In view of the known activity of ifosfamide in recurrent and refractory germ cell tumors and its favorable side effect profile for dose escalation in the BMT setting, investigators at Indiana University added high-dose ifosfamide to the carboplatin/etoposide treatment template (ICE). As a single agent, ifosfamide has been shown to produce responses in patients with recurrent and cisplatin-resistant germ cell cancer.[36] Seven patients were entered into a phase II trial of carboplatin/etoposide in the previously described doses and schedule with the addition of ifosfamide beginning at 10 g/m^2 daily for 5 days with mesna.[37] Patients were treated with one or two courses of HDC. Because of excessive renal toxicity at the first dose level, escalation of the ifosfamide dose was impossible. Renal function declined significantly in four patients, with three of the four requiring hemofiltration or hemodialysis. Serum markers declined in six of the seven patients, indicating a response to treatment, but all responses were brief, perhaps because of the truncated treatment course necessitated by the toxicity encountered.

Recent trials include further attempts to escalate doses of carboplatin and etoposide in patients with refractory germ cell tumors. Escalation has been possible because patients currently undergoing this therapy are much less heavily pretreated than those in the initial phase I trial. Thirty-two patients underwent careful dose escalation of each of these agents. The maximum tolerated dose was carboplatin, 700 mg/m^2, and etoposide, 750 mg/m^2, given on days -6, -5, and -4. Dose-limiting toxicity for this regimen was marked by occurrence of mucositis. There were five treatment-related deaths, four due to sepsis and multiorgan failure and one to central nervous system hemorrhage. Future directions in these patients will focus on attempts to improve the therapeutic index by exploring new agents, both alkylating agents and new platinum analogues, and developing a second "non-cross-resistant" regimen for use in the tandem autologous transplant setting and using newer cytokines to improve supportive care.

In the treatment of acute leukemia, BMT was used initially in end-stage, heavily treated patients with refractory disease. In this setting, a small response rate was observed with few long-term survivors.[38] When this treatment was used in more favorable, less heavily treated patients, toxicity diminished, response rates improved, and more cures were seen. Likewise, the use of HDC with autoBMT in the treatment of multiply relapsed and refractory testicular cancer has resulted in an overall response rate of about 50% and a cure rate of approximately 15–20%. A logical extension of this concept is to begin HDC earlier in the sequence of treatment of recurrent germ cell cancer.

A number of conclusions can be drawn from the series of studies performed at Indiana University. First, HDC can result in cure for a small percentage of patients with multiple relapses of germ cell cancer. Second, the initial attempt to increase the therapeutic ratio of the regimen with the addition of ifosfamide was unsuccessful in this patient population. Furthermore, analysis of prognostic factors from these and other studies suggests that patients with primary mediastinal nonseminomatous germ cell cancer have a particularly poor prognosis and such patients should be entered into clinical trials of more-intense therapy or combinations with newer agents.

Institut Gustave-Roussy Studies

Similar studies from other institutions provide further substantiation of the curative potential of HDC with autoBMT in refractory germ cell cancer. Serial studies at the Institut Gustave-Roussy have demonstrated activity in recurrent germ cell cancer. Droz et al. developed a regimen using cisplatin, 40 mg/m^2, on days 1–5; etoposide, 350 mg/m^2, on days 1–5; and cyclophosphamide, 1600 mg/m^2, on days 2–5 (PEC). Sixteen patients with recurrent germ cell cancer were enrolled.[39] All had received prior therapy with cisplatin-based treatments. Five of the 15 patients evaluable for response were long-term survivors. The ensuing study enrolled untreated patients thought to be at high risk for treatment failure with conventional therapy.[40] Brief conventional induction therapy was followed by a single round of HDC with PEC. Of 32 poor-risk patients entered, 15 (44%) remain free of disease at a median follow-up of 18 months.

Other European Studies

Rosti has expanded the carboplatin/etoposide skeleton with the addition of ifosfamide (ICE).[41] In this study, 21 patients were entered after primary and often secondary chemotherapy had failed. In addition to the carboplatin/etoposide as given at Indiana University, ifosfamide was added at a dose of 12 g/m^2 over 3 days. No significant renal toxicity was encountered in this study. Thirteen of the 21 patients received one course, 7 received two courses, and 1 received three courses. There was one treatment-related mortality (TRM) due to veno-occlusive disease. There were eight CR, ranging from 1 to 33 months. Five CR were ongoing.

A preliminary report from Linkesch et al. in Austria combines features of the PEC protocol and the protocols from Indiana University along with granulocyte-macrophage colony-stimulating factor (GM-CSF).[42] In this study, HDC with carboplatin (2000 mg/m^2), etoposide (1500 mg/m^2), and cyclophosphamide (60 mg/m$^2 \times$ 2) was given to patients with recurrent and refractory germ cell cancer. All patients were deemed to have incurable disease with standard therapy, and 62% had advanced disease by the Indiana University classification system.

Twelve patients in the control group received HDC with autoBMT, and an additional 30 patients (study group) received the same treatment with hematopoietic growth factors. The hematologic toxicity appeared to be successfully modulated by the use of GM-CSF or granulocyte colony-stimulating factor. Of the 12 patients receiving therapy without the growth factors, the median time to an absolute granulocyte count greater than 500/mm^3 was 20 days compared with 13 days for the 30 patients receiving GM-CSF. The median time of isolation was longer in the control group of patients (25 days) than in the study group (18 days). Nonhematologic toxicity included grade 3 and 4 diarrhea in nine patients, renal toxicity in three patients, and liver toxicity in two patients. There was no significant neurotoxicity or cardiac toxicity. There were three TRM.

Response was assessed in 38 patients and reported by state of disease at time of transplantation. In patients with recurrent disease, 11 of 17 patients (65%) obtained a remission, including 5 PR and 6 CR. In patients with refractory disease, 10 of 15 patients (67%) obtained a response, including 7 CR. Of the 6 patients with progressive disease on chemotherapy, only 1 patient obtained a brief PR. Ten of 13 patients obtaining CR remained in CR, with 7 experiencing disease-free survival at greater than 12 months.

HIGH-DOSE CHEMOTHERAPY AS INITIAL SALVAGE TREATMENT

There is now ample evidence that HDC (PEC, high-dose carboplatin/etoposide) can cure disease that is incurable with conventional salvage regimens. In this heavily pretreated population, however, the impact of such therapy has been small (15–20% long-term disease-free survival) and toxicity has been substantial. The next logical step is to consider use of HDC in the course of recurrent disease, prior to the development of bulky drug-resistant disease and when performance status and organ function are maintained.

One of the first reports of such an approach came from the Cancer Control Agency of British Columbia.[43] Barnett et al. report the results of using HDC as part of initial salvage chemotherapy in 18 patients with recurrent or persistent germ cell cancer after cisplatin-based primary therapy. These patients were given conventional induction chemotherapy with cisplatin, etoposide, vincristine, and bleomycin on a weekly schedule or VeIP combinations. At the completion of conventional salvage chemotherapy, consolidation with HDC was given with autoBMT. Patients received high-dose carboplatin/etoposide and either high-dose cyclophosphamide or ifosfamide. There were two toxic deaths; with two patients it was too early to evaluate; and 8 of 14 remained free of progression from germ cell cancer.

In a recent pilot study at Indiana University,[44] 25 patients with cisplatin-sensitive disease were treated with conventional salvage therapy (usually VeIP) for two courses followed by a single course of high-dose carboplatin/etoposide. Several preliminary results of this trial merit emphasis. First, one patient died from acute renal failure associated with sepsis after his first course of VeIP. Thus, there was no TRM in this series. Only 7 of 25 patients did not enter the transplantation portion of the protocol: one VeIP death, two refusals, two with progressive disease, and two patients for whom insurance coverage was denied.

Of the 18 patients completing the protocol, 10 (56%) obtained CR, 1 obtained disease-free status by resection of residual cancer, and 5 (28%) obtained PR, for an overall response rate of 88%. Two of the 18 patients proceeding to transplantation required tandem transplants because of sluggish decline in serum markers. In the seven patients not proceeding to transplantation, there was one CR and one PR, for an overall response rate of 29%. The response rate for all patients entering the protocol was 18 of 25 (72%). Twelve of 25 patients were disease-free at a median follow-up of 19 months. It is unclear whether these results are superior to those obtained with conventional salvage approaches because these patients were highly selected, but the excellent tolerance of therapy and the high response rate are encouraging.

Siegert et al. in Germany reported the results of high-dose ICE in the treatment of recurrent testicular cancer.[45] Patients received a median of six cycles of cisplatin-based chemotherapy. Patients were given two induction courses of conventional-dose cisplatin, etoposide, and ifosfamide prior to receiving escalated therapy. Fifty-five patients received treatment with conventional therapy followed by carboplatin, 1500–2000 mg/m²; etoposide, 1200–2400 mg/

m²; and ifosfamide, 0–10 g/m². There were two TRM. Twelve patients (22%) achieved CR, and 16 patients (29%) obtained marker-negative PR. Twenty-one patients (38%) maintained their response from 3 to 26+ months. Although the precise degree of chemotherapy resistance in this patient population is not given, it is encouraging that a high percentage of recurrent patients remained progression-free.

In 1996, Margolin et al. at the City of Hope Cancer Center reported a trial utilizing high-dose ICE with autologous peripheral blood progenitor cell (PBPC) support in the therapy of recurrent germ cell tumors.[46] In this small trial, 20 patients with recurrent germ cell tumor were entered either with active disease or in the setting of high risk of recurrence after obtaining disease-free status. Patients received ifosfamide, 2 g/m²; carboplatin, 400 mg/m²; and etoposide, 20 mg/kg on days −6, −5, −4 for two cycles of treatment. Additional ifosfamide (2 g/m² on day −3 and 1 g/m² on day −2) was given during the second cycle to those patients with normal renal function. Mesna was given at a dose of 600 mg/m² every 6 hours until 24 hours after the last ifosfamide dose. Overall, the treatment was well tolerated, with no TRM. No patient required hemodialysis, and there was no hematuria or central nervous system toxicity. The most common side effects were abdominal pain, diarrhea, and transient elevation of hepatic enzymes.

This small trial illustrates the difficulty of defining the contribution of HDC to cure in patients with recurrent or high-risk germ cell tumors. Overall, eight of the patients in this study (40%) were continuously disease free and nine patients (45%) were currently disease free at the median follow-up time of 45 months. Many patients, however, were entered while in remission from prior therapy or after isolated central nervous system relapses—situations that have at least a 50% disease-free survival rate without HDC. Although some of these patients almost certainly achieved cure by HDC, the precise impact cannot be measured in this small trial with a heterogeneous patient population.

The limitations of these single-institution experiences notwithstanding, there does appear to be mounting evidence that HDC contributes to the cure rate of patients with recurrent, cisplatin-sensitive testicular cancer. In a study similar to the European trial that defined the role of HDC in the treatment of recurrent lymphoma,[47] the precise contribution of HDC in this setting is rigidly tested in a randomized pan-European trial comparing VeIP as standard salvage therapy with an experimental arm of VeIP plus HDC. The trial is ongoing, and one hopes that accrual will be completed shortly.

HIGH-DOSE CHEMOTHERAPY AS PRIMARY TREATMENT OF GERM CELL CANCER

Memorial Sloan-Kettering Cancer Center began to use HDC in a portion of initial treatment in selected patients.[48] Patients were given conventional chemotherapy (VAB-6 [vinblastine, actinomycin D, bleomycin, cyclophosphamide, cisplatin]), and those patients in whom there was a suboptimal decline in serum HCG or AFP after two to three cycles of treatment were given high-dose carboplatin/etoposide with autoBMT. The majority of patients entered on protocol required transplantation, and there is early evidence of improved outcome relative to a comparable group of patients from earlier trials. Sixteen patients were treated with high-dose carboplatin/etoposide after suboptimal response to VAB-6. Nine patients (56%) obtained CR, and eight were disease-free at 8–27+ months. These reports compare favorably with a similar prognostic group treated with VAB-6 alone, in whom only 14% responded durably to treatment.

A more recent extension of this trial at Memorial Sloan-Kettering Cancer Center enrolled a similar population of poor-risk patients with sluggish declines in serum markers. Patients were begun on eptoposide, ifosfamide, and cisplatin (VIP); if markers failed to decline by predicted half-life, conventional-dose therapy was discontinued and the patient proceeded to two high-dose cycles of carboplatin (1800 mg/m^2), etoposide (1800 mg/m^2), and cyclophosphamide (150 mg/kg). Thirty untreated patients were enrolled, and 16 received VIP alone. In 14, conventional therapy was truncated, and these patients were moved to HDC because of poor marker decline. Overall, 18 of 30 patients (60%) were continuously progression free—a result that compares favorably with a historical group of poor-risk patients from the same institution. Whether this represents a therapeutic advance is being further assessed in a randomized clinical trial with poor-risk patients.[49]

Investigators from Institut Gustave-Roussy have completed a phase III trial testing the addition of HDC to conventional-dose induction therapy for patients with untreated poor-risk germ cell cancer as assigned by the Institut Gustave-Roussy prognostic system. Patients were randomly assigned to receive cisplatin, vinblastine, bleomycin, and etoposide (PVeBV) as described by Ozols et al. or a modified PVeBV regimen for two cycles followed by high-dose intensification with PEC.[50] Preliminary results suggest no benefit for patients receiving high-dose intensification. Of 49 patients randomized to receive four cycles of PVeBV, there were two early deaths and one refusal. Thirty of 49 patients (61%) achieved CR, and 40 patients (82%) were 2-year survivors. In 53 patients randomized to two cycles of modified PVeBV plus consolidation, there were eight early deaths and two refusals. CR was obtained in 21 of 53 patients (41%), and 32 patients (61%) were 2-year survivors. A statistically significant improvement in CR (P = .01) and a trend toward improved survival (P = .1) were seen in the standard arm relative to the "dose-intense" arm.

The trial reported by Institut Gustave-Roussy incorporated principles that were sound at the time of the initiation of the trial; however, subsequent evidence of the ineffectiveness of double-dose cisplatin, the availability and demonstrated activity of high-dose carboplatin, and evidence of the benefit of HDC in patients with refractory disease suggested that it was important to repeat the trial using more modern concepts. Thus, a large intergroup trial has been started in the United States, enrolling patients with poor-risk disease by the new International Prognostic Scoring System and randomizing them to receive either standard therapy (four cycles of cisplatin) or HDC (two cycles of cisplatin). This trial is ongoing and will either support or refute the role of HDC in patients presenting with poor-risk disease.

PROGNOSTIC FACTORS

Throughout the initial studies of HDC in the treatment of germ cell tumors, investigators analyzed outcome in various subgroups in an attempt to better define those who had a significant chance of benefiting from chemotherapy. In initial studies, primary site and degree of chemotherapy resistance appeared to be the most important predictors of outcome. These attempts at defining prognosis were formalized in a large cooperative study by Beyer et al. in 1996.[51] The investigators analyzed clinical data on 310 patients from Berlin, Institut Gustave-Roussy, Austria, and Indiana University who underwent HDC for germ cell tumor. For the group as a whole, the failure-free survival rate was 32%, 30%, and 29% at 1, 2, and 3 years after treatment, respectively. Clinical parameters that obtained significance in the multivariate model were mediastinal primary site, progressive disease prior to treatment, HCG >1000 U/L, refractory disease (response to cisplatin, but progression within 4 weeks), or absolutely refractory disease (no response to cisplatin). The investigators developed three categories of risk using these factors. Good-risk patients experienced a failure-free survival rate of 51% at 3 years compared with 27% and 5% for those with intermediate or poor risk, respectively. Thus, it seems that patients with combinations of cisplatin-resistant disease, mediastinal primaries, high HCG, or progressive disease prior to transplantation have a very poor overall outcome, even with transplantation, and should be considered for less-toxic palliative approaches.

CONCLUSION

New analyses of completed clinical studies on prognostic variables have led to better understanding as to which patients are not likely to benefit from these treatments. Whether HDC will play a major role in the treatment of untreated poor-risk patients or those in whom initial salvage treatments fail, or remain a minor option for rare patients in whom multiple chemotherapies fail, is currently being defined by two large multicenter studies. The results of these ongoing trials will be crucial to planning future investigations of HDC in germ cell tumors.

REFERENCES

1. Drain L: Testicular cancer in California from 1942–1969: the California Tumor Registry experience. Oncology 27:45–51, 1973.
2. Shibley L, Brown M, Schuttinga J, et al: Cisplatin-based combination chemotherapy in the treatment of advanced-stage testicular cancer: cost benefit analysis. J Natl Cancer Inst 82:186–192, 1990.
3. Einhorn L: Treatment of testicular cancer: a new and improved model. J Clin Oncol 8:1777–1781, 1990.
4. Ozols R, Diesseroth A, Javadpour N, et al: Treatment of poor prognosis non-seminomatous testicular cancer with a "high-dose" platinum combination chemotherapy regimen. Cancer 51:1803–1807, 1983.
5. Stoter G, Kaye S, Sleyfer D, et al: Preliminary results of BEP (bleomycin, etoposide, cisplatin) versus an alternating regimen of BEP and PVB (cisplatin, vinblastine, bleomycin) in high volume metastatic testicular non-seminomas: an EORTC study. Proc Am Soc Clin Oncol 5:106, 1986.
6. Bosl G, Geller N, Cirrincione C, et al: Multivariate analysis of prognostic variables in patients with metastatic testicular cancer. Cancer Res 43:3403–3407, 1983.
7. Birch R, Williams S, Cone A, et al: Prognostic factors for favorable

outcome in disseminated germ cell tumors. J Clin Oncol 4(3):400–407, 1986.

8. Horwich A, Stenning S, Mead B, et al: Prognostic factors for survival in advanced non-seminomatous germ cell tumors. Proc Am Soc Clin Oncol 9:132, 1990.

9. Masham S: Medical Research Council Working Party on Testicular Tumours: prognostic factors in advanced non-seminomatous germ-cell testicular tumours: results of a multicentre study. Lancet 1:8–11, 1985.

10. Vaeth M, Schultz HP, Von Der Maase H, et al: Prognostic factors in testicular germ cell tumours: experiences from 1058 consecutive cases. Acta Radiol Oncol 23(4):271–285, 1984.

11. Sledge G, Eble J, Roth B, et al: Relation of proliferative activity to survival in patients with advanced germ cell cancer. Cancer Res 48:3864–3868, 1988.

12. Mead G, Stenning S: Prognostic factors for metastatic germ cell cancers treated with platinum-based chemotherapy: the International Germ Cell Cancer Collaborative Group (IGCCCG) project to standardize risk criteria. Proc Am Soc Clin Oncol 13:251, 1994.

13. Einhorn LH, Williams SD, Loehrer PJ, et al: Evaluation of optimal duration of chemotherapy in favorable-prognosis disseminated germ cell tumors: a Southeastern Cancer Study Group Protocol. J Clin Oncol 7(3):387–391, 1989.

14. Bosl G, Geller N, Bajorin D, et al: A randomized trial of etoposide + cisplatin versus vinblastine + bleomycin + cisplatin + cyclophosphamide + dactinomycin in patients with good-prognosis germ cell tumors. J Clin Oncol 6:1231–1238, 1988.

15. Bajorin DF, Sarosdy MF, Bosl GJ, et al: A randomized trial of etoposide + carboplatin (EC) vs. etoposide (EP) in patients with metastatic germ cell tumors. Proc Am Soc Clin Oncol 10:168, 1991.

16. Loehrer PJ, Elson P, Johnson DH, et al: A randomized trial of cisplatin plus etoposide with or without bleomycin in favorable prognosis disseminated germ cell tumors. Proc Am Soc Clin Oncol 10:169, 1991.

17. Nichols C, Williams S, Loehrer P, et al: Randomized study of cisplatin dose intensity in advanced germ cell tumors: a Southeastern Cancer Study Group and Southwest Oncology Group Protocol. J Clin Oncol 9:1163–1172, 1991.

18. Nichols C, Loehrer P, Einhorn L, et al: Phase III study of cisplatin, etoposide and bleomycin (PVP-16B) or etoposide, ifosfamide, and cisplatin (VIP) in advanced stage germ cell tumors: an intergroup trial. Proc Am Soc Clin Oncol 14:239, 1995.

19. Sampson MK, Rivkin SE, Jones SE, et al: Dose-response and dose-survival advantage for high versus low-dose cisplatin combined with vinblastine and bleomycin in disseminated testicular cancer: a Southwest Oncology Group Study. Cancer 53:1029–1035, 1984.

20. Droz J, Pico J, Biron P, et al: No evidence of a benefit of early intensified chemotherapy (HDC) with autologous bone marrow transplantation (ABMT) in first line treatment of poor risk non-seminomatous germ cell tumors. Proc Am Soc Clin Oncol 11:197, 1992.

21. Fox E, Einhorn L, Weathers T, et al: Outcome analysis for patients with persistent germ cell carcinoma in post chemotherapy (PC) retroperitoneal lymph node dissections (RPLND). Proc Am Soc Clin Oncol 11:198, 1992.

22. Einhorn L, Weathers T, Loehrer P, Nichols C: Second line chemotherapy with vinblastine, ifosfamide, and cisplatin after initial chemotherapy with cisplatin, VP-16 and bleomycin (PVP-16B) in disseminated germ cell tumors (GCT). Proc Am Soc Clin Oncol 11:196, 1992.

23. Motzer R, Cooper K, Geller N, et al: The role of cisplatin + ifosfamide–based chemotherapy as salvage therapy for patients with refractory germ cell tumors. Cancer 66:2476–2481, 1992.

24. Cheson B, Lacerna L, Leyland-Jones B, et al: Autologous bone marrow transplantation: current status and future directions. Ann Intern Med 110:51–65, 1989.

25. Amato R, Hutchinson L, Striegel A: Modulation of dose intensity (DI) by reducing chemotherapy (CHT) intervals in patients (pts) with high volume non-seminomatous germ cell tumors (HV-GCT). Proc Am Soc Clin Oncol 13:253, 1994.

26. Kaye S, Mead G, Fossa S, et al: An MRC/EORTC randomized trial in poor prognosis metastatic teratoma, comparing BEP to BOP-VIP. Proc Am Soc Clin Oncol 14:246, 1995.

27. Wettlaufer JN, Feiner AS, Robinson WA: Vincristine, cisplatin and bleomycin with surgery in the management of advanced metastatic nonseminomatous testis tumors. Cancer 53:203–209, 1984.

28. Daugaard G, Rorth M: High-dose cisplatin and VP-16 with bleomycin,

in the management of advanced metastatic germ cell tumors. Eur J Cancer Clin Oncol 22:477–485, 1986.

29. Horwich A, Brada M, Nicholls J, et al: Intensive induction chemotherapy for poor risk non-seminomatous germ cell tumours. Eur J Cancer Clin Oncol 25(2):177–184, 1989.

30. Bosl GJ, Geller NL, Chan EYW: Stage migration and the increasing proportion of complete responders in patients with advanced germ cell tumors. Cancer Res 48:3524–3527, 1988.

31. Nichols CR, Tricot G, Williams SD, et al: Dose-intensive chemotherapy in refractory germ cell cancer—a phase I/II trial of high dose carboplatin and etoposide with autologous bone marrow transplantation. J Clin Oncol 7:932–939, 1989.

32. Broun E, Nichols C, Kneebone P, et al: Long term outcome of patients with relapsed and refractory germ cell tumors treated with high dose chemotherapy and autologous bone marrow rescue. Ann Intern Med 117:124–128, 1992.

33. Nichols C, Andersen J, Lazarus H, et al: High-dose carboplatin and etoposide with autologous bone marrow transplantation in refractory germ cell cancer: an Eastern Cooperative Oncology Group protocol. J Clin Oncol 10:558–563, 1992.

34. Broun E, Nichols C, Einhorn L, Tricot G: Salvage therapy with high dose chemotherapy and autologous bone marrow support in the treatment of primary nonseminomatous mediastinal germ cell tumors (EGGCT). Cancer 68(7):1513–1515, 1991.

35. Munshi N, Loehrer P, Williams S, et al: Ifosfamide combination salvage chemotherapy in extragonadal germ cell tumors (EGGCT). Proc Am Soc Clin Oncol 10:182, 1991.

36. Wheeler B, Loehrer P, Williams S, Einhorn L: Ifosfamide in refractory male germ cell tumors. J Clin Oncol 4:28–34, 1986.

37. Broun E, Nichols C, Tricot G, et al: High dose carboplatin/VP-16 plus ifosfamide with autologous bone marrow support in the treatment of refractory germ cell tumors. Bone Marrow Transplant 7:53–56, 1991.

38. Thomas E, Buckner C, Banaji M, et al: One hundred patients with acute leukemia treated by chemotherapy, total body irradiation, and allogeneic marrow transplantation. Blood 49:511–533, 1977.

39. Pico J, Droz J, Gouyette A, et al: High dose chemotherapy regimens (HDC) followed by autologous bone marrow transplantation for treatment of relapsed or refractory germ cell tumors. Proc Am Soc Clin Oncol 5:111, 1986.

40. Droz J, Pico J, Ghosn M, et al: High complete remission (CR) and survival rates in poor prognosis (PP) non seminomatous germ cell tumors (NSGCT) with high dose chemotherapy (HDC) and autologous bone marrow transplantation (ABMT). Proc Am Soc Clin Oncol 8:130, 1989.

41. Nichols C, Rosti G: Dose-intensive therapy for germ cell neoplasms. Semin Oncol 19:145–149, 1992.

42. Linkesch W, Krainer M, Wagner A: Phase I/II trial of ultrahigh carboplatin, etoposide, cyclophosphamide with ABMT in refractory or relapsed non-seminomatous germ-cell tumors (NSGCT). Proc Am Soc Clin Oncol 11:196, 1992.

43. Barnett M, Coppin C, Murray N, et al: Intensive therapy an autologous bone marrow transplantation (BMT) for patients with poor prognosis nonseminomatous germ cell tumors. Proc Am Soc Clin Oncol 10:165, 1991.

44. Bhatia S, Cornetta K, Broun R, et al: High-dose chemotherapy with peripheral stem cell autologous bone marrow transplant as initial salvage chemotherapy for testicular cancer. Proc Am Soc Clin Oncol 17:32A, 1998.

45. Siegert W, Beyer J, Weisbach V, et al: High dose carboplatin (C), etoposide (E) and ifosfamide (I) with autologous stem cell rescue (ASCR) for relapsed and refractory non-seminomatous germ cell tumors (NSGCT). Proc Am Soc Clin Oncol 10:163, 1991.

46. Margolin K, Doroshow J, Ahn C, et al: Treatment of germ cell cancer with two cycles of high-dose ifosfamide, carboplatin, and etoposide with autologous stem-cell support. J Clin Oncol 14:2631–2637, 1996.

47. Philip T, Guglielmi C, Hagenbeck A, et al: Autologous bone marrow transplantation as compared with salvage chemotherapy in relapse of chemotherapy-sensitive non-Hodgkin's lymphoma. N Engl J Med 333:1540–1545, 1995.

48. Motzer R, Gulati S, Crown J, et al: High-dose chemotherapy and autologous bone marrow rescue for patients with refractory germ cell tumors: early intervention is better tolerated. Cancer 69:550–556, 1992.

49. Motzer R, Mazumdar M, Lyn P, et al: High dose carboplatin, etoposide

and cyclophosphamide with autologous bone marrow transplantation in first-line therapy for patients with poor-risk germ cell tumors. J Clin Oncol 15:2546–2552, 1997.

50. Ozols RF, Ihde DC, Linehan M, et al: A randomized trial of standard chemotherapy vs. a high-dose chemotherapy regimen in the treatment of poor prognosis nonseminomatous germ-cell tumors. J Clin Oncol 6(6):1031–1040, 1988.

51. Beyer J, Kramar A, Mandanas R, et al: High dose chemotherapy (HDC) as salvage treatment in germ cell tumors (GCT): a multivariate analysis of prognostic variables. J Clin Oncol 14:2638–2645, 1996.

Hematopoietic Stem Cell Transplantation for Treatment of Congenital Immunodeficiencies

Steven Neudorf, M.D., and Alexandra Filipovich, M.D.

The congenital immunodeficiency disorders are a heterogeneous group of diseases. Milder forms of immunodeficiencies (i.e., those predominantly involving antibody deficiencies) can often be corrected by immunoglobulin G supplementation and are compatible with long life. In contrast, many of the combined immunodeficiencies involving T and B lymphocytes are characterized by susceptibility to opportunistic infections and are prematurely lethal. Hematopoietic stem cell transplantation (HSCT) has been shown to be successful for a number of congenital immunodeficiency disorders. The initial reports of successful allogeneic HSCT in the late 1960s were of patients with severe combined immunodeficiency (SCID).[1] HSCT remains the preferred treatment for this group of diseases.

Unlike HSCT for malignancies designed to ablate residual tumor cells, the goal of HSCT as treatment of the immunodeficiencies is to reconstitute an effective immune system. Thus, the least-toxic conditioning therapy that allows persistent engraftment and achieves adequate immunoreconstitution is desirable in the majority of cases. Exceptions include cases in which lymphoproliferative disease, autoreactive (or autoimmune disease), or graft-vs.-host disease (GVHD) has occurred prior to HSCT or diseases (such as Wiskott-Aldrich syndrome [WAS]) that affect several hematopoietic lineages.

This chapter provides guidelines for identifying a rational approach to HSCT for the patient with primary immunodeficiency. We provide a brief description and current references regarding the immunodeficiency disorders correctable by transplantation and relay the current status of the various approaches to transplantation, including conditioning regimens and sources of HSC. Areas of uncertainty and controversy are pointed out. Several issues are specifically addressed: for patients with SCID in whom a graft may be accepted without conditioning, what are the indications for using conditioning therapy? For all immunodeficiencies potentially treated using HSCT, can successful outcomes be achieved without the use of total body irradiation (TBI)? When is T-cell depletion of donor marrow indicated? What is the ideal source of HSC for patients lacking human leukocyte antigen (HLA)-matched sibling donors? These issues are discussed for diseases with which the indications for HSCT have been established and the outcomes of HSCT have been sufficiently well characterized as to be generalizable to other cases.

GENERAL APPROACH TO HSCT FOR PRIMARY IMMUNODEFICIENCIES

Primary immunodeficiency disorders are rare. The genes affected in many of the primary immunodeficiency diseases discussed in this chapter have been identified. Information concerning the function of these gene products is rapidly accumulating. We have learned that immunodeficiencies can arise from a broad range of mutations such as truncations or creation of dominant negative mutations. The best available approach and the likelihood of successful correction of these diseases by HSCT depend on several factors, the first of which is the specific immunodeficiency diagnosis.

For some diseases, such as SCID phenotypes or WAS, the specific genetic defect must be determined so that the plan of therapy can be based on previous experience with HSCT. For other forms of immunodeficiency with which HSCT may be beneficial, such as common variable immunodeficiency, individual cases are heterogeneous with respect to etiology and severity, making accurate prediction of outcomes difficult. For some diseases such as Kostmann syndrome or chronic granulomatous disease, alternative therapies may allow patients to survive for many years without the need for HSCT. A second critical factor is the availability of a suitable HSC donor. Third, the existence of complications that affect the overall clinical status of the patient, such as progressive organ dysfunction (after infections or autoimmune attack) or pre-existing complications such as ongoing infections, GVHD, or lymphoproliferative disease, can compromise the likelihood of success with HSCT.

Such information is currently being analyzed with resources of international cooperation such as the International Bone Marrow Transplant Registry (IBMTR) and National Marrow Donor Program (NMDP) and should increasingly become available in peer-reviewed publications. Additionally, access to physicians and institutions with expertise in mismatched HSCT for these diseases will likely improve the outcome.

The process of correcting a potentially lethal primary immunodeficiency begins with suspicion of such an underlying disorder. In sporadic cases, suspicion is usually raised by history of recurrent infections early in childhood and/or the finding of an opportunistic infection or prolonged respiratory or gastrointestinal infection that leads to one or more hospitalizations. Until the possibility of a life-threatening immunodeficiency is ruled out, the use of non-irradiated blood products should be avoided. Blood products should also be filtered to eliminate leukocytes and reduce the risk of cytomegalovirus or Epstein-Barr virus infections.

A relatively short list of diagnostic studies, taken in conjunction with characteristic presenting symptoms and physical findings, serves to exclude or confirm the majority of severe immunodeficiency diseases that present during the first few years of life. Infection with human immunodeficiency virus (HIV) should be considered part of the differential diagnosis. Key laboratory studies include a complete blood count with differential and peripheral blood smear, quantitative serum immunoglobulins, mitogen proliferation assays, and lymphocyte subset phenotyping. The latter two studies are particularly indicated if SCID is to be ruled out. The use of irradiated blood transfusions rarely interferes with these studies. Erythrocyte transfusions, however, interfere with erythrocyte enzyme analyses for adenosine deaminase or purine nucleoside phosphorylase. Similarly, serum immunoglobulin levels may be affected if significant volumes of plasma have been administered.

Once a primary immunodeficiency has been diagnosed, additional studies should be performed to define the genetic defect (when possible) and, in the case of SCID, rule out GVHD from maternal T cells and determine the level of immune competency (including the presence or absence of natural killer function), which may be useful in predicting the need for conditioning therapy. Maternal T cells are present in as many as 40% of patients with SCID.[2, 3] Maternal cells are often "silent" (i.e., without clinical GVHD). In many cases, maternal T cells are dysfunctional or they result in clinical GVHD, neutropenia, or liver disease.[2–4]

For families with a history of primary immunodeficiency, prenatal diagnosis is possible for many diseases. Ideally, the genetic mutation has already been precisely defined through studies of DNA from the proband. For X-linked disorders in which only one family member has been affected, analysis of maternal DNA may be informative because the mother may be an obligate carrier. At present, prenatal diagnosis of some SCID phenotypes along with HLA typing of the fetus can be used to plan postnatal transplantation. Because there is no evidence that inheritance of primary immunodeficiency leads to irreversible developmental damage prenatally and because results of HSCT in the early postnatal period are exceptionally good, there is currently little rationale for recommending intra-uterine intervention. Discussion of in utero transplantation can be found in Chapter 19. The diagnosis of virtually all primary immunodeficiencies that could benefit from early transplantation can be confirmed after birth (in a matter of hours or several days) using umbilical cord blood samples.

Simultaneously, the search process to identify the donor and source of HSC should be initiated, beginning with serologic and molecular HLA typing of the recipient and immediate family members and followed by searching for potential unrelated bone marrow donors or cord blood donors.

Pretransplantation evaluation of the recipient with pri-mary immunodeficiency should include a vigorous search for infections, potentially infectious pathogens, and occult lymphoproliferative disease. It should include an overall assessment of nutritional and developmental status and vital organ function. Prior to transplantation, aggressive treatment of existing infections, institution of appropriate antimicrobial prophylaxis (e.g., antibiotics and intravenous IgG), and repletion of nutritional status is desirable. The latter may require weeks to months to accomplish. For conditions characterized by histiocytic activation and hemophagocytosis (e.g., hemophagocytic lymphohistiocytosis, Chédiak-Higashi syndrome in accelerated phase, and possibly X-linked lymphoproliferative syndrome), it is beneficial to bring the lymphohistiocytic reaction under control with chemotherapy and/or immunosuppression prior to the start of ablative therapy.

Viral infections (especially cytomegalovirus, adenovirus, or parainfluenza) are a significant risk to patients with SCID awaiting transplantation. Peritransplantation infections with gastrointestinal pathogens (enteroviruses, adenoviruses, rotavirus, and *Clostridium difficile*) are often nosocomially acquired by patients with many forms of primary immunodeficiency and may aggravate gastrointestinal GVHD after the transplantation.[4–8] It is not clear, however, whether laminar air flow facilities provide a significant advantage over strict isolation in reducing the incidence of these infections.

IMMUNODEFICIENCY DISORDERS CORRECTABLE BY STEM CELL TRANSPLANTATION

The primary immunodeficiencies for which HSCT is the treatment of choice are listed in Table 14–1. Table 14–2 lists the other primary immunodeficiency diseases that are curable with HSCT. Median survival with the diseases in Table 14–2 is 10–20 years with the best of available medical therapy. There is evidence, however, to suggest that earlier HSCT in these diseases results in less morbidity and greater long-term success compared with alternative therapies. Table 14–3 lists conditions in which HSCT has the potential to correct the underlying disease but its use remains controversial because alternative therapies exist. The decision to recommend HSCT for such patients must be considered case by case. Ultimately, the decision to perform transplantation depends on the type of donor available as well as the severity of the patient's clinical manifestations.

PRIMARY IMMUNODEFICIENCIES IN WHICH HSCT EARLY IN LIFE IS THE PREFERRED TREATMENT

SCID

Treatment of SCID using HSCT has been extensively applied. Many different genetic defects contribute to SCID (see Table 14–1). In some cases, the specific etiology is not known. Despite differences in the pathogenesis of the disease, the clinical course of patients with SCID is remarkably similar. If untreated by HSCT, most patients die in early childhood from opportunistic infections.

TABLE 14–1. IMMUNODEFICIENCIES IN WHICH HSCT IN EARLY LIFE IS THE PREFERRED TREATMENT

SCID AND SCID VARIANTS*	INHERITANCE	GENE DEFECT	CHARACTERISTIC LABORATORY FINDINGS
Adenosine deaminase (ADA) deficiency SCID with B cells	AR	ADA	Leukopenia, lymphopenia, absent ADA in RBC + WBC
X-linked SCID†	X-linked	IL-2R gamma d-chain[122]	Reduced numbers of T cells, normal B cells, decreased NK function
JAK-3 deficiency	AR	JAK-3[123]	
Lymphopenic SCID†	AR	Rag 1, Rag 2 and other defects[124]	Reduced numbers of T and B cells, NK cells often present
ZAP-70 deficiency	AR	ZAP-70[125]	Decreased CD3 + CD8 + cells, normal B cells
Reticular dysgenesis†	Unknown	Unknown	Pancytopenia,‡ absent T and B cells
Severe MHC class II deficiency	AR	Class II enhancer[126]	Decreased class II expression
Omenn syndrome†	AR	Unknown	Normal T cells, low numbers of B cells, eosinophilia, high IgE
Other immune defects			
Severe leukocyte adhesion deficiency	AR	CD11/18	Leukocytosis
Hemophagocytic lymphohistiocytosis	AR	Unknown	Pancytopenia, absent NK function

*Other rare SCID variants include CD7 deficiencies,[127] N-FAT deficiencies.[128]
†Silent or symptomatic maternal engraftment has been reported.
‡Pancytopenia possibly due to maternal engraftment/graft-versus-host disease.
AR, autosomal recessive; NK, natural killer; MHC, major histocompatibility complex; SCID, severe combined immunodeficiency; RBC, red blood cells; WBC, white blood cells.

HLA-Matched Sibling Donor Transplants for SCID

Most patients with SCID are so severely immunodeficient that they do not need conditioning regimen for engraftment of unmodified marrow from an HLA-identical sibling.[9–12] Reconstitution of both T- and B-lymphocyte function has occurred in the majority of cases. In approximately 10% of cases, reconstitution of only T-lymphocyte function occurs. Complete immunoreconstitution has been achieved by 6 months after HSCT, occurring in the majority of cases within 2–4 months. GVHD has been infrequent, with an incidence of less than 6% grade II and no grade III or IV GVHD. Patients younger than 6 months of age experience statistically better survival compared with older patients. The most frequent cause of death has been infection, present in many cases prior to HSCT. This suggests that an earlier diagnosis of SCID, especially prior to the onset of severe infections, improves the results of HSCT.

Although engraftment of HLA-identical, unmodified marrow occurs without the use of conditioning regimen in the majority of cases of SCID, rare incidences of graft failure have been reported. Some cases of adenosine deami-nase (ADA) deficiency have required multiple infusions of marrow to allow engraftment.[9–13, 25–27] It is hypothesized that transient engraftment may result in improvement in the biochemical abnormalities in ADA deficiency (and improvement in immune function) and thus allow rejection to occur. These observations emphasize the importance of determining the precise etiology of the immunodeficiency prior to HSCT.

Most patients with SCID who have an HLA-identical sibling donor should undergo HSCT without conditioning regimen. Conditioning therapy should be used when the form of SCID is associated with a higher risk of rejection (e.g., ADA deficiency) or in the case of severe autoimmune disease, lymphoproliferative disease, or GVHD. In these cases, conditioning regimen is needed to eliminate alloreactive cells. With HLA-matched donors, T-cell depletion is usually not warranted because the incidence and severity of GVHD is low owing to the age of the patient. For patients who require conditioning regimen, busulfan (4 mg/kg × 4 days) followed by cyclophosphamide (60 mg/kg × 2 days) has been shown to allow engraftment in greater than 95% of cases and results in a less than 10% incidence of transplant-related mortality.[14]

TABLE 14–2. PREMATURELY LETHAL IMMUNODEFICIENCIES THAT HAVE BEEN SUCCESSFULLY TREATED IN LATER CHILDHOOD

DISEASE	INHERITANCE	GENE DEFECT	CHARACTERISTIC LABORATORY FINDINGS
Wiskott-Aldrich syndrome	X	WASP	Microthrombocytopenia
Chédiak-Higashi syndrome	AR	Lyst	Giant leukocyte cytoplasmic granules
X-linked "hyper IgM" syndrome	X	CD40 ligand	Hypogammaglobulinemia with normal or increased IgM, neutropenia
X-linked lymphoproliferative disease	X	Unknown	None
Chronic granulomatous disease	X, AR	NADPH oxidase	Decreased polymorphonuclear chemiluminescence
Kostmann neutropenia	AR	Unknown	Neutropenia
Purine nucleoside phosphorylase (PNP) deficiency	AR	PNP	Reduced numbers of CD3 + CD8 + cells, absent PNP activity

NADPH, nicotinamide-adenine dinucleotide phosphate (reduced form); AR, autosomal recessive.

TABLE 14–3. PRIMARY IMMUNODEFICIENCIES POTENTIALLY CORRECTABLE WITH HSCT WHEN TIMING IS UNCERTAIN

DISEASE	INHERITANCE	GENE DEFECT	CHARACTERISTIC LABORATORY FINDINGS
Common variable immunodeficiency	Unknown	Unknown	Hypogammaglobulinemia variable T-cell defects
X-linked agammaglobulinemia	X	BTK	Absent B cells, hypogammaglobulinemia
Autoimmune lymphoproliferative disease	AR	fas, fas ligand and other defects	Decreased numbers of T cells in blood + lymph nodes

AR, autosomal recessive.

Haploidentical Donors for Treatment of SCID

Haploidentical HSCT has been extensively used to treat patients with SCID.[13, 15–19, 24–27] Haploidentical HSCT requires T-cell depletion of donor marrow to prevent severe, fatal GVHD. Although T-cell depletion of donor marrow has greatly reduced the incidence of GVHD, recipients of haploidentical transplants have a higher incidence of graft rejection. NK cells and/or T cells may mediate rejection. O'Reilly et al. reported the results of mismatched, T-depleted HSCT in 17 patients with SCID.[18, 19] All underwent transplantation without cytoreduction. Ten of 17 experienced engraftment and did not experience GVHD. Graft failure occurred in the remaining seven patients. Patients in whom engraftment did not occur underwent transplantation again using conditioning regimen that resulted in engraftment in five of seven cases. Patients in whom engraftment failed had high NK cell activity against K562 cell targets prior to HSCT, whereas those with sustained engraftment and immunoreconstitution had low NK activity. The link between NK cell activity and graft rejection has been substantiated by a review of SCID cases treated by the European Group for Blood and Marrow Transplantation (EBMT) Working Party on Immunodeficiencies, who likewise found inferior results when patients with SCID had NK cell function.[20] The suggestion that NK cells mediate bone marrow rejection is supported by data using a murine model for mismatched HSCT.[21–23]

T cells have also been implicated in mediating rejection of mismatched marrow. Buckley et al. reported the results of HSCT in 10 patients with SCID.[24] All patients received haploidentical T cell–depleted marrow without cytoreductive therapy. Engraftment occurred in 7 of 10 patients, including two patients with normal NK activity. Rejection was associated with response to mitogens and alloantigens or the presence of low numbers of circulating T cells.

In a review of the European experience using haploidentical donors, graft failure occurred in approximately 25% of cases of SCID[9] and is more common in patients with ADA deficiency.

The use of a non–TBI-containing conditioning regimen is recommended for patients with SCID undergoing haploidentical HSCT and who have lymphoproliferative disease, severe autoimmune disease, or GVHD and for those patients with diseases associated with a higher incidence of rejection (e.g., ADA deficiency). The use of conditioning regimen for patients with other forms of SCID who lack these complications is controversial. Because rejection is more likely in patients with SCID who have circulating T cells, NK cells, or evidence of residual T-cell or NK-cell function, the use of conditioning regimen can be justified. In patients who have life-threatening complications prior to transplantation that are likely to be worsened by conditioning therapy, it is reasonable to attempt transplantation without the use of conditioning regimen while the patient's complications are being controlled. The need for conditioning therapy for patients with SCID who experience silent maternal engraftment (without GVHD) is uncertain. The coexistence of maternal and host cells implies tolerance and would suggest a high likelihood that engraftment of maternal HSC would occur. This was demonstrated in one report in which it was hypothesized that the presence of maternal cells actually hastened the tempo of engraftment.[28] Conditioning regimen should probably be used in cases of maternal engraftment when a donor other than the mother is to be used.

Although it is recommended to proceed to HSCT promptly after a diagnosis of SCID has been established, other therapeutic options need to be considered for ADA-deficient patients. Treatment with commercial preparations of ADA can result in a transient improvement in immune function.[29] Long-term treatment with polyethylene glycol (PEG)-ADA becomes prohibitively expensive, however. The use of PEG-ADA should be considered in ADA-deficient patients who have pre-existing infections or life-threatening complications until the patient's clinical status improves. Similarly, measures to clear infections and improve the clinical status of all patients with primary immunodeficiencies are recommended prior to the initiation of conditioning chemotherapy.

Omenn Syndrome

Omenn syndrome is characterized by exudative dermatitis, lymphadenopathy, hepatosplenomegaly, fever, diarrhea, and eosinophilia.[30] Clinically and histopathologically, cutaneous and gastrointestinal lesions are similar to those in acute GVHD, although there is no evidence of maternal or third-party engraftment in most patients. The underlying gene defect is unknown. HSCT is the only known cure for this disease.[31–34] Gomez et al. reported the results of HSCT in nine patients with Omenn syndrome.[31] Three received grafts from HLA-identical parents and two from HLA-identical sibling donors. A conditioning regimen of cyclophosphamide and antithymocyte globulin (ATG) failed to produce engraftment in one patient. The remaining four patients received conditioning regimens containing busulfan and subsequently experienced engraftment. Of those in whom engraftment succeeded, one died from cytomegalovirus disease and three are alive and well.

MHC Class II Deficiency

In a report of patients who received transplants for major histocompatibility complex (MHC) class II deficiency,[35] seven of whom received non–T cell-depleted grafts from HLA-identical sibling donors, the first patient failed to experience engraftment after a conditioning regimen of cyclophosphamide (50 mg/kg) and antilymphocyte serum. The remaining six patients experienced engraftment using a conditioning regimen of busulfan (20 mg/kg) and cyclophosphamide (200 mg/kg). Patients with MHC class II deficiency have been shown to be capable of experiencing alloreactivity, which can initiate rejection.[36]

Leukocyte Adhesion Deficiency

The CD11/CD18 complex is a heterodimer in which the β-subunit (CD18) is common to all members. There are at least three different α-subunits, called CD11a, CD11b, and CD11c. Patients with leukocyte adhesion deficiency (LAD) lack cell surface CD11/CD18 because of mutations in the CD18 gene.[37, 38] The lack of CD11/CD18 expression results in defective cell-cell interactions that manifest as absent chemotaxis and lack of adhesion by phagocytes. T lymphocytes from patients with LAD show impaired cell-mediated immunity. Severely affected patients have less than 0.2% of normal expression of CD11/CD18 and present with delayed umbilical cord separation, leukocytosis (>50,000/mm³), impaired wound healing, and recurrent skin and respiratory tract infections. Death from infections usually occurs early in childhood. Patients with the mild form of LAD have approximately 5% expression of CD11/CD18 and often survive into adulthood despite recurrent infections.[37] LAD is curable using HSCT.

Thomas et al. reported the results of HSCT for treatment of 14 patients with severe LAD.[39] This series included four patients undergoing transplantation using marrow (not T cell–depleted) from HLA-identical donors. One patient who received busulfan (8 mg/kg) and cyclophosphamide (200 mg/kg) experienced graft rejection. A second transplantation was performed using cyclophosphamide (120 mg/kg) and 8-Gy TBI. Engraftment occurred and the patient was alive 12 years post HSCT. Two patients were given busulfan (16 mg/kg), cyclophosphamide (200 mg/kg), and etoposide (900 mg/m²); all experienced prompt engraftment. A fourth patient who received busulfan (16 mg/kg), cyclophosphamide (200 mg/kg), and thiotepa (10 mg/kg) promptly experienced engraftment as well. One patient died of meningitis at 14 months post HSCT, the other two patients were reported to be alive at 44 months and 18 months after HSCT. Clinical improvement has occurred in patients with LAD who have low levels of donor cells. Interestingly, patients who have undergone HSCT for LAD and show persistence of as little as 3–5% of donor leukocytes remain free of infections.

Hemophagocytic Lymphohistiocytosis

Hemophagocytic lymphohistiocytosis (HLH) is a spectrum of diseases including familial HLH and virus-associated hemophagocytic syndrome. Patients commonly present with fever, failure to thrive, and hepatosplenomegaly. The characteristic histopathologic feature is infiltration of the liver, spleen, marrow, and lymph nodes by histiocytes that are phagocytizing erythrocytes. The pathogenesis is poorly understood. HLH is hypothesized to represent an exaggerated immune response to a viral or other stimulus. Patients have evidence of persistent T-cell activation manifested by increased levels of both soluble interleukin (IL)-2 receptor and soluble CD8. NK cell function is typically absent or reduced. The diagnosis is confirmed by the demonstration of erythrophagocytosis together with pancytopenia, fever, and organomegaly according to guidelines defined by the International Histiocyte Society.[40] HSCT has been shown to be an effective therapy for HLH.

The results of HSCT for 26 cases of HLH have been published in four separate reports.[41–45] Donors included HLA-identical siblings, unrelated donors, and haploidentical donorsy. Conditioning regimens were heterogeneous as well. In those patients undergoing transplantation using HLA-matched sibling donors, the severity of acute GVHD never exceeded grade II. The major causes of death were viral infections and graft failure. The lack of significant GVHD together with occasional instances of graft failure despite the use of conditioning regimen suggests that T-cell depletion of marrow from HLA-identical sibling donors is not warranted for HLH. Not surprisingly, the greatest likelihood for survival was in patients who had quiescent HLH at the time of transplantation.

PRIMARY IMMUNODEFICIENCIES THAT HAVE BEEN SUCCESSFULLY TREATED WITH HSCT LATER IN CHILDHOOD

Wiskott-Aldrich Syndrome (WAS)

WAS is an X-linked recessive disease characterized by eczema, microthrombocytopenia, defects in specific antibody formation, and T-cell dysfunction. WAS is a prematurely fatal disease, with the majority of patients dying from bleeding, infection, or malignancy. The genetic defect has been localized to the short arm of the X chromosome. The WAS protein locus, which encodes a cytoplasmic protein that appears to have multiple functions related to cytoskeletal integrity, signal transduction, and proliferation, is defective in the disease.[46]

Splenectomy may alleviate thrombocytopenia but does not correct the underlying immune deficiency.[47, 48] Most patients who undergo splenectomy still carry a very high risk of death from viral infections or malignancy and autoimmune complications. The projected median survival time with the best available medical management is 15 years.[47, 49] WAS was one of the first diseases corrected by allogeneic HSCT.[50] Engraftment occurred in a majority of 36 patients with WAS who received marrow from HLA-matched sibling donors.[44, 47, 51, 52] Rare instances of graft failure have occurred after use of busulfan and cyclophosphamide and may be due to the rapid clearance of busulfan in young children.[53, 54] Currently, results with unrelated donor HSCT in boys with WAS treated under 5 years of age are comparable to results with matched sibling HSCT.[52]

Chédiak-Higashi Syndrome

Chédiak-Higashi syndrome (CHS) is an autosomal recessive disorder characterized by recurrent infections due to variable immunologic defects and partial oculocutaneous pseudoalbinism. The defective gene, *LYST,* has been identified and shares extensive homology with the *bg* gene in the beige mouse, which is thought to be the murine equivalent of the human disease.[55] Leukocytes contain giant lysosomal inclusions that are diagnostic of this disease.[56] Phagocytes from patients with CHS have defective bactericidal activity and do not respond normally to chemotactic stimulants.[57] In addition, patients with CHS have poor NK cell function.[58] A majority of patients experience an "accelerated phase" manifested by fever, lymphadenopathy, hepatosplenomegaly, and pancytopenia reminiscent of the process that occurs in HLH. Although cytotoxic therapy using corticosteroids or etoposide has resulted in temporary remissions of the accelerated phase, a majority of patients eventually experience relapse and die from bleeding or infection.

Haddad et al. reported the results of HSCT in 10 patients with CHS.[59] Four received grafts from HLA-identical siblings, and three received grafts from HLA-identical parents. The marrow was T cell–depleted in one case. The first patient in this series failed to experience engraftment after cyclophosphamide alone (200 mg/kg). That patient underwent a second, successful HSCT using a conditioning regimen of cyclophosphamide and TBI. The remaining six patients received conditioning regimen prior to HSCT. Four patients who received etoposide (900 mg/m²), cyclophosphamide (200 mg/kg), and busulfan (16 mg/kg) experienced engraftment. One patient who received etoposide (400 mg/m²), cyclophosphamide (200 mg/kg), and busulfan (20 mg/kg) failed to experience engraftment. Failure also followed a second attempt at HSCT using etoposide (400 mg/m²), cyclophosphamide (200 mg/kg), ATG, and busulfan (26 mg/kg), and the patient died. Three patients were mixed hematologic chimeras and still had abnormal leukocyte inclusions in a proportion of their granulocytes. Six of seven patients were reported to be alive and doing well. In all of these instances of graft failure, the grafts were not T cell–depleted. HSCT corrects the life-threatening hematologic defects and eliminates the risk of "accelerated phase" but does not reverse the pseudoalbinism and neurologic damage.[44, 59–61]

X-Linked CD40 Ligand Deficiency: X-Linked Hyperimmunoglobulin M Syndrome

CD40 ligand deficiency affects humoral and, to a variable extent, cell-mediated immunity.[62] CD40 ligand is a 39-kd glycoprotein expressed on activated T cells and is required for proliferation and isotype switching of mature, CD40+ B cells (reviewed in references 63 and 64). Interactions between CD40 and its ligand are also central to activation of other antigen-presenting cells such as monocytes, macrophages, and their derivatives and are important for driving nitric oxide synthesis and IL-12 production, thus promoting the synthesis of type I cytokines (such as IL-2 and interferon-γ) that shape the cell-mediated immune response.[63] In addition to low or absent levels of IgG, IgA, and IgE and normal or elevated levels of serum IgM, many patients with CD40 ligand deficiency demonstrate poor cytotoxic T-cell function. Life-threatening infections are common.

A review of 43 cases confirms the clinical severity of this disorder.[65] Opportunistic infections (*Pneumocystis carinii* and *Cryptosporidium*) are common. Failure to thrive and liver dysfunction are typical. Most patients die of infections in the early decades of life, but liver cirrhosis and hepatocellular carcinoma, sclerosing cholangitis, and bile duct carcinoma occur at a high rate. Several patients have undergone orthotopic liver transplantation.[66, 67] Interestingly, sclerosing cholangitis recurred in two patients, suggesting that liver transplantation is not curative. It is unknown whether HSCT will prevent liver disease. Successful allogeneic HSCT using HLA-identical sibling donors has been reported for CD40 ligand deficiency.[68] Because of the variable clinical severity in patients with this disease (probably due to the large number of different mutations in patients with this disease),[69–73] the decision to proceed to HSCT has been based on a history of poor outcome among other affected family members and the presence of severe T-cell deficiency (e.g., the occurrence of *Pneumocystis carinii*) pneumonia.

X-Linked Lymphoproliferative Syndrome

Patients with X-linked lymphoproliferative syndrome (XLP) are susceptible to life-threatening infections by Epstein-Barr virus (EBV)[74] and other opportunistic infections. Complications of XLP include hyper- or hypo-gammaglobulinemia, fatal infectious mononucleosis, or aplastic anemia after an infection with EBV. Lymphomas, both EBV+ and EBV–, are common. The prognosis is poor, with a median survival time of less than 10 years. The defective gene has been localized to the long arm of the X chromosome.[75] HSCT is the only known cure for XLP.[76, 77]

Chronic Granulomatous Disease

Chronic granulomatous disease (CGD) is characterized by lymphadenopathy with draining nodes, hepatosplenomegaly, pneumonia, and dermatitis, which present by age 2 years. Infections by catalase-positive organisms such as *Staphylococcus aureus, Aspergillus* and *Serratia* species, *Escherichia coli,* and *Pseudomonas* species commonly result in abscess formation, especially in the lung. CGD is caused by the failure of the nicotinamide adenine dinucleotide phosphate (NADPH) oxidase of phagocytes to generate superoxide required for intracellular killing of phagocytized organisms. Defects in the four components of the NADPH oxidase system have been described and can be inherited as X-linked or autosomal recessive.[78] The most common genetic defects are in the gp91-phox component of NADPH oxidase. Abnormalities of gp91-phox occur in virtually all forms of the X-linked CGD and account for 57% of CGD cases. Interferon-γ has been shown to result in clinical improvement in many cases.[79] Leukocyte transfusions have been able to help control life-threatening infections. Although HSCT is the only means to cure CGD,[80, 81] its use is presently considered in cases in which a trial of interferon has failed.

Kostmann Syndrome

Patients with severe, congenital neutropenia (Kostmann syndrome) present with recurrent bacterial infections in infancy. The bone marrow from patients with Kostmann syndrome typically shows an arrest of myelopoiesis at the promyelocyte or myelocyte stage. The defect in Kostmann syndrome is unknown. The use of granulocyte colony-stimulating factor (G-CSF) has resulted in improvement in granulocyte numbers in many patients and improvement in the clinical symptoms.[82] Prior to the use of G-CSF, few patients survived more than 5 years. Patients with Kostmann syndrome have been reported to experience acute myelogenous leukemia.[83, 84] It is unclear whether the development of leukemia is related to the chronic use of G-CSF or represents a spectrum of the disease that has only become apparent as a result of the prolonged survival made possible by the use of G-CSF. Although HSCT has been shown to cure patients with Kostmann syndrome,[85] HSCT is currently recommended only for patients with Kostmann syndrome in whom G-CSF therapy has failed or leukemia has developed.

Purine Nucleoside Phosphorylase Deficiency

Purine nucleoside phosphorylase deficiency is an autosomal recessive disorder of purine metabolism with heterogeneous clinical manifestations (reviewed in reference 86). Qualitative and quantitative T-cell deficiencies (in particular, a disproportional decrease in CD3+CD8+ cells) occur and are progressive over time, leading to recurrent infections. Approximately two thirds of patients have neurologic abnormalities and/or developmental delay. Autoimmune complications are frequent, and there is an increased risk of lymphoma. No patient is known to have survived to age 30 years without HSCT. The few reported cases have required the use of conditioning regimen to achieve prompt engraftment, similar what occurs with ADA deficiency.[24, 87]

ISSUES RELATED TO DONOR SELECTION AND THE NEED FOR CONDITIONING REGIMEN

With the exception of patients with SCID, all other forms of prematurely lethal immunodeficiencies allow sufficient immune function to reject marrow from an HLA-identical sibling and should prompt pre-HSCT conditioning therapy. Busulfan (4 mg/kg/day $\times$ 4 days) followed by cyclophosphamide (60 mg/kg/day $\times$ 2 days) has been widely used as a conditioning therapy for nonmalignant diseases. This regimen has been successfully used in hundreds of cases of thalassemia and is associated with a less than 10% incidence of fatal complications.[14] The main drawback to this regimen is the occasional report of graft failure.[14] According to published series, the incidence of graft failure is less than 10%. Although the incidence is low, graft failure is associated with a high incidence of fatal infections. For these reasons, some have modified the busulfan and cyclophosphamide regimen by adding thiotepa or ATG.[88] The number of patients undergoing transplantation using such regimens is too small to determine whether these maneu-

vers will be successful in reducing the low incidence of graft failures.

With the exception of some cases of SCID, patients who receive a haploidentical transplant require conditioning regimen to prevent rejection. A number of non–TBI-containing conditioning therapies have been reported to result in occasional engraftment of haploidentical grafts in patients with LAD, CHS, WAS, and Omenn syndrome.[9] It is difficult to estimate the incidence of rejection associated with these conditioning regimens because the reported data usually represent selected results from single centers and do not reflect the unsuccessful individual cases, which likely outnumber published reports. In general, patients with immunodeficiencies (other than SCID) treated with haploidentical transplantation require an intensive conditioning regimen similar to that used for patients with malignancies in order for engraftment to occur. Conditioning therapies that result in a high rate of engraftment of haploidentical grafts all contain TBI.[89–92] The relative risks of rejection vary, depending on the use of conditioning regimen, the underlying disease, the HLA disparity between donor and recipient, and the use of T-cell depletion.

Death from post-transplantation EBV-associated lymproliferative disease has also been a major complication in patients with WAS and CHS after haploidentical T-cell–depleted HSCT.[93, 94] This complication tends to be more common in patients in whom T cells have been exhaustively depleted. Data suggest that infusion of donor T cells may be useful in treating this complication.[95]

USE OF UNRELATED DONORS FOR TREATMENT OF PATIENTS WITH IMMUNODEFICIENCIES

Over 3 million potential marrow donors are available through the NMDP. The increased availability of potential donors allows transplantation for nearly all patients lacking a matched sibling donor. Unrelated donors have been successfully used to treat patients with immunodeficiencies.[43, 45, 88, 96, 97] In the earliest series of 12 patients with lethal immunodeficiencies who underwent unrelated donor HSCT, marrows were not T cell–depleted. Of eight patients with SCID (including one patient with Omenn syndrome and one patient with ADA deficiency), two had WAS and two had CHS.[88] All patients received short-course methotrexate, prednisone, and either cyclosporin A or ATG for GVHD prophylaxis. Of three patients with SCID undergoing HSCT without conditioning regimen, engraftment failed in two, who received a second transplant after administration of busulfan, cyclophosphamides, and ATG as conditioning therapy. Both patients subsequently experienced engraftment. Five patients who had unusual variants of SCID and two with WAS received busulfan, cyclophosphamides and ATG as conditioning therapy. All experienced engraftment. Two patients with CHS received conditioning regimens that included TBI and subsequently experienced engraftment. Three of 12 patients had grade III acute GVHD, and one patient had grade II acute GVHD. Chronic GVHD was not observed. All patients had evidence of immunoreconstitution. The actuarial survival rate was 83%, and all of the surviving patients remained clinically well at last report.

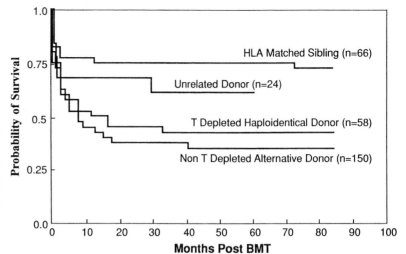

FIGURE 14–1. Probability of survival after HSCT for severe combined immunodeficiency by bone marrow donor type. Data for recipients of HLA-matched sibling BMT (n = 66), T-depleted haploidentical donor BMT (n = 58), and BMT from alternative (related) donors without T-cell–depletion (n = 150) were obtained from the International Bone Marrow Transplantation Registry, Milwaukee. Data for recipients of unrelated donor bone marrow (all non–T cell–depleted) were provided by the National Marrow Donor Program, Minneapolis. (From Filipovich AH: Stem cell transplantation from unrelated donors for correction of primary immunodeficiencies. Immunol Allerg Clin North Am 16:385, 1996.)

An analysis of the first 50 patients who received marrow from unrelated donors (including the earlier-mentioned series) showed that high-risk patients (high-risk = history of a life-threatening complication within 3 months prior to HSCT, n = 25) experienced a 20% long-term survival rate, whereas average-risk patients (n = 25) experienced an 80% long-term survival rate. Exacerbations of infectious or other complications account for the differences in the groups.[98]

Too few patients with SCID have received unrelated donor grafts to know whether conditioning regimen is necessary to facilitate engraftment. Until such data are available, the decision to use conditioning regimen for patients with SCID who receive unrelated donor grafts should be based on whether patients are at risk for exacerbation of ongoing infectious complications or there is a need to ablate host or third-party cells (e.g., autoimmune disease, GVHD, facilitating engraftment of other hematopoietic elements, lymphoproliferative disease).

Patients with SCID variants and other immunodeficiencies appear to need a non–TBI-containing conditioning regimen prior to receiving the non–T cell–depleted graft from an unrelated donor. Data from the IBMTR comparing

survival rates for patients who underwent HSCT using HLA-identical sibling donors, unrelated donors, and haploindentical donors, showed that although the groups are heterogeneous with respect to conditioning regimen, pre-existing complications, and GVHD prophylaxis, the results with unrelated donor HSCT were superior to those with haploidentical donor transplants. The survival of both unrelated and haploidentical-related donor transplants was not as good as that using a matched sibling donor (Fig. 14–1).

Data from 29 patients with WAS who received unrelated donor transplants have been submitted to the NMDP.[98] The overall survival rate was 67% at 3 years post-HSCT (Fig. 14–2). The poor outcome of unrelated donor transplants compared with sibling donor transplants might be explained by a high incidence of GVHD: 50% of patients who received an unrelated or mismatched, related donor transplant had grade II–IV GVHD. In contrast, recipients of matched sibling donor transplants had less than 20% incidence of grade II or higher GVHD. Another factor that may account for the poor survival of unrelated donor transplants is that older recipients of unrelated donor transplants were generally in the terminal stages of their disease

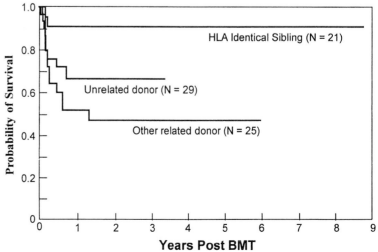

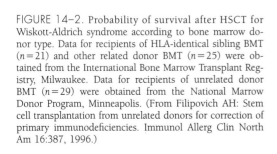

FIGURE 14–2. Probability of survival after HSCT for Wiskott-Aldrich syndrome according to bone marrow donor type. Data for recipients of HLA-identical sibling BMT (n = 21) and other related donor BMT (n = 25) were obtained from the International Bone Marrow Transplant Registry, Milwaukee. Data for recipients of unrelated donor BMT (n = 29) were obtained from the National Marrow Donor Program, Minneapolis. (From Filipovich AH: Stem cell transplantation from unrelated donors for correction of primary immunodeficiencies. Immunol Allerg Clin North Am 16:387, 1996.)

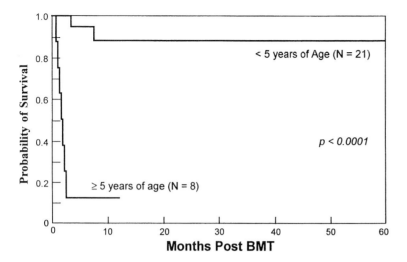

FIGURE 14-3. Probability of survival after unrelated donor BMT for Wiskott-Aldrich syndrome according to recipient age at the time of transplantation. Data from National Marrow Donor Program, Minneapolis. (From Filipovich AH: Stem cell transplantation from unrelated donors for correction of primary immunodeficiencies. Immunol Allerg Clin North Am 16:388, 1996.)

and included two who had a history of prior lymphoma. Patients with WAS who are older than 5 years and more likely to have had life-threatening complications fared poorly when compared with patients receiving transplants at a younger age (Fig. 14-3).

THE USE OF UNRELATED VERSUS HAPLOIDENTICAL DONORS

Both unrelated and haploidentical marrow are good sources of HSC for patients with classic forms of SCID who lack HLA-identical sibling donors. The decision to select one over another source depends on several factors. A center must have access to a T cell–depletion method suitable for removing 2–3 logs of T cells so as to prevent severe GVHD after haploidentical HSCT, whereas HSCT using unrelated donor marrow can be carried out without T-cell depletion. The method used to deplete T cells from haploidentical marrow should also remove B cells capable of transferring EBV from a seropositive donor to a seronegative recipient in order to lower the risk of EBV-associated lymproliferative disease. The risk of EBV-associated lymproliferative disease is higher in recipients of T cell–depleted marrow from mismatched donors than in recipients of non–T cell–depleted grafts.

Although disparity for one class I locus does not appear to adversely affect the outcome of unrelated donor HSCT in children,[99] the use of unmodified, unrelated donor marrow is associated with a high incidence of GVHD compared with HLA-identical sibling donors.[100] The use of T-cell depletion for unrelated donor HSCT is being studied in a multi-institutional, randomized, prospective trial. The results of this trial may provide data to determine whether T-cell depletion should be routinely used for unrelated donor HSCT.

Patients with immunodeficiencies other than SCID are likely to need TBI for engraftment using a haploidentical donor, whereas unrelated donor transplants (not T cell–depleted) can be performed using chemotherapy-based conditioning regimens. Other drawbacks to the use of unrelated donor marrow are the high cost of procurement, the length of time required to identify a donor, and the lack

of donors, particularly for some ethnic minorities. The advantages and disadvantages of haploidentical and unrelated donor transplants are summarized in Table 14–4.

ENGRAFTMENT AND IMMUNORECONSTITUTION

DOCUMENTATION OF ENGRAFTMENT AND IMMUNORECONSTITUTION

For patients who receive conditioning regimen, donor cells are easily detectable as patients recover from the therapy-induced pancytopenia. The most straightforward way is to examine peripheral blood for engraftment of donor T cells. For patients with SCID, flow cytometry should be per-

TABLE 14–4. ADVANTAGES AND DISADVANTAGES OF UNRELATED VERSUS HAPLOIDENTICAL, RELATED MARROW AS A SOURCE OF STEM CELLS

	UNRELATED DONOR	**HAPLOIDENTICAL DONOR**
Advantages	1. Does not require T-cell depletion 2. Engraftment can be achieved without total body irradiation (TBI) in most cases	1. Highly motivated donor usually available
Disadvantages	1. Expensive 2. Requires 2–3 months to identify a donor 3. Not available at every transplant center	1. Requires T-cell depletion* 2. TBI is required for consistent engraftment (patients other than those with severe combined immunodeficiency disease)

*>2.5 logs T-cell depletion and depletion of B cells, which may carry Epstein-Barr virus (EBV) from seropositive donors to non–EBV-exposed recipient, is desirable; marrow manipulation may be costly and not available at many centers.

formed to quantify T-cell numbers after HSCT. The origin of the cells (donor vs. recipient) can be determined with anti-HLA antibodies (in cases of HLA-disparate donors), cytogenetics, or DNA analysis, the latter being the most sensitive. Patients with SCID who receive unmodified marrow from HLA-identical siblings often have lymphoid elements of donor origin in the peripheral blood. Donor peripheral blood T cells can be detected using the polymerase chain reaction as early as 2 weeks post HSCT. Patients with selective engraftment of T cells have been shown to experience engraftment of T-cell progenitors. Subset analysis of CD34+ cells obtained from a patient with SCID undergoing HSCT with haploidentical marrow without conditioning regimen showed a small proportion to be donor-derived and expressing CD2 and CD7. The patient did not have evidence of donor-derived CD34+ cells that expressed myeloid antigens.[101]

Examples of mixed T-cell chimerism, mixed B-cell chimerism, and lymphoid/monocyte chimerism (donor lymphocyte, recipient monocyte) have been reported.[102, 103] An example of mixed megakaryocytic chimerism was reported in a patient with WAS.[104] In cases of mixed chimerism, it is important to document engraftment of donor lymphocytes or those cells that were functionally defective in the underlying immunodeficiency (e.g., platelets in WAS, neutrophils in CHS, cells expressing CD11/CD18 or CD40 ligand in LAD and CD40 ligand deficiency, respectively).

Reconstitution of T-Cell Function

Time to recovery of normal numbers of T cells varies greatly, depending on the use of immunosuppressive drugs to prevent or treat GVHD and HLA disparity between donor and recipient. The influence of GVHD on immunoreconstitution is reviewed elsewhere in this book (see Chapters 39, 45, and 54). Recipients of grafts from HLA-identical siblings typically demonstrate normal numbers of peripheral blood T cells by 2 months after HSCT.[105, 106] Recipients of haploidentical grafts experience delayed reconstitution of T cells compared with recipients of grafts from HLA-identical siblings. The median time for achieving normal numbers of CD3+, CD4+, and CD8+ cells is 10 months post HSCT, with most patients having normal numbers of T cells and subsets by 1 year post HSCT.[24, 107, 108] The responses to phytohemagglutinin (PHA), pokeweed mitogen (PWM), and alloantigen, as tested using the mixed lymphocyte reaction, similarly normalize by 1 year post HSCT in the majority of patients who experience durable engraftment and do not have chronic GVHD. The responses to PWM and alloantigen tend to normalize before the response to PHA. The median times for a normal response to PWM, alloantigen, and PHA were reported to be 4.0, 5.5, and 7.0 months, respectively.[107] The median time for detecting an initial response to PHA was 4 months (range, 1–6 months). There was no difference in the kinetics of reconstitution in patients who received preparative therapy and recipients who did not.

The etiology of delayed immunoreconstitution in patients undergoing mismatched HSCT is not understood. Several hypotheses have been put forth to explain these observations, including the presence of subclinical

GVHD,[109] HLA differences between donor and recipient, and a paucity of donor-derived antigen-presenting cells.[110–112]

Reconstitution of B-Cell Function

Ninety percent of patients with SCID who received grafts from HLA-matched siblings without conditioning regimen experienced reconstitution of B-cell function.[105, 106] Reconstitution of B-cell function has been reported in cases wherein the B cells remain of host origin, suggesting that recipient B cells may be intrinsically normal in many cases of SCID.[106, 113, 114]

In contrast, after HLA-identical transplantation, reconstitution of B-cell function can only be expected in approximately 50% of patients with SCID who receive haploidentical grafts.[24–26, 105, 107, 113, 114] The use of conditioning regimens improves the efficiency of B-cell engraftment but probably does not hasten the tempo of B-cell reconstitution. In recipients of haploidentical grafts, the absolute numbers of peripheral blood B cells normalize 12–15 months post HSCT.[24, 107] In some cases, the normal B-cell numbers have been achieved more than 5 years after HSCT.[107] The median time to normalize B-cell function (production of isohemagglutinins) has been reported to be 18 months after haploidentical HSCT and has been documented to occur as late as 8 years after HSCT.[107] The basis for the low rate of B-cell engraftment and slow functional recovery in recipients of grafts from haploidentical donors is not well understood. In light of the high rate of reconstitution of B-cell function in recipients of grafts from HLA-identical siblings, it is probably not due to the lack of "space." More likely, it is due to persistent defects in cell-cell interaction.

The variable engraftment of B cells has implications for the continued use of intravenous gamma globulin (IVGG) after HSCT. IVGG is commonly used in recipients of allogeneic HSCT to reduce infectious complications and may reduce the incidence of acute GVHD after HSCT.[115] Because B-cell function varies from patient to patient, the duration of IVGG therapy needs to be determined case by case. Determining the isohemagglutinin titer is a useful indicator to document reconstitution of B-cell function.[107] Because isohemagglutinins are of the IgM class and are not in high titer in commercially available preparations of IVGG, the presence of isohemagglutinins in transplant recipients, along with normalization of quantitative serum IgM and IgA levels, is an indicator that B-cell reconstitution is occurring and that IVGG may be discontinued. It is important to monitor endogenous IgG production and specific response to immunizations to confirm full B-cell functional recovery. IVGG should be discontinued at least 4 months prior to immunizing the patient.

SHOULD PATIENTS WITH PARTIAL ENGRAFTMENT UNDERGO RETRANSPLANTATION?

In patients with SCID who did not receive conditioning regimen, the failure to detect donor T cells or donor DNA by 2 months after HSCT suggests that rejection has occurred and warrants conditioning therapy followed by a second transplant. For patients with low levels of engraftment, the decision to perform a second HSCT or "boost" is usually based on the lack of improvement in T-cell function by 5–6 months after HSCT. Significant immunocompetence, as demonstrated by the development of antigen-specific humoral and cell-mediated responses, has occurred in patients with SCID with low percentages of circulating donor cells (<5% in some cases). Because the reconstitution of B-cell numbers and function is highly variable and IVGG therapy is usually effective therapy for hypogammaglobulinemia, most patients in whom B-cell function does not reconstitute do not receive a second transplant.

In cases of LAD and CGD, low levels of donor cells (3–10%) have been associated with freedom from life-threatening infections.[116, 117]

The proportion of donor chimerism can fluctuate with time even in patients who have received conditioning chemotherapy. Patients who demonstrated 10–25% donor cells during the first year post HSCT have gone on to show full donor hematopoietic cells in later years.

FUTURE CONSIDERATIONS

The use of umbilical cord blood as a source of HSC is under active study. Cord blood contains T cells that are relatively naive compared to postnatal cells and may be less likely to produce severe GVHD. The use of cord blood may allow successful partially matched transplants. Another advantage of cord blood is that it may serve as a source of HSC for patients whose HLA types are not well represented in the NMDP. Although the initial reports of cord blood transplants are encouraging,[118, 119] reports of graft failure exist, particularly in patients who received sublethal conditioning regimen,[120] and lethal GVHD has occurred at a number of institutions. We must audit the results of ongoing studies to learn the incidence and severity of GVHD as well as the incidence of graft failure before the use of cord blood cells as a means of correcting immunodeficiencies can be recommended. Additionally, cord blood HSC are collected anonymously and no universally accepted mechanism for retrieving additional HSC from the same donor (i.e., in the case of rejection) currently exists. Also, there is a small chance that cord blood HSC may harbor unrecognized genetic defects. Discussion of cord blood HSC can be found in Chapter 26.

The use of retrovirally mediated gene therapy is also being studied. Persistence of genetically "corrected" cells has been documented in several patients with ADA deficiency, although all recipients continue to receive PEG-ADA treatment.[121] Progress in the development of techniques for gene transduction into HSC has been slow. It is not yet clear whether gene therapy for the primary immunodeficiencies will confer a survival or proliferative advantage to transduced cells. The present limitations to the use of gene therapy for immunodeficiencies are both technical (low rate of transduction efficiency) and theoretical in that the defects underlying many of the immunodeficiencies readily treated by HSCT involve genes whose natural regulatory requirements are still poorly understood. Much remains to be learned before effective gene therapy can be proposed as a promising alternative to HSCT for the majority of patients with primary immunodeficiencies. Gene therapy using HSC is reviewed in Chapter 17.

CONCLUSION

Allogeneic HSCT is the treatment of choice for many congenital immunodeficiencies. When an HLA-matched sibling donor is available, HSCT can be performed in early or late childhood, depending on the disease or condition (see Tables 14–1 and 14–2). Success with HSCT in SCID using haploidentical donors has been reported. The role of T-cell depletion, graft rejection, and conditioning regimens remains to be determined. Currently, the number of patients receiving HSCT using matched unrelated donors is too few for a comprehensive analysis of issues such as conditioning regimens, T-cell depletion, pre-existing complications, and GVHD prophylaxis. Newer forms of therapy are now under active investigation. It is possible to use unrelated cord blood as a source of HSC for allogeneic HSCT. This option is being studied in clinical trials. Infusion of autologous HSC that have been genetically modified to correct for the disease and/or condition may also become possible in the future.

REFERENCES

1. Gatti RA, Meeuwissen HJ, Allen HD, et al: Immunological reconstitution of sex-linked lymphopenic immunological deficiency. Lancet 2:1366–1369, 1968.
2. Pollack M, Kirkpatrick D, Kapoor N, O'Reilly R: Identification by HLA typing of intrauterine derived maternal T cells in four patients with severe combined immunodeficiency. N Engl J Med 307:662–666, 1982.
3. Friedrich W, Muller S, Braumuller H: Engraftment of maternal lymphocytes in SCID: incidence and significance based on an analysis in 86 patients. Presented at the VII Meeting of the European Society for Immunodeficiencies, Goteborg, 1996, Abstract 14.
4. Washington K, Gossage D, Gottfried M: Pathology of the liver in severe combined immunodeficiency and DiGeorge syndrome. Pediatr Pathol 13:485–504, 1993.
5. Jarvis WR, Middleton PJ, Gelfand EW: Significance of viral infections in severe combined immunodeficiency disease. J Infect Dis 2:187–192, 1983.
6. Dagan R, Schwartz RH, Insel RA, Menegus MA: Severe diffuse adenovirus 7a pneumonia in a child with combined immunodeficiency: possible therapeutic effect of human immune serum globulin containing specific neutralizing antibody. Pediatr Infect Dis 3:246–251, 1984.
7. Gilger MA, Matson DO, Conner ME, et al: Extraintestinal rotavirus infections in children with immunodeficiency. J Pediatr 120:912–917, 1992.
8. Stiehm ER, Chin TW, Haas A, Peerless AG: Infectious complications of the primary immunodeficiencies. Clin Immunol Immunopathol 40:69–86, 1986.
9. Fischer A, Griscelli C, Friedrich W, et al: Bone marrow transplantation for immunodeficiencies and osteopetrosis: European survey 1968–1985. Lancet 2:1080–1084, 1986.
10. Fischer A, Landais P, Friedrich W, et al: European experience of bone-marrow transplantation for severe combined immunodeficiency. Lancet 336:850–854, 1990.
11. Bortin M, Rimm A: Severe combined immunodeficiency disease: characterization of the disease and results of transplantation. JAMA 230:591–600, 1977.
12. O'Reilly RJ, Kapoor N, Kirkpatrick D, et al: Transplantation of hematopoietic cells for lethal congenital immunodeficiencies. Birth Defects 19:129–137, 1983.
13. O'Reilly RJ, Keever CA, Small TN, Brochstein J: The use of HLA-

non-identical T-cell-depleted marrow transplants for correction of severe combined immunodeficiency disease. Immununodef Rev 1:273–309, 1989.

14. Lucarelli G, Galimberti M, Polchi P, et al: Bone marrow transplantation in patients with thalassemia. N Engl J Med 322(7):417–421, 1990.

15. Reinherz E, Geha R, Rappaport J, et al: Reconstitution after transplantation with T lymphocyte depleted HLA haplotype mismatched bone marrow for severe combined immunodeficiency. Proc Natl Acad Sci U S A 79:6047, 1982.

16. Vossen JM, Asma GEM, Van Den Bergh RL, et al: HLA-identical and haploidentical bone marrow transplantation for severe combined immunodeficiency: chimerism and immunological reconstitution in vitro and in vivo. In Griscelli G. Vossens J (eds): Progress in Immunodeficiency Research and Therapy I. Amsterdam, Elsevier Science, 1984, pp. 417–424.

17. Fischer A, Durandy A, De Villartay JP, et al: HLA-haploidentical bone marrow transplantation for severe combined immunodeficiency using E-rosette fractionation and cyclosporine. Blood 67:444–449, 1986.

18. O'Reilly R, Brochstein J, Collins N, et al: Evaluation of HLA-haplotype disparate parental marrow grafts depleted of T lymphocytes by differential agglutination with a soybean lectin and E-Rosette depletion for the treatment of severe combined immunodeficiency Vox Sang 51 (Suppl 2):81–86, 1986.

19. O'Reilly R, Keever C, Kernan N, et al: HLA nonidentical T-cell depleted marrow transplants: a comparison of results in patients treated for leukemia and severe combined immnunodeficiency disease. Transplant Proc 19 (Suppl 7):55–60, 1987.

20. Fischer A, Friedrich W, Godthelp B, et al: Bone marrow transplantation. In Fasth A, Bjorkander J (eds): Progress in Immunodeficiency VI. Amsterdam, Elsevier Science, 1996, pp. 111–113.

21. Murphy W, Kumar V, Bennett M: Rejection of bone marrow allografts by mice with severe combined immunodeficiency (SCID) J Exp Med 165:1212–1217, 1987.

22. Murphy W, Kumar V, Bennett M: Acute rejection of murine bone marrow allografts by natural killer cells and T-cells. J Exp Med 166:1499–1509, 1987.

23. Warner J, Dennert G: Bone marrow graft rejection as a function of antibody-directed natural killer cells. J Exp Med 161:563, 1985.

24. Buckley R, Schiff S, Sampson H, et al: Development of immunity in human severe primary T-cell deficiency following haploidentical bone marrow stem cell transplantation J Immunol 136:2398–2407, 1986.

25. Cowan M, Wara D, Weintraub P, et al: Haploidentical bone marrow transplantation for severe combined immunodeficiency disease using soybean agglutinin-negative, T-depleted marrow cells J Clin Immunol 5:370–376, 1985.

26. Friedrich W, Goldmann S, Ebell W, et al: Severe combined immunodeficiency: treatment by bone marrow transplantation in 15 infants using HLA-haploidentical donors Eur J Pediatr 144:125–130, 1985.

27. Kapoor N, Jung L, Engelhard D, et al: Lymphoma in a patient with severe combined immunodeficiency with adenosine deaminase deficiency, following unsustained engraftment of histoincompatible T-cell depleted bone marrow J Pediatr 108:435–438, 1986.

28. Barrett M, Buckley R, Schiff S, et al: Accelerated development of immunity following transplantation of maternal marrow stem cells into infants with severe combined immunodeficiency and transplacentally acquired lymphoid chimerism. Clin Exp Immunol 72:118–123, 1988.

29. Hershfield MS, Buckley RH, Greenberg ML, et al: Treatment of adenosine deaminase deficiency with polythene glycol-modified adenosine deaminase. N Engl J Med. 316:589–596, 1987.

30. Cederbaum SD, Niwayama G, Stiehm ER, et al: Combined immunodeficiency presenting as the Letterer-Siwe syndrome. J Pediatr 85:466–471, 1974.

31. Gomez L, Le Deist F, Blanche S, et al: Treatment of Omenn syndrome by bone marrow transplantation. J Pediatr 127(1):76–81, 1995.

32. Bruckmann C, Lindner W, Roos R, et al: Severe pulmonary vascular occlusive disease following bone marrow transplantation in Omenn syndrome. Eur J Pediatr 150(4):242–245, 1991.

33. Loechelt BJ, Shapiro RS, Jyonouchi H, Filipovich AH: Mismatched bone marrow transplantation of Omenn syndrome: a variant of severe combined immunodeficiency. Bone Marrow Transplant 16:381–385, 1995.

34. Van Leeuwen J, van Tol M, Joosten A, et al: Relationship between patterns of engraftment in peripheral blood and immune reconstitution after allogeneic bone marrow transplantation for (severe) combined immunodeficiency. Blood 84:3936–3947, 1994.

35 Klein C, Cavazzana-Calvo M, Le Deist F, et al: Bone marrow transplantation in major histocompatibility complex class II deficiency: a single-center study of 19 patients. Blood 85(2):580–587, 1995.

36. Knobloch C, Ballas M, Wolpl A, Friedrich W: Allorecognition and T cell repertoire selection in severe combined immunodeficiency lacking HLA class II antigens. Transplantation 53:1295–1301, 1992.

37. Fischer A, Lisowska-Grosspiere B, Anderson C, Springer T: Leukocyte adhesion deficiency: molecular basis and functional consequences. Immunodef Rev. 1:39–55, 1988.

38. Kishimoto TK, Hollander N, Roberts TM, et al: Heterogeneous mutations in the beta subunit common to the LFA-1, Mac-1, and p150,95 glycoproteins cause leukocyte adhesion deficiency. Cell 50(2):193–202, 1987.

39. Thomas C, Le Deist F, Cavazzana-Calvo M, et al: Results of allogeneic bone marrow transplantation in patients with leukocyte adhesion deficiency. Blood 86(4):1629–1635, 1995.

40. Henter JI: Diagnostic guidelines for hemophagocytic lymphohistiocytosis. Semin Oncol 18:29–33, 1991.

41. Hirst WJ, Layton DM, Singh S, et al: Haemophagocytic lymphohistiocytosis: experience at two U.K. centres. Br J Haematol 88(4):731–739, 1994.

42. Bolme P, Henter JI, Winiarski J, et al: Allogeneic bone marrow transplantation for hemophagocytic lymphohistiocytosis in Sweden. Bone Marrow Transplant 15(3):331–335, 1995.

43. Neudorf S, Rybka W, Ball E, et al: The use of counterflow centrifugal elutriation for the depletion of T cells from unrelated donor bone marrow. J Hematother 6:351–359, 1997.

44. Fischer A, Landais P, Friedrich W, et al: Bone marrow transplantation (BMT) in Europe for primary immunodeficiencies other than severe combined immunodeficiency: a report from the European Group for BMT and the European Group for Immunodeficiency. Blood 83(4):1149–1154, 1994.

45. Baker K, DeLaat C, Steinbuch M, et al: Successful correction of hematophagocytic lymphohistiocytosis with related or unrelated bone marrow transplantation. Blood 89:3857–3863, 1997.

46. Derry JM, Ochs HD, Francke U: Isolation of a novel gene mutated in Wiskott-Aldrich syndrome. Cell 78:635–644, 1994.

47. Mullen CA, Anderson KD, Blaese RM: Splenectomy and/or bone marrow transplantation in the management of the Wiskott-Aldrich syndrome: long-term follow-up of 62 cases. Blood 82(10):2961–2966, 1993.

48. Lum LG, Tubergen DG, Blaese RM: Splenectomy in the management of the thrombocytopenia of the Wiskott-Aldrich syndrome. N Engl J Med 302:892–896, 1980.

49. Sullivan KE, Mullen CA, Blaese RM, Winkelstein JA: A multi-institutional survey of the Wiskott-Aldrich syndrome. J Pediatr 125:876–885, 1994.

50. Bach F, Albertini R, Anderson J, et al: Bone marrow transplantation in a patient with the Wiskott Aldrich syndrome. Lancet 2:1364–1366, 1968.

51. Kapoor N, Kirkpatrick D, Blaese RM, et al: Reconstitution of normal megakaryocytopoiesis and immunologic functions in Wiskott-Aldrich syndrome by marrow transplantation following myeloablation and immunosuppression with busulfan and cyclophosphamide. Blood 57:692–696, 1981.

52. Brochstein JA, Gillio AP, Ruggiero M, et al: Marrow transplantation from human leukocyte antigen-identical or haploidentical donors for correction of Wiskott-Aldrich syndrome. J Pediatr 119(6):907–912, 1991.

53. Vassal G, Fischer A, Challine D, et al: Busulfan disposition below the age of three: alteration in children with lysosomal storage disease. Blood 82(3):1030–1034, 1993.

54. Grochow L, Krivit W, Whitley C, Blazar B: Busulfan disposition in children. Blood 75:1723, 1990.

55. Perou CM, Moore KJ, Nagle DL, et al: Identification of the murine beige gene by YAC complementation and positional cloning. Nature Genet 13(3):303–308, 1996.

56. Stiehm R, Fulginiti V (eds): Immunologic Disorders in Infants and Children. Philadelphia, WB Saunders, 1980, p 361.

57. Clark RA, Kimball HR: Defective granulocyte chemotaxis in the Chédiak-Higashi syndrome. J Clin Invest 50:2645–2652, 1971.

58. Katz PA, Zaytoun A, Fauci A: Deficiency of active natural killer cells in the Chédiak-Higashi syndrome: localization of the defect using a single cell assay. J Clin Invest 69:1231–1238, 1982.

59. Haddad E, Le Deist F, Blanche S, et al: Treatment of Chédiak-Higashi syndrome by allogenic bone marrow transplantation: report of 10 cases. Blood 85(11):3328–3333, 1995.

60. Kazmierowski J, Elin R, Reynolds H, et al: Chédiak-Higashi syndrome: reversal of increased susceptibility to infection of bone marrow transplantation. Blood 47:555, 1976.

61. Virelizier JL, Lagrue A, Durandy A, et al: Reversal of natural-killer defect in a patient with Chédiak-Higashi syndrome after bone marrow transplantation. N Engl J Med 6:1055, 1982.

62. Notarangelo LD, Duse M, Ugazio AG: Immunodeficiency with hyper-IgM (HIM). Immunodefic Rev 3:101–122, 1992.

63. Callard RE, Armitage RJ, Fanslow WC: CD40 ligand and its role in X-linked hyper-IgM syndrome. Immunol Today 14:559–564, 1993.

64. Clark EA, Lane PJ: Regulation of human B-cell activation and adhesion. Annu Rev Immunol 9:97–127, 1991.

65. Levy J, Espanol T, Thomas C, et al: Clinical manifestations of 43 European patients with CD40 deficiency. Presented at the VII Meeting of the European Society for Immunodeficiencies, Goteborg, 1996, Abstract No. 38.

66. Caragol I, Hernandez M, Bertran J, et al: Clinical follow up and immunological characterization of hyper-IgM syndrome. Presented at the VII Meeting of the European Society for Immunodeficiencies, Goteborg, 1996, Abstract No. 40.

67. Banatvala N, Davies J, Kanariou M, et al: Hypogammaglobulinaemia associated with normal or increased IgM (the hyper IgM syndrome): a case series review. Arch Dis Child 71(2):150–152, 1994.

68. Thomas C, de Saint Basile G, Le Deist F, et al: Brief report: correction of X-linked hyper-IgM syndrome by allogeneic bone marrow transplantation. N Engl J Med 333(7):426–429, 1995.

69. Korthauer U, Graf D, Mages HW, et al: Defective expression of T-cell CD40 ligand causes X-linked immunodeficiency with hyper-IgM. Nature 361(6412):539–541, 1993.

70. DiSanto JP, Bonnefoy JY, Gauchat JF, et al: CD40 ligand mutations in x-linked immunodeficiency with hyper-IgM. Nature 361(6412):541–543, 1993.

71. Allen RC, Armitage RJ, Conley ME, et al: CD40 ligand gene defects responsible for X-linked hyper-IgM syndrome. Science 259(5097):990–993, 1993.

72. Aruffo A, Farrington M, Hollenbaugh D, et al: The CD40 ligand, gp39, is defective in activated T cells from patients with X-linked hyper-IgM syndrome. Cell 72(2):291–300, 1993.

73. Fuleihan R, Ramesh N, Loh R, et al: Defective expression of the CD40 ligand in X chromosome-linked immunoglobulin deficiency with normal or elevated IgM. Proc Natl Acad Sci USA 90(6):2170–2173, 1993.

74. Purtilo D, Cassel C, Yang J, Harper R: X-linked recessive progressive combined variable immunodeficiency (Duncan's disease). Lancet 1:935–940, 1975.

75. Skare JC, Milunsky A, Byron KS, Sullivan JL: Mapping the X-linked lymphoproliferative syndrome. Proc Natl Acad Sci USA 84(7):2015–2018, 1987.

76. Williams L, Rooney C, Conley M, et al: Correction of Duncan's syndrome by allogeneic bone marrow transplantation. Lancet 342:587–588, 1993.

77. Vowels MR, Po-Tang RL, Berdoukas V, et al: Brief report: correction of X-linked lymphoproliferative disease by transplantation of cord-blood stem cells. N Engl J Med 329:1623–1625, 1993.

78. Segal AW: The electron transport chain of the microbicidal oxidase of phagocytic cells and its involvement in the molecular pathology of chronic granulomatous disease. J Clin Invest 83:1785–1793, 1989.

79. International Chronic Granulomatous Disease Cooperative Study Group: A controlled trial of interferon gamma to prevent infection in chronic granulomatous disease. N Engl J Med 324:509–516, 1991.

80. Kamani N, August C, Campbell DE, et al: Marrow transplantation in chronic granulomatous disease: an update, with 6-year follow-up. J Pediatr 113:697–700, 1988.

81. Hobbs J, Monteil M, McCluskey D, et al: Chronic granulomatous diseases 100% corrected by displacement bone marrow transplantation from a volunteer unrelated donor. Eur J Pediatr 151:806–810, 1992.

82. Boxer L, Hutchinson R, Emerson S: Recombinant human granulocyte-colony stimulating factor in the treatment of patients with neutropenia. Clin Immunol Immunopathol 62:539–546, 1992.

83. Weinblatt ME, Scimeca P, James-Herry A, et al: Transformation of congenital neutropenia into monosomy 7 and acute nonlymphoblastic leukemia in a child treated with granulocyte colony-stimulating factor. J Pediatr 126(2):263–265, 1995.

84. Kalra R, Dale D, Freedman M, et al: Monosomy 7 and activating RAS mutations accompany malignant transformation in patients with congenital neutropenia. Blood 86(12):4579–4586, 1995.

85. Rappaport JM, Parkman R, Newburger PE, et al: Correction of infantile agranulocytosis by allogeneic bone marrow transplantation. Am J Med 68:605–609, 1980.

86. Markert ML: Purine nucleoside phosphorylase deficiency. Immunodefic Rev 3:45–81, 1991.

87. Carpenter PA, Ziegler JB, Vowels MR: Late diagnosis and correction of purine nucleoside phosphorylase deficiency with allogeneic bone marrow transplantation. Bone Marrow Transplant 17(1):121–124, 1996.

88. Filipovich AH, Shapiro RS, Ramsay NK, et al: Unrelated donor bone marrow transplantation for correction of lethal congenital immunodeficiencies. Blood 80(1):270–276, 1992.

89. Aversa F, Tabilio A, Terenzi A, et al: Successful engraftment of T-cell-depleted haploidentical "three-loci" incompatible transplants in leukemia patients by addition of recombinant human granulocyte colony-stimulating factor-mobilized peripheral blood progenitor cells to bone marrow inoculum. Blood 84(11):3948–3955, 1994.

90. Quinones RR, Gutierrez RH, Dinndorf PA, et al: Extended-cycle elutriation to adjust T-cell content in HLA-disparate bone marrow transplantation. Blood 82(1):307–317, 1993.

91. Rummelhart S, Trigg M, Horowitz S, Hong R: Monoclonal antibody T cell depleted HLA haploidentical bone marrow transplantation for Wiskott-Aldrich syndrome. Blood 75:1031–1035, 1990.

92. Henslee-Downey P, Abhyankar S, Parrish R, et al: Use of partially mismatched related donors extends access to allogeneic marrow transplant Blood 89:3864–3872, 1997.

93. Shapiro RS, McClain K, Frizzera G, et al: Epstein-Barr virus associated B cell lymphoproliferative disorders following bone marrow transplantation. Blood 71:1234–1243, 1988.

94. Zutter MM, Martin PJ, Sale GE, et al: Epstein-Barr virus lymphoproliferation after bone marrow transplantation. Blood 72:520–529, 1988.

95. Papadopoulos EB, Ladanyi M, Emanuel D, et al: Infusions of donor leukocytes to treat Epstein-Barr virus-associated lymphoproliferative disorders after allogeneic bone marrow transplantation. N Engl J Med 330(17):1185–1191, 1994.

96. O'Reilly R, Dupont B, Pahwa S, et al: Reconstitution in severe combined immunodeficiency by transplantation of marrow from an unrelated donor. N Engl J Med 297;565–567, 1977.

97. Lenarsky C, Weinberg K, Kohn D, Parkman R: Unrelated donor BMT for Wiskott-Aldrich syndrome. Bone Marrow Transplant 12:145–147, 1993.

98. Filipovich A: Stem cell transplantation from unrelated donors for correction of primary immunodeficiencies. Immunol Allergy Clin North Am (16):377–392, 1996.

99. Davies SM, Shu XO, Blazar BR, et al: Unrelated donor bone marrow transplantation: influence of HLA A and B incompatibility on outcome. Blood 86(4):1636–1642, 1995.

100. Kernan NA, Bartsch G, Ash RC, et al: Analysis of 462 transplantations from unrelated donors facilitated by the National Marrow Donor Program. N Engl J Med 328(9):593–602, 1993.

101. Tjonnfjord G, Steen R, Veiby O, et al: Evidence for engraftment of donor type multipotent CD34+ cells in a patient with selective T lymphocyte reconstitution after bone marrow transplantation for B-SCID. Blood 84:3584–3589, 1994.

102. Bacchetta R, Parkman R, McMahon M, et al: Dysfunctional cytokine production by host-reactive T-cell clones isolated from a chimeric severe combined immunodeficiency patient transplanted with haploidentical bone marrow. Blood 85(7):1944–1953, 1995.

103. Knobloch C, Goldmann SF, Harpprecht J, Friedrich W: Coexistence of donor and host T lymphocytes following HLA-different bone marrow transplantation into a patient with cellular immunodeficiency and nonfunctional CD4+ T cells. Transplantation 52(3):491–496, 1991.

104. Brunel V, Mozziconacci MJ, Sainty D, et al: Lafage-Pochitaloff M. Direct evidence for dissociated megakaryocytic chimaerism in a Wiskott-Aldrich patient successfully allografted. Br J Haematol 90(2):336–340, 1995.

105. Wijnaendts L, Le Deist C, Griscelli C, Fischer A: Development of immunologic functions after bone marrow transplantation in 33 patients with severe combined immunodeficiency. Blood 74:2211–2219, 1989.

106. Kenny A, Hitzig W: Bone marrow transplantation for severe combined immunodeficiency disease Eur J Pediatr 131:155–177, 1979.

107. Dror Y, Gallagher R, Wara DW, et al: Immune reconstitution in severe combined immunodeficiency disease after lectin-treated, T-cell-depleted haplocompatible bone marrow transplantation. Blood 81(8):2021–2030, 1993.

108. Keever C, Flomenberg N, Brochstein J, et al: Tolerance of engrafted donor T cells following bone marrow transplantation for severe combined immunodeficiency. Clin Immunol Immunopathol 48:261–276, 1988.

109. Shearer G, Polisson R: Mutual recognition of parental and F_1 lymphocytes. J Exp Med 151:20–31, 1980.

110. Longo D, Davis M: Early apperance of donor type antigen presenting cell is the thymuses of 1200R radiation induced bone marrow chimeras correlates with self-recognition of donor I region gene products J Immunol 130:2525–2527, 1983.

111. Chu E, Umetsu D, Rosen F, Geha RS: Major histocompatibility restriction of antigen recognition by T cells in a recipient of haplotype mismatched human bone marrow transplantation. J Clin Invest 72(3):1124–1129, 1983.

112. Geha RS: Is the B-cell abnormality secondary to T-cell abnormality in severe combined immunodeficiency? Clin Immunopathol 6:102–106, 1976.

113. Morgan G, Linch D, Knott L, et al: Successful haploidentical mismatched bone marrow transplantation in severe combined immunodeficiency: T-cell removal using CAMPATH-1 monoclonal antibody and E-rosetting Br J Heme 62:421–430, 1986.

114. Griscelli C, Durandy A, Virellizier JL, et al: Selective defect of precursor T cells associated with apparently normal B lymphocytes in severe combined immunodeficiency disease. J Pediatr 93:404–411, 1978.

115. Moen R, Horowitz S, Sondel P, et al: Immunologic reconstitution after haploidentical bone marrow transplantation for immune deficiency disorders: treatment of bone marrow cells with monoclonal antibody CT-2 and complement. Blood 70:664–669, 1987.

116. Geha RS, Rosen FS: The evolution of MHC restrictions in antigen recognition by T cells in a haploidentical bone marrow transplant recipient. J Immunol 143(1):84–88, 1989.

117. Sullivan KP, Kopecky KJ, Jocom J, et al: Immunomodulatory and antimicrobial efficacy of intravenous immunoglobulin in bone marrow transplantation. N Engl J Med 323:705–712, 1990.

118. Wagner JE, Rosenthal J, Sweetman R, et al: Successful transplantation of HLA-matched and HLA-mismatched umbilical cord blood from unrelated donors: analysis of engraftment and acute graft-versus-host disease. Blood 88(3):795–802, 1996.

119. Kurtzberg J, Laughlin M, Graham ML, et al: Placental blood as a source of hematopoietic stem cells for transplantation into unrelated recipients. N Engl J Med 335(3):157–166, 1996.

120. Neudorf SM, Blatt J, Corey S, et al: Graft failure after an umbilical cord blood transplant in a patient with severe aplastic anemia. Blood 85(10):2991–2992, 1995.

121. Hoogerbrugge PM, Vossen JM, Beusechem VW, Valerio D: Treatment of patients with severe combined immunodeficiency due to adenosine deaminase (ADA) deficiency by autologous transplantation of genetically modified bone marrow cells. Hum Gene Ther 3(5):553–558, 1992.

122. Noguchi M, Rosenblatt HM: Interleukin-2 receptor gamma chain mutation results is X-linked severe combined immunodeficiency in humans. Cell 73:147–157, 1993.

123. Macchi P, Villa A, Giliani S, et al: Mutations of Jak-3 gene in patients with autosomal severe combined immune deficiency (SCID). Nature 377:65–68, 1995.

124. Schwarz K, Gauss GH, Ludwig L, et al: RAG Mutations in human B cell-negative SCID. Science 274:97–99, 1996.

125. Chan AC, Kadlecek TA, Elder ME: ZAP-70 deficiency in an autosomal recessive form of severe combined immunodeficiency. Science 264:1599–1601, 1994.

126. Kara JC, Glimcher LH: In vivo footprinting of MHC class II genes: bare promoters in the bare lymphocyte syndrome. Science 252:709–712, 1991.

127. Jung LKL, Fu SM, Hara T, et al: Defective expression of T cell-associated glycoprotein in severe combined immunodeficiency. J Clin Invest 77:940–946, 1986.

128. Castigli E, Pahwa R, Good RA, et al: Molecular basis of a multiple lymphokine deficiency in a patient with severe combined immunodeficiency. Proc Natl Acad Sci U S A 90(10):4728–4732, 1993.

CHAPTER FIFTEEN

Metabolic Diseases

Charles Peters, M.D., and William Krivit, M.D., Ph.D.

The metabolic diseases are a diverse group that includes, but is not limited to, the mucopolysaccharidoses, the leukodystrophies, and disorders of glycoprotein metabolism. A common characteristic is an enzyme deficiency resulting in failure to hydrolyze specific substrate. As a consequence of substrate accumulation, organelle dysfunction occurs and cell destruction ensues. Although the phenotypes of these diseases vary widely, they can be identified by the presence of abnormal cellular metabolites due to the specific enzyme deficiency. Hematopoietic stem cell (HSC) transplantation (HSCT) is either the only therapy or the most effective treatment for selected inborn errors of metabolism.[1]

The objectives of HSCT for progressive, fatal storage diseases are (1) to prolong survival, (2) to improve somatic and, when appropriate, neuropsychologic function, and (3) to enhance quality of life. To promote these objectives, The International Storage Disease Collaborative Study Group was formed. The goals of the Study Group are (1) to establish an international disease-specific database, (2) to facilitate communication among health care professionals, patients, and families, and (3) to support international collaborative basic, translational, and clinical research. After successful engraftment of allogeneic HSC, the recipient acquires a leukocyte enzyme level equal to that of the donor. Indications for and benefits from HSCT vary greatly. In this chapter, each group of diseases is analyzed by presenting the following information, if available: (1) general description and diagnostic criteria, (2) indications and contraindications for transplantation, and (3) guidelines for transplantation and disease-specific outcomes.

This chapter focuses on a subset of these lysosomal and peroxisomal storage diseases (Table 15–1). Storage diseases that are effectively treated by HSCT include mucopolysaccharidoses such as Hurler (MPS I),[2–11] Maroteaux-Lamy (MPS VI),[12, 13] and Sly (MPS VII) syndromes; leukodystrophies such as childhood-onset cerebral X-linked adrenoleukodystrophy (COCALD),[14–19] globoid-cell leukodystrophy (GLD),[17, 20, 21] and metachromatic leukodystrophy (MLD)[1, 15, 17, 20, 22–33]; and glycoprotein disorders such as α-mannosidosis[34] and aspartylglucosaminuria.[1, 35] There are additional diseases for which HSCT is probably effective, such as fucosidosis and Gaucher types 1 and 3,[36–39] as well as diseases for which HSCT is possibly effective, such as Farber lipogranulomatosis, galactosialidosis, GM_1 gangliosidosis, Lesch-Nyhan, mucolipidosis II (I-cell disease),[29, 40–43] multiple sulfatase deficiency, Niemann-Pick types B and C,[44] neuronal ceroid lipofuscinosis, sialidosis, and Wolman disease. Finally, as currently performed, HSCT has proven to be ineffective for three of the mucopolysac-

charidoses—Hunter (MPS II),[20] Sanfilippo (MPS III),[45] and Morquio (MPS IV) syndromes.[46]

MUCOPOLYSACCHARIDOSES

The mucopolysaccharidoses (MPS) are a family of heritable disorders caused by deficiency of lysosomal enzymes needed to degrade glycosaminoglycans. The diseases include Hurler and its variants Hurler-Scheie and Scheie (MPS I), Hunter (MPS II), Sanfilippo (MPS III), Morquio (MPS IV), Maroteaux-Lamy (MPS VI), and Sly (MPS VII) syndromes. All are inherited in an autosomal recessive manner except for MPS II, which is X linked. To date, successes with HSCT have been limited to Hurler, Maroteaux-Lamy, and Sly syndromes. The shortcomings of transplantation for Hunter, Sanfilippo, and Morquio syndromes also are presented.

HURLER SYNDROME

General Description and Diagnostic Criteria

Hurler syndrome (MPS I H) is a progressive inborn error that leads to premature death, usually by 5 years of age. It is the most severe form of MPS I and is distinguishable clinically from Hurler-Scheie (MPS I H/S) and Scheie (MPS IS) syndromes. Deficiency of leukocyte α-L-iduronidase enzyme activity and the consequent accumulation of heparan sulfate and dermatan sulfate substrates contribute to the characteristic facial features, hepatosplenomegaly, cardiac disease, severe skeletal abnormalities or dysostosis multiplex, hydrocephalus, and progressive mental retardation.[47] In 1998, the history of HSCT for Hurler syndrome and the neuropsychological outcomes after transplantation were reviewed.[4, 11]

Indications and Contraindications for Transplantation

The best Hurler syndrome candidates for HSCT have stable cardiopulmonary function and normal intelligence. These characteristics are more likely to be present in a child who is less than or equal to 2 years of age at the time of transplantation.[2, 3] HSCT is not recommended for children with significant cardiopulmonary dysfunction and/or moderate to severe developmental delay. In the former instance, the risks of regimen-related toxicity, such as pulmonary hemorrhage and/or heart failure, are markedly increased.

TABLE 15–1. INBORN ERRORS OF METABOLISM: LYSOSOMAL AND PEROXISOMAL STORAGE DISEASES AND INDICATIONS FOR HEMATOPOIETIC STEM CELL TRANSPLANTATION (HSCT)

DISEASE	HSCT INDICATED?	COMMENTS
Mucopolysaccharidoses (MPS)		
Hurler syndrome (MPS I)	Yes	Preservation of intelligence and improved cardiopulmonary status, skeletal deformities persist
Hunter syndrome (MPS II)	No	Intelligence and somatic status continue to deteriorate despite HSCT for severe MPS II
Sanfilippo syndrome (MPS III)	No	Intelligence continues to deteriorate despite HSCT
Morquio syndrome (MPS IV)	No	Skeletal deformities persist despite HSCT
Maroteaux-Lamy syndrome (MPS VI)	Yes	Significant somatic improvement, especially cardiopulmonary
Sly syndrome (MPS VII)	Yes	Effective in two cases
Leukodystrophies		
Childhood onset cerebral X-adrenoleukodystrophy	Yes	Neuropsychologic and neurologic function can be preserved after HSCT
Globoid-cell leukodystrophy	Yes	Dramatic improvements in neurologic, neuropsychologic, and neurophysiologic function have been noted after HSCT, including cases of infantile onset
Metachromatic leukodystrophy	Yes	Stabilization of central nervous system (CNS) in presymptomatic late infantile, juvenile, and adult onset cases; however, peripheral nervous system disease typically progresses, especially in late infantile cases
Multiple sulfatase deficiency	Possibly	HSCT experience in one case
Glycoprotein disorders		
α-Mannosidosis	Yes	Significant improvement in somatic aspects, including bones after HSCT
Fucosidosis	Probably	Experience still limited; however, HSCT appears to stabilize CNS
Aspartylglucosaminuria	Yes	HSCT very effective in small number of cases
Other Lysosomal Disorders		
Glycogen storage disease, type II (Pompe disease)	No	Enzyme replacement trials in progress
Mucolipidosis II (I-cell disease)	Possibly	Limited HSCT primarily in patients with end-stage disease
Wolman disease	Possibly	One survivor of HSCT
Farber lipogranulomatosis (ceramidase deficiency)	Possibly	Limited HSCT experience
Niemann-Pick	Possibly	HSCT not effective for type A, can be effective for type B, possibly effective for type C
Gaucher	Possibly	HSCT can ameliorate the somatic disease in type 1, though primary therapy is enzyme replacement; is not indicated for type 2; probably effective in type 3
Fabry	No	Enzyme replacement trials in progress
Neuronal ceroid lipofuscinosis (NCL 1: palmitoyl protein thioesterase deficiency and NCL 2: transpeptidase deficiency)	Possibly	Limited HSCT experience for infantile (NCL 1) and late infantile (NCL 2) forms
GM_1 gangliosidosis	Possibly	
Galactosialidosis	Possibly	
GM_2 gangliosidoses	No	

In children with marked developmental delay, the likelihood of achieving independence later in life is minimal.

Guidelines for Transplantation

Guidelines for HSCT in children with Hurler syndrome focus on six areas.

First, a timely diagnosis is important. The progressive developmental delay associated with Hurler syndrome can lead to an insurmountable barrier to successful outcomes. For most affected children, the diagnosis of Hurler syndrome is made during the second year of life, often as a result of one of the following clinical features or problems: pneumonia, cardiac failure or murmur, frequent upper respiratory or ear infections, characteristic somatic abnormalities, or developmental delay.

Second, timing of HSCT is highly dependent on the identification and selection of the optimal donor of HSC. The lowest risk of HSCT-related morbidity and mortality has been associated with human leukocyte antigen (HLA)-identical sibling donors.[3] Less than 25% of children with Hurler syndrome, however, have such a matched, unaffected sibling to donate HSC. Consequently, an expeditious search for an unrelated donor of bone marrow or umbilical cord blood is necessary. The delay in donor identification and processing can decrease the ultimate effectiveness of HSCT because of progression of Hurler syndrome and the associated developmental delay. Although most of the clinical HSCT experience has been with marrow HSC, umbilical cord blood HSC are being used with increasing frequency. When successful, both sources correct the enzymatic deficiency.

Third, the preparation for HSCT and long-term follow-up for a child with Hurler syndrome require the expertise and contributions of a multidisciplinary team. This team should include, but is not limited to, health care professionals in the following areas: HSCT transplant[2-5, 48]; neuropsychology[20, 49]; neurology[49]; radiation therapy[50-53];

pulmonary medicine; cardiology[54, 55]; audiology[56, 57]; endocrinology; ophthalmology[58, 59]; physical, occupational, and speech therapy; orthopedic surgery[60–62]; otolaryngology; anesthesiology[63]; and nursing. Also important are chaplains, social workers, and volunteer staff. The logistics involved in coordinating such care can be daunting. These specialists should assess for disease involvement and potential sites for transplant-related morbidity and provide expert advice and support to patients and families. Furthermore, these patients should be evaluated annually after HSCT because the ultimate impact of enhanced survival for these children includes the need to address ongoing concerns not fully alleviated by HSCT.

Fourth, in the setting of a "timely" HSCT, it is essential that the transplant process causes the least morbidity with the lowest rate of mortality while ensuring the most benefit after donor cell engraftment. The preparation for the transplant must be sufficiently immunosuppressive and myeloablative to enhance the likelihood of donor cell engraftment while minimizing the chance of rejection. Failure to achieve stable engraftment in patients with Hurler syndrome has been a concern after both related and unrelated donor bone marrow transplantation (BMT).[2, 3, 5] A consensus regarding optimal myeloablative and immunosuppressive preparation for BMT in Hurler syndrome awaits future study, as indicated by Peters et al.[2, 3] and Guffon et al.[10] Preliminary work suggests that the hematopoietic microenvironment of Hurler syndrome may be relatively inhospitable to the support of normal hematopoiesis and that affected HSC may be more resistant to myeloablative therapy (C. Verfaillie, personal communication). These areas require further laboratory and clinical investigation. In addition, toxicity to fragile organ systems such as the brain, lungs, and heart should be minimized.

It is clear that children with Hurler syndrome who undergo HSCT are at increased risk for regimen-related complications such as pulmonary hemorrhage and pneumonitis.[64] The etiology of pulmonary hemorrhage remains obscure but may be due, in part, to the effect of radiation and/or chemotherapy on lung parenchyma that contains glycosaminoglycan storage material and activated macrophages. Other important post-transplantation issues include graft-versus-host disease (GVHD), which occurs at an increased frequency and severity in patients with Hurler syndrome undergoing BMT.[2, 3] GVHD is of no clinical benefit to these patients; in fact, Hurler syndrome children who experience grade II acute GVHD or worse after HSCT have significantly poorer cognitive outcomes ($P < .009$).[3]

Fifth, the long-term neurodevelopment of a child with Hurler syndrome depends on the baseline level of function prior to HSCT, the beneficial effects of donor-derived leukocytes and their α-L-iduronidase enzyme product, and the recommendations and individual education programs that result from detailed annual neuropsychologic evaluations after HSCT.[2, 3, 15, 49, 65] HSCT is viewed as an intervention that can lead to the stabilization of intellectual function over 6–12 months after HSCT. It is important to note that donor-derived monocytes can provide a level of enzyme equal to that of the donor and that central nervous system microglia arise from monocytes. The ultimate enzyme level correlates with long-term neuropsychologic function;

higher enzyme levels are associated with better developmental progress.[3]

Sixth, as more children with Hurler syndrome become long-term survivors of HSCT, the concept of "favorable outcome" should evolve. It has been defined as engrafted survival with continuing cognitive development. Today, it should include the concept of independence in activities of daily living as well as a positive quality of life. Mobility, cognitive competence, preservation of sensory ability, independence in daily activities, and the absence of pain are factors that contribute to a positive quality-of-life outcome.[4]

Outcomes After Transplantation

Outcomes after HSCT in patients with Hurler syndrome can and should be assessed from a variety of perspectives. The experience of the North American Storage Disease Collaborative Study Group has been reported for 40 patients undergoing unrelated donor transplantation and for 54 patients undergoing transplantation from related donors.[2, 3] Briefly, these two reports describe the patient characteristics for the largest groups of patients with Hurler syndrome undergoing BMT in the world. Regimen-related complications included significant acute and chronic GVHD as well as mortality. Likelihood of survival with donor-derived engraftment was 73% for related donor transplants and 33% for unrelated donor transplants. The reports concluded that patients with Hurler syndrome, particularly those less than 24 months of age with a baseline Mental Developmental Index (MDI) greater than 70, could achieve a favorable long-term outcome with continuing cognitive development and prolonged survival after successful transplantation. The ultimate enzyme activity level achieved did significantly influence the neuropsychologic outcome. Future protocols must address the high risk of graft rejection or failure and the impact of GVHD in this patient population.

Engraftment after HSCT leads to reduction of substrate in liver, tonsils, conjunctiva, cerebrospinal fluid, and urine.[5, 58, 63, 66, 67] With respect to the brain, successful HSCT can prevent hydrocephalus.[6, 20] In Hurler syndrome, the pathology of the brain shows accumulation of mucopolysaccharide material around the blood vessels in the brain. This is visualized by magnetic resonance imaging (MRI) of the brain. Subsequent to transplantation, these areas are significantly reduced. Opening cerebrospinal fluid pressure as determined by lumbar puncture normalizes after successful engraftment.

The effect of donor enzyme status on neuropsychologic outcome in children with Hurler syndrome who had an MDI over 70 before HSCT has been studied. The correlation of normalized α-L-iduronidase enzyme activity levels with the latest MDI scores for these children was significant.[3] The correlation of the normalized α-L-iduronidase enzyme activity levels with the latest MDI scores for these children was 0.59 ($P = .02$). No child whose ultimate enzyme activity level was low because of either a heterozygous carrier donor or partial engraftment from a homozygous normal donor had normal mental functioning at follow-up. Children who retained fully normal intelligence all experienced complete engraftment from a homozygous enzymatically normal donor.

Hearing has normalized in many patients who have undergone BMT in contrast with the natural progressive loss of hearing in patients who have not undergone BMT.[17] Careful follow-up is indicated. If a significant hearing deficit persists, appropriate intervention such as fitting for hearing aids can be performed. In most instances, sleep apnea resolves after HSCT, and tonsillectomy and adenoidectomy are not required. Otitis media is usually reduced; however, myringotomy with placement of tympanostomy tubes is sometimes needed.

Cardiac failure due to narrowed coronary arteries and myocardial glycosaminoglycan (GAG) accumulation has been common in children with Hurler syndrome who have not undergone BMT.[54, 55] The grave consequences secondary to cardiac problems have been obviated in those experiencing full engraftment for a year after HSCT. The sensitivity of pulsed Doppler during echocardiography has allowed evaluation of the cardiac valves. Murmurs related to mitral and tricuspid insufficiency have been noted along with increased thickening of the respective valves. The relative amount of change in valves is considerably less than in patients not undergoing BMT; however, in long-term survivors, deposition of GAG has been significant, necessitating long-term cardiology follow-up. The implications for possible valve replacement are unclear.

Survival of patients with Hurler syndrome who have experienced engraftment is radically changed from that of patients who have not undergone BMT.[7] Long-term survival data indicate that the lifespan will be extended many decades. This remarkable improvement is directly attributable to persistence of leukocyte α-L-iduronidase enzyme activity. Permanent enzyme expression is due to adoptive transfer of the donor hematopoietic system that includes a new monocyte-phagocyte system.

Although engraftment provides resolution of the lysosomal lesions in most organs of the body after transplantation, this generally does not occur in the skeletal system. The mucopolysaccharide collection in the lysosomes of the chondrocytes persists after engraftment.[60] Direct cell-to-cell contact between the chondrocytes of the recipient and the monocyte-macrophage of the hematopoietic system is limited. Currently, patients with Hurler syndrome who have undergone BMT will likely require orthopedic surgery for carpal tunnel syndrome and trigger digits,[61] genu valgum,[62] hip acetabular dysplasia, and possibly kyphoscoliosis.[48] In contrast, odontoid hypoplasia is corrected by 8–10 years of age with successfully engrafted transplants.[68] This is important because ondontoid hypoplasia can be associated with C1–2 vertebral displacement and consequent paraplegia. We are optimistic that the transplantation of mesenchymal stem cells could decrease this need for orthopedic interventions.[69, 70] In vitro, human mesenchymal stem cells provide progenitors for osteoblasts and chondrocytes. Such differentiated progeny are not supplied by HSC.

Further study of factors and procedures that lead to a better quality of life for patients with Hurler syndrome is needed. The outcomes of quality-of-life assessments based on the perspectives of the parent, child, and physician may differ.[4] Quality of life with respect to health outcomes in patients with long-term engraftment ranges from restricted to near normal from the physician's point of view. Although we think that improved quality of life after HSCT will result from earlier diagnosis and transplantation, preferably during the first year of life, additional study is needed.

Particular attention has been given to analysis of the mutation in the α-L-iduronidase gene and the ability to predict disease severity or phenotype. Although many mutations have been found that result in a spectrum of severity, two mutations, W402X and Q70X, as well as others result in the severe form of the disease.[2, 3, 6, 8–10, 71–75] More than 40 children with phenotypically severe Hurler syndrome from the University of Minnesota underwent mutation analysis by Dr. John Hopwood at Adelaide Children's Hospital in Australia. All children underwent the following evaluations at baseline: MDI, head circumference, height, weight, vision, hearing, skeletal abnormalities, echocardiograms, computed tomographic volumetric studies of liver and spleen (n = 12), and magnetic resonance imaging (MRI) and upper cervical spine. Enzyme level at baseline for all children was less than 0.1 nanomoles/mg of protein/hour. Based on preliminary data, we concluded that mutation type (e.g., W402X, Q70X, or other) at baseline did not allow prediction of a severe phenotype for patients with Hurler syndrome.

The University of Minnesota is examining variables that reflect the child's stage of disease and the transplant process to determine whether they will predict long-term outcomes and quality of life in children who have undergone HSCT for Hurler syndrome. The International Storage Disease Collaborative Study Group and the Correction of Genetic Diseases by Transplantation (COGENT) Society are developing an international registry and database for patients with Hurler syndrome with the assistance of the National Marrow Donor Program, the International Bone Marrow Transplant Registry, and the European Bone Marrow Transplant group. There are plans for an international randomized, clinical trial comparing transplant preparative regimens for rates of engraftment, survival, and neuropsychologic outcome. While we await definitive results from the recent study of human α-L-iduronidase enzyme replacement therapy, HSCT remains the most effective intervention for Hurler syndrome.

HUNTER, SANFILIPPO, AND MORQUIO SYNDROMES

General Descriptions and Diagnostic Criteria

Hunter syndrome comprises two recognized clinical entities, mild and severe, arising from deficiency of lysosomal iduronate sulfatase enzyme activity. The severe form of Hunter syndrome has features similar to those of Hurler syndrome except for the lack of corneal clouding and slower progression of somatic and central nervous system (CNS) involvement. Coarse facial features, short stature, skeletal deformities, joint stiffness, and mental retardation characterize the severe form of Hunter syndrome, with onset between 2 and 4 years of age. The mild form is somewhat analogous to Scheie syndrome (MPS I S), with a prolonged lifespan, minimal to no CNS involvement, and a slow progression of somatic deterioration. An X-linked recessive pattern of inheritance is found in both forms of Hunter syndrome.[47]

Sanfilippo syndrome is composed of four biochemically diverse but clinically similar groups (type A, heparan N-sulfatase; type B, α-N-acetylglucosaminidase; type C, acetyl CoA:α-glucosaminide acetyltransferase; and type D, N-acetylglucosamine 6-sulfatase). The four enzymes are required for the degradation of heparan sulfate. Sanfilippo syndrome is characterized by severe CNS degeneration yet with only mild somatic disease. Onset of clinical features usually occurs between 2 and 6 years of age in a child who previously appeared normal.

Presenting features can include hyperactivity with aggressive behavior, delayed development, coarse facial features, hirsutism, sleep disorders, and mild hepatosplenomegaly. Skeletal involvement is minimal, with only mild dysostosis multiplex, usually normal stature, and mild joint stiffness, which rarely causes loss of function. Recurrent and sometimes severe diarrhea is unexplained but usually improves in older children. Speech development is often delayed, with poor articulation and content. Severe hearing impairment is common. Seizures can occur in older patients. Severe neurologic degeneration occurs in most patients by 6–10 years of age, accompanied by rapid deterioration of social and adaptive skills.[47]

Morquio syndrome is caused by defective degradation of keratan sulfate due to deficiency in either N-acetylgalactosamine 6-sulfatase (MPS IV A) or β-galactosidase (MPS IV B). Both types of Morquio syndrome are characterized by short trunk dwarfism, fine corneal deposits, a skeletal (spondyloepiphyseal) dysplasia distinct from that of the other MPS disorders, and preservation of intelligence. The predominant clinical features of Morquio syndrome are those related to the skeleton and CNS effects. Patients with Morquio syndrome appear normal at birth. The appearance of genu valgum, kyphosis, growth retardation with short trunk and neck, and waddling gait with a tendency to fall are early symptoms of the syndrome. Odontoid hypoplasia is a universal clinical finding with grave medical consequences. Instability of the hypoplastic odontoid process with ligamentous laxity can result in life-threatening atlantoaxial subluxation. Patients with the severe form of Morquio syndrome can experience cervical myelopathy early in life; consequently, they may not survive beyond the third or fourth decades of life. Paralysis from the myelopathy, restrictive chest wall movement, and valvular heart disease all contribute to their shortened lifespan.[47]

Indications and Contraindications for Transplantation

It had been hoped that HSCT would achieve if not identical, at least similar benefits in severe Hunter syndrome as in Hurler syndrome. Unfortunately, HSCT in boys with severe Hunter syndrome has failed to favorably and significantly alter the disease course.[20] Furthermore, at this time, the risk with HSCT would appear to be greater than any possible benefits in mild Hunter syndrome. Unfortunately, the cumulative, long-term follow-up experience of HSCT for MPS III has also been disappointing from a neuropsychologic standpoint.[45] Clearly, this is an area that merits additional study. Finally, HSCT does not ameliorate the severe skeletal deformities that are associated with Morquio syndrome.[20]

Guidelines for Transplantation

HSCT is not recommended for either mild or severe Hunter syndrome because this procedure fails to stabilize intellectual function in the latter case and is not justifiable in the former; HSCT also fails to stabilize intellectual function in children with Sanfilippo syndrome. Unfortunately, HSCT also is not currently recommended for Morquio disease.[20, 45] With the development of mesenchymal stem cell transplants, however, these and other disorders may become amenable to transplantation.

MAROTEAUX-LAMY SYNDROME

General Description and Diagnostic Criteria

Maroteaux-Lamy syndrome is an inborn error due to deficiency of leukocyte arylsulfatase B enzyme activity. Patients with Maroteaux-Lamy syndrome usually exhibit normal mental development, though physical and visual impairments may impede psychomotor performance. The somatic involvement in the severe form of Maroteaux-Lamy syndrome is similar to that in Hurler syndrome. An enlarged head and a deformed chest may be present at birth. Umbilical and/or inguinal hernias are common. Short stature is the rule. Obvious corneal clouding develops in some patients and can result in visual impairment. Restriction of joint movement (knee, hip, and elbow) develops in the first years of life, and the children assume a crouched stance. Claw-hand deformities develop, and carpal tunnel syndrome can occur. Hepatomegaly is common. Cardiac abnormalities characterized by thickening and stenosis of the aortic and mitral valves have been observed. The skeletal changes are similar to those in the dysostosis multiplex of Hurler syndrome. Spinal cord compression from thickening of the dura in the upper cervical spinal canal with resultant myelopathy is frequent in the milder forms of MPS VI.[47] Current methods examining urinary excretion of glycosaminoglycans indicate disease severity.

Indications and Contraindications for Transplantation

Patients should be examined in a comprehensive manner to ensure stable cardiopulmonary function and to establish baseline neuropsychologic function. Particular care must be taken if a patient with advanced-stage disease is to undergo transplantation. Catastrophic pulmonary complications including hemorrhage have been observed with a significant percentage of transplants for MPS VI.

Guidelines for Transplantation and Disease-Specific Outcomes

Reports of the benefits of BMT in Maroteaux-Lamy syndrome have been published.[12, 13] After successful engraftment, arylsulfatase B enzyme activity levels normalized, hepatosplenomegaly decreased, and visual acuity and joint mobility were improved.

SLY SYNDROME

General Description and Diagnostic Criteria

Sly syndrome is characterized by deficiency of leukocyte β-glucuronidase enzyme activity.

Indications and Contraindications for Transplantation

Assessments of cardiopulmonary and neuropsychologic function at baseline are recommended.

Guidelines for Transplantation and Disease-Specific Outcomes

In mice deficient in β-glucuronidase enzyme activity, HSCT reverses the pathology of the cochlea, tympanic membranes, and inner ear as well as the hearing capacity.[76] In two patients with MPS VII, HSCT appeared to be potentially beneficial. Longer follow-up and careful selection of cases for HSCT are needed.

LEUKODYSTROPHIES

The leukodystrophies are a group of progressive degenerative disorders involving myelin of the central and sometimes peripheral nervous systems. The principle diseases to be considered are X-linked adrenoleukodystrophy, globoid-cell leukodystrophy, and metachromatic leukodystrophy.

X-LINKED ADRENOLEUKODYSTROPHY

X-linked adrenoleukodystrophy (ALD) is a disorder that affects the white matter of the nervous system, adrenal cortex, and testes. Its minimum incidence is estimated to be 1:50,000. Although clinical manifestations are most severe in males, approximately 20% of female carriers have mild to moderate disability. At least six distinct phenotypes have been described. They range in severity from the rapidly progressive childhood cerebral form, to more slowly progressive adult forms that affect the spinal cord mainly, to rarer forms in which the nervous system remains intact. Frequently the various phenotypes occur simultaneously within the same family or relatives. The illness does not manifest clinically before the age of 3 years.

Biochemical or genetic studies can diagnose it in the newborn period and prenatally; however, these tests do not permit prediction of the phenotype. The principal biochemical abnormality is the accumulation of saturated very-long-chain fatty acids (VLCFA), due to the impaired capacity to degrade these substances in the peroxisome. The defective gene has been mapped to Xq28 and codes for a peroxisomal membrane protein that is a member of the adenosine triphosphate–binding cassette transporter family and appears to be required for the transport of VLCFA into the peroxisome. The adrenal insufficiency can be readily managed by glucocorticoid and mineralocorticoid replacement therapy. The testicular dysfunction is relatively rare.

CNS involvement, however, is frequent, progressive, and fatal.[77] The only effective therapy for cerebral disease in X-linked ALD is HSCT.[14, 18, 19]

CEREBRAL X-LINKED ADRENOLEUKODYSTROPHY

General Description and Diagnostic Criteria

The childhood-onset cerebral form of X-linked ALD is a demyelinating disorder of the CNS that leads to a vegetative state and death. The symptoms of childhood adrenoleukodystrophy include a variety of neuropsychologic and neurologic manifestations due to demyelination located preferentially in parieto-occipital white matter and pyramidal tracts within the brain stem, less frequently in frontal white matter or the internal capsules.[78, 79]

The disease can progress for 1–3 years; at this stage, patients may have either no neurologic signs or minor changes and subtle neurocognitive defects (visual spatial deficits in the occipital forms, execution and attention deficits in the frontal form). Then, demyelination accelerates, leading to a vegetative state or death within 3 years.[78] This advanced stage corresponds to the onset of inflammatory lesions with accumulation of macrophages and mononuclear cells within the active edge of demyelinating lesions. At this stage, MRI shows marked progression of demyelination and focal disruption of the blood-brain barrier.[78, 79] Prior to the development of a novel brain-sparing total-body irradiation method, allogeneic HSCT had been unsuccessful when performed at an advanced stage of cerebral disease.[80–82] This novel technique is presented later. An early report raised hope that HSCT performed at an earlier stage of disease could stabilize and even reverse demyelination, thus supporting further evaluation of this therapeutic approach.[14]

Indications and Contraindications for Transplantation

The mechanisms by which functional bone marrow cells exert favorable effects on cerebral demyelination in ALD remain unclear. Severe progression of the disease observed in patients with ALD in whom engraftment was unsuccessful after HSCT suggests that myeloablation and immunotherapy are not responsible for the improvement observed after HSCT. Recent observations have raised the possibility of normalization of VLCFA in patients with ALD by pharmacologic approaches.[83, 84] In recent years, however, HSCT has remained the only therapeutic approach of proven benefit in the cerebral form of ALD. It is hoped that better selection of HLA-matched donors will decrease the risk of the procedure.

The clinical experience with HSCT for cerebral X-linked ALD and the natural history of X-linked ALD raise two important questions. First, given the wide phenotypic variation in X-linked ALD, which patients with the biochemical defect of X-linked ALD are likely to experience cerebral demyelination and therefore would be recommended to undergo HSCT? Second, which factors immediately prior to transplantation predict the outcome of HSCT? Because HSCT carries significant risks, these questions are not trivial.

No correlation has been found between the nature of the ALD gene mutation,[85] the biochemical defect,[78] and the clinical phenotype.[86] Consequently, diagnosis of cerebral ALD is difficult in the early stages. Because no definitive biologic marker has been found, careful monitoring with MRI and neuropsychologic tests demonstrate the onset and progression of early cerebral demyelination in boys in whom HSCT is recommended and prognosis is positive. These boys are initially identified by documenting elevated VLCFA levels (identified during family screening) or isolated adrenal insufficiency. All boys in whom adrenal insufficiency is diagnosed before 10 years of age should be tested for X-linked ALD.

MRI site and extent of demyelination, neuropsychologic test results, and rate of progression prior to HSCT are the only predictors of beneficial outcome.[19, 65, 87, 88] Determining the rate of disease progression before HSCT is also crucial, particularly in patients less than 8 years of age who experience a very rapid progression of demyelination. Evaluation of MRI and neuropsychologic decline at intervals of 3–4 months before HSCT provide an estimate of the rate of disease progression. The risk of performing HSCT a few months later, at which time the disease process may accelerate and result in poor outcome, must be balanced with the risk of excluding patients for which HSCT would have been beneficial if performed earlier without assessment of progression rate. This is important given the usual progression of demyelinating lesions during the 6 months following HSCT and the relatively narrow window of opportunity that patients with advanced disease may have before rapid decline. Clearly, biologic markers are urgently needed to help with this decision. A proton magnetic resonance spectroscopy (MRS) study demonstrated a correlation between the neuropsychologic scores and the abnormal choline/creatine and N-acetylaspartate/creatinine ratios in white matter from patients with ALD.[86, 89] Longitudinal studies are needed to determine if these MRS abnormalities are useful markers of disease evolution.

Guidelines for Transplantation

The following are transplantation guidelines for boys and men with cerebral X-linked ALD.

First, the timing of HSCT is critically important. Biochemical diagnosis in patients who are still without signs of the disease by neuropsychologic and/or neurologic evaluation require serial monitoring to identify the onset of cerebral disease.[65] MRI of the brain with determination of the Loes severity score is also informative.[87, 88] When the diagnosis of cerebral X-linked ALD is based on clinical neuropsychologic and/or neurologic abnormalities, HSCT, if it is to be performed, must occur as soon as possible.

Second, we recommend that patients receive dietary therapy and Lorenzo oil for at least 1 month prior to HSCT to achieve normalization of plasma VLCFA. Clinical experience strongly suggests that this greatly reduces the risk of certain life-threatening hemorrhagic complications during and after the transplantation. It is unclear whether there is any benefit from Lorenzo oil and a restricted diet after HSCT.

Third, the optimal source of HSC for these patients is not known. Successes have occurred with both bone marrow and umbilical cord blood transplants. The significance of using a donor who is a carrier for X-linked ALD is not clear. When a sister is HLA-identical and a carrier, we recommend that she be selected as the donor over a noncarrier unrelated or less well-matched donor.

Fourth, the transplant process should be designed to minimize neurotoxicity. For example, busulfan is neurotoxic and can cause seizures.[90] Total-body irradiation (TBI) has typically been delivered to the entire brain. A novel TBI technique has led to sparing of the brain and resulted in improved survival and enhanced neuropsychologic function after HSCT.[19] At some institutions, intravenous intralipid nutrition and benzodiazepines have been avoided on the basis of adverse clinical events or other considerations.

Fifth, long-term follow-up should include assessments of neuropsychologic function, neurologic status, and MRI of the brain. It is recognized that many patients with cerebral disease will have long-term disabilities requiring additional supportive services.[49]

Outcomes After Transplantation

The outcomes following HSCT for cerebral X-linked ALD have been highly variable, depending on disease status at HSCT as well as transplant-related complications. Shapiro et al. reported that BMT can, over an extended period of time, halve the inexorable progressive demyelination and neurologic deterioration.[18] Twelve patients with childhood-onset cerebral ALD who experienced engraftment have been followed for 5–10 years after BMT. MRI and neurologic, neuropsychologic, electrophysiologic, and plasma VLCFA measurements were used to evaluate the effect of this treatment. MRI showed complete reversal in two patients and improvement in one. One patient showed no change from baseline to last follow-up. The condition of all eight patients who showed an initial period of continued demyelination stabilized and remained unchanged thereafter. Motor function remained normal or improved after transplantation in 10 patients.

Verbal intelligence remained within the normal range for 11 patients. Performance abilities (nonverbal) were improved or were stable in seven patients. Decline followed by stability occurred in five patients. Plasma VLCFA levels decreased by 55% and remained slightly above the upper limits of normal. Five- to 10-year follow-up of 12 patients with childhood cerebral adrenoleukodystrophy demonstrated the long-term beneficial effect of BMT when the procedure was performed at an early stage of the disease.[18]

To date, 126 patients have undergone HSCT worldwide for cerebral X-linked ALD. From July 1981 to January 1999, 126 consecutive males with cerebral X-linked ALD and a wide range of disease severity underwent transplantation using HLA-identical matched sibling donors, partially matched related donors, or unrelated donors. HSC sources included bone marrow and umbilical cord blood. Ninety percent of patients experienced engraftment with donor cells. The actuarial probability of survival at 5 years was 55% (95% CI, 42–68%). The leading causes of death were progressive ALD and GVHD. Preliminary results indicate that neurologic and neuropsychologic status did stabilize after engraftment in a large proportion of evaluable survivors in whom engraftment was successful. Severity of disease, as measured by the pretransplantation performance IQ, was the most sensitive indicator of prognosis.[91] Performance IQ evaluates visual perception, spatial, motor, and reasoning abilities.

HCST in severely involved patients with cerebral X-linked ALD presents a significant challenge. One marker of marked disease severity, a performance IQ less than 80 (average range, 85–115), has proven to be a reliable predictor of failure. Patients in this group showed fast rates of disease progression and mortality despite treatment with HCST.[19] Unrelated donors were used to treat most of these severely involved patients because of a lack of unaffected, HLA-matched sibling donors. Engraftment has been a complicating factor as well. To enhance engraftment, several conditioning regimen protocols were compared. Many severely affected patients who received TBI and/or busulfan as part of their conditioning regimen experienced rapid neurologic and neuropsychologic deterioration.[19] Busulfan is neurotoxic[90]; furthermore, it was hypothesized that radiation-induced demyelination was contributing to rapid disease progression immediately after HSCT.[92] Despite favorable rates of engraftment with TBI, significant CNS deterioration and death often followed.

We developed a TBI method whereby the skull, which contains up to 25% of the total bone marrow volume, is irradiated while the underlying brain is spared. Nine patients with severe cerebral ALD as defined by performance IQ were treated with this new regimen. The HSCT conditioning regimen consisted of cyclophosphamide, 60 mg/kg for 2 days, followed by TBI. TBI was given in 7 fractions of 200 cGy over 3.5 days with anteroposterior and posteroanterior fields, with the head turned to the side.

A TBI technique was developed whereby the skull was irradiated but the brain was spared. Five one-half value layer (HVL) blocks were designed to conform to the inner table of the skull. The area of the skull under the blocks was treated with electrons (200 cGy fraction × 7). One-HVL lung blocks were used for each fraction of TBI, and the ribs were boosted with electrons (300 cGy × 2). Prior to HCST, disease severity was based on the Dementia Rating Scale and performance IQ less than or equal to 84. Patient outcome measures included survival, engraftment, dementia rating, and clinical status. Engraftment occurred in eight of nine of the patients given brain-sparing treatment. There were two deaths, one from progressive cerebral X-linked ALD and another from Epstein-Barr virus–associated post-transplantation lymphoproliferative disorder. A comparison was made to 11 patients with severe cerebral ALD who underwent transplantation between January 1993 and June 1996 using different protocols. Only two of these patients survived. Morbidity and mortality have been significantly reduced ($P < .025$) with this new conditioning regimen. Slowing in the rate of disease progression or stabilization in neurologic and cognitive functioning has occurred more readily with this novel regimen. This brain-sparing TBI method appears promising in minimizing CNS injury related to HSCT preparative therapy in boys with rapidly progressing demyelination associated with childhood-onset cerebral X-linked ALD.[19]

This study revealed a significant increase in survival after HCST that included the brain-sparing method as part of the conditioning regimen.[19] In terms of progression of de-

mentia, however, the results were mixed, with four of the seven survivors showing progression of disease. Because of the small number of subjects, we were unable to analyze possible risk factors that may account for this progression, such as performance IQ or baseline brain MRI severity. Although a performance IQ less than 80 has been associated with very high mortality in our comparison group, the brain-sparing method group showed improved survival, thus allowing us to treat more children with severe disease.

GLOBOID CELL LEUKODYSTROPHY

General Description and Diagnostic Criteria

Globoid cell leukodystrophy (GLD) is an autosomal recessive disease due to greatly diminished or absent activity of the lysosomal enzyme galactocerebrosidase. The disease is characterized by progressive loss of central and peripheral myelin, spasticity, dementia, and peripheral neuropathy. It ends in a chronic vegetative state and early death. The more common form begins in early infancy during the first 6 months of life with nonspecific symptoms such as irritability or hypersensitivity to external stimuli, but it soon progresses rapidly, often leading to death by 2 years of age. The late-onset form of the disease has a more insidious onset from childhood to adulthood and progresses, over a period of several years to a decade, to death.[93–95]

Indications and Contraindications for Transplantation

HSCT has been used to treat 20 patients with GLD from throughout the world. In some cases, the anticipated progression of signs and symptoms was arrested after engraftment, supporting the hypothesis that allogeneic HSCT can be effective in GLD. In a 1998 report, five patients with GLD (one with early-onset type, four with late-onset type) were treated by allogeneic HSCT.[96] Evaluations, including leukocyte galactocerebrosidase levels, neurologic examinations, neuropsychologic tests, MRI of the CNS, cerebrospinal fluid protein assays, and neurophysiologic measurements, were performed before and after transplantation with follow-up from 1 to 9 years. Engraftment of donor-derived HSC occurred in all patients and was followed by restoration of leukocyte galactocerebrosidase. In the four patients with late-onset disease, the CNS deterioration was reversed; in the patient with the infantile form, anticipated signs and symptoms have not appeared. MRI has shown a decrease in signal intensity in the three late-onset patients who were assessed before and after transplantation. Cerebrospinal fluid total protein abnormalities were corrected in three patients with late-onset disease and significantly reduced in the patient with the infantile form. CNS manifestations of GLD can be reversed by allogeneic HSCT.[96]

The patients with GLD most likely to benefit from HSCT are those with late-onset disease because the rate of disease progression is slower and the severity of disease is generally less than that encountered in an infant with early-onset GLD. When HSCT has failed, it has been due to either progression of disease in early-onset cases or a transplant-related complication such as GVHD in an adolescent or adult with late-onset GLD.[96]

Guidelines for Transplantation and Disease-Specific Outcomes

The following guidelines are for performing HSCT for patients with both early- and late-onset GLD. First, the extent and severity of disease and its rate of progression should be carefully studied prior to HSCT via neurologic, neuropsychologic, neuroradiologic, and neurophysiologic examinations. A lumbar puncture with determination of cerebrospinal fluid protein and opening pressure can be informative.

Second, the natural history of the disease should be considered together with the time needed to stabilize the disease process. This period includes (1) time to perform HLA typing, (2) donor search, (3) preparative therapy and HSCT, and (4) the 6- to 12-month period following HSCT that is needed to stabilize the GLD through the delivery of donor-derived enzyme-producing cells to the nervous system.

Generally, it has been difficult to arrest the disease course satisfactorily in the early-onset form of GLD; however, for cases of late-onset disease, it has been possible to achieve stability or even improvement in some cases. The limited number of HSCT cases makes generalization difficult.

METACHROMATIC LEUKODYSTROPHY

General Description and Diagnostic Criteria

Metachromatic leukodystrophy (MLD) is an autosomal recessive inherited disorder of myelin metabolism characterized by accumulation of cerebroside sulfate in the white matter of the CNS and in peripheral nerves. MLD is one of the more common lysosomal storage disorders.[97, 98] The estimated incidence has ranged from 1 in 25,000 to 1 in 40,000, with a gene frequency of 0.5%. Documentation of deficiency of arylsulfatase A enzyme activity is necessary but not sufficient to diagnose the disease. The reason is that the arylsulfatase A pseudodeficiency allele is common in the general population; nearly 30% of the general population are carriers. In MLD kindreds, up to 15% of family members are heterozygous for the arylsulfatase A pseudodeficiency allele. Patients with MLD also demonstrate excessive amounts of sulfatides in the urine.

MLD may appear at any age. The late infantile form is first recognized in the second year of life and is fatal within a few years. Juvenile forms present between the ages of 4 and 12 years; the adult form may begin from the mid-teenage years to the seventh decade of life. In each type, gait disturbance, mental regression, and urinary incontinence are among the earliest signs. Other common signs in the childhood forms include blindness, loss of speech, quadriparesis, peripheral neuropathy, and seizures. In the adult with MLD, behavioral disturbances and dementia are the major presenting signs, which are often mistakenly attributed to a psychiatric disorder. The adult form of MLD may progress slowly over decades.

Diagnostic testing should include at least leukocyte arylsulfatase A enzyme activity and measurement of urinary sulfatides. Other evaluations typically include neurologic, neuroradiologic, neuropsychologic, and neurophysiologic examinations as well as a lumbar puncture. A skin biopsy may be performed to conduct radiolabeled sulfatide-loading studies on fibroblasts. Sural nerve biopsy is sometimes performed.[97, 98]

Indications and Contraindications for Transplantation

HSCT is an effective method of providing normal arylsulfatase A enzyme activity to patients with MLD. With long-term engraftment, many patients have experienced amelioration of disease signs and symptoms and prolongation of survival. These patients were treated after a clinical diagnosis was made and supported by biochemical abnormalities. The selection of an appropriate candidate for HSCT must account for an array of factors.

First, symptomatic patients with late infantile MLD have been relatively poor candidates for HSCT because of the propensity for the disease to progress rapidly prior to the time when stabilization can be accomplished by HSCT.[1, 24, 30, 31] Furthermore, the peripheral nervous system disability is relatively refractory to the beneficial effects of HSCT, which are primarily to the CNS. In the cases of juvenile and adult-onset disease, careful neurologic, neuropsychologic, neuroradiologic, and neurophysiologic assessments assist the transplant team in determining the likelihood that a particular patient will derive significant benefit from the transplant.[24, 28, 30, 31]

Second, current worldwide HSCT experience is limited to fewer than 100 cases. Opportunities to intervene with HSCT before the appearance of clinical disease have been few. The advantages include, most importantly, the prevention of clinical symptoms. With a diagnosis of MLD in an older sibling, a patient can be treated by HSCT prior to the onset of clinical signs. A small cohort of patients with MLD has been evaluated and has undergone transplantation prior to development of clinical signs.[30] Several caveats apply. In order to maximize the effectiveness of the transplant therapy, the donor should have homozygous normal arylsulfatase A enzyme activity. When this has not been the case, the results have been less encouraging. Effective GVHD prophylaxis is essential in order to minimize CNS deterioration secondary to damage by activated microglia. Time of transplantation relative to disease onset in the prior affected sibling is critical. As a general rule, at least 1 year should separate the age at which the older sibling experienced clinical signs and the age at transplantation of the younger presymptomatic patient in whom diagnosis has been confirmed biochemically.

Finally, there are plans for several centers to collaborate in an infant screening program for MLD. By examining urinary sulfatides, it may be possible to identify affected children before the onset of symptoms. These clinically unaffected infants could be considered as potential candidates for HSCT. This approach could herald the beginning of a new era in clinical care and management of MLD.

Guidelines for Transplantation and Disease-Specific Outcomes

The following guidelines are for performing HSCT for late infantile, juvenile, and adult-onset MLD.

First, the extent and severity of disease and its rate of progression should be carefully studied prior to HSCT via neurologic, neuropsychologic, neuroradiologic, and neurophysiologic examinations. A lumbar puncture with determination of cerebrospinal fluid protein and opening pressure can be informative.

Second, the natural history of the disease should be considered together with the time needed to stabilize the disease process. This period includes (1) time to perform HLA typing, (2) donor search, (3) preparative therapy and HSCT, and (4) the 6- to 12-month period following HSCT, which is needed to stabilize the MLD through the delivery of donor-derived enzyme-producing cells to the nervous system.

Generally, it has been difficult to arrest the disease course satisfactorily in the late infantile form of MLD; however, for cases of juvenile and adult-onset disease, it has been possible to achieve stability in the CNS in some cases. Presymptomatic patients with biochemical diagnosis of MLD appear to derive the greatest benefit from HSCT. The limited number of HSCT cases makes generalization difficult.[24, 28, 30, 31]

GAUCHER DISEASE

General Description and Diagnostic Criteria

Gaucher disease is a lysosomal glycolipid storage disorder characterized by the accumulation of glucosylceramide (glucocerebroside) due to a deficiency of galactocerebrosidase enzyme activity.[99] Three types of Gaucher disease have been described. Type 1, the most common with a prevalence of 1:40,000, is distinguished from types 2 and 3 disease by the lack of primary CNS involvement. Type 2, the acute neuronopathic form of Gaucher disease, has an early onset with severe CNS involvement and death usually within the first 2 years of life. Type 3, subacute neuronopathic Gaucher disease, has neurologic symptoms with a later onset and a more chronic course than in type 2 disease. Hepatosplenomegaly, bone lesions, and occasionally involvement of lungs and other organs occur in all forms of Gaucher disease.

The quality of life of patients with Gaucher disease can be improved by a variety of medical and surgical procedures such as joint replacement and splenectomy. The accumulation of glucosylceramide and associated clinical manifestations can be reversed by repeated infusions of modified acid β-glucosidase (alglucerase). Enzyme replacement therapy has been used extensively and effectively in type 1 disease and to a lesser extent and with much less efficacy in type 2 and 3 disease. Issues of intravenous access and associated complications, patient comfort and lifestyle, and resources have led to a critical review of the risks and benefits of enzyme replacement therapy. Furthermore, evidence is accumulating that some organs or tissues, such as lungs, lymphoid tissue, and the nervous system,

may derive little benefit from enzyme replacement therapy. In fact, progressive dementia and myoclonic encephalopathy have been observed in patients with type 3 disease who were so treated.[100]

Indications and Contraindications for Transplantation

The indications for HSCT are less clearly defined for Gaucher disease than for other lysosomal storage diseases. The therapeutic successes of enzyme replacement therapy for type 1 Gaucher disease have led to a general reluctance to intervene with a treatment modality with significant morbidity and mortality. However, with persistence or progression of severe bone pain (type 1) (G. Grabowski, personal communication), the expense of enzyme replacement therapy,[101–103] and the progression of neurologic disease (type 3),[100] more careful and critical consideration is being given to the use of HSCT for these disease types and circumstances.

Guidelines for Transplantation and Disease-Specific Outcomes

The HSCT experience is limited in Gaucher disease, partly because of the enthusiasm for enzyme replacement therapy. Cure of type 3 and severe type 1 disease, however, can be achieved by HSCT.[1, 20, 36, 37, 39, 104] The hematologic and visceral effects of HSCT on the disease have been excellent. The children undergoing transplantation have experienced catch-up growth and no further neurologic or mental deterioration. Gene therapy of Gaucher disease using autologous HSC is discussed in Chapter 17.

MANNOSIDOSIS

General Description and Diagnostic Criteria

α-Mannosidosis is an autosomal recessive inherited lysosomal storage disease caused by deficiency of α-mannosidase enzyme activity.[105] This defect in degradation of glycoproteins leads to excretion of mannose-rich oligosaccharides in the urine and accumulation of oligosaccharides in various tissues, including the CNS, liver, and bone marrow.[105] Type 1 (infantile) α-mannosidosis, a more severe form, closely resembles Hurler syndrome. Symptoms arise before age 12 months, with macrocephaly, coarse facial features, hepatosplenomegaly, dysostosis multiplex, loss of previously acquired developmental skills, mental retardation, and recurrent infections. There is progressive deterioration, with death typically occurring between 3 and 12 years of age. Walkley et al. demonstrated that HSCT is effective in the feline model of mannosidosis.[106] They showed that α-mannosidase could be detected in the brain of animals undergoing transplantation.

Indications and Contraindications for Transplantation

Wall et al. described successful HSCT for a 19-month-old child with α-mannosidosis leading to complete resolution of the recurrent sinopulmonary disease and organomegaly, improvement in the bony disease, and stabilization of neurocognitive function.[34] Since this report, at least three additional patients with α-mannosidosis have undergone HSCT. At this time, four of five patients receiving transplants and experiencing engraftment are long-term survivors and have derived significant benefits from HSCT. It should be noted that several patients have experienced significant pulmonary complications from 10 to 20 weeks after transplantation. No infectious etiology could be identified. Patients with storage disease appear to be at increased risk for pulmonary complications, including hemorrhage and/or bronchiolitis obliterans organizing pneumonitis.

Guidelines for Transplantation and Disease-Specific Outcomes

Thorough clinical assessment is indicated for patients with α-mannosidosis prior to HSCT. Generally, patients who undergo transplantation early in their disease course, prior to the onset of significant disease-related complications, are the best candidates.

ASPARTYLGLUCOSAMINURIA

Aspartylglucosaminuria (AGU) is caused by deficiency of aspartylglucosaminidase leading to interruption of the ordered breakdown of glycoproteins in lysosomes.[105] As a consequence of the disturbed glycoprotein catabolism, patients with AGU exhibit severe cell dysfunction, especially in the CNS. The uniform phenotype observed in these patients makes effective evaluation of treatment trials feasible in the future. The medical center in Helsinki has experience with HSCT for three patients with AGU who underwent transplantation at 1.5, 2, and 2.6 years of age.[35] With follow-up ranging from 1 to 5.6 years, serial MRI, biochemical examinations, and clinical examinations were performed. The MR images of six healthy children and five children with AGU who did not undergo transplantation served as controls. The scans of the two patients who underwent transplantation and at least 2 years of follow-up showed nearly normal gray matter/white matter relationships. Neuropsychologic function also appears to have improved.

FUCOSIDOSIS

Fucosidosis is an autosomal recessive disorder resulting from a deficiency of the lysosomal hydrolase, α-fucosidase.[105] The enzyme defect results in the accumulation and excretion of a variety of glycoproteins, glycolipids, and oligosaccharides containing fucoside moieties. Although at least two phenotypes have been described in this disorder, recent experience suggests that the disease may reflect a continuum of severity. Within the first year of life, the more severely affected patients experience the onset of psychomotor retardation, coarse facies, growth retardation, dysostosis multiplex, neurologic retardation, and increase in sweat sodium chloride. Detailed studies of springer span-

iels have revealed that this canine provides a valid animal model for human fucosidosis. Correction of the fucosidase enzyme activity deficiency by allogeneic HSCT after total lymphoid irradiation has been demonstrated with this animal model.[107] There is very limited experience with HSCT in three children. Because of disease variability, a definitive conclusion regarding the benefits of HSCT cannot be reached at this time.

NIEMANN-PICK DISEASE

Niemann-Pick disease types A and B are lysosomal storage disorders resulting from deficient activity of acid sphingomyelinase.[108] Type A is a fatal disorder of infancy characterized by failure to thrive, hepatosplenomegaly, and a rapidly progressive neurodegenerative course culminating in death by 2–3 years of age. HSCT has been shown to be ineffective in preventing the inexorable neurodevelopmental decline.[44] Type B is a phenotypically variable disorder that is usually diagnosed in childhood through the presence of marked hepatosplenomegaly. There is typically no neurologic involvement, and the lifespan can extend into adulthood. HSCT does appear to effectively treat the somatic manifestations of type B Niemann-Pick disease.

Niemann-Pick disease type C is an autosomal recessive lipidosis resulting from a unique error in cellular trafficking of exogenous cholesterol and is associated with lysosomal accumulation of unesterified cholesterol.[109] Type C is biochemically distinct from the primary sphingomyelin lipidoses, types A and B. Most patients with type C disease have progressive neurologic disease, although hepatic injury is prominent in some cases. There is a single case report of a child with type C Niemann-Pick disease undergoing HSCT. At this time, the value of HSCT is unclear.

GM$_2$ GANGLIOSIDOSES (TAY-SACHS, SANDHOFF, AND GM$_2$ ACTIVATOR DEFICIENCY DISEASES)

The GM$_2$ gangliosidoses are a group of inherited disorders caused by excessive accumulation of ganglioside GM$_2$ and related glycolipids in lysosomes, particularly in neuronal cells.[110] There are three forms: (1) Tay-Sachs disease and variants, resulting from mutations of the hexosaminidase A gene and associated with deficient activity of hexosaminidase A but normal hexosaminidase B activity, (2) Sandhoff disease and variants, resulting from mutations of the hexosaminidase B gene and associated with deficient activity of both hexosaminidase A and hexosaminidase B, and (3) GM$_2$ activator deficiency. Clinical phenotypes in the GM$_2$ gangliosidoses vary widely, ranging from infantile onset, rapidly progressive neurodegenerative disease that ends in death by age 4 years (classic Tay-Sachs disease, Sandhoff disease, and GM$_2$ activator deficiency) to later onset, subacute or chronic forms with more slowly progressive neurologic conditions compatible with survival into childhood or adolescence or with long-term survival. HSCT does not appear to successfully treat the GM$_2$ gangliosidoses; however, future therapy that combines a direct CNS intervention with systemic therapy such as HSCT may ultimately prove beneficial in these disorders.[20, 110]

MUCOLIPIDOSIS II (I-CELL DISEASE)

I-Cell disease shows many of the clinical and radiographic features of Hurler syndrome but usually presents earlier and does not demonstrate mucopolysacchariduria.[111] There is severe progressive psychomotor retardation, and death usually occurs in the first decade of life. The deficient enzyme in I-cell disease is a phosphotransferase, which contains a catalytic component as well as a special recognition site for lysosomal enzymes. The experience with HSCT for I-cell disease has been limited, in large part, to patients with advanced-stage disease.[29, 40–43] Assessment of benefit from transplantation has been difficult.

WOLMAN DISEASE

The autosomal recessive inborn error due to deficient activity of lysosomal acid lipase resulting in massive accumulation of cholesteryl esters and triglycerides in most body tissues is called Wolman disease.[112] In 1956, Abramov, Schorr, and Wolman described an infant with abdominal distention, hepatosplenomegaly, and massive calcification of the adrenal glands.[113] The disease occurs in infancy and is nearly always fatal by the first birthday. HSCT has been performed in a small number of patients with Wolman disease. One patient, who experienced engraftment 2 years after unrelated donor BMT at the University of Minnesota, is the only worldwide HSCT survivor with Wolman disease.

NEW APPROACHES: MESENCHYMAL STEM CELL THERAPY

Bone marrow contains both hematopoietic and mesenchymal stem cells. Conventional HSCT has used the former cells for considerable therapeutic benefit in patients, including those with selected lysosomal and peroxisomal storage diseases. Mesenchymal stem cells can give rise to mesenchymal tissues such as bone, cartilage, muscle, ligaments and tendons, endothelium, and marrow stroma.[69, 114–119] Harnessing these cells for therapeutic benefit in a transplant setting could greatly extend the efficacy of transplantation by facilitating engraftment and through disease-specific outcomes (e.g., skeletal abnormalities, peripheral neuropathies).[1]

CONCLUSION

Two decades of clinical experience with HSCT shows that it effectively treats some but not all cases of Hurler, Maroteaux-Lamy, and Sly syndromes; childhood-onset cerebral X-linked adrenoleukodystrophy; globoid-cell leukodystrophy; metachromatic leukodystrophy; α-mannosidosis; and aspartylglucosaminuria. HSCT is probably effective for such diseases as fucosidosis and Gaucher disease types 1 and 3;

HSCT is possibly effective in cases of Farber lipogranulomatosis, galactosialidosis, GM_1 gangliosidosis, Lesch-Nyhan syndrome, mucolipidosis II (I-cell disease), multiple sulfatase deficiency, Niemann-Pick disease, neuronal ceroid lipofuscinosis, sialidosis, and Wolman disease. As currently performed, HSCT has been ineffective for Hunter, Sanfilippo, and Morquio syndromes. HSCT has been most effective when applied early in the disease process or when biochemical diagnosis has been confirmed but the patient is still asymptomatic.

Disease manifestations such as the skeletal deformities of the MPS disorders and the peripheral neuropathies of the leukodystrophies have been relatively refractory to the beneficial effects of HSCT. To overcome these obstacles, novel approaches may be needed. Mesenchymal stem cells, other cellular therapeutic interventions, and enzyme replacement therapy may play evolving roles in the short- and long-term management of these complex, progressive, fatal diseases. Decisions regarding these therapies including HSCT will continue to require a team of knowledgeable clinical investigators who use state-of-the-art laboratory and clinical resources.

REFERENCES

1. Peters C, Krivit W: Hematopoietic stem cell transplantation for inborn errors of metabolism and prospects for gene therapy. J Genet Med, 2000.
2. Peters C, Balthazor M, Shapiro EG, et al: Outcome of unrelated donor bone marrow transplantation in 40 children with Hurler syndrome. Blood 87:4894, 1996.
3. Peters C, Shapiro EG, Anderson J, et al: Hurler syndrome: II. Outcome of HLA-genotypically identical sibling and HLA-haploidentical related donor bone marrow transplantation in fifty-four children. Blood 91:2601, 1998.
4. Peters C, Shapiro EG, Krivit W: Hurler syndrome: past, present, and future. J Pediatr 133:7, 1998.
5. Hobbs J, Hugh-Jones K, Barrett A, et al: Reversal of clinical features of Hurler's disease and biochemical improvement after treatment by bone marrow transplantation. Lancet 2:709, 1981.
6. Whitley C, Belani K, Chang P, et al: Long-term outcome of Hurler syndrome following bone marrow transplantation. Am J Med Genet 46:209, 1993.
7. Krivit W, Henslee-Downey J, Klemperer M, et al: Survival in Hurler's disease following bone marrow transplantation in 84 patients. Bone Marrow Transplant 15:S182, 1995.
8. Hoogerbrugge PM, Brouwer OF, Bordigoni P, et al: Allogeneic bone marrow transplantation for lysosomal storage diseases: the European Group for Bone Marrow Transplantation. Lancet 345:1398, 1995.
9. Vellodi A, Young E, Cooper A, et al: Bone marrow transplantation for mucopolysaccharidosis type I: experience of two British centres. Arch Dis Child 76:92, 1997.
10. Guffon N, Souillet G, Maire I, et al: Follow-up of patients with Hurler syndrome after bone marrow transplantation. J Pediatr 133:119, 1998.
11. Peters C, Shapiro EG, Krivit W: Neuropsychological development in children with Hurler syndrome following hematopoietic stem cell transplantation. Pediatr Transplant 9:250, 1998.
12. Krivit W, Pierpont M, Ayaz K, et al: Bone marrow transplantation in the Maroteaux-Lamy syndrome (mucopolysaccharidosis type VI). N Engl J Med 311:1606, 1984.
13. Krivit W: Maroteaux-Lamy syndrome (mucopolysaccharidosis type VI): treatment by allogeneic bone marrow transplantation in 6 patients and potential for autotransplantation bone marrow gene insertion. Int Pediatr 7:47, 1992.
14. Aubourg P, Blanche S, Jamabaque I, et al: Reversal of early neurologic and neuroradiologic manifestations of X-linked adrenoleukodystrophy by bone marrow transplantation. N Engl J Med 332:1860, 1990.
15. Krivit W, Shapiro E, Lockman L, et al: Bone marrow transplantation treatment for globoid cell leukodystrophy, metachromatic leukodys-

trophy, adrenoleukodystrophy, and Hurler syndrome. *In* Moser H (ed), Neurodystrophies and Neurolipidoses, vol 22, Handbook of Clinical Neurology. Amsterdam, Elsevier Science, 1996, p 87.

16. Krivit W, Lockman LA, Shapiro EG: Childhood onset of cerebral adrenoleukodystrophy: effective treatment by bone marrow transplantation. *In* Steward CG, Hobbs JR (eds), Correction of Genetic Diseases by Transplantation, III. London, COGENT, 1995, p 48.

17. Krivit W, Lockman LA, Watkins PA, et al: The future for treatment by bone marrow transplantation for adrenoleukodystrophy, metachromatic leukodystrophy, globoid cell leukodystrophy and Hurler syndrome. J Inher Metab Dis 18:398, 1995.

18. Shapiro EG, Krivit W, Lockman L, et al: Long-term beneficial effect for twelve patients following bone marrow transplantation for childhood onset of cerebral adrenoleukodystrophy. Lancet, 2000.

19. Ziegler R, Dusenbery K, Peters C, et al: Brain sparing radiation method increases survival rate after hematopoietic stem cell transplantation in severe cerebral adrenoleukodystrophy. Int J Radiat Oncol Biol Phys, In press.

20. Krivit W, Sung JH, Lockman LA, Shapiro EG: Bone marrow transplantation for treatment of lysosomal and peroxisomal storage diseases: focus on central nervous system reconstitution. *In* Rich RR, Fleisher TA, Schwartz BD, et al (eds), Principles of Clinical Immunology, vol 2. St. Louis, Mosby, 1995, p 1852.

21. Arvidsson J, Hagberg B, Mansson JE, Svennerholm L: Late onset globoid cell leukodystrophy (Krabbe's disease)—Swedish case with 15 years of follow-up. [Review]. Acta Paediatr 84:218, 1995.

22. Stillman AE, Krivit W, Shapiro EG, et al: Serial MRI after bone marrow transplantation in two patients with MLD. AJNR Am J Neuroradiol 15:1929, 1994.

23. Pridjian G, Humbert J, Willis J, Shapira E: Presymptomatic late-infantile MLD treated with bone marrow transplantation. J Pediatr 125:755, 1994.

24. Fasth A, Oskarsdottir S, Tulinius M, Manson J-E: Bone marrow transplantation in metachromatic leukodystrophy (MLD): disease progress in a boy despite transplantation two years before expected onset of symptoms. *In* Ringden O, Hobbs JR, Steward CG (eds), Correction of Genetic Diseases by Transplantation IV. Middlesex, UK, COGENT, 1997, p 24.

25. Krivit W, Lockman L, Shapiro E: Metachromatic leukodystrophy. *In* Steward C, Hobbs J (eds), Correction of Genetic Diseases by Transplantation III. Middlesex, UK: COGENT, 1995, p 41.

26. Krivit W, Shapiro E, Kennedy W, et al: Treatment of late infantile metachromatic leukodystrophy by bone marrow transplantation. N Engl J Med 322:28, 1990.

27. Navarro C, Dominguez C, Fernandez JM, et al: Case report: four-year follow-up of bone-marrow transplantation in late juvenile metachromatic leukodystrophy. J Inherit Metab Dis 18:157, 1995.

28. Malm G, Ringden O, Winiarski J, et al: Clinical outcome in four children with metachromatic leukodystrophy treated by bone marrow transplantation. Bone Marrow Transplant 17:1003, 1996.

29. Imaizumi M, Gushi K, Kurobane I, et al: Long-term effects of bone marrow transplantation for inborn errors of metabolism: a study of four patients with lysosomal storage diseases. Acta Paediatr Japon 36:30, 1994.

30. Peters C, Waye JS, Vellodi A, et al: Hematopoietic stem cell transplantation for metachromatic leukodystrophy prior to onset of clinical signs and symptoms. *In* Ringden O, Hobbs JR, Steward CG (eds), Correction of Genetic Diseases by Transplantation IV. London, COGENT, 1997, p 34.

31. Solders G, Celsing G, Hagenfeldt L, et al: Bone marrow transplantation for adult metachromatic leukodystrophy. *In* Ringden O, Hobbs JR, Steward CG (eds), Correction of Genetic Diseases by Transplantation IV. Middlesex, UK, COGENT, 1997.

32. Bayever E, Ladish S, Phioppart M, et al: Bone-marrow transplantation for metachromatic leukodystrophy. Lancet 2:471, 1985.

33. Dhuna A, Toro C, Torres F, Krivit W: Longitudinal neuropsychological studies in a patient with metachromatic leukodystrophy following bone marrow transplantation. Arch Neurol 49:1082, 1992.

34. Wall DA, Grange DK, Goulding P, et al: Bone marrow transplantation for the treatment of alpha-mannosidosis. J Pediatr 133:282, 1998.

35. Autti T, Santavuori P, Raininko R, et al: Bone marrow transplantation in aspartylglucosaminuria: MRI of the brain suggests normalizing myelination. *In* Ringden O, Hobbs JR, Steward CG (eds), Correction of Genetic Diseases by Transplantation. London, COGENT, 1997, p 92.

36. Rappeport JM, Ginns EI: Bone-marrow transplantation in severe Gaucher disease. N Engl J Med 311:84, 1984.

37. Ringden O, Groth C, Erikson A, et al: Long-term results of bone marrow transplantation for Gaucher disease. *In* Steward C, Hobbs J (eds), Correction of Genetic Diseases by Transplantation III. Middlesex, UK, COGENT, 1995, p 57.

38. Ringden O, Groth CG, Winiarski J, et al: Bone marrow transplantation for Gaucher disease. *In* Ringden O, Hobbs JR, Steward CG (eds), Correction of Genetic Diseases by Transplantation. London, COGENT, 1997, p 80.

39. Hobbs J: Juvenile Gauchers: 8 patients 5.6–11.2 years postgraft. *In* Steward C, Hobbs J (eds), Correction of Genetic Diseases by Transplantation III. Middlesex, UK, COGENT, 1995, p 64.

40. Kurobane I, Inoue S, Gotoh Y, et al: Biochemical improvement after treatment by bone marrow transplantation in I-cell disease. Tohoku J Exp Med 150:63, 1986.

41. Kurobane I, Aikawa J-I, Narisawa K, Tada K: Bone marrow transplantation in I-cell disease. *In* Hobbs JR (ed), Correction of Certain Genetic Diseases by Transplantation. London, COGENT, 1989, p 132.

42. Yamaguchi K, Hayasaka S, Hara S, et al: Improvement of tear lysosomal enzyme levels after treatment with bone marrow transplantation in a patient with I-cell disease. Ophthalmic Res 21:226, 1989.

43. Tang X, Hinohara T, Kato S, et al: I-cell disease: report of an autopsy case. Tokai J Exp Clin Med 20:109, 1995.

44. Bayever E, August CS, Kamani N, et al: Allogeneic bone marrow transplantation for Niemann-Pick disease (type IA). Bone Marrow Transplant 10(Suppl 1):85, 1992.

45. Klein KA, Krivit W, Whitley CB, et al: Poor cognitive outcome of eleven children with Sanfilippo syndrome after bone marrow transplantation and successful engraftment. Bone Marrow Transplant 15:S176, 1995.

46. Krivit W, Shapiro E: Bone marrow transplantation for storage diseases. *In* Desnick R (ed), Treatment of Genetic Diseases. New York, Churchill-Livingstone, 1991, p 203.

47. Neufeld E, Muenzer J: The mucopolysaccharidoses. *In* Scriver C, Beaudet A, Sly W, Valle D (eds), The Metabolic and Molecular Bases of Inherited Disease, 7th ed, vol 2. New York, McGraw-Hill, 1995, p 2465.

48. Krivit W, Shapiro E, Balthazor M, et al: Hurler syndrome: outcomes and planning following bone marrow transplantation. *In* Steward C, Hobbs J (eds), Correction of Genetic Diseases by Transplantation III. London, COGENT, 1995, p 25.

49. Shapiro EG, Lockman LA, Balthazor M, Krivit W: Neuropsychological outcomes of several storage diseases with and without bone marrow transplantation. J Inher Metab Dis 18:413, 1995.

50. Kramer J, Crittenden M, Halberg F, et al: A prospective study of cognitive functioning following low-dose cranial irradiation for bone marrow transplantation. Pediatrics 90:447, 1992.

51. Kaleita T, Shields W, Tesler A, Feig S: Normal neurodevelopment in four young children treated with bone marrow transplantation for acute leukemia or aplastic anemia. Pediatrics 83:753, 1989.

52. Smedler A, Bergman H, Holme P: Neuropsychological functioning in children treated with bone marrow transplantation. J Clin Exp Neuropsychol 10:325, 1988.

53. Dusenbery KD, Gerbi BJ: Total body irradiation in conditioning regimens for bone marrow transplantation. *In* Levitt J, Tapley P (eds): Levitt and Tapley's Technological Basis of Radiation Therapy, 3rd ed. Philadelphia, Lippincott Williams & Wilkins, 1999, p 499.

54. Braunlin EA, Hunter DW, Krivit W: Evaluation of coronary artery disease in the Hurler syndrome. Am J Cardiol 62:1487, 1992.

55. duCret RP, Weinberg EJ, Jackson CA, et al: Resting T1–201 scintigraphy in the evaluation of coronary artery disease in children with Hurler syndrome. Clin Nucl Med 19:975, 1994.

56. Schachern P, Shea D, Paparella M: Mucopolysaccharidosis I-H (Hurler's syndrome) and human temporal bone histopathology. Ann Otolaryngol Laryngol 93:65, 1984.

57. Krivit W, Lockman LA, Watkins PA, et al: The future for treatment by bone marrow transplantation for adrenoleukodystrophy, metachromatic leukodystrophy, globoid cell leukodystrophy and Hurler syndrome [Review]. J Inher Metab Dis 18:398, 1995.

58. Summers CG, Purple RL, Krivit W, et al: Ocular changes in the mucopolysaccharidoses after bone marrow transplantation. Ophthalmology 96:977, 1989.

59. Gullingsrud E, Krivit W, Summers C: Ocular abnormalities in the mucopolysaccharidoses following bone marrow transplantation: longer follow-up. Ophthalmology 105:1099–1105, 1997.

60. Field RE, Buchanan JAF, Copplemans MGJ, Aichroth PM: Bone marrow transplantation in Hurler syndrome: effect on skeletal development. J Bone Joint Surg [Br] 76:975, 1994.

61. Van Heest A, House J, Krivit W, Walker K: Surgical treatment of carpal tunnel syndrome and trigger digits in children with mucopolysaccharide storage diseases. J Hand Surg 23:236–243, 1998.

62. Odunusi E, Peters C, Krivit W, Ogilvie J: Genu valgum deformity in Hurler syndrome after hematopoietic stem cell transplantation: correction by surgical intervention. J Pediatr Orthop 19:270, 1999.

63. Belani KG, Krivit W, Carpenter BL, et al: Children with mucopolysaccharidosis: perioperative care, morbidity, mortality, and new findings. J Pediatr Surg 28:403, 1993.

64. Woodard P, Wagner JE, DeFor T, et al: Effect of two hematopoietic stem cell transplant (HSCT) preparative regimens on outcomes in patients with inborn errors of metabolism (IEOM). Blood 92:516a, 1998.

65. Shapiro E, Lockman L, Balthazor M, et al: Neuropsychological and neurological function and quality-of-life before and after bone marrow transplantation for adrenoleukodystrophy. In Ringden O, Hobbs JR, Steward CG (eds), Correction of Genetic Diseases by Transplantation IV. London, COGENT, 1997, p 52.

66. Resnick JM, Krivit W, Snover DC, et al: Pathology of the liver in mucopolysaccharidosis: light and electron microscopic assessment before and after bone marrow transplantation. Bone Marrow Transplant 10:273, 1992.

67. Resnick JM, Whitley CB, Leonard AS, et al: Light and electron microscopic features of the liver in mucopolysaccharidosis. Hum Pathol 25:276, 1994.

68. Hite SH, Peters C, Krivit W: Correction of adontoid dysplasia following bone marrow transplantation and engraftment (in Hurler syndrome MPS 1H). Pediatr Radiol.

69. Prockop DJ: Marrow stromal cells as stem cells for nonhematopoietic tissues. Science 276:71, 1997.

70. Pittenger MF, Mackay AM, Beck SC, et al: Multilineage potential of adult human mesenchymal stem cells. Science 284:143, 1999.

71. Whitley C, Krivit W, Ramsay N, et al: Mutation analysis and clinical outcome of patients with Hurler syndrome (mucopolysaccharidosis type I-H) undergoing bone marrow transplantation. Am J Hum Genet 53:101, 1993.

72. Scott H, Litjens T, Hopwood J, Morris C: A common mutation for mucopolysaccharidosis type I associated with a severe Hurler syndrome phenotype. Hum Mut 1:103, 1992.

73. Moskowitz S, Tieu P, Neufeld E: A deletion/insertion mutation in the IDUA gene in a Libyan Jewish patient with Hurler syndrome (mucopolysaccharidosis I). Hum Mut 2:71, 1993.

74. Bach G, Moskowitz S, Tieu P, Neufeld E: Molecular analysis of Hurler syndrome in Druze and Muslim Arab patients in Israel: multiple allelic mutations of the IDUA gene in a small geographic area. Am J Hum Genet 53:330, 1993.

75. Scott H, Litjens T, Nelson P, et al: Identification of mutations in the alpha-L-iduronidase gene (IDUA) that cause Hurler and Scheie syndromes. Am J Hum Genet 53:973, 1993.

76. Sands MS, Erway LC, Vogler C, et al: Syngeneic bone marrow transplantation reduces the hearing loss associated with murine mucopolysaccharidosis type VII. Blood 86:2033, 1995.

77. Moser H, Smith K, Moser A: X-linked adrenoleukodystrophy. In Scriver C, Beaudet A, Sly W, Valle D (eds), The Metabolic and Molecular Bases of Inherited Disease, vol 2. New York, McGraw-Hill, 1995, p 2325.

78. Moser HW: Adrenoleukodystrophy: phenotype, genetics, pathogenesis and therapy [Review]. Brain 120:1485, 1997.

79. Aubourg P: X-linked adrenoleukodystrophy. In Vinken PJ, Bruyn GW, Moser HW (eds), Handbook of Clinical Neurology: Neurodystrophies and Neurolipidoses. Amsterdam, Elsevier, 1997, p 447.

80. Moser HW, Borel J: Dietary management of X-linked adrenoleukodystrophy [Review]. Ann Rev Nutr 15:379, 1995.

81. Moser HW: Komrower Lecture: Adrenoleukodystrophy: natural history, treatment and outcome [Review]. J Inherit Metabol Dis 18:435, 1995.

82. Moser HW: Adrenoleukodystrophy [Review]. Curr Opin Neurol 8:221, 1995.

83. Kemp S, Wei H-M, Lu J-F: Gene redundancy and pharmacological gene therapy: implications for X-linked adrenoleukodystrophy. Nature Med 4:1261, 1998.

84. Singh I, Pahan K, Khan M: Lovastatin and sodium phenylacetate normalize the levels of very long chain fatty acids in skin fibroblasts of X-adrenoleukodystrophy. FEBS Lett 426:342, 1998.

85. Mosser J, Douar AM, Sarde CO, et al: Putative X-linked adrenoleukodystrophy gene shares unexpected homology with ABC transporters. Nature 361:726, 1993.

86. Rajanayagam V, Balthazor M, Shapiro EG, et al: Proton MR spectroscopy and neuropsychological testing in adrenoleukodystrophy. AJNR Am J Neuroradiol 18:1909, 1997.

87. Loes DJ, Hite S, Moser H, et al: Adrenoleukodystrophy: a scoring method for brain MR observations. AJNR Am J Neuroradiol 15:1761, 1994.

88. Loes DJ, Hite SW, Stillman AE, et al: Childhood cerebral form of adrenoleukodystrophy: short-term effect of bone marrow transplantation on brain MRI observations. AJNR Am J Neuroradiol 15:1767, 1994.

89. Rajanayagam V, Grad J, Krivit W, et al: Proton MR spectroscopy of childhood adrenoleukodystrophy. AJNR Am J Neuroradiol 17:1013, 1996.

90. Vassal G, Deroussent A, Hartman O, et al: Dose dependent neurotoxicity of high-dose busulfan in children: a clinical pharmacological study. Cancer Res 50:6203, 1990.

91. Peters C, Anderson JR, Lockman LA, et al: Treatment of high risk childhood onset cerebral adrenoleukodystrophy (COCALD) with modified hematopoietic stem cell transplantation (HSCT) [Abstract]. Pediatr Res 43:323a, 1998.

92. Peterson K, Rosenblum MK, Powers JM, et al: Effect of brain irradiation on demyelinating lesions. Neurology 43:2105, 1993.

93. Suzuki K, Suzuki Y, Suzuki K: Galactosylceramide lipidosis: globoid-cell leukodystrophy (Krabbe disease). In Scriver C, Beaudet A, Sly W, Valle D (eds), The Metabolic and Molecular Bases of Inherited Disease, vol 2. New York, McGraw-Hill, 1995, p 2671.

94. Kolodny EH: Globoid leukodystrophy. In Moser HW (ed), Handbook of Clinical Neurology: Neurodystrophies and Neurolipidoses, vol 66. Amsterdam, Elsevier, 1996, p 187.

95. Wenger DA, Rafi MA, Luzi P: Molecular genetics of Krabbe disease (globoid cell leukodystrophy): diagnostic and clinical implications [Review]. Hum Mut 10:268, 1997.

96. Krivit W, Shapiro EG, Peters C, et al: Hematopoietic stem-cell transplantation in globoid-cell leukodystrophy. N Engl J Med 338:1119, 1998.

97. Kolodny E, Fluharty A: Metachromatic leukodystrophy and multiple sulfatase deficiency: sulfatide lipidosis. In Scriver C, Beaudet A, Sly W, Valle D (eds), The Metabolic and Molecular Bases of Inherited Disease, vol 2. New York, McGraw-Hill, 1995, p 2693.

98. Kolodny EH: Metachromatic leukodystrophy and multiple sulfatase deficiency: sulfatide lipidosis. In Rosenberg RN, Prusiner SB, DiMauro S, Barchi RL (eds), The Molecular and Genetic Basis of Neurological Diseases, vol 1. Boston, Butterworth-Heinemann, 1996, p 433.

99. Beutler E, Grabowski GA: Gaucher disease. In Scriver CR, Beaudet AL, Sly WS, Valle D (eds), The Metabolic and Molecular Bases of Inherited Disease, vol 2. New York, McGraw-Hill, 1995, p 2641.

100. Schiffmann R, Heyes MP, Aerts JM, et al: Prospective study of neurological responses to treatment with macrophage-targeted glucocerebrosidase in patients with type 3 Gaucher's disease. Ann Neurol 42:613, 1997.

101. Beutler E: Gaucher disease: new molecular approaches to diagnosis and treatment. Science 256:794, 1992.

102. Figueroa ML, Rosenbloom BE, Kay A, et al: A less costly regimen of alglucerase to treat Gaucher's disease. N Engl J Med 327:1632, 1992.

103. Brady RO, Barton NW: Enzyme replacement and gene therapy for Gaucher's disease. Lipids 31 (Suppl):S137, 1996.

104. Erikson A, Mansson J-E: Enzyme infusion therapy of Gaucher disease. In Ringden O, Hobbs JR, Steward CG (eds), Correction of Genetic Diseases by Transplantation. London, COGENT, 1997, p 87.

105. Thomas GH, Beaudet AL: Disorders of glycoprotein degradation and structure: alpha-mannosidosis, beta-mannosidosis, fucosidosis, sialidosis, aspartylglucosaminuria, and carbohydrate-deficient glycoprotein syndrome. In Scriver CR, Beaudet AL, Sly WS, Valle D (eds), The Metabolic and Molecular Bases of Inherited Disease, vol 2. New York, McGraw-Hill, 1995, p 2529.

106. Walkley S, Thrall M, Dobrenis K, et al: Bone marrow transplantation

corrects the enzyme defect in neurons of the central nervous system in a lysosomal storage disease. Proc Natl Acad Sci U S A 91:2970, 1994.

107. Taylor RM, Farrow BRH, Stewart GJ, Healy PJ: Enzyme replacement in nervous tissue after allogenic bone-marrow transplantation for fucosidosis in dogs. Lancet 2:772, 1986.

108. Schuchman EH, Desnick RJ: Niemann-Pick disease types A and B: acid sphingomyelinase deficiencies. *In* Scriver CR, Beaudet AL, Sly WS, Valle D (eds), The Metabolic and Molecular Bases of Inherited Disease, vol 2. New York, McGraw-Hill, 1995, p 2601.

109. Pentchev PG, Vanier MT, Suzuki K, Patterson MC: Niemann-Pick disease type C: a cellular cholesterol lipidosis. *In* Scriver CR, Beaudet AL, Sly WS, Valle D (eds), The Metabolic and Molecular Bases of Inherited Disease, vol 2. New York, McGraw-Hill, 1995, p 2625.

110. Gravel RA, Clarke JTR, Kaback MM, et al: The GM2 gangliosidoses. *In* Scriver CR, Beaudet AL, Sly WS, Valle D (eds), The Metabolic and Molecular Bases of Inherited Disease, vol 2. New York, McGraw-Hill, 1995, p 2839.

111. Kornfeld S, Sly WS: I-cell disease and pseudo-Hurler polydystrophy: disorders of lysosomal enzyme phosphorylation and localization. *In* Scriver CR, Beaudet AL, Sly WS, Valle D (eds), The Metabolic and Molecular Bases of Inherited Disease, vol 2. New York, McGraw-Hill, 1995, p 2495.

112. Assmann G, Seedorf U: Acid lipase deficiency: Wolman disease and cholesteryl ester storage disease. *In* Scriver CR, Beaudet AL, Sly WS, Valle D (eds), The Metabolic and Molecular Bases of Inherited Disease, vol 2. New York, McGraw-Hill, 1995, p 2563.

113. Abramov A, Schorr S, Wolman M: Generalized xanthomatosis with calcified adrenals. J Dis Child 91:282, 1956.

114. Bruder SP, Fink DJ, Caplan AI: Mesenchymal stem cells in bone development, bone repair, and skeletal regeneration therapy. J Cell Biochem 56:283, 1994.

115. Jaiswal N, Haynesworth SE, Caplan AI, Bruder SP: Osteogenic differentiation of purified, culture-expanded human mesenchymal stem cells in vitro. J Cell Biochem 64:295, 1997.

116. Mackay AM, Beck SC, Murphy JM, et al: Chondrogenic differentiation of cultured human mesenchymal stem cells from marrow. Tissue Eng 4:415, 1998.

117. Kadiyala S, Young RG, Thiede MA, Bruder SP: Culture expanded canine mesenchymal stem cells possess osteochondrogenic potential in vivo and in vitro. Cell Transplant 6:125, 1997.

118. Cassiede P, Dennis JE, Ma F, Caplan AI: Osteochondrogenic potential of marrow mesenchymal progenitor cells exposed to TGF-beta 1 or PDGF-BB as assayed in vivo and in vitro. J Bone Miner Res 11:1264, 1996.

119. Bruder SP, Jaiswal N, Ricalton NS, et al: Mesenchymal stem cells in osteobiology and applied bone regeneration. Clin Orthop 355:S247–S256, 1998.

CHAPTER SIXTEEN

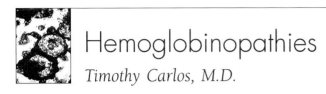

Hemoglobinopathies

Timothy Carlos, M.D.

Abnormalities of hemoglobin are cited as the most prevalent hereditary disorders caused by defects in single genes.[1] In areas of the world where falciparum malaria has been endemic, the incidence of these disorders can reach a frequency such that symptomatic, severe disease affects the health care of a significant portion of the population. For example, the incidence of α-thalassemia is highest in persons originating from southeast Asia or west Africa. In Thailand, where 5–10% of the population carries a defective α-globin gene, approximately 230,000 persons have one of the α-thalassemic phenotypes. Approximately 28% of African Americans lack one of the α-globin genes, and 2% carry α-thalassemia trait (i.e., 2 gene deletion).[2]

Although the frequency of abnormalities of α-globin genes is highest in persons originating from southeast Asia or west Africa, the incidence of β-thalassemia is highest in populations that originated near the Mediterranean basin. In some regions of Italy and Greece, the frequency of these defective genes may rise to 20–30% of the population.[3] Indeed, 3% of the worldwide population carries a defective gene that contributes to a β-thalassemia phenotype. In certain regions of Greece, southeast Asia, and the coastal regions of Italy, the rate of homozygous β-thalassemia births is 1:150–1:200.

The incidence of the genetic mutation for sickle cell anemia in populations across equatorial Africa is relatively constant at 10–20%.[4] In certain populations in east Africa, however, 50% of the people carry the defective gene. Among African Americans and inhabitants of Latin America and the Caribbean, 8% carry the gene, resulting in an expected frequency of 1 in 625 babies being born with sickle cell anemia.[5] Currently, in the United States alone, an estimated 50,000 persons have sickle cell disease.[6]

The clearest example of the effect that a highly prevalent abnormality of hemoglobin could have on a health care system was reported in the 1970s from Cyprus.[7] It was estimated that if no steps were taken to control the frequency of β-thalassemia, in less than 50 years the blood required to treat all of the severely affected children would amount to 78,000 units annually. Forty percent of the population of Cyprus would need to be donors at a total cost to the health care services equaling or exceeding the island's health care budget.

Transplantation of human leukocyte antigen (HLA)-matched allogeneic hematopoietic stem cells (HSC) is the only cure currently available for patients with severe clinical manifestations of the hereditary disorders of hemoglobin. The decision to proceed with this aggressive form of therapy, however, is predicated by the answers to two questions concerning the abnormality of hemoglobin: (1) Is the clinical phenotype of the disease severe enough to justify an aggressive approach? and (2) Does HSC transplantation (HSCT) offer advantages over standard medical care?

Finally, there are clear limitations to the availability of HSCT for hereditary disorders of hemoglobin. A suitable HLA-matched related donor is available to only a minority of patients. The experience with alternative sources of HSC (e.g., cord blood,[8] HLA-matched unrelated donor[9]) or experimental methods of transplantation (e.g., nonmyeloablative transplantation to induce a chimeric state[10, 11]) is limited. The cost of these procedures as well as the availability of these techniques in third-world countries, where the frequency of clinically severe forms of the disease is high enough to justify their use, will probably restrain the dissemination of HSCT as a therapeutic option.

This chapter provides background information on the disorders of hemoglobin for which HSCT is a therapeutic option (i.e., β-thalassemia and sickle cell disease). The usual medical care provided for these patients is discussed. Finally, the characteristics of patients currently being offered allogeneic HSCT and the results of these reports are reviewed.

THALASSEMIAS

PATHOPHYSIOLOGY

Thalassemias are hereditary disorders of hemoglobin synthesis that affect the generation of globin chains. The mechanisms producing these defects include gene deletions that account for the majority of α-thalassemias or point mutations that are the explanation for most β-thalassemias. Over 150 mutations have been reported that affect the transcription or processing of β globin and produce the β-thalassemia phenotype.[12] The clinical severity of the phenotype, however, is determined by the production of normal hemoglobin (Hb A). In some patients, the amount of Hb A produced generates a phenotype of mild to moderate anemia with the infrequent need for transfusions of red blood cells (e.g., thalassemia minor or intermedia). In other patients, no Hb A is generated because of the co-inheritance of defective globin genes from each parent that result in a severe clinical phenotype (i.e., β-thalassemia major, or Cooley's anemia). Worldwide, an estimated 240,000,000 persons are heterozygous for β-thalassemia and an estimated 200,000 infants are born annually with homozygous β-thalassemia.[7] These children would be at risk for manifesting the severe phenotype of β-thalassemia major.

The consequence of diminished globin chain synthesis is the precipitation of unpaired globin chains within the developing red blood cell. Precipitation of globin chains results in oxidative damage to the red blood cell membrane, causing increased cellular rigidity, shortened red blood cell survival, and ineffective erythropoiesis. Unlike unpaired β- or γ-globin chains that can form tetramers of γ or β globin—that is, Hb Bart's (γ_4) or Hb H (β_4), respectively— free α chains present in β-thalassemia are unable to do so, leading to extensive intracellular damage. In addition, lack of generation of β-globin chains leads to the use of γ-globin loci to produce fetal hemoglobin (Hb F). The generation of Hb F further increases the erythropoietic drive because this form of hemoglobin has a high affinity for oxygen. Marrow expansion caused by the accelerated erythropoiesis subsequently leads to skeletal abnormalities and increased iron absorption.[12]

MEDICAL MANAGEMENT

The cornerstone of medical management for severe forms of β-thalassemia is transfusion of red blood cells. Without transfusions, children with β-thalassemia major die within the first 2 years of life.[13] Simple transfusions to alleviate symptoms related to the anemia, however, do not suppress the increased erythropoietic drive or forestall the development of skeletal or metabolic abnormalities. Therefore, children undergo transfusion to maintain an average hemoglobin level between 9 and 11 g/dL. With the adoption of a hypertransfusion program, persons with clinically severe forms of β-thalassemia experience normal growth and development and are now surviving into the third decade of life.

Frequent transfusions have created a second disorder, however—that of iron overload, which remains the major cause of death in patients with β-thalassemia major. Economidou[14] reported in 1982 that only 24% of Greek patients with β-thalassemia major and intermedia were alive by age 28 years. The leading cause of death for this population was heart disease secondary to transfusion-related iron overload. Cardiac failure occurred in 63% of patients with β-thalassemia major by the age of 16, and 50% of the patients died within 1 year of its development. These observations led to a more aggressive approach to iron chelation therapy using deferoxamine.

Oliveri et al. reported that compliance with chelation therapy strongly affected the development of iron-related cardiac failure.[15] Among 97 patients followed for 12 years while receiving both blood transfusions and chelation therapy, 66% of the patients were free of cardiac dysfunction. In contrast with patients who experienced heart disease, this subset of patients had begun chelation therapy at an earlier age, had lower mean serum ferritin levels and, in general, had maintained ferritin levels below 2500 ng/dL. Among the 34% of patients with iron-related cardiac disease, half had died. An important factor in predicting survival free of heart disease was the proportion of serum ferritin levels greater than 2500 ng/dL. The 10-year survival rate in patients in whom less than one-third serum ferritin levels were above this level was 100%. In contrast, patients in whom greater than two-thirds of serum ferritin values

were above this level had a 10-year survival rate of only 38% and a 19 times higher chance of death due to cardiac disease.

The current recommendation regarding chelation therapy is to begin deferoxamine (40 mg/kg/day) when the serum ferritin level rises above 1500 ng/dL. The goal of therapy is to maintain the serum ferritin level less than 1000 ng/dL. Because of the short half-life of deferoxamine, it is recommended that it be administered as a continuous infusion over 8–10 hours. The incidence of side effects from deferoxamine ranges from 2% to 38%, with the main adverse effects involving ocular and auditory abnormalities.

Two major problems limit the utility of chelation therapy. First, the estimated annual cost of chelation therapy in 1991 was calculated to be $32,000, with 60% of the total cost related to the expense of deferoxamine per se. In contrast, the estimated cost of allogeneic HSCT at that time was $175,000.[17] Second, to achieve the goal of iron chelation during ongoing red blood cell support for β-thalassemia major, compliance with chelation therapy is an issue. Less than 70% of older patients with β-thalassemia major have been reported to be compliant with deferoxamine-based chelation therapy.[16] It was initially hoped that oral chelation agents such as deferiprone would supplant the need for daily parenteral administration of deferoxamine. A 1998 study, however, suggested that deferipone is not as efficacious as deferoxamine in reducing total body iron and is associated with an increased risk of hepatic fibrosis.[18]

HEMATOPOIETIC STEM CELL

The first bone marrow transplantation (BMT) for β-thalassemia major was performed successfully in a 16-month-old boy whose parents refused transfusions for religious reasons.[19, 20] In the same year, a 14-year-old patient with β-thalassemia major underwent BMT in Pesaro, Italy but experienced rejection of the graft and reconstitution of the thalassemia phenotype. After these cases, the first large series of BMT for patients with β-thalassemia was reported from Pesaro in 1984.[21] Thirteen patients, 7 of whom underwent transplantation late in the course of disease, received HLA-matched allogeneic marrow after a variety of myeloablative conditioning regimens, including total body irradiation (TBI) with or without busulfan, and with or without cyclophosphamide. Among the 6 deaths, 5 were thought to be related to the conditioning regimen. Five of the remaining 7 patients experienced reconstitution of their β-thalassemia, whereas only 2 patients were long-term survivors and considered cured. From this early experience, the Pesaro group revised both their conditioning regimen and their target population by eliminating TBI and electing to limit transplantation to younger children.

The following year, the Pesaro group reported their findings of allogeneic BMT limited to patients who were less than 8 years of age and who received busulfan and cyclophosphamide as conditioning regimen.[22] Of the patients who received busulfan (16 mg/kg) + cyclophosphamide (200 mg/kg), 3 of 6 died of problems related to transplantation. The next 24 patients received the same dose of cyclophosphamide but a lower amount (14 mg/kg) of busulfan. Only one subsequent death was attributed to the conditioning regimen. The overall survival (OS) rate for the 26 patients was 86%, with a disease-free survival (DFS) rate of 78%. Acute graft-versus-host disease (AGVHD) developed in 23% of the patients despite prophylaxis with methotrexate with or without cyclosporine. Graft rejection was reported to be 12% for the group. By limiting the protocol to younger children and using cyclophosphamide and a lower dose of busulfan as the myeloablative regimen in lieu of TBI, therefore, the researchers lowered the incidence of graft rejection and transplant-related mortality to a level they determined to be acceptable.

A subsequent trial from Pesaro involving 40 older children (8–15 years) with β-thalassemia using busulfan (14 mg/kg) + cyclophosphamide (200 mg/kg) as the conditioning regimen was also successful.[23] OS and DFS rates in this study were 75% and 69%, respectively. Graft rejection and mortality rates remained at about 10%; however, a higher incidence of AGVHD was noted (34%). Thus, age as a factor for transplantation was increased to those younger than 16 years.

In 1990, a retrospective analysis of the first 222 patients less than 16 years of age who underwent allogeneic BMT in Pesaro was reported.[24] Among the entire group of patients, OS and DFS rates were 82% and 75%, respectively. Univariate analysis of factors associated with a poor outcome, however, demonstrated that three conditions adversely affected outcome: (1) the presence of hepatomegaly as defined by enlargement of the liver greater than 2 cm below the costal margin, (2) the presence of liver fibrosis in the pretransplantation liver biopsy, and (3) the quality of chelation therapy received before BMT. The latter was considered adequate when deferoxamine therapy was initiated within 18 months after the first transfusion and was administered subcutaneously for 8–10 hours for at least 5 days weekly. Chelation was considered inadequate if there was any deviation from this requirement. Patients lacking any of these risk factors (i.e., class I) had an OS/DFS rate of 94%:94%. In addition, no patients experienced graft rejection in this group. In patients with one or two risk factors (i.e., class II), the OS and DFS rates were 80% and 77%, respectively, with 9% of patients experiencing graft rejection. Finally, among patients with three risk factors (i.e., class III), OS, DFS, and rejection rates were 61%, 53%, and 16%, respectively. All patients with class I, but only 33% of patients with class II and 8% with class III risk factors, were determined to have received adequate chelation therapy. Thus, the degree of end-organ damage secondary to iron overload was found to be a major contributing factor to outcome.

Although results in children less than 16 years of age continued to improve, the initial experience in BMT for young adults had been less successful.[22] In 1992, the Pesaro group based an adjustment in the concentration of cyclophosphamide from the standard 200 mg/kg to 120–160 mg/kg on the hypothesis that the increased morbidity and mortality observed in older patients primarily was due to cardiac and liver toxicity.[25] The OS, DFS, and rejection rates among 26 adult patients (age range 17–26 years) in this study were 85%, 80%, and 5%, respectively. Mortality related to BMT remained low (3 of 26, or 12%). The benefit of the adjusted dose of cyclophosphamide was also shown in a larger study of 214 patients with class III risk factors.[26]

The OS and nonrejection-related mortality rates for the entire group were 62% and 32%, respectively. Among 95 patients in class III who received the adjusted dose of cyclophosphamide, however, the OS and nonrejection mortality rates were 74% and 24%, respectively. The rejection rate for both groups remained higher than that for patients in class I or II (22% or 35% vs. <10%, respectively). Interestingly, an analysis of risk factors associated with rejection demonstrated that patients in class III who received fewer than 100 transfusions had a 53% incidence of rejection, whereas those who received more than 100 transfusions had a 24% chance of rejection. Thus, in older patients, reducing the dose of cyclophosphamide decreased the mortality in patients with greater transfusion-related (and therefore iron-associated) organ dysfunction. Nonetheless, increased exposure to transfusions appears to diminish the risk of rejection.

At the Third International Symposium on BMT in thalassemia, it was reported that more than 1000 patients have received BMT in centers in Europe, North America, and Asia, with an OS rate of about 80%.[27] Among the surviving patients, nearly 90% have been cured. The latest published summary from the group in Pesaro, involving 826 patients, continues to show the efficacy of BMT in β-thalassemia (Table 16–1). From this summary it is apparent that both OS and DFS diminish with increasing age or class, probably reflecting organ damage mediated by excess iron. Therefore, the group from Pesaro recommends that children with an HLA-matched family donor undergo transplantation while they are in class I. Delaying the BMT until the patient is in class II or higher reduces the success rate and jeopardizes the reversibility of liver and cardiac damage.

Although BMT is a cure for β-thalassemia and obviates the need for further transfusions, moderate to severe iron overload remains in nearly all patients after successful BMT. It has become apparent that although iron utilization and removal improve after BMT, the rate of removal from the heart and liver is slow. It is now recommended that patients have their total iron burden reduced by a program of venesection or deferoxamine beginning 1–2 years after BMT.[29]

Among the 10–20% of patients who did not survive BMT in the Pesaro series, infections were the leading cause of death (38%). Fungal infections accounted for greater than 50% of the fatal infections, whereas viral infections were the cause in 33% of the deaths. Acute and chronic GVHD was the direct or indirect cause of death in about 25% of patients. An unusual cause of mortality in these patients was sudden cardiac tamponade, which occured in 4% of patients.[28]

CONCLUSION

At present, allogeneic BMT from an HLA-matched family donor is the only curative therapy for severe forms of β-thalassemia. Because of the limitations on finding suitable HLA-matched family donors, however, only a minority of current patients can presently be cured by BMT. Alternative strategies of BMT, including the use of mismatched family or matched, unrelated donors as sources for HSC, have met with limited success. There have been only 3 successes

TABLE 16–1. SUMMARY OF ALLOGENEIC BONE MARROW TRANSPLANT EXPERIENCE IN 826 PATIENTS WITH β-THALASSEMIA

POPULATION; AGE (N)	PREPARATIVE REGIMEN	IMMUNOSUPPRESSION	GRAFT REJECTION	SURVIVAL	EFS	NONREJECTION MORTALITY
Class I (121)	Bu (14/kg) Cy (200 mg/kg)	CSA	5%	95%	90%	5%
Class II; <16yr (272)	Bu (14 mg/kg) Cy (200 mg/kg)	CSA	4%	85%	81%	15%
Class III; <16yr (125)	Bu (14 mg/kg) Cy 120–160 mg/kg)	CSA + MTX	33%	78%	54%	19%
Class II; >17 yr (19) *and* Class III; >17 yr (90)	Bu (14 mg/kg) Cy (200 mg/kg) Bu (14 mg/kg) Cy (120–160 mg/kg)	CSA + MTX	4%	67%	63%	35%

EFS, event-free survival; Bu, busulfan; Cy, cyclophosphamide; CSA, cyclosporine; MTX, methotrexate.
Adapted from Lucarelli G, Galimberti M, Giardini C, et al: Bone marrow transplantation in thalassemia: the experience of Pesaro. Ann NY Acad Sci 850:270, 1998.

among 11 attempts at BMT in which the donor was mismatched at 1 antigen and only one success among 7 patients mismatched at more than 1 antigen.[28] There were no successes among the three initial attempts at using unrelated donors.[28] Thus, the use of mismatched or unrelated donors should be attempted only as part of a well-controlled clinical trial.

Because a portion of patients undergoing HSCT for β-thalassemia have experienced stable marrow chimera and remain asymptomatic,[30] alternative approaches to BMT using less-intensive myeloablative regimens with repeated doses of donor HSCT may be a means of both broaching rejection and decreasing transplant-related mortality.[10, 11]

For patients without a donor, the long-term use of transfusions and deferoxamine remains an option.[31] In a recent 14-year follow-up of 1146 patients with β-thalassemia followed at seven teaching hospitals in Italy, 769 patients (67%) were still alive. This survival rate is the same as that of adults receiving BMT in the latest follow-up from Pesaro.[28] Heart disease related to iron overload continued to be the leading cause of mortality, being responsible for 71% of deaths. In contrast with the 1982 report of Economidou,[14] however, in which only 25% of patients reached the age of 25 years, 82% of patients in the cohort born between 1970 and 1974 for whom 25-year follow-up was available were alive. Therefore, chelation therapy with deferoxamine has led to a remarkable improvement in life expectancy. The limitations of this approach are both compliance with chelation therapy and access to a safe blood supply that is free of viruses.

SICKLE CELL DISEASE

PATHOPHYSIOLOGY

Sickle cell disease (SCD) arises from the inheritance of a point mutation within the β-globin gene that substitutes valine for glutamic acid at position six of the globin chain (i.e., β_6 glu → val). The mutation may have been beneficial to those living in areas in which falciparum malaria is endemic and thus is prevalent across a broad belt throughout equatorial Africa and the Arabian and Indian peninsu-

las. Molecular analysis of the β globin gene cluster has shown that this mutation arose spontaneously several times throughout history.[32] Hence, there are at least four DNA haplotypes for the sickle cell gene: a Central African Republic, a Benin, a west African or Senegalese, and an Indian haplotype.

Three disorders of hemoglobin account for the majority of persons with clinical manifestations of SCD. Sickle cell anemia (Hb S) represents the homozygous inheritance of two β globin genes carrying the sickle mutation (β_6 glu → val). Among 3578 persons with SCD in the United States who are followed in the Cooperative Study of Sickle Cell Disease (CSSCD), 67% had sickle cell anemia.[33] The double-heterozygous condition Hb SC reflects the co-inheritance of one β globin gene carrying the sickle mutation and the other β globin gene carrying a second mutation of hemoglobin (β_6 glu → lys). The latter mutation arose in a sharply demarcated zone of west Africa. Twenty-eight percent of the population in regions of northern Ghana and about 3% of African Americans carry the gene for Hb C. In the CSSCD, 23% of patients with SCD had this genotype. The co-inheritance of a sickle gene and a gene for β-thalassemia is a second double-heterozygous condition that produces the sickle cell phenotype. Ten percent of patients followed in the CSSCD have this genotype, with 5% of patients having either S/β⁺- or S/β⁰-thalassemia. Finally, co-inheritance of a sickle gene and other, more rare hemoglobinopathies, such as Hb O^{arab} (β_{121} glu → lys) or Hb D (β_{121} glu → gln), are additional double-heterozygous genotypes that may result in the clinical phenotype of SCD.

In each of these disorders, hemoglobin within the red blood cell can polymerize, leading to the development of a distorted, sickled shape. Hypoxia induces this event. Other factors with mechanisms less clearly defined, however—including infection, stress, menstrual cycles, or changes in ambient temperature—contribute to the generation of sickled red blood cells.[34] In addition to alterations in cell shape, polymerization of sickle hemoglobin leads to a variety of cellular changes, including abnormalities of water and cation homeostasis and alterations in membrane lipids.[35] Increased adhesion of sickle erythrocytes to endothelial cells lining the vasculature also occurs.[36] The latter phenomenon contributes to vascular occlusion and precipitates the typical painful crisis that characterizes SCD.[37]

In contrast with β-thalassemia, SCD is a disorder with variable clinical severity. The frequency of vaso-occlusive episodes varies among the different hemoglobin groups that constitute SCD (e.g., Hb S or S/β^0-thalassemia > Hb SC or S/β$^+$-thalassemia). Repeated episodes of vascular obstruction due to sickle cell crisis, nonetheless, lead to chronic organ damage. The median age of onset of chronic organ damage in patients with Hb S is in the third decade of life.[38] In contrast, the onset of organ damage occurs 15–20 years later for patients with Hb SC, who in general suffer less frequent vaso-occlusive crises. Therefore, the severity of SCD partly depends on the specific hemoglobinopathy inherited.

Even within a group of patients with a specific hemoglobinopathy, however, the severity of clinical disease varies. The CSSCD has defined some of the risk factors associated with severe disease. Patients with prior episodes of acute chest syndrome, seizures, or renal failure or who have an elevated baseline white blood cell count (i.e., >15,000/mm^3) experience earlier mortality.[39] The frequency of painful crises also is a predictor for early death. Patients who experience three or more crises yearly have a median survival of approximately 45 years.[33] Patients with low (<9%) levels of fetal hemoglobin (Hb F) have a worse prognosis.[39] Finally, patients carrying the specific genetic mutation of sickle hemoglobin that arose in the Central African Republic have been shown to have a more severe clinical phenotype.[38] Thus, frequency of painful crises, level of Hb F, DNA haplotype, baseline white blood cell count, and clinical markers (strokes, recurrent episodes of acute chest syndrome) have all be shown in population studies to be markers to predict a phenotype of severe SCD and an earlier death.

Despite these studies demonstrating increased frequencies of vaso-occlusive episodes among patients with certain hemoglobinopathies or with poor prognostic factors, the clinical severity of SCD within each patient over time is uncertain. The majority of patients with SCD have fewer than three vaso-occlusive crises yearly.[33] Thus, predictions of the frequency of crises for an individual are unreliable. Between crises, patients may feel as if they have no disease and may be unwilling to proceed with HSCT. In contrast with an individual with β-thalassemia, whose clinical severity is defined by the frequency of blood transfusions and the resultant iron overload, predicting whether the disease course of an individual patient with SCD will be clinically severe enough to warrant consideration for HSCT is a major challenge.

MEDICAL MANAGEMENT

Acute episodes of vaso-occlusive crisis are managed with oral or intravenous hydration and administration of analgesics.[6] Supplemental oxygen is not thought to reverse sickling of red blood cells and has been reported to decrease reticulocyte production, thus worsening the anemia.[40] Although red blood cell transfusions play a major role in the medical management of β-thalassemia, the need for transfusions and the predictable outcome of iron overload

are not a major feature of SCD. Between vaso-occlusive crises, patients with SCD can maintain a functional level of hemoglobin. Transfusions do not affect the duration of pain during episodes of vaso-occlusive crisis. The clearest indications for transfusions in SCD include aplastic and sequestration crises, preparation of patients for surgery, symptomatic anemia (often with hemoglobin levels of <5–6 g/dL), and in patients who have suffered a stroke.[41–43] Chronic transfusion therapy, such as that given to patients with β-thalassemia, has been reported to decrease the frequency of vaso-occlusive crises.[44] Because of the risk of alloimmunization and iron overload, however, this is not an accepted clinical practice apart from patients who have suffered a stroke and are at risk for a second event.[45]

As stated earlier, between episodes of vaso-occlusive crisis, patients with SCD may feel relatively normal. Supplemental folic acid is generally taken to avoid the risk of aplastic crisis. Hydroxyurea therapy in patients with sickle cell anemia who experience three or more vaso-occlusive crises yearly has been shown to diminish the frequency of crises and the development of acute chest syndrome by 50%.[46] One possible mechanism for this beneficial effect is augmentation of Hb F production induced by the administration of hydroxyurea. Because of the longer survival of erythrocytes containing increased levels of Hb F in patients with SCD, the need for transfusions is decreased. There are, however, unknown risks of mutagenesis and carcinogenesis among patients who may be taking hydroxyurea for decades. A long-term follow-up study involving the Multicenter Study of Hydroxyurea in SCD is presently addressing these questions.

HEMATOPOIETIC STEM CELL TRANSPLANTATION

In 1984, the first attempt at BMT in a patient with sickle cell anemia was reported.[47] The indication for transplantation, however, was not the hemoglobinopathy but acute myelogenous leukemia. The patient, an 8-year-old girl, received an allogeneic BMT from a sibling with sickle cell trait (Hb AS) after myeloablative conditioning with TBI and cyclophosphamide. Although she experienced AGVHD of the skin and gastrointestinal tract, she was doing well at last report.[48]

Later reports of BMT for SCD primarily came from medical centers in western Europe.[49–53] Approximately 43 children with symptomatic SCD underwent BMT from HLA-compatible family donors at centers in Belgium[50, 52] and France[53] (Table 16–2). The usual myeloablative conditioning regimen in these patients has been busulfan (14–16 mg/kg) followed by cyclophosphamide (200 mg/kg). Patients have typically received either cyclosporin alone or cyclosporin with methotrexate as prophylaxis against AGVHD.

The initial reports of BMT in SCD were encouraging.[49, 50] Among the first 10 children who underwent transplantation for symptomatic SCD, no mortality was recorded. GVHD was an infrequent occurrence (20% incidence of AGVHD that was mild [grade I] and 10% incidence of CGVHD). One patient experienced graft rejection, requiring a second attempt at transplantation that was ultimately successful.[49] Thus, BMT was suggested as a viable treatment option for patients with SCD.[49, 50]

TABLE 16–2. SUMMARY OF ALLOGENEIC BONE MARROW TRANSPLANT EXPERIENCE FOR SICKLE CELL DISEASE

AUTHOR	YEAR	NO. OF PATIENTS	GRAFT REJECTION	AGVHD	CGVHD	SURVIVAL	COMMENTS
Johnson et al.[47]	1984	1	0	1	1	1 (100%)	Patient with AML
Vermylen et al.[49]	1988	5	1	2	0	5 (100%)	None
Ferster et al.[50]	1992	5	0	1	0	5 (100%)	2 Patients with recovery of spleen function
Vermylen & Cornu[51]	1993	21*	1	9	3	20 (95%)	5 Patients with recovery of spleen function
Vermylen et al.[52]	1993	28*	3	9	4	27 (96%)	1 Death from GVHD, CMV, and *Aspergillus* infections
Bernaudin et al.[53]	1993	15	1 (2 patients with stable chimerism)	5	3	14 (93%)	1 Death from CGVHD and bronchiolitis obliterans
Walters et al.[58]	1996	22	4 (1 patient with stable chimerism)	2	NS	20 (95%)	1 Death from CGVHD 1 Death from intracranial hemorrhage
Walters et al.[59]	1997	34*	5	6	2	32 (94%)	As above

*Included patients from earlier reports; NS—not stated.
AGVHD, acute graft-versus-host disease; AML, acute myelogenous leukemia; CMV, cytomegalovirus; CGVHD, chronic graft-versus-host disease.

The criteria used to select patients with SCD for transplantation at these centers has been questioned, however.[54–57] The initial entry criteria employed by these centers included symptomatic disease as defined by one episode of vaso-occlusive crisis within the previous year and the need for transfusions.[49, 50] Among the first 10 patients who underwent BMT, the number of crises in the year prior to transplantation ranged from zero to four. An expectant return to Africa—where both the lower standard of medical care and the risk of viral infections associated with unsafe blood products posed threats—was also considered a selection criterion for transplantation. Only 20% of patients had experienced a severe clinical episode (i.e., stroke or acute chest syndrome) in these studies. According to these criteria, 8 of the 26 patients followed at one center were deemed eligible for BMT.[50]

Because of the concerns of performing HSCT with a possible excess in mortality and morbidity in patients with less-severe SCD, guidelines for selection of patients in whom transplantation should be considered were suggested in 1993.[57] Relevant factors to be considered included age 16 years or younger, previous neurologic event, recurrent (two or more) episodes of acute chest syndrome, severe debilitating pain, chronic priapism, retinopathy, and early lung or kidney involvement. Suggested exclusion criteria were lack of an HLA-identical donor and severe lung, liver, or kidney damage.

Continuation of the reports of BMT for SCD from centers in Belgium and France demonstrated that as trials expanded, early mortality, GVHD, and graft rejection were observed.[51–53] Patients included those with clinical markers of severe SCD, including 13 patients (30%) with prior episodes of acute chest syndrome and 5 patients (12%) who had suffered an earlier stroke. The incidence of graft rejection and AGVHD among the 43 patients who underwent transplantation was 10% and 30%, respectively. Five percent of patients died from complications of CGVHD or infection. Interestingly, however, some patients regained splenic function after BMT.[50, 51] A further observation was the occurrence of stable partial engraftment in several patients with amelioration of some of the symptoms of SCD.[53]

The results of a trial of BMT for SCD involving 17 centers in America and Europe have been reported[58] and updated.[59] As opposed to the earlier studies, entry criteria were defined to select patients with debilitating clinical events of SCD. Inclusion criteria were broadened to include patients with other hemoglobinopathies producing vaso-occlusive crises (Table 16–3). Importantly, patients with a severe phenotype of clinical disease (i.e., prior neurologic event or evidence of abnormal neuropsychological function, recurrent episodes of acute chest syndrome, recurrent [two or more] episodes of painful crises for several years) were considered candidates for transplantation. Patients with evidence of advanced end-organ failure (i.e., severe renal, neurologic, or pulmonary dysfunction) were excluded.

Twenty-two children were initially enrolled in this multicenter study, 21 of whom had Hb S and 1 of whom had S/β-thalassemia.[58] Twelve patients had had previous strokes, and five patients had experienced recurrent episodes of acute chest syndrome. As in prior studies of BMT for SCD, the myeloablative conditioning regimen for the majority of the patients consisted of busulfan (14 mg/kg) and cyclophosphamide (200 mg/kg). Therapy for prophylaxis against GVHD included cyclosporin and methotrexate, with 17 patients receiving anti-thymocyte globulin and 5 patients receiving anti-CD52 antibody as further immunosuppression against GVHD and graft rejection.

Among the initial seven patients treated in this trial, four experienced a neurologic event (seizures or intracranial hemorrhages). The protocol was subsequently modified to provide tight control of hypertension and to maintain platelet counts above 50,000/mm³. In addition, continuation of anticonvulsant therapy for the first 6 months after BMT was instituted. With these modifications, no further neurologic events were observed. The most recent update of this trial included 34 children with severe SCD (32 Hb S, 1 S/β-thalassemia, 1 Hb SO^arab).[59] Thirty-two patients survived (93% OS rate, 79% DFS rate), with 6 patients experiencing AGVHD and 14% of patients experiencing graft rejection. As was reported in earlier studies from Europe, one patient who experienced graft rejection maintained 10% expression

TABLE 16–3. SELECTION CRITERIA FOR BONE MARROW TRANSPLANTATION IN SICKLE CELL DISEASE

Inclusion Criteria

Sickle cell disease (Hb SS, Hb SC, S/β-thalassemia

Age <16 years

Available HLA-matched related donor

One or more of the following clinical events:

    Stroke or central nervous system event lasting longer than 24 h

    Acute chest syndrome with recurrent hospitalizations or previous exchange transfusion

    Recurrent (≥2 episodes per year for several years) vaso-occlusive painful crises or recurrent priapism

    Impaired neuropsychological function and abnormal cerebral MRI scan results

    Stage 1 or 2 sickle cell lung disease

    Sickle cell nephropathy (moderate or severe proteinuria or a GFR 30–50% predicted)

    Bilateral proliferative retinopathy or major visual impairment in at least one eye

    Osteonecrosis of multiple joints

    Red blood cell alloimmunization with ≥ 2 antibodies during long-term transfusion therapy

Exclusion Criteria

Age >16 yr

Lack of available HLA-identical donor

One or more of the following clinical situations:

    Karnofsky or Lansky performance score <70

    Acute hepatitis or evidence of moderate or severe portal fibrosis or cirrhosis on biopsy

    Severe renal impairment (GFR <30% predicted value)

    Severe residual neurologic impairment (other than hemiplegia alone)

    Stage 3 or 4 sickle cell lung disease

    Previous history of poor compliance with medical care

    Seropositivity for HIV

GFR, glomerular filtration rate; Hb, hemoglobin; HLA, human leukocyte antigen; MRI, magnetic resonance imaging.

Adapted from Walters MC, Patience M, Leisenring W, et al: Bone marrow transplantation for sickle cell disease. N Engl J Med 335:369, 1996.

of donor cells. At last report, this patient remained asymptomatic with a hemoglobin level of 13 g/dL.

CONCLUSION

As in patients with severe forms of β-thalassemia, allogeneic BMT using an HLA-matched family donor is the only curative therapy for SCD available. In contrast with severe forms of β-thalassemia that require frequent transfusions resulting in predictable iron overload, however, SCD is capricious in nature. Patients may be intermittently symptomatic but, in general, subacute vaso-occlusive events eventually lead to premature end-organ failure, at which point BMT may be associated with increased morbidity. In addition, late BMT may stabilize but not reverse end-organ dysfunction.[60] Choosing the appropriate candidate with SCD for BMT early enough to avoid this situation is the major challenge when considering an approach to therapy. Whether long-term use of hydroxyurea as medical management for SCD is safe and will prevent end-organ damage remains to be determined.

REFERENCES

1. Weatherall DJ, Clegg JB, Higgs DR, Wood WG: The hemoglobinopathies. In Scriver CR, Beaudet AL, Sly WS, Valle D (eds): The Metabolic and Molecular Bases of Inherited Disease, 7th ed. New York, McGraw-Hill, 1995, p 3417.
2. Dozy AM, Kan YW, Embury SH, et al: β-globin gene organization in blacks precludes the severe form of β-thalassemia. Nature 289:605, 1979.
3. Lukens JN: The thalassemias and related disorders: quantitative disorders of hemoglobin synthesis. In Lee GR, Bithell TC, Foerster J, et al (eds): Wintrobe's Clinical Hematology, 9th ed. Philadelphia, Lea & Febiger, 1993, p 1103.
4. Lukens JN, Lee GR: The abnormal hemoglobins: general principles. In Lee GR, Bithell TC, Foerster J, et al (eds): Wintrobe's Clinical Hematology, 9th ed. Philadelphia, Lea & Febiger, 1993, p 1037.
5. Lukens JN: Hemoglobinopathies S, C, D, E, and O and associated diseases. In Lee GR, Bithell TC, Foerster J, et al (eds): Wintrobe's Clinical Hematology, 9th ed. Philadelphia, Lea & Febiger, 1993, p 1062.
6. Management and therapy of sickle cell disease. NIH Publication No. 95-2117, revised December 1995 (3rd ed). National Institutes of Health, National Heart, Lung, and Blood Institute.
7. WHO Working Group on the Community Control of Hereditary Anemias. Bull WHO 61:63, 1983.
8. Wagner JE, Kurtzberg J: Cord blood stem cells. Curr Opin Hematol 4:413, 1997.
9. Sullivan KM, Anasetti C, Horowitz M, et al: Unrelated and HLA-nonidentical related donor marrow transplantation for thalassemia and leukemia: a combined report from the Seattle Marrow Transplant Team and the International Bone Marrow Transplant Registry. Ann N Y Acad Sci 850:312, 1998.
10. Slavin S, Nagler A, Naparstek E, et al: Nonmyeloablative stem cell transplantation and cell therapy as an alternative to conventional bone marrow transplantation with lethal cytoreduction for the treatment of malignant and nonmalignant hematologic diseases. Blood 91:756, 1998.
11. Storb R, Yu Cong, Deeg HJ, et al: Current and future preparative regimens for bone marrow transplantation in thalassemia. Ann NY Acad Sci 850:276, 1998.
12. Rund D, Rachmilewitz E: Advances in the pathophysiology and treatment of thalassemia. Crit Rev Oncol Hematol 20:237, 1995.
13. Piomelli S: Management of Cooley's anaemia. Baillere's Clin Haematol 6:287, 1993.
14. Economidou J: Problems related to treatment of beta-thalassemia major. Pediatrician 11:157, 1982.
15. Oliveri NF, Nathan DG, MacMillan JH, et al: Survival in medically treated patients with homozygous β-thalassemia. N Engl J Med 331:574, 1994.
16. Olivieri NF, Brittenham GM: Iron-chelating therapy and the treatment of thalassemia. Blood 89:739, 1997.
17. Nathan DG: Gene, Blood and Courage. Boston, Harvard University Press, 1995, p 193.
18. Olivieri NF, Brittenham GM, McLaren CE, et al: Long-term safety and effectiveness of iron-chelation therapy with deferipone for thalassemia major. N Engl J Med 339:417, 1998.
19. Thomas ED, Buckner CD, Sanders JE, et al: Marrow transplantation for thalassemia. Lancet 2:227, 1982.
20. Lucarelli G, Giardini C: Bone marrow transplantation in β-thalassemia major: a survey of 13 years activity of a single institute. Forum Trends Exp Clin Med 5:472, 1995.
21. Lucarelli G, Polchi P, Izzi T, et al: Allogeneic marrow transplantation for thalassemia. Exp Hematol 12:676, 1984.
22. Lucarelli G, Polchi P, Galimberti M, et al: Marrow transplantation for thalassemia following busulfan and cyclophosphamide. Lancet 1:1355, 1985.
23. Lucarelli G, Galimberti M, Polchi P, et al: Marrow transplantation in patients with advanced thalassemia. N Engl J Med 316:1050, 1987.
24. Lucarelli G, Galimberti M, Polchi P, et al: Bone marrow transplantation in patients with thalassemia. N Engl J Med 322:417, 1990.
25. Lucarelli G, Galimberti M, Polchi P, et al: Bone marrow transplantation in adult thalassemia. Blood 80:1603, 1992.
26. Lucarelli G, Clift RA, Galimberti M, et al: Marrow transplantation for patients with thalassemia: results in class 3 patients. Blood 87:2082, 1996.
27. Roberts I: Current status of allogeneic transplantation for haemoglobinopathies. Br J Haematol 98:1, 1997.
28. Lucarelli G, Galimberti M, Giardini C, et al: Bone marrow transplantation in thalassemia: the experience of Pesaro. Ann N Y Acad Sci 850:270, 1998.

29. Angelucci E, Muretto P, Lucarelli G, et al: Treatment of iron overload in the "ex-thalassemic": report from the Phlebotomy Program. Ann N Y Acad Sci 850:288, 1998.

30. Andreani M, Manna M, Lucarelli G, et al: Persistence of mixed chimerism in patients transplanted for the treatment of thalassemia. Blood 87:3494, 1996.

31. Borgna-Pignatti C, Rugolotto S, De Stefano P, et al: Survival and disease complications in thalassemia major. Ann NY Acad Sci 850:227, 1998.

32. Nagel RL: Severity, pathobiology, epistatic effects, and genetic markers in sickle cell anemia. Semin Hematol 28:180, 1991.

33. Platt OS, Thorington BD, Brambilla DJ, et al: Pain in sickle cell disease: rates and risk factors. N Engl J Med 325:11, 1991.

34. Embury SH, Hebbel RP, Steinberg MH, Mohandas N: Pathogenesis of vasoocclusion. In Embury SH, Hebbel RP, Mohandas N, Steinberg MH (eds): Sickle Cell Disease: Basic Principles and Clinical Practice. New York, Raven Press, 1994, p 311.

35. Hebbel RP: Beyond hemoglobin polymerization: the red blood cell membrane and sickle cell pathophysiology. Blood 77:214, 1991.

36. Kaul DK, Nagel RL: Sickle cell vasoocclusion: many issues and some answers. Experientia 49:5, 1993.

37. Bunn HF: Pathogenesis and treatment of sickle cell disease. N Engl J Med 337:762, 1997.

38. Powars DR, Chan LS, Schroeder WA: The variable expression of sickle cell disease is genetically determined. Semin Hematol 27:360, 1990.

39. Platt OS, Brambilla DJ, Rosse WF, et at: Mortality in sickle cell disease: life expectancy and risk factors for early death. N Engl J Med 330:1639, 1994.

40. Embury SH, Garcia JF, Mohandas N, et al: Effects of oxygen inhalation on endogenous erythropoietin kinetics, erythropoiesis, and properties of blood cells in sickle cell anemia. N Engl J Med 311:291, 1984.

41. Wayne AS, Kevy SV, Nathan DG: Transfusion management of sickle cell disease. Blood 81:1109, 1993.

42. Davies SC, Roberts-Harewood M: Blood transfusion in sickle cell disease. Blood Rev 11:57, 1997.

43. Vichinsky EP, Haberkern CM, Neumayr L, et al: A comparison of conservative and aggressive transfusion regimens in the perioperative management of sickle cell disease. N Engl J Med 333:206, 1995.

44. Koshy M, Burd L, Wallace D, et al: Prophylactic red-cell transfusions in pregnant patients with sickle cell disease: a randomized cooperative study. N Engl J Med 319:1447, 1988.

45. Cohen AR, Martin MB, Silber JH, et al: A modified transfusion program for prevention of stroke in sickle cell disease. Blood 79:1657, 1992.

46. Charache S, Terrin ML, Moore RD, et al: Effect of hydroxyurea on the frequency on painful crises in sickle cell anemia. N Engl J Med 332:1317, 1995.

47. Johnson FL, Look AT, Gockerman J, et al: Bone-marrow transplantation in a patient with sickle-cell anemia. N Engl J Med 311:780, 1984.

48. Billings FT: Treatment of sickle cell anemia with bone marrow transplantation—pros and cons. Trans Am Clin Climatol Assoc 101:8, 1990.

49. Vermylen C, Fernandez-Robles E, Ninane J, Cornu G: Bone marrow transplantation in five children with sickle cell anemia. Lancet 1:1427, 1988.

50. Ferster A, De Valck C, Azzi N, et al: Bone marrow transplantation for severe sickle cell anemia. Br J Haematol 80:102, 1992.

51. Vermylen C, Cornu G: Bone marrow transplantation in sickle cell anemia. Blood Rev 7:1, 1993.

52. Vermylen C, Cornu G, Ferster A, et al: Bone marrow transplantation in sickle cell anemia: the Belgian experience. Bone Marrow Transplant 12(Suppl 1):116, 1993.

53. Bernaudin F, Souillet G, Vannier JP, et al: Bone marrow transplantation (BMT) in 14 children with severe sickle cell disease (SCD): the French experience. Bone Marrow Transplant 12(Suppl 1):118, 1993.

54. Kirkpatrick DV, Barrios NJ, Humbert JH: Bone marrow transplantation for sickle cell anemia. Semin Hematol 28:240, 1991.

55. Nagel RL: The dilemma of marrow transplantation in sickle cell anemia. Semin Hematol 28:233, 1991.

56. Davies SC: Bone marrow transplantation for sickle cell disease. Arch Dis Child 69:176, 1993.

57. Davies SC: Bone marrow transplantation for sickle cell disease—the dilemma. Blood Rev 7:4, 1993.

58. Walters MC, Patience M, Leisenring W, et al: Bone marrow transplantation for sickle cell disease. N Engl J Med 335:369, 1996.

59. Walters MC, Patience M, Leisenring W, et al: Collaborative multicenter investigation of marrow transplantation for sickle cell disease: current results and future directions. Biol Blood Marrow Transplant 3:310, 1997.

60. Walters MC, Patience M, Leisenring W, et al: Impact of bone marrow transplantation (BMT) for severe sickle cell disease (SCD): long-term follow-up evaluations. Blood 92 (Suppl 1):693a, 1998.

CHAPTER SEVENTEEN

Gaucher Disease

*John A. Barranger, M.D., Ph.D., Erin O'Rourke, M.S., C.G.C.,
Alfred Bahnson, Ph.D., and Edward D. Ball, M.D.*

Gaucher disease is the most common lysosomal storage disorder. In the Ashkenazic Jewish population, the incidence of the disease is 1 in 450, with approximately 1 person in 10 carrying the gene for the disease.[1] In the non-Ashkenazic Jewish population, the carrier frequency is approximately 1 in 100, with 1 person in 40,000 affected.

Persons with Gaucher disease are deficient in glucocerebrosidase, a specialized lysosomal enzyme that hydrolyzes glucosylceramide to glucose and ceramide. As a result of the deficiency, glucosylceramide accumulates in the lysosomes of reticuloendothelial cells to produce the characteristic Gaucher cell.

There are three types of Gaucher disease.[2] Each is the result of glucocerebrosidase deficiency and is inherited in an autosomal recessive manner. The principal difference among the types is the presence and progression of neurologic complications. Type 1 Gaucher disease is the most common and has a chronic, non-neuronopathic course. The age of onset and severity of symptoms vary widely. It is this type of Gaucher disease that has an increased incidence in the Ashkenazic Jewish population. Type 2 Gaucher disease is the acute neuronopathic or infantile form. The average age of onset is 3 months, and neurologic complications are usually apparent by 6 months of age. This type is fatal at an average of 9 months and has no ethnic predilection. Type 3 Gaucher disease is panethnic, but there is a genetic isolate of type 3 disease in the population of northern Sweden. Patients with type 3 Gaucher disease usually present as children and have slowly progressive, neurodegenerative disease. The first neurologic sign is typically oculomotor apraxia, an eye movement disorder.

Gaucher disease is caused by mutations in the gene encoding glucocerebrosidase.[8] The most common genetic mutation causing type 1 disease is a single base-pair substitution in codon 370.[2] It accounts for approximately 70% of the mutant alleles in Ashkenazic Jewish patients with Gaucher disease. The lysosomal enzyme associated with this mutation has reduced activity but is not diminished in concentration in the lysosome.[4] Most patients with the more-severe types of Gaucher disease (types 2 and 3) who present with neurologic complications carry at least one allele with a single base substitution in codon 444. This mutation results in an unstable enzyme with little or no enzymatic activity in the lysosome. More than 150 mutations in the GC gene are known. Most are private alleles occuring in a single kindred.

TREATMENT

The recent success of enzyme replacement therapy has simplified the management of patients with type 1 Gaucher disease. With the isolation and purification of glucocerebrosidase, replacement of the deficient enzyme in persons with Gaucher disease became a possibility.[3] Although initial biochemical results were encouraging, further studies revealed that glucocerebrosidase in its native form was not effectively delivered to the storage macrophages in which glucosylceramide accumulates. Further research established that if the oligosaccharide side chains of the enzyme were degraded to expose mannose residues, the enzyme binds to a mannose-specific receptor on the macrophage plasma membrane and is endocytosed, thus creating a drug delivery system.[4]

Studies in animals showed more than a 10-fold increase in uptake of the modified (mannose-terminated) enzyme by Gaucher cells compared with uptake of native enzyme by the same cells. Periodic infusion of mannose-terminated glucocerebrosidase in patients with Gaucher disease is effective in reaching the target macrophages and reversing disease manifestations. Patients experience an increase in hemoglobin concentration, an increase in platelet count, a reduction in the size of the liver and spleen, and a gradual improvement in bone manifestations.

Enzyme replacement therapy is the first therapeutic breakthrough for the treatment of persons with lysosomal storage disease.[3, 5] The pharmacology of mannose-terminated glucocerebrosidase is complicated, and multiple variables need to be clarified to fine-tune and enhance the success of enzyme replacement therapy. The recommended dosage is 60 U/kg body weight every 2 weeks.[5] The minimum effective dose and the optimal dosage frequency are only beginning to be determined.[5-7] Additional clinical experience and research using cell cultures and transgenic animal models will provide important tools to further evaluate this therapeutic approach.

Given that macrophages are derived from the bone marrow and are the only storage cells in which glucosylceramide accumulates in Gaucher disease, successful bone marrow transplantation (BMT) logically has been curative for this genetic disease. BMT has been reported in several patients with Gaucher disease, who experienced resolution of enzyme deficiency in circulating white blood cells, regression of organomegaly, and improvement in general health. The risk of allogeneic transplantation, however, does not justify the procedure in patients with mild disease. Moreover, transplant-associated risks increase with the severity of the disease and the age of the patient. The advent of enzyme replacement therapy obviously limits the number of patients who are considered for BMT.

The cloning of complementary DNA (cDNA) for the

glucocerebrosidase gene made it possible to consider treating Gaucher disease using somatic cell gene therapy.[8] Initially, it was shown that glucocerebrosidase deficiency can be corrected by transferring the glucocerebrosidase gene into cultured fibroblasts of persons with Gaucher disease.[9] Early studies demonstrated that simplified retroviral vectors carrying the human gene can result in sustained expression of glucocerebrosidase in the hematopoietic stem cells (HSC) of mice.[10, 11]

DEVELOPMENT OF GENE TRANSFER AS A POTENTIAL THERAPY FOR GAUCHER DISEASE

CONSTRUCTION OF MFG-GC

Initial results with N2-derived vectors demonstrated efficient transduction into murine HSC in long-term bone marrow cultures[11] and in irradiated syngeneic recipients of transduced bone marrow.[10] Expression of the transgene was observed in vitro but only minimally in vivo in spleen colonies derived from recipients' transplanted bone marrow transduced with the N2-SV-GC vector. In contrast, sustained long-term expression was achieved in animals undergoing transplantation with bone marrow transduced with the MFG retroviral vector. The features of the MFG-GC vector are that the GC cDNA is transcribed by the retroviral LTR and the start codon of the GC cDNA was placed at the start codon of the deleted envelope protein gene. No internal promoter or dominant selectable marker is included in the construct.[10]

MURINE BONE MARROW TRANSPLANT MODEL

The MFG-GC vector was cotransfected with pSV2neo into the ecotropic ψCRE helper line. After selection in G418 and screening of clones of the supernatants by gene transfer into 3T3 targets, approximately half of 28 G418-resistant clones expressed viral titers in the range of 10^6 integrating copies per mL, and 5 clones expressed titers 5–10 times higher. The titering method was based on a linear correlation observed between enzyme activity in 3T3 targets with Southern blot hybridization intensity calibrated on cell lines of known copy number.[13]

The highest titer ecotropic producer, ψCRE#4, was used to transduce marrow from 5-fluorouracil (5-FU)–treated donor C57BL6/J-GPI[a] mice using 2-day prestimulation followed by 2-day coculture with irradiated producer cells in the presence of interleukin-3 (IL-3), IL-6, and stem cell factor, essentially as outlined by Bodine et al.[14] Irradiated syngeneic recipient mice carried the alternative GPI-1[b] isoenzyme, which permitted estimation of the degree of engraftment of donor cells at various time points after transplantation based on electrophoresis of peripheral blood cell extracts.

The efficiency of transduction and expression of the GC gene in bone marrow cells were estimated by analyzing individual colonies harvested from the spleens of lethally irradiated mice at 12 days after BMT. Eighty-six colonies

from the spleens of mice given MFG-GC transduced cells and 13 colonies from mice reconstituted with marrow infected with N2-SV-GC were analyzed for comparison. Colonies from lethally irradiated mice that underwent transplantation with normal syngeneic marrow were used as controls. Southern blot hybridization revealed that essentially all of the spleen colonies from either group of experimental recipients contained integrated vector at similar copy numbers, but colonies from MFG-GC mice gave enzymatic activities that ranged from two to five times the activity of the controls, whereas the colonies from N2-SV-GC mice were not greater than with the controls.

By 2 months after BMT in mice given 10^6 bone marrow cells, circulating white blood cells were greater than 90% donor type as assessed by GPI and remained greater than 90% until sacrifice. In addition, the majority of circulating white blood cells were positive for the human gene product by immunocytochemical analysis. Animals were sacrificed between 4 and 7 months after BMT. Southern blot test results were positive for the human gene in tissues from the liver, lung, spleen, thymus, lymph nodes, and bone marrow. The enzymatic activity of hematopoietic tissues from mice reconstituted with marrow infected with MFG-GC exceeded the activity of control tissues by an average of three times in spleen and six times in bone marrow. By comparison, the hematopoietic tissues from mice given bone marrow cells infected with N2-SV-GC showed little or no increase above control levels of activity.

The data accumulated on nonhematopoietic tissues (liver, lung) were also informative. These tissues normally are supplied with bone marrow–derived cells on a continuing basis. Under normal physiologic circumstances, bone marrow–derived cells in these tissues are primarily macrophages. In liver, tissue macrophages (Kupffer cells) constitute approximately 15% of the organ. If all of the liver macrophages were replaced in MFG-GC reconstituted animals by the progeny of transduced HSC derived from the bone marrow, the copy number of the vector in the liver should be about 0.15 per cell. The results of Southern blot analyses demonstrated that the MFG-GC vector resulted in a copy number in liver of approximately 0.1 per cell. This result is consistent with a high transduction efficiency of HSC by the MFG-GC vector and the ability of HSC to repopulate the macrophage lineage.

As a further measure of the ability of the MFG-GC vector to transduce self-renewing pluripotent HSC, we performed secondary BMT using bone marrow collected from three long-term reconstituted mice. All secondary spleen colonies from animals sacrificed at 12 days were positive for the human GC gene by Southern blot analyses (n = 27), and the enzymatic activities were two to seven times higher than that of control colony-forming units (spleen). Long-term secondary transplants were maintained for more than 12 months. Assay of peripheral blood leukocytes for GC activity revealed that cells have 4–10 times the background amount of enzyme.

To investigate vector expression in macrophages, bone marrow from sacrificed recipients was expanded in the presence of macrophage colony-stimulating factor (M-CSF), resulting in nearly pure colonies of macrophages that were actively phagocytic as evidenced by the ability to take up latex beads. The enzymatic activity in these cells was on average four times greater than that of control macrophages. Western blots of macrophage extracts showed an intense band of human GC protein not present in control cells cultured from normal mouse bone marrow. The copy number in these cells was approximately 1–2 per cell by Southern blot analyses. Immunochemical staining of these cultured macrophages for the human gene product revealed that most of the cells exhibited positive staining, whereas there was no staining in control cultures. These results demonstrated conclusively that self-renewing pluripotent HSC were transduced, that the transgene was expressed at high levels for the life of the mice, and that macrophages, which are the differentiated cells of therapeutic potential for gene therapy, exhibited robust expression of the GC enzyme at low vector copy numbers.

GENERATION AND CHARACTERIZATION OF AMPHOTROPIC PRODUCER LINES

For preclinical studies and for clinical application, an amphotropic producer cell line was required. Cell surface envelope protein interferes with cross-infection of cells of the same pseudotype, but supernatant from an ecotropic producer can be used to cross-infect an amphotropic packaging cell line to generate stable amphotropic producers and vice versa. In this case, the proviral vector DNA integrates without carriage of plasmid sequences, and transduction efficiency may be high enough to clone candidate producers without selection. The high-titer amphotropic MFG-GC producer, cc-2, was thus generated by cross-infection of ψCRIP packaging cells with supernatant from ψCRE#4. Among 12 isolated clones, 5 yielded significant titer, and 1 clone, cc-2, expressed a titer of about 2×10^7 integrating copies/mL.

The MFG-GC vector was subsequently modified by insertion of a SacII linker immediately downstream of the gag start site, yielding a frame shift to prevent expression of partial gag sequences (incorporated into MFG to retain packaging efficiency). After this change, a set of promising producers was obtained using a two-step process employing the BOSC 23 transient packaging line[19] to produce an ecotropic vector–containing supernatant, which was then used to cross-infect ψCRIP packaging cells. The subsequent titer of a selected ψCRIP producer was highly variable on 3T3 targets, contrasting with human TF-1 cell targets, which remained readily transducible with supernatants from the same producer. Southern blot analysis revealed high copy number in the 3T3 targets, indicating efficient transduction without GC enzyme expression in these targets. More definitively, among a recent set of 15 G418-resistant QCRIP clones cotransfected with the modified MFG-GC vector and pSV2neo, none raised 3T3 target activity as much as 200 U/mg above background, whereas 8 clones yielded elevations of over 500 U/mg in human TF-1 cell targets. These findings reveal unexpected specificity of expression among slightly different forms of the MFG vector (manuscript in preparation) and imply that potentially useful producer clones may have been overlooked because 3T3 target activity was implicitly relied on for titering.

TRANSDUCTION OF CD34+-ENRICHED CELLS

High-titer vector production and efficient expression of the MFG-GC vector facilitated effective supernatant transduction of enriched populations of CD34+ cells obtained from normal cord blood, normal bone marrow, peripheral blood primed with granulocyte colony-stimulating factor (G-CSF) in patients with leukemia, and from bone marrow of patients with Gaucher disease collected during surgical procedures for knee replacement. Enzyme activity in transduced cells was compared with normal and abnormal (Gaucher) enzyme activity levels in nontransduced cells, showing that potentially therapeutic elevation in glucocerebrosidase was readily achieved in transduced cells using this experimental protocol and high-titer cc-2 supernatants.

In the initial protocol, CD34+-enriched cells were prestimulated in medium containing the cytokines, IL-3, IL-6, and stem cell factor, followed by four or five daily exposures to fresh vector-containing supernatants. During the course of these initial studies, experiments indicated that a prestimulation period of 1 day and reduced infection numbers over a shorter time period were equally effective.[13, 15] The rapid appearance of myeloid differentiation antigens on the CD34+ cells over time in culture stressed the importance of minimizing the ex vivo period as much as possible.[15]

Transduction was directly analyzed by Southern blot analysis of *Sst*I digests of genomic DNA from expanded transduced CD34+ cells. Vector proviral DNA hybridization intensity in transduced cells was compared with that of controls consisting of human DNA quantitatively spiked with DNA from a murine fibroblast clone carrying a known vector copy number. Results showed that low copy numbers of the MFG-GC vector (<1 copy per cell) resulted in glucocerebrosidase expression levels that more than compensated for the deficiency of this enzyme in hematopoietic cells in culture of patients with Gaucher disease. Supporting evidence for normal enzyme expression was provided by immunocytochemical staining, which indicated that at least 20% of the expanded cells expressed the transgene and displayed a staining intensity equal to or greater than that of normal bone marrow cells.[13]

CENTRIFUGAL ENHANCEMENT OF TRANSDUCTION

Despite the encouraging results described, variability and reports of lower-than-expected transduction efficiencies when research procedures were applied in clinical practice[16, 17] spurred us to investigate centrifugation as a method to gain additional advantage over the transduction process (R.W. Atchison, personal communication). In part, this effort is based on the assumption that higher observed transduction in progenitor cells will be found to correlate with a higher probability of transduction in the ultimate target, the engrafting pluripotent HSC. This assumption is currently necessary, regardless of the method, because there are no proven assays for this target cell population other than transplantation in human patients.

Initial experiments comparing centrifugal with noncentrifugal transduction of cord blood CD34+-enriched cells demonstrated the potential for improved transduction. In one of the two experiments comparing both methods, polymerase chain reaction (PCR) analysis of granulocyte/macrophage colony-forming cells (CFU-GM) indicated a transduction efficiency of 95% using centrifugation compared with no PCR-positive colonies detected in control cultures of cells transduced in the same experiment at 1 g. A transduction efficiency of 17–20% in the long-term culture initiating cells (LTC-IC) from centrifuged samples was revealed by PCR analysis of CFU-GM taken at 4, 5, and 6 weeks in this experiment. Although these results are among the best reported for retroviral transduction of HSC, lower transduction of LTC-IC compared with CFU-GM points to and reinforces the need for continuing improvement in transduction efficiency.

Additional experiments with cultured human hematopoietic (TF-1) cells indicated that the enhancement effect of centrifugation is directly related to centrifugal force up to 10,000 g and to the time of centrifugation. On the other hand, the effect was inversely related to cell number in a given container, presumably reflecting a requirement for surface area exposure to suspended virus.[18] These variables provide opportunity for further improvement, but for practical application at the present time, we have adopted a procedure using blood bags containing up to 5×10^7 cells per bag centrifuged at 2400 g twice for 2-hour periods with a midpoint change of supernatant. A major advantage of the centrifugation protocol is that it reduces the time the cells must be kept in culture to a minimum. This may be particularly important in light of studies by Peters et al. showing rapid reduction in engraftment potential with increasing time in culture.[24]

TRANSDUCTION OF CD34 CELLS: OPTIMIZATION OF CONDITIONS

Preclinical studies demonstrated efficient transduction in CD34+ cord blood cells as measured by high enzyme activity and positive PCR signals for the glucocerebrosidase transgene in CFU-GM and clonogenic cells arising from LTC-IC cultures in transduced fractions.[25]

Human umbilical cord blood cells were collected after normal deliveries and enriched for the CD34+ fraction using Ceprate columns (CellPro, Inc.). The CD34+-enriched fraction was prestimulated for up to 24 hours with 10 ng/mL each of IL-3, IL-6, and stem cell factor (Pepro Tech) in long-term bone marrow culture media at a concentration of 2×10^5 cells/mL. These cells were transduced with a retroviral vector containing the normal human glucocerebrosidase cDNA three times over the course of 24 hours at a concentration of 10^5/mL using a protocol based on a centrifugation-enhanced technique developed by Bahnson et al.[18] Nontransduced controls were obtained as fractions from each cord blood sample. Data from these experiments demonstrate an average transduction efficiency in the CD34+-enriched fraction of 50% as measured by PCR for the integrated glucocerebrosidase-cDNA in CFU-GM colonies. PCR of CFU-GM harvested from LTC-IC cultures at 6 weeks also indicates transfer of the cDNA to early progenitor cells. Measurements of enzyme activity comparing transduced and nontransduced fractions at 4 or

6 days post transduction indicate an average enzyme increase of six times over nontransduced background levels.

The next question was the stability of the transgene and the ability to sustain expression of a functional enzyme over time. Human cord blood cells would not be appropriate for this assessment because the composition and stability of the CD34+ cell population grown in bulk culture over time is not well defined. The human cell line TF-1, a factor-dependent human erythroleukemia cell line (American Type Culture Collection),[20] was chosen to address this question of stability. TF-1 cultures provide the readily available material in which to optimize a large-scale infection that would be necessary in a clinical trial. These cells were transduced at a concentration of 10^5/mL using the retroviral vector containing the glucocerebrosidase cDNA and maintained in culture for 44 days. With a successful transduction efficiency at a cell concentration of 10^5/mL, the question of increasing cell concentration against efficiency was addressed. Cells from this experiment remained in culture for 35 days. Although a relationship with increasing cell number to decreasing transduction efficiency was observed, both experiments show enzymatic activities in transduced TF-1 cultures that remained at least 25 times above the activity of nontransduced cells throughout a 6-week culture period. The results from this study were used in establishing conditions appropriate for transducing the cells of patients with Gaucher disease in a clinical trial.

PRECLINICAL STUDIES OF CD34+ CELLS FROM PATIENTS WITH GAUCHER DISEASE

Transplantation of CD34+ cells is advantageous for several reasons. First, the number of CD34+ cells required for transplantation is considerably smaller than with a whole bone marrow transplant, consequently reducing the side effects associated with cell transplantation as well those associated with infusion of the cryoprotectant dimethyl sulfoxide. Second, the amount of viral supernatant and cytokines required for transduction and prestimulation is significantly reduced.

We showed previously that a significant number of CD34+ cells can be collected in patients with Gaucher disease, a number adequate for conventional transplantation in the host.[26] These data are reviewed in the following paragraphs.

PATIENTS

Three patients with Gaucher disease were entered into this Institutional Review Board-approved study. Type 1 Gaucher disease was diagnosed in patient No. 1 (JH), aged 48 years, in 1968. He was started on enzyme replacement therapy in September 1993 and is presently on alglucerase (Ceredase), 30 U/kg every 2 weeks. In patient No. 2 (RH), aged 35 years, type 1 Gaucher disease was diagnosed in 1965; this patient has been maintained on alglucerase, 45 U/kg every 2 weeks. In the third patient (IM), aged 49 years, type 1 Gaucher disease was diagnosed in 1954. This patient has been maintained on alglucerase since June

1992. Her present dose was 30 U/kg every 2 weeks. All three patients have responded to enzyme therapy as evidenced by a reduction in organ size and an increase in hematologic indices. Each continues to experience skeletal complications of the disease. The different doses enzyme replacement therapy in these individuals reflect the efforts to reduce the dose from 60 U/kg every 2 weeks to a lower maintenance dose. All patients gave written informed consent.

MOBILIZATION AND LEUKAPHERESIS

Patient No. 1 and patient No. 2 received G-CSF (filgrastim [Neupogen]), 5 μg/kg/day, subcutaneously for 10 days. Patient No. 3 received G-CSF at the dose of 10 μg/kg/day for 10 days. Pre G-CSF laboratory evaluation for each patient involved glucocerebrosidase activity, genotype, complete blood count and differential, platelets, uric acid, alkaline phosphatase, lactate dehydrogenase, and flow cytometric analysis for CD34+ cells. Daily evaluation while the patient was on G-CSF involved complete blood count, platelet count and differential, uric acid, lactate dehydrogenase, alkaline phosphatase, and fluorescence-assisted cell sorting (FACS) analysis for CD34+ cell number.

Leukapheresis was started in the three patients on day 5. A total of five leukaphereses were performed in each patient using the Cobe Spectra device. The total volume of the leukapheresis product was recorded, and samples were removed for cell counts and further analysis. All cell counts were done on the Coulter Counter ZM to determine the total number of white blood cells in the leukapheresis product. The leukapheresis product was washed with RPMI-1640 on the Cobe 2991. The final volume of the washed cell preparation was approximately 150 mL.

After leukapheresis, the total number of white blood cells in the apheresis products averaged 1.6×10^{11} (range, 1.0×10^{11}–2.5×10^{11}), or 2.1×10^9/kg.

ENRICHMENT FOR CD34+ CELLS

Enrichment for CD34+ cells was performed using the CellPro Ceprate system. The washed leukapheresis product was incubated with the biotin-labeled anti-CD34 antibody and 0.1% human serum albumin (25%) for 25 minutes at room temperature with mixing for 15 minutes. After incubation, the cells were washed on the Cobe 2991 and resuspended in phosphate-buffered saline to a volume of 300 mL. Samples were removed for further analysis at this stage, which included cell counts, flow cytometry for CD34 and subset analysis, viability, and clonogenic assays. The cells were processed on the Ceprate SC instrument. The enriched and depleted fractions were collected, and aliquots were removed for further analysis. Sterility testing was also performed on the enriched fraction. The enriched fraction was centrifuged at 1200 rpm for 8 minutes and the supernatant removed. The enriched CD34+ cells were cryopreserved in Media 199 with dimethyl sulfoxide plus 20% autologous plasma using a controlled-rate freezing protocol.

The number of white blood cells in the enriched fractions averaged 6.3×10^8 (range, 4.5×10^8 to $7.9 \times$

10^8), or 9.6×10^6/kg. Using the clinical Ceprate column, enrichments averaging 195 times (range, 4–625 times) were observed. These data demonstrate up to a sixfold increase in the percentage of CD34+ cells in peripheral blood in the three patients.

The recovery varied from a mean of 25.6% (range, 4.9–48.4%), 61.4% (range, 22.4–168.3%), and 36.9% (range, 25–59%), respectively, in the three patients. The total number of CD34+ cells collected was 1.2, 3.5, and 2.1×10^6 cells/kg, respectively.

The CellPro Ceprate system is no longer available commercially. Enrichment of CD34+ cells may be accomplished by other systems, such as Isolex-300i by Nexell. Detailed descriptions of CD34+ cell selection systems can be found in Chapter 28.

FLOW CYTOMETRIC ANALYSIS FOR CD34+ CELLS AND SUBSETS

The procedures described below were designed to apply specifically to this study. A detailed discussion for routine measurement of CD34+ cells by flow cytometry can be found in Chapter 27.

Sample Preparation

The cell concentration was adjusted to 1×10^7 cells/mL in PBS; 100 μL of the cell suspension was then incubated with the labeled monoclonal antibodies. Dual-color staining was performed using the following monoclonal antibodies: CD34 (fluorescein isothiocyanate) combined with either CD38 (phycoerythrin), human leukocyte antigen (HLA)-DR (phycoerythrin), Thy-1 (phycoerythrin), or CD33 (phycoerythrin). Relevent isotype controls were used. A 100-μL aliquot of stained cells was mixed with an equal volume of PBS containing 1% human albumin and 0.1% sodium azide and incubated for 15 minutes at room temperature in the dark. The tubes were then centrifuged for 5 minutes at 250 g and the supernatant decanted. Two milliliters of FACS lysing solution was added to each tube, and the cells were incubated for an additional 10 minutes. The tubes were then centrifuged again for 5 minutes at 250 g, the supernatant decanted, and the pellet resuspended in 500 μL of 1% paraformaldehyde. The suspensions were stored at 4°C in the dark and submitted to flow cytometric analysis in their respective staining solutions.

Samples were acquired on a FACScan flow cytometer (Becton Dickinson, San Jose, CA) equipped with a 15-mW, air-cooled, 488-nm argon-ion laser. Fluorescence data were displayed on a four-decade log scale. Analysis of the bivariate data was performed with LYSYS II software (Becton Dickinson).

Analysis

To obtain total CD34+ cell numbers, samples were analyzed according to CD34 fluorescence intensity within a live cell gate. Gates to identify CD34+ cells were set using the relevant negative isotype control. The CD34+ cells were gated, and the expression of the second antibody was assessed on the CD34+ cells using a dot plot of FL1 versus FL2; 20,000 events were acquired for each sample. To improve the accuracy of subpopulation analysis of those samples in which the CD34+ cell count was low, at least 500 CD34+ events were collected.

We analyzed the percentage of CD34+ cells that coexpressed Thy-1, CD38, HLA-DR, and CD33. The mean percentages of CD34+ cells in peripheral blood that coexpressed Thy-1 was 71.6%, 28.9% and 44.4%, respectively, in the three patients. We noted that there was a trend for the percentage of CD34+/Thy-1+ cells to diminish with enrichment. The reason for this reduction is uncertain and is under investigation. Thy-1 has been shown to be an early hematopoietic marker.[21] Impairment of long-term engraftment by the diminution of these cells is unlikely because CD34+ cells using the CellPro column have been shown to engraft as well as bone marrow.[22] Therefore, the significance of this observation remains unknown at this time. The percentage of other CD34+ subsets remained unaltered with manipulation.

TRANSDUCTION OF HUMAN HEMATOPOIETIC PROGENITORS

We have previously demonstrated high transduction efficiencies using a centrifugation-promoted infection protocol.[18] This method involves centrifugation of small numbers of cells in tubes, which is not feasible in the clinical setting. We have therefore developed a method using blood collection bags for the centrifugation of large numbers of cells applicable to the clinical trial. The patients' CD34+-enriched cells that were frozen were thawed rapidly while being mixed constantly. The cells were washed immediately in long-term bone marrow culture (LTBMC), counted, and resuspended at a concentration of 2×10^5 cells/mL. Prestimulation of the cells was performed using the cytokines IL-3, IL-6, and stem cell factor at concentrations of 10 ng/mL for 16–24 hours. The cell concentration was maintained at 2×10^5/mL throughout the prestimulation procedure. After this, the cells were resuspended at 5×10^6 to 3×10^8 cells in 50 mL of LTBMC. The cytokine concentration was maintained at 10 ng/mL, and protamine sulphate was added to achieve a concentration of 4 μg/mL. A 60-mL syringe was used to inject the cell suspension into a 150-mL capacity blood collection bag. Fifty milliliters of viral supernatant was injected into the same blood collection bag. The air pocket was removed, the bag sealed, and the excess tubing removed. The blood bags were then centrifuged at 2400 g at 24°C for 2 hours. The bags were removed from the centrifuge and transferred to a 50-mL conical tube. The bag was rinsed with 50 mL of LTBMC to remove any adherent cells. The cells were then centrifuged at 2400 g for 5 minutes, the supernatant removed, and the cells resuspended in 25 mL of LTBMC. The cells were counted and subjected to further analysis.

ANALYSIS OF TRANSDUCTION EFFICIENCY

CLONOGENIC ASSAYS. Transduced CD34+ cells were plated at a concentration of 1×10^4 cells/mL in methyl cellulose with IL-3 and GM-CSF. Individual CFU-GM colonies gener-

ated after 14 days were plucked and analyzed by PCR for the GC gene in the retroviral vector.

PCR TECHNIQUE. PCR was carried out on genomic DNA samples in a final volume of 50 μL. The reaction mixture contained 200μM of each deoxynucleotides, 0.5 U Amplitaq (Perkin-Elmer), 2 mM MgCl₂, and 0.2 μM of each primer in Amplitaq buffer. One primer hybridizes within the glucocerebrosidase-cDNA region and the second hybridizes within the viral sequence, yielding a unique 407-bp amplification product (AB1: 5′ ACG GCA TGG CAG CTT GGA TA 3′; AB2: 5′ AGT AGC AAA TTT TGG GCA GG 3′). Thermal cycling was performed on the Gene Amp PCR System 9600 as follows: 94°C × 5 minutes for an initial denaturing cycle, followed by 30 cycles of 94°C × 30 seconds, 58°C × 30 seconds, and 72°C × 30 seconds. The PCR products were resolved on a 6% acrylamide or 2% agarose gel and the bands visualized by ethidium bromide and ultraviolet light.

PCR OF METHYLCELLULOSE COLONIES. Because of the viscosity of the methylcellulose media, extraction of DNA from these CFU-GM colonies required further preparation. Isolated, single colonies were removed and placed into a sterile, nuclease-free microcentrifuge tube. The DNA extraction method is as follows. The lysis solution consists of 1.5 μL of glycogen, 10 μL of 2M sodium acetate (pH 4.5), 20 μL of sterile distilled water, 100 μL of phenol, and 20 μL of chloroform. To each tube, 150 μL of this mixture was added and left to incubate for at least 30 minutes at 4°C. The tubes were then spun in a microcentrifuge at 12,000 g for 10 minutes. The aqueous phase was transferred to a clean tube and precipitated with 100 μL isopropanol at −80°C for at least 3 hours or −20°C overnight. The samples were spun at 12,000 g for 10 minutes; the pellets were washed in cold 70% ethanol, allowed to briefly air dry, and resuspended in 30 μL sterile distilled water. This sample was then ready for PCR analysis. A mean transduction efficiency of 32% was detected.

PCR OF LONG-TERM CULTURE INITIATING CELLS. Long-term bone marrow cultures were maintained as previously described.[23] Transduced CD34+ cells were placed on preformed irradiated allogeneic bone marrow stroma at a minimum concentration of 5×10^5 cells per T25 flask. Half the medium was replaced weekly. The cultures were maintained at a temperature of 33°C. Cells were removed after 4 and 5 weeks and plated in methylcellulose for clonogenic assays. At week 6, nonadherent cells and adherent cells that were removed using trypsin were plated individually in methylcellulose. Individual CFU-GM were plucked at 14 days and analyzed by PCR for the GC gene. A transduction efficiency of 25% for patient #1 and 50% for patient #3 was detected on LTC-IC.

GLUCOCEREBROSIDASE ENZYME ASSAY IN EXPANDED CELLS

The cells were expanded for 6 days in cytokines and assayed for enzyme activity. Up to a 50-fold increase above deficient levels was detected.[13]

CLINICAL TRIAL OF GENE THERAPY FOR GAUCHER DISEASE

DESCRIPTION

Allogeneic BMT has been used successfully to treat several patients with Gaucher disease. Enzyme replacement therapy (ERT) has been available since 1991. More than 1500 patients with type 1 Gaucher disease have been treated and, with few exceptions, the patients experience a reversal of disease symptoms and arrest of the progressive disease.

The risk of mortality associated with allogeneic BMT (~30%), the need for an HLA-matched donor, and the availability of ERT render this approach to treatment of Gaucher disease obsolete. ERT is efficacious, but it involves lifelong infusions and is expensive. Ex vivo gene transfer and autologous BMT could result in a permanent treatment for Gaucher disease without the requirement for a matched donor, the risk of mortality, and the expense of ERT.

Gene therapy involves the insertion of a normal copy of a gene into the cells of a patients with an inherited defect in the corresponding gene. HSC are a pathobiologically important target cell for gene transfer in Gaucher disease because macrophages are derived from the bone marrow. In this approach, HSC are collected, genetically corrected by inserting the gene, and then recolonized in the patient. Gene transfer/autologous BMT avoids the immunologic problems of graft rejection and graft-versus-host disease, which occur with high frequency in allogeneic transplantations. To be successful, gene therapy requires high-efficiency gene transfer into cells followed by persistent expression of the transferred gene at an appropriate level.

In this study, we transduced CD34+ cells obtained from the blood of patients with Gaucher disease using a replication defective retroviral vector called R-GC. The vector carries the human glucocerebrosidase cDNA. Genetically corrected CD34+ cells are returned intravenously to the patient who donated the cells. This process is referred to as ex vivo gene transfer and autologous BMT. The primary aim of the study is to evaluate the safety of this approach. Other aims include estimating the extent of competitive engraftment of genetically corrected CD34+ cells, measuring the endurance of bone marrow engraftment with CD34+ cells, measuring the ability of these genetically corrected cells to sustain expression of glucocerebrosidase, and examining the patients for any clinical response (Fig. 17-1).

The hypothesis of this study is that genetically corrected peripheral blood progenitor cells (PBPC) will engraft and result in the supply of enzymatically competent progeny sufficient to reverse the phenotype in patients with Gaucher disease. The specific aims to be achieved are as follows:

1. Evaluation of the safety and feasibility of correcting the basic genetic defect of Gaucher disease by infusing patients with transduced CD34+ cells
2. Transfer of the human GC gene into PBPC obtained from patients with Gaucher disease
3. Autologous transplantation of transduced PBPC to patients
4. Measurement of the carriage and expression of the trans-

ferred gene and its duration in peripheral blood leukocytes
5. Assessment of the clinical effects of transplanting genetically corrected PBPC in patients with Gaucher disease

The outcome of the study will influence future plans by providing information about the safety and capability of gene transfer using our proposed method. Further developments could influence our decisions about different vectors, different preparations of HSC, and different methods of preparation of patients.

METHODOLOGY

This clinical trial is a phase I study to evaluate the safety and limited efficacy of the gene therapy approach as a treatment for type 1 Gaucher disease. A total of five patients with moderate to moderately severe disease were enrolled.

Patients with type I Gaucher disease were recruited from clinics at the University of Pittsburgh and from referrals. They were counseled and informed of the risks and inconveniences of the study during three separate interviews. They were required to sign a consent form. Both patients who are undergoing ERT and untreated patients were eligible for the study.

G-CSF mobilization (10 μg/kg) was used in patients admitted to the study. Leukapheresis procedures began on day 6 of the G-CSF mobilization and continued until a total of 7×10^8/kg mononuclear cells was obtained. The cells were transduced with the R-GC vector to deliver the GC gene. Patients underwent transplantation with autologous genetically corrected cells at a dose of 2×10^6/kg CD34+ cells. The patient's blood was assessed for the carriage and expression of the transduced gene in peripheral blood leukocytes by PCR. Measurement of glucocerebrosidase activity was used to quantify the extent of restoration of enzyme in these cells. After the restoration of enzymatic activity and carriage of the transferred gene has been established, patients were studied for the clinical responses to the therapy.

We will determine the extent to which CD34+ cells can engraft without a myeloablative conditioning step. Engraftment of CD34+ cells is rapid and occurs within 1 month. Therefore, assay of peripheral blood leukocytes for carriage of the GC gene and glucocerebrosidase activity was performed after that interval of time. The results in these patients will determine the approach to be used in subsequent studies during the first year. If the amount of glucocerebrosidase in leukocytes is not increased two times above the deficient level, it will be concluded that an inadequate number of corrected CD34+ cells have engrafted, and the procedure will be repeated up to a maximum of four times in the first year. After having established the restoration of enzymatic activity and carriage of the transferred gene, patients will be studied for the clinical response to the therapy. This evaluation includes repeated measurements of clinical and laboratory parameters.

The outcome of the study will influence the development plans by providing additional information about the safety and capability of gene transfer using our proposed method. Further developments could influence our decisions about

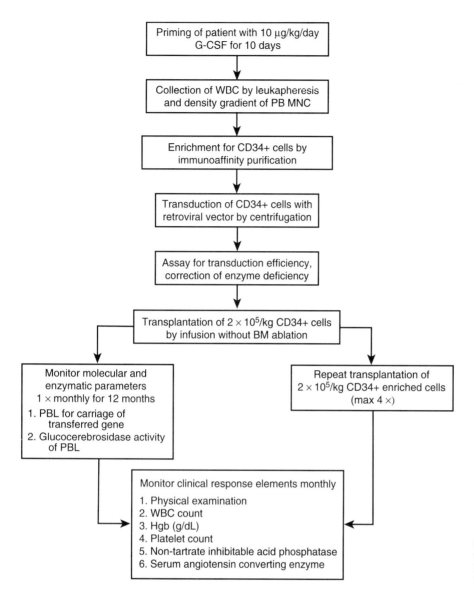

FIGURE 17–1. Flow diagram for the clinical trial of gene therapy for Gaucher disease. BM, bone marrow; PBL, peripheral blood leukocytes; MNC, mononuclear cell.

other vectors, different preparations of hematopoietic stem cells, and different methods of preparation for transplantation. The potential risks associated with the study include those associated with the collection and reinfusion of the patient's CD34+ cells and the minor risks associated with the patient evaluation procedures. We believe, however, that these risks are minimal given the care we have taken in constructing the vector and designing the protocol. We believe that potential risks are outweighed by the critical data we will obtain regarding safety and clinical efficacy. The results of this study will guide the design of future studies in gene therapy for Gaucher disease.

G-CSF PRIMING AND COLLECTION OF A MONONUCLEAR CELL FRACTION

G-CSF mobilization was used in patients with Gaucher disease who are participants in this study to increase the number of CD34+ cells in their blood. Study candidates received G-CSF at a dosage of 10 µg/kg/day by subcutane-

ous injection on consecutive afternoons. Injections were scheduled to begin 5 days prior to the scheduled first leukopheresis procedure. Daily monitoring of white blood cell (WBC) count and differential count was performed. Daily monitoring is essential because the WBC can rise rapidly in response to G-CSF. If the WBC count is greater than 75,000/mL, the G-CSF dose is to be reduced.

Leukapheresis procedures start on day 6 of G-CSF administration and continue on a daily morning schedule until a total mononuclear cell (MNC) yield of 7×10^8/kg is obtained. It is anticipated that two to three collections will be required of the majority of patients to achieve this yield. If a sufficient number of MNCs is not collected, daily G-CSF may be continued at the discretion of the attending physician until an adequate MNC dose is obtained. If cytopenia (WBC <3000/mm^3 or platelets $<50,000$/mm^3) develops during or as a result of leukopheresis, the procedure will be postponed until recovery.

Approximately 15 L of the patient's blood is processed during each leukopheresis procedure. Samples are obtained for hemoglobin, hematocrit, total WBC and differential, platelet count, colony assays, flow cytometry, and microbiologic assays from each leukopheresis product. Each leukapheresis product was enriched for CD34+ cells on the day of collection and pooled.

DOSAGE

Each patient received 2–4 × 10^6 transduced CD34+ cells/kg body weight. This is the dose used to reconstitute the bone marrow in patients who have undergone myeloablation. The dose needed to result in engraftment in an unprepared recipient (one who has not undergone myeloablation) is unknown. Studies of bone marrow transplants in mice and dogs suggest that competitive engraftment in the host animal without preparative myeloablation can be very efficient. We selected a dose of CD34+ cells for this study that has been used to reconstitute the bone marrow in cancer patients who have undergone myeloablation.

INFUSION OF THE TRANSDUCED CELLS

After infection with R-GC, the CD34+ cells were administered to the patient. Aliquots were sampled for biologic activity and tested for adventitious agents.

POSTINFUSION LABORATORY PARAMETERS

In this protocol, the assessment of engraftment of the transduced cells into bone marrow depends on the estimation of carriage of the transgene PCR and enzymatic activity in peripheral blood leukocytes and bone marrow.

At 1 month post infusion, peripheral blood leukocytes from all patients were assayed for glucocerebrosidase activity and carriage of the GC gene. These molecular and enzymatic parameters continued to be monitored according to the schedule. Indicators of clinical response (excluding magnetic resonance imaging, bone marrow biopsy, and radiographs) are conducted monthly for 24 months.

PRELIMINARY FINDINGS

Four study candidates have been entered into the study. One patient experienced a decline in platelet count below 100,000 during G-CSF stimulation. No other unexpected side effects of the procedure were noted in the 4 years of the study. All of the candidates have undergone transplantation at least four times with genetically corrected CD34+ cells at a dose of 2–4 × 10^6/kg. The glucocerebrosidase activity of the corrected cells was 2 to 26 times higher than at their deficient level. Positive signals for the transgene have been noted in the peripheral blood leukocytes of each study subject, and enzymatic activity in circulating WBC has risen to as high as carrier levels in one study subject.

CONCLUSION

The symptoms of Gaucher disease can be ameliorated through the use of ERT. More definitive and permanent benefit can be achieved through the use of BMT. An alternative to allogeneic BMT is described in this chapter. We have shown that successful transduction of hematopoietic progenitor cells with vectors containing the GC gene can be achieved. The clinical trial in progress will test whether transplantation of these genetically altered cells to a patient who has not received any myelosuppressive therapy will result in long-term survival and enzyme expression. Of course, the goal is to achieve expression in cells of sufficient levels of glucocerebrosidase to obviate the need for ERT and to bring about a therapeutic effect. The lessons learned in this clinical trial will be applicable to other diseases with which partial correction of a genetic deficiency may have therapeutic potential.

REFERENCES

1. Zimran A, Gelbart T, Westwood B, et al: High frequency of the Gaucher disease mutation at nucleotide 1226 among Ashkenazic Jews. Am J Hum Genet 49:855–859, 1991.
2. Barranger JA, Ginns EI: Glucosylceramide lipidoses: Gaucher disease. In Scriver CR, Beaudet AL, Sly WS, Valle D (eds): The Metabolic Basis of Inherited Disease, 6th ed. New York, McGraw-Hill, 1989, pp 1677–1698.
3. Barranger JA, Ohashi T, Hong CM, et al: Molecular pathology and therapy for Gaucher disease. Jpn J Inherit Metab Dis 51:45–71, 1989.
4. Furbish FS, Steer CJ, Krett NL, Barranger JA: Uptake and distribution of placental glucocerebrosidase in rat hepatic cells and effects of sequential deglycosylation. Biochim Biophys Acta 673:425–434, 1981.
5. Barton NW, Brady RO, Dambrosia JM, et al: Replacement therapy for inherited enzyme deficiency-macrophage-targeted glucocerebrosidase for Gaucher's disease. N Engl J Med 324:1464–1470, 1991.
6. Fallet S, Sibille A, Mendelson R, et al: Gaucher disease: enzyme augmentation in moderate to life-threatening disease. Pediatr Res 31:496–502, 1992.
7. Beutler E, Kay A, Saven A, et al: Enzyme replacement therapy for Gaucher disease. Blood 78:1183–1189, 1991.
8. Ginns EI, Choudary PV, Martin BM, et al: Isolation of cDNA clones for human β-glucocerebrosidase using the ht11 expression. Biochem Biophys Res Commun 123:574–580, 1984.
9. Choudary PV, Barranger JA, Tsuji S, et al: Retrovirus mediated transfer of the human glucocerebrosidase gene to Gaucher fibroblasts. Mol Biol Med 3:293, 1986.
10. Ohashi T, Boggs S, Robbins P, et al: Efficient transfer and sustained high expression of the human glucocerebrosidase gene in mice and their functional macrophages following transplantation of bone marrow transduced by a retroviral vector. Proc Natl Acad Sci U S A 89:11332–11336, 1992.
11. Nolta JA, Sender LS, Barranger JA, Kohn D: Expression of human glucocerebrosidase in murine long-term bone marrow cultures following retroviral vector-mediated transfer. Blood 75:787–791, 1990.
12. Danos O, Mulligan RC: Safe and efficient generation of recombinant retroviruses with amphotropic and ecotropic host ranges. Proc Natl Acad Sci U S A 85:6460–6464, 1988.
13. Bahnson A, Nimgaonkar M, Fei Y, et al: Transduction of CD34+ enriched cord blood and Gaucher bone marrow cells by a retroviral vector carrying the glucocerebrosidase gene. Gene Therapy 1:176–184, 1994.
14. Bodine DM, Karlsson S, Neinhuis AW: Combination of interleukins 3 and 6 preserves stem cell function in culture and enhances retrovirus-mediated gene transfer into hematopoietic stem cells. Proc Natl Acad Sci U S A 86(22):8897–8901, 1986.
15. Nimgaonkar M, Bahnson A, Boggs S, et al: Transduction of mobilized peripheral blood CD34+ cells with the glucocerebrosidase gene. Gene Therapy 1:201–207, 1994.
16. Dunbar CE, O'Shaughnessy JA, Cottler-Fox M, et al: Transplantation of retrovirally-marked CD34+ bone marrow and peripheral blood cells in patients with multiple myeloma or breast cancer. Blood 82(Suppl 1):217a, 1993.

17. Kohn DB, Weinberg KI, Parkman R, et al: Gene therapy for neonates with ADA-deficient SCID by retroviral-mediated transfer of the human ADA cDNA into umbilical cord CD34+ cells. Blood 82 (Suppl 1):315a, 1993.

18. Bahnson AB, Dunigan JT, Baysal BE, et al: Centrifugal enhancement of retroviral-mediated gene transfer. J Virol Method 54:131–143, 1995.

19. Pear WS, Nolan GP, Scott ML, Baltimore D: Production of high-titer helper-free retroviruses by transient transfection. Proc Natl Acad Sci U S A 90(18):8392–8396, 1993.

20. Kitamura T, Tange T, Terasawa T, et al: Establishment and characterization of a unique human cell line that proliferates dependently on GM-CSF, IL-3, or erythropoietin. J Cell Physiol 140:323, 1989.

21. Murray L, Chen B, Galy A, et al: Enrichment of human hematopoietic stem cell activity in the CD34+Thy-1+Lin3 subpopulation from mobilized peripheral blood. Blood 85(2):368, 1995.

22. Berenson RJ, Bensinger WI, Hill RS, et al: Engraftment after infusion of CD34+ marrow cells in patients with breast cancer or neuroblastoma. Blood 77:1717, 1991.

23. Eaves CJ, Cashman JD, Eaves AC: Methodology of long-term culture of human hematopoietic cells. J Tissue Culture Method 13:55–62, 1991.

24. Peters SO, Kittler ELW, Ramshaw HS, Quesenberry PJ: Ex vivo expansion of murine marrow cells with interleukin-3, interleukin-6, interleukin-11 and stem cell factor leads to impaired engraftment in irradiated hosts. Blood 87:30–37, 1996.

25. Mannion-Henderson J, Kemp A, Mohney T, et al: Efficient retroviral mediated transfer of the glucocerebrosidase gene in CD34+ enriched umbilical cord blood human hematopoietic progenitors. Exp Hematol 23:1623–1632, 1995.

26. Nimgaonkar M, Mierski J, Beeler M, et al: Cytokine mobilization of peripheral blood stem cells in patients with Gaucher disease with a view to gene therapy. Exp Hematol 23:1633–1641, 1995.

Hematopoietic Stem Cell Transplantation for Severe Autoimmune Disease: Know Thyself

Richard K. Burt, M.D.,
Phillip Rowlings, M.B.B.S., M.S., F.R.A.C.P., F.R.C.P.A., and
Ann Traynor, M.D.

Stem cells of the hematopoietic compartment are progenitors of B and T lymphocytes, macrophages, and dendritic cells. These hematopoietic stem cells (HSC) mediate humoral and cellular immunity. Balance between tolerance to self and immunity to foreign antigens is not innate but learned during ontogeny. It has, therefore, been proposed that ablation or near-ablation of a pathologically self-reactive immune system followed by reconstitution of immune ontogeny from either autologous or allogeneic HSC may reintroduce self-tolerance.[1–6] In anecdotal case reports, patients treated by HSC transplantation (HSCT) for a hematologic or neoplastic disease experienced subsequent remission of a coincidental autoimmune disorder.[7–15] In general, most allogeneic and some autologous HSCT have resulted in at least short-term remissions. Because allogeneic HSCT has a higher rate of treatment-related mortality, consensus conferences have recommended initiating autologous HSCT.[1, 3]

CRITERIA FOR AUTOIMMUNE DISEASE

Witebsky classified the evidence for autoimmune disease (later redefined by Rose and Bona) as (1) direct proof, (2) indirect evidence, and (3) circumstantial evidence.[16] Direct proof exists when the disease can be reproduced in a normal person by transfer of antibodies or cells from an afflicted person. Obvious ethical and practical issues limit documentation of direct proof. T-cell response to antigen depends on both the peptide (antigen) and the human leukocyte antigen (HLA) molecule. In order to transfer cellular immunity, pathologic disease-mediating lymphocytes would have to be transferred to an HLA-identical person who is additionally immunosuppressed or otherwise unable to reject the donor's cells. These conditions were accidentally satisfied for juvenile-onset diabetes in a patient undergoing myeloablative conditioning and infusion of HLA-matched marrow from a diabetic sibling donor as therapy for leukemia. Diabetes mellitus developed in the recipient.[17] In contrast, antibody-mediated transfer of disease is not HLA-restricted. Several autoimmune diseases, including myasthenia gravis, polychondritis, and Grave disease, have been transferred transplacentally from mother to child.[18–20]

The majority of human "autoimmune" diseases are assumed to be autoimmune because of circumstantial and indirect evidence. Indirect evidence arises when a similar disease is reproduced in animals by active immunization with autoepitopes or passive transfer of disease-mediating lymphocytes. Circumstantial evidence is based on clinical clues such as amelioration of disease by immunosuppressive therapy. Treatment of autoimmune diseases by HSCT would provide further evidence for an autoimmune pathogenesis. Resolution of disease after HSCT from a normal donor would be direct evidence for autoimmunity.

ETIOLOGY OF AUTOIMMUNE DISEASES

The initiating event or cause of human autoimmune disease is unknown. Animal autoimmune diseases, however, have provided important clues. In general, spontaneous animal autoimmune diseases are genetically preordained. Examples of spontaneously occurring animal autoimmune diseases are a systemic lupus erythematosus–like syndrome in New Zealand black/New Zealand white (NZB/NZW) F1 (B/W) and MRL/lpr mice[21, 22]; a scleroderma-like illness in Tsk mice[23] and UCD L200 chickens[24, 25]; an inflammatory bowel disease in cotton-top tamarin monkeys[26]; and an islet cell inflammatory disease similar to type I diabetes mellitus in NOD mice.[27, 28]

Apoptotic down-regulation of immune cells appears to be one method used to control the immune response. Genetic alterations preventing apoptosis may result in autoimmune disorders. Bcl-2 is a protein located on the inner mitochondrial membrane that inhibits apoptosis. In transgeneic mice with high-level expression of Bcl-2, lupus-like antinuclear antibodies and immune complex glomerulonephritis develop.[29] Mice with the 1pr (lymphoproliferative) mutation have defective expression of the Fas gene. Fas is normally expressed on activated T and B lymphocytes, and ligand binding to Fas induces apoptotic death via signal transduction pathways. Fas-deficient 1pr mice spontaneously experience lupus-like antinuclear antibodies and immune complex glomerulonephritis.[30–32]

MHC genes also play an important role in autoimmunity. The highly polymorphic MHC genes are expressed as membrane proteins on every cell in the body and present small 8- to 14-amino-acid peptides to lymphocytes. The manner in which these peptides are presented determines whether lymphocytes become activated, deleted, or anergic. NZB mice may experience autoimmune anemia but not a lupus-like illness. Mutations at the peptide binding groove (amino acid positions 67, 70, and 71) of the MHC molecule in NZB mice lead to spontaneous development of a lupus-like illness.[33]

In order to characterize genes contributing to autoimmunity, single-sequence–length polymorphisms (SSLP) are being studied. SSLP take advantage of the high degree of variability in repetition of a dinucleotide sequence among persons. For example, the dinucleotide sequence of cytosine/adenine (CA) is variably repeated from two to several times, (CA)n. These repetitions are abundant and randomly distributed throughout the genome. Because of the variability in CA repeats among individuals, polymerase chain reaction (PCR) amplification of SSLP loci using primers to conserved regions outside of the repeated sequence can be used to identify SSLP loci linkage to an autoimmune phenotype. Multiple SSLP loci (called sle-1, sle-2, etc.) contribute independently to a predisposition toward lupus.[34] The identity or function of these genes remains unknown. Probable candidates are genes involved in antigen presentation and subsequent up- or down-regulation of the immune response, including MHC, adhesion, and costimulatory molecules; T-cell–receptor components; immunoglobulin idiotypes; signal transduction kinases and phosphatases; apoptotic pathways; and cytokine genes.

In contrast to spontaneous-onset disease, induced autoimmune diseases are initiated by environmental exposure such as artificial immunization with self-peptides or viral infections. Experimental autoimmune encephalomyelitis (EAE) is an animal model of multiple sclerosis.[35, 36] EAE may be induced in animals by immunization using myelin peptides such as proteolipid protein (PLP) and adjuvant (heat-inactivated *Mycobacterium*). PLP is the most common myelin protein and is confined to the central nervous system. Injection of PLP or immunodominant fragments of PLP without adjuvant does not induce disease. The adjuvant is required to induce costimulatory and/or activation signals at the same time that the T-cell receptor is engaged with PLP peptide. Therefore, it is not the presentation of self but the presentation of self in a proinflammatory environment that induces autoimmunity. Once these self-reactive lymphocytes are primed, EAE may be adoptively transferred to unimmunized animals by transferring CD4 + PLP-primed lymphocytes. Besides EAE, animal autoimmune diseases that arise after immunization with the appropriate self-epitope include collagen-induced arthritis,[37, 38] experimental autoimmune myasthenia gravis,[39, 40] and experimental autoimmune myositis.[41]

A viral animal model of multiple sclerosis is the Theiler murine encephalomyelitis virus (TMEV).[42] This picornavirus is the murine approximation of human poliomyelitis virus. Genetically susceptible mice are unable to clear infection from the central nervous system. As disease progresses, an initial viral infection develops autoimmune features such as splenocyte proliferation to myelin epitopes.[43] This may result from molecular mimicry between myelin and viral proteins. There is no evidence of amino acid homology between myelin and TMEV proteins, however. More likely, the ongoing immune response to the TMEV virus within the central nervous system results in local degradation and presentation of myelin proteins in a proinflammatory environment. That is, infection (in this case, virus) induces a local adjuvant environment for immunization to self.

These observations suggest that some animals are genetically predisposed to autoimmune diseases independent of environmental events. An autologous HSCT would not be anticipated to cure these animals. An allogeneic HSCT from

TABLE 18–1. RESULTS OF BONE MARROW TRANSPLANTATION IN ANIMAL MODELS OF AUTOIMMUNE DISEASE

HUMAN DISEASE APPROXIMATION	ANIMAL MODEL	DISEASE ONSET	TYPE OF BMT	RESULT
Diabetes[44]	NOD mouse	Spontaneous	Allogeneic	Reconstitution of marrow from a resistant strain prevents disease.
Multiple sclerosis[51–55]	Experimental allergic encephalomyelitis	Induced	Syngeneic	BMT before onset of disease prevents disease; after onset of disease BMT arrests disease but does not reverse neurologic deficit.
Myasthenia gravis[50]	Experimental autoimmune myasthenia gravis	Induced	Syngeneic	BMT abolishes immune response to acetylcholine receptor.
Rheumatoid arthritis[48]	Adjuvant induced arthritis (AIA)	Induced	Syngeneic, allogeneic, autologous	Syngeneic, allogeneic, and autologous BMT effective in curing AIA after onset of disease.
Rheumatoid arthritis[49]	Collagen induced arthritis (CIA)	Induced	Syngeneic or allogeneic	BMT before onset of CIA prevented disease; after onset of CIA, BMT decreased progression.
Systemic lupus erythematosus[45–47]	(NZB/NZW) F1, BXSB, MRL/lpr	Spontaneous	Allogeneic	Allogeneic BMT from nonautoimmune prone strain cures or prevents glomerulonephritis and immune and serologic abnormalities.

BMT, bone marrow transplantation.

a nonsusceptible strain, however, might prevent disease. Other animals must encounter environmental stimuli to break self-tolerance. In these cases, a transplant enriched with autologous HSC (lymphocyte depleted) might cure the disease.

Immune ablation and HSC rescue has been attempted in several animal autoimmune disorders[44-55] (Table 18–1). Those that arise spontaneously have been cured by allogeneic bone marrow transplantation (BMT) from a strain resistant to disease. In contrast with spontaneous-onset autoimmune diseases, induced autoimmune disease has been arrested not only by allogeneic but also syngeneic and autologous BMT. Relapse, however, is less frequent after allogeneic HSCT compared with syngeneic or autologous HSCT.

AUTOLOGOUS TRANSPLANTATION FOR HUMAN AUTOIMMUNE DISEASES

Several centers have already reported early results of autologous HSCT for several autoimmune diseases.[56-62] In these reports, transplantation may be accomplished safely with at least short-term benefit. In general, in vivo or ex vivo lymphocyte purging has been attempted to prevent reinfusion of potential disease-causing lymphocytes. It should be cautioned that aggressive lymphocyte depletion of the graft may increase the risk of late opportunistic infection and Epstein-Barr lymphoproliferative disease.[63] At our center, patients are routinely kept on antifungal triazoles and *Pneumocystis carinii* pneumonia prophylaxis for 6 months after transplantation.

The importance of careful patient selection should be emphasized. Autoimmune diseases are a heterogeneous clinical and pathologic spectrum. The disease may wax and wane or be progressive from onset. An acute inflammatory phase may coexist with or progress into a chronic degenerative phase. Prognosis may vary from normal life expectancy with minimal symptoms to severe disease with early mortality. In addition, manifestations of an autoimmune disease may be mimicked by other less-common disorders.

MULTIPLE SCLEROSIS

Multiple sclerosis (MS) is a relatively common disease with a North American prevalence of 1 per 10,000. It generally afflicts young persons 20–40 years old and has a variable natural history: relapsing/remitting, primary progressive, secondary progressive, and relapsing progressive.[64] Adverse prognostic factors are sex = male; onset = polysymptomatic; motor = incomplete recovery; age = more than 40 years old; attack frequency = more than three per year; progression = rapid. Most patients have relapsing/remitting disease (70%) with the same life expectancy as the general population. The majority with secondary or primary progressive MS, however, are wheelchair bound, bedridden, or dead within 10 years of onset of progressive disease. Survival correlates with the level of disability. Less than 6% of patients with an unrestricted activity level are dead within 10 years compared with 70% within 10 years for patients confined to a wheelchair. The cause of death is related to neurologic immobility and immunosuppressive drugs resulting in infection, pulmonary embolus, arrhythmia, or suicide. Possible criteria for an autologous HSCT candidate are shown in Figure 18–1.

End-points for clinical trials are neurologic function and magnetic resonance imaging (MRI). Neurologic function is assessed by relapse frequency and change in disability scores. Two commonly used disability scales are the Kurtzke Extended Status Disability Scale (EDSS) and the Scripps Neurologic Rating Scale (NRS).[65, 66] The EDSS scores a

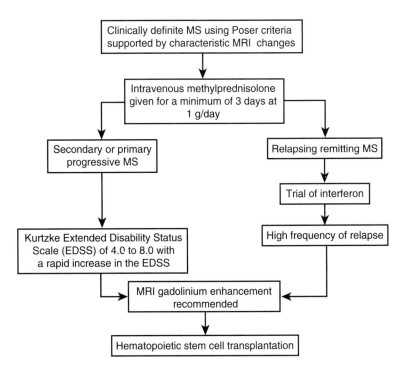

FIGURE 18–1. Algorithm for determining candidacy for stem cell transplantation in the treatment of multiple sclerosis (MS). Criteria are evolving and vary by institution.

TABLE 18–2. SIMPLIFIED KURTZKE EXTENDED STATUS DISABILITY SCALE

```
0 = normal
1–3.5 = abnormalities but fully ambulatory
4.0 = ambulatory < 500 meters
4.5 = ambulatory < 300 meters
5.0 = ambulatory < 200 meters
5.5 = ambulatory < 100 meters
6.0 = ambulatory with a cane
6.5 = ambulatory with a walker
7.0 = wheelchair bound
8.0–8.5 = bedbound with use of arms
9.0–9.5 = bedbound without use of arms
10 = dead
```

patient at half-point intervals from zero (normal) to 10 (dead from neurologic disease) (Table 18–2). A disadvantage of the EDSS is that scoring is heavily weighted by lower-extremity ambulation and is relatively insensitive to cognitive changes, bladder and bowel control, and upper-extremity function. The NRS ranges from 100 (normal) to zero (dead from MS) (Table 18–3). Scoring is more evenly distributed between upper- and lower-extremity function, and 10 points each are available for cognitive ability and bowel/bladder dysfunction. Most studies define improvement as a one-point decline in the EDSS and a 10-point increase in the NRS. MRI allows for assessment of lesion number, total volume, and activity of disease. Lesion en-

hancement after infusion of gadolinium indicates breakdown in the blood-brain barrier from active disease.[67–69]

Strategies for treating MS include limiting demyelination, enhancing remyelination, and improving conduction velocity in demyelinated axons. Immune suppression or modulation is used to limit demyelination. The two most potent immunosuppressive transplant conditioning agents, irradiation and cyclophosphamide, have been used at nontransplant doses to treat multiple sclerosis. Nonmyeloablative doses of total nodal irradiation improve disability scores in progressive MS compared with controls.[70] Cyclophosphamide given 5–10 times below transplant-regimen dosing results in stabilization of disease progression for 2 years.[71]

Even if HSCT is successful in arresting long-term disease progression, recovery of function depends on remyelination of axons and neuronal regeneration. Progress in this area may be achieved with a variety of post-transplantation glial and neuronal growth factors. Axonal potassium ion channel blocking agents improve conduction velocity of demyelinated fibers and may also become useful during post-transplant adjuvant therapy.

Fassas et al.[56] have reported on 15 patients with progressive MS treated by autologous HSCT. BEAM (busulfan [BCNU], etoposide, adriamycin, melphalan) was used as a conditioning regimen.[56] Ex vivo purging of the HSC graft to remove potential disease-reinitiating lymphocytes was not performed. In vivo purging, however, was attempted with cyclophosphamide mobilization prior to HSC collection and with antithymocyte globulin after HSC reinfusion.

TABLE 18–3. SCRIPPS NEUROLOGICAL RATING SCALE (NRS) WORKSHEET*

SYSTEMS EXAMINED	MAXIMUM POINTS	NORMAL	DEGREE OF IMPAIRMENT		
			Mild	**Moderate**	**Severe**
Mentation and mood	10	10	7	4	0
Cranial nerves: Visual acuity	21	5	3	1	0
Fields, discs, pupils		6	4	2	0
Eye movements		5 3	1	0	
Nystagmus		5	3	1	0
Lower cranial nerves	5	5	3	1	0
Motor: RU	20	5	3	1	0
LU		5	3	1	0
RL		5	3	1	0
LL		5	3	1	0
DTRS: UE	5	4	3	1	0
LE		4	3	1	0
Babinski: R:L (2 ea)	4	4	—	—	0
Sensory: RU	12	3	2	1	0
LU		3	2	1	0
RL		3	2	1	0
LL		3	2	1	0
Cerebellar: UE	10	5	3	1	0
LE		5	3	1	0
Gait: trunk and balance	10	10	7	4	0
Special category:					
Bladder/bowel/sexual dysfunction	0	0	−3	−7	−10
Totals	100				

Neurological Rating Scale Score

*Points assigned for each component of the neurologic examination are subtotaled and points for autonomic dysfunction are subtracted, leaving the final (NRS) score.
From Sipe JC, Knobler RL, Braheny SL, et al: A neurologic rating scale (NRS) for use in multiple sclerosis. Neurology 34:1368–1372, 1984.

The patients' median neurologic score as determined by the Kurtzke EDSS and Scripps NRS improved by several points after transplantation. Burt et al. reported on six patients with progressive MS treated with a standard radiation transplant-conditioning regimen of cyclophosphamide and total body irradiation.[57, 62] Total body irradiation was combined with cyclophosphamide and corticosteroids because radiation could penetrate to lymphocytes sequestered within the central nervous system without regard for permeability of the blood-brain barrier. Ex vivo enrichment of CD34 + HSC cells was performed to purge potential autoreactive lymphocytes. Six patients were followed for a median of 8 months after transplantation with stabilization of neurologic deficits despite discontinuation of immunosuppressive medications.

RHEUMATOID ARTHRITIS

Rheumatoid arthritis affects 0.5–1% of the population of the United States. Most patients have a normal life expectancy. Consequently, therapy has traditionally been based on an incremental pyramid scheme of nonsteroidal anti-inflammatory agents and physical therapy, advancing to steroids if nonsteroidal anti-inflammatory agents fail and, finally, disease-modifying antirheumatic drugs such as methotrexate, gold, hydroxychloroquine, or D-penicillamine. The long-held dogma that rheumatoid arthritis does not shorten a person's life expectancy was challenged by Pincus et al., who defined poor prognostic indicators.[72–80] Survival is markedly shortened for any of the following: more than 30 abnormal joints (50% survival at 5 years), time required to walk 25 feet greater than 21 seconds (60% survival at 5 years), time necessary to unbutton and button five buttons greater than 120 seconds (50% survival at 5 years), and limitation of activities of daily living.[57, 58] The activities of daily living questionnaire is composed of 20 questions about the ability to perform daily activities such as walking up stairs, opening a door, or opening a carton of milk[81] (Table 18–4). Significant disability correlates with a survival rate of less than 30% at 5 years. Therefore, a questionnaire on activities of daily living, joint count, and simple functional tests can identify patients at high risk for early mortality who could be potential HSCT candidates. Possible criteria for an autologous HSCT candidate are shown in Figure 18–2.

Primary end-points for clinical trials in rheumatoid arthritis are the number of swollen and tender joints (Table 18–5). Secondary end-points are physician assessment of disease activity, patient assessment of disease activity, patient assessment of pain, activities of daily living questionnaire, and sedimentation rate. Improvement is defined as a 50% decrease in both swollen and involved joints and at least a 20% improvement in three secondary end-points. Other parameters that may be followed include rheumatoid factor, radiographs, and MRI of involved joints and pulmonary function tests to follow subclinical rheumatoid interstitial pneumonitis.

Joske reported on autologous HSCT for one patient with rheumatoid arthritis using a common conditioning regimen for aplastic anemia, cyclophosphamide (200 mg/kg) and

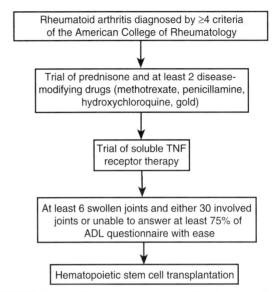

FIGURE 18–2. Algorithm for determining candidacy for stem cell transplantation in the treatment of rheumatoid arthritis. Criteria are evolving and vary by institution. ADL, activities of daily living; TNF, tumor necrosis factor.

antithymocyte globulin (90 mg/kg).[58] The patient went from wheelchair bound to ambulation with ease. Using the same conditioning regimen, Burt et al. reported on two patients with rheumatoid arthritis who were 7 and 4 months post autologous lymphocyte–depleted HSCT with peripheral blood progenitor cell transplantation.[62] Complete remissions were not obtained. Both patients, however, had improved activities of daily living and decreased numbers of swollen joints on less immunosuppressive medications. The conditioning regimen of cyclophosphamide, corticosteroids, and antithymocyte globulin avoids the risk of radiation-associated second malignancy. It also avoids radiation-induced pneumonitis, especially in patients with rheumatoid interstitial lung disease. This regimen, however, is not myeloablative, and other centers are developing protocols using myeloablative regimens.

SYSTEMIC LUPUS ERYTHEMATOSUS

Systemic lupus erythematosus is a multisystem, inflammatory disorder characterized by a variable presentation and clinical course that generally afflicts young women 20–40 years old. Diagnosis depends on fulfilling at least 4 of 11 American Rheumatism Association (ARA) criteria, which are antinuclear antibody, malar rash, discoid rash, photosensitivity, oral ulcers, arthritis, serositis, and a renal, neurologic, hematologic, or immunologic disorder.[82] Ten-year survival has steadily increased with each decade, and the rate is currently 90–93%.[83–91] Improved survival is secondary to more aggressive immunosuppressive intervention with cyclophosphamide (500–1000 mg/m²) and better control of hypertension and hyperlipidemia.[92] As a rule of thumb, 1% of patients with lupus die each year. Within the first 5 years of disease onset, cause of death is usually active disease (e.g., cerebritis, pneumonitis). After 5 years,

TABLE 18–4. RESPONSE FREQUENCIES REGARDING DEGREE OF DIFFICULTY IN PERFORMING ACTIVITIES OF DAILY LIVING USING THE HEALTH ASSESSMENT QUESTIONNAIRE (HAQ) AND A MODIFIED HAQ (MHAQ)

	DEGREE OF DIFFICULTY			
ARE YOU ABLE TO:	**Without Any**	**With Some**	**With Much**	**Unable To Do**
Dressing and grooming				
Dress yourself, including tying shoelaces, and doing buttons?				
Shampoo your hair?				
Arising				
Stand up straight from an armless straight chair?				
Get in and out of bed?				
Eating				
Cut your meat?				
Lift a full cup or glass to your mouth?				
Open a new milk carton?				
Walking				
Walk outdoors on flat ground?				
Climb up five steps?				
Hygiene				
Wash and dry your entire body?				
Take a tub bath?				
Get on and off the toilet?				
Reaching				
Reach and get down a 5-pound object from just above your head?				
Bend down to pick up clothing from the floor?				
Gripping				
Open car door?				
Open jars which have been previously opened?				
Turn faucets on and off?				

TABLE 18–5. SWOLLEN AND TENDER JOINT COUNT

Right			Left	
Tender	Swelling	Joint	Tender	Swelling
		Shoulder		
		Elbow		
		Wrist		
		MCP1		
		MCP2		
		MCP3		
		MCP4		
		MCP5		
		PIP1 thumb		
		PIP2		
		PIP3		
		PIP4		
		PIP5		
		Hip		
		Knee		
		Tarsus		
		MTP1		
		MTP2		
		MTP3		
		MTP4		
		MTP5		

Total # of painful or tender joints = _____.
Total # of swollen/effused joints = _____.
PIP, proximal intraphalangeal joint; MCP, metacarpal phalangeal joint; MTP, metatarsal phalangeal joint.

mortality is secondary to vascular complications of hypertension and hyperlipidemia, such as myocardial infarction or cerebral vascular accidents. Possible criteria for HSCT are listed in Figure 18–3. Clinical nephritis should be documented by biopsy and have a low chronicity (fibrosis, scarring) score and a high activity (acute inflammation) index.[93–96]

Disease activity can be followed by serology (e.g., antinuclear antibodies, anti–double stranded antibodies), response of pretransplantation abnormalities in involved organ systems (e.g., serum creatinine, 24-hour urine protein and creatinine clearance in nephritis; left ventricular ejection fraction in myocarditis; and chest radiograph and pulmonary function tests in pneumonitis), and disease activity indices. These indices can be used to score systemic disease activity in multiple organ systems. Examples are the systemic lupus activity measure (SLAM), lupus activity index (LAI), and systemic lupus erythematosus disease activity index (SLEDAI)[97] (Table 18–6). Improvement is constituted by a 50% improvement in any baseline parameter with no deterioration in any objective parameter.

Marmont et al. reported on a single patient with lupus who had been in remission for more than 1 year after autologous HSCT.[98] Burt et al. reported on two patients with systemic lupus erythematosus who underwent lymphocyte-depleted autologous HSCT.[59, 62] Both patients entered clinical and serologic remissions. The first patient continued in serologic and clinical remission for 1 year after transplantation. Although the conditioning regimen of cyclophosphamide, corticosteroids, and antithymocyte globulin chosen for patients with systemic lupus erythematosus is not myeloablative, enriched CD34+ HSC were reinfused to shorten the duration of severe neutropenia and thrombocytopenia in order to decrease the risk of serious infection and bleeding.

Patients undergoing transplantation for lupus required intense supportive care because of pre-existing renal and pulmonary dysfunction. This fact emphasizes that for autoimmune disease, the usual exclusion criteria of renal, pulmonary, and other end-organ dysfunction do not necessarily apply. An individual who might otherwise be excluded because of organ dysfunction could be included as a candidate if biopsy confirms acute and potentially reversible inflammation.

CROHN DISEASE

Crohn disease is a chronic immunologically mediated disease of the gastrointestinal tract that has a variable course, from mild and intermittently symptomatic to a fulminant illness requiring immunosuppressive therapy, surgery, or both.[99–101] For selected patients, the mortality rate is approximately 1% per year.[102, 103] The risk of early death is increased in patients with most or all of the following: young age at onset, multiple surgical procedures, short bowel/malabsorption, chronic steroid therapy, narcotic addiction, and a history of sepsis. Possible criteria for HSCT are listed in Figure 18–4. Outcome is evaluated by Crohn disease activity index (CDAI) (Table 18–7)[104] and adsorptive indices (e.g., D-xylose kinetics, fecal fat content, Schilling test).[105] To date, no patients have undergone transplantation for Crohn disease. One patient with coincidental Crohn disease treated by autologous transplantation has been described with no evidence of disease 6 months after transplantation.[106]

SYSTEMIC SCLERODERMA

For patients with systemic scleroderma, characterized by fibrosis and vasculopathy, survival is significantly shorter than that of the general population. Patients with renal, cardiac, or pulmonary involvement have the worst prognosis.[107–110] Patients with renal disease, defined as rapidly

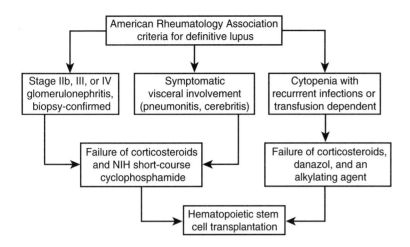

FIGURE 18–3. Algorithm for determining candidacy for stem cell transplantation in the treatment of systemic lupus erythematosus. Criteria are evolving and vary by institution. NIH, National Institutes of Health.

TABLE 18–6. SYSTEMIC LUPUS ERYTHEMATOSUS DISEASE ACTIVITY INDEX (SLEDAI): DATA COLLECTION SHEET

SLEDAI SCORE	DESCRIPTOR	DEFINITION
8	Seizures	Recent onset. Exclude metabolic, infectious, or drug causes.
8	Psychosis	Altered ability to function in normal activity due to severe disturbance in the perception of reality. Include hallucinations, incoherence, marked loose associations, impoverished thought content, marked illogical thinking, bizarre, disorganized, or catatonic behavior. Exclude uremia and drug causes.
8	Organic brain syndrome	Altered mental function with impaired orientation, memory, or other intellectual function, with rapid onset and fluctuating clinical features. Include clouding of consciousness with reduced capacity to focus and inability to sustain attention to environment, plus at least two of the following: perceptual disturbance, incoherent speech, insomnia or daytime drowsiness, or increased or decreased psychomotor activity. Exclude metabolic, infection, or drug causes.
8	Visual disturbance	Retinal changes of SLE. Include cytoid bodies, retinal hemorrhages, serous exudate, or hemorrhages in the choroid or optic neuritis. Exclude hypertension, infection, or drug causes.
8	Cranial nerve disorder	New onset of sensory or motor neuropathy involving cranial nerves.
8	Lupus headache	Severe, persistent headache: may be migrainous but must be nonresponsive to narcotic analgesia.
8	Cerebrovascular accident	New onset of cerebrovascular accident(s). Exclude arteriosclerosis.
8	Vasculitis	Ulceration, gangrene, tender finger nodules, periungual infraction, splinter hemorrhages, or biopsy or angiogram proof of vasculitis.
4	Arthritis	More than two joints with pain and signs of inflammation (i.e., tenderness, swelling or effusion).
4	Myositis	Proximal muscle aching/weakness, associated with elevated creatine phosphokinase/aldolase or electromyogram changes or a biopsy showing myositis.
4	Urinary casts	Heme-granular or red blood cell casts.
4	Hematuria	>5 red blood cells/high-power field. Exclude stone, infection, or other cause.
4	Proteinuria	>0.5 g/24 hours. New onset or recent increase of more than 0.5 g/24 hours.
4	Pyuria	>5 white blood cells/high-power field. Exclude infection.
2	New rash	New onset or recurrence of inflammatory type rash.
2	Alopecia	New onset or recurrence of abnormal, patchy, or diffuse loss of hair.
2	Mucosal ulcers	New onset or recurrence of oral or nasal ulcerations.
2	Pleurisy	Pleuritic chest pain with pleural rub or effusion or pleural thickening.
2	Pericarditis	Pericardial pain with at least one of the following: rub, effusion, or electrocardiogram or echocardiogram confirmation.
2	Low complement	Decrease in CH50, C3, or C4 below the lower limit of normal for testing laboratory.
2	Increased DNA binding	>25% binding by Farr assay or above normal range for testing laboratory.
1	Fever	>38°C. Exclude infectious cause.
1	Thrombocytopenia	<100,000 platelets/mm^3.
1	Leukopenia	<3000 white blood cells/mm^3. Exclude drug causes.

Adapted from Bombardier C, Gladman DD, Urowitz MB, et al: Derivation of the SLEDAI: a disease activity index for lupus patients. Arthritis Rheum 35(6):630–640, 1992.
SLE, systemic lupus erythematosus.

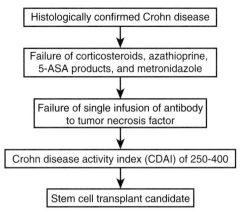

FIGURE 18–4. Algorithm for determining candidacy for stem cell transplantation in the treatment of Crohn disease. Criteria are evolving and vary by institution. 5-ASA, 5-aminosalicylic acid.

TABLE 18–7. CROHN DISEASE ACTIVITY INDEX (CDAI)

VARIABLE	QUANTITY	MULTIPLE
No. of liquid or soft stools per day		2
Abdominal pain	0 = none 1 = mild 2 = moderate 3 = severe	5
General well-being	0 = well 1 = slightly under par 2 = poor 3 = very poor 4 = terrible	7
Number of complications: arthralgias, iritis, erythema nodosum, pyoderma gangrenosa, aphthous ulcerations, anal fissures, anal fistula, anal abscess, fever > 37°C in past week, intestinal obstruction		20
Opiates for diarrhea	Yes = 1 No = 0	30
Abdominal mass	Yes = 5 Questionable = 2 No = 0	10
Deviation of hematocrit < 42% for female, < 47% for male		6
% Deviation from standard weight		1

CDAI < 150 = remission; CDAI > 450 = severely ill.

progressive insufficiency or proteinuria greater than 3.5 g/day, have a 40% 3-year survival rate. Cardiac involvement (pericarditis, congestive heart failure, or arrhythmia) confers a 50% 3-year survival rate. Patients with pulmonary scleroderma diagnosed by interstitial disease on chest radiograph, carbon monoxide diffusing capacity less than 13 mL/min/mm Hg, or pulmonary hypertension on cardiac catheterization or Doppler echocardiogram have a survival rate of 60% at 5 years. Disease may be followed by monitoring affected organ function, serology (e.g., scl-70 titer), and skin elasticity. Tyndall et al. reported marked improvement in one patient with scleroderma after autologous HSCT.[61] Possible criteria for identification of an HSCT candidate are shown in Figure 18–5.

SUMMARY

Autologous HSCT has proven to be feasible, safe, and of short-term benefit. Table 18–8 summarizes published re-

sults on autologous HSCT for human autoimmune diseases. Besides the diseases listed in Table 18–8, several other autoimmune disorders may be treated with HSCT, including myasthenia gravis, pemphigus vulgaris, chronic inflammatory demyelinating polyneuropathy, and juvenile rheumatoid arthritis.

It remains unclear whether autologous transplantation

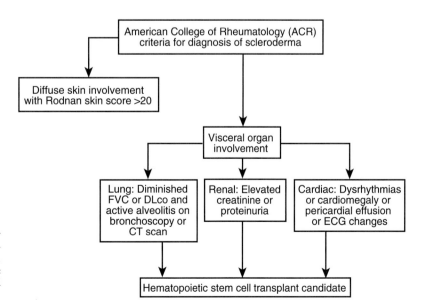

FIGURE 18–5. Algorithm for determining candidacy for stem cell transplantation in the treatment of scleroderma. Criteria are evolving and vary by institution. CT, computed tomography; DLco, carbon monoxide diffusing capacity; ECG, electrocardiogram; FVC, forced vital capacity.

TABLE 18–8. REPORTED EXPERIENCE OF AUTOLOGOUS HEMATOPOIETIC STEM CELL TRANSPLANTATION FOR AUTOIMMUNE DISEASES

DISEASE	NUMBER OF PATIENTS	STEM CELL MOBILIZATION	CONDITIONING REGIMEN	GRAFT MANIPULATION	RESULTS
Multiple sclerosis[56]	15	G-CSF or GM-CSF	BEAM	Antithymocyte globulin post infusion	Improved
Multiple sclerosis[57]	3	G-CSF	TBI and cyclophosphamide	CD34-enriched	Stabilization
Systemic lupus erythematosus[59, 62]	2	Cyclophosphamide and G-CSF	Cyclophosphamide and antithymocyte globulin	CD34-enriched	Complete remission
Systemic lupus erythematosus[98]	1	G-CSF	Thiotepa and cyclophosphamide	T cell–depleted	Complete remission
Rheumatoid arthritis[62]	2	Cyclophosphamide and G-CSF	Cyclophosphamide and antithymocyte globulin	CD34-enriched	Improved
Rheumatoid arthritis[58]	1	G-CSF	Cyclophosphamide and antithymocyte globulin	T cell–depleted	Improved
Systemic scleroderma[61]	1	G-CSF	Cyclophosphamide	CD34-enriched	Improved

BEAM, BCNU (carmustine), etoposide, ara-C, cyclophosphamide; G-CSF, granulocyte colony-stimulating factor; GM-CSF, granulocyte macrophage colony-stimulating factor; TBI, total body irradiation.

establishes self-tolerance or is simply dose-intense immunosuppression. The incidence of disease concordance in identical twins for multiple sclerosis, rheumatoid arthritis, and systemic lupus erythematosus varies between 15% and 50%.[111] This suggests that factors other than genetic predisposition are important for clinically symptomatic autoimmunity. The waxing and waning clinical course of several autoimmune diseases indicates that the immune system is not static but dynamic and may be considered to be in constant flux between tolerance and autoimmunity. Lymphocyte-depleted autologous HSCT may tip the balance toward suppression. It may be, however, that durable remissions will require immune manipulation after transplantation with agents such as interleukin-4 to promote a Th$_2$ phenotype, more aggressive immunoablative regimens, or more complete lymphocyte purging of the autograft before reinfusion. Analysis of the regenerating immune system in terms of T cell–receptor repertoire, lymphocyte flow cytometric phenotype, and cytokine profile in relation to disease status will be important in understanding mechanisms behind disease remission after transplantation.

ALLOGENEIC TRANSPLANTATION

Autoimmune disorders or a subset of patients with autoimmune disease may ultimately require an allogeneic graft from an unaffected sibling for curative therapy. The ability of allogeneic HSCT to cure hematologic malignancy has largely been attributed to an immunologic graft-versus-leukemia effect. This effect results from the cytotoxic effect of the donor's lymphocytes toward the recipient's HSCT cells. In an analogous manner, an allogeneic transplant may result in a graft-versus-autoimmune effect. Such an effect has been noted in animals where induction of allogeneic mixed chimerism in NOD mice from a disease-resistant donor prevented diabetes.[117] Acceptance of allogeneic transplantation for autoimmune diseases, however, will require decreased toxicity, and especially, better methods to control or prevent graft-versus-host disease.

AUTOIMMUNE DISEASE TRANSPLANT REGISTRY

The International Bone Marrow Transplant Registry/American Bone Marrow Transplant Registry (IBMTR/ABMTR) is collecting data on HSCT for autoimmune diseases. Registration and disease-specific data collection forms are being drafted by the IBMTR/ABMTR subcommittee on autoimmune diseases. To ensure scientific accuracy and to facilitate collaboration among international registries, data items collected and definitions should be standardized. A collaborative effort worldwide with such organizations as the European Group for Blood and Marrow Transplant (EBMT) and European League Against Rheumatism (EULAR), which register patients receiving HSCT in Europe, would hasten the acquisition of knowledge. Every center treating autoimmune disease by HSCT is encouraged to submit to these registries.

CONCLUSION

Studies in animals have shown that many autoimmune conditions are mediated by mature lymphocytes. It is possible that ablation of lymphocytes using conditioning regimens similar to those in HSCT for malignancy can prevent further autoimmune-mediated deterioration of normal organ function. Allogeneic HSCT is associated with a high incidence of early mortality and morbidity, and appears not to be justified for use in autoimmune diseases currently because the symptoms are usually not immediately life-threatening. Autologous HSCT can resolve, at least temporarily, autoimmune symptoms in diseases such as multiple sclerosis, rheumatoid arthritis, systemic lupus erythematosus, Crohn disease, and systemic scleroderma. Available clinical data in small trials indicate that long-term disease resolution may be possible by autologous HSCT using mobilized peripheral blood progenitor cells after lymphocyte depletion. Multicenter studies are currently under way to evaluate this possibility. Reporting HSCT results on autoimmune diseases to registries such as IBMTR and EBMT is essential in establishing a database for correlating pretransplant disease status to transplant outcome.

REFERENCES

1. Marmont AM, van Bekkum DW: Stem cell transplantation for severe autoimmune diseases: new proposals but still unanswered questions. Bone Marrow Transplant 16:497–498, 1995.
2. Burt RK, Burns W, Hess A: Bone marrow transplantation for multiple sclerosis. Bone Marrow Transplant 16:1–6, 1995.
3. Marmont AM, Tyndall A, Gratwohl A, et al: Hematopoietic precursor stem cell transplantation for autoimmune diseases. Lancet 345(8955):978, 1995.
4. Burt RK: Bone marrow transplantation for severe autoimmune diseases (SADS): an idea whose time has come. Oncology 11(7):1001–1017, 1997.
5. Krance R, Brenner M: BMT beats autoimmune disease. Nature Med 4(2):153–155, 1998.
6. Slavin S: Treatment of life-threatening autoimmune diseases with myeloablative doses of immunosuppressive agents: experimental background and rationale for ABMT. Bone Marrow Transplant 12:85–88, 1993.
7. Lowenthal RM, Cohen ML, Atkinson K, et al: Apparent cure of rheumatoid arthritis by bone marrow transplantation. J Rheumatol 20(1):137–140, 1993.
8. McKendry RJ, Huebsch L, Leclair B: Progression of rheumatoid arthritis following bone marrow transplantation: a case report with 13 year follow-up. Arthritis Rheum 39(7):1246–1253, 1996.
9. Liu Yin JA, Jowitt SN: Resolution of immune-mediated diseases following allogeneic bone marrow transplantation for leukemia. Bone Marrow Transplant 9:31–33, 1992.
10. McAllister LD, Beatty, PG, Rose J: Allogeneic bone marrow transplantation for chronic myelogenous leukemia in a patient with multiple sclerosis: case study. Bone Marrow Transplant 19(4):395–397, 1997.
11. Salzman P, Tami J, Jackson C, et al: Clinical remission of myasthenia gravis after high dose chemotherapy and autologous transplantation with CD34+ stem cells [Abstract 808]. Blood 84(Suppl 1):206a, 1994.
12. Fastenrath S, Dreger P, Schmitz N: Autologous unpurged bone marrow transplantation in a patient with lymphoma and SLE: short-term recurrence of antinuclear antibodies. Arthritis Rheumatol 38(9):S303, 1995.
13. Euler HH, Marmont AM, Bacigalupo A, et al: Early recurrence or persistence of autoimmune diseases after unmanipulated autologous stem cell transplantation. Blood 88(9):3621–3625, 1996.
14. Lopez-Cubero SO, Sullivan KM, McDonald GB: Course of Crohn's disease after allogeneic marrow transplantation. Gasterenterology 114:433–440, 1998.
15. Meloni G, Capria SD, Vignetti M, Mandelli F: Blast crisis of chronic myelogenous leukemia in long-lasting systemic lupus erythematosus: regression of both diseases after autologous bone marrow transplantation [Letter]. Blood 12:4659, 1997.
16. Rose NR, Bona C: Defining criteria for autoimmune diseases (Witebsky's postulates revisited). Immunol Today 14(9):426–429, 1993.
17. Lampeter EF, Homberg M, Quabeck K, et al: Transfer of insulin-dependent diabetes between HLA identical siblings by bone marrow transplantation. Lancet 341:1243–1244, 1993.
18. Levert AK: In Bona C (ed): Anti-Idiotype Antibodies in Myasthenia Gravis in Biological Application of Anti-Idiotypes. Boca Raton, FL, CRC Press, 1988, pp 20–25.
19. Davis T, Debernardo E: In Davis T (ed): Thyroid Antibodies and Disease: An Overview in Autoimmune Endocrine Disease. New York, John Wiley & Sons, 1983, p 127.
20. Arundel FW, Hasarick JR: Familial chronic atrophic polychondritis. Arch Dermatol 82:439–440, 1960.
21. Cohen PL, Eisenberg RA: The lpr and gld genes in systemic autoimmunity: life and death in the Fas lane. Immunol Today 13(11):427–428, 1992.
22. Drappa J, Brot N, Elkon KB: The Fas protein is expressed at high levels on CD4+ CD8+ positive thymocytes and activated mature lymphocytes in normal mice but not lupus prone strain, MRL lpr/lpr. Proc Natl Acad Sci U S A 90:10340–10344, 1993.
23. Kasturi KN, Shibata S, Muryoi T, et al: Tight-skin mouse: an experimental model for scleroderma. Int Rev Immunol 11:253–271, 1994.
24. Jimenez SD, Christner P: Animal models of systemic sclerosis. Clin Dermatol 12:425–436, 1994.
25. van de Water J, Boyd R, Wick G, et al: The immunologic and genetic basis of avian scleroderma, an inherited fibrotic disease of line 200 chickens. Int Rev Immunol 11:273–282, 1994.
26. Warren BF, Watkins PE: Animal models of inflammatory bowel disease. J Pathol 172:313–316, 1994.
27. Mendez JD, Ramos HG: Animal models in diabetes research. Arch Med Res 25(4):367–375, 1994.
28. Hanfusa T, Miyagawa J, Nakajima H, et al: The NOD mouse. Diabetes Res Clin Pract 24(Suppl):307–311, 1994.
29. Strasser A, Whittingham S, Vaux DL, et al: Enforced BCL2 expression in B-lymphoid cells prolongs antibody responses and elicits autoimmune disease. Proc Natl Acad Sci U S A 88:8661–8665, 1991.
30. Watanabe-Fukunaga R, Brannan CI, Copeland NG, et al: Lympho-proliferation disorder in mice explained by defects in Fas antigen that mediates apoptosis. Nature 356:314–317, 1992.
31. Takahashi T, Tanaka M, Brannan CI, et al: Generalized lymphoproliferative disease in mice caused by a point mutation in the Fas ligand. Cell 76:969–976, 1994.
32. Lynch DH, Watson ML, Alderson MR: The mouse Fas-ligand gene is mutated in gld mice and is part of a TNF family gene cluster. Immunity 1:131–136, 1994.
33. Chiang BL, Bearer E, Ansari S, et al: The BM12 mutation and autoantibodies to dsDNA in NZB.H-2bm12 mice. J Immunol 145:94–101, 1990.
34. Morel L, Rodofsky UH, Longmate JA, et al: Polygenic control of susceptibility to murine systemic lupus erythematosus. Immunity 1:219–229, 1994.
35. Brocke S, Gijbels K, Steinman L: Experimental autoimmune encephalomyelitis in the mouse. In Cohen IR, Miller A (eds): Autoimmune Disease Models: A Guidebook. San Diego, Academic Press, 1994, pp 1–14.
36. Steinman L, Schwartz G, Waldor M, et al: EAE: A Good Model for MS. In Autoimmune Disease Models: A Guidebook. San Diego, Academic Press, 1994, pp 393–397.
37. Hayashida K, Ochi T, Fujimoto M, et al: Bone marrow changes in adjuvant-induced and collagen-induced arthritis. Arthritis Rheum 35(2):241–245, 1992.
38. Durie FH, Fava RA, Noelle RJ: Collagen-induced arthritis as a model of rheumatoid arthritis. Clin Immunol Immunopathol 73(1):11–18, 1994.
39. Patrick J, Lindstrom J: Autoimmune response to acetylcholine receptor. Science 180:871–872, 1973.
40. Vincent A: Experimental autoimmune myasthenia gravis. In Cohen IR, Miller A (eds): Autoimmune Disease Models: A Guidebook. San Diego, Academic Press, 1994, pp 83–106.
41. Rosenberg N: Experimental models of inflammatory myopathies. Baillieres Clin Neurol 2(3):693–703, 1993.
42. Miller SD, Karpus WJ, Pope JG, et al: Theiler's virus-induced demyelinating disease, In Cohen IR, Miller A (eds): Autoimmune Disease Models: A Guidebook. San Diego, Academic Press, 1994, pp 23–36.
43. Miller SD, Vanderlugt CL, Begolka WS, et al: Persistent infection with Theiler's virus leads to CNS autoimmunity via epitope spreading. Nature Med 3(10):1133–1136, 1997.
44. LaFace DM, Peck AB: Reciprocal allogeneic bone marrow transplantation between NOD mice and diabetes-nonsusceptible mice associated with transfer and prevention of autoimmune diabetes. Diabetes 38:894–901, 1989.
45. Ikehara S, Good RA, Nakamura T, et al: Rationale for bone marrow transplantation in the treatment of autoimmune disease. Proc Natl Acad Sci U S A 82:2483–2487, 1985.
46. Himeno K, Good RA: Marrow transplantation from tolerant donors to treat and prevent autoimmune diseases in BXSB mice: immunology. Proc Natl Acad Sci U S A 85:2235–2239, 1988.
47. Ikehara S, Yasumizu R, Inaba M, et al: Long-term observations of autoimmune-prone mice treated for autoimmune disease by allogeneic bone marrow transplantation. Proc Natl Acad Sci U S A 86:3306–3310, 1989.
48. Kamiya M, Sohen S, Yamane T, et al: Effective treatment of mice with type II collagen induced arthritis with lethal irradiation and bone marrow transplantation. J Rheumatol 20:225–230, 1993.
49. Knaan-Schanzer S, Houben P, Kinwel-Bohre EP, et al: Remission

induction of adjuvant arthritis in rats by total body irradiation and autologous bone marrow transplantation. Bone Marrow Transplant 8:333–338, 1991.

50. Pestronk A, Drachman DB, Teoh R, et al: Combined short-term immunotherapy for experimental autoimmune myasthenia gravis. Ann Neurol 14:235–241, 1983.

51. Karussis DM, Vaurka-Karussis U, Lehmann D, et al: Prevention and reversal of adoptively transferred, chronic relapsing experimental autoimmune encephalomyelitis with a single high dose cytoreductive treatment followed by syngeneic bone marrow transplantation. J Clin Invest 92:765–772, 1993.

52. van Gelder M, Kinwel-Bohre EPM, van Bekkum DW: Treatment of experimental allergic encephalomyelitis in rats with total body irradiation and syngeneic BMT. Bone Marrow Transplant 11:233–241, 1993.

53. van Gelder M, van Bekkum DW: Treatment of relapsing experimental autoimmune encephalomyelitis in rats with allogeneic bone marrow transplantation from a resistant strain. Bone Marrow Transplant 16:343–351, 1995.

54. Burt RK, Hess A, Burns W, et al: Syngeneic bone marrow transplantation eliminates v8.2T lymphocytes from the spinal cord of Lewis rats with experimental allergic encephalomyelitis. J Neurosci Res 41:526–531, 1995.

55. Burt RK, Padilla J, Begolka WS, et al: Effect of disease stage on clinical outcome after syngeneic bone marrow transplantation for relapsing experimental autoimmune encephalomyelitis. Blood 91:2609–2616, 1998.

56. Fassas A, Anagnostopoulos A, Kazis A, et al: Peripheral blood stem cell transplantation in the treatment of progressive multiple sclerosis: first results of a pilot study. Bone Marrow Transplant (20):631–638, 1997.

57. Burt RK, Traynor AE, Cohen B, et al: T cell depleted autologous hematopoietic stem cell transplantation for multiple sclerosis: report on the first three patients. Bone Marrow Transplant 21:537–541, 1998.

58. Joske DJL: Autologous bone-marrow transplantation for rheumatoid arthritis [Letter]. Lancet 350:337–338, 1997.

59. Burt RK, Traynor AE, Ramsey-Goldman R: Hematopoietic stem-cell transplantation for systemic lupus erythematosus [Letter]. N Engl J Med 337(24):1777–1778, 1997.

60. Burt RK, Burns WH, Miller SD: Bone marrow transplantation for multiple sclerosis: returning to Pandora's box. Immunol Today 18(12):559–561, 1997.

61. Tyndall A, Black C, Finke J, et al: Treatment of systemic sclerosis with autologous hematopoietic stem cell transplantation [Letter]. Lancet 349:254, 1997.

62. Burt RK, Traynor AE, Pope R, Schroeder J, et al: Treatment of autoimmune disease by intense immunosuppressive conditioning and autologous hematopoietic stem cell transplantation. Blood 92:3505–3514, 1998.

63. Anderson KC, Soiffer R, Delage R, et al: T cell depleted autologous bone marrow transplantation therapy: analysis of immune deficiency and late complications. Blood 76:235–244, 1990.

64. Weinshenker BG: The natural history of multiple sclerosis. Neuro Clin 13(1):119–146, 1995.

65. Kurtzke JF: Rating neurologic impairment in multiple sclerosis: an expanded disability status scale (EDSS). Neurology 33:1444–1452, 1983.

66. Sipe JC, Knobler RL, Braheny SL, et al: A neurologic rating scale (NRS) for use in multiple sclerosis. Neurology 34:1368–1372, 1984.

67. Miller DH: Magnetic resonance in monitoring the treatment of multiple sclerosis. Ann Neurol 36(Suppl):91–94, 1994.

68. Frank JA, Stone LA, Smith ME, et al: Serial contrast-enhaced magnetic resonance imaging in patients with early relapsing-remitting multiple sclerosis: implications for treatment trials. Ann Neurol 36(Suppl):86–90, 1994.

69. Francis GS, Evans AC, Aronold DL: Neuroimaging in multiple sclerosis. Multiple Sclerosis 13(1):147–171, 1995.

70. Cook SD, Devereux C, Trioano R, et al: Effect of total lymphoid irradiation in chronic multiple sclerosis. Lancet 1:1405–1409, 1986.

71. Hauser SI, Dawron DM, Lehrich JR, et al: Intense immunosuppression in multiple sclerosis: a randomized three arm study of high dose intravenous cyclophosphamide, plasma exchange and ACTH. N Engl J Med 308:173–180, 1983.

72. Pincus T, Brooks RH, Callahan LF: Prediction of long-term mortality in patients with rheumatoid arthritis according to simple questionaire and joint count measures. Ann Intern Med 120:26–34, 1994.

73. Pincus T, Callahan LF: Rheumatology function tests: grip strength, walking time, button test and questionnaires document and predict longterm morbidity and mortality in rheumatoid arthritis. J Rheumatol 19(7):1051–1057, 1992.

74. Pincus T: Rheumatoid arthritis: a medical emergency? Scand J Rheumatol 23(Suppl 100):21–30, 1994.

75. Furst DE: Predictors of worsening clinical variables and outcomes in rheumatoid arthritis. Rheum Dis Clin North Am 20(2):309–319, 1994.

76. Corbett M, Dalton S, Young A, et al: Factors predicting death, survival and functional outcome in a prospective study of early rheumatoid disease over fifteen years. Br J Rheumatol 32:717–723, 1993.

77. Wolfe F, Mitchell DM, Sibley JT, et al: The mortality of rheumatoid arthritis. Arthritis Rheum 37(4):481–494, 1994.

78. Myllykangas-Luosujarvi R, Aho K, Kautiainen H, Isomaki H: Shortening of life span and causes of excess mortality in a population-based series of subjects with rheumatoid arthritis. Clin Exp Rheumatol 13:149–153, 1995.

79. Bendtsen P, Bjurulf P, Trell E, et al: Cross-sectional assessment and subgroup comparison of functional disability in patients with rheumatoid arthritis in a Swedish health-care district. Disability Rehabil 17(2):94–99, 1995.

80. Pincus T, Callahan LF: The "side effects" of rheumatoid arthritis: joint destruction, disability and early mortality. Br J Rheumatol 32(Suppl 1):28–37, 1993.

81. Pincus T, Summey JA, Soraci SA Jr, et al: Assessment of patient satisfaction in activities of daily living using a modified Stanford Health Assessment Questionnaire. Arthritis Rheum 26(11):1346–1353, 1983.

82. Tan EM, Cohen AS, Fries JF, et al: The 1982 revised criteria for the classification of systemic lupus erythematosus. Arthritis Rheum 25(11):1271–1277, 1982.

83. Cheigh JS, Kim H, Stenzel KH, et al: Systemic lupus erythematosus in patients with end-stage renal disease: long term follow-up on the prognosis of patients and the evolution of lupus activity. Am J Kidney Dis 16(3):189–195, 1990.

84. Seleznick MJ, Fries JF: Variables associated with decreased survival in systemic lupus erythematosus. Semin Arthritis Rheum 21(2):73–80, 1991.

85. Gladman DD: Prognosis of systemic lupus erythematosus and factors that affect it. Curr Opin Rheumatol 4:681–687, 1992.

86. Cohen MG, Li EK: Mortality in systemic lupus erythematosus: active disease is the most important factor. Aust N Z J Med 22:5–8, 1992.

87. Abu-Shakra M, Urowitz MB, Gladman DD, Gough J: Mortality studies in systemic lupus erythematosus, results from a single center: II. Predictor variables for mortality. J Rheumatol 22(7):1265–1270, 1995.

88. Ward MM, Pyun E, Studens K: Long-term survival in systemic lupus erythematosus. Patient characteristics associated with poor outcomes. Arthritis Rheum 38:274–283, 1995.

89. Gladman DD: Indicators of disease activity, prognosis, and treatment of systemic lupus erythematosus. Curr Opin Rheumatol 5:587–595, 1993.

90. Gulko PS, Reveille JD, Koopman WJ, et al: Anticardiolipin antibodies in systemic lupus erythematosus: clinical correlates, HLA associations, and impact on survival. J Rheumatol 20(10):1684–1693, 1993.

91. Drenkard C, Villa AR, Alarcon-Segovia D, Perez-Vazquez ME: Influence of the antiphospholipid syndrome in the survival of patients with systemic lupus erythematosus. J Rheumatol 21(6):1067–1072, 1994.

92. Boumpas DT, Austin HA, Vaughn EM, et al: Controlled trial of pulse methylprednisolone versus two regimens of pulse cyclophosphamide in severe lupus nephritis. Lancet 340:741–745, 1992.

93. Churg J, Sobin LN: Renal Disease Classification and Atlas, vol 1, Glomerular Diseases. Tokyo, Igaku-Shoin, 1982.

94. Kashgarian M: New approaches to clinical pathologic correlation in lupus nephritis. Am J Kidney Dis 2.164–169, 1982.

95. Austin HA III, Muenz LR, Joyce KM, et al: Prognostic factors in lupus nephritis: contribution of renal histology data. Am J Med 75:382–391, 1983.

96. McLaughlin J, Gladman DD, Urowitz MB, et al: Kidney biopsy in

systemic lupus erythematosus. Arthritis Rheum 34(10):1268–1272, 1991.

97. Bombardier C, Gladman DD, Urowitz MB, et al: Derivation of the SLEDAI: a disease activity index for lupus patients. Arthritis Rheum 35(6):630–640, 1992.

98. Marmont AM, van Lint MT, Gualandi F, Bacigalupa A: Autologous marrow transplantation for severe systemic lupus erythematosus of long duration. Lupus 6:545–548, 1997.

99. Farmer RG., Jawk WA, Turnbull RB: Clinical patterns in Crohn's disease: a statistical study of 615 cases. Gastroenterology 68:627–635, 1975.

100. Ogorek CP, Caroline DF, Fisher RS: Presentation, evaluation, and natural history of inflammatory bowel disease. *In* Macdermott RP, Stenson WF (eds): Inflammatory Bowel Disease. New York, Elsevier, 1992, pp 355–386.

101. Farmer RG, Whelan G, Fazio VW: Long term follow-up of patients with Crohn's disease: relationship of the clinical pattern and prognosis. Gastroenterology 88:1818, 1985.

102. Probert CSJ, Jayanthi V, Wicks ACB, et al: Mortality from Crohn's disease in Leicestershire, 1972–1989: an epidemiological community based study. Gut 33:1226–1228, 1992.

103. Mendelsohn RR, Korelitz BI, Gleim GW: Death from Crohn's disease and lessons from a personal experience. J Clin Gastroenterol 20(1):22–26, 1995.

104. Best WR, Becktel JM, Singleton JW, Kern F: Development of a Crohn's disease activity index: National Cooperative Crohn's Disease Study. Gastroenterology 70:439–444, 1976.

105. Craig RM, Atkinson AJ: D-xylose testing: a review. Gastroenterology 95:223–231, 1988.

106. Drakos PE, Nagler A: Case of Crohn's disease in bone marrow transplantation [Letter]. Am J Hematol 43:157–158, 1993.

107. Bulpitt KJ, Clements PJ, Lachenbruch PA, et al: Early undifferentiated connective tissue disease: III. Outcome and prognostic indicators in early scleroderma (systemic sclerosis). Ann Intern Med 118:602–609, 1993.

108. Lee P, Langevitz P, Alderdice CA, et al: Mortality in systemic sclerosis (scleroderma). Q J Med 82(298):139–148, 1992.

109. Altman RD, Medsger TA, Bloch DA, et al: Predictors of survival in systemic sclerosis (scleroderma). Arthritis Rheum 34(4):403–413, 1991.

110. Silman AJ: Scleroderma-demographics and survival. J Rheumatol 24(Suppl 48):58–61, 1997.

111. Worthington J, Silman AJ: Genetic control of autoimmunity, lessons from identical twins. Clin Exp Immunol 101:390–392, 1995.

112. Li H, Kaufman CL, Baggs SS, et al: Mixed allogeneic chimerism induced by a sublethal approach prevents autoimmune diabetes and reverses insulitis in nonobese diabetic (NOD) mice. J Immunol 156(1):380–388, 1996.

CHAPTER NINETEEN

In Utero Transplantation

Ewa Carrier, M.D.

Many congenital diseases can now be diagnosed prenatally (Table 19–1).[1, 2] Although many of these diseases can be cured by postnatal hematopoietic stem cell (HSC) transplantation (HSCT), serious limitations are associated with its use.[3–7] Only about 25% of patients have a human leukocyte antigen (HLA)–matched sibling donor, and many patients experience graft-versus-host disease (GVHD) with high morbidity and mortality.[8–13] Allogeneic HSCT requires ablation and immunosuppression, which may lead to high-risk, frequently life-threatening, infections. For many congenital metabolic disorders in which the brain is damaged in utero, postnatal HSCT is frequently too late.[3–5] Prenatal therapy can circumvent these difficulties and provide successful therapy for many congenital diseases. To date, over

TABLE 19–1. CONGENITAL DISEASES POTENTIALLY AMENABLE BY IN UTERO TRANSPLANTATION

Inborn Errors of Metabolism
  Mucopolysaccharidoses (MPS)
    Hurler disease (MPS I) (α-iduronidase deficiency)
    Hurler-Scheie syndrome
    Hunter disease (MPS II) (iduronate sulfatase deficiency)
    Sanfilippo B (MPS III B) (α-glycosaminidase deficiency
      syndrome)
    Morquio (MPS IV) (hexosamine-6-sulfatase deficiency
      syndrome)
    Maroteaux-Lamy syndrome (MPS VI) (arylsulfatase B
      deficiency)
  Mucolipidoses
    Fabry disease (α-galactosidase A deficiency)
    Krabbe disease (galactosylceramidase deficiency)
    Niemann-Pick disease (sphingomyelinase deficiency)
    Adrenal leukodystrophy
  Gaucher disease

Congenital Hemoglobinopathies
  Thalassemia major
  Sickle cell anemia
  Diamond-Blackfan syndrome
  Fanconi anemia

Congenital Immunodeficiencies
  Severe combined immunodeficiency disease
  Bare lymphocyte syndrome

Congenital Neutrophil Abnormalities
  Chronic granulomatous disease
  Chédiak-Higashi syndrome
  Wiskott-Aldrich syndrome
  Infantile granulocytosis (Kostmann syndrome)
  Lazy leukocyte syndrome (neutrophil actin deficiency)
  Neutrophil membrane GP-180 deficiency
  Cartilage-hair syndrome

Disorders of Osteogenesis
  Infantile osteoporosis

20 in utero HSCT in humans have been reported worldwide (Table 19–2).

Early in its development, the fetus is incapable of rejecting transplanted allogeneic cells and becomes immunologically tolerant of them.[14, 15] Additionally, the rapidly developing fetal hematopoietic compartment may provide a "niche" for incoming donor cells, especially if they are delivered in large quantity.[16–18] Therefore, the histocompatibility, immunosuppression, and myeloablation associated with postnatal transplantation may not be necessary for in utero transplantation, and potentially every fetal recipient may have a suitable donor.

FETAL HEMATOPOIESIS

Fetal hematopoiesis is a complex process that starts in the yolk sac, proceeds to the fetal liver, and finally ends in the bone marrow.[19–23] In humans, bones develop as a cartilaginous matrix followed by the appearance of osteoblasts by 10 weeks of gestation and other stromal elements at 12 weeks. The first hematopoietic elements from the fetal liver appear at about 15 weeks of gestation, and the process of populating the bone marrow is not finished until week 34 of gestation.[20, 22] Therefore, there is a window of opportunity during which the unpopulated bone marrow stroma supports engraftment of allogeneic HSC without competition from host stem cells. This period is also associated with immune incompetence, which further increases the chance of engraftment of allogeneic cells. Thus, marrow ablation and/or immunosuppression is not needed for allogeneic cell engraftment; however, engraftment of allogeneic HSC in large and small animal models, as well as in humans after in utero transplantation, is minor.

Failure to achieve robust engraftment might be due to defective homing of allogeneic HSC or saturation of the HSC niche. Quesenberry et al. showed that high levels of engraftment can be achieved by multiple injections of high doses of HSC in nonmyeloablated hosts.[16–18] Robust engraftment achieved with multiple doses of allogeneic HSC suggests that only a certain proportion of the marrow stromal HSC niche is available at any given time. Therefore, the bolus of injection of allogeneic HSC in excess of that required to saturate the marrow stromal niche should not increase engraftment.

INDUCTION OF TOLERANCE

Fetal immunologic incompetence provides an opportunity for allogeneic HSC to engraft without the need for immunosuppression.

TABLE 19–2. REPORTED HUMAN CASES IN IN UTERO TRANSPLANTATION

DISEASE	STEM CELL SOURCE	GESTATIONAL AGE (WEEKS)	OUTCOME	PERFORMED BY
Bare lymphocyte syndrome	Fetal liver and thymus	28	Engrafted, lives normal life at home. Requires monthly IvIg.	Touraine et al.[42]
SCID	Fetal liver and thymus	26	Engrafted, well, on monthly IvIg.	Touraine et al.[46]
β-Thalassemia major	Fetal liver	12	Mixed, transient chimerism. Requires transfusion. No evidence of engraftment 1 year posttransplantation.	Touraine et al.[49]
β-Thalassemia major	Fetal liver	19	Fetal bradycardia and death following final infusion of large number of donor cells.	Touraine et al.[49]
β-Thalassemia	T-cell–depleted bone marrow from the sibling	25	No evidence of engraftment.	Slavin et al.[50]
α-Thalassemia	T-cell–depleted maternal bone marrow		Elective pregnancy termination at 24 weeks, postmortem evidence of donor extramedullary hematopoiesis.	Diukman et al.[51]
Chédiak-Higashi disease	T-cell–depleted maternal bone marrow		No evidence of engraftment. Child alive without the disease after postnatal transplantation.	Diukman et al.[51]
Niemann-Pick disease	Fetal liver		No evidence of engraftment	Touraine et al.[49]
X-linked SCID	Paternal CD34 bone marrow cells	16	Alive, well with evidence of T- and B-cell reconstitution.	Flake et al.[47]
X-linked SCID	Paternal CD34 T-cell–depleted bone marrow cells	20	Alive, well. Donor T-cell reconstitution, but not B cell. Requires monthly IvIg.	Wengler et al.[48]

SCID, severe combined immunodeficiency disease; IvIg, intravenous immunoglobulin G.

In 1945, Owen observed that hematopoietic chimerism developed in dizygotic cattle twins that showed cross-placental circulation.[24] Postnatally, they were tolerant of skin or kidney grafts from their siblings.[24, 25] This naturally occurring tolerance was observed in humans and primates as well.[26, 27] This initial observation led Billingham et al. to the "classic" experiment on "actively acquired immunological tolerance," which showed that pre-immune exposure to a foreign antigen results in a specific tolerance to this antigen.[14, 15] This development of specific tolerance after in utero transplantation was shown in both small and large animal models.[28–31] However, the degree of induced tolerance was small.

A decade of research in this area, however, documented only a low degree of engraftment (percentage of donor cells) after in utero transplantation. Recent studies demonstrated the possibility of active immunity by a previously underdeveloped newborn immune system in a mouse model, indicating that tolerance or immunity may develop, depending on the conditions of transplantation.[32] This demonstrates that the neonatal immune system, like an adult's, can be primed to recognize and react to a foreign antigen as long as the antigen is introduced under the right conditions.[32–38]

If allogeneic HSC are recognized by the fetal immune system, they might be rejected. The conditions favorable for tolerance induction to allogeneic HSC may depend on the timing, number, and composition of injected cells, the ratio of T cells to B cells, and the presence of dendritic cells. Further definition of optimal conditions for the development of tolerance should allow for engraftment. On the other hand, the possibility of active immunization against infections and possibly neoplastic diseases is an intriguing concept.

EXPERIENCE IN HUMANS

SEVERE COMBINED IMMUNODEFICIENCY DISORDERS

Severe combined immunodeficiency disorders (SCID) are congenital syndromes that cause abnormal T- and/or B-cell function, leading to increased susceptibility to infections, failure to thrive, low number and function of T lymphocytes, and hypogammaglobulinemia. SCID can be diagnosed prenatally.[39–41] If untreated, these diseases are usually fatal within the first year of life. The following reports describe specific cases of in utero HSCT in humans with special emphasis on the safety of the procedure, extent of donor chimerism, and induction of tolerance.

Case 1

The first reported case of in utero transplantation involved a patient with the Bare lymphocyte syndrome. The transplantation was performed on June 30, 1988, by Touraine et al.[42] The mother's first-born child died of the disease, and the second child's condition was diagnosed at 19 weeks' gestation. The parents were offered three choices: (1) therapeutic abortion, (2) in utero transplantation, or (3) postnatal transplantation with allogeneic fetal liver cells. The mother was informed that this would be the first case of in utero transplantation in humans and that the results were uncertain.

The parents chose prenatal transplantation, which was performed at 28 weeks' gestation. Under direct ultrasound guidance, an injection needle was inserted at the juncture of the umbilical vein and placenta. Five milliliters of fetal blood was removed, and 7 mL of allogeneic fetal liver and fetal thymic epithelial cells were injected using the technique used for intravascular, intrauterine transfusion.[43–45] Liver and thymic cells were obtained from two nonviable fetuses of 7 and 7.5 weeks' gestational age.

After in utero transplantation, no adverse effects were noted in the mother or the baby. At birth, which was uneventful, a diagnosis of Bare lymphocyte syndrome was confirmed, but a small percentage of cells with class I HLA was detected. At 1 month of age, 10% of lymphocytes expressed class I HLA with HLA-A9 donor specificity. Postnatally, this child received seven additional fetal liver transplants from nine different fetal donors without any conditioning. No engraftment of postnatally transferred cells was demonstrated. The proportion of T cells from prenatally transferred cells increased with time, however, and was found to constitute 26% of peripheral blood lymphocytes at 1 year of age. Progressive T-cell maturity and immunologic competence of T cells was demonstrated, as tested by proliferative responses to *Candida,* cytomegalovirus, and tetanus toxoid antigens.

The B cells remained of host origin as demonstrated by persistently low immunoglobulin levels, and the child required monthly intravenous Ig infusion. The patient lived in complete isolation up to 16 months of age, until full immune reconstitution of T cells was demonstrated (Fig. 19–1). At present, this child is 10 years old and is living a normal life at home. This first in utero transplantation proved to be well tolerated by the fetus and resulted in immune reconstitution.

Case 2

The second patient who underwent transplantation for SCID was treated in June 1989 at 26 weeks of gestation by Touraine.[46] In this patient (female), SCID was prenatally diagnosed by complete lack of CD2, CD3, CD4, and CD8

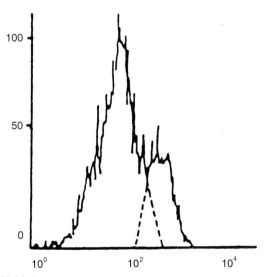

FIGURE 19–1. Evidence of donor lymphocyte engraftment in patient with Bare lymphocyte syndrome (BLS) transplanted in utero. Flow cytometric analysis of peripheral blood mononuclear cells for a human leukocyte antigen (HLA) donor marker showed that 10% of lymphocytes had normal expression of class I HLA antigens. The number of donor cells increased to 26% of peripheral blood lymphocytes at 14 months and has stabilized at 17% since the sixth year of age.

lymphocytes in the blood. Fetal liver cells from a fetal donor of 7.5 weeks' gestation were infused through the umbilical vein under ultrasound guidance. No side effects were noted, and the child was born vaginally without any complications. Chimerism studies showed progressively increasing donor T cells, with a normal response to mitogens. Unfortunately, this girl died recently from complications of liver transplantation surgery for sclerosing cholangitis.

Case 3

The third case was performed by Flake et al. on the son of a 28-year-old woman known to carry X-linked SCID.[47] Her first son died at 7 months of age from this disease. Prenatal diagnosis confirmed the presence of the mutation in the second child at 12 weeks' gestation by chorionic villus sampling. The fetus received three infusions of CD34+ cells enriched from paternal bone marrow between 16 and 18 weeks of gestation. The fetus tolerated the procedure well and was born at term by cesarean section. At birth, the physical examination revealed a maculopapular rash not confirmed by histologic evaluation as GVHD. The rash resolved with a 7-day course of methylprednisolone (1 mg/kg). Analysis of cord-blood mononuclear cells detected cells of donor origin (Fig. 19–2).

At birth, the numbers of B cells and CD8 T lymphocytes were normal and have remained normal. The response to mitogen was increased and fluctuated but, since the age of 6 months, has remained stable and has exceeded that of normal subjects. Patient serum Ig levels were normal except for the absence of IgA. At 7 months of age, after three rounds of vaccination, the patient had detectable IgG antibodies against diphtheria, tetanus, and *Haemophilus.* At 3 months of age, patient lymphocytes reacted to maternal and three unrelated donor lymphocytes but not the paternal cells, suggesting induction of tolerance to paternal cells. The patient has been in excellent health since birth.

Case 4

HSCT was performed by Wengler et al.[48] This patient was a second child of a couple who lost their first child to SCID while awaiting postnatal bone marrow transplantation. At 20 weeks of the second pregnancy, prenatal amniocentesis confirmed the diagnosis of X-linked SCID. CD34+ cells were enriched from paternal bone marrow using the Nexell Isolex system and were further depleted of T-cells by E-rosetting. The cells were given in 2 infusions: 14×10^6 and 4×10^6 at 21 and 22 weeks of gestation, respectively. At 38 weeks' gestation, a 3.6-kg boy was delivered by cesarean section. GVHD was not detected. Since discharge, the baby has lived with his parents at home and is well. At birth, cord-blood analysis showed that 20% of cells were of donor origin. There were no B cells of donor origin, and serum IgA was undetectable, with low IgM levels (0.09 g/L). The child requires monthly intravenous Ig infusions. Immune reconstitution in this child after in utero transplantation is shown in Figure 19–3.

CHRONIC GRANULOMATOUS DISEASE

In 1992, a patient with chronic granulomatous disease received two infusions of fetal liver cells by Touraine.[49]

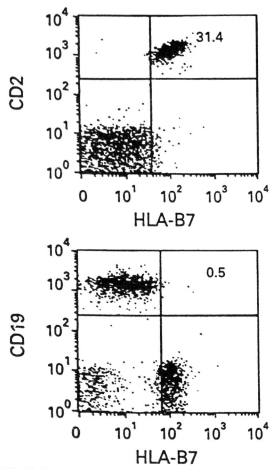

FIGURE 19–2. Flow cytometry analysis of cord blood of a child with severe combined immunodeficiency who underwent transplantation with CD34+ paternal bone marrow cells. Human leukocyte antigen B7 is a donor-specific marker. The lineage-positive cells of donor origin are shown in upper right quadrant. All CD2+ cells (T lymphocytes) were of donor origin, and there were no donor cells in CD19+ cells (B lymphocytes).

The first infusion was carried out uneventfully by umbilical vein infusion at 17 weeks of gestation, but the number of cells available for infusion was considered insufficient. A second infusion was attempted at 21 weeks' gestation but resulted in fetal bradycardia (possibly related to the rapid infusion of a large number of donor cells) and fetal death within 1 hour. No engraftment was detected at birth or postnatally. Another case of prenatal transplantation for chronic granulomatous disease was reported by Harrison (unpublished data). Paternal CD34+, Thy-1–positive, lineage-negative bone marrow cells were infused intraperitoneally during the second trimester. The child was born uneventfully at term. Flow cytometry analysis of cord blood and subsequent peripheral blood samples of functional nicotinamide adenine dinucleotide phosphate oxidase activity did not show any enzyme activity. These cases demonstrate the lack of engraftment in fetal hosts with intact hematopoiesis.

CONGENITAL HEMOGLOBINOPATHIES

Touraine performed a prenatal transplantation for homozygous β-thalassemia.[49] Cells were infused at 12 weeks' gesta-

tional age. In this case, very low engraftment of donor cells was documented, which was insufficient for the correction of hemolytic anemia. In another case reported by Touraine, allogeneic fetal liver cell infusion was attempted by cord-blood infusion at 17 weeks of gestational age.[49] Four milliliters of blood were removed, and 10 mL of fetal cells containing medium were infused. Fetal bradycardia, possibly related to the relatively rapid infusion of a large number of donor cells, resulted in fetal death.

Four cases of prenatal transplantation for congenital hemoglobinopathies (α-thalassemia [two cases], sickle cell anemia [one case], and β-thalassemia [one case]) have been reported by Westgren et al. (Table 19–3).[50] Two to seven fetal liver donors were used per recipient. Cell infusion was performed between 13 and 31 weeks of gestation. No evidence of donor cells was demonstrated in any of these cases. Similarly, no engraftment was detected in a β-thalassemic fetus following in utero transplantation with T-cell depleted bone marrow from the sibling.[51] An α-thalassemic fetus transplanted in utero with maternal T-cell depleted marrow cells was terminated at 24 weeks due to the lack of engraftment.[52]

A fetus homozygous for α-thalassemia-1 was given haploidentical paternal CD34+ cells at 13, 19, and 24 weeks' gestation and supported throughout pregnancy with blood transfusion. The pregnancy was normal, with adequate growth and development, and no hydrops fetalis was detected. Prenatal blood sampling for HLA and α-globin DNA did not show evidence of donor cells. Analysis of

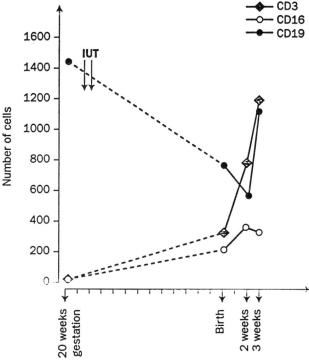

FIGURE 19–3. Evidence of immune reconstitution in patient with X-linked severe combined immunodeficiency who underwent transplantation in utero with CD34+ T-cell–depleted paternal cells. The absolute numbers of CD3, CD16, and CD19 were measured at birth, 2 weeks, and 3 weeks of age. There is evidence of immune reconstitution by increasing numbers of CD3 (T lymphocytes), CD16 (natural killer cells), and CD19 (B lymphocytes) after in utero transplantation in this patient.

TABLE 19–3. IN UTERO TRANSPLANTATION FOR CONGENITAL HEMOGLOBINOPATHIES

DIAGNOSIS	GESTATIONAL AGE (WEEKS)	SEX	ROUTE	CELL DOSE × 10^8/kg	NO FETAL LIVERS
α-Thalassemia	15	M	IP	20.4	7
α-Thalassemia	31	M	IV	1.2	6
Sickle cell anemia	13	F	IP	16.7	5
β-Thalassemia	18	F	IV	8.6	5

IP, intraperitoneal; IV, intravenous.

cord blood at birth and bone marrow at 3 months of age demonstrated cells of donor origin. Tolerance studies of the infant's blood mononuclear cells showed small proliferative and no cytotoxic response to donor cells, with full response to third-party cells. Additional paternal CD34 + cells were infused at 3 months of age, but this did not reduce the transfusion requirement. Although there was evidence of tolerance to donor cells, the postnatal infusion did not increase the level of chimerism. Infants induced to tolerance in utero would be ideal candidates for repeated infusion of paternal CD34 + cells in an effort to boost paternal cell engraftment.

INBORN ERRORS OF METABOLISM (GLOBOID CELL LEUKODYSTROPHY)

Bambach et al. performed transplantation in a female patient with globoid cell leukodystrophy during the first trimester of gestation using selected paternal bone marrow CD34 + cells.[53] CD34 + selection allowed a substantially greater number of HSC to be transplanted. The fetus died 7 weeks after the procedure (during week 20 of gestation). The cause of death appeared to be overwhelming donor engraftment and leukostasis, with paternal myeloid cells infiltrating most tissues. No histologic evidence of GVHD was detected. This indicates that infusion of a large number of HSCs may cause lethal paternal cell proliferation. This suggests that the window of opportunity may be not only time-dependent but dose-dependent, with upper and lower limits on cell number.

PRENATAL GENE THERAPY

The Third Gene Therapy Policy Conference on Prenatal Gene Transfer: Scientific, Medical and Ethical Issues, sponsored by the National Institutes of Health, was held January 7–9, 1999, specifically to address the following questions:

1. What is known about fetal immune competence?
2. What is known about the induction of fetal immune tolerance?
3. What is known about prenatal transgene expression/ vector dissemination?
4. What is known about germline gene transduction and expression?
5. What are the genotypic/phenotypic correlations for diseases diagnosed prenatally?
6. What are the ethical/legal issues related to fetal therapy?

7. What are the international regulations regarding prenatal gene therapy?

Following are summaries of preclinical data, ethical considerations, and international regulations regarding prenatal gene therapy.

ANIMAL MODELS OF PRENATAL GENE THERAPY

Sheep

Porada et al. reported on ex vivo and in vivo gene transfer in sheep fetuses.[54] In the first experiment, an autologous retroviral vector/HSC transplantation protocol was used to introduce a bacterial NeoR gene into preimmune fetal sheep at 1–2 months before birth. Of the 10 recipient sheep, 6 exhibited G418-resistant hematopoietic progenitors in the bone marrow, 2 showed vector DNA sequences, and 1 had neomycin phosphotransferase activity.

In two other separate studies involving 31 sheep fetuses, a direct vector injection protocol was used in preimmune sheep about 3 months before birth. Although 10–15% of hematopoietic progenitors were G418 resistant, expression of the NeoR gene was detected in only 1% of white blood cells, 0.6% of lymphocytes, and 4% of granulocytes/macrophages in the peripheral blood. Fourteen animals continued to exhibit presence of the transgene in the blood and bone marrow 2–6 years after in vivo gene transfer. The analysis of maternal blood exhibited only transient presence of the vector sequences by polymerase chain reaction. Vector distribution was widespread in the tissues but not detected in purified sperm. Breeding experiments, which included experimental animals with expression of the transgene, failed to demonstrate germline involvement.

Mice

Snyder et al. described the results of prenatal ex vivo gene transfer in mice with β-glucuronidase (β-GUS)–deficient mucopolysaccharidosis VII (Sly disease).[55] Lysosomal accumulation of glycosaminoglycans occurs in the brain and other tissues, causing a fatal progressive degenerative disorder, including mental retardation. Fetal liver cells and β-GUS cells expressing multipotent neural progenitor were transduced ex vivo and transplanted prenatally into cerebral ventricles of newborn mice. β-GUS activity was expressed along the entire neuraxis, resulting in widespread correction of lysosomal storage in neurons and glia of affected mice.

ETHICAL DISCUSSIONS

Prenatal gene therapy is purely an experimental approach. There are not enough experimental data to properly assess the efficacy and safety of this procedure. If such therapy is offered to the patient, the consent form should specifically address the following:

1. Fetal and maternal safety
2. Discussion of other available treatments for the condition
3. Selection of a condition that has a predictable severe phenotype
4. Discussion of germline transduction during the procedure
5. Abortion option to be presented prior to introduction of prenatal therapy

INTERNATIONAL REGULATIONS REGARDING PRENATAL GENE THERAPY

France was one of the first countries to adopt a national regulation regarding biomedical research with its ethical, legal, and social aspects. It formed La Comité Consultatif National d'Ethique in 1983 and established a law concerning the protection of human beings who agree to be "under biomedical research" in 1988 and laws for the respect of the human body, in vitro fertilization, and prenatal diagnosis in 1994. Special concerns were raised about fetal integrity, possibly inadvertent germline integration, informed consent, and stringent evaluation of risks and benefits in every case. French law permits only somatic gene therapy. Every clinical trial, including prenatal in vivo gene transfer, that can affect the germline is prohibited in France at present.

In November 1998, the United Kingdom Gene Therapy Advisory Committee (GTAC) issued a report on the use of gene therapy in utero. The New and Emerging Technologies Subgroup of the GTAC, based on the United Kingdom Codes of Practice related to the use of fetuses in research, concluded that, because of unresolved specific scientific and ethical considerations, direct in utero gene therapy will not be used at present. The specific concerns were related to the modification of the germline and other nontarget effects. They concluded, however, that transplantation of genetically modified stem cells into fetuses would be ethically acceptable when clear advantage over postnatal therapy can be demonstrated. It must be specified that the treated disorder is life threatening or associated with severe disability and that no other adequate therapy exists.

FUTURE CONSIDERATIONS

In recent years, approximately 5 successful in utero transplantations in humans have been reported for SCID. Clinical success has only been achieved for conditions with an immunologic deficit and when a proliferative advantage for donor cells exists. Rapidly proliferating fetal HSC pose a barrier to successful engraftment of allogeneic cells. In its current form, in utero transplantation is not successful in diseases with intact endogenous hematopoietic and immune systems. At present, the only indication for prenatal stem cell therapy should be SCID. Recent reports demonstrate the possibility of active immune reaction to prematurely injected allogeneic cells in immunologically intact fetuses.[56] Further research is needed.

SAFETY OF THE PROCEDURE

The risks of in utero transplantation include the following:

1. Risk associated with prenatal diagnosis
2. Risk associated with the in utero procedure
3. Other risks

The risk of fetal loss with chorionic villus sampling was well documented and is below 1%.[57] The risk of the in utero procedure associated with intraperitoneal or intravenous infection is unknown at this time but could be compared to the risk associated with intrauterine transfusion for fetal rhesus factor disease.[43–45] There may, however, be more risks associated with this procedure than with in utero transplantation, such as a fetus compromised by anemia, the use of large-volume transfusions, and the use of a 16-gauge needle. For in utero transplantation, a 22-gauge spinal needle is used and the volume infused is very small. The estimated and observed risk for intravascular prenatal transfusions is 0.8%; for intraperitoneal transfusions, the risk is 3.5%. The risk related to in utero transplantation may be between these two figures.

Nonprocedural risks to the mother and fetus include the risk of transmitted infectious disease (especially with the use of fetal liver as a source of donor cells) and GVHD. The primary difficulty in the use of fetal liver is that there are no quality controls on donor screening, procurement, or preparation of cells.[55] With adult sources of HSC, standard protocols and procedures can be used and a high level of quality control established, which can reduce the risk of viral contamination to less than 1 in 10,000 and virtually eliminate clinically relevant bacterial and fungal contamination. The risk of GVHD depends on the source of cells used. The experience with postnatal infusion of marrow cells suggests that the use of more than 1×10^5 T cells/kg is associated with increased risk of GVHD. Existing experience in humans with prenatal transplantation for SCID suggests that CD34+ cell selection, which is associated with T-cell depletion, reduces the risk of GVHD to almost zero.[47, 48]

ETHICAL CONSIDERATIONS

The use of human fetal tissue and the treatment of the fetus has generated heated ethical discussion. Although there is no doubt that scientific research using fetal tissue has enormous potential, different governments have imposed varying restrictions on its use. In France, fetal tissue banking is nationally regulated. In England, an advisory group was asked to consider the ethical, medical, social, and legal implications of using fetuses and fetal material for research. The Peel Report,[59] followed by the Polkinghorne Report,[60] recommended that research should be allowed on fetuses that weigh less than 300 g provided the mother fully agrees with the research and an ethical committee of the institution fully approves all procedures used in the research.

One of the principal concerns of the opponents of fetal research is that women might be pressured into terminating pregnancy in order to provide fetal material. One of the recommendations of the Peel Report is that the doctors involved in performing an abortion be completely separated from the scientists performing fetal research. Another recommendation is that ethical committees of each institution be actively involved and oversee and regulate activities related to the fetal research. Finally, the informed consent should specifically state that the woman decided not to abort the sick fetus prior to knowing about the in utero transplantation treatment option.

In 1994, a study was conducted on the attitudes of women toward fetal tissue research.[61] Regardless of their past experience, the women were overwhelmingly in favor of research using fetal tissue (94%). They made little distinction between basic research and research with obvious clinical relevance. Women who underwent abortion were significantly more likely to approve of all types of research, including that aimed at improving methods of abortion and research using live fetuses in utero.

Because of the experimental nature of in utero transplantation, it is important that the ethical framework and public policy used to counsel patients and guide clinical decisions be further developed.[62] McCullough and Chervenak argued that the fetus has no independent moral or legal status.[63, 64] They postulated that the fetus is fully dependent on its mother and on her autonomous decisions. Therefore, they recommended that only the mother can consent to prenatal HSC therapy. Because of the experimental nature of in utero transplantation, however, the mother has no obligation to subject her fetus to this procedure. Thus, the clinical investigator proposing in utero transplantation must respect the mother's autonomous right to make this decision and not pressure her. Important in this process is accurate and nondirective counseling in the informed consent form.

Fetal therapy has been sensationalized by the media and therefore has created unrealistic expectations and hope.[65] Parents who have just received information that their unborn child is affected are unusually susceptible to investigator bias and optimism. Additionally, emotional detachment is difficult when considering the treatment of the affected child. Many risks and potential benefits are undefined and therefore subject to interpretation and bias by the investigator and patient. It is, therefore, extremely important that each couple considering in utero transplantation therapy receive extensive independent counseling. Specifically, families at risk should receive counseling before conception.

After prenatal diagnosis, the options include termination of pregnancy, prenatal transplantation, and postnatal therapy. The key part of counseling should be to ensure that the parents understand the risks and benefits of all options. The mother must understand that after the in utero transplantation procedure, she has a right to terminate the pregnancy at any time prior to the legal gestational limit for abortion.

CONCLUSION

In utero, HSCT has the potential to correct certain congenital disorders without the risks of a myeloablative and immunosuppressive conditioning regimen. Cases of engraftment and detectable postnatal chimerism have been reported, however, and success is not universal. Limiting the infused T-cell dose in the HSC grafts, either by CD34 + cell selection and/or T-cell depletion, appears to be necessary. Similar conclusions were published in a recent review.[66] Additional trials are currently in progress to study questions such as diseases and conditions that will be amenable for treatment by in utero HSCT, CD34 + cell dose, and timing of HSC infusion, as well as postnatal boosts with donor cells. In addition to the medical and technical hurdles, ethical and moral considerations such as donation of fetal tissues and the informed consent process must be addressed.

REFERENCES

1. Modell M, Wonke B, Anionwu E, et al: A multidisciplinary approach for improving services in primary care: randomized controlled trial of screening for haemoglobin disorders. BMJ 317(7161):788, 1998.
2. Alter BP: Advances in the prenatal diagnosis of hematologic disease. Blood 64(2):329, 1984.
3. Krivit W, Shapiro E, Kennedy W, et al: Treatment of late infantile metachromatic leukodystrophy by bone marrow transplantation. N Engl J Med 322(1):28, 1990.
4. Krivit W, Pierpont ME, Ayaz K, et al: Bone-marrow transplantation in the Maroteaux-Lamy syndrome (mucopolysaccharidosis VI): biochemical and clinical status 24 months after transplantation. N Engl J Med 311(25):1606, 1984.
5. Parkman R: The application of bone marrow transplantation to the treatment of genetic diseases. Science 232(4756):1373, 1986.
6. Sullivan KM: Current status of bone marrow transplantation. Transplant Proc 21(3 Suppl 1):41, 1989.
7. Clark J: The challenge of bone marrow transplantation. Mayo Clin Proc 65(1):111, 1990.
8. Sasazuki T, Juji T, Morishima Y, et al: Effect of matching of class I HLA alleles on clinical outcome after transplantation of hematopoietic stem cells from an unrelated donor: Japan Marrow Donor Program. N Engl J Med 339(17):1177, 1998.
9. Exner BG, Acholonu I, Ildstad ST: Hematopoietic chimerism, tolerance induction and graft-versus-host disease: considerations for composite tissue transfer. Transplant Proc 30(6):2718, 1998.
10. Ellison C, Gartner J: Acute, lethal graft-versus-host disease in a F1-hybrid model using grafts from parental-strain, T-cell receptor-delta gene knockout donors. Scand J Immunol 48(3):272, 1998.
11. Asplund S, Gramlich TL: Chronic mucosal changes of the colon in graft-versus-host disease. Mod Pathol 11(6):513, 1998.
12. Nagler A, Condiotti R, Nabet C, et al: Selective CD34 + -T cell depletion does not prevent graft-versus-host disease. Transplantation 66(1):138, 1998.
13. Klingebiel T, Schlegel PG: GVHD: overview on pathophysiology, incidence, clinical and biological features. Bone Marrow Transplant 21(Suppl 2):S45, 1998.
14. Billingham RE, Brent L, Madawar PB: Actively acquired tolerance of foreign cells. Nature 4379:603, 1953.
15. Billingham R, Brent L, Madawar PB: Quantitative studies on tissue transplantation immunity: actively acquired tolerance. Philos Trans R Soc Lond B Biol Sci 239:357, 1956.
16. Stewart FM, Crittenden RB, Lowery PA, et al: Long-term engraftment of normal and post-5-fluorouracil murine bone marrow into normal nonmyeloablated mice. Blood 81:2566, 1993.
17. Quesenberry PJ, Crittenden RB, Lowry P, et al: In vitro and in vivo studies of stromal niches. Blood Cells 20(1):97, 1994.
18. Quesenberry PJ, Ramshaw H, Crittenden RB, et al: Engraftment of normal murine marrow into nonmyeloablated host mice. Blood Cells 20(2–3):348, 1994.

19. Tavassoli M: Embryonic and fetal hemopoiesis: an overview. Blood Cells 17(2):269, 1991.
20. Bessler H, Djaldetti M: Ultrastructural studies on bone marrow development in embryonic mice. Biol Neonate 61(4):243, 1992.
21. Djaldetti M, Ovadia J, Bessler O, et al: Ultrastructural study of the erythropoietic events in human embryonic livers. Biol Neonate 28(5–6):367, 1975.
22. Sminia T, Djkstra CD: The origin of osteoclasts: an immunohisto-chemical study on macrophages and osteoclasts in embryonic rat bone. Calcif Tissue Int 39(4):263, 1986.
23. Hann IM, Bodger MP, Hoffbrand AV: Development of pluripotent hematopoietic progenitor cells in the human fetus. Blood 62(1):118, 1983.
24. Owen RD: Immunogenetic consequences of vascular anastomoses between bovine cattle twins. Science 10:400, 1945.
25. Cragle RG, Stone WH: Preliminary results of kidney grafts between cattle chimeric twins. Transplantation 5:328, 1967.
26. van Dijk BA, Boomsma DI, de Man AJ: Blood group chimerism in human multiple births is not rare. Am J Med Genet 61(3):264, 1996.
27. Picus J, Aldrich WR, Letvin NL: A naturally occurring bone-marrow-chimeric primate. I: Integrity of its immune system. Transplantation 39(3):297, 1985.
28. Hajdu K, Tanigawara S, Mclean LK, et al: In utero allogeneic hematopoietic stem cell transplantation to induce tolerance. Fetal Diagn Ther 11(4):241, 1996.
29. Kim HB, Shaaban AF, Yang EY, et al: Donor specific tolerance in a murine model of in utero stem cell transplantation requires hematopoietic microchimerism and is dependent on donor cell source. Blood 1618:95a, 1997.
30. Carrier E, Lee TH, Busch MP, Cohen MJ: Recruitment of engrafted donor cells postnatally into the blood with cytokines after in utero transplantation in mice. Transplantation 64(4):627, 1997.
31. Carrier E, Lee TH, Busch MP, Cowan MJ: Induction of tolerance in non defective mice after in utero transplantation of major histocompatibility complex mismatched fetal hematopoietic stem cells. Blood 86(12):4681, 1995.
32. Sarzotti M, Robbins DS, Hoffman PM: Induction of protective CTL responses in newborn mice by a murine retrovirus. Science 271(5256):1726–1728, 1996.
33. Kappler JW, Roehm N, Marrack P: T cell tolerance by clonal elimination in the thymus. Cell 49(2):273, 1987.
34. Fuchs EJ, Matzinger P: B cells turn off virgin but not memory T cells. Science 258:1156, 1992.
35. Matzinger P: Tolerance, danger, and the extended family. Annu Rev Immunol 12:991, 1994.
36. Ridge JP, Fuchs EJ, Matzinger P: Neonatal tolerance revisited: turning on newborn T cells with dendritic cells. Science 271(5256):1723, 1996.
37. Lehmann PV, Forsthuber T, Miller A, Sercarz EE: Spreading of T-cell autoimmunity to cryptic determinants of an autoantigen. Nature 358(6382):155, 1992.
38. Forsthuber T, Yip HC, Lehmann PV: Induction of TH1 and TH2 immunity in neonatal mice. Science 271(5256):1728, 1996.
39. Puck JM, Stewart CC, Nussbaum RL: Maximum-likelihood analysis of human T-cell X chromosome inactivation patterns: normal women versus carriers of X-linked severe combined immunodeficiency. Am J Hum Genet 50(4):742, 1992.
40. Puck JM, Conley ME, Bailey LC: Refinement of linkage of human severe combined immunodeficiency (SCIDX1) to polymorphic markers in Xq13. Am J Hum Genet 53(1):176, 1993.
41. Puck JM, Pepper AE, Bedard PM, Laframboise R: Female germ line mosaicism as the origin of a unique IL-2 receptor gamma-chain mutation causing X-linked severe combined immunodeficiency. J Clin Invest 95(2):895, 1995.
42. Touraine JL, Raudrant D, Royo C, et al: In utero transplantation of stem cells in bare lymphocyte syndrome. Lancet 1(8651):1382, 1989.

43. Berkowitz RL, Chitkara U, Wilkins I, et al: Technical aspects of intravascular intrauterine transfusions: lessons learned from thirty-three procedures. Am J Obst Gynecol 157(1):4, 1987.
44. Bowman JM: Hemolytic disease (erythroblastosis fetali S). In Creasy R, Resnick R (eds): Maternal and Fetal Medicine: Principles and Practice. Philadelphia, WB Saunders, 1994, p 730.
45. Moise KJ Jr: Intrauterine transfusion with red cells and platelets. West J Med 159(3):318, 1993.
46. Touraine JL: Treatment of human fetuses and induction of immunological tolerance in humans by in utero transplantation of stem cells into fetal recipients. Acta Hematol 96(3):115, 1996.
47. Flake AW, Roncarolo MG, Puck JM, et al: Treatment of X-linked severe combined immunodeficiency by in utero transplantation of paternal bone marrow. N Engl J Med 335(24):1806, 1996.
48. Wengler GS, Lanfranchi A, Fruscat T, et al: In utero transplantation of parental CD34 haematopoietic progenitor cells in a patient with X-linked severe combined immunodeficiency (SCID XI). Lancet 348(9040):1484, 1996.
49. Touraine JL: In utero transplantation of fetal liver stem cells into human fetuses. J Hematother 5(2):195, 1996.
50. Westgren M, Ringden O, Eik-Nes S, et al: Lack of evidence of permanent engraftment after in utero fetal stem cell transplantation in congenital hemoglobinopathies. Transplantation 61(8):1176, 1996.
51. Slavin S, Naparstek E, Ziegler M: Clinical application of intrauterine bone marrow transplantation for treatment of genetic disease—feasibility studies. Bone Marrow Transplant 1:189, 1992.
52. Duikman R, Golbus MS: In utero stem cell therapy. J Reprod Med 37:515, 1992.
53. Bambach BJ, Moser HW, Blakemore K, et al: Engraftment following in utero bone marrow transplantation for globoid leukodystrophy. Bone Marrow Transplant 19(4):399, 1997.
54. Porada CD, Tran N, Eglitis M, et al: In utero gene therapy: transfer and long-term expression of bacterial neo(r) gene in sheep after direct injection of retroviral vectors into preimmune fetuses. Hum Gene Ther 9(11):1571, 1998.
55. Snyder EY, Taylor RM, Wolfe JH: Neural progenitor cell engraftment corrects lysosomal storage throughout the MPS VII mouse brain. Nature 374(6520):367, 1995.
56. Orlandi F, Giambona A, Messana F, et al: Evidence of induced non-tolerance in HLA-identical twins with neuroglobinopathy after in utero fetal transplantation. Bone Marrow Transplant 18(3):637, 1996.
57. Rhoads GG, Jackson LG, Schlesselman SE, et al: The safety and efficacy of chorionic villus sampling for early prenatal diagnosis of cytogenetic abnormalities. N Engl J Med 320(10):609, 1989.
58. Mychaliska GB, Muench MO, Rice HE, et al: The biology and ethics of banking fetal liver hematopoietic stem cells for in utero transplantation. J Pediatr Surg 33(2):394, 1998.
59. The Peel Report. Chairman, Sir Jonathan Peel: The Use of Fetuses and Fetal Material for Research. London, HMSO, 1972.
60. The Polkinghorne Report. Chairman, the Rev. Dr. John Polkinghorne: Review of the Guidance on the Research of Fetuses and Fetal Material. London, HMSO, 1989.
61. Anderson F, Glasier A, Ross J, Baird DT: Attitudes of women to fetal tissue research. J Med Ethics 20(1):36, 1994.
62. Fletcher JC: Fetal therapy, ethics and public policies. Fetal Diagn Ther 7(2):158, 1992.
63. McCullough LB, Chervenak FA: Ethics in Obstetrics and Gynecology. New York, Oxford University Press, 1994.
64. Chervenak FA, McCullough LB: Does obstetric ethics have any role in the obstetrician's response to the abortion controversy? Am J Obstet Gynecol 163(5 Pt 1):1425, 1990.
65. Kingman S, Yamauchi H, Donozyski A, et al: Fetal tissue research around the world. BMJ 304(6831):591, 1992.
66. Flake AW, Zanjani ED: In utero hematopoietic stem cell transplantation: ontogenic opportunities and biological barriers. Blood 94:2179, 1999.

Evaluation of the Transplant Candidate

CHAPTER TWENTY

Evaluation of Patients Before Hematopoietic Stem Cell Transplantation

David J. Oblon, M.D.

Evaluation of a patient before hematopoietic stem cell transplantation (HSCT) has two purposes: to define the patient's health/physical status and the status of the disease. This chapter focuses on the recipient/patient and how the evaluation affects the decision of whether HSCT should be offered and the care plan after HSCT. Other parts of the text discuss such factors as diagnosis, biology of the disease, staging, and indications for HSCT.

The pretransplantation evaluation has three primary objectives. The first is the identification of conditions that increase the risk of serious morbidity or death as a result of the procedure. The second is the diagnosis of potential diseases or circumstances for which prophylaxis or surveillance with early intervention can lower the risk of transplant complications. The third is the estimation of the probability that the patient will comply with medical instructions.

BACKGROUND

Pretransplantation evaluation has its roots in the anecdotal experience of the early transplant centers and in the study design process of the clinical trials. The first attempts at HSCT using bone marrow in the late 19th century and the 20th century concentrated on the technical barriers to allogeneic transplantation but ignored the role of the recipient/patient.[1–5] The elucidation of the human leukocyte antigen (HLA) system and the development of serologic methods for tissue typing improved the success rate of bone marrow transplantation (BMT). Studies in animals documented the need for a conditioning regimen with sufficient immunosuppressive properties to prevent graft rejection. There was also a theoretical need to provide space within the marrow where the graft could proliferate. The treatment of malignant diseases requires agents with sufficient cytotoxic activity to completely eradicate the tumor. The combination of high-dose cyclophosphamide and single-fraction total body irradiation (TBI) met these criteria.[6, 7] Santos et al.[8] developed the combination of busulfan and cyclophosphamide, which satisfied the essential criteria for immunosuppression, space, and cytotoxicity and obviated the need for TBI.[8, 9] Variations of these early regimens are still the most commonly used conditioning regimens in allogeneic HSCT. The first report of successful BMT in a child with an inherited immunodeficiency disorder proved the feasibility of the procedure, and reports of successful engraftment in patients with malignancy followed rapidly.[10, 11] The seminal paper by Thomas et al. demonstrated the potential for BMT to cure patients with refractory acute leukemia.[7]

As the number of allogeneic BMT increased, there was a growing awareness of the toxic effects on normal tissues of the recipient/patient. The search for improvement evolved along two lines of investigation. One was the modification of the conditioning regimens to decrease toxicity. For example, fractionated TBI helped reduce pulmonary damage.[12, 13] The other approach was selection of the recipient/patient. Two paradigms, namely, the experience at transplant centers and the inclusion or exclusion criteria of clinical trials, led rapidly to guidelines that included or excluded patients according to age and tests of organ function. These criteria, however, were institution-specific, and industry-wide standards were lacking.

The development of cryopreservation procedures led to the application of autologous BMT.[14–16] Many centers applied similar pretransplantation evaluation standards used for allogeneic transplants to autologous patients. Most of these selection criteria remained static for over a decade.

Recent developments, both in allograft and in autograft technologies, have forced a re-evaluation of selection criteria. The widespread use of peripheral blood progenitor cells (PBPC) has decreased the time spent in aplasia after infusion of the grafts. The more rapid hematologic recovery has correlated with less normal tissue toxicity. The result has been lower mortality rates in the period immediately following HSCT. Newer chemotherapy-based conditioning regimens have obviated the need for TBI. These regimens have either lessened toxicity or have shifted the toxicity to organs with more regenerative capacity. Nonmyeloablative strategies have further decreased the risk of extramedullary toxicity.[17–19] This approach has shifted the focus from cytotoxicity of the conditioning regimen to reliance on the graft-versus-tumor effect. By design, the main benefactor has been the normal tissue of recipient/patient. Less toxic regimens have made HSCT available to older people or to those with comorbid conditions, which contraindicates a more traditional myeloablative conditioning regimen. The impact of these developments on the time-tested pretransplantation evaluation has been substantial. The rapid evolution in technologies has resulted in a "moving target." Patients who might have been rejected a few years ago may be candidates for these novel strategies. Any discussion of the pretransplantation evaluation has to recognize the changing nature of the field and the paucity of published data.

An important function for pretransplantation evaluation is guidance of the informed consent process. For example, the identification of a comorbid condition, which heretofore would have been a contraindication to transplantation, may now be an indicator of increased risk. This added risk becomes an element within the equation of disease, the probability the transplant will lead to cure or long-term palliation, and the toxicity profile of the conditioning regimen. The physician can present the information about the identified risk and advise the patient to make an informed decision.

PARAMETERS FOR EVALUATION

There are four broad categories within the pretransplantation evaluation: patient demographics, psychosocial characteristics, individual organ system assessments, and evaluation of systemic conditions, both active and latent.

PATIENT DEMOGRAPHICS

Age

Age is the most important demographic factor. Increasing age is associated with greater morbidity and mortality. Both regimen-related toxicity and incidence of severe graft-versus-host disease (GVHD) increase with age.[20–22] Because older age is also associated with a diminished organ reserve, the toxic effects of myeloablative conditioning regimens are more pronounced. The improvements in supportive care and the refinement in chemotherapeutic agents have made transplants in older people more feasible. The emphasis has shifted from chronologic age to the less-defined "physiologic age." This semiquantitative judgment relies heavily on the absence of defined comorbid disease(s) and a history of an active lifestyle. It is common sense that older patients with good muscle tone and an energetic attitude are more likely to recover quickly from the toxicity of HSCT. As centers gain more experience with older patients, more objective measures of physiologic age may become available to more precisely predict the probability of morbid events.

Gender

The gender of the recipient and the donor play a role in the risk of GVHD.[21, 22] Female donor to male recipient confers the greatest risk. Very few sibling transplants, however, have the luxury of a choice in the gender of donors. The expanded donor pool for matched unrelated donors occasionally allows for the choice of gender.

Because many HSCT candidates are in their reproductive years, birth control, sterility, induction of early menopause, and hormone replacement therapy often become issues during the pretransplantation evaluation. Currently practiced at most centers, and incorporated into the Standards in the Foundation for the Accreditation of Hematopoietic Cell Therapy (FAHCT), is the requirement that female patients have a negative pregnancy test result. The hazards of conditioning regimens and post-transplantation immune suppression mandate use of a reliable contraceptive method.

Myeloablative doses of TBI and alkylating agents result in sterility for most males. For example, one study examined semen of 323 men who received a TBI-containing conditioning regimen. Five men (<2%) experienced return of spermatogenesis.[23] Another trial reported a high incidence of sexual dysfunction defined as erectile failure, ejaculation problems, and decreased libido in 51 men after allogeneic BMT.[24] Sperm banking before administration of conditioning regimen is an option unless the disease or earlier exposure to chemotherapeutic agents has reduced the sperm count to an unacceptable level.

For females, the impact of conditioning regimens on ovarian function is more variable. A few women maintain regular menstrual cycles; others experience transient amenorrhea, and some experience the induction of early menopause. The ultimate effect on reproductive function depends on the conditioning regimen, patient age, and previous exposure to chemotherapy. For example, long-term follow-up of women receiving a total of 200 mg/kg of cyclophosphamide for aplastic anemia documented resumption of menses in all patients less than 26 years old (median time to recovery, 0.75 years); 12 of 19 women between ages 26 and 38 resumed regular menses. None of 50 women conditioned with busulfan and cyclophosphamide recovered ovarian function after 1–2 years following BMT. Longer follow-up of women conditioned with TBI showed that 3% of the patients recovered ovarian function at a median of 5 years (range, 3–7 years).[23–27] The pretransplantation evaluation presents an opportunity to discuss possible effects on gonadal function and to begin discussion of the options for hormone replacement if early menopause does occur.

PSYCHOSOCIAL EVALUATION

A successful outcome, especially for allogeneic HSCT, depends on patient compliance. Living with immune suppression mandates a rigorous adherence to medications, diet, and a lifestyle that reduces the risk of post-transplantation complications. The psychosocial assessment is a systematic approach to evaluating the ability of the patient and those around the patient to provide the necessary adherence to medical care.

The evaluation has three components. The first is to identify a caregiver who can assist and observe the patient outside the transplant center. The second is to identify any psychiatric disorders and/or social behaviors that may exclude the patient from HSCT. The third is to assess the dynamics of the patient, family, and support system. The psychosocial profile should allow development of a psychosocial care plan, which can prevent development of psychosocial crisis after HSCT.

The requirements for the specialist who performs the psychosocial evaluation vary among HSCT centers. Most include a social worker with expertise in interviewing and counseling. This individual is the focal point of the routine psychosocial care. A psychiatrist or psychologist should be available for more in-depth evaluation of patient and the family. Whether the psychiatrist interviews each candidate or not depends on institutional resources, policies, and reimbursement patterns. Some programs use a psychiatric evaluation when initial screening identifies a potential problem, such as substance abuse or a personality disorder. Most importantly, the psychosocial consultants must appreciate and understand the physical and psychological rigors of HSCT.

Institutions with a hospital chaplain may include a formal spiritual evaluation. The chaplain's involvement should go beyond a simple identification of people for whom religion is an important part of life. The chaplain can educate the community pastor or spiritual counselor about the physical stresses of HSCT on the patient and the family. Preparation of spiritual counselors, especially those with no previous experience dealing with patients undergoing HSCT, can improve their interactions with and the potential to comfort the patient.

A number of programs include art or music therapists. Their evaluations can help find useful ways to reduce patient stress.

Caregiver

The evaluation should identify a caregiver as a critical member of the outpatient team. This person is usually a family member or close friend. A small group, however, can be as effective and allows each member to maintain employment and attend to family obligations. The critical issue is to assess each caregiver's ability to perform the necessary tasks such as central line care and dressing changes. More importantly, the caregiver should learn how to contact the transplant team, receive clear answers to questions, and respond in an emergency. If the person is not suited for the role, a substitute must be identified before committing to the HSCT procedure.

The length of service often determines who can participate as a caregiver. As autologous HSCT shifts from the inpatient to the outpatient setting, more demands are placed on the patient and caregiver during aplasia and the early period of engraftment. Prompt hematologic recovery and a lower risk of life-threatening complications permit less of a time demand on the primary caregiver. The complexities of an allogeneic transplant require a caregiver for a longer period. Most centers recommend participation up to day +100.

Psychiatric Disorders and/or Social Behaviors Contraindicated for HSCT

Current literature offers little guidance, and most lessons have come from the solid organ transplant experience.[28, 29] A psychiatrist should assist with this phase of the workup. Most programs consider psychopaths, sociopaths, and borderline personality disorders as a contraindication to HSCT. Obtaining consistent compliance from these individuals is usually impossible. Many of these persons are highly manipulative and frequently wreak psychological havoc with the staff. Sociopaths and psychopaths may exhibit violent behavior, which places the staff at an unnecessary risk of physical harm. Others, however, have taken a less restrictive approach.[30] If a center decides to perform transplantation with such a person, it is imperative to institute close psychiatric follow-up with defined criteria for interventions before initiation of the procedure. The institution must also take the necessary precautions to ensure the safety of the staff.

The diagnosis of a psychotic disorder such as schizophrenia or bipolar disorder is not a contraindication to transplantation. The decision to offer HSCT to these patients depends on a variety of factors. Considerations usually include the response to medication, the history of compliance with psychotropic drugs, comorbid conditions such as active substance abuse, and the strength of the patient's support system.

Potential HSCT candidates with a history of substance abuse pose a dilemma.[29–31] Both drug and alcohol abuse are frequently associated with comorbid conditions and personality traits that can make transplantation dangerous. The decision to offer HSCT to potential patients is usually based on multiple factors. The following is a partial list of issues to be evaluated:

- Substance being abused
- Frequency and severity of the abuse
- Past history or other episodes of abuses of the same or other substance(s)
- Current status of the abuse, if still active
- Changes in social and psychological surroundings that may alleviate or deepen the abuse
- Strength of support system
- Prior history of compliance or noncompliance with medical care
- Comorbid conditions frequently associated with the abuse

Evaluation of these factors can guide the decision to include or exclude a patient.

INDIVIDUAL ORGAN ASSESSMENT

The primary purpose of the organ system evaluation is to identify conditions that have reduced organ reserve and place the patient at high risk for complications. Many of the tests are screening tools. An abnormal result often highlights the need for more extensive examinations. The test data are combined to guide medical judgment. Few prospective studies have been published that correlate the value of a given organ function test with post-transplantation mortality and morbidity. The Foundation for Accreditation of Hematopoietic Cell Therapy (FAHCT) has specific guidelines for the assessment of patients prior to HSCT (see Chapter 65).

Eyes

The history and physical examination is sufficient for screening. Sight-impaired and blind patients can undergo HSCT as long as the support system is strong. Most other ocular conditions, such as glaucoma, can be controlled with medication and do not place the patient at higher risk.

Oral Cavity

A careful dental examination and dental radiographs are part of the pretransplantation work-up. Routine preparative care includes a thorough dental cleaning and repair of cavities or damaged fillings, which may lead to oral infection. The abnormalities most likely to lead to post-transplantation complications are impacted third molars, failed endodontics, and periapical pathoses with nonvital, non-endodontically treated teeth. The decision to extract third molars depends on the risk of local infection. Generally, if the distal gingiva is in the occlusal one third of the crown, the tooth should be extracted.[32, 33] It is important to consider that as the duration of neutropenia lessens, the risk of infection and the need for extraction also decreases.[32, 33] If tooth extraction or oral surgery is performed, most patients need approximately 2 weeks for tissues to heal before undergoing HSCT.

Oral mucositis after transplantation is associated with blood infections and an increased risk of mortality. Rapoport et al. prospectively studied 202 HSCT recipients and did not identify any pretransplantation predictors of severe oral mucositis.[34] Strategies under active investigation currently emphasize prophylaxis with agents such as glutamine, interleukin-11, and keratinocyte growth factor rather than identification of risk factors in recipients/patients.[35–37]

Lungs

Pulmonary complications are a major contributor to transplant morbidity and mortality. Recent advances such as fractionated TBI and cytomegalovirus prophylaxis have reduced the risk of respiratory failure; however, the pretransplantation evaluation is limited in its ability to prospectively identify patients who will experience respiratory failure.

The primary screening tools are the history, physical examination, and pulmonary function tests (PFT). Crawford and Fisher prospectively collected data on 1297 patients (82% allogeneic, 18% autologous) undergoing transplant for malignant diseases.[38] Univariate and multivariate analyses identified abnormal test results for gas exchange as a predictor of fatal outcome. Both diffusing capacity and arterial oxygenation remained independent risk factors even after adjustments for age and active malignancy. It is noteworthy that many of the deaths were the result of nonpulmonary or infectious causes. Both the authors of the paper and an accompanying editorial comment emphasized that the PFT results should be used as a part of the informed consent process but that abnormal PFT values are not a contraindication to HSCT.[38, 39]

Spuriously abnormal diffusing capacity results are possible in patients with anemia. Although many laboratories performing PFT routinely correct the measured diffusing capacity for the patient's hematocrit, some do not. It is important to document that the laboratory has performed the calculation for anemic patients.

Obstructions to airflow as evidenced by abnormal forced expiratory volume/forced vital capacity are not a predictor of an adverse pulmonary event. Three analyses have been unable to document a relationship between obstructive lung disease and adverse outcomes.[40] These studies could not separate cigarette use from other competing causes of lung diseases. Many centers, however, take a common-sense approach by recommending reduction or cessation of smoking as part of a broader effort at improving pulmonary toilet before HSCT.

Patients with mild to moderate asthma controlled with medication can undergo HSCT without excessive risk. Input from the pulmonary specialist is useful to coordinate the asthma drug therapy, monitor drug levels, and develop prospective contingency plans for an exacerbation. It is wise to avoid drugs in the conditioning regimen that have a high probability of pulmonary toxicity, such as BCNU. Patients with severe asthma require careful case-by-case evaluation.

Heart

Cardiac complications account for approximately 5% of early transplant-related fatalities. The challenge for pretransplantation evaluation is to identify patients at highest risk for cardiac complication. The history, physical examination, electrocardiogram (EKG), and radionuclide scan are the principal screening tools. The two broad categories of heart disease are electrical and structural abnormalities.

The history and EKG may suggest a rhythm disturbance. Further testing with 24-hour continuous monitoring and, on rare occasions, electrophysiologic studies diagnose most arrhythmias. Additional tests to rule out causes such as pericardial disease, coronary artery disease, atrial abnormalities, or myocardial dysfunction are essential. Documentation of a serious arrhythmia during the pretransplantation evaluation is rare, however.

Structural abnormalities are more likely to become apparent during the evaluation. Radionuclide scanning is the most commonly employed test to detect myocardial dysfunction. Bearman et al. screened 136 patients identified as high-risk by history and EKG testing.[20] Total anthracycline dose did not predict for a decreased ejection fraction or for transplant-related mortality. Radionuclide scanning identified only 14 patients (10%) with ejection fractions less than 50%. Two of 10 patients experienced grade III or IV cardiac toxicity. In contrast, 5 of 116 patients with an ejection fraction greater than 50% suffered severe cardiac complications. The small number of patients with a low (<50%) ejection fraction precluded firm conclusions, but the trend raised serious concerns.[41]

Hertenstein et al. studied 150 patients undergoing allogeneic HSCT and 20 patients undergoing autologous transplant with radionuclide scanning.[42] Eight patients suffered cardiac complications, with three classified as life-threatening. Although 38 patients (22%) had detectable abnormalities, a low ejection fraction did not predict for life-threatening toxicity but did predict a cardiac complication. A history of clinically documented congestive heart failure has a strong association with fatal cardiac toxicity.[20] This experience is similar to published reports in non–transplant recipients. Survivors of anthracycline-induced congestive heart failure experienced fatal exacerbations of heart failure as a result of a physiologic stress such as infection.[43]

A few general principles can be derived from the studies:

1. Routine radionuclide scanning for every patient is not necessary.
2. An ejection fraction below 50% predicts cardiac complications but is not an absolute contraindication to HSCT.
3. A history of congestive heart failure is a contraindication to HSCT unless there are compelling mitigating circumstances.

The major cause of cardiac complications is the conditioning regimen. Cyclophosphamide is most commonly associated with cardiac toxicity.[44, 45] The advent of newer regimens such as the nonmyeloablative strategies may reduce the cardiac risks, especially for patients with low ejection fractions.

Liver

The liver is a major source of post-transplantation morbidity and mortality. Pretransplantation evaluation can identify a variety of abnormalities that affect patient selection and management. The history and physical examination, serum transaminases, bilirubin, and serologic studies for hepatitis A, B, and C viruses are the primary screening tests for liver disease. Neither computed tomography nor magnetic resonance imaging is part of the screening evaluation, but these modalities may add valuable anatomic information when more detailed testing becomes necessary.

Elevation of the transaminases before transplantation is a powerful predictor of severe veno-occlusive disease (VOD). A seemingly trivial elevation carries an increased risk of VOD. The higher the level of the transaminases, however, the greater the risk of fatal complications.[46–49] A study of 355 patients found that hepatitis was a predictor of fatal liver complications (with a relative risk 4.6).[50] Many conditions may cause hepatitis, manifested as elevated liver function test results, with or without clinical symptoms. The diagnosis of acute viral hepatitis is usually straightforward. HSCT must be deferred until the hepatitis is resolved because of the high risk of fatal complications.[51] Other causes of hepatitis may be much more difficult to diagnose with certainty. Drug-induced hepatitis is often a diagnosis of exclusion. Discontinuation of all drugs is important. Postponing transplantation until the transaminases return to normal levels is the safest course.

Chronic hepatitis, especially with hepatitis C virus (HCV), is a difficult issue. Therapy with agents such as interferon and ribavirin rarely results in rapid improvement. Deferral of HSCT for many months may not be practical. Although patients with HCV-induced chronic hepatitis can undergo transplantation, they face a high risk of complications, which include VOD, acute fulminant hepatitis, and progression to cirrhosis. A study of 62 patients with HCV infection before transplantation found severe VOD in 22 (48%) of 46 evaluable patients, compared with 150 (14%) of 229 patients without HCV infection.[50] Interestingly, the presence of HCV and normal trans-

aminases did not increase the risk of VOD. The risk of fulminant hepatitis is 1% or less. The published literature is limited to case reports.[51, 52] Progression to cirrhosis is a much greater risk. Strasser et al. studied 3721 patients who survived more than 1 year after transplantation: 31 experienced cirrhosis. Hepatitis C was a factor in 25 of 31 patients and in 15 of 16 patients followed for more than 10 years after transplantation.[51]

Carriers of hepatitis B virus (HBV) have a small risk of fulminant hepatitis. The risk is approximately 5%.[53, 54] Limited data suggest that a transplant from an HBV-immune donor may eradicate HBV from the recipient.[53–55] Cirrhosis of the liver is a contraindication to HSCT because of the high rate of regimen-related mortality. Liver complications after HSCT are discussed in Chapter 46.

Kidney

The history, serum creatinine, and 24-hour urine collection for creatinine clearance are the primary screening tests for renal function. Because serum creatinine can vary considerably from person to person, borderline or elevated values merit quantification with a creatinine clearance. An excretion of greater than 60 mL/min has been a traditional threshold for HSCT. Patients with impaired renal function (<60 mL/min) can undergo transplantation. Meticulous attention must be paid to drug-selection details in order to avoid nephrotoxic agents. For example, platinum compounds should be excluded from the conditioning regimen. If possible, exclusion of aminoglycosides from antibiotic choices and a liposomal formulation of amphotericin B should be considered. There are no prospective data to predict renal complications with the newer, less-intense conditioning regimens, however.

Gastrointestinal Tract

The history and physical examination are the best screening tools for gastrointestinal (GI) disorders. There are no simple tests to screen for excessive risk of GI complications. The best predictors of GI toxicity are (1) GI symptoms and (2) the known toxicity profile of agents in the conditioning regimen. Prophylactic strategies aimed at specific known toxicities may abrogate some of the morbidity. For example, propantheline can reduce oral mucositis associated with high-dose etoposide.[56, 57]

Pretransplantation symptoms of upper GI abnormalities such as esophageal pain, heartburn, dysphagia, epigastric pain, and unexplained nausea and vomiting may indicate mucosal ulceration. Ulceration is a risk factor for gastrointestinal bleeding during aplasia. Upper GI endoscopy can detect both ulceration and unsuspected infectious causes. Common infectious agents include herpes simplex virus, cytomegalovirus (CMV), and fungal organisms.

Lower intestinal diseases, such as Crohn disease and ulcerative colitis, should be evident from the history. Colonoscopy can diagnose active disease. A follow-up examination is important to document ulcer healing, which reduces the risk of GI tract bleeding. Interestingly, immunosuppressive therapy may cause the underlying autoimmune disease to remit.[58, 59]

More acute symptoms such as diarrhea merit investigation to exclude pathogens. Common infecting agents are *Clostridium difficile,* CMV, and *Entamoeba histolytica.* Therapy prior to transplantation is essential. One organism, *Strongyloides,* deserves special mention. This parasite may disseminate and kill the immunosuppressed patient. Infestation may not cause symptoms, and persistent eosinophilia may be the only clue.[60] Careful examination of several fresh stool specimens for parasites is important. Therapy eradicates the organism and permits HSCT.

Central Nervous System

The evaluation examines two categories: (1) primary neurologic disorders and (2) tumor invasion within the central nervous system (CNS). The neurologic examination and scanning with computed tomography or magnetic resonance imaging (MRI) are the primary tools to evaluate CNS anatomy and to exclude metastatic tumors. MRI, with and without gadolinium enhancement, is currently the most sensitive modality. Lumbar puncture with a cytologic examination can detect spread of leukemia, lymphoma, or carcinoma to the meninges.

Patients with seizure disorders controlled by medication can undergo HSCT with active monitoring of antiepileptic drug levels. Whenever possible, the conditioning regimen should avoid agents such as busulfan that lower the seizure threshold. Progressive degenerative diseases contraindicate HSCT. Autoimmune disorders such as multiple sclerosis, however, may improve after immune suppressive therapy, and HSCT for multiple sclerosis is currently an area of active clinical investigation.[59]

Involvement of the CNS with carcinoma is a contraindication to HSCT. The poor outcomes for patients with meningeal carcinomatosis or with parenchymal lesions do not justify transplantation with current technology. An exception is enrollment in a clinical trial designed to explore new HSCT techniques for controlling CNS metastases. Leukemic involvement of the CNS is associated with a poor prognosis but does not contraindicate allogeneic HSCT. Most centers recommend intrathecal chemotherapy to clear the central spinal fluid of detectable leukemia cells before proceeding to transplantation; specific regimens are discussed in other chapters.

SYSTEMIC DISEASES

Infection

The pretransplantation testing for systemic processes, especially infections, can affect patient selection and/or post-transplantation management. Active infections before HSCT are associated with a very high mortality rate. The diagnosis of most acute bacterial infections is straightforward. Therapeutic success must be documented because partially treated infections can become exacerbated during aplasia.

Fungal infections present a more difficult diagnostic problem. *Aspergillus* species and *Candida* species are the most common organisms that infect transplant recipients. Systemic aspergillosis detected after allogeneic HSCT has a mortality rate in excess of 90%. Aggressive pretransplantation work-up including biopsy may be necessary for diag-

nosis. Intensive antifungal therapy can suppress reactivation.

Aspergillus gains access through the nasal and sinus passages. Nasal cultures can detect colonization prior to transplantation. The impact of pre-emptive therapy is uncertain, however. A number of newer antifungals are in clinical trials and may prove useful for prophylaxis or pre-emptive therapy of *Aspergillus* colonization.

The pretransplantation assessment can detect a number of viruses for which effective prophylaxis exists. Serologic testing for the hepatitis viruses, CMV, herpes simplex virus, varicella zoster virus, and human immunodeficiency virus (HIV) identifies patients with prior exposure. The recent recognition of human herpesvirus 6 as a post-transplantation pathogen has stimulated investigation.[61–63] Routine serologic tests are not yet available.

Documentation of CMV status affects two areas of post-transplantation management: (1) antiviral therapy and (2) transfusion support. Patients seropositive for CMV may experience reactivation of the virus after immunosuppression. Either antiviral prophylaxis or surveillance with early intervention markedly reduces the risk of fatal CMV infections.[64–67] Patients without CMV antibodies may acquire the virus from blood transfusions. Blood component therapy with CMV-safe products (i.e., leukodepletion of red blood cells and platelets) can abrogate viral transmission.[68, 69]

Post-transplantation herpes simplex virus infections range from painful oral lesions to fatal pneumonia. Prophylaxis with antiviral drugs such as acyclovir is effective (Chapter 36). Varicella zoster virus infections are usually a later complication for which we lack a simple prophylactic strategy. Early interventions with antivirals are effective, however. Surveillance for relapse with unusual clinical manifestations is important (Chapter 43).[70]

Most centers consider HIV infection a contraindication to HSCT. Early experience with marrow transplantation to restore immune competency yielded mixed results.[71, 72]

Previous Chemotherapy

Many patients arrive at HSCT centers after a history of one or more courses of various chemotherapy regimens. The systemic effects on normal tissues are protean. Exposure to multiple cycles of cytotoxic drugs is a well-recognized predictor of post-transplantation complications. Identification of this increased risk is important for the informed consent process but is not reason to exclude a patient unless there is severe damage to a vital organ.

CONCLUSION

The pretransplantation evaluation is the opportunity for the transplant team to identify conditions that increase the risk of a complication after transplantation. Identification of risk factors allows selection of patients for prophylaxis or early intervention. These strategies include accrual of patients to clinical trials that investigate novel therapies. The pretransplantation evaluation highlights psychosocial issues, which the transplant team must address to improve the probability of a positive outcome. Finally, the pretransplantation evaluation is evolving as transplant technology changes.

REFERENCES

1. Billings J: Therapeutic use of extract of bone marrow. Bull Johns Hopkins Hosp 5:115–117, 1894.
2. Osgood EE, Riddle MC, Matthews TJ: Aplastic anemia treated with daily transfusion and intravenous marrow: case report. Ann Intern Med 13:358–367, 1939.
3. Morrison M, Samwick AA: Intramedullary (sternal) transfusion of human bone marrow. JAMA 115:1708–1711, 1940.
4. Mathe G: Transfusions et greffes de moelle ossene homologue chez des humains irradies a huate dose accident effement. Fr Etudes Clin Biol 4:226–238, 1959.
5. Bortin MM: A compendium of reported human bone marrow transplants. Transplantation 9(6):571–587, 1970.
6. Thomas ED, Buckner CD, Cheever MA, et al: Marrow transplantation for leukemia and aplastic anemia. Transplant Proc 8(4):603–605, 1976.
7. Thomas ED, Buckner CD, Banaji M, et al: One hundred patients with acute leukemia treated by chemotherapy, total body irradiation, and allogeneic marrow transplantation. Blood 49(4):511–533, 1977.
8. Santos GW, Tutschka PJ, Brookmeyer R, et al: Marrow transplantation for acute nonlymphocytic leukemia after treatment with busulfan and cyclophosphamide. N Engl J Med 309(22):1347–1353, 1983.
9. Buckner CD, Clift RA, Fefer A, et al: Marrow transplantation for the treatment of acute leukemia using HL-A-identical siblings. Transplant Proc 6(4):365–366, 1974.
10. Gatti RA, Meuwissen HJ, Allen HD, et al: Immunological reconstitution of sex-linked lymphopenic immunological deficiency. Lancet 2(7583):1366–1369, 1968.
11. Thomas E, Storb R, Clift RA, et al: Bone-marrow transplantation (first of two parts). N Engl J Med 292(16):832–843, 1975.
12. Wara WM, Phillips TL, Margolis LW, Smith V: Radiation pneumonitis: a new approach to the derivation of time-dose factors. Cancer 32(3):547–552, 1973.
13. Peters LJ, Withers HR, Cundiff JH, Dicke KA: Radiobiological considerations in the use of total-body irradiation for bone-marrow transplantation. Radiology 131(1):243–247, 1979.
14. Barnes BD, Loutit JF: The radiation recovery factor: preservation by the Polge-Smith-Parkes technique. J Natl Cancer Inst 15:901–905, 1954.
15. Dicke KA, McCredie KB, Spitzer G, et al: Autologous bone marrow transplantation in patients with adult acute leukemia in relapse. Transplantation 26(3):169–173, 1978.
16. Appelbaum FR, Herzig GP, Ziegler JL, et al: Successful engraftment of cryopreserved autologous bone marrow in patients with malignant lymphoma. Blood 52(1):85–95, 1978.
17. Giralt S, Estey E, Albitar M, et al: Engraftment of allogeneic hematopoietic progenitor cells with purine analog-containing chemotherapy: harnessing graft-versus-leukemia without myeloablative therapy. Blood 89(12):4531–4536, 1997.
18. Slavin S, Nagler A, Naparstek E, et al: Nonmyeloablative stem cell transplantation and cell therapy as an alternative to conventional bone marrow transplantation with lethal cytoreduction for the treatment of malignant and nonmalignant hematologic diseases. Blood 91(3):756–763, 1998.
19. Khouri IF, Keating M, Korbling M, et al: Transplant-lite: induction of graft-versus-malignancy using fludarabine-based nonablative chemotherapy and allogeneic blood progenitor-cell transplantation as treatment for lymphoid malignancies. J Clin Oncol 16(8):2817–2824, 1998.
20. Bearman SI, Appelbaum FR, Back A, et al: Regimen-related toxicity and early posttransplant survival in patients undergoing marrow transplantation for lymphoma. J Clin Oncol 7(9):1288–1294, 1989.
21. Weisdorf D, Hakke R, Blazar B, et al: Risk factors for acute graft-versus-host disease in histocompatible donor bone marrow transplantation. Transplantation 51(6):1197–1203, 1991.
22. Bross DS, Tutschka PJ, Farmer ER, et al: Predictive factors for acute graft-versus-host disease in patients transplanted with HLA-identical bone marrow. Blood 63(6):1265–1270, 1984.
23. Sanders JE: The impact of marrow transplant preparative regimens on subsequent growth and development: the Seattle Marrow Transplant Team. Semin Hematol 28(3):244–249, 1991.
24. Baruch J, Benjamin S, Treleaven J, et al: Male sexual function following bone marrow transplantation. Bone Marrow Transplant 7 (Suppl 2):52, 1991.
25. Jacobs P, Dubovsky DW: Bone marrow transplantation followed by normal pregnancy. Am J Hematol 11(2):209–212, 1981.
26. Sanders JE, Buckner CD, Amos D, et al: Ovarian function following marrow transplantation for aplastic anemia or leukemia. J Clin Oncol 6(5):813–818, 1988.
27. Schmidt H, Ehninger G, Dopfer R, Waller HD: Pregnancy after bone marrow transplantation for severe aplastic anemia. Bone Marrow Transplant 2(3):329–332, 1987.
28. Surman OS: Psychiatric aspects of organ transplantation [published erratum appears in Am J Psychiatry 1989 Nov;146(11):1523]. Am J Psychiatry 146(8):972–982, 1989.
29. Frierson RL, Lippmann SB: Heart transplant candidates rejected on psychiatric indications. Psychosomatics 28(7):347–355, 1987.
30. Futterman AD, Wellisch DK, Bond G, Carr CR: The Psychosocial Levels System: a new rating scale to identify and assess emotional difficulties during bone marrow transplantation. Psychosomatics 32(2):177–186, 1991.
31. Mai FM, McKenzie FN, Kostuk WJ: Psychiatric aspects of heart transplantation: preoperative evaluation and postoperative sequelae. Br Med J 292(6516):311–313, 1986.
32. Heimdahl A, Mattsson T, Dahllof G, et al: The oral cavity as a port of entry for early infections in patients treated with bone marrow transplantation. Oral Surg Oral Med Oral Pathol 68(6):711–716, 1989.
33. Woo S-B, Matin K: Off-site dental evaluation program for prospective bone marrow transplant recipients. J Am Dental Assoc 128:189–193, 1997.
34. Rapoport A, Watelet LFM, Linder T, et al: Analysis of factors that correlate with mucositis in recipients of autologous and allogeneic stem-cell transplants. J Clin Oncol 17(8):2446–2453, 1999.
35. Anderson PM, Ramsay NK, Shu XO, et al: Effect of low-dose oral glutamine on painful stomatitis during bone marrow transplantation. Bone Marrow Transplant 22(4):339–344, 1998.
36. Orazi A, Du X, Yang Z, et al: Interleukin-11 prevents apoptosis and accelerates recovery of small intestinal mucosa in mice treated with combined chemotherapy and radiation. Lab Invest 75(1):33–42, 1996.
37. Serdar C, Heard R, Prathikanti R, et al: Safety, pharmacokinetics and biologic activity of rHuKGF in normal volunteers: results of a placebo-controlled randomized double-blind phase I study. Blood 90(172a):761, 1997.
38. Crawford SW, Fisher L: Predictive value of pulmonary function tests before marrow transplantation [see comments]. Chest 101(5):1257–1264, 1992.
39. Krowka MJ: Lung function and the complications of bone marrow transplantation [editorial; comment]. Chest 101(5):1186–1187, 1992.
40. Krowka MJ, Staats BA, Hoagland HC: A prospective study of airway reactivity before bone marrow transplantation. Mayo Clin Proc 65(1):5–12, 1990.
41. Bearman SI, Petersen FB, Schor RA, et al: Radionuclide ejection fractions in the evaluation of patients being considered for bone marrow transplantation: risk for cardiac toxicity. Bone Marrow Transplant 5(3):173–177, 1990.
42. Hertenstein B, Stefanic M, Schmeiser T, et al: Cardiac toxicity of bone marrow transplantation: predictive value of cardiologic evaluation before transplant. J Clin Oncol 12(5):998–1004, 1994.
43. Moreb JS, Oblon DJ: Outcome of clinical congestive heart failure induced by anthracycline chemotherapy. Cancer 70(11):2637–2641, 1992.
44. Steinherz LJ, Steinherz PG, Mangiacasale D, et al: Cardiac changes with cyclophosphamide. Med Pediatr Oncol 9(5):417–422, 1981.
45. Goldberg MA, Antin JH, Guinan EC, Rappeport JM: Cyclophosphamide cardiotoxicity: an analysis of dosing as a risk factor. Blood 68(5):1114–1118, 1986.
46. McDonald GB, Sharma P, Matthews DE, et al: Venocclusive disease of the liver after bone marrow transplantation: diagnosis, incidence, and predisposing factors. Hepatology 4(1):116–122, 1984.
47. Jones RJ, Lee KS, Beschorner WE, et al: Venocclusive disease of the liver following bone marrow transplantation. Transplantation 44(6):778–783, 1987.
48. Ganem G, Saint-Marc Girardin MF, Kuentz M, et al: Venocclusive disease of the liver after allogeneic bone marrow transplantation in man. Int J Radiat Oncol Biol Phys 14(5):879–884, 1988.

49. McDonald GB, Hinds MS, Fisher LD, et al: Veno-occlusive disease of the liver and multiorgan failure after bone marrow transplantation: a cohort study of 355 patients. Ann Intern Med 118(4):255–267, 1993.

50. Strasser SI, Myerson D, Spurgeon CL, et al: Hepatitis C virus infection and bone marrow transplantation: a cohort study with 10-year follow-up. Hepatology 29(6):1893–1899, 1999.

51. Strasser SI, Sullivan KM, Myerson D, et al: Cirrhosis of the liver in long-term marrow transplant survivors. Blood 93(10):3259–3266, 1999.

52. Kanamori H, Fukawa H, Maruta A, et al: Case report: fulminant hepatitis C viral infection after allogeneic bone marrow transplantation. Am J Med Sci 303(2):109–111, 1992.

53. Locasciulli A, van't Veer L, Bacigalupo A, et al: Treatment with marrow transplantation or immunosuppression of childhood acquired severe aplastic anemia: a report from the EBMT SAA Working Party. Bone Marrow Transplant 6(3):211–217, 1990.

54. Reed EC, Myerson D, Corey L, Meyers JD: Allogeneic marrow transplantation in patients positive for hepatitis B surface antigen. Blood 77(1):195–200, 1991.

55. Chen PM, Fan S, Liu CJ, et al: Changing of hepatitis B virus markers in patients with bone marrow transplantation. Transplantation 49(4):708–713, 1990.

56. Ahmed T, Engelking C, Szalyga J, et al: Propantheline prevention of mucositis from etoposide. Bone Marrow Transplant 12(2):131–132, 1993.

57. Oblon DJ, Paul SR, Oblon MB, Malik S: Propantheline protects the oral mucosa after high-dose ifosfamide, carboplatin, etoposide and autologous stem cell transplantation. Bone Marrow Transplant 20(11):961–963, 1997.

58. Marmont AM: Stem cell transplantation for severe autoimmune diseases: progress and problems. Haematologica 83(8):733–743, 1998.

59. Burt R, Traynor A, Pope R, et al: Treatment of autoimmune disease by intense immunosuppressive conditioning and autologous hematopoietic stem cell transplantation. Blood 92:3505–3514, 1998.

60. Walzer PG, Genta RM: Parasite Infections in the Compromised Host. New York, Marcel Dekker, 1989.

61. Lau YL, Peiris M, Chan GC, et al: Primary human herpes virus 6 infection transmitted from donor to recipient through bone marrow infusion. Bone Marrow Transplant 21(10):1063–1066, 1998.

62. Cone RW, Huang ML, Corey L, et al: Human herpes virus 6 infections after bone marrow transplantation: clinical and virologic manifestations. J Infect Dis 179(2):311–318, 1999.

63. Carrigan DR, Drobyski WR, Russler SK, et al: Interstitial pneumonitis associated with human herpesvirus-6 infection after marrow transplantation. Lancet 338(8760):147–149, 1991.

64. Prentice HG, Gluckman E, Powles RL, et al: Long-term survival in allogeneic bone marrow transplant recipients following acyclovir prophylaxis for CMV infection: the European Acyclovir for CMV Prophylaxis Study Group. Bone Marrow Transplant 19(2):129–133, 1997.

65. Goodrich JM, Bowden RA, Fisher L, et al: Ganciclovir prophylaxis to prevent cytomegalovirus disease after allogeneic marrow transplant. Ann Intern Med 118(3):173–178, 1993.

66. Ippoliti C, Morgan A, Warkentin D, et al: Foscarnet for prevention of cytomegalovirus infection in allogeneic marrow transplant recipients unable to receive ganciclovir. Bone Marrow Transplant 20(6):491–495, 1997.

67. Zaia JA, Schmidt GM, Chao NJ, et al: Preemptive ganciclovir administration based solely on asymptomatic pulmonary cytomegalovirus infection in allogeneic bone marrow transplant recipients: long-term follow-up. Biol Blood Marrow Transplant 1(2):88–93, 1995.

68. Bowden RA, Slichter SJ, Sayers M, et al: A comparison of filtered leukocyte-reduced and cytomegalovirus (CMV) sero-negative blood products for the prevention of transfusion-associated CMV infection after marrow transplant [see comments]. Blood 86(9):3598–3603, 1995.

69. Pamphilon DH, Rider JR, Barbara JA, Williamson LM: Prevention of transfusion-transmitted cytomegalovirus infection. Transfus Med 9(2):115–123, 1999.

70. Oblon DJ, Elfenbein GJ, Rand K, Weiner RS: Recurrent varicella-zoster infection after acyclovir therapy in immunocompromised patients. South Med J 79(2):256–257, 1986.

71. Holland HK, Saral R, Rossi JJ, et al: Allogeneic bone marrow transplantation, zidovudine, and human immunodeficiency virus type 1 (HIV-1) infection: studies in a patient with non-Hodgkin lymphoma. Ann Intern Med 111(12):973–978, 1989.

72. Lane HC, Zunich KM, Wilson W, et al: Syngeneic bone marrow transplantation and adoptive transfer of peripheral blood lymphocytes combined with zidovudine in human immunodeficiency virus (HIV) infection. Ann Intern Med 113(7):512–519, 1990.

Donor Selection and Evaluation

CHAPTER TWENTY-ONE

Histocompatibility

*Gayle Rosner, Ph.D., Joan Martell, B.S., and
Massimo Trucco, M.D.*

The major histocompatibility complex (MHC), located on the short arm of human chromosome 6, contains numerous closely linked genes integral to the immune response. These genes encode heteromeric cell surface glycoproteins, which were originally identified on leukocytes[1, 2] and hence were called human leukocyte antigens (HLA).[3, 4]

Molecules encoded by the MHC allow the organism to distinguish between "self" and "nonself." Data from early experience in solid organ transplantation showed that graft rejections were correlated with disparity between the HLA molecules of the donor and recipient.[5, 6] The use of posttransplant immunosuppression allowed recipients to tolerate HLA disparity without rejection.[7, 8] The recipient's immune system, although clinically suppressed by medication, remains intact.

In allogeneic hematopoietic stem cell (HSC) transplantation (HSCT), however, the recipient's immune system is completely ablated, leaving the patient immunologically incompetent. In addition, the graft, derived from bone marrow or mobilized peripheral blood, contains substantial quantities of immunologically competent cells (e.g., monocytes, T cells) capable of recognizing and responding to the recipient's HLA molecules. The resulting graft-versus-host disease (GVHD) is a major cause of mortality and morbidity.[9–11]

The degree of HLA disparity has been shown to be directly correlated with incidence and severity of GVHD. HLA disparity in allogenic HSCT is also associated with graft failure.[12] Thus, unlike solid organ transplantation, HLA identity between the donor and recipient has markedly prolonged graft survival (and hence patient survival) and lessened GVHD. The clinical relevance and scientific basis for HLA matching between donors and recipients have evolved from recent discoveries in MHC biochemistry, molecular genetics, and immunology. A review of these findings facilitates our understanding of how HLA genetics has moved so quickly from "bench to bedside."

THE HLA COMPLEX AND THE SPECIFIC IMMUNE RESPONSE

The genetics of histocompatibility were initially based on animal experiments. Transplantation of tissue from an unrelated animal of the same species (i.e., an *allogeneic* animal) was rejected as foreign, whereas that from a *syngeneic* animal (i.e., one inbred to be genetically identical) was accepted. Rejection of the tissue graft by the recipient was found to be strictly correlated with differences among histocompatibility molecules between the donor and recipient.[13, 14]

Later on, identification of recipient antibodies against allogeneic leukocytes underscored the importance of the MHC as immunologically relevant molecules (i.e., targets of an immune response).

The physiologic function of the MHC molecule is fully elucidated now that techniques in protein biochemistry have matured. Crystallization of the first HLA molecule and characterization of its tertiary structure provided unquestionable evidence that the MHC combines with processed peptides derived from foreign tissues to trigger a specific immune reaction.[15] Macrophages, monocytes, dendritic cells, or mature B cells are capable of efficiently phagocytosing the foreign molecules, capture the nonself proteins, and enzymatically cleave them into smaller peptides. These peptides are transported to the cell surface of the antigen-presenting cells by HLA molecules structurally compatible with peptides. The function of this site, or peptide-binding groove, was clearly determined once the interpretation of the crystal structure of the HLA molecule was completed.[16]

The HLA/peptide complex exposed at the cell surface is recognized and engaged by the T-cell receptor (TCR) complex, thereby initiating the activation of the T lymphocyte, leading to mitosis and secretion of specific factors necessary to promote proliferation and differentiation of other cells involved in the immune response.[17] The signal from the engaged TCR is transmitted inside a cell by a chain of molecules, including the CD3 complex, that ultimately activates the enzymes necessary to stimulate cell division, receptor exposure, and lymphokine production[18, 19] (Fig. 21–1). Lymphokines are secreted cellular hormones that can inhibit or stimulate other cells to become activated. Therefore, the T cells producing "helper" factors are known as T-helper (TH) cells. Based on preferential secretion of certain lymphokines, TH cells are divided into TH_1 and TH_2 subgroups.[20] TH_2 cells promote activation of B lymphocytes and subsequent antibody production via secretion of interleukins 4, 5, 6, and 10.[21] TH_1 cells, which preferentially secrete interleukin-2, interferon-γ, and tumor necrosis factor β, potentiate other T cells, already committed to killer T-cell lineage, to proliferate.[22] These cytotoxic T cells

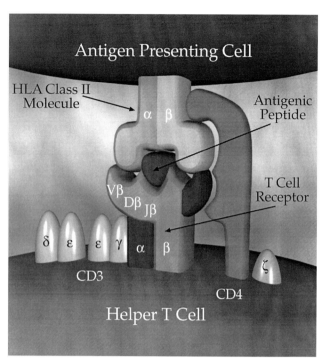

FIGURE 21–1. The human leukocyte antigen (HLA) class II molecule, expressed at the surface of an antigen-presenting cell, is schematically shown to interact with the processed antigenic peptide, lodged in the Björkman groove of the molecule, and the α/β T-cell receptor (TCR) molecule, present on the cell membrane of a helper T cell. The co-receptor, accessory molecule CD4, stabilizes the binding of the TCR with the HLA molecule. CD4 fulfills signaling and antigen-specific T-cell activation functions that are independent from those mediated by CD3. The CD3 complex, composed of δ, ε, and γ molecules, transfers the signal of the successfully engaged TCR into the cytoplasm of the T cell. The ζ molecule is also part of the CD3 complex but is functionally separated by the other CD3 subunits. (Modified from Conrad B, Trucco M: Superantigens as etiopathogenetic factors in the development of insulin dependent diabetes mellitus. Diabetes Metab Rev 10:309–338, 1994).

recognize and destroy cells carrying the original peptides that initiated the chain of reactions.

TH cells can easily be recognized and distinguished from cytotoxic T cells by differences in surface receptor expression and MHC restriction. CD4 and CD8 are T-cell surface molecules that stabilize the TCR/antigenic peptide/MHC molecule complex while recognition is being carried out (see Fig. 21–1). In general, CD4+ T cells preferentially recognize MHC class II molecules that have bound peptides derived from internalized, exogenous proteins, whereas CD8+ T cells react with MHC class I molecules bound to cell-derived endogenous peptides.

HLA CLASSIFICATION, STRUCTURE, AND POLYMORPHISM

HLA molecules are grouped into two classes based on their structure, function, and cellular expression. Class I (HLA-A, -B, and -C molecules) are characterized by a heavy α-chain with three domains (α_1, α_2, and α_3) encoded by the MHC on chromosome 6 (Fig. 21–2). This chain dimerizes with β_2-microglobulin, a short (12-kD) protein, encoded by a gene on chromosome 15, which provides the fourth

domain necessary to stabilize the HLA molecule.[23] Class I molecules are expressed on nearly all white blood cells and platelets and are anchored via the transmembrane portion and the short cytoplasmic tail of the α-chain. Class II molecules (HLA-DR, -DQ, and -DP) consist of MHC-encoded α and β chains, each with two domains, that are anchored by both chains, each of which can communicate across the membrane with cytoplasmic structures (see Fig. 21–2). Class II molecules are expressed primarily on B lymphocytes, activated T cells, and endothelial cells. Both class I and class II HLA molecules need to be typed for allogeneic HSCT.

The two outermost domains of each molecule (α_1 and α_2 in class I; α_1 and β_1 in class II) fold together to form the cleft in which the antigenic peptide can lodge (see Fig. 21–2). This antigen-combining site (also known as the Björkman groove) is composed of a β-pleated sheet with eight antiparallel strands forming the floor of the groove and the sides assuming the shape of α-helices (Fig. 21–3). The amino acid residues forming this cleft are very polymorphic and are relevant in the α-helical regions. This first external domain (for DR and DQ molecules) is encoded by the second exon of the gene and is approximately 90 amino acids, or 270 base pairs, in length. The polymorphic regions of the second exon are clustered into three or four discrete hypervariable regions, which become obvious when the nucleotide sequence of the alleles are aligned (Fig. 21–4). As the protein folds into its tertiary structure (Fig. 21–5), some of the hypervariable regions assume a location pointing into the cleft (i.e., an optimal position for interaction with the processed antigen). Other hypervariable segments are located on the external part of the molecule and constitute the determinants potentially involved with TCR recognition. These same hypervariable regions form the molecular basis of alloreactivity in transplantation (i.e., donor differences in these amino acids are recognized as "foreign" by the recipient). For class I molecules, the polymorphism is more extensive, being encoded by the third as well as the second exon.

The genes encoding the HLA class I and class II molecules constitute the most highly polymorphic genetic system in humans. In a population, a stable, inherited polymorphism within a gene gives rise to alternative forms of the protein (i.e., *alleles*). Nearly all the HLA genes have different alleles. At least 75 HLA-A, 161 HLA-B, 41 HLA-C, 158 HLA-DR, and 28 HLA-DQ alleles have been reported.[24] New alleles are being identified every year. The molecular basis for HLA gene polymorphism resides in nucleotide sequence differences present in the coding regions of the HLA genes. Although most HLA alleles occur in all ethnic groups, the frequency of any particular HLA allele may vary between individuals of different ethnicity. The ethnic background of transplant donor and recipient should be identical before further HLA matching is initiated.

GENETICS OF THE HLA COMPLEX

The genomic organization of the genes included in the HLA complex is shown in Figure 21–6. The 4000 kilobase (kb) long DNA segment encompassing this complex can be subdivided into three major regions, which encode class I

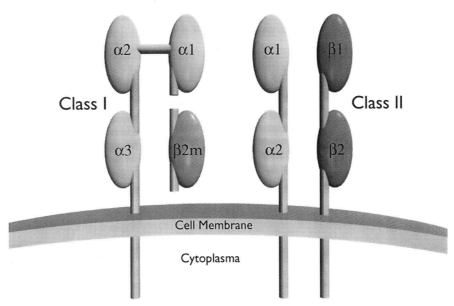

FIGURE 21–2. Secondary structure of human leukocyte antigen class I and class II molecules in comparison. As with immunoglobulins, peptidic sequences that show similarities and are present more than once in the same polypeptidic chain are called "domains." α_1, α_2, and α_3 constitute the domains of the class I α-chain, whereas α_1 and α_2 are the domains of the class II α-chain and β_1 and β_2 are the domains characteristic of the class II β-chain. Both class I and class II heterodimers (i.e., molecules formed by noncovalently bound and somewhat different α- and β-chains) form, at their most external end, a peptide combining site composed of the α_1 and α_2 domains for class I, and α_1 and β_1 domains form them for class II molecules. The β_2-microglobulin completes the structure of class I molecules. (Modified from Trucco M: To be, or not to be Asp 57, that is the question. Diabetes Care 15:705–715, 1992.)

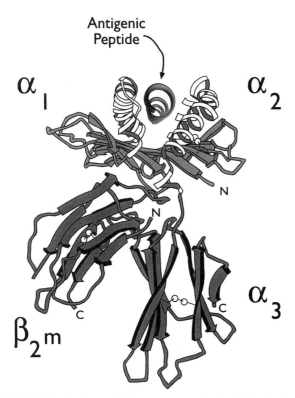

FIGURE 21–3. The human leukocyte antigen class I molecule is shown from the side. The most external domains (α_1 and α_2) form the antigen combining site in which the processed antigenic peptide finds the correct position to be presented to a T cell able to recognize the complex with its T-cell receptor molecule. (See also Fig. 21–5.) (Modified from Faas SJ, Trucco M: Major histocompatibility locus and other genes that determine risk of development of insulin-dependent diabetes mellitus. *In* LeRoith D, Taylor S, Olefsky JM (eds): Diabetes Mellitus: A Fundamental and Clinical Text. Philadelphia, JB Lippincott, 1996, pp 326–333.)

molecules (2000 kb), class III molecules (1000 kb), and class II molecules (1000 kb).[25] The physical location (i.e., *locus*) of each HLA gene determines their order on chromosome 6, although the nomenclature chronologically recapitulates the characterization of the genes at the various loci. The A locus is the most distant from the centromere and was the first to be characterized. The characterization of the B locus immediately followed that of the A locus. A and B, however, are geographically separated by the C locus, which was the last to be characterized. Class II loci, DR, DQ, and DP, were characterized after the class I loci and are in the same physical order on chromosome 6, closer to the centromere than class I loci (see Fig. 21–6). The class I and class II regions are physically separated on the chromosome by genes encoding MHC class III molecules. Class III proteins include components of the complement cascade, tumor necrosis factor, and heat shock proteins and are not related in the HLA-matching process.

The class I genes encode molecules that can efficiently present antigenic peptides. The class I region also contains nonfunctional genes (i.e., pseudogenes) and genes that are potentially functional but the products of which are not yet known.[25] The class II region includes genes encoding proteins involved in antigen processing and in peptide transport from the cytoplasm to the cell surface.[25] Besides LMP and TAP genes, other genes are present in this region, and their physiologic function awaits determination.

The class II molecules are heterodimers (i.e., they consist of two MHC-encoded polypeptide chains): the α (encoded by "A" genes), which is noncovalently bound to the β (encoded by "B" genes) (see Fig. 21–2). For DQ molecules, only the DQA1 and DQB2 gene products are known to be expressed as functional DQ α/β heterodimers. The DQA2 and DQB2 genes are pseudogenes (see Fig. 21–6). Likewise, only the DPA1 and DPB1 genes encode the chains of

This page presents a nucleotide sequence alignment (IMGT/HLA style) of HLA-DQB1 alleles. Codon position numbers (1, 10, 20, 30 in the upper block; 40, 50, 60 in the lower block) appear above the reference codon row. Dashes (–) indicate identity to the reference sequence, asterisks (*) indicate positions not sequenced, and letters indicate nucleotide substitutions.

Upper block (codons 1–33)

```
               1                                           10                                          20                                      30
               AGA GAC TCT CCC GAG GAT TTC GTG TAC CAG  TTT AAG GGC CTG TGC TTC ACC AAC GGG  ACG GAG CGC GTG CGG GGT GTG ACC AGA CAC  ATC TAT AAC CGA
DQB1*0501      --- --- *** *** *** *** *** *** *** ---  *** *** *** *** *** *** *** *** **-  --- --- --- --- --- --- --- --- --- ---  --- --- --- ---
DQB1*0502      --- --- *** *** *** *** *** *** *** ---  *** *** -C- A-- *** *** *** *** **-  --- --- --- --- -T- TA- --- --- --- T--  --- --- --- ---
DQB1*05031     --- --- *** *** *** *** *** *** *** ---  *** *** -C- A-- *** *** *** *** **-  --- --- --- --- -T- TA- --- --- --- T--  --- --- --- ---
DQB1*05032     --- --- *** *** *** *** *** *** *** ---  *** *** --- --- *** *** *** *** **-  --- --- --- --- --- --- --- --- --- ---  --- --- --- ---
DQB1*0504      -A- --- C-- *** *** *** *** *** CT- ---  *** *** -C- A-- *** *** *** *** **-  --- --- --- --- -T- CT- --- -A- --- T--  --- --- --- ---
DQB1*06011     --- --- G-- *** *** *** *** *** -T- ---  *** *** -C- A-- *** *** *** *** **-  --- --- --- --- -T- CT- -A- --- --- T--  --- --- --- ---
DQB1*06012     --- --- G-- *** *** *** *** *** --- ---  *** *** -C- A-- *** *** *** *** **-  --- --- --- --- -T- CT- -A- --- --- T--  --- --- --- ---
DQB1*0602      --- --- --- --- --- --- --- --- --- ---  --- --- --- A-- --- --- --- -T- ---  --- --- --- --- -T- CT- -A- --- --- T--  --- --- --- ---
DQB1*0603      --- --- --- --- --- --- --- --- --- ---  --- --- --- A-- --- --- --- --- ---  --- --- --- --- -T- CT- -A- --- --- T--  --- --- --- ---
DQB1*0604      --- --- --- --- --- --- --- --- --- ---  --- --- --- A-- --- --- --- --- ---  --- --- --- --- -T- CT- -A- --- --- T--  --- --- --- ---
DQB1*06051     --- --- *** *** *** *** *** *** *** ---  *** *** --- A-- *** *** *** *** **-  --- --- --- --- -T- CT- -A- --- --- T--  --- --- --- ---
DQB1*06052     --- --- *** *** *** *** *** *** *** ---  *** *** --- A-- *** *** *** *** **-  --- --- --- --- -T- CT- -A- --- --- T--  --- --- --- ---
DQB1*0606      --- --- *** *** *** *** *** *** *** ---  *** *** --- A-- *** *** *** *** **-  --- --- --- --- -T- CT- -A- --- --- T--  --- --- --- ---
DQB1*0607      --- --- *** *** *** *** *** *** *** ---  *** *** --- A-- *** *** *** *** **-  --- --- --- --- -T- CT- -A- --- --- T--  --- --- --- ---
DQB1*0608      --- --- *** *** *** *** *** *** *** ---  *** *** --- A-- *** *** *** *** **-  --- --- --- --- -T- TA- --- -A- --- T--  --- --- --- ---
DQB1*0609      --- --- *** *** *** *** *** *** *** ---  *** *** --- A-- *** *** *** *** **-  --- --- --- --- -T- CT- --- -A- --- T--  --- --- --- ---
DQB1*0201      -A- AT- --- --- --- --- --- --- --- ---  --- *** -C- --- --- --- --- --- ---  -A- --- --- --- --- --- --- --- --- AG-  --- --- --- ---
DQB1*0202      -A- AT- --- --- --- --- --- --- --- ---  --- *** -C- --- --- --- --- --- ---  -A- --- --- --- --- --- --- --- --- AG-  --- --- --- ---
DQB1*0301      --- --- --- --- --- --- --- --- --- ---  --- --- --- --- --- --- --- --- ---  --- --- --- --- --- --- --- --- --- ---  --- --- --- ---
DQB1*0302      --- CA- --- --- --- --- --- --- --- ---  --- --- --- --- --- --- --- --- ---  --- --- --- --- --- --- --- --- --- ---  --- --- --- ---
DQB1*03032     --- CA- --- --- --- --- --- --- --- ---  --- --- --- --- --- --- --- --- ---  -C- --- --- --- --- --- --- --- --- ---  --- --- --- ---
DQB1*0304      --- CA- --- --- --- --- --- --- --- ---  --- --- --- --- --- --- --- --- ---  -C- --- --- --- --- --- --- --- --- ---  --- --- --- ---
DQB1*0305      --- --- *** *** *** *** *** *** *** ---  *** *** --- A-- *** *** *** *** **-  -C- --- --- T-- --- --- --- --- --- ---  --- --- --- ---
DQB1*0401      --- --- C-- --- --- --- --- --- -T- ---  --- --- --- A-- --- --- --- --- ---  -C- --- --- --- --- TA- --- --- --- T--  --- --- --- ---
DQB1*0402      --- --- C-- --- --- --- --- --- -T- ---  --- --- --- A-- --- --- --- --- ---  --- --- --- --- --- --- --- --- --- T--  --- --- --- ---
```

Lower block (codons ~34–68)

```
               GAG GAG TAC GTG CGC TTC GAC AGC GAC  GTG GGG GTG TAC CGG GCA GTG ACG CCG CAG  GGG CCT CGG GTT GCC GAG TAC TGG AAC AGC  CAG AAG GAA GTC CTG
                                 40                                     50                                          60
DQB1*0501      --- --- --- --- --- --- --- --- ---  --- --- --- --- --- -G- --- --- --- ---  --- --- --- AGC --- --- --- --- --- ---  --- --- --- --- ---
DQB1*0502      --- --- --- --- --- --- --- --- ---  --- --- --- -T- --- -G- --- --- --- ---  --- --- --- --- --- --- --- --- --- ---  --- --- -C- -A- ---
DQB1*05031     --- --- G-- --- --- --- --- --- ---  --- --- --- -T- --- -AC --- --- --- ---  --- --- --- --- --- --- --- --- --- ---  --- --- -C- -A- ---
DQB1*05032     --- --- G-- --- --- --- --- --- ---  --- --- --- --- --- -G- --- --- --- ---  --- --- --- AGC --- --- --- --- --- ---  --- --- -C- -A- ---
DQB1*0504      -A- --- --- --- --- --- --- --- ---  --- --- --- --- -C- -G- --- --- --- ---  --- --- --- -AC --- --- --- --- --- ---  --- --- --- --- ---
DQB1*06011     --- --- --- --- --- --- --- --- ---  --- --- --- --- -C- -G- --- --- --- ---  --- --- --- -A- --- --- --- --- --- ---  --- --- -C- -A- ---
DQB1*06012     --- --- --- --- --- --- --- --- --C  --- --- --- --- --- -G- --- --- --- ---  --- -T- --- -A- --- --- --- --- -T- ---  --- --- -C- -A- ---
DQB1*0602      --- --- --- --- --- --- --- --- ---  --- --- --- -T- --- -G- --- --- --- ---  --- --- --- --- --- --- --- --- -T- ---  --- --- --- --- ---
DQB1*0603      --- --- --- --- --- --- --- --- ---  --- --- --- -T- --- -A- --- --- --- ---  --- --- --- --- --- --- --- --- -T- ---  --- --- --- --- ---
DQB1*0604      --- --- --- --- --- --- --- --- ---  --- --- --- --- --- -G- --- --- --- ---  --- --- --- --- --- --- --- --- --- ---  --- --- --- --- ---
DQB1*06051     --- --- --- --- --- --- --- --- ---  --- --- --- --- --- -G- --- --- --- ---  --- --- --- --- --- --- --- --- -T- ---  --- --- --- --- ---
DQB1*06052     --- --- --- --- --- --- --- --- ---  --- --- --- --- --- -G- --- -C- --- ---  --- --- --- -C- --- --- --- --- -T- ---  --- --- --- --- ---
DQB1*0606      --- --- --- --- --- --- --- --- ---  --- --- --- --- --- -G- --- --- --- ---  --- --- --- --- --- --- --- --- --- ---  --- --- --- --- ---
DQB1*0607      --- --- --- --- --- --- --- --- ---  --- --- --- --- -C- -G- --- -C- --- ---  --- --- --- -A- --- --- --- --- --- ---  --- --- --- --- ---
DQB1*0608      --- --- --- --- --- --- --- --- ---  --- --- --- --- --- -G- --- --- --- ---  --- --- --- --- --- --- --- --- --- ---  --- --- --- --- ---
DQB1*0609      --- --- --- --- --- --- --- --- ---  --- A-- --- --- --- -G- --- --- --- ---  --- --- --- -A- --- --- --- --- --- ---  --- --- -C- -A- ---
DQB1*0201      -A- --- AT- --- --- --- --- --- ---  --- --- --- -T- --- -G- --- -T- T-- ---  --- -T- --- -CC --- --- --- --- -T- ---  --- --- -C- -A- ---
DQB1*0202      -A- --- AT- --- --- --- --- --- ---  --- A-- --- -T- --- -G- --- -T- T-- ---  --- --- --- -CC --- --- --- --- -T- ---  --- --- -C- -A- ---
DQB1*0301      --- --- --- --- --- --- --- --- ---  --- A-- --- --- --- -G- --- -C- --- ---  --- -C- --- -AC --- --- --- --- -T- ---  --- --- --- --- ---
DQB1*0302      --- --- --- --- --- --- --- --- ---  --- --- --- -T- --- -G- --- -C- --- ---  --- -C- --- -CC --- --- --- --- -T- ---  --- --- --- --- ---
DQB1*03032     --- --- --- --- --- --- --- --- ---  --- --- --- -T- --- -G- --- -C- --- ---  --- -C- --- -CC --- --- --- --- -T- ---  --- --- --- --- ---
DQB1*0304      --- --- --- --- --- --- --- --- ---  --- --- --- --- --- -G- --- -C- --- ---  --- -C- --- -CC --- --- --- --- -T- ---  --- --- --- --- ---
DQB1*0305      --- --- --- --- --- --- --- --- ---  --- A-- --- --- --- -G- --- -C- --- ---  --- -C- --- -CC --- --- --- --- -T- ---  --- --- --- --- ---
DQB1*0401      --- --- --- --- --- --- --- --- ---  --- --- --- -T- --- -AC --- --- --- ---  --- -T- -T- -AC -T- --- --- --- --- ---  --- --- -C- -A- ---
DQB1*0402      --- --- --- --- --- --- --- --- ---  --- --- --- -T- --- -AC --- --- --- ---  --- -T- -T- -AC -T- --- --- --- --- ---  --- --- -C- -A- ---
```

```
                  70                                      80                                      90                                     100
DQB1*0501    GAG GGG GCC CGG GCG TCG GTG GAC AGG GTG TGC AGA CAC AAC TAC GAG GTG GCG TAC CGC GGG ATC CTG CAG AGG AGA GTG GAG CCC ACA GTG ACC ATC TCC
DQB1*0502    --- --- --- --- --- --- --- --- --A --- --- --- --- --- --- --- --- --- --- --- --- --- --- --- --- --- --- --- --- --- --- --- --- ---
DQB1*05031   --- --- --- --- --- --- --- --- --A --- --- --- --- --- --- --- --- --- --- --- --- --- --- --- --- --- --- --- --- --- --- --- --- ---
DQB1*05032   --- *** *** *** *** *** *** *** *** *** *** *** *** *** *** *** *** *** *** *** *** *** *** *** *** *** *** *** *** *** *** *** *** ***
DQB1*0504    --- -A- -A- --- --- --- --- --- --- --- --- --- --- --- -** *** *** *** *** *** *** *** *** *** *** *** *** *** *** *** *** *** *** ***
DQB1*06011   --- A-- A-- --A --- GA- T-- --- -C- --- --- --- --- --- --- --- --- --- -T- --- --- --- T-- --- --- --- --- --- --- --- --- --- --- ---
DQB1*06012   --- A-- A-- --A --- GA- T-- --- -C- --- --- --- *** *** *** *** *** *** *** *** *** *** *** *** *** *** *** *** *** *** *** *** *** ***
DQB1*0602    --- --- A-- --- --- GA- T-- --- -C- --- --- --- --- --- --- --- --- --- -T- --- --- --- T-- --- --- --- --- --- --- --- --- --- --- ---
DQB1*0603    --- --- A-- --- --- GA- T-- --- -C- --- --- --- --- --- --- --- --- --- -T- --- --- --- T-- --- --- --- --- --- --- --- --- --- --- ---
DQB1*0604    --- A-- A-- --- --- GA- T-- --- -C- --- --- --- --- --- --- --- --- -G- --- --- --- --- --- --- --- --- --- --- --- --- --- --- --- ---
DQB1*06051   --- A-- A-- --- --- GA- T-- --- -C- --- --- --- --- --- --- --- --- -G- --- --- --- --- --- --- --- --- --- --- --- --- --- --- --- ---
DQB1*06052   --- A-- A-- --- --- GA- T-- --- -C- *** *** *** *** *** *** *** *** *** *** *** *** *** *** *** *** *** *** *** *** *** *** *** *** ***
DQB1*0606    --- A-- A-- --- --- G-- --- --- --- --- *** *** *** *** *** *** *** *** *** *** *** *** *** *** *** *** *** *** *** *** *** *** *** ***
DQB1*0607    --- A-- A-- --- --- GA- T-- --- -C- --- --- --- --- --- -** *** *** *** *** *** *** *** *** *** *** *** *** *** *** *** *** *** *** ***
DQB1*0608    --- --- A-- --- --- GA- T-- --- -C- --- --- --- --- --- -** *** *** *** *** *** *** *** *** *** *** *** *** *** *** *** *** *** *** ***
DQB1*0609    --- A-- A-- --- --- GA- T-- --- -C- --- --- --- --- --- --- --- --- -G- --- --- --- --- --- --- --- --- -** *** *** *** *** *** *** ***
DQB1*0201    --- A-- AAA --- --- G-- --- --- --- --- --- --- --- --- --- C-- T-- -A- CT- --- AC- -C- T-- --- C-- C-- --- --- --- --- --- --- --- ---
DQB1*0202    --- A-- AAA --- --- G-- --- --- --- --- --- --- --- --- --- C-- T-- -A- CT- --- AC- -C- T-- --- C-- C-- --- --- --- --- --- --- --- ---
DQB1*0301    --- A-- A-- --- --- GA- T-- --- -C- --- --- --- --- --- --- C-- T-- -A- CT- --- AC- -C- T-- --- C-- C-- --- --- --- --- --- --- --- ---
DQB1*0302    --- A-- A-- --- --- GA- T-- --- -C- --- --- --- --- --- --- C-- T-- -A- CT- --- AC- -C- T-- --- C-- C-- --- --- --- --- --- --- --- ---
DQB1*03032   --- A-- A-- --- --- GA- T-- --- -C- --- --- --- --- --- --- C-- T-- -A- CT- --- AC- -C- T-- --- C-- C-- --- --- --- --- --- --- --- ---
DQB1*0304    --- A-- A-- --- --- GA- T-- --- -C- --- --- --- --- --- --- C-- T-- -A- CT- --- AC- -C- T-- --- C-- C-- --- --- --- --- --- --- --- ---
DQB1*0305    --- A-- A-- --- --- GA- T-- --- -C- --- --- --- --- --- --- C-- T-- -A- CT- --- AC- -C- T-- --- C-- C-- --- --- --- --- --- --- --- ---
DQB1*0401    --- -A- -A- --- --- --- --- --- -CC --A --- --- --- --- --- C-- T-- -A- CT- --- AC- -C- T-- --- C-- C-- --- --- --- --- --- --- --- ---
DQB1*0402    --- -A- -A- --- --- --- --- --- -CC --A --- --- --- --- --- C-- T-- -A- CT- --- AC- -C- T-- --- C-- C-- --- --- --- --- --- --- --- ---
```

FIGURE 21–4. Allelic nucleotide sequences of the human leukocyte antigen DQB1 gene. The most polymorphic (i.e., hypervariable) regions between allelic DQB1 polypeptidic chains are encoded by nucleotides contained in the second exon of the gene (i.e., nucleotides 1–270) and are expressed as differences in the amino-acid composition of the most external domain of the molecule (i.e., the first 90 amino acids).

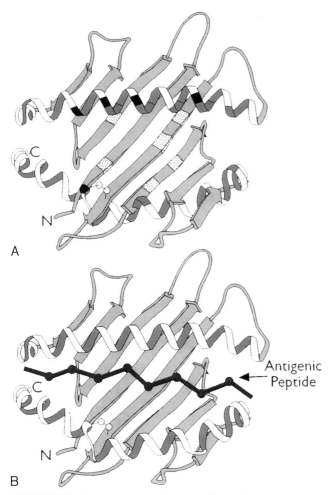

FIGURE 21–5. The two outermost domains of human leukocyte antigen (HLA) class I and class II molecules fold together to form their antigen-combining sites in which the antigenic peptide can find appropriate lodging. *A*, The polymorphic regions of the HLA molecule as seen from the top, present on the floor and on the α-helices of its groove, are indicated in different nuances of color from gray to black. *B*, A schematic, 9-amino-acid-long peptide is shown in the groove of the molecule. The antigenic peptides found in HLA class I molecule grooves are normally of this same size, whereas the antigenic peptides most frequently associated with HLA class II molecules are longer than 9 amino acids and can vary considerably in size. (Modified from Trucco M: To be or not to be Asp 57, that is the question. Diabetes Care, 15:705–715, 1992.)

functional DP molecules. More than one type of DR molecule can be encoded by the same chromosome, however, and all are coexpressed at the surface of the same cell. Different DRB genes are present in different numbers and in different combinations on chromosome 6 in different individuals (see Fig. 21–6; Fig. 21–7). Each type of DRβ-chain pairs with the single nonpolymorphic α-chain encoded by the DRA1 gene (see Fig. 21–6).[26] HLA-typing techniques include methods to evaluate the HLA molecule on the cell surface (i.e., serologic typing) as well as the genes encoding these proteins (i.e., molecular typing).

At any single HLA locus, an individual has one maternal and one paternal allele. If the maternal allele and the paternal allele differ, as they often do, the person is said to be *heterozygous* at the HLA locus. If the inherited maternal and paternal alleles happen to be the same, the person is *homozygous* at the locus. Because the maternal and paternal

alleles are expressed codominantly, each cell of an individual will express both alleles (e.g., two HLA-A molecules, two HLA-B molecules). The combined expression of all HLA molecules constitutes the HLA *phenotype* of an individual. For clinical purposes, the most-sensitive, high-resolution HLA methods must be used to determine both alleles at a given locus.

Because of the relative proximity of the HLA genes, recombination events between loci within a region, or even between regions, are possible but limited. In addition, a selective pressure also contributes to maintain the genes of each established HLA haplotype together—that is, in *linkage disequilibrium.*[27] Therefore, the HLA *haplotype* defines the genetic unit inherited from one or the other parent. The haplotype includes the class I, II, and III regions of each chromosome 6 of an individual. Each HLA haplotype is transmitted from the parent to the child in mendelian fashion so that each child shares one haplotype with each parent (Fig. 21–8). Thus, each parent and child are *haploidentical.* The HLA *genotype* of an individual is composed of one paternal and one maternal HLA haplotype.

Within a family, one can find siblings who share two haplotypes (i.e., they are HLA identical), one haplotype (i.e., they are HLA haploidentical), or no haplotypes (i.e., they are HLA different) with the probability of each being 25%, 50%, and 25%, respectively. Recombination may occur during parental gametogenesis by crossing-over during meiosis. Because of the tight linkage disequilibrium and the very close proximity of the HLA genes on the chromosome, however, an HLA haplotype composed in part of the paternal and in part by the maternal genes (i.e., a *recombinant* haplotype) presents as a rare event (see Fig. 21–8). Family studies are recommended, both to confirm the alleles present in each of the patient's haplotypes and to rule out the possibility of recombination. Only a family study and the analysis of allele segregation can positively elucidate the genotype of an individual.

CLINICAL HISTOCOMPATIBILITY TESTING

Determining the HLA phenotype of an individual is the goal of histocompatibility testing (i.e., tissue typing) and can be achieved using serologic and/or molecular techniques (see later). By typing members of a family, one can easily track all four haplotypes through the family and consequently deduce the genotype of the patient, resolve homozygosity versus heterozygosity at each locus and, most importantly, determine who in the family is a suitable donor for a particular recipient. Generally, a sibling who is HLA-identical to the recipient constitutes the first choice as a donor, although transplants from haploidentical donors are being performed. With the declining birth rate in the United States and western Europe, the likelihood of finding a genotypically identical sibling has dwindled. An estimated 65–75% of persons requiring HSCT do not have a suitable donor in their family.[28]

Alternative sources for HSC are sought from phenotypically HLA-matched unrelated donors. As of November 1998, the National Marrow Donor Program has facilitated over 7500 HSCT with matched unrelated donors.[29] Transplantation using umbilical cord blood instead of bone mar-

HLA Complex

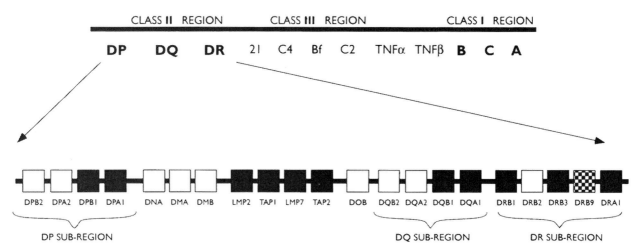

FIGURE 21–6. The human leukocyte antigen (HLA) complex present on human chromosome 6 can be subdivided into three regions. The genes present in each region encode class I, class III, and class II molecules, respectively. The class II region, closest to the centromere of the chromosome, is conventionally subdivided into three additional subregions. Among the genes contained in each subregion, are some that encode functional molecules (in *black*), genes that are not functioning, i.e., pseudogenes (in *white*), or genes that encode proteins not yet characterized (also in *white*). Although DQA1 and DQB1 genes encode for the α and the β chains of a functional HLA-DQ molecule (like DPA1 and DPB1 genes for the chains of a functional HLA-DP molecule), the DRA1 gene encodes for an α-chain able to pair with the products of each of the functional DRB genes. In the example, a DR3-positive haplotype of an individual is shown. DRB1 gene encodes for the DR3 allele, DRB2 is a pseudogene, and DRB3 encodes for the so-called DR52 molecule, which is always associated with DR3. The DRB9 gene has not been well studied yet but seems to be able to encode for a nonfunctionally stable protein chain. Transporter associated with antigen processing (TAP)1 and 2 genes are cytoplasmic transporters of antigenic peptides, whereas LMP 2 and 7 are genes encoding proteasome subunits. Both these molecules are involved in the antigenic peptide transport from the cytoplasm to the cell surface. TNF, tumor necrosis factor. (Modified from Luppi P, Rossiello MR, Faas S, Trucco M: Genetic background and environment synergistically contribute to the onset of autoimmune diseases. J Mol Med 73:381–393, 1995.)

row from HLA-matched and partially mismatched unrelated donors has been performed with success.[30] Discussion of cord blood transplantation can be found in Chapter 26.

Unlike related donors who match at all loci within the shared haplotypes, unrelated donors can match at some, but not all loci. Therefore, precise HLA typing at the class I and class II loci becomes essential. Although clinical experience in HSCT using matched unrelated donors has proved that long-term survival in some patient populations is achievable, the risks of graft failure and serious acute GVHD are higher than those of matched-sibling HSCT. One plausible explanation for the increased incidence and severity of GVHD is that, unlike the case with genotypically identical HLA-matched siblings, who are "identical by descent" for HLA, other poorly characterized MHC or non-MHC (i.e., minor) histocompatibility antigens[31] exist, and mismatches in the antigens can contribute to the alloreactivity. Furthermore, recent advances in MHC molecular genetics have revealed polymorphism at the genetic level that is detectable only with DNA-based technology. These differences may have functional and clinical relevance. The failure to identify these differences using serologic and/or cellular techniques suggests that unrelated donor/recipient pairs thought to be phenotypically matched actually were mismatched.[32]

METHODS OF HISTOCOMPATIBILITY TESTING

Histocompatibility testing for HSCT presents unique challenges and problems to clinicians and to the laboratory. A variety of serologic, cellular, biochemical, and molecular techniques are available. Important parameters include sources of HSC (e.g., marrow, cord blood), the degree of resolution and turnaround time needed, the number of samples, and the level of expertise of the institution in different techniques.

SEROLOGIC METHODS OF HLA TYPING

Tissue typing refers to determination of the class I and class II specificity (i.e., the HLA phenotype) of the potential donor(s) and recipient. Finding the best donor generally means finding a "six-antigen" match by looking at each of the two alleles at HLA-A, -B, and -DR. In practice, however, HLA-C and -DQ are also typed and often considered. Until recent years, HLA typing has been performed largely by the microlymphocytotoxicity assay.[33] In this technique, the lymphocytes are incubated with a panel or alloreactive antisera and complement (C′). The anti-HLA antibodies in the various sera are specific for the individual structural determinants that characterize the polymorphism of the HLA antigens. When a specific antigen-antibody complex is formed, C′ activation results in cell lysis. After addition of a vital dye, the percentage of dead versus live cells can be visualized by phase-contrast microscopy. A reaction is positive when at least half of the cells are killed. The HLA type is assigned by interpreting the patterns of reactivity of dozens of sera of specificity.

Most antisera are obtained from donors who have been inadvertently immunized with cells bearing foreign HLA

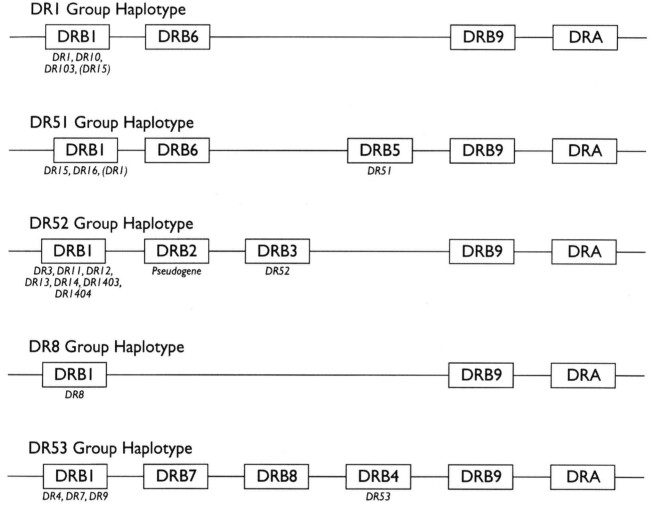

FIGURE 21–7. DRB genes are present in different numbers and in different combinations on chromosome 6 of different individuals. Although the DRB1 gene encodes the serologically best-defined DR alleles, DRB3, DRB4, and DRB5 encode for three molecules (DR52, DR53, and DR51, respectively) always found associated with certain DRB1 alleles like DR3, DR4, and DR1, respectively. It is perhaps noteworthy to stress that DR51, DR52, and DR53 are then not allelic forms at a certain locus, like the DRB1 alleles, but are proteins, each encoded by a specific gene only present in certain haplotypes. (Modified from Dupont B, Yang SY: Histocompatibility. *In* Forman S, Blume K, Thomas ED (eds): Bone Marrow Transplantation. Oxford, England, Blackwell, 1994, pp 22–40.)

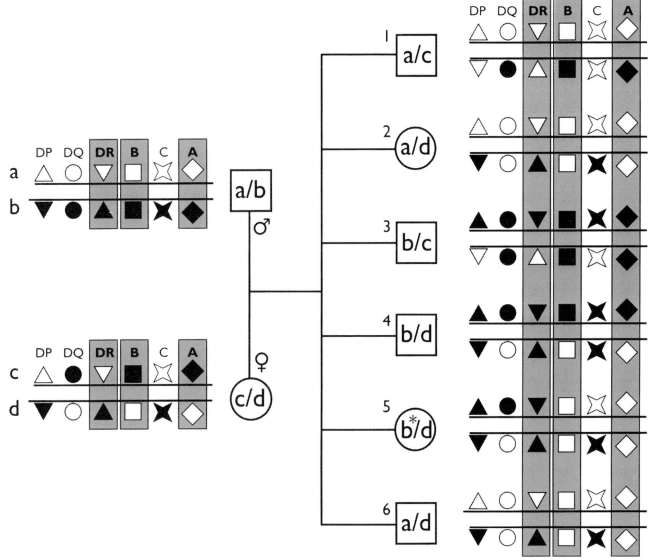

FIGURE 21–8. The study of the segregation of human leukocyte antigen (HLA) alleles through the family is based on the determination of the HLA phenotypes on at least the two parents and a child or on three HLA-different members of the same family. Segregation analysis allows the definition of the four haplotypes (normally called a, b, c, and d) present in the family, and, consequently, the definition of individuals heterozygous or homozygous at certain loci (e.g., sibling 1 is homozygous at DP, DR, and C, both alleles are white; but heterozygous at DQ, B, and A loci, 1 white and 1 black allele), together with the recognition of individuals who share one haplotype only (e.g., siblings 1, 2, and 6 share the "a" haplotype), or two haplotypes (e.g., siblings 1 and 6 share the "a" and the "d" haplotypes), or none (e.g., siblings 2 and 3). A bone marrow transplant always offers the best chance of success if it is performed between HLA-identical siblings like sibling 2 and sibling 6 of this family. "Six antigen matching" refers to the situation in which two individuals share both alleles at the locus A, B, and DR (gray background). In our simplistic example, father and mother of the family are sharing the alleles at the A, B, and DR loci and constitute a 6 antigen matching pair although they can be not HLA-"identical" because their haplotypes are different. Although it is considered a rare event, it is possible to find individuals, represented here by sibling 5, in which a crossing-over between class I and class II gene regions, involving the paternal and maternal haplotypes of the father, cause the a-b recombination, flagged here with an asterisk (b*).

molecules, through transfusion or multiple pregnancies.[34, 35] It is the responsibility of the tissue typing laboratory to procure, test, and maintain quality control of the antisera. Sera can be obtained locally or through national or international exchange programs. Commercial trays with well-characterized sera are most widely used. All accredited laboratories are required to adhere to rigorous standards regarding reagents, protocols, and quality assurance set forth by the American Society for Histocompatibility and Immunogenetics (ASHI). In addition, most laboratories participate in proficiency testing programs administered by agencies such as the College of American Pathologists (CAP).

Even with reagent standardization and proficiency testing, many problems still confound the serologic results. Serology is encumbered by the requirement for relatively pure populations of viable lymphocytes, which has the greatest impact on class II typing because DR and DQ molecules are expressed on B lymphocytes, which make up about 20% of the peripheral blood lymphocyte population. Hence, a relatively large quantity of blood (30 mL) from each individual (frequently a child) must be processed in order to obtain enough B cells to complete typing. Also, if the cells are not 100% viable at the beginning (which can occur because of malignant disease and/or chemotherapy), subsequent procedures (e.g., density gradient centrifugation, separation of T and B cells) may further increase cell death, leading to a high background such that specific killing becomes indistinguishable. Also, serology cannot be used to type patients recently treated with anti-CD3 antibodies because the antibodies are cytotoxic in the presence of C'. Finally, the C' can be a source of variability because the rabbit serum can be cytotoxic, which can be alleviated by preparing large batches of the reagent and maintaining good quality control.

In many leukemic conditions (e.g., chronic myelogenous leukemia), insufficient numbers of B cells and/or reduced antigen expression can preclude class II testing. Although Epstein-Barr virus transformation and a variety of other procedures have been developed in attempts to procure sufficient numbers of B cells for testing, they can be labor intensive, time consuming, and expensive, and they are often unproductive.[36] A major drawback to Epstein-Barr virus transformation is that the transformed B cells are overly sensitive to C' activity. Although complement preadsorption with each cell line to be tested can avoid this problem, such treatment is impractical for widespread clinical use.

Cross-reactivity (i.e., lack of specificity) of antisera still remains an unsolved problem for serologic typing. The HLA types defined by serologic methods are often not directly correlated with single alleles. Certain class I antigens belong to cross-reactive groups that share distinct immunogenic epitopes, called *public*, or broad, specificities.[37] All the cells sharing a public epitope react with the same antiserum. Furthermore, the antisera used for class II typing are not naturally class II specific. These sera are frequently "contaminated" with class I antibodies, which may cause false-positive reactions. Although extensive absorption with platelets (which express class I but not class II proteins) can provide a relatively pure preparation of

anti–class II antibodies, the antisera are generally of poorer quality and in greater demand than class I antisera.

The need for ongoing screening programs to replenish sera is further complicated in that two donors (e.g., two polygravidae) never have exactly the same specificity, only 200 mL of blood can legally be collected post partum, and even serum obtained from the same donor after subsequent pregnancies can differ with respect to titer or range of reactivity. Standardization of reagents and implementation of standard procedures have been problematic, although agencies such as ASHI have developed standards and guidelines to ameliorate these problems. It is well known, however, that accurate serologic HLA typing largely depends on the experience, and extensive knowledge of protocols and reagents, of specialized HLA laboratory personnel.

Scarcity of reagents for some antigens, particularly, for those preferentially expressed on the cells of non-Caucasian individuals (despite ongoing efforts of 12 International Histocompatibility Workshops), and the inability to recognize clinically relevant microvariation within the serologically defined specificities are further limitations to this technique. Individual, or *private*, specificities[37] recognized by alloantibody binding often prove to be closely related antigens that can be "split" into allelic subtypes of variants as newly discovered reagents become available and/or by newer techniques. In recent years, several groups have developed panels of monoclonal antibodies for serologic testing[38] in attempts to increase specificity, but their use is not yet widespread because of the limited number of recognized epitopes. Despite its limitations, the microlymphocytotoxicity test remains the most popular test for clincial use to provide class I and class II typing at a moderate level of resolution within 1 working day.

CELLULAR METHODS OF HLA TYPING

Other alleles, including those at HLA-C, -DQ, -DP, and perhaps other loci, are not strongly immunogenic (i.e., they do not elicit antibodies in large quantity or with high affinity). The first successful cellular approach was the unidirectional mixed lymphocyte culture (MLC). The MLC is a cellular cross-match predominantly triggered by class II antigens that do not define an individual HLA type. In this test, lymphocytes from two individuals (thought to be compatible by serologic techniques) are incubated for several days together in tissue culture. If the two individuals are disparate for a class II allele or for a non-MHC, minor histocompatibility antigen undetectable by serology, both cell types undergo lymphoblastogenesis, leading to DNA synthesis and proliferation. In the presence of ³H thymidine, the degree of newly synthesized DNA can be estimated. Cells that are HLA-identical are nonreactive in MLC, with little or no incorporation of ³H thymidine above the values from controls.

In order to separately monitor the response of the recipient (host-versus-graft) and the donor (graft-versus-host), two separate unidirectional mixed lymphocyte reactions are simultaneously performed. The cells chosen to stimulate but not respond (i.e., the *stimulators*) are inactivated by irradiation. Every MLC is set up as a complicated matrix of many one-way reactions, including three unrelated HLA-mismatched individuals used for positive controls to determine the maximum proliferative ability of the responder cells. Cells from each donor are mixed with every possible combination of cells from other donors, acting as both the stimulator and the responder. In addition, autologous controls (i.e., each individual's cells incubated with its own irradiated cells) are used to normalize the response of each cell type to its stimulators. The results are expressed as a relative response or as a stimulation index. Ideally, when two individuals are HLA-identical, the proliferative responses are less than 20% of the positive controls.[39]

The MLC test was developed primarily to help select the most compatible (i.e., least stimulatory) donor when several compatible family members are available.[40] It is used for confirmation of genotypic identity in siblings, especially when a complete haplotype could not be determined (e.g., one parent is unavailable for testing) or one appears to be serologically homozygous for DR or DQ. Both in vitro, as the MLC response, and in vivo, DR is thought to have dominance over DQ, perhaps because the expression at the cell surface of DR is 10 times higher than with DQ. The role of DP, which expresses 100 times fewer molecules than DR per single cell, remains controversial. The cellular antigens recognized in the MLC were originally designated as HLA-Dw "antigens" but were eventually recognized to be immunogenic combinations of HLA-DR, -DQ, and/or -DP determinants recognized as such by alloreactive T cells but not necessarily by alloantisera. The HLA-Dw determinants also recognized by certain antisera were then defined as D-related (DR) alleles.

A variation of this test can be performed in which the target lymphocytes are used as responders in an MLC in which a battery of defined homozygous typing cells are used as irradiated stimulators. Although the HLA-Dw specificity can be defined with this approach, the homozygous typing cells themselves are difficult and costly to procure, and the results of the testing are sometimes difficult to interpret. Other available but not commonly used cellular tests include the primed lymphocyte test, frequently performed to better identify DP antigens, and the cell-mediated lympholysis test, which primarily reflects the stimulatory and effector functions of cytotoxic T lymphocytes in culture.[41, 42]

Until recent years, the convention was to use HLA-A, -B, and -DR serology (i.e., six antigen matching) to select a donor with the MLC as the final arbiter of donor-recipient compatibility. In addition, a pretransplantation cross-match of patient's serum against donor lymphocytes ensures that there is no recipient presensitization to donor HLA, which could prevent engraftment.

The MLC was criticized,[43] however, mainly because of its lack of sensitivity and specificity, particularly when used for patients with hematologic disorders. Spontaneous proliferation of malignant blast cells in culture and/or poor HLA expression can contribute to false-positive or false-negative results. The MLC is technically difficult, and as many as 40% of test results are uninterpretable.[43] Furthermore, it does not have predictive value for either rejection or GVHD. Therefore, despite being the only functional test for assessing class II histocompatibility, the National Marrow Donor Program no longer requires its performance in matched unrelated HSCT, and the MLC has been largely abandoned by most clinical histocompatibility laboratories, including our own.

MOLECULAR METHODS OF HLA TYPING

The practical limitations of both serologic and cellular assays, as well as their inability to resolve clinically relevant subtypes, prompted the rapid development of molecular techniques for HLA typing. Molecular techniques can precisely define differences missed by serologic typing and/or those suggested by an incompatible MLC result. In the 1980s, molecular biology techniques (including gene cloning and sequencing) became easier. This facilitated the isolation and characterization of the HLA genes at different loci from hundreds of persons. By comparing DNA sequence variations from person to person, the structure and location of the polymorphic regions of the HLA complex were revealed.

Restriction Fragment Length Polymorphism

The first attempts to perform molecular HLA typing, although generating more precise and more complete results than serologic typing, were limited by the complexity of adapting difficult and frequently cumbersome techniques to which the personnel of a clinical HLA typing laboratory were not accustomed (i.e., restriction fragment length polymorphism [RFLP] analysis).[44] RFLP testing uses a specific DNA probe to recognize a certain HLA gene distributed on a different set of DNA fragments. These fragments are generated by digesting genomic DNA with a particular set of commercially prepared, bacterial restriction endonucleases (i.e., restriction enzymes) that recognize short, specific nucleotide sequences. The resulting array of restriction fragments are separated on agarose gels by electrophoresis, transferred by capillary action to a nitrocellulose or nylon membrane (Southern blotting), and sequentially hybridized with radiolabeled DNA probes specific for each HLA locus.[44] The radioactive probes present on the membranes were revealed by exposing them to x-ray film for 1 or 2 days, resulting in an autoradiogram revealing one or more fragments per sample that could be sized by comparison with known-molecular-weight DNA standards.

In some laboratories, the use of radioactivity posed a problem or a high-quality Southern blot could not be achieved, and the turnaround time for even a small number of tests was long. Furthermore, the necessary expertise in molecular biology and the need for additional equipment, especially to prepare and label adequate amounts of DNA probes, made performing these DNA tests nearly impossible in a clinical setting.

In an attempt to address these problems and to identify DNA class II sequence variation on a global scale, the Tenth International Histocompatibility Workshop was organized with the specific aim of transferring RFLP technology to laboratories specializing in HLA serology.[45, 46] All laboratories shared a common set of homozygous lymphoid cell lines as controls and a battery of DNA probes. The lack of quality control in expanding and purifying DNA probes, however, together with failures in probe labeling and hybridization, transferring DNA segments from gels to membranes, and reading the autoradiograms, made interpretation of band patterns, and the consequent allele assignments, extremely subjective. For this reason, a large part of the proceedings of this workshop, published in 1987, was devoted to establishing standards for RFLP analysis of class II loci. Although the collective data revealed strong associations between certain DR and DQ alleles and the RFLP, they were not definitive, largely because of strong homology and, hence, cross-reactivity between loci.[46, 47] These restriction fragments result from the presence or absence (due to polymorphism) of restriction sites that could be located nearby, and in linkage disequilibrium with, but *not* within, the HLA coding sequences.[44] Because other techniques that directly analyze HLA polymorphism were being developed, RFLP analysis was quickly deemed unsuitable for general clinical use.

Polymerase Chain Reaction and Sequence-Specific Oligonucleotide Probe

The polymerase chain reaction (PCR) obviated many of these limitations and revolutionized HLA molecular typing.[48, 49] PCR is a powerful and versatile technique for generating millions of copies of specific genomic DNA fragments from minute amounts of starting material once the nucelotide sequence of a certain gene is known. Amplification is accomplished automatically in a DNA thermal cylcer by incubating nanogram quantities of DNA, isolated from any possible source, in solution with buffer, free deoxynucleotide triphosphates (dNTP), specific (i.e., able to specifically recognize the target DNA segments) oligonucleotide primers, and thermostable DNA polymerase (Fig. 21–9). After approximately 30 cycles of denaturation of template DNA into single strands, annealing of specific primer pairs to conserved (i.e., ubiquitous) sequences outside the HLA polymorphic target regions, and extension of the primers by DNA polymerase, enough DNA is available for subsequent analysis.

The most common analyses are performed by dot blotting. A few microliters of the amplified material is spotted onto replicate nylon membranes, each of which is denatured in sodium hydroxide and then hybridized with a labeled sequence-specific oligonucleotide probe (SSOP) with an attached reporter moiety. After the unbound excess is washed away, the retention of specific probe can be visualized by a variety of methods (Fig. 21–10a). The most common method involves autoradiography of ^{32}P-labeled probes. This approach allowed typing of hundreds of samples with a relatively small number of SSOP to determine, for example, that variants of sequences involving codon 57

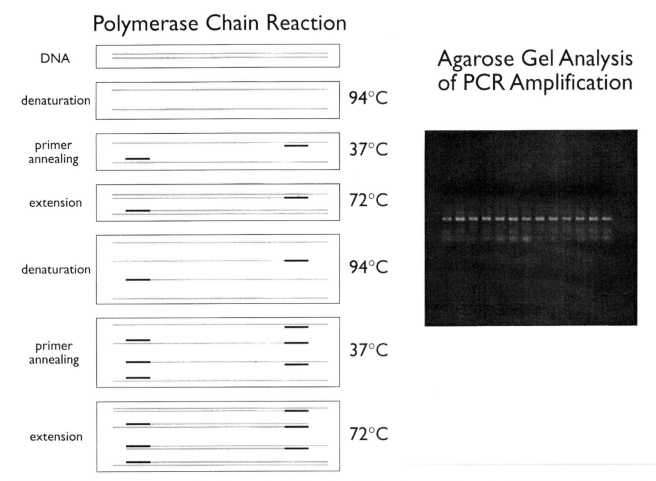

Polymerase Chain Reaction

DNA

denaturation — 94°C

primer annealing — 37°C

extension — 72°C

denaturation — 94°C

primer annealing — 37°C

extension — 72°C

Agarose Gel Analysis of PCR Amplification

FIGURE 21–9. Schematic representation of the three steps involved in each cycle of a polymerase chain reaction (PCR). Thirty cycles are normally sufficient to amplify a certain DNA segment more than 100,000 times. (Modified from Trucco M: To be or not to be Asp 57, that is the question. Diabetes Care 15:705–715, 1992.)

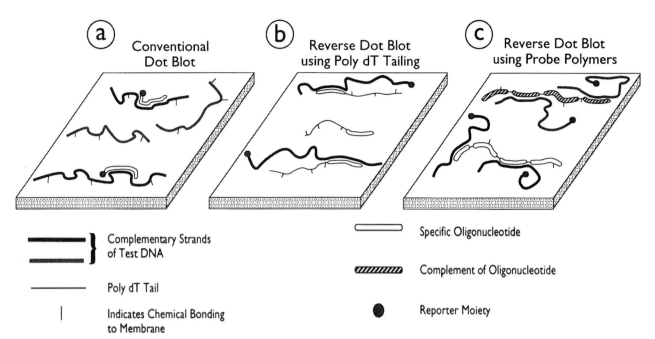

FIGURE 21–10. Conventional dot blot used in specific oligonucleotide probe typing (a) is compared with reverse dot blot after poly (d)T tailing of the various probes (b) and with reverse dot blot of polymeric probes (c). (Modified from Rudert WA, Trucco M: A novel approach for a rapid HLA class II molecular typing. *In* Tsuji K, Aizawa M, Sasazuki T (eds): Histocompatibility Testing, 1991. Oxford, England, Oxford University Press. 1992, pp 352–356.)

of the second exon of the HLA-DQB1 gene were reliable markers of susceptibility to insulin-dependent diabetes mellitus.[50, 51] As the extremely large sequence diversity of the class II gene second exon was revealed, the possibility of using this technique for complete HLA class II typing seemed difficult yet feasible. This daunting task was promoted and organized by the Eleventh International Histocompatibility Workshop, which provided standardized conditions and a battery of 140 SSOP to each of its participant laboratories.

The advantages of this technique, often called *oligotyping*, are many. The requirement for viable, purified lymphocytes expressing HLA is eliminated. Reagents can be standardized and synthesized in unlimited quantities. Functionally relevant subtypes and polymorphisms as small as one nucleotide substitution can be precisely defined because stringent conditions for hybridization can be perfected for each probe. In HSCT, in which patient cells may be limited or phenotypically deficient with respect to HLA expression, oligotyping can provide accurate HLA typing.

To provide the high-resolution HLA typing required for HSCT, up to seven separate PCR amplifications may be needed for DRB and DQB typing alone. A complete set of results, no matter how large or small, requires 4–5 days to be finalized. Major drawbacks to this technique are its labor intensiveness and time requirements. In particular, the labeling and manipulation of over 100 probes (each of which has to be washed at a different temperature that must be empirically determined) is not well suited for routine clinical applications in which a relatively small number of samples are tested in comparison with the number of probes and membranes required. The use of tetramethylammonium chloride nearly obviates the need for specific conditions for each probe, and an alternative detection system can eliminate use of radioactivity. Such

methods involve incorporation of a molecule recognizable by an antibody-enzyme conjugate into the probe followed by incubation with a substrate to the enzyme. The cleaved substrate can be recognized colorimetrically or by chemoluminescence.[52, 53] Yet other limitations, including the high cost of reagents, level of expertise required, and problems with reproducibility, make SSOP oligotyping impractical for all but a handful of clinical HLA laboratories.

Other Techniques

Our research laboratory was the first to introduce RFLP analysis on PCR-amplified DNA for HLA typing.[54] In this method, specific HLA-encoding gene segments are amplified, then cut with restriction endonucleases that recognize polymorphic sequences *within* the HLA genes themselves. The number and the size of the generated fragments revealed in an agarose gel allow the attribution of the different alleles.[55, 56] Although this approach has the advantage of being more rapid than SSOP analysis and more practical for testing one or a few samples at a time, it is still too complex for routine laboratories.

A different format called the *reverse dot blot* has proven advantageous in reducing the amount of technical manipulation and in improving turnaround time.[57, 58] Reverse dot blots feature a pre-made membrane to which the entire battery of probes has been fixed. An individual test DNA incorporates the reporter moiety during amplification, followed by hybridization against the probes present on a single membrane. Advantages include labeling one or few DNA samples instead of more than 100 probes, performing an entire test in only one container and obtaining results in 1 working day.

The canonical size of specific oligonucleotides normally used as probes is about 20 nucleotides, a size that has been determined as best for discriminating even one base pair change while still guaranteeing a sufficiently high signal with an appropriate detection system. For the reverse dot blot, the direct attachment of probes this size is inefficient and involves formations of chemical bonds to portions of the probe, resulting in reduced hybridization capability. These difficulties have been solved by enzymatically adding a large number of thymidine nucleotides to the end of the probe (poly dT tailing).[57] The increased length facilitates binding efficiency and allows formation of chemical bonds only in the poly dT tails, not in the sequence-specific parts of the probe (Fig. 21–10b). This approach is being used in some commercial kits for HLA typing.[57]

A new method developed in our research laboratory uses a different approach to bind nucleotide probes to the membrane.[58] Long polymers, usually greater than 25 repeats of the specific nucleotide sequence, are synthesized and bound to the membrane with high efficiency.[59] Although chemical bonds between the membrane and the DNA prevent hybridization to some sequences, theoretically, a single bond in one unit of probe sequence per polymer will sufficiently anchor the molecule. The result is that many more sequences are available (i.e., higher probe concentration), which consequently allows use of shorter hybridization times and/or less-sensitive detection methods. Another important advantage of this method is that both complementary strands of probe sequence are bound to the membrane (i.e., the probes are double-stranded), which allows both strands of amplified DNA (Fig. 21–10c) to hybridize to the probe, further increasing the sensitivity of this assay. Finally, more polymers of the same size can be generated from those cloned into plasmid vectors. This level of reproducibility is not obtainable with poly dT tailing and would permit standardization of this technique for intralaboratory use. Other "reverse" techniques involve fixing probes to 96-well plastic trays with either colorimetric or fluorescent detection.[53, 60]

A technique recently developed by a number of groups that has been widely adapted for clinical use is based on a series of sequence-specific primers (SSP) and PCR.[61–63] An aliquot of each primer pair, capable of amplifying one or a group of specific alleles, is used to amplify only the specific segment. The PCR products are then loaded onto an agarose gel. After electrophoresis and staining with ethidium bromide (which intercalates between the DNA bases and becomes fluorescent under ultraviolet [UV] light), the presence and length of the specifically amplified DNA segments can be visualized on a UV lightbox. Another primer pair designed to amplify the same (frequently non-HLA) fragment in every tube acts as an internal positive control to monitor the integrity of the DNA added to each reaction. The SSP method offers the possibility of obtaining moderate to high-resolution HLA typing in a few hours. Techniques for DRB molecular typing using 32 sequence-specific pairs of primers and DQB typing using 14 primer pairs have been published.[61, 62] Several commercial companies offer SSP testing kits.

Class I Molecular Typing

Both SSP and SSOP methods have been applied to class I typing, which is a formidable task because of the high degree of polymorphism compared with the class II genes and technical problems caused by the presence of pseudogenes. One method of SSP typing uses nine coding-strand and seven non–coding-strand primers in various combinations to generate HLA-A specific amplification products.[64] The specificity of PCR priming is increased by taking advantage of the amplification refractory mutation system, in which nonspecific reactions are inhibited by introducing a nucleotide mismatch near the 3′ end of the primer.[65] Fifteen HLA-A groups can be successfully characterized using this method, which appears to be comparable to routine serology with respect to identification and resolution of HLA-A alleles. Subtypes of each group can be more specifically resolved using additional primer pairs.[66]

Low-resolution typing of the HLA-B alleles using a similar approach has also been described.[67] Twenty-four PCR reactions using 34 primers are sufficient to determine the majority of, but not all, serologically defined alleles at the B locus. It is likely, however, that the number of alleles identified by this approach will expand with the implementation of new or slightly modified primers and/or by performing a "two-tiered" assay that incorporates a second round of PCR with additional primer sets.

Amplification refractory mutation system PCR has been used to detect alleles at the HLA-C locus, although the limited characterization of this locus at the serologic level makes the comparison between serologic and molecular typings of these genes difficult.[68] This approach, however, can reproducibly detect all of the HLA-C alleles for which there is sequencing information and has been used to identify new alleles.

The SSP approach is especially amenable to use in clinical laboratories that do not have molecular biology experience because the equipment and special techniques required are minimal. Reliable and easily interpretable results can be generated in less than 4 hours. The gel-based method is particularly well suited for clinical laboratories analyzing only a small number of samples. For laboratories performing large-scale molecular typing, however, a strategy combining the high-throughput advantages of SSOP with the speed, high resolution, and relative ease of SSP analysis is recommended.

We have used the SSP approach together with a modification of a recently described method that permits amplification *and* direct detection of specific target DNA with no requirement for postamplification hybridization or gel analysis steps.[69, 70] This assay takes advantage of the 5′ to 3′ exonuclease activity of the Taq DNA polymerase normally used in PCR DNA amplification. An oligonucleotide probe, labeled at the 5′ end with a reporter fluorescent dye and at the 3′ end with a "quencher" fluorescent dye, is premixed in each PCR reaction with the allele-specific primers. The annealing of the probe to one of the PCR template strands during amplification generates a substrate suitable for exonuclease attack. Cleavage of the hybridized probe generates smaller fragments that physically release the reporter from the quenching residue, enabling its detection by an increase in sample fluorescence (Fig. 21–11). The fluorescence signal is read directly from the PCR reaction mixture via a luminescence spectrometer. The sequence-specific priming and exonuclease released fluores-

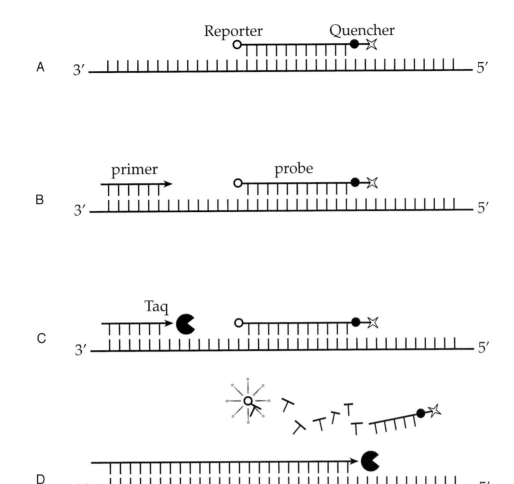

FIGURE 21–11. Schematic representation of sequence-specific priming and exonuclease-released fluorescence (SSPERF) detection. *A,* Hybridization of a doubly labeled fluorogenic probe to the target DNA sequence. The reporter (○) and the quencher (●) dye portions are indicated. The 3′ phosphate added to inhibit the primer function of the probe is indicated with a star (☆). *B,* The annealing of the primer to the DNA template follows the annealing of the probe to it because its size is shorter than one of the probes. *C,* Taq polymerase catalyzes the extension of the primer. *D,* Taq polymerase exerts its exonuclease function once it encounters the double-stranded template formed by the hybridization of the probe to one of the strands of the DNA to be amplified. The cleavage of the probe physically separates the reporter from the quencher dye, promoting an increase in reporter fluorescence. (From Faas SJ, Menon R, Braun ER, et al: Sequence-specific priming and exonuclease-released fluorescence detection of HLA-DQB1 alleles. Tissue Antigens 48:97–112, 1996.)

cence (SSPERF) assay is a highly specific, sensitive, and rapid method already successfully tested for the detection of HLA-A, HLA-B, DQB1, DQA1, and DRB alleles.[70–72] This approach offers all the advantages of the conventional approach based on SSP-PCR without the need of agarose gel preparations to read the results (Fig. 21–12).

Although the preparation and purification of fluorescent probes is more time consuming than the synthesis and labeling of conventional fluorescent or radioactive probes for SSOP-based typing, the probes, once validated, can be generated in large scale (1–10 μM), which provides sufficient reagents for more than 200,000 reactions. The doubly labeled probes, together with SSP primers, buffer, dNTP, and MgCl₂, can be aliquotted and stored indefinitely at −20°C in PCR strip tubes. Subsequent use would involve manual addition of extracted DNA and Taq polymerase to each tube. The rest is automated. A simple machine that serves as both a DNA thermocycler and a spectrometer has been made commercially available from PE Applied Biosystems (ABI PRISM 7700 Sequence Detection System).

In addition to SSOP, reverse dot blotting, RFLP, SSP, or SSPERF, other PCR-based techniques include PCR-heteroduplex analysis, PCR-SSCP (sequence-specific conformational polymorphism) analysis, and PCR-direct sequencing.[73–75] Unlike serologic testing, in which one test method predominates, the vast choice of available molecular techniques can be confusing at first. Each laboratory can choose whatever method or methods best meet the needs to fulfill the requirements of the HSCT programs. For the 16 contract laboratories of the National Marrow Donor Program (NMDP), the SSOP method is generally used for HLA-DRB typing to screen thousands of potential donors per week. The NMDP presently requires that all patients undergoing HSCT and their donors be typed and matched prospectively at the allele level using DNA methods for DRB typing. Many believe that, in the near future, molecular typing for HLA-A, -B, and perhaps -C will be required as well. Our laboratory performs molecular DR and DQ testing using "in-house" SSOP and SSP methods for all patients, family members, and unrelated donors. Molecular A, B, or C

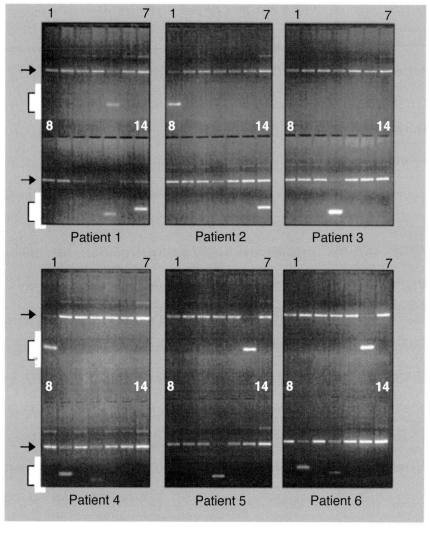

A

	1	2	3	4	5	6	7	8	9	10	11	12
A	0.086	335.443	59.513	343.912	28.915	40.681	32.562	37.637	86.009	26.563	32.231	31.888
B	72.882	248.266	79.573	297.952	80.964	82.198	69.151	68.510	64.126	46.699	57.824	66.677
C	69.948	68.503	73.595	78.290	79.028	79.086	42.544	47.964	47.027	169.938	43.837	204.938
D	71.047	72.601	75.268	77.989	78.420	78.001	57.393	65.390	50.436	60.848	64.018	63.130
E	79.592	77.426	79.496	85.706	84.346	84.484	89.333	97.923	347.519	92.204	327.134	87.711
F	115.771	78.758	78.591	81.537	82.790	82.682	202.683	53.055	51.826	56.942	54.991	51.504
G	85.046	83.323	84.531	85.061	302.259	337.683	81.629	89.281	84.558	89.006	82.657	86.816
H	87.855	90.420	87.383	92.537	87.922	89.869	200.142	236.200	84.960	93.976	89.677	82.533

B p: 1   2   3   4   5   6   1   2   3   4   5   6

FIGURE 21–12. An example of results obtained by sequence-specific priming typing of human leukocyte antigen DQB1 alleles of six patients' DNA revealed by ethidium bromide–labeled bands in an agarose gel (*A*) or as FAM fluorescence values determined by a TaqMan spectrometer (*B*). FAM, 6-carboxy-fluorescein. (From Faas SJ, Menon R, Braun ER, et al: Sequence-specific priming and exonuclease-released fluorescence detection of HLA-DQB1 alleles. Tissue Antigens 48:97–112, 1996.)

typing is also performed when resolution or sensitivity of the serologic typing is insufficient. In the last few years, many types of commercial reagents for class II molecular typing have become available.

CLINICAL SIGNIFICANCE OF HLA MOLECULAR TYPING

A possible criticism of DNA typing is that it provides "too much" information. Although it has been hypothesized that even one nucleotide difference, and hence one amino acid disparity, can result in increased risk of alloreactivity in vivo, many nucleotide substitutions do not cause amino acid changes.[76] Given the huge number of detectable alleles at the various loci, it would be important to determine which mismatches are allowable and which ones are relevant to clinical outcome. A number of studies have attempted to determine the clinical impact of HLA matching in matched unrelated HSCT. Many reports have shown that the incidence of both acute GVHD and rejection are significantly higher among patients undergoing transplantation with phenotypically matched HSC from unrelated donors compared with cells from genotypically identical siblings when only serologic techniques are used for HLA typing.[10–12, 25, 30] Furthermore, the incidence and severity tend to increase with increasing HLA mismatch, except in very young patients, in whom mismatch in one HLA locus can be tolerated.[11, 77] With the advent of DNA-based HLA typing, it has been proved that unrelated donors with apparent serologically HLA-identical types were not matched at the DNA level. Recent studies using DNA methods for both class I and class II typing have shown that molecular matching may reduce the risks of acute GVHD and mortality, although it remains unclear whether molecular matching for HLA-C and -DP may contribute to improving clinical outcome.[78–80]

The likelihood of finding a matched unrelated donor also depends on whether the patient has a common or a rare HLA genotype. Not only are some alleles more common within a particular ethnic or racial group, but because of linkage disequilibrium, certain alleles can give rise to different haplotypes within different populations. The National Institutes of Health and ASHI have recently sponsored an African American Workshop whose main goal is to define HLA alleles and extended haplotypes and their frequencies in African Americans using both serologic and molecular techniques. The data will be used to assess whether African American donor identification/recruitment is as expected according to the HLA characteristics of the population. This and other studies of different minority groups will help increase the likelihood that patients requiring HSCT can find a more suitable HLA-matched donor.

Even considering all the possible genotypically identical sibling donors and the large number of potential donors enrolled in the NMDP registry, a substantial number of patients will not be able to find an HLA-matched donor. Also, with the discovery of new loci and alleles, the odds of finding a complete match will decrease further. Therefore, one of the more important areas in HSCT is a precise definition of HLA mismatches that are clinically permissible

in terms of rejection, GVHD, and overall mortality and morbidity.

The following is the current protocol for identifying a suitable histocompatible donor at the University of Pittsburgh Medical Center for patients requiring allogeneic HSCT. The process of donor selection includes identification and evaluation of all potential donors and selection of the best donor when more than one donor seems appropriate.

All patients undergo HLA typing, which includes the following:

- Serologic class I typing (HLA-A, -B, -C)
- High-resolution DNA class II typing (HLA-DR, -DQ)
- DNA class I typing (HLA-A, -B, -C) as needed to resolve serologic typing
- Family studies, including typing both parents, whenever possible

Related potential donors (i.e., siblings or other family members) undergo the following:

- Serologic class I typing (HLA-A, -B, -C)
- If A and B match (four of four antigens) or match at three of four antigens, DNA class II typing is performed
- A preliminary search in the NMDP if no related donor is found

Unrelated potential donors undergo the following:

- Review of preliminary HLA typing data from the NMDP registry
- Activation of formal search if a potential match is identified
- Confirmatory serologic class I typing (HLA-A, -B, -C)
- Confirmatory high-resolution DNA class II typing (HLA-DR, -DQ)
- DNA class I typing as needed
- Leukocyte cross-match between patient serum and potential donor cells as needed to facilitate donor selection

CONCLUSION

Although histocompatibility is the primary factor in donor selection, other issues, including donor cytomegalovirus status, age, gender and parity, ABO blood type, and risk of marrow harvest, should be considered. We recommend that the HLA laboratory personnel and the HSCT team (including clinicians and nurse coordinators) review all of these factors continually to assess and select the best donor for each patient.

REFERENCES

1. Ivanyi P, Dausset J: Allo-antigens and antigenic factors in human leukocytes: a hypothesis. Vox Sanguinis 11:326, 1966.
2. Bodmer J, Bodmer WF, Payne R, et al: Leucocyte antigens in man: a comparison of lymphocytotoxic and agglutination assays for their detection. Nature 210:28, 1966.
3. Amos DB: Human histocompatibility locus HL-A. Science 159:659, 1968.
4. Ceppellini R, van Rood JJ: The HL-A system: I. Genetics and molecular biology. Semin Hematol 11:233, 1974.

5. van Rood JJ: Transplantation antigens in man: their recognition and relevance in clinical organ transplantation. Br J Haematol 17:310, 1969.

6. Zmijewski CM, Amos DB: A model of leukocyte typing and donor selection for human renal transplantation. Vox Sanguinis 11:377, 1966.

7. Cho Y, Terasaki P, Graver B: Fifteen year kidney graft survival. In Terasaki P (ed): Clinical Transplants. Los Angeles, UCLA Tissue Typing Laboratory, 1989, p 325.

8. Markus BH, Duquesnoy RJ, Gordon RD, et al: Histocompatibility and liver transplant outcome: does HLA exert a dualistic effect? Transplantation 46:372, 1988.

9. Ferrara JLM, Deeg HJ: Graft-versus-host-disease. N Engl J Med 324:667, 1991.

10. Anasetti C, Beatty PG, Storb R, et al: Effect of HLA incompatibility on graft-versus-host disease, relapse and survival after marrow transplantation for patients with leukemia or lymphoma. Hum Immunol 29:79, 1990.

11. Beatty PG, Anasetti C, Hansen JA, et al: Marrow transplantation from unrelated donors for treatment of hematologic malignancies: effect of mismatching for one HLA locus. Blood 81:249, 1993.

12. Anasetti C, Amos D, Beatty PG, et al: Effect of HLA compatibility on engraftment of bone marrow transplants in patients with leukemia or lymphoma. N Engl J Med 320:197, 1989.

13. Snell GD: The H-2 locus of the mouse: observations and speculations concerning its comparative genetics and its polymorphism [Review]. Folia Biol 14:335, 1968.

14. Summerell JM, Davies DA: Physical properties of mouse H-2 transplantation alloantigens. Biochimi Biophys Acta 207:92, 1970.

15. Bjorkman P, Saper M, Samraoui W, et al: Structure of the human class I histocompatibility antigen, HLA-A2. Nature 329:506, 1987.

16. Bjorkman P, Saper M, Samraoui B, et al: The foreign antigen binding site and T cell recognition regions of class I histocompatibility antigens. Nature 329:512, 1987.

17. Davis MM, Bjorkman PJ: T-cell antigen receptor genes and T-cell recognition. Nature 334:395, 1988.

18. Jorgensen PAR, Ehrich EW, Davis MM: Molecular components of T-cell recognition. Annu Rev Immunol 10:835, 1992.

19. Weiss A: T cell antigen receptor signal transduction: a tale of tails and cytoplasmic protein-tyrosine kinases. Cell 73:209, 1993.

20. Romagnani S: Induction of Th21 and Th2 responses: a key role for the "natural" immune response? Immunol Today 13:379, 1992.

21. Tony, HP, Parker DC: Major histocompatibility complex-restricted, polyclonal B cell responses resulting from helper T cell recognition of anti-immunoglobulin presented by small B lymphocytes. J Exp Med 161:223, 1985.

22. Mosmann TR, Cherwinski H, Bond MW, et al: Two types of murine helper T cell clones: I. Definition according to profiles of lymphokine activities and secreted proteins. J Immunol 136:2348, 1986.

23. Grey HM, Kubo RT, Colon SM, et al: The small subunit of HLA antigens is beta-2 microglobulin. J Exp Med 138:1608, 1973.

24. Marsh S: Nomenclature for factors of the HLA system, update April 1996. Tissue Antigens 48:69, 1996.

25. Campbell RD, Trowsdale J: Map of the human MHC. Immunol Today 14:349, 1993.

26. Dupont B, Yang SY: Histocompatibility. In Forman S, Blume K, Thomas ED (eds): Bone Marrow Transplantation. Oxford, England, Blackwell Science, 1994, pp 22–40.

27. Bodmer WF: Population genetics of the HL-A system: retrospect and prospect. In Dausset J, Colombani J (eds): Histocompatibility Testing. Copenhagen, Munksgaard, 1972, p 611.

28. Kernan NA, Bartsch G, Ash RC, et al: Analysis of 462 transplantations from unrelated donors facilitated by the National Marrow Donor Program. N Engl J Med 328:593, 1993.

29. Perkins HA, Kollman C, Howe CW: Unrelated-donor marrow transplants: the experience of the National Marrow Donor Program. Clinical Transplants, 1994, pp 295–301.

30. Kurtzberg J, Laughlin M, Graham ML, et al: Placental blood as a source of hematopoietic stem cells for transplantation into unrelated recipients. N Engl J Med 335:157, 1996.

31. Goulmy E, Schipper R, Pool J, et al: Mismatches of minor histocompatibility antigens between HLA-identical donors and recipients and the development of graft-versus-host disease after bone marrow transplantation. N Engl J Med 334:281, 1996.

32. Nademanee A, Schmidt GM, Parker P, et al: The outcome of matched unrelated donor bone marrow transplantation in patients with hematologic malignancies using molecular typing for donor selection and graft-versus-host disease prophylaxis regimen of cyclosporine, methotrexate, and prednisone. Blood 86:1228, 1995.

33. Takasugi M, Sengar DP, Terasaki PI: Microassays in transplantation immunology. Am J Med Technol 37:470, 1971.

34. Ceppellini R, Connard GD, Coppo F, et al: Transplantation antigens: introductory symposium. Mixed leukocyte cultures and HL-A antigens: I. Reactivity of young fetuses, newborns and mothers at delivery. Transplant Proc 3:58, 1971.

35. Payne R, Bodmer WF, Troup GM, Walford RL: Serologic activities and specificities of eleven human leukocyte antisera produced by planned immunization. Transplantation 5:597, 1967.

36. Trucco M, Garotta G, Stocker JW, Ceppellini R: Murine monoclonal antibodies against HLA structures. Immunol Rev 47:219, 1979.

37. Klein J: Private and public antigens of the mouse H-2 system. Nature 229:635, 1971.

38. Trucco M, Stocker JW, Ceppellini R: Monoclonal antibodies against human lymphocyte antigens. Nature 273:666, 1978.

39. Meo T, Vives J, Miggiano V, Shreffler D: A major role for the Ir-1 region of the mouse H-2 complex in the mixed leukocyte reaction. Transplant 5:377, 1973.

40. Bach FH, Albertini RJ, Amos DB, et al: Mixed leukocyte culture studies in families with known HL-A genotypes. Transplant Proc 1:339, 1969.

41. Dormoy A, Urlacher A, Tongio MM: Complexity of the HLA-DP region: RFLP analysis versus PLT typing and oligotyping. Hum Immunol 34:39, 1992.

42. Yamamoto M, Sugihara K, Ohtsuki F, et al: Generation of self HLA-DR-specific CD3+ CD4− CD8+ cytotoxic T cells in chronic graft-versus-host disease. Bone Marrow Transplant 14:525, 1994.

43. Mickelson EM, Bartsch GE, Hansen JA, Dupont B: The MLC assay as a test for HLA-D region compatibility between patients and unrelated donors: results of a National Marrow Donor Program involving multiple centers. Tissue Antigens 42:465, 1993.

44. Turco E, Fritsch R, Trucco M: Use of immunologic techniques in gene analysis. In Herberman R, Mercer DW (eds): Immunodiagnosis of Cancer, ed 2, vol 53. New York, Marcel Dekker, 1990, pp 205–222.

45. Cascino I, Rosenshire S, Turco E, et al: Relationship between DQ alpha and DQ beta RFLP and serologically defined class II HLA antigens. J Immunogenet 13:387, 1986.

46. Carsson B, Wallin J, Bohme J, Moller E: HLA-DR-DQ haplotypes defined by restriction fragment length analysis: correlation to serology. Hum Immunol 20:95, 1987.

47. Trucco M, Ball E: RFLP analysis of DQ-beta chain gene: workshop report. In Dupont B (ed): Histocompatibility Testing 1987, vol 1. New York, Springer-Verlag, 1989, p 860.

48. Mullis KB, Faloona FA: Specific synthesis of DNA in vitro via a polymerase-catalyzed chain reaction. In Diego RW (ed): Methods in Enzymology. San Diego, Academic Press, 1987, p 335.

49. Saiki RK, Gelfand OH, Stoffel S, et al: Primer-directed enzymatic amplification of DNA with a thermostable DNA polymerase. Science 239:487, 1989.

50. Todd JA, Bell JI, McDevitt HO: HLA-DQ-beta gene contributes to susceptibility and resistance to insulin-dependent diabetes mellitus. Nature 329:559, 1987.

51. Morel P, Dorman J, Todd J, et al: Aspartic acid at position 57 of the HLA DQ-beta chain protects against type I diabetes: a family study. Proc Natl Acad Sci U S A 85:8111, 1988.

52. Scharf SJ, Griffith RL, Erlich HA: Rapid typing of DNA sequence polymorphism at the HLA-DRB1 locus using the polymerase chain reaction and nonradioactive olignocleotide probes. Hum Immunol 30:190, 1991.

53. Giorda R, Lampasona V, Kocova M, Trucco M: Non-radioisotopic typing of human leukocyte antigen class II genes on microplates. Biotechniques 15:918, 1993.

54. Trucco G, Fritsch R, Giorda R, Trucco M: Rapid detection of IDDM susceptibility, using amino acid 57 of the HLA-DQ beta chain as a marker. Diabetes 38:1617, 1989.

55. Hsia S, Tong JY, Parris GL, et al: Molecular compatibility and renal graft survival: the HLA DRB1 genotyping. Transplantation 55:395, 1993.

56. Tong JY, Hsia S, Parris GL, et al: Molecular compatibility and renal graft survival: the HLA DQB1 genotyping. Transplantation 55:390, 1993.

57. Saiki RK, Walsh PS, Levenson CH, Erlich HA: Genetic analysis of amplified DNA with immobilized sequence-specific oligonucleotide probes. Proc Natl Acad Sci U S A 86:6230, 1989.
58. Rudert WA, Trucco M: Rapid detection of sequence variations using polymers of specific oligonucleotides. Nucl Acid Res 5:1146, 1992.
59. Rudert WA, Trucco M: DNA polymers of protein binding sequences generated by PCR. Nucl Acid Res 18:6460, 1990.
60. Chia D, Terasaki P, Chan H, et al: Direct detection of PCR products for HLA class II typing. Tissue Antigens 42:146, 1993.
61. Olerup O, Aldener A, Fogdell A: HLA-DQB1 and -DQA1 typing by PCR amplification with sequence-specific primers (PCR-SSP) in 2 hours. Tissue Antigens 41:119, 1993.
62. Olerup O, Zetterquist H: HLA-DR typing by PCR amplification with sequence-specific primers (PCR-SSP) in 2 hours: an alternative to serological DR typing in clinical practice including donor-recipient matching in cadaveric transplantation. Tissue Antigens 39:225, 1992.
63. Bunce M, Taylor CJ, Welsh KI: Rapid HLA-DQB typing by eight polymerase chain reaction amplifications with sequence-specific primers (PCR-SSP). Hum Immunol 37:201, 1993.
64. Browning MJ, Krausa P, Rowan A, et al: Tissue typing the HLA-A locus from genomic DNA by sequence-specific PCR: comparison of HLA genotype and surface expression on colorectal tumor cell lines. Proc Natl Acad Sci U S A 90:2842, 1993.
65. Newton CR, Graham A, Heptinstall LE, et al: Analysis of any point mutation in DNA: the amplification refractory mutation system (ARMS). Nucleic Acids Res 17:2503, 1989.
66. Karusa P, Bodmer JG, Browning MJ: Defining the common subtypes of HLA A9, A10, A28 and A19 by use of ARMS/PCR. Tissue Antigens 42:91, 1993.
67. Sadler AM, Petronzelli F, Krausa P, et al: Low-resolution DNA typing for HLA-B using sequence-specific primers in allele- or group-specific ARMS-PCR. Tissue Antigens 44:148, 1994.
68. Bunce M, Welsh KI: Rapid DNA typing for HLA-C using sequence-specific primers (PCR-SSP): identification of serological and non-serologically defined HLA-C alleles including several new alleles. Tissue Antigens 43:7, 1994.
69. Holland PM, Abramson RD, Waton R, Gelfand DH: Detection of specific polymerase chain reaction product by utilizing the 5′ to 3′ exonuclease activity of Thermus aquaticus DNA polymerase. Proc Natl Acad Sci U S A 88:7276–7280, 1991.
70. Faas SJ, Menon R, Braun ER, et al: Sequence-specific priming and exonuclease-released fluorescence detection of HLA-DQB1 alleles. Tissue Antigens 48:97–112, 1996.
71. Rudert WA, Braun ER, Faas SJ, et al: Double-labeled fluorescent probes for 5′ nuclease assays: purification and performance evaluation. BioTechniques 22:1140–1145, 1997.
72. Menon R, Rudert WA, Faas SJ, et al: Sequence-specific priming and exonuclease-released fluorescence assay for a rapid and reliable HLA-A molecular typing. Mol Diagn 2:99–111, 1997.
73. D'Amato M, Sorrentin R: A simple and economical DRB1 typing procedure combining group-specific amplification, DNA heteroduplex and enzyme restriction analysis. Tissue Antigens 43:295, 1994.
74. Carrington M, Miller T, White M, et al: Typing of HLA-DQA1 and DQB1 using DNA single-strand conformation polymorphism. Hum Immunol 33:208, 1992.
75. Santamaria P, Reinsmoen NL, Lindstrom AL, et al: Frequent HLA class I and DP sequence mismatches in serologically (HLA-A, HLA-B, HLA-DR) and molecularly (HLA-DRB1, HLA-DQA1, HLA-DQB1) HLA-identical unrelated bone marrow transplant pairs. Blood 83:280, 1994.
76. Fleischhauer K, Kernan NA, O'Reilly RJ, et al: Bone marrow-allograft rejection by T lymphocytes recognizing a single amino acid difference in HLA-B44. N Engl J Med 323:1818, 1990.
77. Davies SM, Shu XO, Blazar BR, et al: Unrelated donor bone marrow transplantation: influence of HLA A and B incompatibility on outcome. Blood 86:1636, 1995.
78. Speiser DE, Tiercy J-M, Rufer N, et al: High resolution HLA matching associated with decreased mortality after unrelated bone marrow transplantation. Blood 87:4455, 1996.
79. Petersdorf EW, Longton GM, Anasetti C, et al: The significance of HLA-DRB1 matching on clinical outcome after HLA-A, B, DR identical unrelated donor marrow transplantation. Blood 86:1606, 1995.
80. Petersdorf EW, Smith AG, Mickelson EM, et al: The role of HLA-DPB1 disparity in the development of acute graft-versus-host disease following unrelated donor marrow transplantation. Blood 81:1923, 1993.

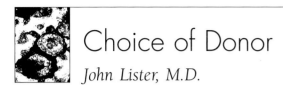

CHAPTER TWENTY-TWO

Choice of Donor

John Lister, M.D.

Criteria for donor selection remain poorly defined and validated despite extensive experience with hematopoietic stem cell (HSC) transplantation (HSCT). There is a subtle interplay among donor availability, transplant indication, and recipient status that makes it difficult to define absolute rules for donor selection. Nonetheless, given sufficient information, experienced HSCT physicians can rapidly triage possible donors.

This chapter does not attempt to exhaustively review all relevant data concerning donor selection. Rather, it addresses donor selection from the standpoint of the following questions. Once allogeneic HSCT is determined as the best treatment option for a patient, how does one select the most suitable donor from those available? The use of DNA-based typing is emphasized in this chapter. Furthermore, it addresses, selection among family donors and discusses when an extended family search might be reasonable. With respect to autologous donation, this discussion focuses on identifying candidates unlikely to achieve an adequate collection from either a blood or a bone marrow source. Selection of matched unrelated donors and umbilical cord blood units is also discussed. The final topic is a speculation about future development in the field as it might influence the decision regarding the choice of the most appropriate donor.

ALLOGENEIC HSCT

In situations in which allogeneic HSCT is preferred, a fully human leukocyte antigen (HLA)-matched sibling is the best donor when graft rejection, graft-vs.-host disease (GVHD), and transplant-related mortality are the primary concerns. If more than one family member is fully HLA-matched and does not have a transmissible infectious disease, other factors such as the sex, age, cytomegalovirus (CMV) status, ABO type, venous access for peripheral blood progenitor cell (PBPC) collection, and the presence of comorbid conditions should be considered in the selection process. The relative importance of these factors or any combination of them has not been accurately quantified. Factors that can be used in the process of selecting a donor from among those available are listed in Table 22–1.

The data are often conflicting, as illustrated by published reports on the influence of donor-recipient sex difference. Gratwohl et al., reviewing the European experience before 1990, concluded that male donors who were recipients of female marrow HSC conferred a worse survival and that recipients who received cyclosporine for GVHD prophylaxis experienced improved survival.[1] Hagglund et al., how-

ever, reported no adverse effect of female-to-male transplantation when analyzing 291 HLA-matched sibling transplants between 1975 and 1993.[2] Przepiorka et al. reported the results of allogeneic PBPC transplantation in 160 cases and found that a donor-recipient sex difference was not a determinant of more severe GVHD or worse survival.[3] These investigators also found that the use of cyclosporin and a high CD34+ cell dose were associated with a higher incidence of grade 2–4 acute GVHD.

These differences are more likely to be accounted for by technique (marrow vs. PBPC) and the introduction of tacrolimus for GVHD prophylaxis. Carlens et al. found that chronic GVHD developed more frequently in male recipients receiving HSC from immune female donors.[4] In the absence of definitive data, most clinicians would prefer the youngest donor who is CMV-negative, ABO-matched, nulliparous, and readily available. Our practice specifically targets the CMV status of the donor, if the recipient has negative CMV serology. In recipients with positive CMV serology, age, ABO-matching, and sex-matching are used as primary triage parameters.

Any donor who is acutely ill is deferred until the illness has resolved. When the donor experiences a minor illness on the collection day or shortly before, the illness is treated and the donation proceeds. Serious illness must be dealt with individually.

EXTENDED FAMILY DONOR SEARCH

Family members other than siblings can be used as HSCT donors. Given the general preference for related donors, when might an extended family search be undertaken? Patients without a sibling match but with large numbers of first and second cousins, common haplotypes, and homozygosity for HLA loci represent ideal situations for extended family searching. With knowledge of antigen frequency, linkage disequilibrium, and the size of the donor pool, it should be possible to predict the chance of finding a

TABLE 22–1. FACTORS INFLUENCING THE CHOICE OF ALLOGENEIC DONOR

Age of donor
Sex of donor and recipient
Cytomegalovirus serologic status of donor and recipient
ABO type of donor and recipient
Co-morbid condition in donor
Adequacy of venous access for peripheral blood stem cell collection

matched family donor within the extended family. Schipper et al. reported a statistical procedure for calculating the probability of finding an appropriate donor within the extended family. They codified their work in a computer program (EXTFAM).[5] A similar approach has been advocated by Kaufman.[6, 7] A rule of thumb for extended family searching that has not been validated is that, for any patient with 30 or more first and second cousins, an extended family search might be undertaken. Obviously, recombination events within the HLA complex and a multiracial pedigree might greatly reduce the chance of finding a family donor. Hence, a full family study including parental typing should be performed before second-degree relatives are typed.

HLA TYPING IN UNRELATED DONORS

When searching for an unrelated donor, molecular typing of HLA-A, -B, -C, -DR, and -DQ should be performed in all cases.[8] Recent analysis clearly shows that GVHD is greater with donor-recipient HLA-DRB1 mismatches; HLA-A, -B, and -C mismatch; and perhaps HLA-DQB1 mismatch.[9–15] Retrospective analysis of HLA-DRB1 mismatches did not include molecular class 1 typing. Therefore, enhancement of GVHD by class 1 molecular mismatch is a distinct possibility.

Recent publications revealed conflicting results on the contribution to GVHD of specific allele mismatches to GVHD.[9, 16] Sasazuki et al. reported the Japanese experience with unrelated donor transplantation when analyzed by high-resolution DNA-based typing.[9] Mismatch at HLA-A and -B was associated with an increased incidence of GVHD and decreased survival. With HLA-C mismatch, there was an increased incidence of GVHD but a balancing decrease in disease relapse that caused no difference in overall survival. Surprisingly, there was no adverse effect of mismatching at HLA-DRB1, -DQA1, -DQB1, -DPA1, and -DPB1. It is clear, however, that multilocus mismatching is associated with increased graft failure, GVHD, and transplant-related mortality.[15] The conflicting results between the Japanese and American analyses suggests that other factors are probably important in causing GVHD. The most likely candidates are minor histocompatibility antigens. Some have been more fully characterized.

Routine testing for minor histocompatibility antigens has not been extended to clinical practice. The possibility that minor histocompatibility antigens might be involved in the pathogenesis of GVHD has been considered since a female cytotoxic T-cell response was demonstrated against the H-Y antigen.[17] Subsequently, the ability of this antigen to provoke GVHD has been demonstrated.[18–21] Other antigens have been identified that may be relevant in GVHD and graft rejection.[22, 23] An understanding of the interplay between minor antigens and HLA might provide more-specific risk assessment for GVHD and allow a more-sophisticated choice among available donors. Examples of specific HLA alleles that presumably present minor antigen determinants have been published.[24–26] With the cloning of the alleles of the minor histocompatibility antigen HA-1, it is now possible to determine the alleles present in the donor and the recipient at the DNA level using a polymerase

chain reaction technique.[27] Identification of minor antigens and knowledge of their interaction with HLA molecules might allow a better typing strategy that would more accurately predict the risk of GVHD, graft rejection, and graft-vs.-tumor effects.

As a general rule, the donor and recipient should match for HLA-DRB1. Probably, HLA-A and -B alleles would be the next most important, with HLA-C and HLA-DQB1 of third priority for matching in persons of white racial background. The Japanese data suggest that HLA class 1 antigens should hold first priority for matching. The influence of HLA-DPB1 and other polymorphic genes within the HLA region is uncertain at this time. Much more remains to be learned before more specific rules for donor selection can be advanced. This is particularly true for non-white populations.

GVHD AND THE GRAFT-VERSUS-TUMOR EFFECT

In recent years, allogeneic HSCT has been increasingly employed for its immunologically mediated antitumor effect.[28–32] The immunogenetic mechanism of the graft-versus-tumor effect remains poorly understood, however. Although there is a definite association with the occurrence of GVHD, the ability to separate graft-vs.-tumor effects from GVHD still eludes us. It is tantalizing to postulate that there may be specific HLA and minor histocompatibility antigen mismatches that permit graft-vs.-tumor effects without provocation of severe GVHD. The Japanese data on HLA-C mismatching are the most encouraging to date.[9]

The many methods available for T-cell depletion have the capacity to abrogate GVHD even in the haploidentical sibling situation.[33–43] Thus, graft engineering has the potential to completely change the rules with respect to donor selection. Discussion of T cell depletion can be found in Chapter 30.

In clinical situations in which the relapse rate is very high, the choice of a less well matched donor might be associated with less risk of relapse. Aversa et al. reported results of haploidentical family donor HSCT in patients with high-risk acute leukemia.[33] All patients received highly T cell–depleted, granulocyte colony-stimulating factor (G-CSF)-mobilized PBPC (n = 43) and, in 28 cases, a bone marrow graft that was also T cell depleted. Despite a profound cellular immune deficit and the lack of GVHD, the rate of relapse was no higher and was possibly reduced in patients with acute myelogenous leukemia compared with the authors' previous experience with matched donor transplantation. Furthermore, there is a suggestion that the reconstituted natural killer and T-cell repertoire might preferentially exert a graft-versus-leukemia effect in the absence of GVHD. Unfortunately, a randomized comparison among related, unrelated, and mismatched donor HSCT in patients with high-risk malignancy is not available; however, existing data suggest that a lower relapse risk is associated with matched unrelated donor (MUD) HSCT for leukemia.[35, 44–46] These data reflect serologic HLA-typing of class 1 alleles and limited DNA-based typing of class 2 alleles. Retrospectively, DNA-based typing of donor-recipient pairs has shown that many pairs were mismatched at the allele level.[47, 48] Thus, the decreased relapse rate reported with MUD transplantation might simply be an effect of HLA mismatch. More accurate DNA-based typing might be expected to yield a higher rate of relapse, although this remains to be demonstrated. Analysis of the incidence and severity of GVHD and graft rejection suggests that the advent of DNA-based typing has reduced these complications.[9, 14–16, 44, 46, 49] Nevertheless, MUD HSCT cannot be routinely recommended for patients with a fully matched sibling.[50]

TRANSPLANTATION OF UMBILICAL CORD BLOOD HSC

Matching umbilical cord blood (UCB) units with the recipient should follow the same general rules as those applied to MUD transplantation, although there is the suggestion that UCB may have less potential to cause acute GVHD.[51–58] The ultimate incidence of chronic GVHD in the adult population after UCB HSCT remains to be defined because the majority of UCB transplantations have been performed in younger patients, who experience less GVHD. We also do not know whether specific allele mismatch has the same magnitude of effect on GVHD. Discussion of cord blood HSCT can be found in Chapter 26.

HEMATOPOIESIS IN ALLOGENEIC DONORS

Abnormal hematopoiesis in the potential donor is an absolute contraindication to donation. In the allogeneic setting, very few cases of donors with abnormal hematopoiesis have been reported, but the cases are instructive. At least one reported case of transmission of myelodysplastic hematopoiesis has been documented.[59] The donor later developed refractory anemia with del(20q) after giving HSC to her HLA-identical sister. Post-transplantation myelodysplastic hematopoiesis with identical characteristics was identified in both the donor and the recipient. The myelodysplastic HSC did not seem to be deficient in their ability to reconstitute hematopoiesis. The authors speculated that in autologous transplantation, myelodysplastic HSC have no competitive disadvantage with respect to engraftment and that if they contaminate a graft, disease relapse will occur. Barquinero et al. reported data on transplantation from donors with Down syndrome (n = 4), heterozygosity for the Fanconi syndrome (n = 4), and the 47,XXX abnormality (n = 2).[60] These were the only donors with the specified chromosomal abnormalities identified among 8488 allogeneic transplants. Poor graft function or graft failure occurred in six of eight donors with Down syndrome or heterozygosity for the Fanconi syndrome. The two 47,XXX grafts functioned normally.

The frequency of abnormal hematopoiesis is low among young allogeneic donors, certainly far less than 1%. From this standpoint alone, the testing of hematopoietic function beyond a routine complete blood count and careful review of the peripheral blood film might seem unwarranted. Nevertheless, the potential impact of transferring abnormal hematopoiesis to the recipient has continued to force us to perform a diagnostic bone marrow aspirate and biopsy on all allogeneic donors. The reader is referred to Chapter 20 for additional considerations with donor evaluation.

AUTOLOGOUS HSCT

The autologous donor may have a damaged hematopoietic reserve that prevents collection of a graft sufficient for rapid and sustained engraftment. Parameters that predict for poor graft quality include low collection-day platelet count, cytogenetic abnormalities, morphologic myelodysplasia, and extensive prior myelotoxic therapy. Table 22–2 lists factors that can be used to predict or are associated with failure to achieve an adequate stem cell collection. Visani et al. reported that patients with acute myelogenous leukemia who had received fludarabine in the treatment regimen had a markedly impaired capacity to mobilize HSC.[61] Morton et al. reported that a low collection-day platelet count, previous radiation therapy, and alkylating agent therapy impaired the ability to collect PBSC.[62] Bone marrow that is frankly myelodysplastic should preclude autologous donation. A clonal cytogenetic abnormality should also be an absolute contraindication to autologous donation, unless the abnormality is constitutional and benign. Certainly, genetic abnormalities associated with marrow dysfunction should preclude donation. The presence of pancytopenia is often a measure of the marrow reserve and predicts for a poor mobilizing capacity and ability to reconstitute hematopoiesis. All of these adverse factors are more likely to be present when the history includes extensive prior myelotoxic therapy.

Data that indirectly support these contraindications come from patients undergoing HSCT for lymphoma who experienced myelodysplasia post transplantation. There was concordance of cytogenetic abnormalities before and after autologous transplantation, which suggested that the myelodysplasia was a consequence of cytotoxic therapy received before transplant conditioning was given.[63–66] Our own experience at the Western Pennsylvania Cancer Institute shows that chemotherapy given in conjunction with G-CSF for HSC mobilization causes a variable increase in peripheral blood CD34 count. Collections performed on days when the peripheral blood CD34 count was $>25/mm^3$ or greater reliably gave a total of at least 10^6 CD34+ cells/kg of recipient body weight.[67] It is our practice to limit leukapheresis to days when this target is reached. Similar analyses of CD34+ cell kinetic data allow optimization of PBPL collection.[68–73] The reader is referred to

TABLE 22–2. FACTORS INFLUENCING THE SUCCESS OF AUTOLOGOUS DONATION

Extent of prior myelotoxic therapy
Peripheral blood counts (pancytopenia)
Myelodysplasia on bone marrow examination
Clonal cytogenetic abnormality
Type of mobilization regimen
  Growth factor alone
  Chemotherapy + growth factor
  Escalated growth factor dose
  Intensified chemotherapy regimen

Chapter 25 for a detailed discussion of HSC mobilization and collection.

Bone marrow harvesting to supplement inadequate PBPC collections and vice versa does not seem to make up for an inadequate collection.[74] Some patients may benefit from an additional collection, but engraftment is delayed and the long-term outcome, particularly the incidence of myelodysplasia and secondary leukemia, is not known.[75, 76] Preliminary data suggest that a second attempt at stem cell mobilization with more-intensive chemotherapy might be worthwhile in selected patients.[77, 78] Other investigators have reported successful mobilization with increased doses of G-CSF or a combination of GM-CSF and G-CSF after a first failed attempt.[79, 80] Hasegawa et al.[81] reported control of hematopoietic progenitor cell mobilization by loci on chromosomes 2 and 11 in mice. Identification of similar loci in humans might allow for specific methods of mobilization based on these as yet unidentified traits.

CONCLUSION

Autologous HSCT should only be performed when an adequate graft is collected. The graft should provide rapid reconstitution of hematopoiesis that should be sustained. The most important factor that prevents adequate collection of HSC is extensive myelotoxic therapy prior to mobilization. This fact would argue for the earlier application of autologous HSCT in any malignant disease course, before cytotoxic therapy has compromised marrow function.

Fully HLA-matched related donors are preferred for allogeneic transplantation. With graft T cell–depletion techniques, however, it is possible to perform mismatched transplantation up to the haploidentical family member. The effect of mismatching at HLA loci and at minor antigen loci opens up the possibility of immunogenetic manipulation of the graft-versus-tumor effect. This effect might be strengthened or perhaps dependent on specific HLA-allele or minor antigen mismatch. In high-risk malignancy, a mismatched graft might offer improved disease-free survival if infectious and other complications were more effectively prevented. The relationship of malignant disease biology, particularly the presentation of novel tumor antigens, to the immunogenetics of HLA and minor antigen matching remains largely undefined.

REFERENCES

1. Gratwohl A, Hermans J, Lyklema A, Zwaan FE: Bone marrow transplantation for leukaemia in Europe. Folia Haematol Int Mag Klin Morphol Blutforsch 116:353, 1989.
2. Hagglund H, Bostrom L, Remberger M, et al: Risk factors for acute graft-versus-host disease in 291 consecutive HLA-identical bone marrow transplant recipients. Bone Marrow Transplant 16:747, 1995.
3. Przepiorka D, Smith TL, Folloder J, et al: Risk factors for acute graft-versus-host disease after allogeneic blood stem cell transplantation. Blood 94:1465, 1999.
4. Carlens S, Ringden O, Remberger M, et al: Risk factors for chronic graft-versus-host disease after bone marrow transplantation: a retrospective single centre analysis. Bone Marrow Transplant 22:755, 1998.
5. Schipper RF, D'Amaro J, Oudshoorn M: The probability of finding a suitable related donor for bone marrow transplantation in extended families [see comments]. Blood 87:800, 1996.
6. Kaufman R: HLA prediction model for extended family matches. Bone Marrow Transplant 15:279, 1995.

7. Kaufman R: A generalized HLA prediction model for related donor matches. Bone Marrow Transplant 17:1013, 1996.
8. Hurley CK, Wade JA, Oudshoorn M, et al: Histocompatibility testing guidelines for hematopoietic stem cell transplantation using volunteer donors: report from The World Marrow Donor Association—Quality Assurance and Donor Registries Working Groups of the World Marrow Donor Association. Bone Marrow Transplant 24:119, 1999.
9. Sasazuki T, Juji T, Morishima Y, et al: Effect of matching of class I HLA alleles on clinical outcome after transplantation of hematopoietic stem cells from an unrelated donor. Japan Marrow Donor Program [see comments] [published erratum appears in N Engl J Med 1999 Feb 4;340(5):402]. N Engl J Med 339:1177, 1998.
10. Petersdorf EW, Smith AG, Mickelson EM, et al: The role of HLA-DPB 1 disparity in the development of acute graft-versus-host disease following unrelated donor marrow transplantation. Blood 81:1923, 1993.
11. Petersdorf EW, Longton GM, Anasetti C, et al: The significance of HLA-DRB1 matching on clinical outcome after HLA-A, B, DR identical unrelated donor marrow transplantation. Blood 86:1606, 1995.
12. Petersdorf EW, Longton GM, Anasetti C, et al: Definition of HLA-DQ as a transplantation antigen. Proc Natl Acad Sci U S A 93:15358, 1996.
13. Petersdorf EW, Longton GM, Anasetti C, et al: Association of HLA-C disparity with graft failure after marrow transplantation from unrelated donors. Blood 89:1818, 1997.
14. Petersdorf E, Anasetti C, Servida P, et al: Effect of HLA matching on outcome of related and unrelated donor transplantation therapy for chronic myelogenous leukemia. Hematol Oncol Clin North Am 12:107, 1998.
15. Petersdorf EW, Mickelson EM, Anasetti C, et al: Effect of HLA mismatches on the outcome of hematopoietic transplants. Curr Opin Immunol 11:521, 1999.
16. Petersdorf EW, Gooley TA, Anasetti C, et al: Optimizing outcome after unrelated marrow transplantation by comprehensive matching of HLA class I and II alleles in the donor and recipient. Blood 92:3515, 1998.
17. Goulmy E, Termijtelen A, Bradley BA, van Rood JJ: Y-antigen killing by T cells of women is restricted by HLA. Nature 266:544, 1977.
18. Goulmy E, Blokland E, van Rood J, et al: Production, expansion, and clonal analysis of T cells with specific HLA-restricted male lysis. J Exp Med 152:182s, 1980.
19. Goulmy E, Gratama JW, Blokland E, et al: A minor transplantation antigen detected by MHC-restricted cytotoxic T lymphocytes during graft-versus-host disease. Nature 302:159, 1983.
20. Goulmy E, Schipper R, Pool J, et al: Mismatches of minor histocompatibility antigens between HLA-identical donors and recipients and the development of graft-versus-host disease after bone marrow transplantation [see comments]. N Engl J Med 334:281, 1996.
21. Perreault C, Decary F, Brochu S, et al: Minor histocompatibility antigens. Blood 76:1269, 1990.
22. Balduini CL, Noris P, Giorgiani G, et al: Incompatibility for CD31 and human platelet antigens and acute graft-versus-host disease after bone marrow transplantation. Br J Haematol 106:723, 1999.
23. den Haan JM, Meadows LM, Wang W, et al: The minor histocompatibility antigen HA-1: a diallelic gene with a single amino acid polymorphism. Science 279:1054, 1998.
24. Pierce RA, Field ED, den Haan JM, et al: Cutting edge: the HLA-A*0101-restricted HY minor histocompatibility antigen originates from DFFRY and contains a cysteinylated cysteine residue as identified by a novel mass spectrometric technique. J Immunol 163:6360, 1999.
25. Rufer N, Wolpert E, Helg C, et al: HA-1 and the SMCY-derived peptide FIDSYICQV (H-Y) are immunodominant minor histocompatibility antigens after bone marrow transplantation. Transplantation 66:910, 1998.
26. Tseng LH, Lin MT, Hansen JA, et al: Correlation between disparity for the minor histocompatibility antigen HA-1 and the development of acute graft-versus-host disease after allogeneic marrow transplantation. Blood 94:2911, 1999.
27. Wilke M, Pool J, den Haan JM, Goulmy E: Genomic identification of the minor histocompatibility antigen HA-1 locus by allele-specific PCR [see comments]. Tissue Antigens 52:312, 1998.
28. Giralt S, Estey E, Albitar M, et al: Engraftment of allogeneic hematopoietic progenitor cells with purine analog-containing chemotherapy: harnessing graft-versus-leukemia without myeloablative therapy. Blood 89:4531, 1997.

29. Khouri IF, Keating M, Körbling M, et al: Transplant-lite: induction of graft-versus-malignancy using fludarabine-based nonablative chemotherapy and allogeneic blood progenitor-cell transplantation as treatment for lymphoid malignancies. J Clin Oncol 16:2817, 1998.

30. van Besien KW, de Lima M, Giralt SA, et al: Management of lymphoma recurrence after allogeneic transplantation: the relevance of graft-versus-lymphoma effect. Bone Marrow Transplant 19:977, 1997.

31. Kapelushnik J, Or R, Slavin S, Nagler A: A fludarabine-based protocol for bone marrow transplantation in Fanconi's anemia. Bone Marrow Transplant 20:1109, 1997.

32. Slavin S, Nagler A, Naparstek E, et al: Nonmyeloablative stem cell transplantation and cell therapy as an alternative to conventional bone marrow transplantation with lethal cytoreduction for the treatment of malignant and nonmalignant hematologic diseases. Blood 91:756, 1998.

33. Aversa F, Tabilio A, Velardi A, et al: Treatment of high-risk acute leukemia with T-cell-depleted stem cells from related donors with one fully mismatched HLA haplotype [see comments]. N Engl J Med 339:1186, 1998.

34. Gajewski J, Gjertson D, Cecka M, et al: The impact of T-cell depletion on the effects of HLA DR beta 1 and DQ beta allele matching in HLA serologically identical unrelated donor bone marrow transplantation. Biol Blood Marrow Transplant 3:76, 1997.

35. Hessner MJ, Endean DJ, Casper JT, et al: Use of unrelated marrow grafts compensates for reduced graft-versus-leukemia reactivity after T-cell-depleted allogeneic marrow transplantation for chronic myelogenous leukemia. Blood 86:3987, 1995.

36. Reisner Y, Bachar-Lustig E, Li HW, et al: The role of megadose CD34+ progenitor cells in the treatment of leukemia patients without a matched donor and in tolerance induction for organ transplantation. Ann N Y Acad Sci 872:336, 1999.

37. Henslee-Downey PJ, Gluckman E: Allogeneic transplantation from donors other than HLA-identical siblings. Hematol Oncol Clin North Am 13:1017, 1999.

38. Henslee-Downey PJ, Abhyankar SH, Parrish RS, et al: Use of partially mismatched related donors extends access to allogeneic marrow transplant. Blood 89:3864, 1997.

39. Bishop MR, Henslee-Downey PJ, Anderson JR, et al: Long-term survival in advanced chronic myelogenous leukemia following bone marrow transplantation from haploidentical related donors. Bone Marrow Transplant 18:747, 1996.

40. Fleming DR, Henslee-Downey PJ, Romond EH, et al: Allogeneic bone marrow transplantation with T cell–depleted partially matched related donors for advanced acute lymphoblastic leukemia in children and adults: a comparative matched cohort study. Bone Marrow Transplant 17:917, 1996.

41. Godder K, Pati A, Abhyankar S, et al: Partially mismatched related donor transplants as salvage therapy for patients with refractory leukemia who relapse post-BMT. Bone Marrow Transplant 17:49, 1996.

42. O'Reilly RJ: Bone marrow transplants in patients lacking an HLA-matched sibling donor. Pediatr Ann 20:682, 1991.

43. O'Reilly RJ: T-cell depletion and allogeneic bone marrow transplantation. Semin Hematol 29:20, 1992.

44. Heslop HE: Haemopoietic stem cell transplantation from unrelated donors. Br J Haematol 105:2, 1999.

45. Beatty PG, Anasetti C, Hansen JA, et al: Marrow transplantation from unrelated donors for treatment of hematologic malignancies: effect of mismatching for one HLA locus. Blood 81:249, 1993.

46. Hansen JA, Petersdorf E, Martin PJ, Anasetti C: Hematopoietic stem cell transplants from unrelated donors. Immunol Rev 157:141, 1997.

47. Prasad VK, Kernan NA, Heller G, et al: DNA typing for HLA-A and HLA-B identifies disparities between patients and unrelated donors matched by HLA-A and HLA-B serology and HLA-DRB1. Blood 93:399, 1999.

48. Mytilineos J, Lempert M, Scherer S, et al: Comparison of serological and DNA PCR-SSP typing results for HLA-A and HLA-B in 421 black individuals: a Collaborative Transplant Study report. Hum Immunol 59:512, 1998.

49. Kernan NA, Bartsch G, Ash RC, et al: Analysis of 462 transplantations from unrelated donors facilitated by the National Marrow Donor Program [see comments]. N Engl J Med 328:593, 1993.

50. Szydlo R, Goldman JM, Klein JP, et al: Results of allogeneic bone marrow transplants for leukemia using donors other than HLA-identical siblings. J Clin Oncol 15:1767, 1997.

51. Abecasis MM, Machado AM, Boavida G, et al: Haploidentical cord blood transplant contaminated with maternal T cells in a patient with advanced leukemia. Bone Marrow Transplant 17:891, 1996.

52. Arcese W, Guglielmi C, Iori AP, et al: Umbilical cord blood transplant from unrelated HLA-mismatched donors in children with high risk leukemia. Bone Marrow Transplant 23:549, 1999.

53. Elia L, Arcese W, Torello M, et al: HLA-C and HLA-DQB1 compatibility in unrelated cord blood transplants. Haematologica 84:530, 1999.

54. Gluckman E, Rocha V, Boyer-Chammard A, et al: Outcome of cord-blood transplantation from related and unrelated donors. Eurocord Transplant Group and the European Blood and Marrow Transplantation Group. N Engl J Med 337:373, 1997.

55. Kato S, Nishihira H, Sako M, et al: Cord blood transplantation from sibling donors in Japan: report of the national survey. Int J Hematol 67:389, 1998.

56. Kurtzberg J, Laughlin M, Graham ML, et al: Placental blood as a source of hematopoietic stem cells for transplantation into unrelated recipients [see comments]. N Engl J Med 335:157, 1996.

57. Nishihira H, Ohnuma K, Ikuta K, et al: Unrelated umbilical cord-blood stem cell transplantation: a report from Kanagawa Cord Blood Bank, Japan. Int J Hematol 68:193, 1998.

58. Wagner JE, Rosenthal J, Sweetman R, et al: Successful transplantation of HLA-matched and HLA mismatched umbilical cord blood from unrelated donors: analysis of engraftment and acute graft-versus-host disease. Blood 88:795, 1996.

59. Mielcarek M, Bryant E, Loken M, et al: Haemopoietic reconstitution by donor-derived myelodysplastic progenitor cells after haemopoietic stem cell transplantation. Br J Haematol 105:361, 1999.

60. Barquinero J, Witherspoon R, Sanders J, et al: Allogeneic marrow grafts from donors with congenital chromosomal abnormalities in marrow cells. Br J Haematol 90:595, 1995.

61. Visani G, Lemoli RM, Tosi P, et al: Fludarabine-containing regimens severely impair peripheral blood stem cells mobilization and collection in acute myeloid leukaemia patients. Br J Haematol 105:775, 1999.

62. Morton J, Morton A, Bird R, et al: Predictors for optimal mobilization and subsequent engraftment of peripheral blood progenitor cells following intermediate dose cyclophosphamide and G-CSF. Leuk Res 21:21, 1997.

63. Abruzzese E, Radford JE, Miller JS, et al: Detection of abnormal pretransplant clones in progenitor cells of patients who developed myelodysplasia after autologous transplantation. Blood 94:1814, 1999.

64. Sobecks RM, Le Beau MM, Anastasi J, Williams SF: Myelodysplasia and acute leukemia following high-dose chemotherapy and autologous bone marrow or peripheral blood stem cell transplantation. Bone Marrow Transplant 23:1161, 1999.

65. Traweek ST, Slovak ML, Nademanee AP, et al: Myelodysplasia and acute myeloid leukemia occurring after autologous bone marrow transplantation for lymphoma. Leuk Lymphoma 20:365, 1996.

66. Amigo ML, del Canizo MC, Rios A, et al: Diagnosis of secondary myelodysplastic syndromes (MDS) following autologous transplantation should not be based only on morphological criteria used for diagnosis of de novo MDS. Bone Marrow Transplant 23:997, 1999.

67. Shadduck RK, Zeigler ZR, Andrews DF, et al: Mobilization and transplantation of peripheral blood stem cells. Stem Cells 16:145, 1998.

68. Armitage S, Hargreaves R, Samson D, et al: CD34 counts to predict the adequate collection of peripheral blood progenitor cells [see comments]. Bone Marrow Transplant 20:587, 1997.

69. D'Arena G, Musto P, Cascavilla N, et al: Circulating CD34+ absolute cell number is the best single parameter to predict the quality of leukapheretic yield [Letter; Comment]. Bone Marrow Transplant 22:215, 1998.

70. de Fabritiis P, Gonzalez M, Meloni G, et al: Monitoring of CD34+ cells during leukapheresis allows a single, successful collection of hemopoietic progenitors in patients with low numbers of circulating stem cells. Bone Marrow Transplant 23:1229, 1999.

71. Elliott C, Samson DM, Armitage S, et al: When to harvest peripheral-blood stem cells after mobilization therapy: prediction of CD34-positive cell yield by preceding day CD34-positive concentration in peripheral blood. J Clin Oncol 14:970, 1996.

72. Le Corroller AG, Moatti JP, Chabannon C, et al: Optimization of peripheral blood stem cell collection by leukapheresis: interaction between economic and clinical assessment of an innovation. Int J Technol Assess Health Care 15:161, 1999.

73. Leibundgut K, von Rohr A, Brulhart K, et al: The number of circulating CD34+ blood cells predicts the colony-forming capacity of leukapheresis products in children. Bone Marrow Transplant 15:25, 1995.

74. Watts MJ, Sullivan AM, Leverett D, et al: Back-up bone marrow is frequently ineffective in patients with poor peripheral-blood stem-cell mobilization. J Clin Oncol 16:1554, 1998.

75. Scott MA, Ager S, Jestice HK, et al: Failure to mobilise and harvest PBPC does not necessarily preclude the use of high-dose therapy and autologous stem cell rescue [Letter]. Bone Marrow Transplant 15:487, 1995.

76. Aurran-Schleinitz T, Chabannon C, Faucher C, et al: Bone marrow and blood cells as alternative sources of hematopoietic progenitors after failure of a first collection: a single institution retrospective study. Transplantation 61:518, 1996.

77. Klein J, Rey P, Dansey R, et al: Cyclophosphamide and paclitaxel as initial or salvage regimen for the mobilization of peripheral blood progenitor cells. Bone Marrow Transplant 24:959, 1999.

78. Reiser M, Josting A, Draube A, et al: Successful peripheral blood stem cell mobilization with etoposide (VP-16) in patients with relapsed or resistant lymphoma who failed cyclophosphamide mobilization. Bone Marrow Transplant 23:1223, 1999.

79. Gazitt Y, Freytes CO, Callander N, et al: Successful PBSC mobilization with high-dose G-CSF for patients failing a first round of mobilization. J Hematother 8:173, 1999.

80. Bashey A, Corringham S, Gilpin E, et al: Simultaneous administration of G-CSF and GM-CSF for re-mobilization in patients with inadequate initial progenitor cell collections for autologous transplantation. Cytotherapy 2:195, 2000.

81. Hasegawa M, Baldwin TM, Metcalfe D, Foote SJ: Progenitor cell mobilization by granulocyte colony-stimulating factor controlled by loci on chromosomes 2 and 11. Blood 95:1872–1874, 2000.

Vascular Access

CHAPTER TWENTY-THREE

Long-Term Venous Access During Hematopoietic Stem Cell Transplantation

Joshua Rubin, M.D.

INDICATIONS FOR CATHETER INSERTION

Patients undergoing hematopoietic stem cell transplant (HSCT) require multiple intravenous agents during their prolonged and intensive period of treatment. They require the placement of multilumen central venous catheters to facilitate the administration of cytotoxic drugs, fluids, antibiotics, antiemetics, parenteral nutrition, and blood products.[1, 2]

CATHETER TYPES AND THEIR SELECTION

There are several types of central venous catheters, differing in design, gauge, number of lumens, and material of construction. These differences determine which device is most appropriate for a particular patient.

Short-term central venous access can be established by the placement of single- or multiple-lumen polyurethane or polyethylene catheters. These are not suited for use beyond about 7 days because they are relatively stiff and are not designed with a Dacron cuff, which adds to long-term stability. For patients who require venous access for a longer period of time, a soft silicone catheter can be placed through the cephalic, subclavian, external jugular, or internal jugular vein and can remain in place for up to 4 weeks (as per the manufacturer). A percutaneous indwelling central catheter line is an alternative to central venous catheter placement. This single- or double-lumen catheter is advanced centrally via an antecubital vein and can remain in place for 1 month. All of these catheters can be placed using local anesthesia without x-ray guidance.

Patients who require venous access for longer than 4 weeks may be more appropriately treated with a tunneled central venous Hickman[1] or Groshong catheter or a subcutaneous port.[2] These implants can be left in place for more than a year with appropriate care. Their insertion is more complicated, however, because fluoroscopic guidance is recommended and a subcutaneous pocket or tunnel must be fashioned. These catheters are surgically implanted in an operating or special procedure room and usually administered under IV sedation in addition to local anesthesia.

What distinguishes tunneled catheters from subcutaneous ports is the presence or absence of an external component. It is important to select the most appropriate device for each patient. Both Hickman and Groshong catheters are placed through a subcutaneous tunnel with the catheter exiting the skin over the chest anteriorly. The catheter is connected directly to IV tubing for the administration of medications or it can be accessed with a needle for blood collection. Ports are buried in a subcutaneous pocket over the anterior upper chest and can only be accessed percutaneously with a noncoring Huber needle. These two types of long-term venous catheters are generally recommended for patients who will rarely, if ever, be disconnected from an IV infusion, including patients with hematologic malignancy who are expected to require antibiotics, parenteral nutrition, intravenous fluids, or intensive blood product support for the duration of their extended hospital stay. External tunneled catheters are also better suited for coagulopathic or thrombocytopenic patients who are likely to bleed into the subcutaneous pocket of a port.

Several potential advantages are associated with ports. Patients are not encumbered by an external catheter that requires at least some protection, lest it be pulled out. Ports require flushing only once every 4 weeks in order to maintain their patency, unlike external catheters, which should be flushed with heparin every 1–7 days. Although patients must exercise some care with external catheters during bathing, no precautions are required for patients with ports. We generally recommend ports to patients with limited venous access who require intermittent or limited continuous venous access over a long period of time. These devices are ideally suited for patients who need weekly or monthly chemotherapy and frequent phlebotomy.

Other differences among venous catheters are important for patient selection. Catheters may be open-ended or valved. The lumen of the latter is isolated from the bloodstream by a two-way valve located on the side of the catheter rather than the tip. The theoretical advantage of a valve is that blood cannot make its way into the catheter, obviating the need for heparin flushes to maintain catheter patency. Neither we nor others have noted a significant advantage to the use of these valved, or Groshong, catheters.[3, 4]

Catheters are available with one, two, or three lumens. Subcutaneous ports are only available as one- or two-lumen catheters. One should recommend the smallest number of lumens thought to be necessary for treatment because multiple lumens are associated with a slightly higher incidence of infection and venous thrombosis.[5]

Patients undergoing autologous HSCT will require a large-bore pheresis catheter to facilitate peripheral blood apheresis. A large-gauge (13 French) double-lumen catheter allows adequate blood flow and can be used for the subsequent administration of high-dose chemotherapy and supportive care medications. Patients undergoing allogeneic HSCT require a triple-lumen Hickman or Groshong catheter to allow the administration of multiple pharmaceutical agents, blood products, and fluids.

PREOPERATIVE PREPARATION

Percutaneous indwelling central catheter lines and Hohn catheters are almost always placed at the bedside using local anesthesia. More-permanent catheters are usually inserted in an operating room or a special procedure unit because fluoroscopy is recommended for their safe and reliable placement. In addition to local anesthesia, we prefer to administer IV sedation to patients undergoing long-term catheter placement in order to make the procedure less unpleasant.

Before any of these devices is placed, a review of pertinent systems, past medical history, and physical examination is indicated to minimize the risk of procedure-related complications. Previous mastectomy, a history of chest wall radiation therapy, previous axillary dissection, or the presence of a breast prosthesis could affect the technique of catheter placement. Subcutaneous ports should be placed on the side opposite an irradiated chest wall because radiation therapy may impair healing of the subcutaneous pocket. Mastectomy flaps may be thin and interfere with the creation of an adequate pocket for a port. If possible, the port should be placed on the side opposite the mastectomy. Previous axillary dissection may impair lymphatic drainage of the anterior chest wall and could predispose to infection. A breast implant, particularly one that rides high on the chest wall, could make placement of a subcutaneous port or an external tunneled catheter difficult, and the prosthesis could be inadvertently injured during the procedure. For this reason, one should avoid placing a device on the side of a breast implant. Anatomic deformities such as previous head trauma or neck dissection could make percutaneous placement of a venous catheter dangerous or technically challenging. Catheters may be placed more safely in these patients by venous cutdown. We and others find ultrasound guidance for routine catheter placement unnecessary and no safer than using anatomic landmarks or venous cutdown.[6] Other conditions of potential importance include spinal metastases or a severe cold.

A history of central venous catheterization is important because occult venous thrombosis or scarring could have developed. Patients should be asked about arm edema or documented venous thrombosis, both of which should prompt a noninvasive evaluation of the veins prior to catheter placement. A history of difficult central venous catheter placement or a technical complication resulting from its placement might alter the surgeon's usual approach to placing these devices.

Patients with a history of heparin-induced thrombocytopenia are perhaps better treated through a valved central venous catheter, which purportedly can be flushed with normal saline alone. Patients who have recently been treated with chemotherapy should be evaluated for neutropenia, if appropriate, before catheter insertion, because neutropenia is an independent risk factor for catheter-related infection.[1] It is prudent to delay placement of a long-term catheter in patients whose neutropenia is thought to be reversible. Patients with an ongoing coagulapathy can safely undergo placement of a tunneled central venous catheter, but placing subcutaneous ports should be avoided because the risk of bleeding into the pocket is probably increased.

Unless the catheter is being placed for long-term administration of antibiotics, patients should be evaluated for ongoing infection. Physical examination should include a detailed evaluation of the skin in search of abscesses or cellulitis. Patients with an unexplained cough should be evaluated for pneumonia if clinically appropriate. Unexplained fever should prompt evaluation in order to identify heretofore unrecognized infection. This can be difficult in the setting of tumor-related fever or fever in patients with leukemia. Clinical judgment should be exercised in differentiating this from infection so as to avoid unnecessary delay of therapy. In febrile patients with leukemia, placement of a central venous catheter is occasionally undertaken after a short course of antibiotics when such patients need urgent chemotherapy. For patients with infection who require venous access even for the administration of antibiotics, a temporary central venous catheter can be placed for several days in order to eradicate the infection with antibiotics. Later, the temporary catheter is removed and a more-permanent catheter is placed at another site, provided the patient remains afebrile.

Arm or facial edema noted on physical examination could be a manifestation of venous occlusion resulting from lymphadenopathy or scarring as a result of previous central venous catheters. This finding should be evaluated by Doppler ultrasonography of the great veins of the chest and neck prior to catheter placement. Clinical suspicion of superior vena cava obstruction due to lymphadenopathy in patients with lymphoma should prompt evaluation of the chest by computed tomography in order to determine whether the superior vena cava is patent. Superior vena cava syndrome is a contraindication to placement of a central venous catheter, and a venous access catheter should be inserted in the femoral vein until the superior caval obstruction is eliminated.

The risk of bleeding complications increases in patients with an ongoing coagulapathy. Findings of petechiae or ecchymosis on physical examination or clinical settings associated with coagulation disorders should prompt further evaluation of the patient's platelet count, prothrombin time, and international normalized ratio. There is little agreement concerning preoperative treatment of thrombocytopenia or coagulopathy. Many surgeons recommend platelet transfusions for patients whose platelet count is less than 50,000. It is also recommended that patients with an international normalized ratio exceeding 1.5 be treated with fresh frozen plasma or vitamin K prior to placement of a central venous catheter. Obviously, the risk of bleeding complications in these patients must be reconciled with the skill of the practitioner who is placing the catheter and the urgency of establishing venous access. Some reports suggest that central venous catheters can be safely placed with thrombocytopenia or coagulation disorders far worse than these arbitrary guidelines just listed, and we commonly place catheters in patients with leukemia whose platelet counts are close to 20,000.

Preprocedure laboratory evaluation should be based on the history, physical examination, and level of clinical suspicion regarding the presence of either infection or a coagulation disorder. For patients with dysuria, a urinalysis should be obtained in order to rule out urinary tract infection.

TECHNIQUE OF CATHETER PLACEMENT

The technique of catheter placement has been well described in a variety of sources and is dealt with only briefly here. Percutaneous indwelling central catheter lines and Hohn catheters can be inserted using local anesthesia. Long-term tunneled catheters and ports can either be placed percutaneously through any of the major chest or neck veins or be placed by venous cutdown. The latter approach makes pneumothorax or inadvertent injury to a major vascular structure unlikely. Percutaneous placement of a catheter into the subclavian, internal jugular, external jugular, or even the cephalic veins is much quicker than venous cutdown and, in experienced hands, the risks of major vascular injury and pneumothorax are exceedingly small.[5] We generally reserve venous cutdown for patients whose subclavian vein cannot be easily identified for percutaneous catheter placement or for patients who cannot lie supine. It is also useful for patients with deformities of the chest or neck in whom percutaneous access may be difficult or dangerous.

We recommend intravenous sedation for patients who require placement of a tunneled catheter or a port so that anesthesia is more adequate. Tunneled catheters and subcutaneous ports are placed under fluoroscopic guidance in order to ensure that the tip of the catheter is situated in the very distal superior vena cava. We also use fluoroscopy to monitor placement of the introducer sheath and dilator because these devices are stiff and can easily result in major vascular injury if their progress during insertion is not closely monitored.

The catheter exit site for an external catheter and the subcutaneous pocket for a port should be positioned well away from the breast and particularly the nipple so that movement of the device is minimal and a dressing can be applied without placement of adhesive over the nipple. All patients should be evaluated by upright chest radiograph after insertion of a central venous catheter in order to document the position of the catheter and to rule out the presence of a pneumothorax. In patients whose ports will be used soon after placement, the device should be accessed with a Huber needle intraoperatively while the skin is still anesthetized. This obviates the need to manipulate the tender operative site soon after the procedure.

COMPLICATIONS

The number of described complications resulting from placement of a venous access device is large and varies with the expertise of the surgeon and the technique of catheter placement. Fortunately, their incidence is exceedingly small. Pneumothorax occurs when the insertion needle is placed underneath the clavicle at too acute an angle. This is rarely recognized intraoperatively unless air is aspirated from the syringe in the course of the procedure. Most pneumothoraces are identified on the postoperative chest radiograph, although they may not present for several days. Patients with clinically significant pneumothoraces generally experience chest pain, shoulder pain, or shortness of breath. Rarely, untreated pneumothoraces progress to tension pneumothorax, a life-threatening lesion requiring emergency therapy. Attention to orientation of the needle in relation to the clavicle should make this complication very infrequent; it never occurs when catheters are placed by venous cutdown. The use of ultrasound guidance during placement of a venous access catheter via the subclavian vein is no protection against this complication. A pneumothorax in excess of 20% or progressive pneumothorax should be treated by placement of a percutaneous catheter under local anesthesia. The air leak usually resolves within several days, provided the lung is fully expanded.

Bleeding rarely complicates placement of central venous catheters. Puncture of the subclavian artery by the needle is not common and is usually of little consequence in patients who are not coagulopathic. Placement of a large dilator and introducer sheath into the subclavian artery, however, is more likely to be associated with clinically significant arterial injury and may require operative repair. This applies to the carotid artery as well when catheter placement is attempted through the neck. Arterial injury at the time of arterial puncture should always be recognized by the surgeon because the aspirated blood is usually more red and its flow is pulsatile. Findings on postoperative chest radiograph that might suggest arterial injury include an apical cap or mediastinal widening.

Other intraoperative misadventures include venous injury due to inappropriate use of the guidewire or unmonitored advancement of the dilator. Major venous injury is usually well tolerated because the intravascular pressure is low. Findings on postoperative chest radiograph might include widening of the mediastinum. This is usually self-limited, and therefore initial therapy consists of avoiding the supine position and obtaining serial chest radiographs. Early postoperative bleeding in patients with subcutaneous ports can create a hematoma in the pocket. This often stops spontaneously and sometimes can be treated expectantly. More-substantial bleeding should be managed by re-exploration of the subcutaneous pocket and establishment of hemostasis.

Catheter malfunction may be due to a variety of conditions. One of the most common causes is kinking of the external limb of the catheter, which is more common with stiffer polyurethane catheters. Repositioning the catheter invariably corrects this problem. If sutures are used to hold the catheter in place, they may compromise the catheter lumen and obstruct it. Replacing the suture with one tied less tightly is usually enough to correct this problem unless the catheter has been fractured.

Placement of a central venous catheter via the subclavian vein should be performed lateral to the costoclavicular ligament. More-medial placement can predispose to compression of the catheter between the clavicle and the first rib.[8] This may lead to inflow or outflow occlusion in certain cases. More-chronic compression has led to catheter fracture and embolism of the venous limb of the catheter into the right ventricle. The contour of the catheter should be evaluated intraoperatively under fluoroscopy, and if the catheter is compressed, it should be repositioned at that time. Minor degrees of compression can probably be tolerated and are of little clinical significance.

The position of the catheter tip can affect catheter function. It is advised that the tip of the catheter be placed in the distal superior vena cava. Some surgeons suggest that the softer catheters can be safely placed at the atriocaval junction or perhaps just within the right atrium. Postoperative catheter migration into the azygos vein and internal jugular vein has occurred and can lead to either vascular injury or catheter malfunction. We generally recommend to patients that malpositioned catheters be reoriented. This can usually be accomplished percutaneously by an interventional radiologist.

External catheters, particularly Hickman and Groshong catheters, cannot be easily dislodged when traction is applied to their external limb because they are fashioned with a Dacron cuff, which stabilizes them after 1 or 2 months because of scar tissue. A catheter that becomes dislodged, however, should be removed if the cuffs are externalized. If not, the position of the catheter should be evaluated by chest radiograph. The catheter can still be used if its tip is in reasonably good position.

Catheter fracture can result from several circumstances. External catheters are fashioned with clamps in order to occlude the catheter when not in use. These clamps should be secured on the catheter in the designated position, not too close to the hub. Placement of the clamp close to the hub can actually fracture the catheter at this site. External catheters can also be fractured if undue tension is applied to them. Finally, catheters can be fractured if flushed with excessive force. It is recommended that nothing smaller than a 10- mL syringe be used to flush central venous catheters. Smaller syringes generate pressures within the catheter that may exceed the tensile strength of the catheter wall.

The most common late catheter-related complications are catheter occlusion and infection. Inability to aspirate through the central venous catheter is most commonly due to either lumenal clot or a fibrin sheath that lines the catheter surface, extends beyond its tip, and acts as a one-way valve when negative pressure is applied to the lumen of the catheter.[9] Constant care must be taken to prevent this complication by regularly flushing ports and catheters with heparinized saline solution. It is recommended that external catheters be flushed daily and that ports be flushed at least monthly. There is no good evidence that these complications are less frequent in patients with valved catheters. Low doses of warfarin (1 mg/day) have been shown to significantly decrease the incidence of catheter-related thrombosis and venous occlusion.[10]

Dysfunctional catheters should be evaluated by chest radiograph early on to document migration of the catheter tip or compression of the catheter between the first rib and clavicle. As mentioned earlier, catheters can be repositioned percutaneously under fluoroscopic guidance. Catheters

caught between the clavicle and rib should be replaced if they do not function well.

Treatment of catheter thrombosis or a fibrin sheath is generally suboptimal. The catheter can be flushed using tissue plasminogen activator (TPA). TPA has replaced urokinase, which is currently unavailable. TPA, in a volume adequate to fill the catheter lumen, is allowed to dwell for 30 minutes and is then aspirated. This procedure can be repeated until good blood return is established. If this treatment is unsuccessful, refer the patient to interventional radiology for catheter stripping. To accomplish this, a snare is passed through the femoral vein and is used to grasp the central venous catheter to strip it free of clot. Stripping is also useful for management of a fibrin sheath. Unfortunately, these approaches usually result in transient correction of the problem, and a fibrin sheath or intraluminal clot frequently recurs. The decision to place a new catheter can be difficult and must account for the expected period of time that the catheter will be required as well as the risk of catheter placement.

Extravasation of infusate is an unusual complication. It can occur if the Huber needle migrates out of a subcutaneous port. The use of transparent dressings to dress subcutaneous ports when vesicants are being administered can aid in the early recognition of this complication. It is also important to document good blood flow by aspirating on a port prior to drug administration. A less-common cause of extravasation is the presence of a fibrin sheath surrounding the catheter and its tip.[11] This can lead to retrograde flow of infusates between the sheath and the external wall of the catheter. It may manifest itself as a sensation of pain or coolness in the subcutaneous tunnel of the catheter. Any suspicion of extravasation should prompt a dye study of the catheter under fluoroscopy. Catheter stripping can temporarily eradicate this problem.

The incidence of catheter-related venous thrombosis is high and depends somewhat on the underlying disease, the size of the catheter, and the period of time the catheter has been in place.[12] Venous thrombosis may manifest itself as arm edema or pain. Diagnosis can usually be established noninvasively with Doppler ultrasonography or computed tomography employing IV contrast. Although the risk of pulmonary embolism is thought to be low,[13] a 3-month course of anticoagulation is recommended for the treatment of venous thrombosis. If the central venous catheter is still necessary, it may be left in place. The thrombus will resolve as a result of anticoagulation despite the presence of the catheter. Anticoagulation can be continued beyond 3 months if the catheter is still required because venous thrombosis is almost certain to recur once anticoagulation is stopped in the presence of a foreign body.

The incidence of catheter infection increases over time. The number of lumens and the quality of catheter care are also directly related to infection risk. External catheters can become infected at the catheter exit site, and ports can become superficially infected at the point of needle insertion. These infections can usually be eliminated by a course of antibiotics. Ports should not be accessed in the presence of overlying or nearby cellulitis.

A subcutaneous tunnel can also become infected. It was thought that the Dacron cuff and silver-impregnated collagen cuff on external catheters would serve as effective barriers to infection, but this is not supported by clinical experience.[12–15] Tunnel infections are more difficult to treat and may not resolve with a course of antibiotics. Removal of the catheter and antibiotics for treatment of these infections in immunocompromised patients is generally recommended. The subcutaneous pocket housing a port, when infected, requires operative removal of the port. The skin is incised directly over the port so that the underlying abscess can be drained and packed postoperatively. These incisions should not be closed because another abscess would be very likely.

Catheter infection may present as systemic sepsis. This is usually due to contamination of the lumen of the catheter, which usually results from introduction of bacteria through the port during infusion of medication or when accessing the device. This complication sometimes manifests as rigors and fever only when the catheter is flushed. Some reports suggest that catheters can be sterilized by treating all lumens with a prolonged course of antibiotics, with or without urokinase.[16–18] The catheter should always be removed for persistent sepsis or fever despite appropriate choice of antibiotics administered for 24–48 hours. Recurrent infection shortly after the course of antibiotics is finished should also prompt removal of the catheter. Never place a new catheter at the same time that an infected catheter is removed.

CATHETER USE AND CARE

After insertion of a subcutaneous port, it is important that the incisions be kept dry until fully healed. External catheters should also be protected from moisture. Waterproof dressings should be applied prior to showering. Although there are few prescribed activities for patients with a subcutaneous port, they should refrain from vigorous activity that could result in chest wall trauma.

As stated earlier, ports and external catheters should be flushed regularly with heparinized saline. Particular attention should be paid to the technique of catheter flushing. It is common practice to instill the entire volume of heparinized saline into the catheter or port and then remove the needle. This may lead to the drawback of blood into the tip of the catheter as the needle is withdrawn and can subsequently serve as the nidus for intracatheter clot. It is recommended that the needle be slowly withdrawn from the catheter or the port while the last 1 mL of heparinized saline is being infused, which may prevent or delay the development of intracatheter clot.

CATHETER REMOVAL

Elective catheter removal is usually advised when the device is no longer needed or is no longer functional. Percutaneous indwelling central catheter lines and Hohn catheters can be removed at the bedside without local anesthesia after the stay sutures have been cut. The distal 1 inch of the catheter should be cut using sterile scissors and placed in a sterile container for culture and sensitivity testing if there is any suspicion of infection. If a catheter is being removed because of suspected infection, the skin sur-

rounding the exit site should be prepared and draped in sterile fashion to avoid contaminating the tip of the catheter with skin bacteria.

The removal of tunneled catheters and ports is more complicated. Generally, tunneled catheters can be removed at the bedside. After the stay sutures are cut, gentle traction is applied to the catheter until it is liberated from the Dacron cuff. One must take care not to fracture the catheter in the process of removing it. If undue pain is experienced or if the catheter cannot be dislodged, one should cut down directly over the palpable Dacron cuff and release it from the surrounding tissues operatively. Some argue that the Dacron cuff should always be removed this way because a retained Dacron cuff may serve as a nidus of infection.[19, 20]

Ports require operative removal, and this can usually be performed under local anesthesia in the operating room or a special procedure unit. It is helpful to have electrocautery available for hemostasis. The previous incision can be used, or a separate incision over the most prominent portion of the port can be employed. The port can be easily delivered through the incision once the stay sutures have been cut. Little if any traction should be required to remove the catheter. Obliterate the subcutaneous tunnel with a stitch to prevent back-bleeding and formation of a hematoma within the subcutaneous pocket. Unless the port is being removed for infection, always close the skin with subcuticular stitches.

Whenever a central venous catheter has been removed, one should always check to see that it has been removed intact. If there is any suspicion that the catheter fractured during its removal, as manifested by a venous limb that appears to be too short or ragged, a chest radiograph should be obtained to make sure the catheter has not embolized to the right ventricle or pulmonary artery. Fortunately, fractured catheters that embolize to the heart can almost always be easily removed percutaneosly under fluoroscopic guidance.

As mentioned earlier, catheters being removed for presumed infection should be removed urgently. The tip of the catheter should be sent for culture and sensitivity testing as described earlier. For ports, the subcutaneous pocket should be swabbed for culture and for sensitivity testing. Infected pockets usually contain an exudate, and the lining of the pocket does not have a typical smooth and shiny appearance. If a port is being removed for presumed infection, the subcutaneous pocket should not be closed because an abscess is likely. Rather, the pocket should be treated with twice-daily wet to dry dressing changes until it has closed and epithelialized.

ALTERNATIVE APPROACHES TO VENOUS ACCESS

Rarely, patients are not candidates for placement of central venous catheters through the veins of the chest, upper extremities, or neck. This poses a clinically important dilemma with patients who require very long-term venous access, such as those with sickle cell disease. Short-term venous access can be accomplished by placement of a catheter through the right or left femoral vein. This approach is associated with increased risk of deep vein thrombosis of the lower extremities and infection.[21, 22] Therefore, these catheters should be removed in a timely fashion. Patients should probably be placed on subcutaneous heparin or a low dose of warfarin to decrease the chances of this complication.

Longer-term venous access can be accomplished by placement of inferior vena cava catheters through a translumbar approach.[23] The subcutaneous port is then positioned over the right flank or the right lower quadrant. This procedure is performed using interventional radiology under fluoroscopic guidance and can be accomplished with very little morbidity.

CONCLUSIONS

Most patients undergoing HSCT require venous access devices. Venous access devices can be placed with very little morbidity as long as well-described precautions are heeded. Catheters have been responsible for a variety of complications that can almost always be effectively managed if they are recognized early. Catheters should be removed soon after they are no longer needed in order to avoid these complications.

REFERENCES

1. Hickman RO, Buckner CD, Clift RA, et al: A modified right atrial catheter for access to the venous system in marrow transplant recipients. Surg Gynecol Obstet 148:8871–8912, 1979.
2. Niederhuber JE, Ensminger W, Gyves JW, et al: Totally implanted venous and arterial access system to replace external catheters in cancer treatment. Surgery 92:706–712, 1982.
3. Haire WD, Lieberman RP, Lund GB, et al: Thrombotic complications of silicone rubber catheters during autologous marrow and peripheral stem cell transplantation: prospective comparison of Hickman and Groshong catheters. Bone Marrow Transplant 7:57–59, 1991.
4. Pasquale MD, Campbell JM, Magnant CM: Groshong versus Hickman catheters. Surg Gynecol Obstet 174:408–410, 1992.
5. Eastridge BJ, Lefor AT: Complications of indwelling venous access devices in cancer patients. J Clin Oncol 13:233–238, 1995.
6. Mansfield PF, Hohn DC, Fornage BD, et al: Complications and failures of subclavian-vein catheterization. N Engl J Med 331:1735–1738, 1994.
7. Howell PB, Walters PE, Donowitz GR, Farr B: Risk factors for infection of adult patients with cancer who have tunneled central venous catheters. Cancer 75:1367–1375, 1995.
8. Hinke DH, Zandt-Stastny DA, Goodman LR, et al: Pinch-off syndrome: a complication of implantable subclavian venous access devices. Radiology 177:353–356, 1990.
9. Raad I, Luna M, Khalil SM, et al: The relationship between the thrombotic and infectious complications of central venous catheters. JAMA 271:1014–1016, 1994.
10. Bern MM, Lokich JJ, Wallach SR, et al: Very low doses of warfarin can prevent thrombosis in central venous catheters. Ann Intern Med 112:423–428, 1990.
11. Gemlo BT, Rayner AA, Swanson RJ, et al: A serious complication of the split-sheath introductor technique for venous access. Arch Surg 123:490–492, 1988.
12. Raad I, Davis S, Becker M, et al: Low infection rate and long durability of nontunneled silastic catheters: a safe and cost-effective alternative for long-term venous access. Arch Intern Med 153:1791–1843, 1993.
13. Leiby JM, Purcell H, De Maria JJ, et al: Pulmonary embolism as a result of Hickman catheter-related thrombosis. Am J Med 86:228–231, 1989.
14. Groeger JS, Lucas AB, Coit D, et al: A prospective, randomized evaluation of the effect of silver impregnated subcutaneous cuffs for preventing tunneled chronic venous access catheter infections in cancer patients. Ann Surg 218:206–210, 1993.
15. Andrivet P, Bacquer A, Nogc CV, et al: Lack of clinical benefit from subcutaneous tunnel insertion of central venous catheters in immunocompromised patients. Clin Infect Dis 18:199–206, 1994.
16. Ascher DP, Shoupe BA, Maybee D, Fischer GW: Persistent catheter-related bacteremia: clearance with antibiotics and urokinase. J Pediatr Surg 28:627–629, 1993.
17. Jones GR, Konsler GK, Dunaway RP, et al: Prospective analysis of urokinase in the treatment of catheter sepsis in pediatric hematology-oncology patients. J Pediatr Surg 28:350–357, 1993.
18. Mueller BU, Skelton J, Callender DPE, et al: A prospective randomized trial comparing the infectious and noninfectious complications of an externalized catheter versus a subcutaneously implanted device in cancer patients. J Clin Oncol 10:1943–1948, 1992.
19. Al-Wali WI, Wilcox MH, Thickett KJ, et al: Retained Hickman cuff as a source of infection. J Infect 26:199–201, 1993.
20. Ruppel LJ, Brown RA, Borson RA, Whitman ED: Retained Hickman catheter cuff as an infectious source following allogeneic bone marrow transplant. Bone Marrow Transplant 14:169–171, 1994.
21. Harden JL, Kemp L, Mirtallo J: Femoral catheters increase risk of infection in total parenteral nutrition patients. Nutr Clin Pract 10(2):60–66, 1995.
22. Trottier SJ, Veremakis C, O'Brien J, Auer AI: Femoral deep vein thrombosis associated with central venous catheterization: results from a prospective, randomized trial. Crit Care Med 23:52–58, 1995.
23. Lund GB, Lieberman RP, Haire WD, et al: Translumber inferior vena cava catheters for long-term venous access. Radiology 174:31–35, 1990.

Graft Procurement

 # Bone Marrow Harvesting

Barbara Rutecki, R.N., M.S.N., M.P.H., and John Lister, M.D.

The procedure for harvesting bone marrow from human donors was first described in 1970[1] and has not changed significantly throughout the years. The collection of cells from the marrow space is performed in the sterile environment of an operating suite. The physician uses large-bore aspiration needles to pierce the bony cortex of the iliac crest, delivers the cells into an anticoagulant, filters particulate bony matter and fat, and transfers the cell suspension into a holding bag. The advancements in the harvesting procedure over time have included the use of disposable aspiration needles; use of a sterile, disposable, closed collection and filtering system; and the exclusive use of the posterior iliac crests as the sites for bone marrow harvesting. In the early years, marrow cells were collected from the sternum, anterior iliac crests, and posterior iliac crests. The use of numerous harvest sites prolonged the procedure, increased the duration of anesthesia, and resulted in increased pain for the donor.

Bone marrow harvesting has become less common at this time in the evolution of the field of hematopoietic stem cell transplantation (HSCT). Peripheral blood progenitor cell (PBPC) collection via leukapheresis has emerged as an alternative method of obtaining hematopoietic stem cells. Hematopoietic cell recovery occurs more rapidly after both autologous and allogeneic transplantation of PBPC compared with bone marrow.[2, 3] With the increased use of PBPC for hematopoietic cell support or transplantation, the bone marrow harvest procedure may become obsolete or may be used in selected situations to supplement an inadequate PBPC collection. This chapter describes the donor preoperative evaluation, the bone marrow harvest procedure, and the donor experience.

PREOPERATIVE DONOR EVALUATION

After the bone marrow donor has been selected based on human leukocyte antigen (HLA)-matching (see Chapters 21 and 22), a complete medical examination is required to establish that the donor is physically and emotionally fit for anesthesia and the harvest (Chapter 20). A complete blood count, blood chemistry panel, and infectious disease tests for hepatitis B (hepatitis B surface antigens, HbsAg, and anti–core antibody) and hepatitis C, cytomegalovirus, human T-cell leukemia virus type I/II (HTLV-I/II), human immunodeficiency virus (HIV-1 and -2, HIV-p24), and syphilis are obtained. The presence of HbsAg, HIV-1/2, HTLV-I/II, and syphilis contraindicates the use of the donor

for allogeneic transplantation. The panel of tests currently required for autologous recipients and allogeneic donors is published by national and international organizations such as the American Association for Blood Banks (AABB), Foundation for the Accreditation for Hematopoietic Cell Therapy (FAHCT), and National Marrow Donor Program (NMDP). A complete history and physical examination, chest radiograph, and electrocardiogram are also obtained. If the donor has a significant past medical history, additional testing and/or consultation may be indicated. Unrelated bone marrow donors are to remain anonymous to the recipient and family and, if female, must not be pregnant. In addition, the unrelated donor evaluation, harvest procedure, and necessary medical follow-up should be at a center distinct from the transplant center treating the bone marrow recipient.

Written informed consent must be obtained from the donor before the bone marrow recipient begins the pretransplantation conditioning regimen. The risks of the bone marrow harvest procedure should be thoroughly reviewed (as described later in this chapter). The benefits of being a bone marrow donor are limited to the knowledge that the donor has assisted another person (family member or unrelated person) in a unique way. In the case of autologous transplantation, the marrow harvest is part of the treatment plan. At the time of consenting, the donor should be counseled regarding his or her role as donor, which is limited to the collection of marrow only. The outcome of the recipient and the transplantation is in no way the donor's responsibility or fault.

Approximately 1 week prior to the marrow harvest, one or two autologous units of blood may be collected from the donor. This blood will be used after the harvest if needed by the donor. Avoiding the use of homologous blood decreases the risk of transfusion-related infections to the donor. If an autologous donor does not have adequate red blood cell mass prior to the harvest, homologous blood may be transfused during or after the harvest. These units of packed red blood cells must be leukocyte-reduced and irradiated to minimize alloimmunization and transmission of viable lymphocytes capable of causing graft-versus-host disease.

BONE MARROW HARVEST PROCEDURE

The marrow harvest is usually a same-day surgery procedure, avoiding an overnight hospital stay.[4] The bone marrow donor arrives approximately 2 hours prior to the scheduled procedure. The donor meets with the anesthesiologist and signs consent for the plan of anesthesia. General anesthesia is used most frequently, though spinal and epidural anesthesia may be considered. The newer anesthetic agents have shorter half-lives, allowing more-rapid recovery from general anesthesia and thus fewer adverse effects. In addition, use of intraoperative analgesics can avoid postoperative analgesics in a majority of donors, allowing discharge to home with oral analgesics.

The harvest procedure must be performed by trained medical and nursing staff, generally members of the HSCT team. Usually, two physicians perform the procedure together. Other required operating room personnel include an anesthesiologist or nurse anesthetist, an operating room technician, and an operating room registered nurse to circulate the area to assist throughout the procedure.

After induction of anesthesia in the operating suite, an indwelling urinary catheter is placed if the harvest is expected to last longer than 1 hour, as is usual in an autologous bone marrow harvest. The donor is then placed in the prone position onto a supportive frame allowing the posterior iliac crests to be prominent. Care must be taken to ensure that the donor's head, breasts, genitalia, and extremities are positioned correctly with minimal pressure to bony prominences and soft tissues. The posterior iliac crest area is washed with a sterile provodone-iodine solution followed by a sterile saline rinse. The surrounding area is draped with sterile towels and sheets, allowing easy access to the posterior iliac crests.

The choice of harvest needle is one of personal or institutional preference. The needle should be very sharp and have a comfortable gripping handle and an easily removable trochar. Harvest needles are available in varying lengths and gauges. The smallest needle size should be used as determined by the size and weight of the donor. The needle with trochar is inserted through the skin and into the iliac crest bone, using a slight rotary motion. When the needle is firmly in place, the trochar is removed and a heparinized 20- or 50-mL syringe is attached to the needle hub. Five to 10 mL of bone marrow blood is aspirated while the needle is rotated. The majority of bone marrow cells is collected with the initial aspirate pull. If greater than 10 mL per aspirate are collected, significant blood dilution is likely. After the bone marrow aspirate is obtained, the syringe is handed to an operating room technician to empty into a heparinized collecting bag. Approximately 100 mL of normal saline (or tissue culture medium, which is not approved for infusion) containing heparin (50 U/mL) should be in the collection bag to prevent clotting of the aspirated marrow cells. In addition, the collection bag should be agitated by gentle squeezing throughout the harvest to ensure uniform distribution of anticoagulant. Citrate (ACD) may be used (10 mL ACD per 70 mL of marrow) instead of heparin.

Bone marrow cells are aspirated from the entire posterior iliac crest using two to eight skin sites per side. After each aspirate, the needle is reinserted at the same skin site but repositioned to a new bone site. After approximately 500 mL of bone marrow has been collected, a 1-mL syringe sample from the collecting bag is obtained to measure the nucleated cell count. This sample is sent to a hematology laboratory, where the number of nucleated cells is measured. This number is used to determine the volume of marrow harvest, using the recipient's body weight as a reference.[5] The present recommended number of total nucleated cells to be collected to achieve engraftment is as follows: for an HLA-matched sibling and unrelated graft, a minimum total of 3×10^8 cells/kg; for an autologous graft, a minimum of $1.5–2.0 \times 10^8$ cells/kg; if the allogeneic marrow is to be T cell–depleted or if an ABO-mismatch exists between donor and recipient, a minimum of 4×10^8 cells/kg is required; if tumor cell purging (using monoclonal antibodies + complement, CD34+ cell selection, or chemotherapeutic agents) is to be performed on an autologous harvest, 6×10^8 cells/kg may be needed.[6, 7] If insufficient numbers of nucleated cells are harvested, PBPC may be collected at a later date and added to the marrow harvest.

Upon completion of the marrow harvesting procedure, the physician assists the operating room technician with the filtration of the cell suspension. A sterile closed system (Baxter bone marrow collection kit with flexible prefilter and inline filters) is preferred because the aspirated heparinized marrow is not exposed to air and the risk of spillage is lessened. The aspirated marrow flows via gravity through two inline filters into a large blood-holding bag. The filtered marrow in the holding bag is properly labeled with donor and recipient identification and taken to the processing laboratory for enumeration of nucleated cell and CD34+ cells, microbiologic culturing, and any further processing as required for a particular product.

As the marrow is being filtered, the nurse applies manual pressure to the harvest sites on the patient to aid hemostasis. The sites are then cleansed with sterile normal saline. An antibacterial ointment is applied to each site, followed by a bulky dry sterile pressure dressing to the entire posterior iliac crest area. Anesthesia is tapered off, and intraoperative analgesic medication is given to the donor. The general guideline for intravenous fluid replacement during a bone marrow harvest is 3 L of crystalloid intravenous fluid to 1 L marrow aspirated. The bone marrow harvest procedure can last from 30 minutes with a normal healthy donor up to several hours with an autologous donor who has received prior therapies that may have decreased bone marrow cellularity.

After the application of a pressure dressing, the donor is repositioned to the supine position and anesthesia is discontinued. Assuming the procedure and anesthesia have been without complication, the donor arrives in the postanesthesia recovery area responsive to simple commands and breathing independently with assistance of oxygen via mask. Oxygen support is maintained until the donor is fully awake, breathing normally, and has a normal pulse oximeter reading. Intravenous hydration continues until the donor is taking adequate fluids orally and begins eating small amounts of food as tolerated. The donor's hemoglobin and hematocrit are measured upon arrival at the recovery area. If necessary, previously drawn autologous units of packed red blood cells are transfused to the donor. Homologous packed red blood cell units may be transfused to the autologous patient as needed. Harvest site pain is initially controlled with intravenous medication in the recovery area. Oral pain medication is prescribed to all donors prior to discharge to home. To avoid masking postoperative fever, antipyretics should be avoided. Medications such as codeine, hydrocodone/acetaminophen (Vicodin), or oxycodone are frequently used.

DONOR EXPERIENCE

Bone marrow harvesting is a safe procedure with minimal risk of complications. Review of over 3000 records of histocompatible bone marrow donors by the International Bone Marrow Transplant Registry and the Marrow Transplant team at Fred Hutchinson Cancer Research Center determined that the overall incidence of life-threatening complications associated with the harvest procedure was 0.27%.[8, 9] The reported life-threatening complications included nonfatal cardiac arrest during anesthesia, aspiration pneumonia, pulmonary embolus, infection at the harvest sites, intravenous thrombosis, ventricular tachycardia, and cerebral infarction. Five of these seven reported complications can be attributed to the risk of general anesthesia. All donors had pain at the harvest sites for several days postoperatively, though less than 0.5% of donors experienced pain persisting for a week or more. In donors experiencing prolonged pain, there appeared to be hematoma formation at the harvest sites, sciatic nerve pain, displaced cortical fractures of the anterior iliac crests, or hip pain of uncertain cause that resolved within 3 weeks. Other consequences of normal donor bone marrow harvest included fever of unknown origin, anemia of sufficient magnitude to require transfusion, one case of a broken aspiration needle tip requiring surgical removal (which was believed to be due to a defect in the needle), transient episodes of hypotension, and laryngospasm. Fewer than 1% of the donors were over 60 years of age. Increasing donor age was associated with a reduction in the harvested marrow cellularity.

Autologous bone marrow harvesting is also associated with low morbidity and mortality. In a review of 224 marrow harvests from 200 patients with various malignant diseases,[10] a total of 36 (17.4%) complications were associated with marrow harvesting, including two (0.97%) life-threatening complications. Postoperative fever accounted for 23 of 34 incidences of minor complications. It was concluded that the incidence of complications with autologous harvesting did not significantly differ from that observed in a normal donor harvest experience. A second review of 166 patients who underwent 170 autologous bone marrow harvest procedures[11] revealed a higher morbidity than with harvesting from normal donors. The complications were reversible and of little consequence to the patient, however. Both reviews concluded that the autologous bone marrow harvest procedure is safe and does not interfere with planned high-dose chemotherapy followed by autologous bone marrow transplantation.

A telephone survey conducted by the National Marrow Donor Program addressed the incidence of complications and long-term consequences of bone marrow donation.[12] After harvest, 493 unrelated HLA-matched donors were surveyed several times. Acute complications occurred in 5.9% of the surveyed persons, including hypotension with episodes of syncope, fever, prolonged nausea, pain at harvest sites, phlebitis at peripheral intravenous sites, postspinal headache, and an apneic episode during spinal anesthesia. At 2 weeks after the harvest, approximately 25% of the 430 surveyed donors continued to experience fatigue, pain at harvest sites, and low back pain. A majority of donors had recovered from the harvest procedure within 19 days; however, 12.6% of the donors indicated they had not completely recovered by 30 days. At a 1-year post-harvest follow-up survey of 359 responding donors, 11.1% indicated that they had suffered a side effect or complication secondary to the bone marrow harvest procedure.

Bone marrow donor outcome was correlated with the volume of marrow collected per unit of donor weight, the duration of anesthesia, and the duration of the harvest procedure. All of these variables are interdependent, and all correlated positively with at least some donor complications. Only the duration of the harvest procedure significantly correlated with donor recovery time.

An investigation of the psychosocial effects of bone marrow harvest, which was performed on the same 493 participants, also revealed that the longer the harvest procedure, the more negative the memory of stressful psychosocial effects.[13] Regardless of complications, the majority of unrelated bone marrow donors felt that the experience was positive and said they would be willing to donate marrow again in the future.

CONCLUSION

Bone marrow harvesting is performed much less frequently in the current era of HSCT. Presently, marrow sources are used primarily in the allogeneic donor setting. It is likely that allogeneic PBPC grafts will be used more widely in the future. The widespread movement to use PBPC for autologous transplants has nearly eliminated autologous marrow harvesting. Though bone marrow harvesting may not remain the preferred method to obtain hematopoietic stem cells, it is a procedure still in practice and requiring expertise. It is important for transplant teams to be familiar with the procedure itself and the donor experience.

REFERENCES

1. Thomas ED, Storb R: Technique for human marrow grafting. Blood 36(4):507–515, 1970.
2. Liberti G, Pearce R, Taghipour G, et al: Comparison of peripheral blood stem-cell and autologous bone marrow transplantation for lymphoma patients: a case-controlled analysis of the EBMT Registry data. Ann Oncol 5 (Suppl 2):S151–S153, 1994.
3. Repka T, Weisdorf D: Peripheral blood versus bone marrow for hematopoietic cell transplantation. Curr Opin Oncol 10(2):112–117, 1998.
4. Ordemann R, Holig K, Wagner K, et al: Acceptance and feasibility of peripheral stem cell mobilisation compared to bone marrow collection from healthy unrelated donors. Bone Marrow Transplant 21 (Suppl 3):S25–S28, 1998.
5. Thorne AC, Stewart M, Gulati SC: Harvesting bone marrow in an

outpatient setting using newer anesthetic agents. J Clin Oncol 11(2):320–323, 1993.

6. Jones R, Burnett AK: How to harvest bone marrow for transplantation. J Clin Pathol 45:1053–1057, 1992.

7. Voak D, Cann R, Finney RD, et al: Guidelines for the collection, processing and storage of human bone marrow and peripheral stem cells for transplantation. Transfus Med 4:165–172, 1994.

8. Bortin MM, Buckner CD: Major complications of marrow harvesting for transplantation. Exp Hematol 11(10):916–921, 1983.

9. Buckner CD, Clift RA, Sanders JE, et al: Marrow harvesting from normal donors. Blood 64(3):630–634, 1984.

10. Jin NR, Hill RS, Petersen FB, et al: Marrow harvesting for autologous marrow transplantation. Exp Hematol 13:879–884, 1985.

11. Kessinger A, Armitage JO: Harvesting marrow for autologous transplantation from patients with malignancies. Bone Marrow Transplant 2:15–18, 1987.

12. Stroncek DF, Holland PV, Bartch G, et al: Experiences of the first 493 unrelated marrow donors in the National Marrow Donor Program. Blood 81(7):1940–1946, 1993.

13. Butterworth VA, Simmons RG, Bartsch G, et al: Psychosocial effects of unrelated bone marrow donation: experiences of the National Marrow Donor Program. Blood 81(7):1947–1959, 1993.

Peripheral Blood Progenitor Cell Mobilization and Collection

Thomas A. Lane, M.D.

Hematopoietic stem (HSC) cells collected from mobilized peripheral blood progenitor cells (PBPC) are increasingly used for both autologous and allogeneic transplantation after myeloablative or nonmyeloablative therapies.[1, 2] Advantages of PBPC include rapid and durable trilineage hematologic engraftment, improved tolerance of the harvesting procedure (without general anesthesia), and possibly diminished tumor contamination in the autologous setting.[3–5] The ability of autologous mobilized PBPC to provide long-term reconstitution suggested that PBPC grafting might also be successful for allogeneic transplantation. Early reports in animals and syngeneic transplants in humans supported this hypothesis.[6–8] The first patient receiving allogeneic PBPC in modern ages from a human leukocyte antigen (HLA)-matched sibling donor experienced engraftment, but sustained engraftment could not be evaluated because the patient died of *Aspergillus* infection.[9]

In recent years, hundreds of patients have undergone transplantation using mobilized PBPC allografts instead of bone marrow. Reports on these patients demonstrated that hematopoietic recovery is rapid, complete (all lineages), and durable, the latter demonstrated by cytogenetics or molecular markers.[10–14] Neutrophil recovery (>500/mm³) and platelet recovery (>20,000/mm³) is typically between 9 and 15 days[15, 16] in matched sibling transplants, but longer engraftment times (16–33 days) have been reported in mismatched transplants.[17] Only 1 graft failure was reported in 62 patients receiving mobilized PBPC allografts; the patient had previously experienced failed allogeneic marrow transplantation from the same donor.[17]

Although allogeneic PBPC from matched sibling donors are increasingly supplanting marrow as the graft of choice, PBPC collected from matched unrelated donors are currently under clinical investigation. Intensive efforts have focused on methods to optimize the mobilization and collection of PBPC from healthy persons. Widespread successful utilization of allogeneic PBPC depends on a variety of factors, including ethical considerations, which impel physicians to harvest allogeneic PBPC using regimens with the least possible risk, discomfort, and expense to the patient/donor and the highest quality of the grafts, which is determined by the content of primitive as well as committed hematopoietic cells.

This chapter reviews the current practices and controversies regarding mobilization and collection of PBPC from patients for autologous transplantation and from normal donors for allogeneic transplantation.

ELIGIBILITY

Both autologous and allogeneic marrow and PBPC donors must be evaluated to determine the risks of donation and possible risk to the recipient after receiving the cells. Evaluation for eligibility includes a limited history, physical examination, and laboratory testing. In general, eligibility requirements for autologous PBPC donation are less strict than for allogeneic donation because the donation risks are balanced by direct clinical benefits as well as the fact that the autologous graft cannot transmit a new exogenous virus. Autologous evaluation includes an assessment of the need to use a catheter for vascular access, the likelihood of achieving the cell dose after mobilization and collection, and the possibility of the patient requiring transfusion (especially platelet) support during multiple apheresis procedures. For both autologous and allogeneic donation, laboratory testing includes assays to ensure the safety of the donor during apheresis (blood counts, electrolytes, calcium, magnesium) and for infectious diseases that may be transmitted by blood.

The donor history is relevant to the type of collection procedure performed. Whereas a history of active asthma may be a relative contraindication to bone marrow harvesting under general anesthesia, the same condition is not a contraindication for PBPC harvesting by leukapheresis. Likewise, patients with severe low back pain are more suited to PBPC collection. In contrast, patients with poor peripheral veins require the placement of a central catheter for PBPC apheresis. The consideration of vascular access is relevant to both autologous and allogeneic donors. Autologous donors are at increased risk for catheter complications of infection and bleeding. For allogeneic donors who require catheters, marrow harvesting may be preferred. A history of allergy to hematopoietic growth factors is a contraindication for mobilization. Additional contraindications to mobilization may include patients with inflammatory ocular conditions, autoimmune diseases with an inflammatory component, risk of thrombotic complications or, in normal donors, risk of hematologic malignancy. In general, persons who are eligible to donate blood or platelets by apheresis should be eligible for mobilization and collection of PBPC.

Eligibility for PBPC donation does not differ from marrow collection in the requirements for infectious disease testing. All donors must be tested for hepatitis (hepatitis B surface antigen, hepatitis B core antibody, hepatitis C virus), human immunodeficiency virus (HIV)-1/2, HIV-p24 antigen, human T-cell lymphotropic virus I/II, syphilis, and cytomegalovirus. Whether additional testing (e.g., nucleic acid testing for HIV and hepatitis C virus) will be required in the future is unclear, but because these tests will soon be implemented in normal blood donors, it seems reasonable to expect that they will be required in allogeneic PBPC donors as well. The list is mandated by national and international organizations such as the American Association of Blood Banks (AABB), Foundation for the Accreditation of Hematopoietic Cell Therapy (FAHCT), and National Marrow Donor Program (NMDP). In contrast with the case of blood donors, a positive test result (especially a false-positive result) for one of these agents may not be a contraindication to autologous transplantation. The tests are performed primarily to ensure that the patient is a candidate for the transplantation procedure (e.g., HIV or hepatitis B virus), to ensure the safety of laboratory and health care workers, and to minimize cross-contamination of other products during processing and storage. A positive or false-positive test result for some viruses in an allogeneic donor may not be a contraindication to donation, but this decision is made individually, with full disclosure to the patient/recipient.

AUTOLOGOUS MOBILIZATION

HSC are found in peripheral blood of healthy persons. Their numbers, however, are insufficient to permit collection of an adequate graft by standard leukapheresis.[9, 18] Fortunately, a variety of methods have been discovered to increase the circulation of progenitor and stem cells by "mobilizing" them from the marrow into the peripheral blood. For autologous transplantation, hematopoietic stem/progenitor cells may be mobilized into the peripheral blood (1) during the rebound phase of the leukocytes after transient leukopenia induced by myelosuppressive chemotherapy, (2) by hematopoietic growth factors, or (3) by a combination of both.

CHEMOTHERAPY

HSC mobilization into peripheral blood was first described as a procedure following myelosuppressive therapy.[19] A variety of myelosuppressive chemotherapy regimens can mobilize hematopoietic stem and progenitor cells into the peripheral blood. Commonly used regimens include cyclophosphamide alone, in single doses of 4–7 g/m^2, or other agents, such as Adriamycin (doxorubicin), carboplatin, Taxol (paclitaxel), etoposide, ifosfamide, daunorubicin, cytosine arabinosides 6-thioguanine, either alone or in combination, have been employed.[19–23] The regimens induce a transient but profound myelosuppression in patients, with white blood cell (WBC) counts dropping below 100 cells/mm^3 7–14 days after chemotherapy. This is typically followed on day 10–21 by rapid reappearance of leukocytes in the peripheral blood and frequently a "rebound" increase of the circulating leukocytes above baseline levels. As the leukocyte count rises, hematopoietic progenitor cells also begin to appear in the peripheral blood and rapidly increase.

With chemotherapy alone, 20- to 40-fold increases in the number of colony-forming units granulocyte macrophages (CFU-GM) are typically observed compared with premobilization levels, and the increased levels persist for several days, during which the PBPC can be collected.[22, 24, 25] Some investigations have observed a positive correlation between the extent of PBPC mobilization and the intensity of the myelosuppressive treatment.[22, 24, 26] Ideally, the patient's malignancy also is sensitive to the agents used, and thus the chemotherapy also provides effective antitumor therapy, diminishing the likelihood of cancer cells being "mobilized" into the peripheral blood. Sometimes mobilization is preceded by one or more cycles of "chemotherapeutic debulking" or "in vivo purging" to diminish the probability of tumor contamination of the PBPC product.[27–29] Disadvantages of employing chemotherapy alone for mobilization include the necessity to submit the patient to the potential side effects of transient myelosuppression (principally infection and hemorrhage), uncertainty regarding optimal timing for collection, wide variability in the extent and duration of myelosuppression, and inability to predict the success of mobilization in a given patient.

HEMATOPOIETIC GROWTH FACTORS

Growth factors have been used alone to mobilize PBPC in autologous transplant recipients as first described by Socinski et al.[30] Duhrsen et al. performed an extensive, dose-response study of the mobilization of hematopoietic progenitors in 30 patients with a variety of malignancies.[31] G-CSF, 0.3–60 μg/kg/day for 4 days SC or IV, increased the number of CFU-GM by a mean of 20 times on day 5. Similar increases were observed with CFU-erythrocyte (CFU-E) and megakaryocyte colonies. There was no clear dose-response effect for IV administration, and the highest SC dose used, 10 μg/kg/day, resulted in stimulation of progenitors equal to that of IV use. Other investigators have reported similar kinetics of mobilized PBPC.[32–34] Kroger et al. studied the effect of split dosing of G-CSF (10 μg/kg/day vs. 5 μg/kg twice a day) on PBPC mobilization in 57 patients with high-risk breast cancer. The twice-daily schedule resulted in significantly higher yields of CD34 + cells and CFU at each leukapheresis and decreased numbers of procedures required to achieve the target cell dose. There were no differences in engraftment after high-dose chemotherapy in the two groups.[35]

Other studies have compared the collection of PBPC mobilized by G-CSF versus GM-CSF. Peters et al. compared the mobilization of CFU-GM and CD34 + cells in 48 patients with breast cancer or melanoma treated with G-CSF or GM-CSF prior to three leukapheresis procedures.[36] Increases in PBPC over baseline were not evaluated, but at similar schedule and dose (8 μg/kg/day for 8 days), approximately five times more CD34 + cells were collected after G-CSF administration compared with GM-CSF administration. In contrast, approximately the same number of CFU-GM was collected for both drugs. Increasing the dose of GM-CSF twofold resulted in an increased CD34 + cell collection to nearly that of G-CSF, but a longer schedule of administration of GM-CSF (14 days) before apheresis was associated with lower collections of CD34 + cells and CFU.

These findings have since been confirmed by other investigators.[37, 38]

New combinations of growth factors show promise. Begley et al. randomized 62 patients with early-stage breast cancer to receive combined stem cell factor (SCF, in escalating doses) and G-CSF versus G-CSF alone. SCF acted to sustain the levels of PBPC after cessation of growth factor, and levels of PBPC were elevated 100-fold at later time-points compared with G-CSF alone. The maximum levels of PBPC were increased approximately 5 times at day 5 of growth-factor administration. PBPC levels in blood and yield in leukapheresis products were further increased.[39] Weaver et al. reported similar findings in 48 patients with ovarian cancer.[40]

CHEMOTHERAPY AND HEMATOPOIETIC GROWTH FACTORS

Socinski et al. were also the first to demonstrate that the administration of GM-CSF after chemotherapy increased circulating CFU-GM.[30] In their study, 13 patients with sarcoma were treated with GM-CSF alone, at 4–64 µg/kg/day IV for up to 7 days. One week after return of blood counts to normal, three of the same patients were treated with a myelosuppressive dose of combination chemotherapy followed by the same dose of GM-CSF on day 5 through the leukocyte nadir (phase 2). After return of blood counts to baseline, the same three patients were treated with the same regimen of chemotherapy but without GM-CSF (phase 3). Compared with the pretreatment assays, GM-CSF resulted in a 13-fold increase in blood CFU-GM, the combination of chemotherapy and GM-CSF resulted in a 63-fold increase, and chemotherapy alone resulted in a 2-fold increase in blood CFU-GM. No clear dose-response was observed for GM-CSF. This small study employed a suboptimal schedule of GM-CSF, but the data indicated that GM-CSF treatment resulted in significant progenitor mobilization, and treating patients with GM-CSF during the rebound from chemotherapy had additive effects.

Many investigators have since reported that mobilization employing a combination of chemotherapy and followed by growth factor (GM-CSF or G-CSF) administration is more effective than either chemotherapy or growth factor alone.[20, 24, 40–51] The combination typically results in a 50- to 75-fold increase in circulating CFU-GM and 10- to 50-fold increase in CD34+ cells.[24, 30, 40, 42, 44] Direct comparisons show that chemotherapy and growth factors resulted in a mean 3.5-fold greater peak number of circulating CFU-GM (range, 0 to 6.8 times greater) versus chemotherapy or growth factor alone.[22, 24, 40–43, 45, 46] Studies have demonstrated no advantage to increasing GM-CSF from 10 to 16 µg/kg[47] and no difference in the efficacy of G-CSF compared with GM-CSF.[48, 49] Other regimens (e.g., chemotherapy followed by sequential IL-3 and G-CSF) have been described.[50] Meisenberg et al. found that a combination of cyclophosphamide and sequential GM-CSF (5 µg/kg/day) and G-CSF (10 µg/kg/day, each for 5 days) resulted in 66% of patients with breast cancer reaching a target 4 × 10^6 CD34+ cells/kg in a single leukapheresis session, compared with 14% who received G-CSF alone (10 µg/kg/day

× 5 days). The mean number of sessions required to reach the target cell dose was also reduced by the combination regimen. As expected, engraftment was similar in both cohorts of patients, although the cost of mobilization was reduced by 25% for the combined regimen.[50] Not all studies have shown additive effects between chemotherapy and growth factors,[25] and mobilization using combination chemotherapy and growth factor is not 100% effective.[51]

It is not possible to define an optimal regimen of mobilization given the great variability in the studies with respect to patient populations, prior treatment, chemotherapy used for mobilization (which varies by disease), dose, schedule, and type of growth factor and laboratory methods available for study of progenitors.

FACTORS AFFECTING AUTOLOGOUS MOBILIZATION

The definition of a "poor mobilization" differs from one institution to another but is typically defined as inability to collect at least 2 × 10^6 CD34+ cells/kg or at least 20 × 10^4 CFU-GM/kg. Inability to obtain a sufficient number of HSC for grafting may be due to a variety of factors other than the mobilization regimen, such as inadequate vascular access for apheresis and inadequate apheresis technique during collection. This discussion, however, focuses on the mobilization regimen and patient variables.

Several investigators have attempted to define relationships among patient characteristics, drug and dosing regimens, and the ability to mobilize hematopoietic progenitors (Table 25–1). Factors affecting PBPC mobilization in autologous transplant recipients include the extent of prior chemotherapy and radiotherapy; diagnosis (e.g., lymphoma vs. breast cancer); presence and extent of bone marrow involvement; type of chemotherapy as a mobilizing regimen and the intensity of myelosuppression; type, dose, and schedule of growth factors; and patient sex and age. Some examples will be examined in greater detail.

Schneider et al. studied 17 patients with breast and ovarian cancer who received variable schedules of G-CSF or GM-CSF, with or without chemotherapy.[52] The extent of CFU-GM mobilization was significantly increased by chemotherapy and G-CSF versus either regimen alone and was diminished by a history of prior chemoradiotherapy. Bensinger et al. studied 54 patients with breast cancer, lymphoma, myeloma, and other cancers who received 16

TABLE 25–1. FACTORS REPORTED TO AFFECT THE MOBILIZATION OF PERIPHERAL BLOOD PROGENITOR CELLS

1. Mobilization technique
   Chemotherapy—degree of transient myelosuppression
   Growth factors—type, schedule, dose
   Use of combined chemotherapy and growth factors
2. Extent and type of prior chemotherapy/radiotherapy
3. Patient age
4. Presence of marrow disease or metastases
5. Patient diagnosis
6. Patient gender

μg/kg/day of G-CSF, SC for 4–7 days, prior to two to six leukapheresis procedures targeted to collect 10^9 mononuclear cells/kg.[53] They found that the number of collected CD34+ cells was inversely correlated with age, the presence of marrow disease, and prior radiation or chemotherapy.

Haas et al. studied 61 patients with lymphoma who received chemotherapy and G-CSF (300 μg/m²/day), followed by leukaphereses to collect either 0.4×10^9 nucleated cells or 5×10^6 CD34+ cells/kg.[54] Patients with Hodgkin disease had lower CD34+ cell yields, but most of these patients had received extensive radiation therapy. They found no correlation between leukapheresis yields to age, sex, and disease status (active vs. remission). Too few patients had involved marrow to permit evaluation of this parameter. A history of prior chemotherapy or more-than-local radiotherapy was associated with a poor yield of CD34+ cells. On regression analysis, each cycle of chemotherapy was associated with a decrement in each leukapheresis of 0.2×10^6 CD34+ cells/kg and radiotherapy was associated with a loss of 1.8×10^6 CD34+ cells/kg.

Ho et al. prospectively investigated the effect on mobilization of three successive courses of myelosuppressive chemotherapy designed to mobilize PBPC, each lasting 20 days and spaced approximately 1 month apart.[44] They found a marked, significant decrease in peak mobilization of CFU-GM and CD34+ cells between courses 1 (19.5-fold and 10-fold increases over baseline CFU-GM and CD34+ cells, respectively) and 2 (7.5-fold and 4.6-fold increases, respectively), with a smaller decline between course 2 and 3 (6.7-fold and 5.5-fold increases, respectively). Kotasek et al. studied predictors of optimal harvesting in 60 patients mobilized with chemotherapy. Correlations were identified with increased mobilization dose, longer interval from last chemotherapy, and higher premobilization CFU-GM level. The patient's age, presence of marrow disease, type of malignancy, and number of prior chemotherapy cycles were not predictive.[55] Moskowitz et al. found that PBPC mobilization and harvesting (median of three procedures) in 58 patients with lymphoma using G-CSF after chemotherapy were superior to mobilization and harvesting using G-CSF alone.[46] In addition, patients who had received prior "stem cell–toxic" chemotherapy (nitrogen mustard, procarbazine, melphalan, carmustine or more than 7.5 g of cytarabine) mobilized less well than others (2.0 vs. 6.0×10^6 CD34+ cells/kg), and patients who had received more than 10 cycles of any chemotherapy mobilized poorly (2.6 vs. 6.7 $\times 10^6$ CD34+ cells/kg). Similar adverse effects of prior chemotherapy on mobilization and collection have been reported by others.[54, 56]

Demirer et al. investigated different mobilization regimens in variably pretreated patients with myeloma. By linear regression, they found that the extent of marrow involvement and the extent of prior chemotherapy and prior radiation therapy were significantly associated with diminished mobilization. They also found that a mobilizing regimen containing a combination of cyclophosphamide, etoposide, and G-CSF was associated with higher yields of CD34+ cells than G-CSF or GM-CSF alone or in combination with only cyclophosphamide.[57]

It is noteworthy that some[57, 58] but not all studies have demonstrated an effect of the degree of marrow involvement on mobilization.[59] Bolwell et al. found no relationship between the extent of CFU-GM mobilization as a function of drug schedule (daily vs. twice-daily GM-CSF), patient age, and history of prior chemotherapy/radiation therapy.[37] Kessinger et al. found no difference in the mobilization of CFU-GM or their collection in a heterogeneous group of 70 patients with hematologic malignancy and solid tumors. These patients were mobilized with GM-CSF at a dose of 250 μg/m²/day, either by continuous IV infusion or by a single SC dose.[60] Chatta et al. prospectively studied the effect of age on mobilization. Nineteen young (age, 20–30 years) and elderly (age, 70–80 years) healthy subjects were administered G-CSF, 30 or 300 μg/kg/day SC, for 14 days. Young subjects mobilized two times more CFU-GM ($P <$ .05) after 5 days at the higher, but not at the lower, dose.[61] Some, but not other, retrospective studies have identified age-dependent differences in PBPC mobilization.[53–55, 62]

The timing of collection after myelosuppressive chemotherapy is critical but not always predictable. Peak levels of PBPC as measured by colony-forming assays have been reported to occur when the circulating leukocyte count reaches approximately 1000–5000/mm³ or during the exponential increase in the circulating WBC count, and these parameters are widely employed.[24, 25, 63] A relevant practical limitation is that leukapheresis is difficult to initiate with WBC counts of less than 1000/mm³ because the visible leukocyte "interface" will not be apparent.[64] The mobilization of progenitors in response to G-CSF appears to be more reliable, with most studies indicating maximum levels of circulating progenitors on days 5–7. The optimal time course using GM-CSF appears to be somewhat longer, at 5–11 days.[64–66] Another technique that has been shown to recruit PBPC into the circulation and maximize yields is to simply increase the duration of leukapheresis and therefore the volume of blood processed during a given procedure, although not all investigators have found this technique useful.[64, 67]

MANAGEMENT OF POOR MOBILIZERS

There is no universally accepted means to manage poorly mobilizing patients, and success in this endeavor has been variable. Prince et al. studied second mobilization attempts in a group of previously treated patients with multiple myeloma who experienced a poor initial mobilization. These authors reported that the only significant variable in the first mobilization attempt was the extent of prior chemotherapy and that repeat collections using a similar mobilization protocol were universally unsuccessful.[59] Weaver et al. reported that second attempts to mobilize patients who had experienced poor initial mobilizations using chemotherapy and/or G-CSF successfully achieved the target dose of CD34+ cells (2.5×10^6/kg) in 48% of 119 patients.[68]

In some cases it may be possible to collect sufficient PBPC by repeat mobilization using a modified regimen. Lie et al. found that in 6 of 10 patients, simply increasing the dose of G-CSF by 5 μg/kg daily resulted in collection of sufficient CD34+ cells for autologous transplantation.[69] Russell et al. reported that, in myeloma patients, the use of G-CSF alone was consistently effective and that some patients in whom previous mobilization with cyclophosphamide and G-CSF had failed were successfully remobilized with G-CSF alone.[70] Likewise, Lie et al. reported that increasing the dose of chemotherapy during a second mobilization attempt also increased the yield of CFU-GM in a heterogeneous group of six patients.[71] Similar findings were reported by Goldschmidt et al., who studied 32 patients with multiple myeloma randomized to receive 4 or 7 g/m² of cyclophosphamide followed by G-CSF to collect autologous PBPC.[72] Recognizing the difficulty in predicting apheresis yields because of the heterogeneity of patients and mobilization regimens, investigators have sought methods to predict the yield of PBPC prior to the initiation of apheresis. Haas et al. found that the preleukapheresis level of blood CD34+ cells correlated with the total number collected; specifically, a count of 50 CD34+ cells/mm³ was associated with a yield of greater than 2.5×10^6 CD34+ cells/kg, a dose correlated with rapid engraftment.[54, 73] The observation was not confirmed by other investigators.[74] Armitage et al. also found that a blood CD34+ count of greater than 20 CD34+ cells/mm³ was 94% predictive that a single apheresis, performed the following day, would contain at least 2×10^6 CD34+ cells/kg.[75]

FACTORS AFFECTING ENGRAFTMENT

Speed of engraftment is an important clinical end-point that affects the overall success of transplantation[76–89] and has been reported to depend on the extent of prior chemotherapy/radiation therapy and, most importantly, cell dose (Table 25–2).[90–95] Tricot et al. found a striking negative relationship between the extent of prior therapy and likelihood of rapid engraftment at any given dose of CD34+ cells.[90] Patients exposed to prior chemotherapy for 24 months or more required higher doses of CD34+ cells (5 vs. 2×10^6/kg) to ensure rapid engraftment. Haas et al. performed transplantation with 42 patients who received PBPC mobilized with chemotherapy plus G-CSF and found that a dose of CD34+ cells above 2.5×10^6/kg predicted rapid, complete, and sustained engraftment of platelets and neutrophils (both in less than 14 days), but below this dose, both neutrophil and platelet engraftment was delayed (absolute neutrophil count > 500/mm³ at 17 days, platelet count > 20,000/mm³ at 31 days).[54] Most[53, 89–91, 93–95] but not all other studies have confirmed this relationship,[53] and good correlation between engraftment and CD34+ cells or CFU-GM dose has also been observed[23, 89, 92] or denied.[53] Ketterer et al. reported that patients who received relatively high doses of CD34+ cells not only had shorter engraftment times but also fewer platelet transfusions and

TABLE 25–2. FACTORS REPORTED TO AFFECT THE SPEED OF ENGRAFTMENT BY PERIPHERAL BLOOD PROGENITOR CELLS (PBPC)

1. Use of mobilized PBPC
2. Use of post-transplantation growth factor
3. Extensive prior chemotherapy/radiation therapy
4. Dose of CD34+ cells infused
5. Diagnosis

antibiotic treatments, as well as shorter hospital stay.[94] An adverse effect of extensive prior chemotherapy or radiotherapy on engraftment of neutrophils and platelets has been reported in several studies.[46, 86, 93, 95]

ALLOGENEIC MOBILIZATION

Although a variety of regimens are effective in mobilizing sufficient numbers of PBPC for autografting, chemotherapy cannot be ethically administered to healthy persons. An ideal regimen would, after a single administration of the drug, rapidly and reliably mobilize a sufficient number of primitive and committed HSC to be collected, and, upon infusion into an allogeneic transplant recipient, result in rapid and sustained long-term engraftment. The number of contaminating mature leukocytes and platelets would be minimal. Harvesting would be accomplished with a single collection of a small volume (i.e., <500 mL) of blood from the donor, who would experience minimal discomfort and suffer no long-term effects. Such a regimen does not exist currently, but several growth factor regimens are considered adequate to accomplish this goal. Mobilization of PBPC in healthy persons for allogeneic transplants has most frequently been accomplished by administering recombinant human G-CSF.

DOSING OF G-CSF

G-CSF administered subcutaneously for 4–6 days results in reliable mobilization of CD34+ cells and CFU-GM.[10–14, 62, 95, 98] Several investigators have reported that mobilization of CD34+ cells by G-CSF is dose-dependent over the range of 2.5–10 μg G-CSF/kg/day given as a single dose subcutaneously and that the higher peak levels of blood CD34+ cell resulting from higher G-CSF doses were associated with a significantly higher yield of CD34+ cells.[62, 98–101] The marked individual variation in CD34+ cell mobilization is highlighted by Stroncek et al., who reported a significant relationship between G-CSF dose and the yield of CD34+ cells.[96] Because of the wide variability, however, the authors could not demonstrate any statistically significant difference in CD34+ cell yields from healthy subjects treated with 7.5 μg G-CSF/kg/day for 5 days ($4.1 \pm 2.5 \times 10^8$ CD34+ cells, n = 21) vs. those treated with 10 μg G-CSF/kg/day for 5 days ($4.7 \pm 3.2 \times 10^8$ CD34+ cells, n = 27).[96]

Brown et al. reported that baseline blood CD34+ cell counts varied over a 10-fold range in normal persons.[16] They also found that donors receiving less than 650 μg total G-CSF had only a 25% chance of achieving the targeted CD34+ cell dose of 5×10^6/kg recipient weight in a single apheresis, compared with a probability of 70% for donors receiving greater than 650 μg and 86% for those receiving greater than 850 μg G-CSF. Because the patients who received the lower doses were also smaller in weight and donor weight correlated poorly with CD34+ cell yields, the authors hypothesized that smaller donors may require higher doses of G-CSF, per kilogram of body weight, to achieve adequate mobilization.[16] Because the correlation between G-CSF dose (hence body weight) and pre-apheresis (or premobilization) blood levels of CD34+ cells was poor ($r^2 = 0.27$), the likelihood that such a strategy will be successful is unclear.

Administration of doses of G-CSF higher than 10 μg/kg/day has not been extensively studied in randomized trials with allogeneic donors. In a retrospective analysis of allogeneic PBPC donors, Luider et al. found that administration of more than 10 μg G-CSF/kg/day to 12 subjects for 3 days (apheresis on day 4 after G-CSF injection) did not lead to any increase in the yield of CD34+ cells; compared with 24 subjects treated with 4–10 μg G-CSF/kg/day.[101] Waller et al. reported that twice-daily subcutaneous administration of 10 or 12 μg G-CSF/kg (total of 20 or 24 μg G-CSF/kg/day) to normal donors for 7 days was associated with a trend toward higher circulating leukocytes and higher yields of CD34+ cells (per liter of blood processed) on days 4–7 than administration of 10 μg G-CSF/kg once daily, but the levels of CD34+ cells or CFU in blood were not measured and the differences in apheresis yields were not significant.[102] The finding that the target value of 3.5 × 10⁶ CD34+ cells/kg was achieved after two aphereses in 11 of 14 subjects who received the 20–24 μg/kg dose, compared with only one of five who received the 10 μg/kg/day dose, suggests a benefit with the higher-dose regimen.

Majolino et al. administered 10 μg G-CSF/kg/day for 5 days to five normal donors and 16 μg G-CSF/kg b.i.d. to six donors for 4 days prior to collection.[103] They found no difference between the two groups with respect to peak levels of blood CD34+ cells, the yield of CD34+ cells per liter of blood processed, or the total CD34+ cells/kg recipient weight, and that a single apheresis sufficed in 80% of all donors to reach the target dose of 4 × 10⁶ CD34+ cells/kg.[103] Thus, doses of G-CSF higher than 10–12 μg/kg/day have been associated with higher peak circulating levels of CD34+ cells and apheresis yields of CD34+ cells in some but not all studies in healthy donors.

In view of the large individual variability, it appears that additional randomized studies enrolling more donors will be required to resolve this issue. The routine use of high doses of G-CSF (>10 μg/kg/day) must be balanced against potential risks of growth factor administration to healthy subjects[104] and diminished donor tolerance because Stroncek et al. have reported that side effects experienced by donors also depend on G-CSF dose (and to some extent donor gender—see later).[96]

G-CSF is typically administered once each day by subcutaneous injection, but several centers had used twice-daily dosing, presumably because of the short (3- to 4-hour) circulating half-life of G-CSF.[105] Many of the biologic effects of G-CSF, however, are prolonged for at least 24 hours,[106] and it is not clear whether the twice-daily dosing schedule is advantageous compared with single administration of the same total G-CSF dose. Grigg et al. reported no benefit in the level of blood CD34+ cells by continuous infusion of G-CSF dose at 3 μg/kg/day compared with a single subcutaneous injection.[99] Yano et al. reported no difference in the number of CD34+ cells or CFU collected by a single apheresis and in the tolerance of healthy subjects using two G-CSF dosing regimens: 5 μg/kg twice daily for 5 days versus a single injection of 10 μg/kg/day.[107] Likewise Majolino et al. treated normal donors with either a single dose of 10 μg/kg/day for 4 days or 16 μg/kg/day in two equal doses (8 μg/kg twice a day) and found no difference in (1) the peak level of blood CD34+ cells or CFU, (2) the apheresis yield of CD34+ cells, or (3) donor tolerance.[103]

In 1998, however, Arbona et al. compared three different regimens of G-CSF dosing in normal persons: A single daily dose of 10 μg/kg/day, vs. 6 or 8 μg/kg/12 hours each × 5 days. The latter two regimens resulted in a significantly higher blood CD34+ cell count (83.3 and 121 per mm³, respectively) than 10 μg/kg/day (72 per μL) as a single dose. The two twice-daily regimens were also associated with a significantly higher yield of CD34+ cells by a single apheresis (6.30 and 6.56 vs. 3.05 × 10⁶ CD34+ cells/kg of donor weight, respectively).[108]

The time interval between G-CSF administration (a single daily subcutaneous dose) and apheresis collection has also been studied.[66, 109] Sato et al. systematically studied G-CSF administration to groups of seven normal subjects and observed changes in CFU over 1, 2, 4, 6, 24, and 30 hours.[66] They found that the CFU count increased by day 3 and that the increases occurred continuously during G-CSF dosing. CFU were highest between 24 and 30 hours post G-CSF injection after 5 days of treatment. Thus, these investigators concluded that the most appropriate time for PBPC collection was 24–30 hours after the last injection of G-CSF. Because the difference between the 4- and 24-hour postinjection CFU values was considered to be of little clinical significance after a 5-day regimen, apheresis can be started as early as 4 hours after 5 days of G-CSF dosing.[66] In contrast, after only 3 days of G-CSF administration, the 4-hour postinjection CFU level was considerably lower than that at 24 or 30 hours; hence, apheresis should be delayed for 24 hours if a 3-day dosing regimen is used.

DURATION OF G-CSF

The optimal (minimum) duration of G-CSF administration prior to collection of mobilized PBPC has been studied by several investigators. It is important to recognize that the kinetics of PBPC mobilization is distinctly different from the kinetics of granulocytosis caused by G-CSF administration. Elevated leukocyte count does not necessarily translate into an elevated level of blood CD34+ cells. After a single injection of G-CSF, blood granulocytes increase as early as 2–4 hours, peak at 12–24 hours,[66, 110] and remain elevated for the duration of G-CSF administration.[99, 109] In contrast, increases in CD34+ cells and CFU generally occur no earlier than 48–72 hours after the first administration of G-CSF. The maximum level of blood CD34+ cells is typically reached after 5 or 6 days of G-CSF administration.[65, 96, 99] The day of peak blood CD34+ cells, however, varies considerably among individuals (e.g., from day 4 to day 8). The increase in CD34+ cells is typically paralleled by increases in CFU.[62, 65, 98, 111]

Matsunaga et al. studied the effect of prolonged administration of G-CSF in three healthy subjects given 2.5 μg G-CSF/kg/day for 6 days, followed by 5 μg/kg/day of G-CSF for 4 days (for a total of 9 consecutive days of G-CSF). The level of blood CD34+ cells peaked on day 6 or 7 followed by a decline to baseline values despite the continued administration of G-CSF. There were no differences in the kinetics of mobilization of CD34+/CD33− and CD34+/CD33+ cells, and there was no appreciable difference in the mobilization kinetics of CFU-GM and BFU-E (burst-forming unit—erythroid). This small study thus suggested that PBPC mobilization occurred over a finite time course.[111] In a later study, Stroncek et al. administered G-CSF to healthy persons once daily in doses ranging from 2 to 7.5 μg/kg/day for up to 10 days.[96] They reported that the level of blood CD34+ cells peaked at day 6 (range, day 4–8) and began to decline in most subjects by day 8 despite continued G-CSF administration. The apheresis yield of CD34+ cells was also lower in the cohort of subjects when collection was performed after 10 days of G-CSF administration. Similar results were reported by Grigg et al.[99] These studies indicated that (1) G-CSF results in maximal levels of blood CD34+ cells and CFU after 4–6 days of treatment and (2) prolonged administration of G-CSF does not enhance PBPC mobilization.

FACTORS AFFECTING ALLOGENEIC MOBILIZATION

Despite receiving the same G-CSF regimen, different individuals mobilize CD34+ cells over a tenfold range. The ability to define a reliable method to mobilize PBPC increases the likelihood of collecting the target cell dose with a minimum number of apheresis procedures. Several groups have investigated potential factors that might account for the variability of mobilization and thereby attempt to identify predictive correlation among PBPC collection, donor characteristics, and G-CSF regimens.

Age

Older persons are reported to have normal blood counts.[112] An age-dependent decrease in marrow cellularity has been reported[113] along with a diminished yield of nucleated cells in harvested marrow[114] and responsiveness of myeloid precursors to cytokines.[115] Retrospective analyses in autologous mobilization and collections have not identified age-dependent factors,[37, 54, 55, 116, 117] but differences were found among normal donors. In a prospective study of healthy persons by Chatta et al., 19 young (age, 20–30 years) and elderly (age, 70–80 years) subjects were administered G-CSF, 30 or 300 μg/day, for 14 days. Young subjects mobilized two times more CFU-GM than older subjects did after 5 days of G-CSF administration at the higher dose, and the older group did not respond to the lower dose at all.[61] Similar negative effects of increasing age on PBPC mobilization have been identified by some[61, 118, 119] but not all[96, 120] investigators. Thus, older persons might require higher doses of G-CSF to achieve a given level of PBPC mobilization, but those over the age of 60 years can still effectively serve as PBPC donors.[121]

Gender

Several studies have demonstrated a lack of association between donor sex and CD34+ cell mobilization and collection.[16, 54, 96, 118, 119] In contrast, Miflin et al. reported that, with the same G-CSF regimen (10 μg/kg/day for 4 days), the apheresis yield of CD34+ cells from 10 male donors (4.96 × 10⁶/kg donor weight for a 12-L apheresis) was significantly higher than that from 7 female donors (2.79 × 10⁶/kg).[117] In addition, the target cell yield of 4 × 10⁶ CD34+ cells was achieved by a single apheresis in 9 of the 10 males but in only 1 of the 7 females. Notably, the males were significantly heavier than the females (mean, 90 vs. 60 kg), but the calculations of cell yield were corrected for this difference. Wiesneth et al. also reported diminished mobilization and CD34+ cell yields after similar mobilization regimens in female donors.[119]

Obesity

In one study, a weak positive correlation was found between the presence of morbid obesity (>150% ideal body weight) and the apheresis yield of CD34+ cells.[118] This finding was attributed to the disproportionately smaller increase in extracellular fluid and hematopoietic tissue in obese subjects compared with body weight. This would result in obese subjects receiving a relatively higher dose of G-CSF per unit weight of hematopoietic tissue when G-CSF is administered on a per-kilogram of body weight basis.[118] Whether this effect might have also played a role in the improved cell yields achieved by Miflin et al. is unclear because peak levels of blood CD34+ cell were not reported.[117]

Premobilization Characteristics

The possibility that a readily measurable parameter in the laboratory prior to mobilization might predict the apheresis yield of CD34+ cells has been of great interest. Brown et al. reported that the level of premobilization blood CD34+ cells correlated, but only poorly, with the apheresis yield of CD34+ cells ($r^2 = 0.24$) and accounted for less than 50% of the variability in CD34+ cell collection. Therefore, other as-yet-unidentified factors play a more important role in mobilization efficacy.[16] A relationship between premobilization blood CD34+ cells and the apheresis yield of CD34+ cells has not been confirmed by other groups.[74, 118] Anderlini et al. retrospectively examined which premobilization characteristics might predict the apheresis yield of CD34+ cells in normal persons.[118] Apart from the weak correlation in donor age, they reported a small association with baseline leukocyte count but not with baseline CD34+ counts. A very weak relationship between the percentage of marrow CD34+ cells and the apheresis yield of CD34+ cells has been reported in autologous transplant recipients.[122] Thus, at this time there are no readily available laboratory or clinical parameters that permit prediction of how an individual donor will respond to growth factor in the mobilization of CD34+ cells.

GROWTH FACTOR COMBINATIONS

The marked interdonor variability in mobilization after G-CSF administration remains a problem. A variety of strategies have been suggested to mitigate this problem, including higher doses of G-CSF,[100] the use of different cytokines[65, 123] or cytokine combinations,[65, 124–127] or, in the investigational setting, the use of monoclonal antibodies to adhesion molecules.[128, 129] Little information is available regarding alternative regimens to mobilize CD34+ cells in allogeneic transplant donors. Corringham and Ho described an allogeneic transplant donor who failed to mobilize with 10 μg G-CSF/kg/day but who mobilized well after administration of GM-CSF, 10 μg/kg/day for 3 days, followed by G-CSF administration at the same dose until completion of apheresis.[14] Recipient engraftment was rapid and durable. Lane et al. investigated a variety of combinations of GM-CSF and G-CSF administration in normal persons.[65, 130] They identified several alternative regimens employing combinations of GM-CSF and G-CSF that were equally well tolerated by donors as G-CSF was, yielded equal numbers of CD34+ cells, and mobilized greater numbers of primitive CD34+ subsets than G-CSF alone.[65, 130, 131] Additional studies of optimal methods to reliably mobilize large numbers of PBPC from normal donors with tolerable side effects are needed.

DONOR TOLERANCE

The ability of healthy persons to tolerate G-CSF and PBPC collection strongly influences the success of achieving the target cell dose.[16] An optimal mobilization protocol should minimize adverse effects on short- or long-term donor safety. Specific issues include effects on hematologic parameters and function, organ function, complications of apheresis, possible contraindications to G-CSF administration, and the potential late effect of G-CSF for carcinogenesis or HSC exhaustion.[132]

The administration of G-CSF in doses ranging from 5 to 10 μg/kg/day to normal persons has been associated with a predictable array of side effects (Table 25-3). The most common was bone pain, experienced by 77–90% of subjects, most commonly located in the back, hips, pelvis, or extremities but sometimes in the chest; this pain could be alarming to some subjects.[96] Headaches are the next most common symptom, found in 44–70% of subjects. Other symptoms include body aches, fatigue, and "flu-like" symptoms, which occur in 15–50% of subjects. Less common are gastrointestinal abnormalities (anorexia, nausea, vomiting), fever and/or chills, inflammation at the injection site, and a variety of rare reactions.[98] Generalized skin rash was uncommon (2 of 241 reported subjects) but is of considerable importance because it might require discontinuation of G-CSF[96] (Lane, unpublished observation).

Symptoms appeared in most subjects within hours of the first injection of G-CSF and tended to persist or increase throughout the course of G-CSF administration. Most donors (62–81%) require analgesics for symptomatic relief, and the treatment was at least partially effective in nearly all donors. One report suggested that an antihistamine drug prevented severe bone pain in an autologous transplant recipient mobilized with G-CSF.[133] Prednisone, 1 μg/kg, has been reported to be of no benefit in preventing the side effects of G-CSF.[16] Stroncek et al. systematically studied the tolerability in 102 normal persons mobilized using G-CSF in doses ranging from 2.5 to 10 μg/kg/day for 5–10 days.[96] They found that increased doses of G-CSF were associated with an increased incidence of side effects (chiefly bone and body aches) as well as the use of analgesics; however, Waller et al., who administered 20–24 μg G-CSF/kg/day for up to 7 days to sibling donors, reported that most donors experienced only mild to moderate bone pain.[102] In addition, only 1 of 14 donors in this report required G-CSF dose reduction, a proportion similar to the 9 of 85 donors in the group of Stroncek et al., who received 5–10 μg G-CSF/kg/day for 5 days.[98, 105] This suggests that highly motivated family members may tolerate G-CSF higher than 10 μg/kg/day. Stroncek et al. also reported that women were more likely than men to experience side effects such as fatigue, gastrointestinal problems, fever, sweats, or flu-like symptoms; were more likely to require dose reduction; or were more likely to be unable to complete the study.[96] Symptoms were not affected by the age of the subject. Anderlini et al. found that most symptoms lasted no longer than 2–4 days post treatment, but some subjects complained of residual bone pain for up to 7 days.[132] Taken together, these data indicated that a majority of healthy persons can tolerate G-CSF dosages of 5–10 μg/kg/day for 4–6 days without the need for dose reduction or omission.[62, 65, 96, 98, 120, 122]

Hematologic Effects

G-CSF administration results in dose-dependent granulocytosis with a left shift.[61, 132, 135] The leukocytosis peaks approximately 12 hours after each dose of G-CSF, but the leukocyte count tends to increase progressively during the course of G-CSF administration.[99, 110, 134, 136] In a preclinical study in which primates were treated with doses of G-CSF of 1150 μg/kg/day or more for up to 18 days, the investigators observed 15- to 28-fold increases in peripheral leukocyte counts, neutrophil-infiltrated hemorrhagic foci in the cerebrum and cerebellum, neurologic symptoms, and death in five of eight animals (Neupogen package insert). Thus,

TABLE 25-3. PERCENTAGE OF SUBJECTS REPORTING SYMPTOMS DURING A COURSE OF G-CSF ADMINISTRATION FOR PERIPHERAL BLOOD PROGENITOR CELL MOBILIZATION

STUDY	REF. NO.	N	BONE PAIN*	HEADACHE	FEVER/CHILLS	FLU-LIKE	GI	FATIGUE	LOCAL
Dreger et al., 1994	62	9	77	n/a	n/a	n/a	n/a	n/a	n/a
Stroncek et al., 1996	96	102	83	39	7	57	12	14	7
Anderlini et al., 1996	132	40	82	70	0	n/a	10	20	7
Lane et al., 1999	130	49	90	59	0	51	29	49	11
Bishop et al., 1997	120	41	83	44	27	n/a	22	n/a	n/a

*Numbers refer to percentage of subjects who reported the symptom during the course of growth factor administration.

it has been recommended that the dose of G-CSF be reduced in normal donors if the leukocyte count exceeds 70,000/mm³. Excessive leukocytosis is uncommon in humans treated with 5–10 μg G-CSF/kg/day. G-CSF administration also increases the number of blood lymphocytes and monocytes.[8, 111, 137, 138]

A relationship between the dose of G-CSF administered to normal subjects and the extent of increase in peripheral blood T lymphocytes has been reported by one study[96] but not in others.[62, 98] Most studies agreed on a lack of change in lymphocyte subsets with increasing doses of G-CSF.[98, 135] Eosinophils and basophils do not appear to be increased by G-CSF administration.

Depression of platelet counts has been observed in both patients[138] and healthy persons during G-CSF administration.[134] Other investigators, however, reported no change in platelet counts.[62, 65–96, 135] More important from the perspective of donor safety is the predictable 30–50% decrease in platelet counts that accompanies large-volume apheresis collection of PBPC after mobilization.[139, 140] Typically, platelet counts return to normal values within 4–6 days after a single apheresis procedure for platelet collection.[3] It has been reported that normal granulocyte donors receiving daily G-CSF during a series of apheresis procedures have lower mean platelet counts than donors who did not receive G-CSF.[141] In addition, a longer time is required for the platelet counts of allogeneic PBPC donors mobilized with G-CSF to return to baseline (approximately 7–10 days), suggesting that G-CSF may suppress platelet production.[96, 135]

Moderate thrombocytopenia is a recognized (although occasional) complication in normal apheresis platelet donors and is not considered a cause for concern or deferral.[142] During PBPC collection, both physical loss of platelets and platelet activation may play a role in the thrombocytopenia.[143] Thrombocytopenia was not severe enough to cause a delay in scheduling apheresis for allogeneic PBPC collection in G-CSF–mobilized donors.[62, 132] Okamoto et al. reported an allogeneic PBPC donor with markedly depressed platelet count (47,000/mm³) and prolonged thrombocytopenia (11 days) after mobilization with 10 μg G-CSF/kg/day for 5 days and two 6-L apheresis procedures.[144] Luider et al., who employed large-volume apheresis, reported that procedures were delayed or canceled in 3 of 85 donors because of postapheresis thrombocytopenia (30,000–50,000 platelets/mm³) after one to three collections.[101] Ordemann et al. studied 40 unrelated healthy donors who received 10 μg/kg/day G-CSF × 5 days followed by two aphereses. There was a significant decrease in platelet count (242,000/mm³ before, 98,000/mm³ after aphereses). Autologous platelets were transfused after the second aphereses in four donors.[145]

Wiesneth et al. studied the mobilization of CD34+ cells in 96 healthy family member donors, ranging in age from 17 to 76 years, after administration of G-CSF ranging from 6 to 17 μg/kg. After a median of two apheresis procedures, transfusion of autologous platelets after apheresis was necessary in 16% of the donors because of a platelet count below 80,000/mm³.[119] It has been proposed to separate and re-infuse platelets from the PBPC products of donors whose postdonation platelet counts fall below 100,000/mm³.[145–147] All donors who become thrombocytopenic should be cau-

tioned regarding activities and medications that might pose a bleeding risk, and apheresis should not be performed if the preapheresis platelet count is less than 70,000/mm³.[96, 134]

Platelet activation in healthy subjects after G-CSF administration has been reported. The effects were indicated by increased platelet expression of P-selectin,[148] blood thromboxane B2, and AT-III complex levels.[149] G-CSF enhances platelet aggregation to collagen and adenosine diphosphate,[114] presumably by a G-CSF receptor–mediated priming event.[150] There have been two reports of arterial thrombosis in two patients with cancer who were receiving G-CSF after chemotherapy.[151, 152] Concern has been expressed regarding induction of a possible prethrombotic state in some normal donors,[149, 153] and such risk was suggested in two cases. The first involved a 54-year-old, apparently healthy female donor mobilized with G-CSF who experienced a cerebrovascular accident 2 days after an uneventful apheresis. The second involved a 64-year-old male with a history of coronary artery disease who experienced a myocardial infarction after PBPC collection.[134] The role of G-CSF and/or PBPC collection in these cases is unclear.

The possible adverse effects of apheresis platelet collection on lymphocyte loss (1–50 × 10⁶ per procedure) and immunologic responsiveness after repeated procedures have been of some concern. Strauss et al. reported no long-term adverse effects of such procedures in normal donors but recommended limiting lymphocyte losses to less than 10¹¹ and delaying apheresis when donor lymphocyte counts fell to less than 500/mm³.[154] Korbling et al. investigated the effects of G-CSF mobilization (6 μg/kg twice daily for 3–5 days, followed by apheresis on day 4 or 5) on lymphocyte subsets.[155] They found that lymphocytes (and CD34+ cells) decreased after apheresis to a nadir at day 7 after apheresis, returned to normal levels by day 30, and were slightly diminished at day 100. Kadar et al. studied 13 allogeneic family donors mobilized with 5 μg/kg G-CSF twice daily and two large-volume apheresis procedures as well as bone marrow collection.[156] The authors reported that loss of T cells (3 × 10¹⁰ CD3+ cells) was much greater with apheresis procedures than with marrow harvesting, but they noted no long-term decrement in lymphocyte counts in seven of the donors who were followed for a mean of 209 days.

Transient neutropenia (absolute neutrophil count < 1500/mm³) persisting for at least 7–10 days has been reported in 2 of 13 allogeneic donors mobilized with 6 μg G-CSF/kg twice daily for 3 or 4 days followed by a three-times blood volume apheresis. Neutropenia was asymptomatic and resolved within 8–45 days.[105] The implications of this observation are unclear, and the authors did not recommend routine monitoring of postapheresis leukocyte counts. Splenomegaly has been reported after high-dose G-CSF administration to primates and other species (Neupogen package insert). Of note, Becker et al.[157] reported a case of spontaneous splenic rupture in an allogeneic donor 4 days after a 6-day regimen of G-CSF.

Nonhematologic Effects

Perhaps the most serious concern in mobilization and collection of PBPC in normal persons, apart from those relating to the administration of G-CSF or other cytokines, relates to the possible consequences of apheresis. Specifically, the placement of large-bore catheters into persons with inadequate venous access has raised medical and ethical issues. Apheresis for component collection is reported to be at least as safe as blood donation and is occasionally associated with mild hypocalcemia due to the infusion of citrate.[158] Approximately 5–20% of healthy donors, however, have inadequate venous access for apheresis without a central venous catheter.[16, 120, 132, 134]

Some institutions consider the requirement for catheter use to perform apheresis to be a contraindication to PBPC collection.[116, 132] The use of catheters appears to vary widely among institutions collecting PBPC for allografting.[11, 13, 14, 16, 62, 96, 101, 120, 132] For example, Anderlini et al.[132] reported that 3 of 43 allogeneic donors had inadequate venous access, a proportion similar to that reported by Urbano-Ispizua et al. (3 of 30).[100] At the other end of the spectrum, the protocol employed by Russell et al. specified the use of central venous catheters for all 10 allogeneic donors.[159] Although few complications and only one pneumothorax have been reported in normal donors to date,[100] catheter use has been associated with such complications as infection, pneumothorax, and bleeding in up to 1% of autologous collections.[160, 161] Other apheresis complications, such as citrate toxicity or electrolyte disturbances, may be mitigated by electrolyte infusion or the addition of heparin to limit citrate use.[123]

Additional adverse reactions to G-CSF administration include the following. Snowden et al. reported that rheumatoid flare occurred in a minority of patients with rheumatoid arthritis who were being mobilized with G-CSF at 5–10 μg/kg/day.[162] Cho et al. reported a patient who experienced a psoriasiform eruption during treatment with GM-CSF or G-CSF.[163] Cases of episcleritis and iritis have also been reported to accompany G-CSF mobilization,[125, 164] and it seems reasonable to assume that patients mobilized with this or any cytokine will be at risk (albeit small) for any of the known reported side effects and adverse effects of these agents.

The metabolic effects of G-CSF administration in both patients with cancer and healthy persons have been reported.[62, 96, 132] G-CSF administration to normal subjects has been associated with transient two- to three-fold increases in serum levels of alkaline phosphatase and lactate dehydrogenase as well as smaller increases in alanine aminotransferase and uric acid. Serum gamma-glutamyl transferase and creatine phosphokinase remain unaltered, suggesting that the noted changes in alkaline phosphatase and lactate dehydrogenase are due to an expanding myeloid mass.[134] Moderate decreases in blood urea nitrogen, glucose, bilirubin, potassium, and occasionally magnesium have been reported. These changes appear to be of no clinical consequence except for the possible need for electrolyte supplementation during large-volume leukapheresis.[165]

Long-Term Safety Considerations

Use of G-CSF in normal donors for granulocyte collection has become a common practice.[141, 166] Despite the apparent safety of short-term courses of G-CSF, data are minimal regarding the long-term safety of G-CSF or other growth factors.[134] Specific concerns have been raised regarding the potential for single or repeated courses of G-CSF and apheresis collection of PBPC leading to exhaustion of HSC. Although no large long-term studies are available, several small studies suggest that stem cell exhaustion does not occur with limited follow-up duration. Harada et al. found no abnormalities in the blood counts of nine donors 1½ years after administration of 10 μg of G-CSF/kg/day for 5 days.[97] In a preliminary report, Kunkel et al. reported no difference after 1 year in the baseline hematologic values of 46 subjects who had been mobilized with G-CSF alone or in combination with GM-CSF.[167] In a subgroup of 11 subjects who underwent a second course of mobilization using one of the three different regimens 1 year later, the apheresis yields of CD34+ cells were not different between the first and the second collection. Similar findings have been reported by others.[168, 169] These studies are encouraging, but they are too small and too short in terms of follow-up to ensure that no adverse effects on hematopoiesis will be encountered as a rare event after a longer time period, and it has been proposed that each institution periodically follow mobilized PBPC donors.[134]

Because of the ability of G-CSF to stimulate the growth of leukemic cells ex vivo,[170, 171] another concern for normal PBPC donors is the leukemogenic, or more generally, the neoplastic potential of G-CSF. The peak serum levels of G-CSF after a single administration of 10 μg/kg (approximately 1 ng/mL) are reported to be approximately 1.5 times higher than mean endogenous G-CSF levels during infection and equal to the upper quartile of values reported (approximately 1–3 ng/mL).[172, 173] Thus, it seems doubtful that a short course of G-CSF would pose a significant risk. Only anecdotal data, however, attest to the lack of leukemic potential in normal donors at this time.[174] G-CSF has also been employed in patients with severe congenital neutropenia for several years.[175, 176] Although cases of leukemia and myelodysplasia have been reported in patients with severe congenital neutropenia and aplastic anemia,[175, 177–180] patients with these diseases appear to be predisposed to these malignancies[181, 182] and it cannot be ascertained that the use of G-CSF has altered the natural history of the diseases. Thus, data are insufficient to evaluate the possible leukemogenic risk of G-CSF or even to indicate that such a risk exists. Moreover, it is doubtful that meaningful clinical data regarding the safety of G-CSF will become available in the near future.

Hasenclever and Sextro have estimated that in order to ascertain even a 10-fold increase in leukemia risk in normal donors, it will be necessary to follow 2000 subjects for 10 years.[183] The control group for such a study would require careful definition because HLA-matched family members of patients with leukemia may also have an inherently increased risk of leukemia compared with the general population.[183, 184] A preliminary report on the follow-up of marrow donors supports this possibility.[185]

ALLOGENEIC MARROW VERSUS PBPC

Donor preferences and safety considerations play an important role in choosing marrow versus PBPC. Kadar et al.

studied the effect of combined PBPC mobilization with 5 μg/kg of G-CSF given twice daily and two large-volume leukapheresis procedures versus bone marrow collection from the same donors in 13 family donors for allogeneic transplantation. Overall, 12 of the 13 donors preferred PBPC collection.[156] Participants in a 1996 workshop concluded that the short-term safety profile of G-CSF appears to be acceptable enough that most healthy persons can be PBPC donors, especially family donors.[132] In view of our limited knowledge of the possible unusual adverse effects of G-CSF, however, a variety of relative or possible contraindications to mobilization with G-CSF and PBPC apheresis should be considered.

Some centers consider inadequate venous access to be a contraindication to PBPC collection because of the risk of catheter-related complications. The decision to harvest marrow rather than inserting a catheter should include an assessment of all the possible risks for marrow harvesting (e.g., general anesthesia) and the possibility of homologous transfusion. For example, PBPC collection might be safer for an HLA-matched sibling donor with poor veins but with a higher anesthetic risk (e.g., active asthma). Likewise, for donors older than 65 years, it might be preferable to collect PBPC because age has little effect on the apheresis yield of CD34+ cells and a 1995 study reported a high rate (22%) of homologous blood transfusion in older marrow donors.[186] PBPC collection might be preferable in donors who have severe back pain because exacerbation of this condition has been reported in marrow harvesting.[185] Clearly, patients who have a known allergy to G-CSF are candidates for marrow harvesting because generalized allergic dermatitis has occurred after G-CSF administration[96] (Lane, unpublished observation). Marrow harvesting might be preferred in donors who have a history of inflammatory eye disorders because cases of episcleritis and iritis during G-CSF administration have been reported.[125, 187] Potential donors who are at risk for venous or arterial thrombosis or who have vascular disease may be at increased risk for complications due to PBPC mobilization in view of the effects of G-CSF on hemostasis. Whether marrow harvesting poses a lower risk than G-CSF administration and PBPC apheresis in such patients is also uncertain. Potential PBPC donors with a history of autoimmune disorders may be at increased risk for flare (e.g., systemic lupus erythematosis with serositis and/or myalgia, rheumatoid arthritis, multiple sclerosis).[162–168]

Whether marrow obtained from donors who have been administered G-CSF is as efficacious in promoting early engraftment is clear, but if this technique proves to be effective, increasing numbers of normal marrow donors will also be exposed to G-CSF.[188] PBPC mobilization and collection might be approached more cautiously in donors with a history of malignancy treated with chemotherapy/radiation therapy, premalignant conditions, or a strong family history of myelodysplasia or leukemia (other than the intended recipient). Morbid obesity may also be a relative contraindication to marrow harvesting and would make PBPC collection preferable.[117] Additional considerations should include the recipient's conditions.

Numerous studies have reported no significant difference in the incidence and severity of acute graft-versus-host disease (GVHD) in patients undergoing allografting with PBPC (57%) compared with bone marrow (45%) despite the 10- to 20-fold higher numbers of T cells given with PBPC.[11, 13, 15, 100] Some preliminary reports, however, suggest that the incidence of chronic GVHD was increased in recipients of PBPC compared with marrow.[12, 189] Consequently, a patient considered to be at high risk for complications associated with chronic GVHD (and who has a disease that does not benefit from the graft-versus-leukemia effect) might be a better candidate for marrow grafting. Alternatively, administration of T cell–depleted PBPC allografts has been associated with only mild acute GVHD and limited chronic GVHD.[190]

The costs (approximately \$14,000–\$15,000) of PBPC mobilization and collection in 37 donors who did not require central venous lines were reported to be comparable to those associated with marrow harvest in 33 donors.[132]

LEUKAPHERESIS

PBPC collection can be performed with one of several commercially available devices (e.g., Fenwal CS3000, COBE Spectra, Fresenius 104) with varying levels of automation. Typical collection procedures use an input blood flow rate of 50–80 mL/minute (depending on the height and weight of patients), blood-to-anticoagulant ratio of 12:1 to 14:1, and processed blood volume of 10–12 L (or twice the blood volume). Total collection time is 2–3 hours. Cell separation is based on physical parameters such as cell size and density. Detection of interface between plasma and red blood cells is an integral part of the collection devices. Nontarget blood components such as plasma, red blood cells, and leukocytes of higher densities (granulocytes) are returned to the donor or patient. Product volume depends on the machine and the procedure (50–200 mL). Concurrent plasma is usually collected for possible storage of product before processing and the preparation of cryoprotectant (see Chapter 28).

Typical product contains mainly lymphocytes and monocytes, although high proportions of granulocytes (>50%) are sometimes unavoidable because of the use of chemotherapy and/or growth factors. Enrichment of CD34+ cells using only the apheresis devices has not been successful because the range of density and size of CD34+ cells overlapped with those of lymphocytes and monocytes. A new dual-stage, automated collection system that requires less user input is reported to be associated with equivalent yield, increased collection efficiency, lower platelet contamination, and smaller product volume compared with a previous version that required subjective operator evaluation of the effluent hematocrit.[191]

INITIATION OF LEUKAPHERESIS

The timing of leukapheresis for the collection of the mobilized PBPC after myelosuppressive chemotherapy is not always predictable. Peak levels of PBPC, as measured by colony-forming assays, have been reported to occur when the circulating leukocyte count reaches approximately 1000–5000/mm³ or during the exponential increase in the circulating leukocyte count, and these parameters are widely employed.[24, 25, 62] A relevant practical limitation is that leukapheresis is difficult to perform with leukocyte counts less than 1000/mm³ because the visible leukocyte "interface" is usually not apparent below this count.[64] The mobilization of PBPC in response to G-CSF appears to be more reliable, with most studies indicating maximum levels of circulating progenitors on days 5–7. The optimal time course of mobilization with GM-CSF appears to be somewhat longer at 5–11 days.[34, 64–66]

Attention has also been focused on the extent to which post-treatment measurements can predict either the level of mobilization or the apheresis yield of CD34+ cells. Although a preapheresis leukocyte count less than 5000/mm³ was reported to predict poor leukapheresis yields, the leukocyte count itself is a poor predictor of CD34+ cell yield.[192] Excellent correlations have been reported between the blood level of CD34+ cells on the day of apheresis and the yield of CD34+ cells in normal persons mobilized with G-CSF for allogeneic transplantation in some[12, 98, 99] but not all[101] studies.

Several investigators have proposed guidelines for the timing of apheresis after mobilization.[54, 193–198] Some reported that, using 10-L apheresis, greater than 10 CD34+ cells/mm³ on the day of apheresis predicts collection of greater than 0.5×10^6 CD34+ cells/kg,[193] less than 20 CD34+ cells/mm³ predicted less than 4×10^6 CD34+ cells/kg,[194] greater than 20 CD34+ cells/mm³ predicted collection of greater than $2–2.5 \times 10^6$ CD34+ cells/kg after one or two procedures,[195] greater than 50 CD34+ cells/mm³ predicted collection of either greater than 2.5×10^6 CD34+ cells/kg[54] or greater than 4×10^6 CD34+ cells/kg.[194]

Protocols that employ direct measurements of circulating CD34+ cells on the day of apheresis require a rapid laboratory turnaround. Investigators have attempted to identify more readily available predictors of CD34+ cell yield. Although some have identified a correlation between the preapheresis leukocyte count and the yield of CD34+ cells,[118] others have not[122] and, at best, the correlations are so weak that they are of no practical value.[36, 54] Others have proposed the measurement of circulating immature myeloid cells on the day of apheresis to predict the yield of CD34+ cells, but the correlation with this parameter was also weak (r² = 0.59).[196]

Alternatively, measurement of blood CD34+ cells on the day prior to apheresis has been reported to correlate with the yield of CD34+ cells (r² = 0.71) and mitigates the need for rapid turnaround in the CD34+ cell measurements.[195] Because the day of peak blood CD34+ cells varies between 4 and 8 days after G-CSF administration, the peak's prediction cannot be based on premobilization criteria or dosing schedule, and "real time" CD34+ counts are not available in most institutions, the decision as to when to initiate leukapheresis in allogeneic PBPC donors is arbitrary and varies among institutions. In most centers, apheresis is initiated 3–4 hours after the fourth to fifth injection of G-CSF (approximately 72–96 hours after the initial injection) in order to permit a second procedure, if necessary, on the following day, when the level of blood CD34+ cells is still likely to be high.

Anderlini et al. compared initiating leukapheresis on day 4 versus day 5 in similar groups of normal allogeneic

donors mobilized with 6 μg of G-CSF/kg twice daily (until completion of apheresis). CD34+ cells were collected using large-volume apheresis procedures.[104] Peak blood CD34+ cell levels were not measured, but the 5-day group had higher levels of blood mononuclear cells. The 5-day mobilization group was significantly more likely to achieve the target CD34+ cell dose (4×10^6/kg recipient weight) after a single procedure (30 of 32) than the 4-day group (30 of 45). The 5-day group, however, also had greater numbers of symptoms and higher leukocyte counts; consequently, the investigators elected to use the 4-day regimen in order to minimize G-CSF exposure to the normal donors.[104]

Bishop et al. investigated the optimal timing of apheresis in 41 allogeneic donors using 5 μg of G-CSF/kg/day until completion of apheresis initiated on day 4 and continued through day 6.[120] They found that collections on day 6 yielded the highest number of CD34+ cells and that 93% of the combined yields from apheresis on days 5 and 6 were adequate for transplantation (3×10^6 CD34+ cells/kg recipient weight), compared with 83% of the combined yields of days 4 and 5. A fourth apheresis was required to achieve the CD34+ cell dose in 15% of donors, however. Thus, the number of apheresis procedures in collecting allogeneic PBPC typically varies from one to more than four, starting on day 3–5, and the amount of donor blood processed per procedure may vary from two to four times the blood volumes, depending on the efficacy of mobilization, the target dose of CD34+ cells desired, the adequacy of venous access, the donor tolerance of the procedure, the time of day apheresis is performed, and the need to perform ex vivo manipulations that will result in the loss of CD34+ cells (e.g., T-cell depletion).

Termination of leukapheresis requires close communication between the apheresis, processing laboratory, and transplant physicians. Most institutions have adopted a target CD34+ cell dose for transplantation.[1, 64, 199] Minimum dose is usually $1–2 \times 10^6$ CD34+ cells/kg; the optimal dose at least 5×10^6 CD34+ cells/kg. When a sufficient quantity of PBPC has been collected, the processing laboratory should notify the transplant physician to make the decision to stop further collection. For allogeneic transplantation, additional cells might be needed for donor lymphocyte infusion after myeloablative or nonablative therapy and PBPC infusion. If the donor is in a different geographic location, one or two more apheresis sessions may be required to collect the cells, which are then cryopreserved for donor lymphocyte infusion.

LARGE-VOLUME LEUKAPHERESIS

Another technique to optimize the apheresis yield of CD34+ cells is to increase the volume of blood processed during the procedure.[67, 197, 198, 201] Processing blood volume is increased from 10 L to as high as 40 L. Total number of collected leukocytes is proportional to the volume of processed blood.[195, 197, 201] Studies show that CD34+ cells are recruited into the circulation during leukapheresis but that the overall number of CD34+ cells diminishes.[202] The increased amount of infused anticoagulant necessitates calcium replacement, either orally or intravenously. The start of laboratory processing (e.g., for cryopreservation, CD34+ cell selection) is delayed because of the lengthening in apheresis time (as long as 8 hours). Storage of product for overnight or longer alleviates the technologist's time spent in laboratory processing (see Chapter 28). For patients with good mobilization, large-volume leukapheresis (LVL) can decrease the number of apheresis sessions required to achieve the target CD34+ cell dose. For poorly mobilized patients, even with the application of LVL, target or minimum CD34+ cell dose was not achieved in a substantial portion of patients.[203] Despite the increase in total leukocytes collected by LVL, engraftment, especially for platelet recovery, might be delayed because of the poor quality of PBPC.[204] The overall utility of LVL must be balanced against the frequent requirement for central venous catheter placement,[205] calcium depletion, platelet loss, length of time for collection, and postcollection processing.

PLATELET LOSS

Depressed platelet count after PBPC collection in healthy donors of allogeneic transplants is not uncommon and has been discussed. The decrease in platelet counts during apheresis for autologous transplant recipients can be substantial, especially for those heavily pretreated patients mobilized with chemotherapy plus growth factor. Platelet transfusion should be considered when the postapheresis count drops below 20,000/mm³. The threshold should be individualized and depends on the status of the patient (inpatient vs. outpatient), the history of platelet recovery after chemotherapy, the amount of infused anticoagulant (hence the number of prior apheresis sessions within the same mobilization and collection series), and whether apheresis will be performed the next day. It is possible to separate platelets from the PBPC product using a low-speed centrifugation procedure. The platelets may be infused fresh or cryopreserved for later infusion.[206, 207] The platelet cryopreservation procedure, however, has not been universally accepted.[208] Furthermore, the PBPC product of patients with a low platelet count and who require transfusion typically does not contain enough platelets to warrant processing (Lane, unpublished observation).

CONCLUSION

Mobilization of PBPC for autologous transplantation appears to be a reliable method of obtaining a graft with the consistent ability to support rapid, trilineage engraftment in a majority of patients. The choice of regimen and dose of agents used to mobilize PBPC, however, are highly individual and should be based on several considerations, including the patient's diagnosis, disease status, extent of prior chemotherapy/radiation therapy, marrow infiltration with tumor, previous and response to mobilization, as well as whether extensive cell loss during processing is anticipated. Given the CD34+ cell losses that are obligatory with increasing use of postmobilization manipulation (e.g., positive and negative selection), the mobilization of an "adequate" dose of CD34+ cells is an ever-changing goal. Progress has also been made in identifying persons who

are likely to be "poor mobilizers," and several potential approaches are available to enhance PBPC mobilization in such persons. The poorly mobilizing patient, however, remains a serious impediment to delivery of high-dose chemotherapy/radiation therapy with stem cell support, and continued investigation should be focused on more-reliable methods of managing such cases.

It is now possible to reliably obtain sufficient PBPC from most normal donors to perform allogeneic transplantation, with tolerable side effects, by the administration of a single daily dose of G-CSF at 7.5–10 μg/kg subcutaneously for 4–6 days, followed by one to three apheresis procedures starting on day 3–5. There is, however, wide variability among individuals with respect to the extent of mobilization achieved by the regimen and the optimal timing of apheresis. Studies suggest that the likelihood of obtaining an adequate harvest of CD34+ cells, as defined locally, may be enhanced by employing higher doses or different schedules of G-CSF, monitoring the mobilization and/or collection of PBPC, and using apheresis procedures processing at least twice the blood volume. An optimal regimen for mobilization and harvesting for all donors has not yet been identified, however, and a small percentage of donors may not mobilize adequately with G-CSF alone. Alternative regimens employing combinations of G-CSF and GM-CSF are available that may prove useful in such cases, and novel cytokines that are even more effective than G-CSF in mobilizing HSC are eagerly awaited. Based on the currently available experience with several hundred normal donors, the short-term safety of G-CSF appears to be acceptable, although there are several scenarios in which marrow harvesting may be preferable to G-CSF mobilization and apheresis collection of PBPC.

REFERENCES

1. Lane TA: Allogeneic marrow reconstitution using peripheral blood stem cells: the dawn of a new era. Transfusion 36:585–589, 1996.
2. Giralt S, Estey E, Albitar M, et al: Engraftment of allogeneic hematopoietic progenitor cells with purine analog-containing chemotherapy: harnessing graft-versus-leukemia without myeloablative therapy. Blood 89:4531–4536, 1997.
3. Lasky LC, Lin A, Kahn RA, McCullough J: Donor platelet response and product quality assurance in plateletpheresis. Transfusion 21(3):247–260, 1981.
4. Moss TJ, Sanders DG, Lasky LC, Bostrom B: Contamination of peripheral blood stem cell harvests by circulating neuroblastoma cells. Blood 76:1879–1883, 1990.
5. Sharp JG, Joshi SS, Armitage JO, et al: Significance of detection of occult non-Hodgkin's lymphoma in histologically uninvolved bone marrow by a culture technique. Blood 79:1074–1080, 1992.
6. Fliedner TM, Flad HD, Bruch C, et al: Treatment of aplastic anemia by blood stem cell transfusion: a canine model. Haematologica 61(2):141–156, 1976.
7. Molineux G, Pojda Z, Hampson IN, et al: Transplantation potential of peripheral blood stem cells induced by granulocyte colony-stimulating factor. Blood 76:2153–2158, 1990.
8. Weaver CH, Buckner CD, Longin K, et al: Syngeneic transplantation with peripheral blood mononuclear cells collected after the administration of recombinant human granulocyte colony-stimulating factor. Blood 82:1981–1984, 1993.
9. Kessinger A, Smith DM, Strandjord SE, et al: Allogeneic transplantation of blood-derived, T cell–depleted hemopoietic stem cells after myeloablative treatment in a patient with acute lymphoblastic leukemia. Bone Marrow Transplant (6):643–646, 1989.
10. Russell NH, Hunter A, Rogers S, et al: Peripheral blood stem cells as an alternative to marrow for allogeneic transplantation [Letter]. Lancet 341(8858):1482, 1993.

11. Bensinger WI, Weaver CH, Appelbaum FR, et al: Transplantation of allogeneic peripheral blood stem cells mobilized by recombinant human granulocyte colony-stimulating factor. Blood 85(6):1655–1658, 1995.

12. Korbling M, Przepiorka D, Huh YO, et al: Allogeneic blood stem cell transplantation for refractory leukemia and lymphoma: potential advantage of blood over marrow allografts. Blood 85(6):1659–1665, 1995.

13. Schmitz N, Dreger P, Suttorp M, et al: Primary transplantation of allogeneic peripheral blood progenitor cells mobilized by filgrastim (granulocyte colony-stimulating factor). Blood 85(6):1666–1672, 1995.

14. Corringham RET, Ho AD: Rapid and sustained allogeneic transplantation using immunoselected CD34+ selected peripheral blood progenitor cells mobilized by recombinant granulocyte- and granulocyte-macrophage colony stimulating factors. Blood 86:2052–2054, 1995.

15. Pavletic ZS, Bishop MR, Tarantolo SR, et al: Hematopoietic recovery after allogeneic blood stem-cell transplantation compared with bone marrow transplantation in patients with hematologic malignancies. J Clin Oncol 4:1608–1616, 1992.

16. Brown RA, Adkins D, Goodnough LT, et al: Factors that influence the collection and engraftment of allogeneic peripheral-blood stem cells in patients with hematologic malignancies. J Clin Oncol 15(9):3067–3074, 1997.

17. Russell JA, Desai S, Herbut B, et al: Partially mismatched blood cell transplants for high-risk hematologic malignancy. Bone Marrow Transplant 19(9):861–866, 1997.

18. Bender JG, Unverzagt KL, Walker DE, et al: Identification and comparison of CD34-positive cells and their subpopulations from normal peripheral blood and bone marrow using multicolor flow cytometry. Blood 77:2591–2596, 1991.

19. Richman CM, Weiner RS, Yankee RA: Increase in circulating stem cells following chemotherapy in man. Blood 47:1031–1039, 1976.

20. Siena S, Bregni M, Brando B, et al: Circulation of CD34+ hematopoietic stem cells in the peripheral blood of high-dose cyclophosphamide-treated patients: enhancement by intravenous recombinant human granulocyte-macrophage colony-stimulating factor. Blood 74:1905–1914, 1989.

21. Stiff PJ, Murgo AJ, Wittes RE, et al: Quantification of the peripheral blood colony forming unit-culture rise following chemotherapy. Transfusion 23:500–503, 1983.

22. To LB, Haylock DN, Kimber RJ, Juttner CA: High levels of circulating haemopoietic stem cells in very early remission from acute non-lymphoblastic leukaemia and their collection and cryopreservation. Br J Haematol 58:399–410, 1984.

23. To LB, Roberts MM, Haylock DN, et al: Comparison of haematological recovery times and supportive care requirements of autologous recovery phase peripheral blood stem cell transplants, autologous bone marrow transplants and allogeneic bone marrow transplants. Bone Marrow Transplant 9:277–284, 1992.

24. Pettengell R, Testa NG, Swindell R, et al: Transplantation potential of hematopoietic cells released into the circulation during routine chemotherapy for non-Hodgkin's lymphoma. Blood 82:2239–2248, 1993.

25. Sutherland HJ, Eaves CJ, Lansdorp PM, et al: Kinetics of committed and primitive blood progenitor mobilization after chemotherapy and growth factor treatment and their use in autotransplants. Blood 83:3808–3814, 1994.

26. Craig JI, Parker AC, Anthony RS: The effects of various chemotherapy regimes on the levels of peripheral blood stem cells in patients with lymphoma. Bone Marrow Transplant 5 (Suppl 1):30–31, 1990.

27. Gee A: Purging of peripheral blood stem cell grafts. Stem Cells 13 (Suppl 3):52–62, 1995.

28. Tarella C, Zallio F, Caracciolo D, et al: Hemopoietic progenitor cell mobilization and harvest following an intensive chemotherapy debulking in indolent lymphoma patients. Stem Cells 17(1):55–61, 1999.

29. Fischer T, Neubauer A, Mohm J, et al: Chemotherapy-induced mobilization of karyotypically normal PBSC for autografting in CML. Bone Marrow Transplant 21(10):1029–1036, 1998.

30. Socinski MA, Elias A, Schnipper L, et al: Granulocyte-macrophage colony stimulating factor expands the circulating haemopoietic progenitor cell compartment in man. Lancet 1:1194–1198, 1988.

31. Duhrsen U, Villeval JL, Boyd J, et al: Effects of recombinant human granulocyte colony-stimulating factor on hematopoietic progenitor cells in cancer patients. Blood 72(6):2974–2981, 1988.

32. DeLuca E, Sheridan WP, Watson D, et al: Prior chemotherapy does not prevent effective mobilisation by G-CSF of peripheral blood progenitor cells. Br J Cancer 66(5):893–899, 1992.

33. Haas R, Ho AD, Bredthauer U, et al: Successful autologous transplantation of blood stem cells mobilized with recombinant human granulocyte-macrophage colony-stimulating factor. Exp Hematol 18:94–98, 1990.

34. Bensinger W, Singer J, Appelbaum F, et al: Autologous transplantation with peripheral blood mononuclear cells collected after administration of recombinant granulocyte stimulating factor. Blood 81:3158–3163, 1993.

35. Kroger N, Zeller W, Hassan H, et al: Schedule-dependency of granulocyte colony-stimulating factor in peripheral blood progenitor cell mobilization in breast cancer patients. Blood 91:1828, 1998.

36. Peters WP, Rosner G, Ross M, et al: Comparative effects of granulocyte-macrophage colony-stimulating factor (GM-CSF) and granulocyte colony-stimulating factor (G-CSF) on priming peripheral blood progenitor cells for use with autologous bone marrow after high-dose chemotherapy. Blood 81:1709–1719, 1993.

37. Bolwell BJ, Goormastic M, Yanssens T, et al: Comparison of G-CSF with GM-CSF for mobilizing peripheral blood progenitor cells and for enhancing marrow recovery after autologous bone marrow transplant. Bone Marrow Transplant 14:13–18, 1994.

38. Spitzer G, Adkins D, Mathews M, et al: Randomized comparison of G-CSF + GM-CSF vs G-CSF alone for mobilization of peripheral blood stem cells: effects on hematopoietic recovery after high-dose chemotherapy. Bone Marrow Transplant 20(11):921–930, 1997.

39. Begley CG, Basser R, Mansfield R, et al: Enhanced levels and enhanced clonogenic capacity of blood progenitor cells following administration of stem cell factor plus granulocyte colony-stimulating factor to humans. Blood 90(9):3378–3389, 1997.

40. Weaver A, Chang J, Wrigley E, et al: Randomized comparison of progenitor-cell mobilization using chemotherapy, stem-cell factor, and filgrastim or chemotherapy plus filgrastim alone in patients with ovarian cancer. J Clin Oncol 16(8):2601–2612, 1998.

41. Gianni AM, Siena S, Bregni M, et al: Very rapid and complete haematopoitic reconstitution following myeloablative treatments: the role of circulating stem cells harvested after high-dose cyclophosphamide and GM-CSF. In Dicke KA, Spitzer G, Jagannath S, Evinger-Hodges MJ (eds): Bone Marrow Transplantation, 4th ed. Austin, University of Texas Press, 1989, pp 723–731.

42. Haas R, Hohaus S, Egerer G, et al: Recombinant human granulocyte-macrophage colony-stimulating factor (rhGM-CSF) subsequent to chemotherapy improves collection of blood stem cells for autografting in patients not eligible for bone marrow harvest. Bone Marrow Transplant 9(6):459–465, 1992.

43. Teshima T, Harada M, Takamatsu Y, et al: Granulocyte colony-stimulating factor (G-CSF)-induced mobilization of circulating haemopoietic stem cells. Br J Haematol 84:570–573, 1993.

44. Ho AD, Glück S, Germond C, et al: Optimal timing for collections of blood progenitor cells following induction chemotherapy and granulocyte-macrophage colony-stimulating factor for autologous transplantation in advanced breast cancer. Leukemia 7:1738–1746, 1993.

45. Mohle R, Pforssich M, Fruehauf S, et al: Filgrastim post-chemotherapy mobilizes more CD34+ cells with a different antigenic profile compared with use during steady-state hematopoiesis. Bone Marrow Transplant 14:827–832, 1994.

46. Moskowitz CH, Glassman JR, Wuest D, et al: Factors affecting mobilization of peripheral blood progenitor cells in patients with lymphoma. Clin Cancer Res 4(2):311–316, 1998.

47. Kurekci AE, Kiss JE, Koehler M: Mobilization of peripheral blood progenitor cells using 16 versus 10 µg/kg/d G-CSF in children with malignancies. Pediatr Transplant 2(2):160–164, 1998.

48. Hohaus S, Martin H, Wassmann B, et al: Recombinant human granulocyte and granulocyte-macrophage colony-stimulating factor (G-CSF and GM-CSF) administered following cytotoxic chemotherapy have a similar ability to mobilize peripheral blood stem cells. Bone Marrow Transplant 22(7):625–630, 1998.

49. Demuynck H, Delforge M, Verhoef G, et al: Comparative study of peripheral blood progenitor cell collection in patients with multiple myeloma after single-dose cyclophosphamide combined with rhGM-CSF or rhG-CSF. Br J Haematol 90(2):384–392, 1995.

50. Meisenberg B, Brehm T, Schmeckel A, et al: A combination of low-dose cyclophosphamide and colony-stimulating factors is more cost-effective than granulocyte-colony-stimulating factors alone in mobilizing peripheral blood stem and progenitor cells. Transfusion 38(2):209–215, 1998.

51. Bellido M, Sureda A, Martino R, et al: Collection of peripheral blood progenitor cells for autografting with low-dose cyclophosphamide plus granulocyte colony-stimulating factor. Haematologica 83(5):428–431, 1998.

52. Schneider JG, Crown JP, Wasserheit C, et al: Factors affecting the mobilization of primitive and committed hematopoietic progenitors into the peripheral blood of cancer patients. Bone Marrow Transplant 14:877–884, 1994.

53. Bensinger WI, Longin K, Appelbaum F, et al: Peripheral blood stem cells (PBSCs) collected after recombinant granulocyte colony stimulating factor (rhG-CSF): an analysis of factors correlating with the tempo of engraftment after transplantation. Br J Haematol 87(4):825–831, 1994.

54. Haas R, Mohle R, Fruhauf S, et al: Patient characteristics associated with successful mobilizing and autografting of peripheral blood progenitor cells in malignant lymphoma. Blood 83(12):3787–3794, 1994.

55. Kotasek D, Shepherd KM, Sage RE, et al: Factors affecting blood stem cell collections following high-dose cyclophosphamide mobilization in lymphoma, myeloma and solid tumors. Bone Marrow Transplant 9(1):11–17, 1992.

56. Dreger P, Looss M, Petersen B, et al: Autologous progenitor cell transplantation: prior exposure to stem cell-toxic drugs determines yield and engraftment of peripheral blood progenitor cell but not of bone marrow grafts. Blood 86:3970, 1995.

57. Demirer T, Rowley S, Buckner CD, et al: Peripheral-blood stem-cell collections after paclitaxel, cyclophosphamide, and recombinant human granulocyte colony-stimulating factor in patients with breast and ovarian cancer. J Clin Oncol 13(7):1714–1719, 1995.

58. Bensinger W, Appelbaum F, Rowley S, et al: Factors that influence collection and engraftment of autologous peripheral-blood stem cells. J Clin Oncol 13(10):2547–2555, 1995.

59. Prince HM, Imrie K, Sutherland DR, et al: Peripheral blood progenitor cell collections in multiple myeloma: predictors and management of inadequate collections. Br J Haematol 93(1):142–145, 1996.

60. Kessinger A, Bishop MR, Anderson JR, et al: Comparison of subcutaneous and intravenous administration of recombinant human granulocyte-macrophage colony-stimulating factor for peripheral blood stem cell mobilization. J Hematother 4:81–84, 1995.

61. Chatta GS, Price TH, Allen RC, Dale DC: Effects of in vivo recombinant methionyl human granulocyte colony-stimulating factor on the neutrophil response and peripheral blood colony-forming cells in healthy young and elderly adult volunteers. Blood 84:2923–2929, 1994.

62. Dreger P, Haferlach T, Eckstein V, et al: G-CSF-mobilized peripheral blood progenitor cells for allogeneic transplantation: safety, kinetics of mobilization, and composition of the graft. Br J Haematol 87(3):609–613, 1994.

63. To LB, Haylock DN, Dowse T, et al: A comparative study of the phenotype and proliferative capacity of peripheral blood (PB) CD34+ cells mobilized by four different protocols and those of steady-phase PB and bone marrow CD34+ cells. Blood 84:2930–2939, 1994.

64. To LB: Mobilizing and collecting blood stem cells. In Gale RP, Juttner CA, Henon P, (eds): Blood Stem Cell Transplants. Cambridge, Cambridge University Press, 1994, pp 56–74.

65. Lane TA, Law P, Maruyama M, et al: Harvesting and enrichment of hematopoietic stem cells mobilized into the peripheral blood of normal donors by granulocyte-macrophage colony stimulating factor (GM-CSF) or G-CSF: potential role in allogeneic marrow transplantation. Blood 85:275–282, 1995.

66. Sato N, Sawada K, Takahashi TA, et al: A time course study for optimal harvest of peripheral blood progenitor cells by granulocyte colony-stimulating factor in health volunteers. Exp Hematol 22:973–978, 1994.

67. Hillyer CD: Large volume leukapheresis to maximize peripheral blood stem cell collection. J Hematother 2(4):529–532, 1993.

68. Weaver CH, Tauer K, Zhen BO, et al: Second attempts at mobilization of peripheral blood stem cells in patients with initial low CD34+ cell yields. J Hematother 7:241–249, 1998.

69. Lie AK, Hui CH, Rawling T, et al: Granulocyte colony-stimulating factor (G-CSF) dose-dependent efficacy in peripheral blood stem cell mobilization in patients who had failed initial mobilization with chemotherapy and G-CSF. Bone Marrow Transplant 22(9):853–857, 1998.

70. Russell NH, McQuaker G, Stainer C, et al: Stem cell mobilisation in lymphoproliferative diseases. Bone Marrow Transplant 22(10):935–940, 1998.

71. Lie AK, Rawling TP, Bayly JL, To LB: Progenitor cell yield in sequential blood stem cell mobilization in the same patients: insights into chemotherapy dose escalation and combination of haemopoietic growth factor and chemotherapy. Br J Haematol 95(1):39–44, 1996.

72. Goldschmidt H, Hegenbart U, Haas R, Hunstein W: Mobilization of peripheral blood progenitor cells with high-dose cyclophosphamide (4 or 7 g/m²) and granulocyte colony-stimulating factor in patients with multiple myeloma. Bone Marrow Transplant 17(5):691–697, 1996.

73. Fruehauf S, Haas R, Conradt C, et al: Peripheral blood progenitor cell (PBPC) counts during steady-state hematopoiesis allow to estimate the yield of mobilized PBPC after filgrastim (R-metHuG-CSF)-supported cytotoxic chemotherapy. Blood 85:2619–2626, 1995.

74. Roberts A, Begley C, Grigg A, Basser R: Do steady-state peripheral blood progenitor cell (PBPC) counts predict the yield of PBPC mobilized by filgrastim alone? [Letter]. Blood 86:2451, 1995.

75. Armitage S, Hargreaves R, Samson D, et al: CD34 counts to predict the adequate collection of peripheral blood progenitor cells. Bone Marrow Transplant 20(7):587–591, 1997.

76. Nemunaitis J, Rabinowe SN, Singer JW, et al: Recombinant granulocyte-macrophage colony-stimulating factor after autologous bone marrow transplantation for lymphoid cancer. N Engl J Med 3224:1773–1778, 1991.

77. Sheridan WP, Morstyn G, Wolf M, et al: Granulocyte colony-stimulating factor and neutrophil recovery after high-dose chemotherapy and autologous bone marrow transplantation. Lancet 2:891–895, 1989.

78. Rowe JM, Ciobanu N, Ascensao J, et al: Recommended guidelines for the management of autologous and allogeneic bone marrow transplantation. Ann Intern Med 120:143–158, 1994.

79. American Society of Clinical Oncology: American Society of Clinical Oncology recommendations for the use of hematopoietic colony-stimulating factors: evidence-based, clinical practice guidelines. J Clin Oncol 12:2471–2508, 1994.

80. Chao NJ, Schriber JR, Grimes K, et al: Granulocyte colony-stimulating factor "mobilized" peripheral blood progenitor cells accelerate granulocyte and platelet recovery after high-dose chemotherapy. Blood 81(8):2031–2035, 1993.

81. Kessinger A, Armitage JO, Smith DM, et al: High-dose therapy and autologous peripheral blood stem cell transplantation for patients with lymphoma. Blood 74:1260–1265, 1989.

82. Juttner CA, To LB, Haylock DN, et al: Circulating autologous stem cells collected in very early remission from acute nonlymphoblastic leukemia produce prompt but incomplete haemopoietic reconstitution after high dose melphalan or supralethal chemoradiotherapy. Br J Haematol 61:739–745, 1985.

83. Gianni AM, Siena S, Bregni M, et al: Granulocyte-macrophage colony-stimulating factor to harvest circulating haemopoietic stem cells for autotransplantation. Lancet 2(8663):580–585, 1989.

84. Bishop MR, Anderson JR, Jackson JD, et al: High-dose therapy and peripheral blood progenitor cell transplantation: effects of recombinant human granulocyte-macrophage colony-stimulating factor on the autograft. Blood 83(2):610–616, 1994.

85. Elias AD, Ayash L, Anderson KC, et al: Mobilization of peripheral blood progenitor cells by chemotherapy and granulocyte-macrophage colony stimulating factor for hematologic support after high-dose intensification for breast cancer. Blood 79:3036–3044, 1992.

86. Lowenthal RM, Fabaeres C, Marit G, et al: Factors influencing haemopoietic recovery following chemotherapy-mobilised autologous peripheral blood progenitor cell transplantation for haematological malignancies: a retrospective analysis of a 10-year single institution experience. Bone Marrow Transplant 22(8):763–770, 1998.

87. Smith TJ, Hillner BE, Schmitz N, et al: Economic analysis of a randomized clinical trial to compare filgrastim-mobilized peripheral-blood progenitor-cell transplantation and autologous bone marrow transplantation in patients with Hodgkin's and non-Hodgkin's lymphoma. J Clin Oncol 15(1):5–10, 1997.

88. Sheridan WP, Begley CG, Juttner CA, et al: Effect of peripheral-blood progenitor cells mobilised by filgrastim (G-CSF) on platelet recovery after high-dose chemotherapy. Lancet 339(8794):640–644, 1992.

89. Schwartzberg L, Birch R, Blanco R, et al: Rapid and sustained hematopoietic reconstitution by peripheral blood stem cell infusion alone following high-dose chemotherapy. Bone Marrow Transplant 11(5):369–374, 1993.

90. Tricot G, Jagannath S, Vesole D, et al: Peripheral blood stem cell transplants for multiple myeloma: identification of favorable variables for rapid engraftment in 225 patients. Blood 85:558–596, 1995.

91. Kiss J, Rybka W, Winkelstein A, et al: Relationship of CD34+ cell dose to early and late hematopoiesis following autologous peripheral blood stem cell transplantation. Bone Marrow Transplant 19:303, 1997.

92. Reiffers J, Bernard P, David B, et al: Successful autologous transplantation with peripheral blood hemopoietic cells in a patient with acute leukemia. Exp Hematol 14(4):312–315, 1986.

93. Marit G, Thiessard F, Faberes C, et al: Factors affecting both peripheral blood progenitor cell mobilization and hematopoietic recovery following autologous blood progenitor cell transplantation in multiple myeloma patients: a monocentric study. Leukemia 12(9):1447–1456, 1998.

94. Ketterer N, Salles G, Raba M, et al: High CD34+ cell counts decrease hematologic toxicity of autologous peripheral blood progenitor cell transplantation. Blood 91:3148–3155, 1998.

95. Bernstein S, Nademanee A, Vose J, et al: A multicenter study of platelet recovery and utilization in patients after myeloablative therapy and hematopoietic stem cell transplantation. Blood 91:3509–3517, 1998.

96. Stroncek DF, Clay ME, Petzoldt ML, et al: Treatment of normal individuals with G-CSF: donor experiences and the effects on peripheral blood CD34+ cell counts and the collection of peripheral blood stem cells. Transfusion 36:601–610, 1996.

97. Harada M, Nagafuji K, Fujisaki T, et al: G-CSF-induced mobilization of peripheral blood stem cells from healthy adults for allogeneic transplantation. J Hematother 5:63–72, 1996.

98. Hoglund M, Smedmyr B, Simonsson B, et al: Dose-dependent mobilisation of haematopoietic progenitor cells in healthy volunteers receiving glycosylated rHuG-CSF. Bone Marrow Transplant 18:19–27, 1996.

99. Grigg AP, Roberts AW, Raunow H, et al: Optimizing dose and scheduling of filgrastim (granulocyte colony-stimulating factor) for mobilization and collection of peripheral blood progenitor cells in normal volunteers. Blood 86(12):4437–4445, 1995.

100. Urbano-Ispizua A, Solano C, Brunet S, et al: Allogeneic peripheral blood progenitor cell transplantation: analysis of short-term engraftment and acute GVHD incidence in 33 cases. Bone Marrow Transplant 18:35–40, 1996.

101. Luider J, Brown C, Selinger S, et al: Factors influencing yields of progenitor cells for allogeneic transplantation: optimization of G-CSF dose, day of collection, and duration of leukapheresis. J Hematother 6:575–580, 1997.

102. Waller CF, Bertz H, Wenger MK, et al: Mobilization of peripheral blood progenitor cells for allogeneic transplantation: efficacy and toxicity of a high-dose rhG-CSF regimen. Bone Marrow Transplant 18(2):279–283, 1996.

103. Majolino I, Scime R, Vasta S, et al: Mobilization and collection of PBSC in healthy donors: comparison between two schemes of rhG-CSF administration. Eur J Haematol 57(3):214–221, 1996.

104. Anderlini P, Przepiorka D, Huh Y, et al: Duration of filgrastim mobilization and apheresis yield of CD34+ progenitor cells and lymphoid subsets in normal donors for allogeneic transplantation. Br J Haematol 93(4):940–942, 1996.

105. Anderlini P, Przepiorka D, Seong D, et al: Transient neutropenia in normal donors after G-CSF mobilization and stem cell apheresis. Br J Haematol 94(1):155–158, 1996.

106. Pollmacher T, Korth C, Mullington J, et al: Effects of granulocyte colony-stimulating factor on plasma cytokine and cytokine receptor levels and on the in vivo host response to endotoxin in healthy men. Blood 87(3):900–905, 1996.

107. Yano T, Katayama Y, Sunami K, et al: G-CSF-induced mobilization of peripheral blood stem cells for allografting: comparative study of daily single versus divided dose of G-CSF. Int J Hematol 66(2):169–178, 1997.

108. Arbona C, Prosper F, Benet I, et al: Comparison between once a day vs twice a day G-CSF for mobilization of peripheral blood progenitor cells (PBPC) in normal donors for allogeneic PBPC transplantation. Bone Marrow Transplant 22(1):39–45, 1998.

109. Fischer J, Unkrig C, Ackermann M, et al: Intra-day CD34+ cell counts depend on the time to application and correlate with the resulting G-CSF plasma level after steady-state mobilization of PBPC by filgrastim [Abstract]. Blood 84 (Suppl 1):23a, 1994.

110. de Haas M, Kerst JM, van der Schoot CE, et al: Granulocyte colony-stimulating factor administration to healthy volunteers: analysis of the immediate activating effects on circulating neutrophils. Blood 84(11):3885–3894, 1994.

111. Matsunaga T, Sakamaki S, Kohgo Y, et al: Recombinant human granulocyte colony stimulating factor can mobilize sufficient amounts of peripheral blood stem cells in healthy volunteers for allogeneic transplantation. Bone Marrow Transplant 11:103–108, 1993.

112. Zaino EC: Blood counts in the nonagenarian. N Y State J Med 81(8):1199–1200, 1981.

113. Lipschitz DA, Udupa KB, Milton KY, Thompson CO: Effect of age on hematopoiesis in man. Blood 63(3):502–509, 1984.

114. Buckner CD, Clift RA, Sanders JE, et al: Marrow harvesting from normal donors. Blood 64(3):630–634, 1984.

115. Chatta GS, Andrews RG, Rodger E, et al: Hematopoietic progenitors and aging: alterations in granulocytic precursors and responsiveness to recombinant human G-CSF, GM-CSF, and IL-3. J Gerontol 48(5):M207–212, 1993.

116. Bensinger W, Appelbaum F, Rowley S, et al: Factors that influence collection and engraftment of autologous peripheral-blood stem cells. J Clin Oncol 13(10):2547–2555, 1995.

117. Miflin G, Charley C, Stainer C, et al: Stem cell mobilization in normal donors for allogeneic transplantation: analysis of safety and factors affecting efficacy. Br J Haematol 95(2):345–348, 1996.

118. Anderlini P, Przepiorka D, Seong D, et al: Factors affecting mobilization of CD34+ cells in normal donors treated with filgrastim. Transfusion 37:507–512, 1997.

119. Wiesneth M, Schreiner T, Friedrich W, et al: Mobilization and collection of allogeneic peripheral blood progenitor cells for transplantation. Bone Marrow Transplant 21 (Suppl 3):S21–24, 1998.

120. Bishop MR, Tarantolo SR, Jackson JD, et al: Allogeneic-blood stem-cell collection following mobilization with low-dose granulocyte colony-stimulating factor. J Clin Oncol 15(4):1601–1607, 1997.

121. Anderlini P, Przepiorka D, Lauppe J, et al: Collection of peripheral blood stem cells from normal donors 60 years of age or older. Br J Haematol 97(2):485–487, 1997.

122. Passos-Coelho JL, Braine HG, Davis JM, et al: Predictive factors for peripheral-blood progenitor-cell collections using a single large-volume leukapheresis after cyclophosphamide and granulocyte-macrophage colony-stimulating factor mobilization. J Clin Oncol 13(3):705–714, 1995.

123. Moskowitz CH, Stiff P, Gordon MS, et al: Recombinant methionyl human stem cell factor and filgrastim for peripheral blood progenitor cell mobilization and transplantation in non-Hodgkin's lymphoma patients—results of a phase I/II trial. Blood 89(9):3136–3147, 1997.

124. Glaspy JA, Shpall EJ, LeMaistre CF, et al: Peripheral blood progenitor cell mobilization using stem cell factor in combination with filgrastim in breast cancer patients. Blood 90:2939–2951, 1997.

125. Huhn RD, Yurkow EJ, Tushinski R, et al: Recombinant human interleukin-3 (rhIL-3) enhances the mobilization of peripheral blood progenitor cells by recombinant human granulocyte colony-stimulating factor (rhG-CSF) in normal volunteers. Exp Hematol 24(7):839–847, 1996.

126. Basser RL, Rasko JE, Clarke K, et al: Randomized, blinded, placebo-controlled phase I trial of pegylated recombinant human megakaryocyte growth and development factor with filgrastim after dose-intensive chemotherapy in patients with advanced cancer. Blood 89(9):3118–3128, 1997.

127. Papayannopoulou T, Nakamoto B, Andrews RG, et al: In vivo effects of Flt3/Flk2 ligand on mobilization of hematopoietic progenitors in primates and potent synergistic enhancement with granulocyte colony-stimulating factor. Blood 90(2):620–629, 1997.

128. Papayannopoulou T, Nakamoto B: Peripheralization of hemopoietic progenitors in primates treated with anti-VLA4 integrin. Proc Natl Acad Sci U S A 90(20):9374–9378, 1993.

129. Craddock CF, Nakamoto B, Andrews RG, et al: Antibodies to VLA4

integrin mobilize long-term repopulating cells and augment cytokine-induced mobilization in primates and mice. Blood 90:4779–4789, 1997.

130. Lane TA, Ho AD, Bashey A, et al: Mobilization of blood-derived stem and progenitor cells in normal subjects by granulocyte-macrophage and granulocyte-colony stimulating factor. Transfusion 39:39–47, 1999.

131. Ho AD, Young D, Maruyama M, et al: Pluripotent and lineage committed CD34+ subsets in leukapheresis products mobilized by G-CSF, GM-CSF versus a combination of both. Exp Hematol 24:1460–1468, 1996.

132. Anderlini P, Przepiorka D, Seong D, et al: Clinical toxicity, laboratory effects and analysis of charges for filgrastim mobilization and blood stem cell apheresis from normal donors. Transfusion 36:590–595, 1996.

133. Gudi R: Astemizole in the treatment of granulocyte colony-stimulating factor–induced pain. Ann Intern Med 123:236–237, 1995.

134. Anderlini P, Korbling M, Dale D, et al: Allogeneic blood stem cell transplantation: considerations for donors [Editorial]. Blood 90(3):903–908, 1997.

135. Stroncek DF, Clay ME, Smith J, et al: Changes in blood counts following the administration of G-CSF and the collection of peripheral blood stem cells from healthy donors. Transfusion 36:596–600, 1996.

136. Liles WC, Huang JE, Llewellyn C, et al: A comparative trial of granulocyte-colony-stimulating factor and dexamethasone, separately and in combination, for the mobilization of neutrophils in the peripheral blood of normal volunteers. Transfusion 37(2):182–187, 1997.

137. Gabrilove JL, Jakubowski A, Fain K, et al: Phase I study of granulocyte colony-stimulating factor in patients with transitional cell carcinoma of the urothelium. J Clin Invest 82(4):1454–1461, 1988.

138. Sica S, Rutella S, Di Mario A, et al: rhG-CSF in healthy donors: mobilization of peripheral hemopoietic progenitors and effect on peripheral blood leukocytes. J Hematother 5(4):391–397, 1996.

139. Hillyer CD, Tiegerman KO, Berkman EM: Increase in circulating colony-forming units-granulocyte-macrophage during large-volume leukapheresis: evaluation of a new cell separator. Transfusion 31:327, 1991.

140. Malachowski ME, Comenzo RL, Hillyer CD, et al: Large-volume leukapheresis for peripheral blood stem cell collection in patients with hematologic malignancies. Transfusion 32:732, 1992.

141. Bensinger WI, Price TH, Dale DC, et al: The effects of daily recombinant human granulocyte colony-stimulating-factor administration on normal granulocyte donors undergoing leukapheresis. Blood 81:1883–1888, 1993.

142. Rogers RL, Johnson H, Ludwig G, et al: Efficacy and safety of plateletpheresis by donors with low-normal platelet counts. J Clin Apheresis 10(4):194–197, 1995.

143. Gutensohn K, Maerz M, Kuehnl P: Alteration of platelet-associated membrane glycoproteins during extracorporeal apheresis of peripheral blood progenitor cells. J Hematother 6(4):315–321, 1997.

144. Okamoto S, Ishida A, Wakui M, et al: Prolonged thrombocytopenia after administration of granulocyte colony-stimulating factor and leukapheresis in a donor for allogeneic peripheral blood stem cell transplantation [Letter]. Bone Marrow Transplant 18(2):482–483, 1996.

145. Ordemann R, Heolig K, Wagner K, et al: Acceptance and feasibility of peripheral stem cell mobilisation compared to bone marrow collection from healthy unrelated donors. Bone Marrow Transplant 21 (Suppl 3):S25–S28, 1998.

146. Link H, Arseniev L, Bahre O, et al: Transplantation of allogeneic CD34/cells. Blood 87:4903, 1996.

147. Bensinger WI, Buckner CD, Shannon-Dorcy K, et al: Transplantation of allogeneic CD34+ peripheral blood stem cells in patients with advanced hematologic malignancy. Blood 88:4132–4138, 1996.

148. Avenarius HJ, Freund M, Kleine HD, et al: Granulocyte colony-stimulating factor enhances the expression of CD62 on platelets in vivo. Int J Hematol 58(3):189–196, 1993.

149. Kuroiwa M, Okamura T, Kanaji T, et al: Effects of granulocyte colony-stimulating factor on the hemostatic system in healthy volunteers. Int J Hematol 63:311–316, 1996.

150. Shimoda K, Okamura S, Harada N, et al: Identification of a functional receptor for granulocyte colony-stimulating factor on platelets. J Clin Invest 91(4):1310–1313, 1993.

151. Conti JA, Scher HI: Acute arterial thrombosis after escalated-dose methotrexate, vinblastine, doxorubicin, and cisplatin chemotherapy with recombinant granulocyte colony-stimulating factor: a possible new recombinant granulocyte colony-stimulating factor toxicity. Cancer 70(11):2699–2702, 1992.

152. Kawachi Y, Watanabe A, Uchida T, et al: Acute arterial thrombosis due to platelet aggregation in a patient receiving granulocyte colony-stimulating factor. Br J Haematol 94(2):413–416, 1996.

153. Falanga A, Marchetti M, Oldani E, et al: Changes of hemostatic parameters in healthy donors administered G-CSF for peripheral blood progenitor cells (PBPC) collection (Abstract). Bone Marrow Transplant 17:S72, 1996.

154. Strauss RG: Effects on donors of repeated leukocyte losses during plateletpheresis. J Clin Apheresis 9(2):130–134, 1994.

155. Korbling M, Anderlini P, Durett A, et al: Delayed effects of rhG-CSF mobilization treatment and apheresis on circulating CD34+ and CD34+ Thy-1dim CD38− progenitor cells, and lymphoid subsets in normal stem cell donors for allogeneic transplantation. Bone Marrow Transplant 18(6):1073–1079, 1996.

156. Kadar JG, Arseniev L, Schnitger K, et al: Technical and safety aspects of blood and marrow transplantation using G-CSF mobilized family donors. Transfus Sci 17(4):611–618, 1996.

157. Becker PS, Wagle M, Matous S, et al: Spontaneous splenic rupture following administration of granulocyte colony-stimulating factor (G-CSF): occurrence in an allogeneic donor of peripheral blood stem cells. Biol Blood Marrow Transplant 3(1):45–49, 1997.

158. Huestis DW: Adverse effects in donors and patients subjected to hemapheresis. J Clin Apheresis 2(1):81–90, 1984.

159. Russell JA, Bowen T, Brown C, et al: Second allogeneic transplants for leukemia using blood instead of bone marrow as a source of hemopoietic cells. Bone Marrow Transplant 18(3):501–505, 1996.

160. Goldberg SL, Mangan KF, Klumpp TR, et al: Complications of peripheral blood stem cell harvesting: review of 554 PBSC leukaphereses. J Hematother 4(2):85–90, 1995.

161. Meisenberg BR, Callaghan M, Sloan C, et al: Complications associated with central venous catheters used for the collection of peripheral blood progenitor cells to support high-dose chemotherapy and autologous stem cell rescue. Support Care Cancer 5(3):223–227, 1997.

162. Snowden JA, Biggs JC, Milliken ST, et al: A randomised, blinded, placebo-controlled, dose escalation study of the tolerability and efficacy of filgrastim for haemopoietic stem cell mobilisation in patients with severe active rheumatoid arthritis. Bone Marrow Transplant 22(11):1035–1041, 1998.

163. Cho SG, Park YM, Moon H, et al: Psoriasiform eruption triggered by recombinant granulocyte-macrophage colony stimulating factor (rGM-CSF) and exacerbated by granulocyte colony stimulating factor (rG-CSF) in a patient with breast cancer. J Korean Med Sci 13(6):685–688, 1998.

164. Parkkali T, Volin L, Siren MK, Ruutu T: Acute iritis induced by granulocyte colony-stimulating factor used for mobilization in a volunteer unrelated peripheral blood progenitor cell donor. Bone Marrow Transplant 7(3):433–434, 1996.

165. Anderlini P, Przepiorka D, Champlin R, Korbling M: Biologic and clinical effects of granulocyte colony-stimulating factor in normal individuals. Blood 88(8):2819–2825, 1996.

166. Caspar CB, Seger RA, Burger J, Gmur J: Effective stimulation of donors for granulocyte transfusions with recombinant methionyl granulocyte colony-stimulating factor. Blood 8:2866–2871, 1993.

167. Kunkel LA, Samia SA, Ioli M, et al: Normal donor follow-up after second cytokine mobilization of peripheral blood stem cells [Abstract]. Blood 88 (Suppl 1):398a, 1996.

168. Anderlini P, Lauppe J, Przepiorka D, et al: Peripheral blood stem cell apheresis in normal donors: feasibility and yield of second collections. Br J Haematol 96(2):415–417, 1997.

169. Stroncek D, Clay ME, Herr G, et al: Blood counts in healthy donors one year following the collection of granulocyte-colony-stimulating factor–mobilized progenitor cells and the results of a second mobilization and collection. Transfusion 37:304–308, 1997.

170. Baer MR, Bernstein SH, Brunetto VL, et al: Biological effects of recombinant human granulocyte colony-stimulating factor in patients with untreated acute myeloid leukemia. Blood 87:1484–1494, 1996.

171. Matsushita K, Arima N, Ohtsubo H, et al: Granulocyte-colony stimulating factor-induced proliferation of primary adult T-cell leukaemia cells. Br J Haematol 96(4):715–723, 1997.

172. Morstyn G, Lieschke GJ, Sheridan W, et al: Clinical experience with recombinant human granulocyte colony-stimulating factor and granulocyte-macrophage colony-stimulating factor. Semin Hematol 26 (Suppl 2):9–13, 1989.

173. Kawakami M, Tsutsumi H, Kumakawa T, et al: Levels of serum granulocyte colony-stimulating factor in patients with infections. Blood 76:1962–1964, 1990.

174. Sakamaki S, Matsunaga T, Hirayama Y, et al: Haematological study of healthy volunteers 5 years after G-CSF [Letter]. Lancet 346(8987):1432–1433, 1995.

175. Imashuku S, Hibi S, Nakajima F, et al: A review of 125 cases to determine the risk of myelodysplasia and leukemia in pediatric neutropenic patients after treatment with recombinant human granulocyte colony-stimulating factor [Letter]. Blood 84:2380–2381, 1994.

176. Freedman MH, Bonilla MA, Boxer L, et al: MDS/AML in patients with severe chronic neutropenia (SCN) receiving G-CSF [Abstract]. Blood 88 (Suppl 1):448a, 1996.

177. Kojima S, Tsuchida M, Matsuyama T: Myelodysplasia and leukemia after treatment of aplastic anemia with G-CSF [Letter]. N Engl J Med 326(19):1294–1295, 1992.

178. Bonilla MA, Dale D, Zeider C, et al: Long-term safety of treatment with recombinant human granulocyte colony-stimulating factor (R-metHuG-CSF) in patients with severe congenital neutropenias. Br J Haematol 88:723–730, 1994.

179. Dong F, Brynes RK, Tidow N, et al: Mutations in the gene for the granulocyte colony-stimulating-factor receptor in patients with acute myeloid leukemia preceded by severe congenital neutropenia [see comments]. N Engl J Med 333(8):487–493, 1995.

180. Imashuku S, Hibi S, Kataoka-Morimoto Y, et al: Myelodysplasia and acute myeloid leukaemia in cases of aplastic anaemia and congenital neutropenia following G-CSF administration. Br J Haematol 89(1):188–190, 1995.

181. Gilman PA, Jackson DP, Guild HG: Congenital agranulocytosis: prolonged survival and terminal acute leukemia. Blood 36(5):576–585, 1970.

182. de Planque MM, Bacigalupo A, Wursch A, et al: Long-term follow-up of severe aplastic anaemia patients treated with antithymocyte globulin: Severe Aplastic Anaemia Working Party of the European Cooperative Group for Bone Marrow Transplantation (EBMT). Br J Haematol 73(1):121–126, 1989.

183. Hasenclever D, Sextro M: Safety of AlloPBPCT donors: biometrical considerations on monitoring long term risks. Bone Marrow Transplant 17 (Suppl 2):S28–S30, 1996.

184. Bortin MM, D'Amaro J, Bach FH, et al: HLA associations with leukemia. Blood 70:227–232, 1987.

185. Gluckman E, Socie G, Guivarch C, et al: The long time forgotten HLA identical bone marrow donor: result of a survey on 818 patients [Abstract]. Blood 88 (Suppl 1):612a, 1996.

186. Doney K, Buckner CD, Storb R: Marrow harvesting from donors > 65 years of age [Abstract]. Exp Hematol 23:861a, 1995.

187. Fassas A, Anagnostopoulos A, Kazis A, et al: Peripheral blood stem cell transplantation in the treatment of progressive multiple sclerosis: first results of a pilot study. Bone Marrow Transplant 20:631–638, 1997.

188. Damiani D, Fanin R, Silvestri F, et al: Randomized trial of autologous filgrastim-primed bone marrow transplantation versus filgrastim-mobilized peripheral blood stem cell transplantation in lymphoma patients. Blood 90(1):36–42, 1997.

189. Majolino I, Saglio G, Scime R, et al: High incidence of chronic GVHD after primary allogeneic peripheral blood stem cell transplantation in patients with hematologic malignancies. Bone Marrow Transplant 17(4):555–560, 1996.

190. Urbano-Ispizua A, Rozman C, Martinez C, et al: Rapid engraftment without significant graft-versus-host disease after allogeneic transplantation of CD34+ selected cells from peripheral blood. Blood 89(11):3967–3973, 1997.

191. Ravagnani F, Siena S, De Reys S, et al: Improved collection of mobilized CD34+ hematopoietic progenitor cells by a novel automated leukapheresis system. Transfusion 39:48–55, 1999.

192. Yu J, Leisenring W, Bensinger WI, et al: The predictive value of white cell or CD34+ cell count in the peripheral blood for timing apheresis and maximizing yield. Transfusion 39:442–450, 1999.

193. Schots R, Van Riet I, Damiaens S, et al: The absolute number of circulating CD34+ cells predicts the number of hematopoietic stem cells that can be collected by apheresis. Bone Marrow Transplant 17(4):509–515, 1996.

194. Papadopoulos KP, Ayello J, Tugulea S, et al: Harvest quality and factors affecting collection and engraftment of CD34+ cells in patients with breast cancer scheduled for high-dose chemotherapy and peripheral blood progenitor cell support. J Hematother 6(1):61–68, 1997.

195. Elliott C, Samson DM, Armitage S, et al: When to harvest peripheral-blood stem cells after mobilization therapy: prediction of CD34-positive cell yield by preceding day CD34-positive concentration in peripheral blood. J Clin Oncol 14(3):970–973, 1996.

196. Hollingsworth KL, Zimmerman TM, Karrison T, et al: The CD34+ cell concentration in peripheral blood predicts CD34+ cell yield in the leukapheresis product. Cytotherapy 1:141–146, 1999.

197. Teshima T, Sunami K, Bessho A, et al: Circulating immature cell counts on the harvest day predict the yields of CD34+ cells collected after granulocyte colony-stimulating factor plus chemotherapy-induced mobilization of peripheral blood stem cell [Letter]. Blood 89(12):4660–4661, 1997.

198. Gillespie TW, Hillyer CD: Peripheral blood progenitor cells for marrow reconstitution: mobilization and collection strategies. Transfusion 36(7):611–624, 1996.

199. Bender JG, To LB, Williams S, Schwartzberg LS: Defining a therapeutic dose of peripheral blood stem cells. J Hematother 1(4):329–341, 1992.

200. Mavroudis D, Read E, Cottler-Fox M, et al: CD34+ cell dose predicts survival, posttransplant morbidity, and rate of hematologic recovery after allogeneic marrow transplants for hematologic malignancies. Blood 88(8):3223–3229, 1996.

201. Smolowicz AG, Villman K, Tidefelt U: Large-volume apheresis for the harvest of peripheral blood progenitor cells for autologous transplantation. Transfusion 37(2):188–192, 1997.

202. Smolowicz AG, Villman K, Berlin G, Tidefelt U: Kinetics of peripheral blood stem cell harvests during a single leukapheresis. Transfusion 39:403–409, 1999.

203. Law P, Lane TA, Ward DM, et al: Application of large volume leukapheresis (LVL) to collect sufficient quantities of peripheral blood progenitor cells (PBPC) for inadequately mobilized patients. Blood 90(10) (Suppl 1):329b, 1997.

204. Bashey A, Lane TA, Mullen M, et al: Value of percentage of CD34 positive cells in leukapheresis product as a predictor of platelet engraftment in autologous transplants. Blood 90(10) (Suppl 1):370a, 1997.

205. Shariatmadar S, Noto TA: Femoral vascular access for large-volume collection of peripheral blood progenitor cells. J Clin Apheresis 13(3):99–102, 1998.

206. Schiffer CA, Aisner J, Dutcher JP: Platelet cryopreservation using dimethyl sulfoxide. Ann N Y Acad Sci 411:161–169, 1983.

207. Schiffer CA, Aisner J, Dutcher JP, et al: A clinical program of platelet cryopreservation. Prog Clin Biol Res 88:165–180, 1982.

208. Law P: The tolerance of human platelets to osmotic stress. Exp Hematol 10:351–357, 1983.

CHAPTER TWENTY-SIX

Cord Blood Stem Cells

Jeffrey McCullough, M.D., Mary Clay, M.S., and John E. Wagner, M.D.

Hematopoietic stem cell (HSC) transplantation (HSCT) has proved to be a successful therapy for a variety of diseases.[1] Most transplantations are performed using bone marrow or peripheral blood progenitor cells from human leukocyte antigen (HLA)-matched siblings.[2] It has also been established that transplantation can be successful using marrow from properly matched unrelated persons.[3] Graft failure and graft-versus-host disease (GVHD), however, remain substantial issues in successful HSCT, especially when the donor is not related to the patient. Therefore, there has been considerable interest in alternative sources of HSC that might reduce or eliminate these problems and increase the availability of transplantation for patients who lack HLA-identical siblings. Although more than 2 million HLA-A, -B, and -DR-typed donor specimens currently are registered in marrow donor registries worldwide, 50% of all patients requiring transplant therapy are still unable to find an available, suitably HLA-matched donor.[4] Furthermore, patients of racial and ethnic populations of non–Northern European descent have an even lower probability of finding a suitable donor.[4] To potentially alleviate the shortage of suitable donors and reduce the length of the donor search process, Placental Blood Banking Programs were initiated in 1993.[5] As of December 1999, approximately 25,000 HLA-A, -B, and -DR-typed cord blood grafts had been collected, tested, and cryopreserved for clinical use in transplantation worldwide.

Human umbilical cord blood contains pluripotent HSC,[6, 7] and successful hematopoietic reconstitution has been accomplished using cord blood stem cells.[8–16] Initial success using cord blood from donors with two or three HLAs mismatched with the recipient, the apparent ease of engraftment, and the lack of GVHD suggest that cord blood stem cells might have advantages over bone marrow in a wider variety of situations, especially for transplants between unrelated persons. In addition, cord blood has the potential advantages over marrow of being free of contamination with latent viruses (cytomegalovirus, Epstein-Barr virus) and having a low number of GVHD-producing T lymphocytes.[6, 7, 17]

In 1992, the International Cord Blood Transplant Registry was established as a repository of clinical data on outcomes observed in patients undergoing transplantation with placental-umbilical cord blood (P-UCB) in an attempt to more quickly discern the true risks and benefits of this new hematopoietic stem cell source. In 1993, a similar registry was developed in Europe as part of the European Research Project on Cord Blood Transplantation (EuroCord Transplant Registry).

SIBLING DONOR PLACENTAL-UMBILICAL CORD BLOOD TRANSPLANTATION

Data on patients receiving P-UCB transplants from sibling donors for the treatment of malignant and nonmalignant disorders have been reported previously.[11, 14, 15] As of March 1997, transplant outcomes in 74 patients had been reported to the International Cord Blood Transplant Registry by 22 transplant teams. Patients were a median of 4.9 years old (range, 0.5–16.3 years). Fifty-six patients received HLA-matched (zero to one antigen) grafts and 18 received HLA-mismatched (two to three antigens) grafts. Prophylaxis for acute GVHD varied but most often consisted of cyclosporine alone or in combination with methylprednisolone or an anti–T-cell antibody. Hematopoietic growth factors were used early after the infusion of P-UCB in half of the patients by study design.

For recipients of HLA-matched (zero to one antigen) sibling donor P-UCB grafts (n = 62), the actuarial probability of hematopoietic recovery at 60 days after transplantation was 0.91 ± 0.02. The median times to neutrophil recovery (defined as time to achieve an absolute neutrophil count of >500/mm³) and platelet recovery (defined as platelet count of >500,000/mm³ untransfused for 7 days) were 22.0 days (range, 9–46) and 51 days (range, 15–117), respectively. Four patients never had signs of hematopoietic recovery, and one patient experienced early recovery but the cells were entirely host in origin. Of the five patients without donor cell engraftment, four had undergone P-UCB transplantation for the treatment of a bone marrow failure syndrome and one for the treatment of Hunter syndrome. Similar results have been reported by Gluckman et al. for the EuroCord Transplant Registry.[14, 18] Although the engraftment rate is high for the group as a whole, there is a trend toward greater risk of graft failure in recipients with a prior history of a bone marrow failure syndrome, hemoglobinopathy, or storage disease, as with marrow transplant recipients. Multivariate analyses with larger patient numbers are required to determine what factors are important in engraftment after sibling donor P-UCB transplantation.

Notably, no one has detected a correlation between nucleated cell count or hematopoietic progenitor cell content of the P-UCB graft and time to neutrophil recovery or probability of engraftment in the sibling donor setting. Moreover, the use of hematopoietic growth factor early after transplantation has not shortened the time to neutrophil recovery after P-UCB transplantation. Whether these observations are due to unique attributes of the neonatal HSC or simply to small patient numbers or patient selection bias is unknown at this time.

Remarkably, acute GVHD has occurred only rarely in recipients of HLA-matched (zero to one antigen) P-UCB transplants. The actuarial probabilities of grades II–IV and grades III–IV GVHD at 100 days after transplantation remain 0.03 ± 0.02 and 0.02 ± 0.02, respectively. Despite the fact that the risk of acute GVHD is lower in young children, the incidence of acute GVHD appears to be lower compared with similar-aged patients (ages 0–7 years) undergoing transplantation with HLA-identical marrow from sibling donors. Similar results have been reported by Gluckman et al.[14] Of the entire cohort of patients with an HLA-disparate (zero to one antigen) sibling donor, chronic GVHD has been reported in only three patients to date, and no patients had extensive disease.

Interestingly, moderate to severe GVHD has also been observed infrequently in 15 evaluable patients with haploidentical sibling donors (three recipients of HLA-disparate [two to three antigens] sibling donor P-UCB were not evaluable because of graft failure or early death). Of the 15 evaluable patients, 2 were mismatched for two antigens and 13 were mismatched for three antigens. Although patient numbers are small, donor-recipient pairs mismatched at the noninherited maternal allele did appear to be less likely to experience grades II–IV GVHD than donor-recipient pairs mismatched at the paternal allele. This observation supports the hypothesis that partial tolerance to the noninherited maternal allele may develop during gestation.

At a median follow-up of 2.0 years, the actuarial probability of survival for recipients of HLA-matched (zero to one antigen) grafts was 0.61 ± 0.12. Causes of death were multifactorial, including graft failure, relapse, interstitial pneumonitis/adult respiratory distress syndrome, veno-occlusive disease, intracranial hemorrhage, and early bacterial sepsis. For the entire cohort, GVHD was listed as a cause of death in only one patient with an HLA-mismatched (three antigens) donor graft. The actuarial probability of disease-free survival in those treated for malignancy was 0.41 ± 0.11. Relapse was observed in two patients with relapsed neuroblastoma and in one patient with relapsed acute myelocytic leukemia after prior autologous HSCT, in two patients with juvenile myelomonocytic leukemia, in three patients with acute lymphocytic leukemia (one in first complete remission but with the 9;22 translocation; two in second complete remission), and in one patient with adult-type chronic myelogenous leukemia.

In summary, analysis of Registry data and other case reports in the literature[7–10, 19–28] demonstrates that engraftment occurs in most patients, with the risk of graft failure possibly greater in patients with nonmalignant diseases. Moreover, the data suggest that GVHD occurs infrequently in recipients of P-UCB, with results in haploidentical P-UCB transplants supporting the postulate of partial tolerance to the noninherited maternal allele. Although patient age has clearly been shown to be an important predictor of GVHD, it does not fully explain the very low incidence of grades II–IV disease in patients undergoing transplantation with P-UCB. Properties of the neonatal immune system that might account for the relative absence of a GVH reaction are currently being explored and have already been outlined. Importantly, these data also suggest that maternal cell contamination of the P-UCB at the time of collection may be of limited clinical importance.

UNRELATED DONOR P-UCB TRANSPLANTATION

As a result of the early successes with P-UCB transplantation from sibling donors, pilot programs for the banking of unrelated donor P-UCB were initiated in many countries around the world. Known benefits of banked P-UCB include (1) rapid availability, (2) absence of donor risk, (3) absence of donor attrition, and (4) very low risk of transmissible infectious diseases, such as cytomegalovirus and Epstein-Barr virus. Although this source of hematopoietic stem cells may allow us to expand the available donor pool in targeted ethnic and racial minorities, this remains to be proven.

To date, very few reports have been published on the use of unrelated donor P-UCB transplantation. The largest series to date was reported by Rubinstein et al.[16] The clinical results with unrelated donor P-UCB transplantation at Duke University and the University of Minnesota, the two largest single-center experiences, are summarized in the following paragraphs.[12, 13]

At Duke University and the University of Minnesota, 144 patients underwent transplantation with unrelated donor P-UCB between 1993 and 1997. Although the median age of recipients was 7.2 years (range, 0.2–58), 19 patients were older than 18 years. The median weight of patients was 21.6 kg (range, 4.8–92), and the median cell dose was 3.5 × 10^7/kg (range, 0.7–33.8).

In this analysis, all unrelated donor P-UCB grafts were identified at the Placental Blood Program of the New York Blood Center. Prior to transplantation, confirmatory HLA typing of patient and cryopreserved donor specimens was performed using standard serologic techniques for identifying all World Health Organization (WHO)-recognized specificities for HLA-A and -B and using serologic level or high-resolution DNA techniques for HLA-DR. Units were selected to deliver the highest cell dose with the closest matched unit, prioritizing matching at HLA-DR over HLA-A or -B. For purposes of this analysis (in contrast with that reported for the EuroCord Transplant Registry), HLA typing was based on high-resolution oligotyping of DRB1.

HEMATOPOIETIC RECOVERY AND ENGRAFTMENT

For the 111 recipients eligible for this analysis, the median volume collected, nucleated cell dose, and colony-forming unit–granulocyte-macrophage (CFU-GM) dose in the P-UCB graft at the time of collection were 84 mL (40–214), 3.5 × 10^7/kg (0.7–33.8), and 1.6 × 10^4/kg (0.1–23), respectively, as reported by the New York Blood Center. The median CD34+ and CD3+ cell doses, as determined at the transplant centers at the time the P-UCB graft was thawed, were 1.6 × 10^5 (0.1–32.9) and 8.0 × 10^6/kg (0.4–101), respectively.

The overall probabilities of neutrophil recovery by day 42 and of platelet recovery by 6 months were 0.83 (0.76–0.90) and 0.76 (0.69–0.88), respectively. The median times required to achieve an absolute neutrophil count exceeding 500/mm³ and a platelet count exceeding 500,000/mm³ were 23 days (12–59) and 2.4 months (1–8), respectively. For both neutrophil and platelet recovery, there was no difference in probability of recovery between patients with HLA disparity of zero to one antigen and patients with HLA disparity of two to three antigens. In contrast with previous reports of sibling donor P-UCB transplantation, time to neutrophil recovery strongly correlated with the dose of cryopreserved nucleated cells (correlation coefficient, -0.40 [P < .01]), CFU-GM, and the dose of thawed CD34 + cells.

In univariate analysis, the rate of neutrophil and platelet recovery was significantly faster in recipients of a regimen that did not include total body irradiation or that included a higher graft cell dose content (nucleated cells, CD34 + cells, CFU-GM). A trend could be discerned for more rapid recovery in recipients of prophylactic granulocyte colony–stimulating factor (G-CSF). Among continuous variables in Cox regression analysis, nucleated cell dose, CFU-GM dose, and CD34 + cell dose were the only factors significant for predicting neutrophil recovery by day 42 and platelet recovery by 6 months.

GRAFT-VERSUS-HOST DISEASE

The overall respective probabilities of grades II–IV and grades III–IV acute GVHD for the entire group of patients were 0.35 (0.26–0.44) and 0.12 (0.06–0.18) by day 100 after unrelated donor P-UCB transplantation. In univariate analysis, no factor was significantly associated with risk of acute GVHD, including CD3 + cell dose and degree of HLA disparity. The respective probability of acute GVHD for HLA disparity of zero to one antigen and for two to three antigens was 0.29 (0.16–0.42) and 0.40 (0.27–0.53). Moreover, there was no difference in the probability of acute GVHD between patients treated with cyclosporine plus high-dose methylprednisolone (n = 54, 0.34 [0.21–0.47]) versus lower dose methylprednisolone (n = 38, 0.36 [0.20–0.52]) versus other regimens (n = 19, 0.36 [0.13–0.60]) (P = NS). The only factor that approached significance in univariate analysis was nucleated cell dose (<3 versus >3 × 10⁷/kg, P = .09). In Cox regression analysis, no risk factor was identified for acute GVHD. Notably, the probability of extensive chronic GVHD was 0.04.

RELAPSE

The probability of relapse in patients with malignant disease was 0.10 (0.03–0.17) at 1 year and 0.14 (0.05–0.23) at 2 years after P-UCB transplantation. In univariate analysis, only prophylactic use of G-CSF was associated with a lower risk of relapse (P < .01). Notably, risk of relapse was not significantly different between standard and high-risk patients (0.16 versus 0.10, respectively). In Cox regression analysis, however, no factor predicted higher risk of relapse.

SURVIVAL

With a median follow-up of 1 year, the probability of survival at 2 years after unrelated donor UCB transplantation was 0.44 (0.32–0.56). In univariate analysis, younger recipient age (<2 years, P = .05), harvested graft nucleated cell dose (>3 × 10⁷/kg, P < .01), and thawed graft CD34 + cell dose (>2 × 10⁵/kg, P < .01) were associated with improved survival. In Cox regression analysis, however, CD34 + cell dose and age were the most favorable risk factors for survival.

At these two centers, 26 patients over 18 years of age have undergone transplantation with unrelated donor P-UCB. Notably, overall probabilities of neutrophil recovery, grades II–IV acute GVHD, and survival were no different than that for the group as a whole.

SUMMARY

The results reported by Gluckman et al.[14] for the EuroCord Registry and Rubinstein et al.[16] for the New York Blood Center database are consistent with the Duke/University of Minnesota Database in terms of rate of hematopoietic recovery and engraftment and risk of grades II–IV acute GVHD. The reasons for differences in survival between the EuroCord Registry and Duke University/University of Minnesota data are not readily apparent but may be due to differences in patient selection. Importantly, all data sets have independently documented the importance of cell dose in predicting engraftment and survival. Although degree of HLA-A, -B, and -DRB1 disparity has not affected survival according to the EuroCord Registry and Duke University/University of Minnesota data, this may reflect limited patient sample sizes. More recent data from the New York Blood Center[16] indicate that degree of HLA disparity may affect survival, with survival being poorer in patients with greater degrees of HLA disparity.

In order to carry out larger clinical trials to establish the role of cord blood cells in transplantation, it is necessary to establish "banks" of stored cord blood stem cells. Many issues must be resolved, specific procedures developed, and requirements defined as these banks are established[29–39] (Table 26–1).

CORD BLOOD BANK START-UP ACTIVITIES

The implementation and operation of an unrelated umbilical cord blood bank is analogous to the establishment of a new blood collection/banking program. First, the objectives and goals of the umbilical cord blood bank must be defined in order to estimate the bank size and/or unit criteria required to meet those objectives. For instance, the selection of hospital(s) as potential collection sites may be based on their ability to fulfill goals such as the distribution of HLA types or ethnic diversity of the donors. Next, responsibility for crucial umbilical cord blood bank functions must be determined. Examples of these activities include (1) establishing professional and administrative relationships and activities for umbilical cord blood collection at the selected site(s), (2) preparing the necessary docu-

TABLE 26-1. POLICIES AND PROCEDURES (ISSUES) IN ESTABLISHING A CORD BLOOD BANK

Informational material provided
Obtaining consent
Determination of the suitability of cord blood for placement in an
   allogeneic bank
   Donor medical history
   Donor laboratory testing for infectious diseases
   Laboratory testing for genetic diseases
   Contamination of cord blood stem cells with maternal blood
Cord blood collection and preservation
   Collection
   Containers for cord blood
   Anticoagulant for short-term storage
   Short-term storage conditions
   Freezing and long-term storage
Red blood cell depletion or other processing
Histocompatibility testing
Transplant-related testing specimens
Data, information, and labeling
Transportation conditions
Cord blood testing of suitability for transplantation
Confidentiality

Adapted from McCullough J: Transfusion Medicine. New York, McGraw-Hill, 1998.

ments and program materials, (3) donor recruitment, education, and obtaining consent, (4) performing umbilical cord blood unit collection, processing, cryopreservation, storage, transportation, unit searches, unit infusions, and data collection activities, and (5) providing in-service education and training programs for umbilical cord blood bank staff.

The necessary supplies and equipment must be obtained. Collection supplies and equipment include disposable gowns, gloves, barrier pads, face masks, collection bags, syringes, clamps, alcohol swabs, iodine swabs, test tubes, collection frames, and blood bag mixer (tipper) scales. Much of the necessary capital equipment may already be part of an HSC processing facility, which includes biosafety hoods, centrifuges, programmable freezers, storage containers for cryopreserved HSC, monitoring equipment with alarms, a liquid nitrogen supply, refrigerators/freezers for storage of reagents and media, water baths, and CO_2 incubators. Space for the processing, short-term (quarantine) storage, and long-term storage must be arranged and computer equipment (software and hardware) obtained for data collection/management and donor search activities.

Next, it is essential to determine what standard operating procedures are necessary for the function of the P-UCB bank and who will develop them. The qualifications of personnel carrying out the various functions associated with the P-UCB bank should be defined, and the capabilities of personnel hired should be commensurate with job responsibilities. The major activities of the P-UCB bank can be divided as follows: medical affairs, quality assurance, program management/supervision, donor education/recruitment, and P-UCB bank operations (collection, processing, cryopreservation, storage, data collection/management, and donor searches). There must be a written training program that includes training in the guidelines of good manufacturing practices as well as the specific management or operational activities.[40] Thereafter, compe-

tence should be demonstrated through an ongoing program of performance monitoring or proficiency testing.

Finally, start-up and continuing operational costs must be determined and sources of funding secured. Once again, these costs depend on how the bank is structured in terms of size and how the various operational activities are carried out. In general, our experience and that of others[32] has indicated that the establishment of an unrelated cord blood bank requires approximately $150,000–$250,000 to initiate the start-up activities as described, including the collection of umbilical cord blood units for staff training and establishment of quality control parameters.

ESTABLISHING HOSPITAL COLLECTION SITES

The use of staff dedicated to the collection of cord blood standardizes the collection procedure and maintains a standardized process for a variety of procedures as discussed in the following paragraphs. This necessitates the staffing of a laboratory or a collection site in hospitals and means that the recruitment and consent process is focused on physicians admitting to that obstetrics ward.

The desired number and ethnic mix of the P-UCB units that make up the bank determine the hospital collection sites that must be established to meet the goals of the program. Once the initial and ongoing composition of the P-UCB bank has been determined, a variety of exclusionary factors (Table 26–2) can be used to calculate the number of potential P-UCB units (i.e., births) necessary to provide the desired number of P-UCB units in the bank.[41] By applying this analysis, the most appropriate and cost-effective hospital collection sites can be identified. This must specifically consider the number of collection sites, the number of days or shifts when collections are performed, and the proximity of the collection sites to the processing

TABLE 26-2. FACTORS THAT CONTRIBUTE TO THE NUMBER OF UMBILICAL CORD BLOOD UNITS THAT CAN BE COLLECTED VERSUS THOSE AVAILABLE FOR TRANSPLANT FROM A HOSPITAL COLLECTION SITE

PRECOLLECTION

Total number of annual births
Racial mix of annual births
Number of days of week collections are performed
Number of shifts per day collections are performed
Previous donor history of hepatitis or HIV infection or exposure
Complication of delivery or previous history of a high-risk birth
Current pregnancy of >1 fetus
Problem with retrieval and/or preparation of the placenta or cord

POSTCOLLECTION

Inadequate volume of CD34+ cells
Problem with processing procedure, quality control, or reagents
Donor exclusion
   Did not meet eligibility criteria
   Consent or blood sample not obtained within 24 hours
Positive infectious disease results
Other problems (human leukocyte antigen/ABO typing discrepancies)

Adapted from Peterson RK, Clay M, McCullough J: Unrelated cord blood banking. *In* Broxmeyer HE (ed): Cellular Characteristics of Cord Blood and Cord Blood Transportation. Bethesda, MD, AABB Press, 1998.

center/bank facility, which are the major contributing factors to individual unit and overall costs of operation for the P-UCB bank.

Once a hospital collection site has been selected, it is necessary to develop and maintain working relationships with obstetricians, nurses, delivery suite personnel, and hospital administrators at the participating collection sites. A smoothly functioning system for the identification of potential P-UCB donors and obtaining of consent for donation must be implemented in order to collect P-UCB units, using protocols that conform to standard obstetric practice. These activities require numerous meetings, good communication skills, and ongoing supportive efforts to establish and maintain the proper collection of P-UCB in an area not routinely designed or designated for standard volunteer blood collection.

DONOR RECRUITMENT AND OBTAINING CONSENT

The collection of P-UCB is a multistep procedure that begins with donor recruitment. Donor recruitment would optimally occur in the physician's office while a women receives prenatal care and is in a comfortable, nonthreatening environment. Information would be conveyed to mothers and informed consent obtained prior to the onset of labor. Although this approach has been used to a limited extent, a potential disadvantage is the unavailability of some women who do not seek or receive prenatal care. The situation is especially acute among minorities. Because one potential advantage of P-UCB is to address shortages of bone marrow donors in these populations, an alternative recruitment and consent pathway should be developed; for instance, seeking P-UCB donation upon admission for delivery or after delivery has occurred.[42] Although obtaining consent in such an environment may introduce issues of donation under possible physical and/or emotional duress, such circumstances can be avoided by involving the obstetrician and nursing staff. Some investigators have approached mothers to obtain consent for donation after collection of the P-UCB.[30] This procedure, however, has raised concerns of P-UCB collection without consent. In the ideal situation, consent is obtained while the mother is in the hospital, well rested, comfortable, and not in active labor.

It is necessary to give mothers adequate information regarding P-UCB donation and banking. Although the P-UCB is of fetal origin and ethically belongs to the neonate, the mother can give consent by proxy. An information brochure should be written for the layman, available in the language used commonly by the potential donor, and must include background on the uses of P-UCB, describe the method of collection, and explain the risks and benefits. Donation must be voluntary and confidential without compensation. Consent for infectious disease testing on blood drawn from the mother, as well as for genetic disease testing, if required, should be specifically included on the P-UCB donation consent form.

Some investigators have postulated that informed consent is not necessary to collect and store P-UCB. Presently, umbilical cord blood is considered medical waste and disposed of at the hospital's discretion. This discarded material could be salvaged for potential public health benefit. There are, however, several reasons for gaining consent, including the ability to ensure safety through maternal and P-UCB testing, the ability to gather follow-up information in the future, and the respect for individual rights inherent in informed consent.

In addition, the process of P-UCB banking involves obtaining a medical history from the mother; review of the medical records of pregnancy, labor, and delivery; obtaining blood samples from the mother and testing these for transmissible diseases; and possibly testing the cord blood for inherited disease. These activities all require consent.

Although several reports have been published about obtaining consent for P-UCB donation and banking,[31, 33, 35, 43] several other situations involve donation of tissues that could provide experience applicable to P-UCB. These include donation of blood, organs, and tissues from cadavers, fetal tissue from abortion, bone from living donors, and marrow.

CONSENT FOR DONATION OF ORGANS, TISSUES, AND BLOOD

Although the Uniform Anatomical Gift Act allows an individual to make an anatomic bequest before death, organ donation programs cannot ethically base organ removal on an individual's actions during his or her lifetime. Instead, consent from the next of kin is obtained shortly after brain death is pronounced. Hence, the next of kin must be approached and give consent while in an extremely emotional state because of the loss, a situation compounded by the fact that, in most cases, an accident is the cause of death. Despite the extreme circumstances, however, most family members agree to donate their loved one's organs in the United States. It is clear that the consent rate for donation increases when the family is approached by a person trained specifically in the aspects of organ transplantation who is comfortable in the surrounding of death and grieving and who is chosen for his or her communication style and empathy.

Cadaver tissue programs involve collection of skin, bone, cartilage, fascia, dura, corneas, and heart valves recovered several hours after cessation of cardiorespiratory activity. Legislation passed in 1987 requires that hospital personnel approach the family of all patients who meet established criteria at the time of death about whether they wish to give consent for donation of tissues from the deceased. Usually, a few key nurses in each hospital are trained in the consent process and meet with the family of the deceased to discuss donation. The nurse also obtains a brief medical history using specific questions developed to meet donation guidelines.

Because of the high demand for bone for allografting in orthopedic and other surgical procedures, banks have been developed to store bone removed during routine surgery.[44] Potential living bone donors are mostly healthy persons undergoing elective surgery such as total hip replacement, during which some bone will be removed. Consent for use of this otherwise discarded tissue is sought at the hospital in which the surgery is performed, usually on the morning of surgery. In most situations, the hospital nurse approaches the patient and poses the option of donation, discusses the procedure, and obtains a brief medical history to determine whether the patient meets donation criteria before consent is signed. The consent to donate may be given at a stressful time because patients are asked to give consent a few hours before surgery.

In fetal tissue donation, consent is obtained from the mother only, immediately after unexpected and unplanned pregnancy loss. Usually, hospital nurses make the initial approach to expectant mothers because procurement of the fetal tissue may occur at any time. Nursing and medical staff provide potential candidates with education regarding the donation requirements as well as guidance and support. With this system in place, women under extreme emotional duress are able to make decisions about donation. The mother must give consent for the entire fetus, not merely a portion of medical waste as in P-UCB donation.

Another example of obtaining consent involves matched, unrelated marrow donors. Marrow donation poses potential risks (general anesthesia, as well as other factors associated with the collection of a substantial volume of marrow[45, 46]), yet approximately 1200 individuals in the United States annually proceed to donate. In this situation, the donor consents to making an anatomic gift with potential risks substantially higher than that of P-UCB collection. Currently, a multilevel phased approach for recruitment and consent of bone marrow donors is used. Initially, platelet apheresis donors are approached about donating bone marrow. Persons give verbal consent to be put on the potential list after carefully reading two brochures about bone marrow donation. Subsequently, signed written consents for each stage of the process, including initial HLA typing, confirmatory HLA typing, and infectious disease testing, are obtained. The donor signs a written consent for actual marrow harvest just before the recipient starts to receive the myeloablative conditioning regimen. Marrow collecting facilities may require additional consents before the surgical procedure.

WHOLE BLOOD AND APHERESIS DONATION

For the donation of whole blood, written consent is obtained but the risks and complications of blood collection are not explained in detail, nor are they listed on the consent document. The interview process for whole blood donors is not designed to include a structured discussion of the risk, and most donors probably are not aware of the risks of blood collection despite the written consent. When new apheresis donors are recruited, they are given educational material that includes a description of the procedure and side effects. The donors are required to give written consent for each apheresis collection. During the predonation interview, however, there is typically no structured discussion of the potential risks.

EXPERIENCE WITH CONSENT FOR CORD BLOOD DONATION

The largest P-UCB bank in the world, the New York Blood Center, approaches women after delivery and seeks permission to discuss P-UCB donation. A verbal consent is generally obtained prior to delivery, and full consent is obtained after delivery.[30] The amount of education and information provided to women before delivery varies because some of the mothers have received little or no prenatal care. Guidelines issued by the New York State Department of Health state that "whenever possible" consent should be obtained prior to delivery.[47] A discussion of ethical issues in P-UCB banking[43] recommends that "informed consent of parents must be obtained before harvesting P-UCB." The American Medical Association Work Group on Ethical Issues in Cord Blood Banking has recommended that "in general . . . obtain written informed consent before labor and delivery, followed by an affirmation of this consent after delivery."[43] Most P-UCB banks do not obtain consent from all fathers, and some, such as the New York Blood Center, collect P-UCB before securing consent from the mothers. Still other P-UCB banks provide information about P-UCB and banking in obstetricians' offices and prenatal education classes, which leads to a modest effort to obtain written consent before labor and delivery, and collect the P-UCB from all suitable women at delivery regardless of whether written consent has been given. Postdelivery consent is also obtained in this model. The father's consent is not considered to be necessary.

In summary, current practice shows that consent for P-UCB donation can be obtained at several times during pregnancy: prenatally (during a visit to the obstetrician or prenatal class), before delivery but during labor (intralabor), or after delivery (postpartum).

In the *prenatal model,* women receive information during pregnancy via brochures about P-UCB banking, the collection process, medical history requirements, laboratory tests, and other important features of the program. The brochure includes a phone number for questions or additional information. Prenatal instructors are educated about cord blood donation. Consent can be obtained by the obstetrician or obstetrics nurse.

In the *predelivery intralabor model,* educational material is made available in obstetricians' offices (as in the prenatal model). Questions are answered by the obstetrician and by P-UCB bank staff. When the expectant mother has settled in the delivery unit, the hospital nurse determines whether the woman is able to consider donating P-UCB according to preestablished criteria, such as frequency of contractions, centimeters of cervical dilation, and presence or absence of certain complicating conditions. The nurse's assessment is reviewed with the obstetrician or midwife as part of the admission process, and a final decision is made by the obstetrician or midwife. After the approval of the obstetrician or midwife, the nurse asks the expectant mothers whether they would like to speak to a P-UCB counselor. Interested women speak to the counselor about P-UCB donation. This discussion is brief and involves only the collection of the P-UCB immediately after delivery. If the woman consents, the P-UCB is collected. After she recovers from the delivery process and is not under the influence of medication, the counselor engages the mother about full consent for donating the stored P-UCB to the bank. This is a more extensive discussion and involves all aspects of the banking, including all testing (HLA and infectious disease) and storage for future transplantation.

In the *postdelivery model,* the expectant mother receives information about P-UCB donation from her obstetrician or midwife during pregnancy as described earlier but is not approached by a P-UCB bank counselor until after delivery. The advantage of this model is that the mother is in a relatively stable condition and there is ample time to provide education, answer questions, and carry out a thorough and thoughtful process of informed consent. In addition, this procedure is solely performed by trained P-UCB bank personnel so that recruitment costs are minimized and no additional burden is placed on the obstetricians and staff. The major disadvantage is that the P-UCB material has already been collected.

It is clear that several parties could obtain informed consent for P-UCB donation: the obstetrician and/or staff, the hospital delivery room nurse, or the trained P-UCB counselor. The latter is most knowledgeable about donation and banking, but the obstetrics staff or midwife is more familiar with the patient. The most appropriate model in terms of the exact role of each of these legal, economic, and medical considerations remains to be determined and depends on the ethics and location of each P-UCB bank.

MODEL OF PHASED CONSENT FOR P-UCB DONATION AND BANKING

We propose that the consent process should involve three phases: during pregnancy, during labor, and after delivery. In the prenatal phase, information about P-UCB donation, banking, and transplantation is provided to the expectant mother at the obstetrician/midwife offices and through childbirth education programs. A more extensive set of material, including answers to commonly asked questions, should be provided to the obstetricians/midwives and their staff. Women are encouraged to contact the P-UCB bank counselor for more complicated and/or technical questions.

The second phase of the process begins when the expectant mother is admitted to the labor/childbirth unit. As part of the initial assessment of the woman, a determination is made (by the obstetrician/midwife after consultation with the hospital nurse), as discussed earlier, as to whether she should be approached about P-UCB donation. In our experience, about 80% of women were deemed suitable for the approach. The expectant mother is asked by the P-UCB counselor if she is aware of the information about P-UCB banking. If so, she is given an additional one-paragraph document describing P-UCB collection and a commitment not to place the P-UCB in the bank without her written consent. The third phase of the process is carried out after delivery, when the mother has recovered. A counselor from the P-UCB bank meets with the mother, provides detailed information about the P-UCB bank, answers questions and, if the woman agrees, obtains the signed consent for P-UCB processing, storage, and transplantation.

A possible disadvantage of the three-phase model is that expectant mothers are approached during labor; however, consent processing during stress is not uncommon for organ, tissue, bone, and fetal tissue collection. In our experience, almost all women who are deemed suitable by the nurse and obstetrician/midwife to discuss P-UCB banking give consent to donate their P-UCB for research. The deci-

sion about approaching the expectant mother rests with the attending obstetrician or midwife and is based on established criteria. This ensures that women will not be pestered by overzealous P-UCB bank staff. We believe that a major advantage of the three-phase process is that consent is obtained for each step and no action is taken (such as collecting the P-UCB) without written permission.

DETERMINATION OF THE SUITABILITY OF P-UCB FOR PLACEMENT IN AN ALLOGENEIC BANK

Many steps are necessary to ensure that P-UCB units placed in a bank will be as safe as possible and will provide long-term sustained hematopoietic recovery after transplantation. Requirements for the decision include relevant medical history of the mother, laboratory testing results of the mother, and laboratory testing results of the P-UCB.[30, 31] The medical history requirements and laboratory tests used for allogeneic blood or marrow donors can be used as a model.

The requirements include those designed to protect the safety of the recipient and those designed to protect the safety of the donor. Recipient safety information should be used with little or no changes, whereas donor safety issues can be modified. In addition, a history of potential risk of genetically inherited diseases from both parents' families and the meeting of some criteria relating to the pregnancy and delivery are also needed. In marrow collection, in addition to the infectious diseases testing, the adequacy of hematopoietic cells to sustain engraftment is usually assessed. The medical history review and laboratory tests must ensure the absence of HSC defects. A sample medical history is shown in Table 26–3. The pregnancy and delivery history must also be evaluated, and examples of these criteria are shown in Table 26–4.

Laboratory testing for infectious diseases could be carried out on peripheral blood of the infant and/or mother. In any disease involving viremia in the mother, the virus can potentially cross the placenta. Examples of this are varicella virus, cytomegalovirus, hepatitis B virus, and HIV. Because immunoglobulin G antibodies cross the placenta, however, infectious disease tests that detect these antibodies may falsely react with cord blood because of maternal antibody, not necessarily because of the infection status of the infant. Therefore, the tests are same as those presently performed for blood donors (Table 26–5) to minimize the risk of transmitting an infectious disease. If a test result is positive, the mother must be notified and, if required, proper public health authorities must also be notified so that early treatment could be initiated, if indicated. If indicated, steps should be taken to minimize the transmission of disease to contacts of the infant or mother.

The testing of the P-UCB for genetic diseases is a complex issue that is presently unresolved. It is possible to consider genetic diseases in three categories (Table 26–6); however, testing has only been done for a limited number of diseases that may manifest in a P-UCB transplant recipient. P-UCB contains some maternal cells, which could cause GVHD in the transplant recipient. The number of such cells is few and, in the absence of additional data,

TABLE 26–3. UMBILICAL CORD BLOOD DONATION MEDICAL HISTORY QUESTIONS

Have you ever:
1. Been refused as a blood donor or told not to donate blood?
2. Had cancer, convulsions, a blood disease, or a bleeding problem?
3. Been given growth hormone or taken Tegison for psoriasis?
4. Had Chagas disease or babesiosis?
5. Had yellow jaundice, liver disease, hepatitis, or a positive test result for hepatitis?
6. Had AIDS or a positive test result for AIDS virus; had sex, even once, with anyone who has?
7. Used a needle, even once, to take any drug (including steroids)?
8. Taken clotting factor concentrations for a bleeding problem, such as hemophilia?
9. At any time since 1977 taken money for drugs or sex?

In the last 3 years have you:
1. Been outside the United States or Canada?
2. Had malaria or taken antimalarial drugs?

In the last 12 months have you:
1. Received blood or had an organ or a tissue transplant?
2. Received a tattoo, ear or skin piercing, acupuncture, or an accidental needle stick?
3. Had close contact with a person with yellow jaundice or hepatitis, or have you been given hepatitis B immune globulin?
4. Had or been treated for syphilis or gonorrhea or had a positive test result for syphilis?
5. Given money or drugs to anyone to have sex with you?
6. Had sex with anyone who has ever taken money or drugs for sex?
7. Had sex with anyone who has used a needle, even once, to take any drug (including steroids)?
8. Had sex with anyone who has taken clotting factor concentrates for a bleeding disorder such as hemophilia?
9. Had a major illness or surgery?
10. Had any shot or vaccinations?
11. Had sex with a man who has had sex with another man, even once, since 1977?

Have you:
1. Taken any pills or medications in the last 4 weeks?
2. Do you understand that if you have the AIDS virus, you can give it to someone else, even though you may feel well and have a negative AIDS test result?

Adapted from Peterson RK, Clay M, McCullough J: Unrelated cord blood banking. *In* Broxmeyer HE (ed): Cellular Characteristics of Cord Blood and Cord Blood Transportation. Bethesda, MD, AABB Press, 1998.

routine testing for contaminating maternal blood is not recommended.[7, 29]

P-UCB COLLECTION AND PRESERVATION

P-UCB can be collected while the placenta is in the uterus; however, this must be done by the obstetrics staff, or P-UCB bank personnel must be in the delivery area. It is generally preferable to harvest P-UCB after the placenta has been delivered. This can be done outside of the delivery area to avoid intruding on the emotion of the birth setting. The placenta is quickly taken after delivery and transferred to trained P-UCB bank personnel. The P-UCB collection area should be clean and stocked with all necessary supplies and equipment.

P-UCB is easily recovered from the umbilical vein. The preferred method, as described by Rubinstein et al.,[48] is to collect the P-UCB into a sterile collection bag with citrate-phosphate-dextrose-adenine (CPDA) after cannulating the umbilical vein. Because the umbilical vein and its tributaries easily collapse under external or negative pressure, the

TABLE 26–4. PREGNANCY AND DELIVERY MEDICAL HISTORY CRITERIA FOR DETERMINATION OF UMBILICAL CORD BLOOD SUITABILITY

Full-term pregnancy
Absence of known infectious disease in mother
Lack of signs for infection in the neonate
No history of prolonged rupture of membranes
No clinically observable birth defects in the infant
Absence of genetic disease history
Birth weight greater than 2500 g
Duration of labor less than 24 hours
Five-minute APGAR score greater than 8
Lack of significant resuscitation efforts for the infant

vein should be suspended with the umbilical cord hanging down. The umbilical cord is cleansed with disinfectant and the umbilical vein cannulated. Blood drains via gravity into the P-UCB collection bag. The blood is collected into a plastic double-bag system, which should contain 22.5 mL of the anticoagulant, which is sufficient for up to 160 mL of P-UCB. Plastic bag sets designed specifically for the collection and processing of P-UCB are commercially available. The time involved in an expedient process should not result in any significant loss of hematopoietic cells, but a delay of more than 10–15 minutes could result in a decreased volume of P-UCB and, thus, a decreased number of hematopoietic cells. The collection procedure should be carried out by trained P-UCB bank personnel. Collection by hospital or obstetrics staff is not recommended because it would introduce uncontrollable variability to the product.

SHORT-TERM STORAGE CONDITIONS FOR P-UCB

The P-UCB usually is not be processed immediately after collection because deliveries occur at all hours and in locations with varying distances from the laboratory. It is necessary to specify the maximum duration between collection and cryopreservation of the P-UCB and the conditions under which the P-UCB should be maintained. Lasky et al.[49] showed that the number of marrow hematopoietic progenitors was well maintained for 24–36 hours when stored in a refrigerator. Berbolini and colleagues[50] have shown that P-UCB can be stored up to 36 hours at room temperature without a significant loss of hematopoietic progenitors. In studies of P-UCB, Broxmeyer et al.[6] reported that the hematopoietic cells could be stored at 4°C for at least 24 hours without a significant decrease in progenitors. Current guidelines stated that the P-UCB could

TABLE 26–5. TESTS FOR INFECTIOUS DISEASES CARRIED OUT ON MATERNAL BLOOD

Human immunodeficiency virus 1 and 2 (HIV-1, HIV-2)
Human T-cell lymphotropic virus 1 and 2 (HTLV-1, HTLV-2)
Anti–hepatitis B core (anti-HBc)
Hepatitis B surface antigen (HBsAg)
Anti-hepatitis C virus (anti-HCV)
Cytomegalovirus immunoglobulin M (CMV IgM) antibody
Syphilis

TABLE 26–6. A POSSIBLE STRUCTURE FOR CONSIDERING TESTING CORD BLOOD FOR GENETIC DISEASES

Genetic diseases unlikely to affect recipient
 Fragile X syndrome
 Hemochromatosis
 Gaucher disease
 Lesch-Nyhan syndrome
 Erythrocyte enzymopathies
 Ataxia-telangiectasia
Genetic diseases treated by transplantation
 Mucopolysaccharidosis types I–VII
 X-linked agammaglobulinemia (Bruton disease)
 X-linked severe combined immunodeficiency disease
 Adenosine deaminase deficiency
 Wiskott-Aldrich syndrome
Genetic diseases for which testing is recommended
 Sickle cell disease
 α-Thalassemia
 Hemoglobin E disease
 Hemoglobin C disease
 G-6PD deficiency
 Hereditary spherocytosis and elliptocytosis
Genetic diseases for which effect on recipient is unknown
 Huntington disease
 Spinocerebellar ataxia (SCA 1, 2, 3, 6, 7)

be maintained at 1–6°C and processed within 24 hours after collection.

Autologous marrow grafts are generally cryopreserved using dimethyl sulfoxide and controlled-rate freezing. This same method is also used for P-UCB,[51] and the units can be stored in the liquid nitrogen or vapor-phase liquid nitrogen storage freezer. Storage in liquid nitrogen has been associated with the transmission of hepatitis B from marrow grafts.[52] The observation is causing a trend to store in the vapor phase; P-UCB units should be stored in quarantine. The P-UCB should be placed in the active bank for long-term storage only after all documentation of consent, maternal medical history, infectious disease, and quality control of the unit is complete and deemed medically satisfactory. P-UCB stored in this manner has not shown significant loss in cell viability for periods up to 7–10 years.[53–55]

RED BLOOD CELL DEPLETION OR OTHER PROCESSING

It is desirable to enrich the hematopoietic cells, remove red blood cells to avoid hemolysis, and reduce the volume of stored P-UCB. This processing may reduce the costs of storage and the volume of infused dimethyl sulfoxide.[56] A red blood cell depletion step can be accomplished successfully prior to freezing. In the future, the positive selection of CD34+ cells may be possible.

QUALITY CONTROL TESTING OF P-UCB

An effective and comprehensive quality assurance program is essential for the operation of a P-UCB bank. The procedures should be designed along the guidelines of FDA

Good Manufacturing Practices and good tissue practice. The program should include the following sections:

1. Standard operating procedures
2. Personnel qualifications, job descriptions, and training requirements
3. Appropriateness of ancillary reagents and materials used for processing, with verification procedures or vendors'/suppliers' qualifications
4. Equipment performance criteria, calibration, validation, repair, and preventive maintenance schedules
5. Process flow diagrams, critical control points, process controls, and change control
6. Product definition, quarantine criteria, labeling procedures, and release criteria
7. Facilities maintenance and monitoring

The general quality assurance system should be supplemented with a quality control program specifically designed for P-UCB (Table 26–7). This might include measurement of initial P-UCB volume, total white blood cells, mononuclear cells, CD34+ cells, hematocrit, bacterial and fungal cultures, HLA type, and infectious disease test results.

TRANSPORTATION, THAWING, AND ADMINISTRATION OF P-UCB

The transportation, thawing, and transfusion of P-UCB are similar to those for marrow and peripheral blood progenitor cell grafts. Small containers, "coolers," or "dry" shippers that maintain low temperature (below −135°C) have been successfully used for transportation. It is important that the presence of liquid nitrogen be verified in the container, both at shipment from the P-UCB bank and on arrival at the transplant center.

The procedure used for thawing and preparing the umbilical cord blood unit[57] is similar to that used for marrow and peripheral blood progenitor cell grafts. The unit is placed into a sterile plastic Zip-Loc bag, closed, submerged in a 37°C water bath, and gently agitated while thawing. If leaks are present, the site is located and clamped with a sterile hemostat. The P-UCB unit is removed once it is completely thawed and weighed to determine infused volume. Leaking units should be placed into a sterile laminar flow hood and transferred to a 300-mL transfer pack and the volume measured. The thawed unit is then diluted with a 50% volume of half 10% dextran and half 5% albumin. For example, if the P-UCB volume is 120 mL, 60 mL of 10% dextran and 60 mL of 5% albumin are used. These fluids are each mixed into the P-UCB over 5 minutes (10 minutes total). The diluted unit is allowed to rest for an additional 5 minutes, transferred to a labeled 300-mL or

TABLE 26–7. QUALITY CONTROL TESTING OF CORD BLOOD

Volume	Bacteriologic cultures
ABO Rh	CD34+ cell counts
Hematocrit	Colony-forming unit assays
Nucleated cell count	

600-mL transfer pack, and centrifuged at 250 g for 10 minutes at 10°C. The supernatant is carefully removed to avoid cell loss, and the cell pellet should be gently resuspended with 50 mL of 10% dextran and 50 mL of 5% albumin, added individually with continual mixing. Two 0.6-mL samples should be drawn for confirmatory bacterial and fungal cultures, and the unit should be allowed to rest for an additional 10 minutes. Information required for the transfusion service may be recorded during this rest period.

After the P-UCB unit is administered, specific data regarding the transfusion should be recorded. This could include the date, location, unit number, number of nucleated and CD34 + cells, time of transfusion, and transfusing physician's name along with any problems encountered during thawing or administration. Engraftment outcome (absolute neutrophil count and platelets) and other transplantation-related events should be documented at the transplant facility and reported to the P-UCB bank in a timely fashion.

CONCLUSION

Transplantation of P-UCB from HLA-matched related and unrelated donors has led to long-term sustained engraftment. Because of the limited volume and hence cell numbers, P-UCB transplantation has been used primarily in pediatric patients, although success in adults has been reported. Compared with that for matched unrelated donor marrow grafts, engraftment time for platelets is typically longer for P-UCB transplantation, but the incidence and severity of GVHD appear to be lower. The initial success of P-UCB transplants has led to the establishment of many P-UCB banks. These banks have the potential to collect P-UCB from ethnic minorities, which are underrepresented in the National Marrow Donor Program. Many issues, such as timing of informed consent, acceptability of P-UCB by volume and cell number, post-thaw manipulation, and expansion of HSC in banked P-UCB units, remain to be examined.

REFERENCES

1. Bortin MM, Horowitz MM, Rimm AA: Increasing utilization of allogeneic bone marrow transplantation. Ann Intern Med 116:505–512, 1992.
2. O'Reilly RJ: Allogeneic bone marrow transplantation: current status and future directions. Blood 62:941–964, 1983.
3. Kernan NA, Bartsch G, Ash RC, et al: Analysis of 462 transplantations from unrelated donors faciliated by the national marrow donor program. N Engl J Med 328:593–602, 1993.
4. Confer DL: Unrelated marrow donor registries. Curr Opin Hematol 4:408–412, 1997.
5. Wagner JE, Kurtrzberg J: Allogeneic umbilical cord blood transplantation. In Broxmeyer HE (ed): Cellular Characteristics of Cord Blood and Cord Blood Transplantation. Bethesda, MD, AABB Press, 1998, pp 113–146.
6. Broxmeyer HE, Douglas GW, Hangoc G, et al: Human umbilical cord blood as a potential source of transplantable hematopoietic stem/progenitor cells. Proc Natl Acad Sci U S A 86:3828–3832, 1989.
7. Broxmeyer HE, Kurtzberg J, Gluckman E, et al: Umbilical cord blood hematopoietic stem and repopulating cells in human clinical transplantation. Blood Cells 17:313–329, 1991.
8. Gluckman E, Broxmeyer HE, Auerbach AD, et al: Hematopoietic reconstitution in a patient with Fanconi's anemia by means of umbili-

cal cord blood from an HLA-identical sibling. N Engl J Med 321:1174–1178, 1989.
9. Wagner J, Broxmeyer HE, Byrd RL, et al: Transplantation of umbilical cord blood after myeloablative therapy: analysis of engraftment. Blood 79:1874–1881, 1992.
10. Pahwa RN, Fleischer A, Sue T, Good RA: Successful hematopoietic reconstitution with transplantation of erythrocyte-depleted allogeneic human umbilical cord blood cells in a child with leukemia. Proc Natl Acad Sci U S A 91:4485–4488, 1994.
11. Wagner JE, Kernan NA, Steinbuch M, et al: Allogeneic sibling umbilical cord blood transplantation in children with malignant and nonmalignant disease. Lancet 346:214–219, 1995.
12. Kurtzberg J, Laughlin M, Graham ML, et al: Placental blood as a source of hematopoietic stem cells for transplantation into unrelated recipients. N Engl J Med 335:157–166, 1996.
13. Wagner JE, Rosenthal J, Sweetman R, et al: Successful transplantation of HLA-matched and HLA-mismatched umbilical cord blood from unrelated donors: analysis of engraftment and acute graft-versus-host disease. Blood 88:795–802, 1996.
14. Gluckman E, Rocha V, Boyer-Chammard A, et al: Outcome of cord-blood transplantation from related and unrelated donors. N Engl J Med 337:373–381, 1997.
15. Cairo MS, Wagner JE: Placental and/or umbilical cord blood: an alternative source of hematopoietic stem cells for transplantation. Blood 90:4665–4678, 1997.
16. Rubinstein P, Carrier C, Scaradavou A, et al: Outcomes among 562 recipients of placental-blood transplants from unrelated donors. N Engl J Med 330:1565–1577, 1998.
17. Wagner JE: Umbilical cord blood stem cell transplantation. Am J Pediatr Hematol Oncol 15(2):169–174, 1993.
18. Rubinstein P, Rosenfield RE, Adamson JW, Stevens CE: Stored placental blood for unrelated bone marrow reconstitution. Blood 81:1679–1690, 1993.
19. Vilmer E, Sterkers G, Rahimy C, et al: HLA-mismatched cord blood transplantation in a patient with advanced leukemia. Transplantation 53:1155–1157, 1992.
20. Vanlemmens P, Plouvier E, Amsallem D, et al: Transplantation of umbilical cord blood in neuroblastoma. Nouv Rev Fr Hematol 34:243–246, 1992.
21. Kernan NA, Schroeder ML, Ciavarella D, et al: Umbilical cord blood infusion in a patient for correction of Wiskott-Aldrich syndrome. Blood Cells 20:242–244, 1994.
22. Kurtzberg J, Graham M, Casey J, et al: The use of umbilical cord blood in a mismatched related and unrelated hematopoietic stem cell transplantation. Blood Cells 20:275–284, 1994.
23. Bogdanic V, Nemet D, Kastelan A, et al: Umbilical cord blood transplantation in a patient with Philadelphia-chromosome positive chronic myeloid leukemia. Transplantation 56:477–479, 1993.
24. Vowels MR, Lam-PO-Tang R, Berdoukas V, et al: Brief report: correction of X-linked lymphoproliferative disease by transplantation of cord-blood stem cells. N Engl J Med 329:1623–1625, 1993.
25. Kohli-Kumar M, Shahidi NT, Broxmeyer HE, et al: Haematopoietic stem/progenitor cell transplant in Fanconi anaemia using HLA-matched sibling umbilical cord blood cells. Br J Haematol 85:419–422, 1993.
26. Issaragrisil S, Visuthisakchai S, Suvatte V, et al: Transplantation of cord blood stem cells into a patient with severe thalassemia. N Engl J Med 332:367–369, 1995.
27. Neudorf SML, Blatt J, Corey S, et al: Graft failure after an umbilical cord blood transplant in a patient with severe aplastic anemia [Letter]. Blood 85:2991–2992, 1995.
28. Miniero R, Busca A, Roncarolo MG, et al: HLA haploidentical umbilical cord blood stem cell transplantation in a child with advanced leukemia: clinical outcome and analysis of hematopoietic blood (UCB): outcomes and analysis of risk factors. Blood 90:398a, 1997.
29. Rubinstein P, Rosenfield RE, Adamson JW, Stevens CE: Stored placental blood for unrelated bone marrow reconstitution. Blood 81:1679–1690, 1993.
30. Rubinstein P, Taylor PE, Scaradavou A, et al: Unrelated placental blood for bone marrow reconstitution: organization of the placental blood program. Blood Cells 20:587–600, 1994.
31. McCullough J, Clay ME, Fautsch S, et al: Proposed policies and procedures for the establishment of a cord blood bank. Blood Cells 20:609–626, 1994.
32. Meny GM: Issues in the development of a local cord blood bank. J Hematother 5:129–133, 1996.

33. Sugarman J, et al: Ethical aspects of banking placental blood for transplantation. JAMA 74(22):1784, 1995.

34. Silberstein LE, Jefferies L: Placental-blood banking—a new frontier in transfusion medicine. N Engl J Med 335:199–200, 1996.

35. Sugarman J, Kaalund V, Kodish E, et al: Ethical issues in umbilical cord blood banking. JAMA 278:938–943, 1997.

36. Haley R, Harvath L, Sugarman J: Ethical issues in cord blood banking: summary of a workshop. Transfusion 38:867–873, 1998.

37. Vawter DE: An ethical and policy framework for the collection of umbilical cord blood stem cells: the meaning and importance of respecting donors. In Weir RF (ed): Stored Tissue Samples: Ethical, Legal, and Public Policy Implications. Iowa City, IA, University of Iowa Press, 1998.

38. Wagner J, Kurtzberg J: Banking and transplantation of unrelated donor umbilical cord blood: status of the National Heart, Lung, and Blood Institute sponsored trial [Editorial]. Transfusion 38:807–809, 1998.

39. Fraser JK, Cairo MS, Wagner EL, et al: Cord blood transplantation study (COBLT): cord blood bank standard operating procedures. J Hematother 7:521–561, 1998.

40. Zuck TF: The applicability of cGMP to cord blood cell banking. J Hematother 5:135–137, 1996.

41. McCullough J, Herr G, Lennon S, et al: Factors influencing the availability of umbilical cord blood for banking and transplantation. Transfusion 38:508–510, 1998.

42. Lazazari L, Corsini C, Curioni C, et al: The Milan cord blood bank and the Italian cord blood network. J Hematother 5:117–122, 1996.

43. AMA Council on Ethical and Judicial Affairs: "2.165 Fetal Umbilical Cord Blood," Code of Medical Ethics: Current Opinions with Annotations, 1996–97 ed. Chicago, American Medical Association, 1997.

44. Jacobs NJ, Kline WE, McCullough JJ: Bone transplantation, bone banking, and establishing a surgical bone bank. In Bradford DS, Lonstein JE, Moe JH, et al (eds): Moe's Textbook of Scoliosis and Other Spinal Deformities. Philadelphia, WB Saunders, 1987, pp 592–607.

45. Bortin MM, Buckner CD: Major complications of marrow harvesting for transplantation. Exp Hematol 11:916, 1983.

46. Buckner CD, Clift RA, Sanders JE, et al: Marrow harvesting from normal donors. Blood 64:630, 1984.

47. New York State Council on Human Blood and Transfusion Services: Guidelines for Collection, Processing and Storage of Cord Blood Stem Cells. Albany, New York State Department of Health, 1997.

48. Rubinstein P, Carrier C, Taylor P, Stevens CE: Placental and umbilical cord blood banking for unrelated marrow reconstitution. In Brecher ME, Lasky LC, Sacher RA, Issitt LA (eds): Hematopoietic Progenitor Cells: Processing, Standards, and Practice. Bethesda, MD, American Association of Blood Banks, 1995, pp 1–17.

49. Lasky LC, McCullough J, Zanjani ED: Liquid storage of unseparated human bone marrow: evaluation of hematopoietic progenitors by clonal assay. Transfusion 26:331–334, 1986.

50. Bertolini F, Gibelli N, Lanaz A, et al: Effects of storage temperature and time on cord blood progenitor cells [Letter]. Transfusion 38:615–616, 1998.

51. Wagner WE, Broxmeyer HE, Cooper S: Umbilical cord and placental blood hematopoietic stem cells: collection, cryopreservation, and storage. J Hematother 1:167–173, 1992.

52. Gorin NC: Cryopreservation and storage of stem cells. In Areman EM, Deeg HJ, Sacher RA (eds): Bone Marrow and Stem Cell Processing: A Manual of Current Techniques. Philadelphia, FA Davis, 1995, pp 298–299.

53. Broxmeyer HE, Hangoc G, Cooper S, et al: Growth characteristics and expansion of human umbilical cord blood and estimation of its potential for transplantation of adults. Proc Natl Acad Sci U S A 80:4109–4113, 1992.

54. Harris DT, Schumacher MJ, Rychlik S, et al: Collection, separation, and cryopreservation of umbilical cord blood for use in transplantation. Bone Marrow Transplant 13:135–143, 1994.

55. Broxmeyer HE, Cooper S: High efficiency recovery of immature hematopoietic progenitor cells with extensive proliferative capacity from human cord blood cryopreserved for ten years. Clin Exp Immunol 107:45–53, 1997.

56. Stroncek DF, Fautsch SK, Lasky LC, et al: Adverse reactions in patients transfused with cryopreserved marrow. Transfusion 31:521–527, 1991.

57. Rubinstein P, Dobrila L, Rosenfield RE, et al: Processing and cryopreservation of placental/umbilical cord blood for unrelated bone marrow reconstitution. Proc Natl Acad Sci U S A 92:10119–10122, 1995.

CHAPTER TWENTY-SEVEN

Stem Cell Quantification: The ISHAGE Guidelines for CD34+ Determination—Applications in Autologous and Allogeneic Hematopoietic Stem Cell Transplantation

D. Robert Sutherland, M.Sc., Michael Keeney, A.R.T., F.I.M.L.S., Andrew Pecora, M.D., and Ian Chin-Yee, M.D.

A variety of studies in recent years have established that the 1–3% of cells in the bone marrow that express the cell-surface antigen CD34,[1, 2] are capable of long-term, multilineage hematopoietic reconstitution after myeloablative therapy.[3, 4] CD34+ cells are also found in the peripheral circulation of normal persons but are extremely rare (range, 0.01–0.1%). CD34+ cells, however, can also be mobilized from the marrow to the peripheral circulation in far greater numbers by chemotherapy and/or recombinant hematopoietic cytokines.[5, 6]

The increased use of peripheral blood progenitor cells (PBPC) versus marrow for autografting has been driven by a number of factors. The initial impetus for autologous transplantation involved mobilized PBPC as a potentially less tumor-contaminated product than autologous marrow. Time to engraftment is shorter with PBPC transplants, resulting in significant cost savings. Increased use of recombinant cytokines (singly or in combination) has elevated the level of peripheral blood CD34+ cells and decreased the number of leukapheresis procedures needed for an adequate graft. Currently, PBPC collections are preferred over autologous marrow for transplantation.[7–11] The PBPC product may be more amenable to ex vivo manipulations such as CD34+ cell selection,[3, 4, 11, 12] tumor purging,[13] and gene therapy.[14, 15] Mobilized PBPC collections (using granulocyte colony-stimulating factor) are also replacing marrow in the allogeneic setting.[16, 17] With this increased use of PBPC, standardized methods are required for the accurate, sensitive, and reproducible assessment of the engraftment potential of the collections.

GRAFT ASSESSMENT BY COLONY-FORMING UNIT ASSAYS

Few hematopoietic stem cell (HSC) transplantation centers still rely on an increase in the peripheral white blood cell count to initiate leukapheresis. In the past, the most widely used method to assess PBPC grafts relied on colony-forming unit (CFU) assays, which measure the relatively late and lineage-committed hematopoietic progenitors. Unfortunately, the results are at best indirectly, associated with long-term engraftment potential and other problems have limited its use as a standard method. These include variations in the procedure used for CFU assays among different centers, particularly the widely differing culture conditions and different cytokine cocktails.[18] Consequently, the minimum number of CFU per kilogram of patient body weight has not yet been established. The most serious limitation of CFU assays, however, remains the 10- to 14-day interval required for readout, which precludes using the assay in the analysis of PBPC content to optimize timing of apheresis and in the "on-line" quantitation of PBPC yield during apheresis. Furthermore, the CFU assays do not assess the more-primitive precursors and true HSC that mediate long-term engraftment.

GRAFT ASSESSMENT BY FLOW CYTOMETRY

ENUMERATING CD34+ CELLS

Recently, re-infusion of purified CD34+ cells has resulted in hematopoietic recovery after myeloablative conditioning.[3, 4, 11] Hence, quantitation of cells bearing this cell surface molecule can provide a rapid means to measure graft potential.[19] The CD34+ population is heterogeneous, encompassing the earliest quiescent HSC as well as the maturing, lineage-committed progenitors.[1, 2, 20, 21] By using multiparameter flow cytometry, it is possible to address not only quantitative aspects of the graft—that is, the total number of CD34+ cells present—but also the qualitative composition of the PBPC product. A flow cytometry–based approach, because it can be completed within 1 hour, would be suitable for the determination of optimal timing for apheresis collections in heavily pretreated patients and possibly "on-line" evaluation of the apheresis product. A standardized procedure should be capable of generating data that are directly comparable among transplant centers so that valuable information regarding the dose of CD34+ cells required for rapid, sustained engraftment can be summarized without bias.[22] Finally, when "positive selection" techniques are employed to purify CD34+ cells, the ability to accurately enumerate the CD34+ cells as a percentage of a well-defined cell population such as total nucleated white blood cells is of critical importance in calculating the efficiency of the CD34+ cell purification technique.

CD34 ANTIGEN: STRUCTURAL CONSIDERATIONS

The CD34 antigen is a highly glycosylated structure containing both complex-type N-linked glycans and numerous sialylated O-linked glycans that cluster in an extended mucin-like amino-terminal domain.[2, 23, 24] These features suggested that CD34 may be a substrate for a proteolytic enzyme from *Pasteurella haemolytica* that cleaves glycoproteins rich in O-linked structures.[25] The sensitivity of CD34 epitopes to sialidase[26] and glycoprotease[27] allowed the classification of epitopes into three broad categories. Of the seven CD34 antibodies designated at the IVth Leukocyte Differentiation Antigens Workshop, those that bind to epitopes sensitive to sialidase (*Vibrio cholera* neuraminidase) and glycoprotease were designated class I antibodies (BI.3C5, 12.8, My 10, and ICH3). Antibodies to epitopes resistant to sialidase but sensitive to the glycoprotease were designated class II (QBEnd10). Epitopes detected by antibodies TUK3 and 115.2 and the non-Workshop antibody 8G12 were insensitive to both enzymes and thus designated class III. This scheme was subsequently adopted by the Vth International Leukocyte Differentiation Antigens Workshop as a standard for the classification of 14 new CD34 antibodies.[2, 27] The latter Workshop studies also confirmed that the enzyme chymopapain cleaves class I and class II epitopes.[20]

Because of their dependence on carbohydrate moieties (sialic acids) and inability to detect all glycoforms of the CD34 antigen, class I antibodies fail to detect the CD34 antigen expressed on some forms of leukemia and leukemic cell lines.[2, 20, 28] These observations raise the possibility that subsets of CD34+ cells in normal hematopoiesis may display glycoforms of CD34 that escape detection by class I antobodies. Indeed, present evidence suggests that class I epitope expression is variable[29] (Sutherland, unpublished observations). The lower avidity of class I antibodies and their general inability to retain reactivity after conjugation with fluorochrome, such as fluorescein isothiocyanate (FITC) or phycoerythrin (PE), further reduces their utility in enumeration of CD34+ cells. Thus, to develop a reliable flow-cytometry method for unmanipulated samples, it is important to use class II or class III CD34 antibodies.

GENERATING AN ABSOLUTE CD34+ CELL COUNT

The determination of the absolute CD34+ cell count in peripheral blood and apheresis products requires an accurate quantitation of the target cell measured by flow cytometry and an accurate nucleated cell count from a hematology analyzer (two-instrument platform). Alternatively, by incorporating fluorescent beads or volume measurement in flow cytometry, an absolute CD34+ cell count can be generated with a single instrument. Although a number of flow-cytometry methods for CD34+ cells have been described,[19, 31–38] a consensus means for "rare event" analysis for CD34+ cells has only recently begun to emerge.[39] Choice of anti-CD34 monoclonal antibody, use of live/dead discriminator dyes, and isotype controls vary among the proposed methods. Not all CD34 antibodies and their conjugates detect all CD34+ cells in different clinical samples with equal efficiency. The practice of using isotype-matched control antibodies to set the "positive" analysis region for CD34+ cells can result in the erroneous enumeration of CD34+ cells. Furthermore, sample variability is a significant problem with respect to numbers of red blood cells, platelets, platelet aggregates, nonspecifically stained adherent cells, and cellular debris, all of which may be recorded by flow cytometers. To include all nucleated cells, some investigators have used dyes, such as LDS-751[34, 40] and SY-III-8,[41] in three-color methods; however, SY-III-8 is detectable in FL-1, and a different fluorochrome conjugate to CD45 (detectable in FL-3 or FL-4) must be used. Thus, the choice of CD34 antibody conjugate, denominators, gating strategies, and methods of calculating absolute CD34+ cell numbers, have contributed to the divergent data.[42]

EARLY FLOW METHODS

Siena et al.[19] were the first to describe a flow cytometric method based on indirect fluorescence to measure "%CD34+ cells." The subsequent development of what is now called the Milan protocol[31] was due to the availability, around 1990, of class III CD34 antibodies, such as 8G12, that could be conjugated with FITC without loss of reactivity. The gating strategy utilizes forward-angle (FSC) versus side-angle (SSC) light scatter to set a denominator, and an isotype-matched control to set the positive analysis region for CD34+ events. In the CD34 antibody-stained sample, the number of events that stain brigher than the control and exhibit low to intermediate SSC are counted and used as the numerator in the calculation of "%CD34+ cells." The total number of events counted is 50,000 or a minimum number of 50 "CD34+" events. The Nordic group further modified the basic Milan protocol by gating the CD34+ cells as a single bright cluster of events. In its latest version, the same gating region is used to analyze the isotype control sample, and any non-specifically stained events are subtracted from the CD34 result.[32]

The first multiparametric strategy was developed by Bender et al.,[33] in which CD45-FITC is used in addition to CD34-PE. CD45 staining is used to establish a more stable denominator by including only nucleated white blood cells in the analysis. CD45+ events are then analyzed in a similar manner to that of the Milan protocol, using an isotype and CD34 staining versus SSC analysis to enumerate CD34+ cells. The Dutch protocol[34] utilizes the laser dye solution LDS-751, which stains DNA and, to a lesser degree, RNA, to identify nucleated cells (the "denominator") during listmode data collection. Monocytes and granulocytes are excluded from the analysis using FITC-conjugated antibodies to CD14 and CD66e, and CD34+ cells are identified using a class III antibody labeled with PE. A control tube containing LDS-751, CD14, CD66e, and a PE-labeled isotype control are analyzed, and any events stained by the isotype are subtracted from the positive-analysis tube. In another approach, Owens and Loken[35] incorporate the nuclear dye 7-amino actinomycin D (7-AAD) to exclude dead cells, a CD14 antibody to exclude monocytes, and a CD34 antibody to identify CD34+ cells. A plot of CD14-FITC versus SSC is generated from the live cell gate (7-AAD negative events) to exclude monocytes. From this histogram, a third plot of CD34-PE versus SSC is generated and compared to an IgG PE control, versus SSC, as is used in the Milan protocol. Both dim and bright CD34+ events are included in the calculation. CD34+ events are expressed as a percent of total nucleated cells (live plus dead) based on an FSC versus SSC plot.

FLOW-CYTOMETRIC CD34+ CELL ENUMERATION USING CD45/CD34 AND SEQUENTIAL GATING

In early attempts to circumvent problems in analyzing CD34+ cells from heterogeneous clinical samples, we simultaneously stained mobilized PBPC using antibodies against CD45 and CD34. CD45-FITC was chosen as a counterstain because it stained all nucleated white blood cells. Although nucleated red blood cells and fully mature plasma cells are not stained by CD45-FITC, these cells are not generally found in PBPC and do not affect the utility of "CD45+" events to generate a stable "denominator" in the calculation of the absolute CD34+ value. By including only CD45+ events in the analysis, flow-cytometric events present in PBPC, such as red blood cells and their nucleated precursors, platelets, and cellular debris, are excluded.[38] Additionally, Shah et al.,[43] Stelzer et al.,[44] and Borowitz et al.[45] showed that primitive normal and leukemic blast cells that exhibit light-scatter properties similar to those of lymphocytes express lower levels of CD45 on their surfaces, thus providing a means of delineating nonspecifically stained lymphocytes from normal or leukemic blast cells using this surface marker.

On flow-cytometric analysis of CD45 staining versus side scatter (granularity), three major populations of CD45+ cells can be identified (Fig. 27–1, *plot 1*); lymphocytes (low SSC and bright CD45 staining), monocytes (slightly lower CD45 staining and intermediate side scatter), and granulocytes (low CD45 staining and high side scatter). CD45− events, which by light-scatter analysis and microscopic observation consist mainly of unlysed red blood cells and platelet debris, are excluded. When the CD45+ cells in region R1 are analyzed for CD34 phycoerythrin (PE) staining (*plot 2*), a population of CD34+ events can be detected

in region R2. The events in R2 are then displayed on CD45 versus side-scatter dot-plot (*plot 3*), and true CD34+ cells gated from region R2 form a discrete cluster (R3), which is characterized by low side scatter and dim CD45 staining. Nonspecifically stained events in R2 are excluded from R3. Cells in R3 exhibited a relatively restricted range of (medium) size and are found within the blast/lymphocyte region R4 when analyzed by side scatter and forward scatter (*plot 4*). Statistical analysis of the gated populations showed the number of CD34+ cells to represent 0.53% of the nucleated white blood cells (CD45+) identified by R1. CD34+ events were not detected in the CD45− fraction of this sample nor in other similar analyses (*data not shown*). When an appropriate panleukocyte antibody is used, all subsets of mobilized nonmalignant peripheral blood CD34+ cells express CD45, albeit at lower levels than normal lymphocytes.

The essential components of this gating strategy were shown to generate accurate CD34+ cell data from a variety of normal and abnormal hematopoietic samples.[38] Indeed, the original impetus to develop an accurate and reliable CD34+ cell enumeration method arose from an inability to quantitate CD34+ cells in bone marrow aspirates from which we were purifying CD34+ cells using the glycoprotease technique.[27, 46] To calculate the recovery of CD34+ cells, their initial numbers in the unseparated marrow had to be accurately quantitated. Marrow CD34+ cells, unlike their peripheral blood counterparts, vary broadly in size from small lymphocytes, to intermediate-size blast cells, to large megakaryoblast/granulomonocyte progenitors. Additionally, the cells exhibit a wider range of granularity or side-scatter characteristics as they mature into lineage-committed progenitors. Finally, the detected spectrum of CD34 staining intensities is large compared with that of the peripheral blood CD34+ cells. In contrast with single-parameter flow-cytometry procedures,[31, 32, 37] the gating strategy outlined above generates data on marrow, peripheral blood and cord blood that is similar to that observed by fluorescence microscopy.[38]

THE ISHAGE GUIDELINES

After publication of the above CD34+ cell detection method, the International Society of Hematotherapy and Graft Engineering (ISHAGE) established a Stem Cell Enumeration Committee to validate this procedure in a multicenter study. The mandate of the committee was to construct clinical guidelines for the quantitation of CD34+ cells in PBPC and to design a multicenter study to assess whether reproducible data could be generated using prestained/fixed samples distributed to the participating centers. The committee sought to establish the utility and reproducibility of the guidelines with different flow cytometers. It also sought to develop guidelines to optimize timing of apheresis collections and establish recommendations for a threshold CD34+ cell dose for rapid and sustained engraftment. By incorporation of a third antibody conjugate (such as CD33, CD38, or CD90), the qualitative aspects (primitive and committed subsets) of CD34+ cells can be determined.[47]

By April 1995, the first draft of the clinical guidelines

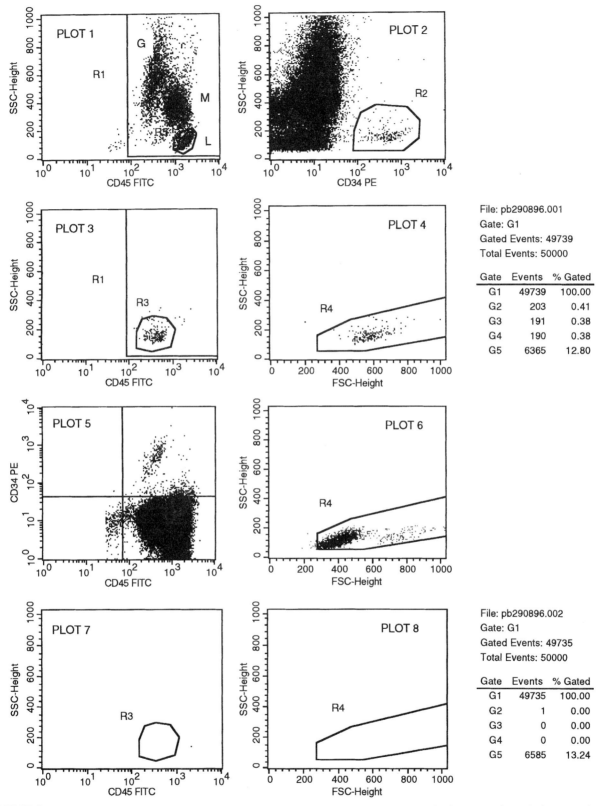

File: pb290896.001
Gate: G1
Gated Events: 49739
Total Events: 50000

Gate	Events	% Gated
G1	49739	100.00
G2	203	0.41
G3	191	0.38
G4	190	0.38
G5	6365	12.80

File: pb290896.002
Gate: G1
Gated Events: 49735
Total Events: 50000

Gate	Events	% Gated
G1	49735	100.00
G2	1	0.00
G3	0	0.00
G4	0	0.00
G5	6585	13.24

FIGURE 27–1. Enumeration of CD34+ cells in an apheresis sample (pb290896.001) using CD45-FITC (J33)/CD34-PE (QBEnd10). Precise details of the cumulative four dot-plot gating strategy are described in reference 50. *Plots 1–6,* analysis of sample stained with CD34/PE/CD45/FITC. Plot 1 is gated on all events. Plot 2 is gated on region R1 events. Plot 3 is gated on R1 and R2 events, and Plot 4 is gated on R1, R2, and R3 events. Plot 5 is gated on all events and Plot 6 is lymphocytes back-gated from region R5 to ensure optimal placement of lymph-blast region R4 as described in references 64 and 65. Plots 7 and 8 showed analysis of same sample stained with isotype PE/CD45-FITC (pb290896.002). Only the last two plots (equivalent to Plots 3 and 4) are shown for the isotype control sample. Cell clusters marked L, M, and G represent lymphocytes, monocytes, and granulocytes, respectively. Analysis was performed on a BD FACScan using Cellquest software.

had been produced (Chin-Yee I, et al.: *Enumeration of Hematopoietic Stem Cells in Peripheral Blood: Guidelines for the Performance of CD34+ Cell Determination* [draft]). Although this 35-page document was originally produced for the use of participants in the ISHAGE validation study and was not intended for formal publication, it was widely circulated both directly and indirectly to a large number of clinical and research laboratories around the world. The basic protocol was included in other studies in Canada[48] and Australia[49] that had started prior to the availability of the *Guidelines,* and results generated with this protocol showed greater concordance over multiple sites compared with data generated using other procedures. Partly because of the feedback received from transplant centers, the basic protocol was significantly updated and was published in 1996.[50]

ANTIBODY SELECTION

CD45 ANTIBODIES

Selection of an appropriate CD45 antibody is important because all epitopes of CD45 are not expressed on all white blood cells.[51–53] Because of the differential splicing of the single CD45 pre-mRNA species, a variety of CD45 isoforms (polypeptides) can be synthesized and differentially glycosylated to produce a large number of unique glycoforms.[51, 52] "Restricted" epitopes (CD45 "R") are not expressed on all leukocytes. During the screening process, one "CD45" reagent (clone ALB12, Immunotech) was found that not only required sialic acids for its binding but was sensitive to *Pasteurella* glycoprotease cleavage (unpublished observations). Thus, although the epitope detected by this reagent was likely determined by exon 3, common to all isoforms of CD45, it was variably expressed on white blood cells and poorly expressed on primitive (CD34+) precursors. Thus, CD45 antibodies that detect not only all isoforms but also all glycoforms of this structure are required. The following CD45 antibodies are produced by current Good Manufacturing Processes (cGMP) and can be used with confidence: HLE-1 (Becton Dickinson), and J33 (Immunotech/Coulter). Of these reagents, J33 is particularly useful because it retains its high signal-to-noise ratio in all its conjugated forms. Although other CD45 antibodies can probably be used, it is important to know that the selected antibody is a bona fide pan-CD45 reagent and that its epitope is resistant to both sialidase and glycoprotease.

CD34 ANTIBODIES

Phycoerythrin Conjugates

As indicated earlier, antibodies that detect class II or class III epitopes are required. To identify rare events such as CD34+ cells, it is advantageous to use an antibody conjugated to the brightest fluorochrome (i.e., phycoerythrin). After parallel analysis of a large number of samples of normal blood, mobilized peripheral blood, cord blood, and marrow, as well as CD34+ cell lines that fail to express some class I CD34 epitopes, cGMP-produced PE conjugates

of QBEnd10 (Immunotech/Coulter), 8G12 (HPCA2, Becton Dickinson), and 581 (class III, Immunotech/Coulter) work interchangeably in the procedures described in the ISHAGE *Guidelines.*[50]

FITC Conjugates

If the basic protocol is modified to incorporate a third conjugated antibody in a three-color analysis,[47, 50] the use of FITC conjugates (with an increased net negative charge from FITC) can have unexpected consequences for at least some class II CD34 antibodies. For example, although unconjugated and PE-conjugated forms of the QBEnd10 appear to bind to all glycoforms of CD34, binding of the FITC antibody is reduced because the epitope is nested between the clusters of similarly negatively charged (sialylated) O-linked carbohydrates in the most distal amino-terminal domain of the CD34 molecule.[50, 54] Additionally, FITC conjugates of CD34 antibodies can stain nonviable cells in some samples, and QBEnd10 (a murine monoclonal antibody containing lambda light chains) may be problematic.[55, 56] As discussed in greater detail elsewhere,[56] this hypothesis explains why a number of published studies using FITC-conjugated class II antibodies yielded divergent results.[55, 57, 58] If FITC conjugates of CD34 antibodies have to be used, class III reagents, such as 8G12 and 581, are recommended because parallel analyses of clinical samples (FITC and PE-CD34) using the ISHAGE *Guidelines* reported similar results.

Other Fluorochromes

The PE-CY-5 "tandem" or "tricolor" conjugate of 581, emitting in the third (far-red) fluorescence channel, can be used in three-color analyses. A recent report of the Fcγ1 receptor–mediated binding of such conjugates to monocytes and neutrophils suggested that additional care must be taken with data interpretation.[59] Using the gating strategy of the *Guidelines,* however, eliminates this concern. In contrast, PE-CY-5 conjugates of some other class III CD34 antibodies we have assessed were found to stain CD64+ cells in this assay and should be carefully evaluated before use (unpublished observations).

HPCA2 conjugated to the far red–emitting dye PerCP (peridinium chlorophyll protein complex) can be excited by argon lasers, but PerCP conjugates generally have reduced emission efficiencies compared with PE or PE-Cy-5 tandem conjugates. Moreover, their use is not recommended on sorters with high-power argon lasers, which can cause rapid quenching of this fluorochrome. For cytometers equipped with an appropriate laser, allophycocyanin (APC) conjugates of both HPCA2 and 581 can be utilized with confidence. Overall, the above observations not only underline the importance of selecting an appropriate CD34 antibody clone, but also of selecting one that retains the high specificity and avidity of its binding after conjugation to the designated fluorochrome.

ISOTYPE CONTROLS

Because every monoclonal antibody has slightly different "nonspecific" binding characteristics, appropriate isotype controls for rare-event analysis do not exist. Use of an isotype control to set a positive analysis region for rare-event analysis can result in either the inclusion of "nonspecifically" stained events in the CD34+ cell analysis region or it can mask the staining of rare, bona fide CD34+ cells.[60]

Use of isotype control antibodies requires titration, as with other monoclonal reagents. At the appropriate concentration, the isotype control should give the same level of fluorescence staining on a CD34− leukocyte population (e.g., lymphocytes) as exhibited by the CD34-PE reagent. Staining histograms of CD34− events generated by the two reagents should be very similar. Even at the optimum concentration, however, some isotype control antibodies can stain more leukocytes (nonspecifically) than the CD34-PE antibody can. These events are "gated out" by the other characteristics of true CD34+ cells specified in the *Guidelines*. If any such isotype-positive events appear in R4, they are simply subtracted from the CD34+ cell numbers enumerated in the CD45/CD34 tube(s). In contrast with traditional practice, gating regions in the *Guidelines* are established on the "positive analysis" tube (CD45/CD34) as shown in Figure 27–1. The nonspecifically stained events are enumerated for the CD45/isotype control tube using exactly the same gating regions.[50]

An alternative to the traditional isotype-matched control is to add a large excess of unlabeled CD34 antibody to a duplicate tube containing CD34-PE/CD45-FITC conjugates and enumerate nonspecifically stained events as described earlier.[37] Other than the increased expense, this approach may not be available for all appropriate CD34 clones.[39] It is also possible that the unlabeled antibody would not necessarily "block" all nonspecific staining of its conjugated counterpart. This could be particularly problematic when FITC-conjugated CD34 antibodies have been employed on a sample containing nonviable cells. Recent evidence suggests that isoclonic controls appear to block not just specific staining of CD34 PE to the target cells, but also "nonspecific" staining. As recently reviewed,[61] alternative methods, such as analyzing cellular autofluorescence, analyzing negative cell populations within the same test sample, or using sequential boolean gating for rare event analysis, provide more reliable information than that generated with isotype/isoclonic controls.

SENSITIVITY

We have analyzed a large number of peripheral blood and PBPC samples. If 100,000 events are collected in listmode on the flow cytometer, we can readily detect 10–20 events as a cluster in R3 and R4, translating into a sensitivity of 0.01–0.02%. In the validation studies, the first stained/fixed sample sent out for multicenter analysis contained 0.04% CD34+ cells. The centers that followed the *Guidelines* were able to accurately detect these cells with a high degree of reliability. Even with this sensitivity, it is recommended that a minimum of 100 CD34+ events be collected to maintain precision and reliability.

ABNORMAL CLINICAL SAMPLES

The gating strategy at the heart of the *Guidelines* has been able to detect abnormalities of the CD34+ cell compart-ment in some clinical samples. In one case, a bone marrow sample from a supposedly healthy donor contained approximately 14% CD34+ cells as assessed by microscopy, and about half of the CD34+ cells contained granular cytoplasm. Flow-cytometry analysis using CD45/CD34 confirmed these findings, with the CD34+ cells exhibiting a wide range of granularity. Interestingly, the subsequent clinical diagnosis of myelodysplastic syndrome/refractory anemia with excess blasts explains these observations because refractory anemia may predate the onset of overt acute myeloblastic leukemia. The most prevalent type of myeloid leukemia in these patients is FAB M2, the brief clinical definition of which is "blasts with differentiation."

In other studies, perturbations in the CD34 compartment of atopic persons were detected, and the increased numbers of CD34+ cells detected in the marrow and blood of such samples correlated with a specific increase in the numbers of basophil/eosinophil colony-forming cells.[62]

CALCULATION OF THE ABSOLUTE CD34+ CELL NUMBER

TWO-INSTRUMENT PLATFORM

The *Guidelines* analysis is simple and can be performed on most single-laser instruments. Requiring only routine settings and basic software, it is suitable for routine analysis in flow-cytometry laboratories. Sample variability with respect to the number of red blood cells, dead cells, platelets, platelet aggregates, and other cellular debris is minimized by the sequential gating strategy. The results can be expressed as percentage of CD45+ cells or by incorporating a leukocyte count determined by hematology analyzer in the calculation as an absolute CD34+ cell count. In the following example, the number of nonspecific events in R4 from the isotype control tube is subtracted from the average total number of events in the duplicate CD34-stained tubes. This corrected number of CD34+ cells is the numerator, and the average number of CD45+ events from the CD45-FITC/CD34-PE sample is the denominator. This value is multiplied by the absolute white blood cell (WBC) count as determined by the hematology analyzer to calculate the absolute CD34+ stem/progenitor cell numbers.

$$\text{Absolute WBC count/mm}^3 \times \frac{\text{(CD34+ events)}}{\text{(CD45+ events)}}$$

$$= \text{Absolute CD34+ cells/mm}^3$$

Example:

421 (average corrected CD34+ events):
75,000 (CD45+ events):
5200/mm³ (absolute WBC count):

$$5200 \times \frac{421}{75,000} = 29.1/\text{mm}^3$$

To determine the absolute CD34+ cell number in the apheresis product, the number in the example is multiplied by the volume and any dilution factor used.

ABSOLUTE CD34+ CELL COUNTING USING FLUORESCENT BEADS

In a recent development based on the *Guidelines* fluorescent microspheres were added to generate an absolute CD34+ cell count on a single-instrument platform.[63] Fluorescent beads (at a known concentration) are added to the stained sample after red blood cell lysis. The number of CD34+ cells are identified using the basic *Guidelines* and compared with the total number of beads counted in the third (or fourth) fluorescence channel of the cytometer,[63] or as more recently modified, by counting the beads using time versus forward scatter parameters.[64] This simple modification eliminates the need to perform an absolute leukocyte count on hematology analyzer, thus eliminating a possible source of error in the calculation of absolute CD34+ cell count.

Another benefit of including an internal reference bead in a three (or four) color analysis is that the CD45 positivity is no longer used as the denominator in the calculation. Thus, earlier controversial issues of "true denominator," nucleated WBC (CD45+ events), or total nucleated cells (DNA dye-positive events) can be avoided.[65] Instead, the CD45 expression is used solely as part of the sequential gating strategy to accurately identify bona fide CD34+ cells. This modification also eliminates the potential errors in calculating the absolute CD34+ cell count because the operator does not need to be concerned about the presence of nucleated red blood cells (that express little or no CD34/CD45) that are counted as leukocytes by hematology analyzers. An example of the use of such beads in the *Guidelines* is shown in Figure 27–2. The calculation of an absolute CD34+ cell count per liter is

$$\frac{\text{No. of CD34 + events (gate 4)}}{\text{No. of beads counted (gate 5)}}$$

$$\times \text{ bead concentration} \times \text{cell dilution factor}$$

This value is multiplied by the volume (in liters) to convert this value to an absolute CD34+ cell number $\times$ 10^6 in the apheresis product.

Example (from Fig. 27–2):

1681 (average corrected CD34+ events) (G4)
1600 beads (G7)
Bead concentration (from manufacturer) $1.024 \times 10^{-3}/$ mm^3
Cell dilution factor 1/50
Pack volume 4.9×10^4/mm^3

$$\frac{1681}{1600} \times 1024 \times 50 \times 4.9 \times 10^4 \times 10^6 = 2636/\text{mm}^3$$

LIVE/DEAD CELL DISCRIMINATION

The original *Guidelines* gating strategy[50] does not control for the presence of nonviable cells directly and because live cells cannot be reliably distinguished from dead cells according to light-scatter properties alone, some centers

have added nuclear dyes that can pass freely through the disrupted membranes of dead cells for staining and analysis. 7-Actinomycin D (7-AAD)[35, 66] emits in the far-red spectrum and can be used in combination with the CD45-FITC and CD34-PE reagents. Propidium iodide, however, is not optimal for three-color analysis on single-laser instruments because it is difficult to compensate the near-red emissions that spill over into the FL2 channel. Recent studies have confirmed the compatibility of 7-AAD with the basic protocol and additionally demonstrated that dead non-CD34+ cells (that can stain nonspecifically with CD34 and CD45 antibodies) are efficiently excluded by the sequential gating strategy. However, for samples in less-than-pristine condition, the use of 7-AAD is recommended to exclude dead CD34+ cells. 7-AAD is especially useful when incorporated into the single platform variant of the ISHAGE protocol because of the increased debris and "electronic noise" present in such samples consequent to lyse-no-wash sample processing. Using this modification allows an absolute viable CD34+ cell count to be obtained using only a flow cytometer.[63] This capability is particularly useful when analyzing samples that are not in good condition due, for example, to shipping, purging, or other ex vivo manipulations. Many of the technical innovations of the modified single-platform protocol have been adopted by the European Working Group in Clinical Cell Analysis in their recently published Guidelines for Stem Cell Enumeration.[67] Furthermore, the essential components and fine technical details of the single-platform protocols are embodied in the Basic Protocol recently devised for *Current Protocols in Cytometry.*[64]

CD34+ CELL SUBSET ANALYSIS

As outlined in detail elsewhere,[21, 47, 50] more-sophisticated analysis is possible using the basic method. For example, it is possible using the third fluorescence channel of the cytometer to assess other surface antigens, such as Thy-1 (CD90)[68, 69] or CD109, the coexpression of which is associated with the primitive HSC subsets of CD34+ cells.[70] Alternatively, the lack of expression of lineage-associated antigens (Lin−), such as CD38, CD71, or human leukocyte antigen (HLA)-DR, can also be used to assess similarly primitive subsets. It has been shown that the CD90 subset of CD34+ cells in PBPC samples were enriched for the primitive colony-forming cells currently detectable in long-term cultures. Furthermore, the human CD90+ subset was capable of multilineage engraftment in immune-deficient mice.[68] Other reports suggested that increased numbers of CD33-negative subset of CD34+ cells might correlate with faster engraftment.[71, 72] Possibly, some regimens will prove more efficient than others at mobilizing the primitive HSC subset of CD34+ cells, particularly in heavily pretreated patients. Thus, though there may be fewer *total* CD34+ cells, than is desirable, a sufficient number of these primitive cells may be present to effect (at least delayed) engraftment. Given the increasing numbers of growth factors that can be used to stimulate hematopoiesis in vivo, it may be possible to obtain an adequate autograft from fewer CD34+ cells than the minimum dose currently advocated (about 2×10^6 cells/kg body weight). Recent studies from

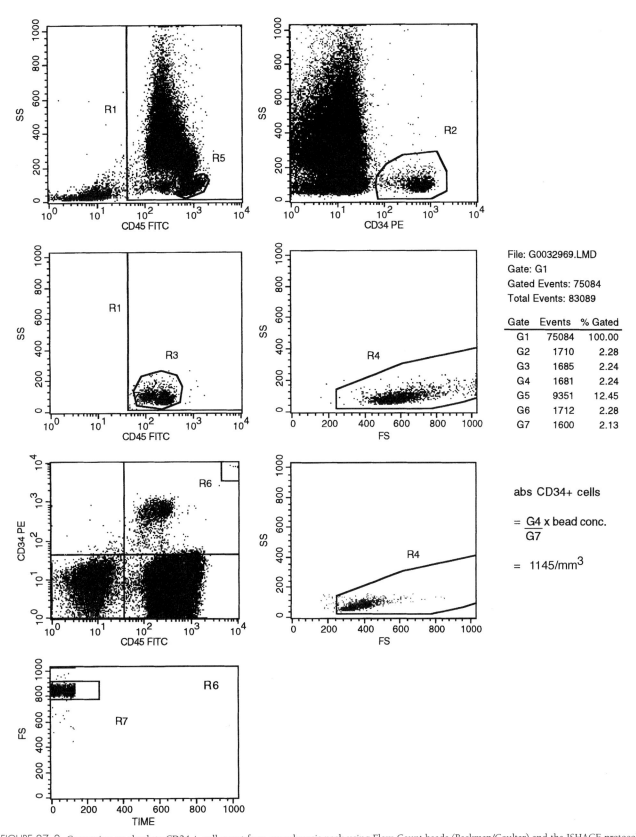

FIGURE 27–2. Generating an absolute CD34+ cell count from an apheresis pack using Flow-Count beads (Beckman/Coulter) and the ISHAGE protocol. Listmode data collected on Coulter EPICS XL and analyzed using FACSConvert and Cellquest software. Gating regions 1–4 on CD45 FITC (J33)/CD34 PE (581) stained sample (G003269.LMD) established as in Figure 27–1, with region R1, is drawn to include all CD45+ events and beads, which although not visible are in the very top right corner of Plot 1. Total and singlet beads gated in regions R6 and R7, respectively, as described.[64, 65] Plot 6 is included as described[63, 64] to ensure optimal placement of lymph-blast region R4.

Negrin et al. suggest that rapid multilineage engraftment can occur with as few as 8×10^5 highly purified Lin−/CD90+/CD34+ PBPC-derived cells.[73]

A variety of fluorochrome conjugates of CD90 are available for three-color analysis in combination with CD34 and CD45. Several of the recommended CD45 clones are available in a variety of conjugated forms, and FITC, PE, and PE-CY-5 conjugates of J33, for example, can all be used with confidence in any three-reagent cocktail. The recent availability of HPCA2 PerCP and 581 PE-CY-5 also facilitates subset analysis. The CD90-1 antibody clone 5e10 (Pharmingen Inc.) is available in FITC-, PE-, and PE-CY-5-conjugated forms. Because CD90 is present in low density on candidate HSC, however, the FITC conjugate is not recommended for this assay.

Although recent tests have shown that a J33-FITC/5e10-PE/581PE-CY-5 cocktail can be used with confidence, all potential combinations of antibodies and fluorochromes have not been tested. A majority of our experiments has used a combination of CD45-PE-CY-5 (J33), CD34-FITC (581), and CD90-PE (5e10). An example of such a three-color analysis is shown in Figure 27–3. Two sample tubes are set up containing CD45 and CD34 antibodies and either IgG1–PE isotype control or CD90-PE reagent. CD34+ cells, identified in the control tube using the *Guidelines* gating strategy in R4, are analyzed for staining with the isotype control to determine the positive analysis region for CD34+ cells stained with the CD90 antibody in the second tube.

The modified approach was used in 12 patients with myeloma in a study in which peripheral blood samples were taken daily after chemotherapy and during mobilization with granulocyte macrophage colony-stimulating factor (GM-CSF).[47] The data indicated that the level of CD34+/CD90+ cells was highest even before collection would normally be scheduled if an increase in WBC count or a predetermined duration was used as timing criterion. Thus, the primitive CD90+ subsets enter the peripheral circulation first[68, 69] and are most numerous relative to other CD34+ cells before an increase in WBC is detectable. Consequently, a window of opportunity for optimal collection may exist, and the application of serial measurements of the CD34+/CD90+ cell concentration in the circulation to define early collection days may be advantageous in certain clinical settings.[47] This approach may be especially useful for those heavily pretreated patients with myeloma with reduced likelihood of successful collection, given the recently reported increase in malignant cell contamination of apheresis products noted on later collection days,[74] if this window of opportunity is missed while awaiting an increase in WBC.[75] Analysis of the results also indicated that the frequency of circulating CD34+ cells not only best predicted the apheresis CD34+ cells and CFU-granulocytic macrophage (CFU-GM) but was the only predictor of the apheresis CD34+/CD90+ cell count.[47]

Another potential use for optimized timing of collections is in the chronic myeloid leukemia (CML) setting. In early chronic phase, prior to the onset of accelerated and blast crisis phases, there is good evidence that normal hematopoiesis is maintained alongside leukemogenic hematopoiesis. A number of autologous HSCT have been performed during the early chronic phase, and recent studies suggest that the first wave of CD34+ cells to enter the peripheral circulation after chemotherapy and cytokine stimulation are enriched for the primitive CD34+/CD90+ subset.[76] In another development, it was demonstrated that although the CD34+/CD90+/Lin− fraction of marrow affected by CML still contained a few Philadelphia chromosome–positive (Ph+) leukemia cells, virtually all the candidate normal (Ph−) hematopoietic stem cell activity is in this subset.[77] On later collection days, a majority of peripheral blood CD34+ cells plated in colony-forming cell assays generated Ph+ colonies. Thus, daily monitoring of the CD34+/CD90+ subset to optimize the timing of collection of nonleukemogenic CD34+ cells in CML may provide the most useful indicator of the likelihood of obtaining sufficient normal CD34+ cells to effect engraftment.

USING THE GUIDELINE IN ALLOGENEIC TRANSPLANTATION

In allogeneic HSCT, regardless of the source of donor cells (bone marrow or mobilized blood collections), the number of T lymphocytes in the graft has to be carefully adjusted to prevent graft-versus-host disease (GVHD). At the same time, sufficient T cells have to be retained to facilitate engraftment and graft-versus-tumor effects.[16, 17] By incorporating a third fluorescent conjugate of a CD3 antibody into the basic *Guidelines* procedure, the number of CD34+ cells and CD3+ T cells can be assessed at the same time.

In the example shown in Figure 27–4, CD34+ cells were selected from normal marrow using the CellPro system. Analysis of this fraction using the basic *Guidelines* demonstrated the fraction to contain approximately 72% CD34+ cells (G4). A cluster of cells accounting for a further 9.14% of the total CD45+ events was readily visible, however, exhibiting the bright CD45 staining/low side-scatter characteristics of lymphocytes (G5). By gating this fraction (R5) and analyzing these cells for expression of CD3, it was shown that 8.23% of the total CD45+ events were in fact T cells (G6). The fraction enriched with CD34+ cells was further processed to remove T cells using CD2-conjugated immunomagnetic beads, and the fraction was analyzed once more with identical antibody cocktail. The numbers of contaminating lymphocytes and T lymphocytes were reduced to 0.9% and 0.27%, respectively. Concomitantly, the CD34+ cells increased to over 85% (*not shown*). The ability to accurately quantitate not just CD34+ cells but also T lymphocytes should greatly facilitate the ability to engineer the most-appropriate composition of the donor cell suspension.

RECENT DEVELOPMENTS

As detailed elsewhere,[64, 67, 78] a number of commercial kits have recently been marketed based on single-platform methodologies. A three-color kit (ProCount), developed by Becton Dickinson, utilizes a nuclear dye in combination with CD45 PerCP and CD34 PE. The inclusion of a calibrated number of Trucount fluorescent beads in a lyse-no-wash protocol allows the absolute number of CD34+

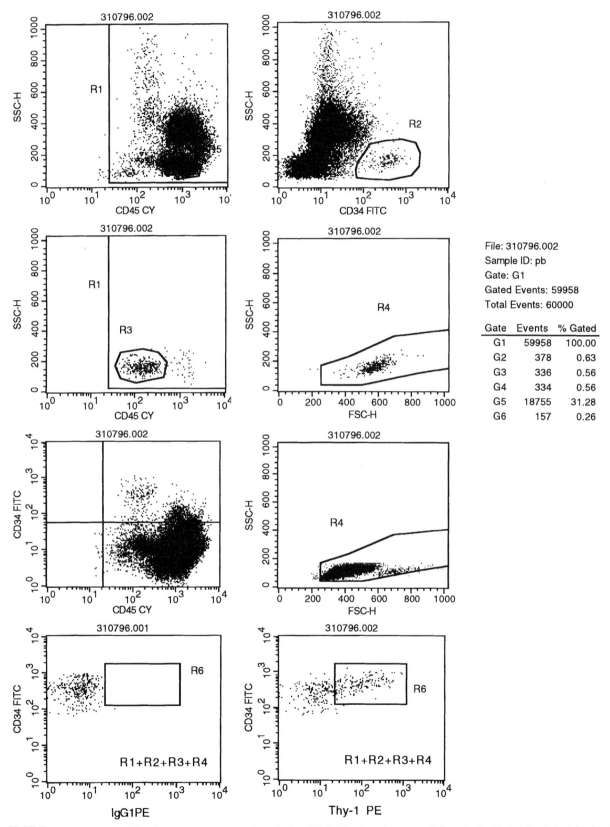

FIGURE 27–3. Enumerating candidate hematopoietic stem cells with the CD34hi/Thy-1+ phenotype. Cells stained with CD45-PE-CY-5 (J33)/CD34-FITC (HPCA2) and either IgG1-PE (*bottom left*) or Thy-1-PE (5e10) (*bottom right*). CD34+ cells are quantitated through gating regions 1–4 as in Figure 27–1. IgG1-PE control sets the positive analysis region R6 for CD34+/Thy-1+ cells. Sample analyzed on BD FACScan running Cellquest software.

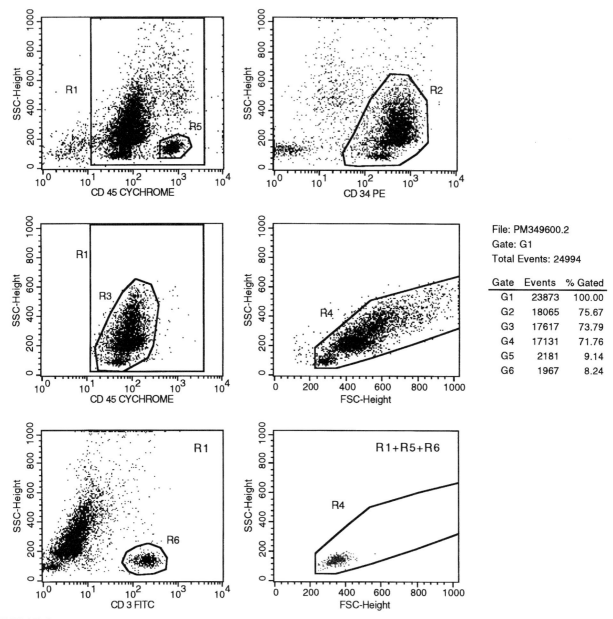

FIGURE 27–4. Assessing the CD34+ cell purity and residual T-lymphocyte content in a CD34+ fraction selected on a CellPro Ceprate device. Sample stained with CD45-PE-CY-5 (J33)/CD34-PE (HPCA2)/CD3-FITC (UCHT1) combination. CD34+ cells are quantitated through gating regions 1–4 as in Figure 27–1. Residual lymphocytes are identified by bright CD45/low side scatter (region R5), and the gated cells are assessed for staining with CD3 FITC (region R6, *bottom left*). Gate statistics show that the sample contains 71.76% CD34+ cells, 9.14% lymphocytes, and 8.24% T cells.

cells to be enumerated directly from the flow cytometer.[65] Because the beads are smaller than the smallest leukocytes, the threshold is set on events stained by the nuclear dye. Although a prototype of this assay was published previously,[41] specialized software has been developed for semi-automated data acquisition and analysis.[79] In manual mode, 60,000 (dye-positive) events are acquired. CD34 + cells have to satisfy the simultaneous criteria of DNA dye-positive, CD45 dull/negative, and CD34 +. An isotype control tube is used to assess the levels of nonspecific staining, but any such events satisfying the above gating criteria for CD34 + cells are not subtracted from the positive analysis tube. This product is only intended for use on fresh peripheral blood and apheresis products in good condition, as the presence of nonviable cells, and platelet aggregates in particular, are problematic.

A volumetry-based system for absolute CD34 + cell counting—the IMAGN 2000 microvolume fluorimeter STELLer assay, has been developed by Biometric Imaging (Mountain View, CA, now distributed by Becton Dickinson). Although not a flow cytometer, this instrument uses a CY5 conjugated CD34 antibody (581) and a helium-neon laser at 633 nm to scan, image and identify fluorescent cells present in the precisely known volume of sample contained in a capillary tube.[80] Data comparing this new technology with traditional flow cytometric methods have shown a very good correlation on mobilized blood samples.[81, 82] As only 2 μL of sample is analyzed, samples containing less than 20 CD34 + cells/mm³ show reduced precision. As indicated above for the ProCount kit, this product has only been validated for analysis of fresh peripheral blood and apheresis products in good condition. The effects of dead cells, platelet aggregates, and other debris on this system have not been published.

The Stem-Kit (Immunotech/Beckman-Coulter) utilizes Flow-Count fluorescent beads and *Guidelines* gating criteria to identify CD34 + cells. The kit also contains a novel CD45-FITC/CD34 (Isoclonic) control to enumerate nonspecifically stained events, as discussed above.[37] However, given the selectivity of the sequential gating strategy utilized in this protocol, which takes into account both positivity and intensity of antigen expression, the isoclonic control may be redundant.[61, 64, 67] In a recent study,[63] only three samples exhibited background staining with the isoclonic control above one event per mm³. Additionally, Stem-Kit also includes Stem-Trol control cells, KG1a cells that have been modified to present the CD34 and CD45 epitopes at densities similar to those found on normal CD34 + hematopoietic cells.[83] The inclusion of Stem-Trol cells is useful in determining and monitoring the accuracy of the pipetting steps of the single-platform method. As this material can be diluted in peripheral blood, it can also be used as a "process control," undergoing staining and lysis exactly as performed on the test samples.[63, 64] The staining pattern with respect to CD34/CD45 reagents can be used as an extra internal control to ensure that the FL1, FL2, and light scatter parameters of the cytometer are adequately set. This kit can be used on both Becton Dickinson and Beckman/Coulter flow cytometers, and it is entirely compatible with the use of the viability dye 7-AAD. As recently described in technical detail, however, some platform-specific differ-ences exist in the way that the instruments are set up and events are acquired.[63, 64]

The single-platform variant of the *Guidelines,* including viability dye 7-AAD, forms the Basic Protocol of the technical manual recently published in *Current Protocols in Cytometry.*[64] This method is in routine use in the authors' laboratories for the analysis of blood and apheresis samples for autologous and allogeneic HSCT as well as for the assessment of normal marrow samples in the allotransplant setting. Furthermore, it is also routinely used to enumerate absolute viable CD34 + cells in cord blood samples for the local cord blood bank. Absolute counting of subsets is also possible using the Flow-Count fluorescent beads and the three-color subset assay described above.

Regarding subsets, published data on CD34 + cell subset quantitation have used a variety of different gating strategies to identify CD34 + cell subsets in marrow, cord blood, and peripheral blood.[47, 71, 72] As recently reviewed,[78] while the utility of CD34 + subset analysis as a clinical predictor of rapid engraftment requires further investigation, subset analysis of rare populations of CD34 + cells adds to the complexity of flow cytometric assay. To address this issue, we have described a standardized method based on the original *Guidelines* for the identification and quantitation of CD34 + cell subsets in a three-color assay, the technical details of which are also contained in the recent document produced for *Current Protocols in Cytometry.*[69]

CONCLUSION

The studies described earlier show that the two-color sequential gating strategy[50] is extremely flexible and can be used to analyze CD34 + cells in a variety of hematologic tissues and in different clinical situations. Using three- and four-color flow cytometers, the third and/or fourth fluorescence channel can be used to assess, in an autologous HSCT setting, the qualitative composition of the CD34 + cell fraction, especially the quantitation of subsets of candidate hematopoietic stem cells. Furthermore, the addition of a known concentration of internal standard beads converts the flow-cytometric CD34 + cell assay into a single-instrument platform for the absolute CD34 + cell count determination. By incorporating 7-AAD into this assay, nonviable cells can be efficiently excluded. Additionally, in an allogeneic HSCT setting, the addition of a T-cell marker such as CD3 can be used alongside the CD34/CD45 combination to accurately quantitate T lymphocytes. These modifications to the ISHAGE *Guidelines* should allow investigators to select panels required to accurately quantitate and qualitatively define the harvested PBPC product.

REFERENCES

1. Civin C, Trischman T, Fackler MJ, et al: Summary of CD34 cluster workshop section. *In* Knapp W, et al (eds): Leucocyte Typing IV. Oxford, Oxford University Press, 1989, p 818.
2. Sutherland DR, Keating A: The CD34 antigen: structure, biology and potential clinical applications. J Hematother 1:115, 1992.
3. Andrews RG, Bryant EM, Bartelmez SH, et al: CD34 + marrow cells, devoid of T and B lymphocytes, reconstitute stable lymphopoiesis and myelopoiesis in lethally irradiated baboons. Blood 80:1693, 1992.
4. Shpall EJ, Jones RB, Franklin W, et al: Transplantation of autologous

CD34+ hematopoietic progenitor cells into breast cancer patients following high-does chemotherapy. J Clin Oncol 12:28, 1994.

5. Juttner CA, To LB, Haylock DN, et al: Circulating autologous stem cells collected in very early remission from acute non-lymphoblastic leukemia produce prompt but incomplete hematopoietic reconstitution after high-dose melphelan or supralethal chemoradiotherapy. Br J Haematol 61:739, 1985.

6. Siena S, Bregni M, Brando B, et al: Circulation of CD34+ hematopoietic stem cells in the peripheral blood of high-dose cyclophosphamide-treated patients: enhancement by intravenous recombinant human granulocyte-macrophage colony-stimulating factor. Blood 74:1905, 1989.

7. Kessinger A, Armitage JO: The evolving role of autologous peripheral stem cell transplantation following high-dose therapy for malignancies. Blood 77:211, 1989.

8. Henon PR: Peripheral blood stem cell transplantation: past present and future. Stem Cells 11:154, 1993.

9. To LB, Maylock DN, Simmons PJ, Juttner CA: The biology and clinical uses of blood stem cells. Blood 89:2233, 1997.

10. Chao NJ, Schriber JR, Grimes K, et al: Granulocyte colony-stimulating factor "mobilized" peripheral blood progenitor cells accelerate granulocyte and platelet recovery after high-dose chemotherapy. Blood 81:2031, 1993.

11. Brugger W, Henschler R, Heimfeld S, et al: Positively selected autologous blood CD34+ cells and unseparated peripheral blood progenitor cells mediate identical hematopoietic engraftment after high-dose VP16, Ifosfamide, Carboplatin, and Epirubicin. Blood 84:1421, 1994.

12. Tricot G, Jagannath S, Vesole DH, et al: Peripheral blood stem cell transplants for multiple myeloma: identification of favourable variables for rapid engraftment in 225 patients. Blood 85:588, 1995.

13. Freedman AS, Nadler LM: Developments in purging in autotransplantation. Hematol Oncol Clin North Am 7:687, 1993.

14. Bregni M, Magni M, Siena S, et al: Human peripheral blood hematopoietic progenitors are optimal targets of retroviral-mediated gene transfer. Blood 80:1418, 1992.

15. Dunbar CE, Nienhuis AW, Stewart FM, et al: Amendment to clinical research projects: genetic marking with retroviral vectors to study the feasibility of stem cell gene transfer and the biology of hematopoietic reconstitution after autologous transplantation in multiple myeloma, chronic myelogenous leukemia, or metastatic breast cancer. Hum Gene Ther 4:205, 1993.

16. Russell NH, Hunter AE: Peripheral blood stem cells for allogeneic transplantation [Editorial]. Bone Marrow Transplant 13:353, 1994.

17. Goldman JM: Peripheral blood stem cell for allografting [Editorial]. Blood 85:1413, 1995.

18. Wunder E, Sovolat H, Fritsch G, et al: Report on the European workshop on peripheral blood stem cell determination and standardisation—Mulhouse, France. J Hematother 1:131, 1992.

19. Siena S, Bregni M, Belli N, et al: Flow cytometry for clinical estimation of circulating hematopoietic progenitors for autologous transplantation in cancer patients. Blood 77:400, 1991.

20. Greaves MF, Titley I, Colman SM, et al: Report on the CD34 cluster workshop. In Schlossman S, et al (eds): Leukocyte Typing V, 1995, p 840.

21. Sutherland DR, Yeo EL, Stewart AK, et al: Identification of CD34+ subsets following glycoprotease selection: engraftment of CD34+/Thy-1+/Lin− stem cells in fetal sheep. Exp Hematol 24:795–806, 1996.

22. Bender JG, To LB, Williams S, et al: Defining a therapeutic dose of peripheral blood stem cells. J Hematother 1:329, 1992.

23. Sutherland DR, Watt SM, Dowden G, et al: Structural and partial amino acid sequence analysis of the human haemopoietic progenitor cell antigen CD34. Leukemia 2:743, 1988.

24. Simmons DL, Satterthwaite AB, Tenen DG, Seed B: Molecular cloning of a cDNA encoding CD34, a sialomucin of human hematopoietic stem cells. J Immunol 148:267, 1992.

25. Sutherland DR, Abdullah KM, Cyopick P, Mellors A: Cleavage of the cell-surface O-sialoglycoproteins CD34, CD43, CD44 and CD45 by a novel glycoprotease from *Pasteurella haemolytica*. J Immunol 148:1458, 1992.

26. Watt SM, Karhi K, Gatter K, et al: Distribution and epitope analysis of the cell membrane glycoprotein (HPCA-1) associated with human haemopoietic progenitor cell. Leukemia 1:417, 1987.

27. Sutherland DR, Marsh JCW, Davidson J, et al: Differential sensitivity of CD34 epitopes to cleavage by *Pasteurella haemolytica* glycoprotease:

implications for purification of CD34-positive progenitor cells. Exp Hematol 20:590, 1992.

28. Titley I, Healy LE, Grimsley PG, et al: Discordant CD34 epitope expression. In Schlossman S, et al (eds): Leukocyte Typing V. Oxford, Oxford University Press, 1995, p 858.

29. Titely I, Healy LE, Scott M, et al: Extent of variability inherent in measurements of CD34-positive cells in different human haematopoietic tissues. Bone Marrow Transplant 16:611, 1995.

30. Civin CI, Tischmann T, Kadan NS, et al: Highly purified CD34+ cells reconstitute hematopoiesis. J Clin Oncol 14:2224, 1996.

31. Siena S, Bregni M, Di Nicola M, et al: Milan protocol for clinical CD34+ cell estimation in peripheral blood for autografting in patients with cancer. In Wunder E, Sovolat H, Henon PR, Serke S (eds): Hematopoietic Stem Cells: The Mulhouse Manual. Alphamed Press, Dayton, Ohio, 1994, p 23.

32. Johnsen H, Knudsen LM: Nordic flow cytometry standards for CD34+ cell enumeration in blood and apheresis products: report from the second Nordic workshop. J Hematother 5:237–245, 1996.

33. Bender J, Unverzagt K, Walker D: In Wunder E, et al (eds): Hematopoietic Stem Cells: The Mulhouse Manual. Dayton, Alphamed Press, 1994, pp 31–43.

34. Gratama JW, Kraan J, Levering W, et al: Analysis of variation in results of CD34+ hematopoietic progenitor cell enumeration in a multicentre study. Cytometry 30:109–117, 1997.

35. Owens MA, Loken MP (eds): Peripheral blood stem cell quantitation. In Flow Cytometry Principles for Clinical Laboratory Practice. New York, Wiley-Liss, 1995, pp 111.

36. Trischmann TM, Schepers KG, Civin CI: Measurement of CD34+ cells in bone marrow by flow cytometry. J Hematother 2:305, 1993.

37. Kreissig C, Kirsch A, Serke S: Characterization and measurement of CD34-expressing hematopoietic cells. J Hematother 3:263, 1994.

38. Sutherland DR, Keating A, Nayar R, et al: Sensitive detection and enumeration of CD34+ cells in peripheral and cord blood by flow cytometry. Exp Hematol 22:1003, 1994.

39. Marti G, Johnsen H, Sutherland R, Serke S: A convergence of methods for a worldwide standard for CD34+ cell enumeration [Letter]. J Hematother 7:105, 1998.

40. Himmelfarb J, Hakim RM, Holbrook DG, et al: Detection of granulocyte reactive oxygen species formation in whole blood using flow cytometry. Cytometry 13:83, 1992.

41. Chen CH, Lin W, Shye S, et al: Automated enumeration of CD34+ cells in peripheral blood and bone marrow. J Hematother 3:3, 1994.

42. Brecher ME, Sims L, Schmitz JL, et al: North American multicenter study on flow cytometric enumeration of CD34+ hematopoietic stem cells. J Hematother 5:227, 1996.

43. Shah VO, Civin CI, Loken MR: Flow cytometric analysis of human bone marrow IV: differential quantitative expression of T200 common leukocyte antigen during normal hemopoiesis. J Immunol 140:1861, 1988.

44. Stelzer GT, Shults KE, Loken MR: CD45 gating for routine flow cytometric analysis of human bone marrow specimens. Ann N Y Acad Sci 677:265, 1993.

45. Borowitz MJ, Guenther KL, Schults KE, et al: Immuno-phenotyping of acute leukemia by flow cytometry: use of CD45 and right angle light scatter to gate on leukemic blasts in three color analysis. Am J Clin Pathol 100:534, 1993.

46. Marsh JCW, Sutherland DR, Davidson J, et al: Retention of progenitor cell function in CD34+ cells purified using a novel O-sialo-glycoprotease. Leukemia 6:926, 1992.

47. Stewart AK, Imrie K, Keating A, et al: Optimizing the CD34+ Thy-1+ stem cell content of peripheral blood collections. Exp Hematol 23:1619, 1995.

48. Chin-Yee I, Keeney M, Anderson L, et al: Quality assurance of stem cell enumeration by flow cytometry. Cytometry 30:1, 1997.

49. Chang A, Ma DDF: The influence of gating strategy on the standardisation of CD34+ cell quantitation: an Australian multicenter study. J Hematother 5:605, 1996.

50. Sutherland DR, Anderson L, Keeney M, et al: The ISHAGE Guidelines For CD34+ Cell Determination By Flow Cytometry. J Hematother 3:213, 1996.

51. Streuli M, Hall LR, Saga Y, et al: Differential usage of three exons generates at least five different mRNAs encoding human leukocyte common antigens. J Exp Med 166:1548, 1987.

52. Thomas ML: The leukocyte common antigen family. Annu Rev Immunol 7:339, 1989.

53. Lansdorp PM, Sutherland HJ, Eaves CJ: Selective expression of CD45 isoforms on functional subpopulations of CD34 + hemopoietic cells from human bone marrow. J Exp Med 172:363, 1990.

54. Tseng-Law J, Szalay P, Guillermo R, et al: Identification of a peptide directed against the anti-CD34 antibody, 9C5, by phage display and its use in hematopoietic stem cell selection. Exp Hematol 27:936, 1999.

55. Hughes K, Bell DN: Nonspecific binding of anti-CD34 antibody QBEnd10 to nonviable cells [Letter]. Exp Hematol 23:968, 1995.

56. Sutherland DR, Anderson L, Keeney M, et al: re: QBEnd10 (CD34) antibody is unsuitable for routine use in the ISHAGE CD34 + cell determination assay [Letter]. J Hematother 5:601, 1996.

57. Sienna S, Bregni M, Brando B, et al: Flow cytometry to estimate circulating hematopoietic progenitors for autologous transplantation: comparative analysis of different CD34 monoclonal antibodies. Haematologica 76:330, 1991.

58. Steen R, Tjonnfjord G, Gaudernack G, et al: Differences in the distribution of CD34 epitopes on normal progenitor cells and leukemic blast cells. Br J Hematol 94:597, 1996.

59. van Vugt MJ, van den Herik-Oudijk IE, van de Winkel JGJ: Binding of PE-CY5 conjugates to the human high-affinity receptor for IgG (CD64) [Letter]. Blood 88:2358, 1996.

60. Sutherland DR, Anderson L, Keeney M, et al: Towards a worldwide standard for CD34 + enumeration? J Hematother 6:85, 1997.

61. Keeney M, Chin-Yee I, Gratama JW, et al: Perspectives: Isotype controls in the analysis of lymphocytes and CD34 + stem/progenitor cells by flow cytometry—time to let go! Cytometry 34:280–283, 1998.

62. Sehmi R, Howie K, Sutherland DR, et al: Increased levels of CD34 + hematopoietic progenitors in atopic subjects. Am J Respir Cell Mol Biol 15:645, 1996.

63. Keeney M, Chin-Yee I, Weir K, et al: Single platform flow cytometric absolute CD34 + cell counts based on the ISHAGE guidelines. Cytometry 34:61–67, 1998.

64. Gratama JW, Keeney M, Sutherland DR: Enumeration of CD34 + hematopoietic stem and progenitor cells. In Current Protocols in Cytometry, New York, Wiley & Sons, unit 6.4.1–6.4.22. 1999.

65. Knape CC: Standardization of absolute CD34 cell enumeration. J Hematother 5:211, 1996.

66. Schmid I, Krall WJ, Uittenbogaart C, et al: Dead cell discrimination with 7-actinomycin D in combination with dual color immunofluorescence in single-laser flow cytometry. Cytometry 13:204, 1992.

67. Gratama JW, Orfao A, Barnett D, et al: Flow cytometric enumeration of CD34 + hematopoietic stem and progenitor cells. Cytometry (Comm Clin Cytometry) 34:128–142, 1998.

68. Murray L, Chen B, Galy A, et al: Enrichment of hematopoietic stem cell activity in the CD34 + Thy-1 + Lin − subpopulation from mobilized peripheral blood. Blood 85:368, 1995.

69. Haas R, Mohle R, Pforsich M, et al: Blood-derived autografts collected during granulocyte colony-stimulating factor–enhanced recovery are enriched with early Thy-1 + hematopoietic progenitor cells. Blood 85:1936, 1995.

70. Murray LJ, Bruno E, Uchida N, et al: CD109 is expressed on a subpopulation of CD34 + cells enriched in hematopoietic stem and progenitor cells. Exp Hematol 27:1282, 1999.

71. Dercksen MW, Rodenhuis S, Dirkson MKA, et al: Subsets of CD34 + cells and rapid hematopoietic recovery after peripheral blood stem cell transplantation. J Clin Oncol 13:1922–1932, 1995.

72. Pecora AL, Preti RA, Gleim GW, et al: CD34 + CD33 − cells influence the days to engraftment and transfusion requirements in autologous blood stem-cell recipients. J Clin Oncol 16:2093–2104, 1998.

73. Negrin RS, Tierney D, Stockerl-Goldstein KE, et al: Rapid hematopoietic engraftment following transplantation of purified CD34 + Thy-1 + cells in patients with metastatic breast cancer. Blood 90(suppl 1):593, 1997.

74. Gazitt Y, Tian E, Barlogie B, et al: Differential mobilization of myeloma cells and normal hematopoietic stem cells in multiple myeloma following treatment with cyclophosphamide and GM-CSF. Blood 87:805, 1996.

75. Prince HM, Imrie K, Sutherland DR, et al: Peripheral blood progenitor cell collections in multiple myeloma: predictors and management of inadequate collections. Br J Haematol 93:142–145, 1996.

76. Carella AM, Podesta M, Frassoni F, et al: Collection of "normal" blood repopulating cells during early hematopoietic recovery after intensive conventional chemotherapy in chronic myeloid leukemia. Bone Marrow Transplant 12:267, 1993.

77. Van Den Berg D, Wessman M, Murray L, et al: Leukemic burden in subpopulations of CD34 + cells isolated from the mobilised peripheral blood of α-interferon-resistant or -intolerant patients with chronic myeloid leukemia. Blood 87:4348–4357, 1996.

78. Sutherland DR, Filshie R, Keeney M, et al: Quantitation and Phenotypic Characterization of Hematopoietic Progenitor Cells. In Read EJ, Gee A, Collins N (eds): Cellular Therapy: A Clinical Laboratory Approach. Oxford, ISIS Medical Media (in press).

79. Verwer BJH, Ward DM: An automated classification algorithm for PROCOUNT flow cytometric acquisition and analysis (abstract). J Hematother 6:169, 1997.

80. Dietz LJ, Dubrow RS, Manian BS, et al: Volumetric capillary cytometry: a new method for absolute cell determination. Cytometry 23:177–186, 1996.

81. Sims LC, Brecher ME, Gertis K, et al: Enumeration of CD34 + stem cells: evaluation and comparison of three methods. J Hematother 6:213–226, 1997.

82. Read EJ, Kunitake ST, Carter CS, et al: Enumeration of CD34 + hematopoietic progenitor cells in peripheral blood and leucapheresis products by microvolume fluorimetry: a comparison with flow cytometry. J Hematother 6:291–301, 1997.

83. Roth P, Maples J, Hall J, et al: Use of control cells to standardize enumeration of CD34 + stem cells. Ann NY Acad Sci 770:370–372, 1996.

Graft Engineering

CHAPTER TWENTY-EIGHT

Graft Processing, Storage, and Infusion

Ping Law, Ph.D.

Hematopoietic stem cells (HSC) and progenitor cells contribute a small portion (<5%) of the cells in bone marrow (BM) or peripheral blood progenitor cell (PBPC) grafts. For autologous transplantation, the graft, whether BM or PBPC, needs to be cryopreserved while the patient receives conditioning regimen. For allogeneic transplantation, processing may be required to deplete plasma, to reduce red blood cell (RBC) content and—in some centers, prior to cryopreservation—to ensure the collection of an adequate dose of HSC or other cell types before initiation of myeloablative or nonablative conditioning regimen. Graft processing is divided into "simple" and "complex" procedures for discussion in this chapter. Simple procedures are defined as those that separate cells and components by their physical properties; do not require specifically designed equipment; and are not dependent on cell surface characteristics, intracellular metabolism, or other biochemical pathways. Complex procedures are defined as those that separate different cell types by their surface markers or biochemical characteristics and/or require specially designed systems. In recent years, HSC from cord blood collection have been used for sibling and mismatched unrelated transplantation. Processing is required before cord blood collections are cryopreserved (see Chapter 26).

SIMPLE PROCEDURES

Table 28–1 is a list of commonly used simple procedures for graft processing. Typically, autologous PBPC grafts require little or no processing before cryopreservation. Depending on the leukapheresis device or the procedures used to collect cells, PBPC may need to be concentrated (by centrifugation) before cryopreservation to minimize infusion of cryoprotectant and to conserve space in the liquid nitrogen storage freezer. Buffy coat processing is usually performed for autologous BM grafts for volume reduction.[1, 2] The procedure has been adapted to apheresis or cell washing devices for semiautomated processing.[3–8] Little or no loss in white blood cells (WBC) and/or CD34+ cells was reported. Buffy coat concentration of BM WBC has also been used for debulking before subsequent density gradient separation or other complex procedures.[7] Manual centrifugation is often used when the packed RBC volume is too small for machine processing.[9] Sedimentation of RBC

can be achieved using hydroxyethyl starch.[10] The procedure is hardly performed because PBPC have all but replaced BM as the autograft of choice.

Several simple procedures are routinely used for allograft processing. For minor ABO-mismatched transplants, the plasma volume in the graft should be reduced according to standard transfusion practice. The limit of incompatible plasma is usually set to less than 500 mL to avoid hemolytic reactions. Plasma reduction can be achieved by single-step low-speed centrifugation of BM or PBPC grafts and replacement of the plasma with saline and human serum albumin. For allogeneic PBPC grafts, care should be taken to include all leukapheresis collections in the estimation of the allowable plasma volume. For major ABO-mismatched transplantation, packed RBC volume should be reduced to less than 50 mL,[6, 8] which can be achieved by density gradient centrifugation of BM and PBPC grafts using commercially available material such as Ficoll-Paque or Percoll. Low-density mononuclear cells are washed to remove residual gradient material before infusion. The procedure has also been adapted to cell-washing devices.[3, 6, 8, 11–17] ABO-mismatched marrow grafts are typically processed through the buffy-coat procedure before density gradient separation.[6, 7] Overall WBC recovery of the processing (buffy-coat and density gradient centrifugation) is between

TABLE 28–1. SIMPLE GRAFT PROCESS PROCEDURES

PROCEDURE	APPLICATION	HSC SOURCE
Centrifugation (for plasma depletion)	Minor ABO mismatched allograft; concentrating cells for cryopreservation	BM, PBPC
Buffy coat	Volume reduction for cryopreservation or subsequent manipulation	BM
RBC sedimentation	RBC depletion and/or volume reduction	CB, BM
Density gradient separation of mononuclear cells	For RBC depletion in major ABO mismatched allotransplantation or debulking for subsequent manipulations	BM, PBPC, CB

BM, bone marrow; HSC, hematopoietic stem cell; PBPC; peripheral blood progenitor cell; CB, cord blood.

15% and 50%, and CD34+ cell recovery is 50–100%. A closed disposable density gradient system (BDS-60, based on Percoll) has been developed for this purpose.[18] The system has been tested in clinical trials with acceptable outcomes.

Cord blood products are collected at delivery and cryopreserved by the cord blood banks. Two types of cord blood banks are currently in operation. Private banks are funded by charges to the family of the newborns from which cord blood products are collected. The cord blood product is specifically stored for the newborn. Cost typically includes an initial collection/processing/cryopreservation fee and an annual charge for liquid nitrogen and storage space. Public banks are funded by charges to the patients/recipients (or third-party payers) of the cord blood product. The donor of the cord blood and the recipient are shielded from each other, with procedures and guidelines similar to those of the National Marrow Donor Program.[101] Most operating cord blood banks employ procedures for RBC reduction to obtain a uniform volume for each cord blood unit.[19] RBC reduction has been achieved by sedimentation in hydroxyethyl starch,[19] gelatin,[20] or density gradient.[21] Currently, most cord blood products are processed by the hydroxyethyl starch sedimentation procedure developed by New York Blood Center and adopted by the cord blood banks sponsored by the National Institutes of Health.[19, 101]

COMPLEX PROCEDURES

The goal of most complex procedures is to remove unwanted cell populations from the products while maintaining the quantity of the HSC. Currently, the most common method for determining the adequacy of HSC collection is the flow cytometric determination of CD34+ cells (see Chapter 27).[84, 86] The minimum dose of CD34+ cells is usually greater than or equal to 1×10^6/kg recipient weight (see Graft Assessment). Recently, primitive CD34− HSC have been reported in animals and humans.[33–40] In utero xenograft transplantation of human CD34− cells into sheep has demonstrated that such cell populations appear to have superior long-term engraftment potential compared with the CD34+ cells.[33, 38] The clinical relevance of this discovery is still unknown. Most recent results in mice suggest that activation (such as fluorouracil treatment) induces expression of CD34 from CD34− cells,[103, 104] and that the activated primitive self-renewing CD34+ cells can revert to the CD34− phenotype.

Table 28–2 is a list of common complex procedures for graft processing. Allograft manipulation using positive selection of CD34+ cells and/or T-cell depletion is discussed in Chapter 30. Clinical trials in autologous and allogeneic transplantation of enriched CD34+ cells have resulted in prompt and sustained engraftment.[22–27] Parallel comparisons of different CD34+ cell selection systems have been published.[28–32] A comparison of the commonly use systems is shown in Table 28–3.

For autologous transplantation, disease relapse is a major cause of treatment failure. Relapse can be caused by residual disease in vivo or the infusion of occult tumor cells not easily detected in the HSC collection. Tumor cell purging is discussed in detail in Chapter 29. Selection of CD34+ cells may be used as a passive procedure for tumor cell depletion.

Expansion of HSC can reduce the difficulty of collecting a minimal HSC dose for transplantation. A minimal dose of 1×10^6 CD34+ cells/kg recipient weight is usually achieved by harvesting greater than or equal to 1 L of BM (for adults) or two to five sessions of apheresis collection

TABLE 28–2. COMPLICATED GRAFT PROCESSING PROCEDURES

PROCESS	METHODOLOGY	STATUS	MORE INFORMATION	COMMENTS
Enrichment for CD34+ cells	Incubation with biotinylated antibody; capture on avidin column; release by mechanical disruption of antibody	Approved in U.S. and Europe	Shpall et al[22, 23]	CellPro has developed the system. The company no longer exists.
	Incubation with CD34 MAb; capture with paramagnetic beads and magnets; release by competitive displacement	Approved in U.S. and Europe	Strauss et al,[96] Civin et al,[97] Hardwick et al[98]	Approved by Food and Drug Administration and marketed by Nexell
	Incubation with microbeads coated with CD34 MAb; capture on enhanced magnetic fields; microbeads not released from target cells	Approved in Europe	Radbruch et al,[99] Miltenyi et al[100]	Not yet approved in U.S. Supported by Miltenyi Biotec.
Purging of tumor cells	Pharmacologic killing using 4-HC or mafosfamide	IND	Rowley et al,[7] Chap 29	
	Antibody-directed complement mediated lysing	IND	Chap 29	
	Immunomagnetic depletion	IND	Hardwick et al[98]	
Expansion of HSC	Stroma containing culture device	IND	Chap 32	
	Cytokine-mediated culture	IND	Chap 32	

HSC, hematopoietic stem cells; IND, investigational new drug exemption.

TABLE 28–3. COMPARISON OF COMMON CD34+ CELL SELECTION SYSTEMS

	CELLPRO CEPRATE	NEXELL ISOLEX-300i	MILTENYI CLINIMACS
Capture of CD34+ cells	Indirect*	Indirect*	Direct†
Release of captured cells	Mechanical disruption	Competitive displacement	No release process (beads left on cell surface)
Automated procedure	Yes	Yes	Yes
Cell washing steps	Performed separately	Incorporated	Performed separately
Purity of enriched cells	~50%	~85%	>90%
CD34+ cell yield	~20–50%	~50%	~70%
Capacity	>6 × 10¹⁰ WBC‡	~4 × 10¹⁰ WBC§	~8.9 × 10¹⁰#

*Cells must be sensitized with antibody and washed before capturing on substrate.
†Antibody is attached to microbeads, and no presensitization of cells is necessary.
‡Based on calculation of capture capacity on the avidin column.
§Calculated from the following assumption: 1% CD34+ cells in peripheral blood progenitor cell product, 2 beads per target cell needed for magnetic capture, 1 out of every 5 beads bound to target cells, and total of 4 × 10⁹ beads provided in each reagent kit.[98]
#See Schumm et al.[102]

of PBPC. Cord blood transplantation is primarily limited to pediatric patients because of the size of each cord blood product. Expansion of HSC can reduce the amount of harvested BM or number of sessions in PBPC apheresis; such expansion can also extend the utility of cord blood products to adult patients. Expansion of HSC is discussed in detail in Chapter 32. Currently, purging procedures and expansion processes are not approved for routine clinical use by national regulatory agencies.

GRAFT STORAGE

The increased complexity of processing has led to lengthy processing time. Also, large-volume leukapheresis, processing 20–40 L of blood (see Chapter 25), increases the collection time and hence delays the start of processing, and cryopreservation of autologous PBPC products. Storage of products for overnight or longer periods, especially PBPC, becomes logistically necessary. Parameters for product storage, such as temperature, cell concentration, buffer, and pH, have not yet been fully and systematically investigated. Published studies demonstrated that PBPC grafts can be stored at ambient (20°–24°C) or refrigerated (2°–6°C) temperatures for 24 hours before processing.[41–44] Viability (assessed using membrane compromise dyes, such as trypan blue or propidium iodide), proportion of CD34+ cells, and cloning efficiencies of colony-forming hematopoietic progenitor cells are maintained. Stored cells can be used for complex processing procedures such as CD34+ cell enrichment without any apparent decrease in separation

TABLE 28–4. CONDITIONS FOR OVERNIGHT STORAGE OF PBPC PRODUCTS BEFORE PROCESSING

TEMPERATURE	ADVANTAGES	DISADVANTAGES
Ambient (20–24°C)	Little or no change to platelet or granulocyte function	Control of cell concentration to ≤1.5 × 10⁸/mL
Refrigerated (2–6°C)	No apparent limit on cell concentration	Possible platelet activation; possible granulocyte disintegration

PBPC, peripheral blood progenitor cell.

efficiency.[26, 44] The neutrophil and platelet engraftment times of PBPC products cryopreserved after storage, once thawed and infused into patients, are not different from those cryopreserved without storage.[26, 44] The advantages and disadvantages for storage at either ambient or refrigerated temperature are listed in Table 28–4. Each transplant program is encouraged to validate center-specific parameters before adopting a standard policy and procedure.

There are reports suggesting that PBPC products can be stored in liquid state without cryopreservation for autologous infusion after myeloablative therapy.[45–48] The feasibility of the storage procedure should be validated before it is adopted as standard procedure.

CRYOPRESERVATION

SOLUTION EFFECT AND INTRACELLULAR ICE FORMATION

The theory of freeze-thaw damage in single-cell suspensions has not changed since the publication of Mazur in 1970.[49] When cell survival was studied as a function of cooling rate, a biphasic response was observed for different cell types. If cells are cooled slowly, ice crystals are formed mainly in the extracellular solution. As the temperature decreases, the solute concentration increases in the extracellular space (Fig. 28–1A). Cells shrink in response to the osmotic imbalance—hence the reference to "solution effect."[49] After a minimum volume (depending on the cell type) is reached, further cell shrinkage becomes impossible, resulting in membrane tension that leads to cell damage.[50–53] When cells are cooled slowly, water loss created by extracellular freezing and the increase of intracellular solution prevents ice nucleation from forming inside the cells. As cooling rate increases, less time is available for dehydration, making the intracellular solution more dilute than the extracellular compartment. If the cooling rate is fast enough, small intracellular ice crystals can form through homogeneous nucleation. The small ice crystals recrystallize during thawing, leading to rupture of cell membranes and disruption of intracellular organelles, resulting in cell death (Fig. 28–2).

Intracellular freezing is generally a lethal event, although the extent of recrystallization can be minimized by rapid

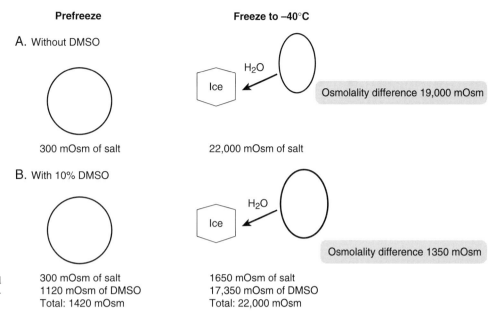

FIGURE 28–1. Solution effect and colligative cryoprotector. DMSO, dimethylsulfoxide.

thawing.[54] The optimal cooling rate is a kinetic balance at which dehydration is not sufficient for cell damage but has caused sufficient increase in intracellular solute concentration to prevent nucleation inside the cells. The rate depends on the cell type and is a complex function of the water permeability, isotonic cell volume, minimum cell volume, protein and other cellular contents, and membrane structure (types of phospholipids, membrane protein, intracellular and extracellular skeleton). For example, the mouse colony-forming unit–granulocyte macrophage has an optimal cooling rate of about 1°–10°C/minute; the rate for human RBC is greater than 100°C/minute.[49] Even at the optimal rate, the portion of cells surviving the freeze-thaw process is very small (<5%).[49] Cryoprotection is necessary to ensure high viability.

COLLIGATIVE PROTECTION

Damage resulting from the solution effect during slow cooling can be reduced by the addition of a permeable solute.[51] A nonpermeable solute increases extracellular osmolality and dehydrates cells just as effectively as ice formation. As illustrated in Figure 28–1B, the presence of cryoprotectant inside and outside of a cell dramatically reduces the osmotic stress on the cell membrane; the total solute concentration remains the same with or without the cryoprotectant. For human RBC, glycerol is a good cryoprotectant because the erythrocyte has a facilitated transport mechanism for this chemical.[55, 56] Dimethylsulfoxide (DMSO) is an excellent cryoprotectant for most types of cells and tissues. The chemical has a high coefficient of permeability

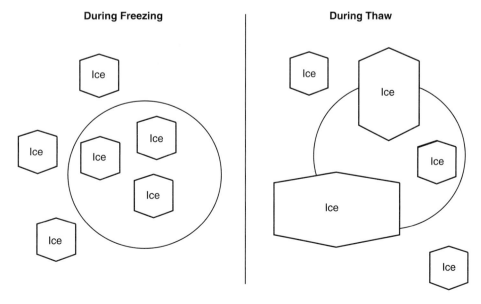

FIGURE 28–2. Rapid freezing injury.

to cell membrane[57–61] and is relatively nontoxic at low temperature (4°C), even with the intermediate concentration (10% or 1.2 M) necessary for cryoprotection. DMSO can broaden the optimal cooling rate peak into a plateau by decreasing the amount of dehydration or solution effect at the slow-cooling side and by reducing the risk of intracellular ice formation at the rapid-cooling side by increasing the intracellular solute concentration. Its rapid penetration into and out of cells and tissues minimizes the osmotic shock associated with its introduction and removal.

Certain high-molecular-weight polymers can also be used as cryoprotectant. Hydroxyethyl starch and polyvinylpyrrolidone are the two most commonly used agents.[62, 63] The chemicals do not permeate into the cells but, as temperature decreases during extracellular freezing, these high-molecular-weight polymers exert their cryoprotective effect by forming a relatively impermeable and highly viscous glassy layer of solution around the cells. Further loss of water and dehydration is prevented, and cell viability is maintained.

CONTROLLED RATE VERSUS SIMPLE STEP COOLING

Cryoprotectant and HSC Products

Cryopreservation of BM or PBPC products is traditionally achieved by controlled rate freezing at −1°C/minute.[64, 65] DMSO is prepared in cold (0°–4°C) as a 20% solution in tissue culture medium with 5–20% autologous plasma or human serum albumin. Because tissue culture media are not approved for infusion into humans, different varieties of saline (approved for infusion), such as normal saline, Normosol, Plasmalyte, or an equivalent, are used to replace tissue culture medium. Anticoagulant (heparin or acid citrate dextrose [ACD]) may be added to prevent platelet clumping during the thawing process. The solution is then added slowly to the HSC suspension at a 1:1 ratio in cold for a final DMSO concentration of 10%. Because the mixing of DMSO and water causes an exothermic reaction, care must be taken to ensure that (1) the 20% DMSO solution is cold before adding it to the HSC suspension and (2) the 20% DMSO and the HSC cell suspension are thoroughly mixed in cold. It is more advisable to add 20% DMSO solution to the HSC suspension than vice versa to minimize osmotic shock to the cells. Although early cryopreservation procedures typically require the nucleated cell concentration to be less than 1×10^8/mL, more recent methods have increased cell concentrations to as high as 5×10^8 without any compromise in post-thaw engraftment kinetics.[66]

Preparation of Bags and Controlled-Rate Cooling

The HSC product containing 10% DMSO is then distributed into special bags constructed with material capable of withstanding the temperature range of freezing and thawing. The thickness of the filled bags should not exceed 7.5 mm so that the entire suspension is cooled at a similar rate. All air trapped in the bag and transfer tubing must be removed. It is possible for the residual air inside the bag to liquefy during freezing and storage and to vaporize during thawing, which cause rapid volume expansion leading to breakage of the bag. Each bag is wiped dry and placed into a metal cassette to ensure rapid and homogeneous heat transfer to the entire bag. Condensation left on the outside of the bag forms ice during freezing, and the solid ice particles can potentially puncture the bag, which becomes brittle at low temperatures, especially during the thawing process, when the bag is removed from the cassette before immersion into water bath (see later). If more than one cassette is cryopreserved at the same time, the cassettes should be placed in the freezing chamber with ample space between each unit. Cooling is controlled via computer or microprocessor by adjusting the speed of liquid nitrogen infusion into the freezing chamber. The programmed cooling rate typically consists of the following steps: allow time to allow the HSC/DMSO mixture to reach the starting temperature (typically between 4°C and 0°C), super-cool to −10° to −15°C, suddenly decrease temperature to induce ice nucleation, allow time for the dissipation of the heat of fusion, and control the rate of cooling (−1°C/minute) to −80°C or −100°C. The cassettes are then transferred to a storage freezer.

Single-Step Cryopreservation

Single-step cryopreservation was developed by Stiff et al.[10, 67, 68] The cryoprotective solution consists of 10% DMSO and 12% hydroxyethyl starch in combined electrolyte solution (Normosol) with human serum albumin. The solution is added to the HSC suspension at a 1:1 ratio as described earlier, and the mixture is distributed into cryopreservation bags, which are then placed in metal cassettes. Final concentrations of the cryoprotectant are 5% DMSO and 6% hydroxyethyl starch. The cassettes are placed horizontally in a freezer set at −80°C. The same precautions of limiting the bag thickness, removing trapped air, wiping off condensation, and ensuring sufficient space for heat transfer in each cassette (as discussed earlier) should be observed. The geometry of the arrangement and the temperature difference between the HSC/DMSO–hydroxyethyl starch mixture and the −80°C environment inside the freezer ensure that the cooling rate will not be too fast for intracellular ice formation. HSC products can be stored in the −80°C freezer or in a liquid nitrogen storage freezer. This method takes advantage of the broadened optimal cooling rate plateau of using cryoprotectant and has been used successfully with BM and PBPC products. Infusion of thawed products has resulted in prompt and sustained engraftment.[68]

Cryopreservation of Vials of HSC

Vials (two to four) containing 1 to 4 mL of the same HSC product and cryoprotectant (DMSO or DMSO–hydroxyethyl starch) should be cryopreserved at the same time. These vials should be processed and stored under similar conditions as used for the bags, and the vials may be used later. Situations in which the vials may be thawed include confirmation of microbiologic contamination, assessment of tumor cell markers, and reassessment of HSC or other cell contents.

INVENTORY AND STORAGE

Cryopreserved products are typically stored in liquid nitrogen freezers in either the vapor or the liquid phase. All storage freezers should have continuous temperature monitoring, printout of temperature history at regular intervals, and an alarm system in case of failure or temperatures exceeding preset limits. Assess to the freezers should be restricted. Current regulatory requirement has specified the standards for the management of storage freezers (see Chapter 65). Although the liquid phase of liquid nitrogen provides a homogeneous and stable ultralow temperature ($-196°C$), there is a possibility of cross-contamination from products that have tested positive for an infectious agent.[69–72] The risk for cross-contamination can be avoided by keeping untested products in a quarantine freezer. The products should be transferred to the regular freezer once negative test results are obtained. The quarantine freezer can also be used to store products that have tested positive for infectious disease markers but must be collected and kept for medical reasons.

Storage in the vapor phase can avoid the potential risk of cross-contamination. Temperature in the vapor phase of the freezer, however, can vary between $-100°$ and $-190°C$, depending on the distance to the liquid surface, frequency of opening and closing of the lid, and quality of insulation of the freezer. A1 least one temperature probe should be placed close to the lid of the freezer to monitor the highest possible temperature inside the storage chamber. The upper limit of the temperature detected by this probe should be set below $-120°C$ to avoid any phase transition of the HSC suspension/cryoprotectant mixture.[64]

HSC products cryopreserved by the single-step freezing procedure can be stored at $-80°C$ for extended periods of time without compromising the engraftment potential.[10, 67, 68] Because colligative cryoprotection takes place in a nonequilibrium state, storage in vapor or liquid nitrogen phase is preferred.[64] Other arguments for liquid nitrogen freezers are that most freezers set at $-80°C$ are mechanical devices more prone to malfunction, and temperature maintenance at ultralow level is better with liquid nitrogen freezers.

Commercially available freezers can be equipped with a racking and inventory system. The use of such a system allows easy access to the cryopreserved cassettes. A new ultralow temperature storage system has been developed with a bar-code reader and robotic arm controlled by a computerized inventory-manipulation mechanism.[101] The system is currently used in some cord blood banks.

THAWING AND INFUSION

THAWING

Cryopreserved BM or PBPC products are usually thawed rapidly at bedside and infused immediately.[64, 65] Rapid thawing can reduce recrystallization of intracellular ice, as discussed earlier, and decrease exposure time to osmotic imbalance, which is more important during thaw because the cells may have sustained some damage during the freezing phase. In actual practice, the water bath is thoroughly cleaned and disinfected. Sterile water or saline is heated to 37°–45°C. Cryopreserved products are transported to the nursing station in a dry-shipper. Each bag is carefully removed from the cassette, put into a second bag, and then immersed completely in water with gentle massage. A secondary bag is used as a safety precaution. If the bag containing the HSC product is compromised during thawing, cells that leak out can be collected and infused if necessary. The bag is taken out from the water bath when ice and liquid are both in the bag. Care must be taken not to overheat the BM or PBPC product. The cells are immediately infused by gravity or using a syringe. The thawing process on the second bag should not be initiated until the first bag has been infused completely. Prolonged exposure to DMSO after thawing has been shown to decrease colony formation of cryopreserved BM products.[73, 74] Adverse reactions during infusion should be carefully monitored and recorded. If the graft contains a large quantity of bags (>10), more than 1 day of infusion may be required.

Neutrophil and platelet engraftment days are reported to the processing laboratory to fulfill the regulatory requirement of outcome tracking (see Chapter 65). Any adverse events should be discussed in patient-care meetings together with apheresis and processing laboratory staff to ensure a continuum of quality service by the transplant program. Toxicity resulting from infusion of thawed BM or PBPC products has been low[75–77] and is mainly due to fluid overload, the quantity of infused DMSO, and/or RBC stroma induced by the freeze-thaw process. Infusion of enriched CD34 + cells from BM has been shown to have reduced side effects compared with unmanipulated product.[23]

POST-THAW MANIPULATION

Some clinical study protocols require post-thaw manipulation of BM or PBPC products.[78–80] The procedures must be clearly defined and validated before clinical trials are initiated. The HSC of BM and PBPC have been shown to behave differently when cultured in interleukin-2 for 24 hours after thawing.[78] In contrast, cord blood products are routinely washed to remove DMSO before infusion (see Chapter 26).[19] Such a procedure appears to reduce the side effects of infusion, especially for pediatric patients.

OTHER ISSUES FOR THE PROCESSING LABORATORY

GRAFT ASSESSMENT

Viability

Viability of collected BM or PBPC is usually measured by vital dyes such as trypan blue or fluorescence stains such as acridine orange/propidium iodide and fluorescein diactate/ethidium bromide. Scoring is performed visually under a microscope or fluorescence microscope. Fluorescent dyes such as propidium iodide can be used in conjunction with CD34 + cell staining and measurement is performed under fluorescence microscopy or by flow cytometry (see Chapter 27).[81–84] The assay measures only the integrity of the cell membrane and does not indicate cell function. Because the proportion of HSC in BM or PBPC is seldom greater than 2%, the measurement without specific staining has little or no bearing on HSC. Testing of membrane compromise viability, however, is easy and rapid and provides a good indication of the general condition of the product. The determination is especially important when the processing laboratory and the collection facility are not close to each other (noncontiguous locations) and products have to be transported.

CD34 + Cells

Flow cytometric measurement of CD34 + cells has become the standard of evaluating HSC grafts (see Chapter 27). Current data suggest that autograft engraftment kinetics correlates with CD34 + cell dose when a minimum of about 2×10^6/kg is not achieved.[81] Some studies have shown that quality of the autograft, measured by the percentage of CD34 + cells, may correlate with platelet engraftment.[85] Because the assay can be completed within hours after receipt of the product in the processing laboratory, most transplant centers have used this assessment to determine the adequacy of leukapheresis collection of PBPC.

Early studies reported large variations among different laboratories measuring CD34 + cells from the same sample.[82, 86] Recent efforts by cooperative workshops, study groups, academic societies, and companies developing clinical grade reagents and automated acquisition and analysis procedures have alerted investigators to the importance of sample preparation, calibration of equipment, and standardization of the acquisition and analysis procedures. Discrepancies among well-trained laboratories have become much smaller because of the attention.[86, 87]

Subsets and Other Leukocytes

Subsets of CD34 + cells can determine the proportions of HSC that are primitive or committed to different lineages of maturation.[88–92] One study has reported that engraftment kinetics is correlated with the dose of CD34 + CD33 − cells.[93] Correlation of engraftment with other CD34 + cell subsets has not been successful.[84] CD34 + determination should be sufficient for determination of HSC dose for grafts subjected only to simple processing procedures.

Measurement of other leukocyte populations is necessary for allografts and for tracking purposes when an autograft is processed through complex procedures (see Chapter 30). Common markers include T cells, B cells, monocytes, and natural killer cells. If purging is performed, a tumor marker becomes desirable (see Chapter 29).

Colony Culture

Hematopoietic progenitor colony formation is sometimes used to measure the HSC content of each product.[7, 73, 94] It is a functional determination of the ability of the committed progenitors to grow in vitro. The assay requires 14 days to complete and depends on the growth factor combination, serum or protein supplement, and subjective scoring of the laboratory technologists. The most commonly used assay is the culture of colony-forming unit–granulocyte macrophage (CFU-GM) progenitor cells. It can be impractical because of the culture time. Some autografts may have already been infused before the CFU-GM results are known. It is also not possible to use the CFU-GM assay to determine the number of apheresis PBPC products needed for an adequate graft. Colony assay becomes desirable as a quality assurance parameter for complex procedures of processing because an increase in manipulation time and steps could lead to compromise of the functional status of the HSC products. Commercially available premixed culture medium has decreased the variability of the CFU-GM assay among different laboratories.

MICROBIAL CONTAMINATION

A small fraction of each product is used for assessment of microbial contamination. The sample should be removed prior to distribution to the cryopreservation bags to account for all manipulation procedures. Only assays approved by regulatory agencies should be used. If a laboratory outside the transplant center is used, the facility should be properly licensed or accredited by regulatory agencies or professional organizations. If the assessment yields negative results, the products are not completely free of contamination because only a small fraction of the product is sampled and cultured. If results are positive attending physicians should be immediately notified and confirmation tests should be initiated using vials of cells cryopreserved separately from the same product (see earlier). The decision of whether a potentially contaminated product should be infused is made by the attending physician and the transplant team after careful consideration of such parameters as disease status and condition of the patient, total number of HSC collected, the type(s) of organism(s) and, if bacteria contamination is reported, the sensitivity of the organisms to antibiotics.

TRANSPORTATION

BM or PBPC products may be shipped in a liquid or cryopreserved state.[95] A matched unrelated donor BM graft is transported fresh in the liquid state. The National Marrow Donor Program (NMDP) has strict standards for the transportation that involve using a designated carrier from the collection center to the transplant center. Extra precaution is essential because the patient has already undergone myeloablative conditioning. It is possible, although rare, that an allograft from a matched or mismatched related donor may be collected in a geographic location different from that of the transplant facility and that product transportation is required. The NMDP standards for transportation should be adopted in such situations. Viability, flow cytometry, and other functional assessment of the product may become necessary before shipment and after receipt.

Cryopreserved autografts should be transported in a liquid nitrogen dry-shipper. Liquid nitrogen will not spill from the dry-shipper because the fluid is absorbed into the insulation lining material. The dry-shipper should be equilibrated with a sufficient amount of liquid nitrogen according to the manufacturer's instructions. Temperature inside the shipper should be verified at pickup and delivery. The products may be transported using reliable commercial carriers. The Foundation for the Accreditation of Hematopoietic Cell Therapy (FAHCT) has developed standards pertaining to the transportation of BM or PBPC grafts in a liquid or cryopreserved state.

DISCARD OF PRODUCTS

BM or PBPC products from deceased patients or that are no longer needed medically should be discarded. For example, the products may be collected and cryopreserved as backup, or the extra HSC may be intended for a second transplant while the patient is not medically suitable for receiving the graft. The discarded product should be considered potentially hazardous and must be disposed according to governmental (federal, state, and local) and institutional regulations. The FAHCT has developed standards for product removal. Important considerations include confirmation of patient death or documentation of the conditions in which the products are no longer needed, review by the laboratory facility's medical director and consultation with attending physicians, verification of product and patient identification, and a record of how the products are disposed.

CONCLUSION

Processing and cryopreservation of autologous BM and PBPC products has become standard practice in transplant centers. Although the steps are written into standard operating procedure, a clear understanding of both the mechanisms of freeze-thaw damage and the rationale of the techniques is important to avoid overlooking critical features. Simple procedures are used for cell concentration, plasma removal, or RBC depletion. Complex procedures are designed for enrichment or depletion of specific cell populations. During freezing, cell damage is osmotic and can be minimized by the use of cryoprotectants such as DMSO and hydroxyethyl starch. Cryopreserved products should be stored below $-120°C$. Thawing and infusion should be performed as rapidly as possible. Graft adequacy may be assessed by leukocyte count, cell viability, flow cytometry measurement of CD34+ cells, and/or colony formation. It is important for the processing laboratory to monitor the regulatory requirements so that standard operating procedures can be updated to include the latest revisions and so that sufficient record-keeping is maintained. Good communication from the processing laboratory to other services of the HSC transplant program is essential so that deviations from standard operating procedures and adverse events can be properly investigated in a timely fashion.

REFERENCES

1. Davis JM, Rowley SD, Braine HG, et al: Clinical toxicity of cryopreserved bone marrow graft infusion. Blood 75:781, 1990.

2. Elliott C, McCarthy D: A survey of methods of processing and storage of bone marrow and blood stem cells in the EBMT. Bone Marrow Transplant 14:419, 1994.

3. Gilmore MJML, Prentice HG, Corringham RE, et al: A technique for the concentration of nucleated bone marrow cells for in vitro manipulation or cryopreservation using the IBM 2991 blood cell processor. Vox Sang 45:294, 1983.

4. Angelini A, Dragani A, Iacone A, et al: Human bone marrow processing using Cobe 2991 and CS3000 blood cell separators for further ex-vivo manipulation. J Artif Organs 43:57, 1988.

5. Areman E: Automated isolation of mononuclear cells using the Fenwal CS3000 blood cell separator. In Gross SR, Gee A (eds): Bone Marrow Purging and Processing, vol 33. New York, Alan R Liss, 1990, p 379.

6. Jin N, Hill R, Segal G, et al: Preparation of red-blood-cell-depleted marrow for ABO-incompatible marrow transplantation by density-gradient separation using the IBM-2991 Blood Cell Processor. Exp Hematol 15:93, 1987.

7. Rowley SD, Davis JM, Piantadosi S, et al: Density gradient separation of autologous bone marrow grafts before ex vivo purging with 4-hydroperoxycyclophosphamide. Bone Marrow Transplant 6:321, 1990.

8. Braine HG, Sensenbrenner LL, Wright SK, et al: Bone marrow transplantation with major ABO blood group incompatibility using erythrocyte depletion of marrow prior to infusion. Blood 60:420, 1982.

9. Hartl ML: Bone marrow processing with the Haemonetics V50 Plus. In Gee AP (ed): Bone Marrow Processing and Purging: A Practical Guide. Boca Raton, FL, CRC Press, 1991, pp 39–51.

10. Stiff PJ, Koester AR, Weidner MK, et al: Autologous bone marrow transplantation using unfractionated cells cryopreserved in dimethylsulfoxide and hydroxyethyl starch without controlled-rate freezing. Blood 70:974, 1987.

11. Beaujean MF, Gordin MF, Farcet JP, et al: Separation of large quantities of mononuclear cells from human blood using a blood processor. Transfusion 25:152, 1985.

12. English D, Lamderson R, Graves V, et al: Semiautomated processing of bone marrow grafts for transplantation. Transfusion 29:12, 1989.

13. Faradji A, Andreu G, Pillier-Loriette C, et al: Separation of mononuclear bone marrow cells using the Cobe 2997 Blood Cell Processor. Vox Sang 55:133, 1988.

14. DeWitte T, Plas A, Vet J, et al: A simple method to obtain low density marrow cells for human transplantation. Vox Sang 55:221, 1987.

15. Humblet Y, Lefebvre P, Jacques JL, et al: Concentration of bone marrow progenitor cells by separation on a Percoll gradient using the Haemonetics model 30. Bone Marrow Transplant 3:63, 1988.

16. Gilmore MJML, Prentice HG, Blacklock HA, et al: A technique for rapid isolation of bone marrow mononuclear cells using Ficoll-metrizoate and the IBM-2991 blood cell processor. Br J Haematol 50:619, 1982.

17. Law P, Alsop P, Dooley DC, et al: Density gradient isolation of peripheral blood mononuclear cells using a blood cells processor. Transfusion 28:145–150, 1988.

18. Przepiorka D, Van Vlasselaer P, Huynh L, et al: Rapid debulking and CD34 enrichment of filgrastim-mobilized peripheral blood stem cells by semiautomated density gradient centrifugation in a closed system. J Hematother 5:497, 1996.

19. Rubenstein P, Dobrilla L, Rosenfield RE, et al: Processing and cryopreservation of placental/umbilical cord blood for unrelated bone marrow reconstitution. Proc Natl Acad Sci U S A 92:10119, 1995.

20. Lazzari L, Corsini C, Curioni C, et al: The Milan Cord Blood Bank and the Italian Cord Blood Network. J Hematother 5(2):117–122, 1996.

21. Harris DT, Shumacher MJ, Rychlik S, et al: Collection, separation, and cryopreservation of umbilical cord blood for use in transplantation. Bone Marrow Transplant 13:135, 1994.

22. Shpall EJ, Jones RB, Bearman SI, et al: Transplantation of CD34+ hematopoietic progenitor cells. J Hematother 3:145, 1994.

23. Shpall EJ, Jones RB, Bearman SI, et al: Transplantation of enriched CD34-positive autologous marrow into breast cancer patients following high-dose chemotherapy: influence of CD34-positive peripheral-blood progenitors and growth factors on engraftment. J Clin Oncol 12:28, 1994.

24. Kawano Y, Takaue Y, Watanabe A, et al: Partially mismatched pediatric transplants with allogeneic CD34+ blood cells from a related donor. Blood 92:3123, 1998.

25. Kawano Y, Takaue Y, Law P, et al: Clinically applicable bulk isolation of blood CD34+ cells for autografting in children. Bone Marrow Transplant 22(10):1011, 1998.
26. Chabannon C, Cornetta K, Lotz JP, et al: High-dose chemotherapy followed by reinfusion of selected CD34+ peripheral blood cells in patients with poor-prognosis breast cancer: a randomized multicentre study. Br J Cancer 78(7):913, 1998.
27. Socié G, Cayuela JM, Raynal B, et al: Influence of CD34 cell selection on the incidence of mixed chimaerism and minimal residual disease after allogeneic unrelated donor transplantation. Leukemia 12(9):1440, 1998.
28. de Wynter FA, Coutinho LH, Pei X, et al: Comparison of purity and enrichment of CD34+ cells from bone marrow, umbilical cord, and peripheral blood (primed for apheresis) using five separation systems. Stem Cells 13:524, 1995.
29. McNiece I, Briddell R, Stoney G, et al: Large-scale isolation of CD34+ cells using the Amgen cell selection device results in high levels of purity and recovery. J Hematother 6:5, 1997.
30. Stainer CJ, Mifflin G, Anderson S, et al: A comparison of two different systems for CD34+ selection of autologous or allogeneic PBSC collections. J Hematother 7:375, 1998.
31. Björkstrand B, Sundman-Engberg B, Christensson B, Kumlien G: A controlled comparison of two different clinical grade devices for CD34+ cell selection of autologous blood stem cell grafts. J Hemtother 8:75, 1999.
32. McNiece IK, Stoney GB, Kern BP, Briddell RA: CD34+ cell selection from frozen cord blood products using the Isolex-300i and CliniMACS CD34 selection device. J Hematother 7:457, 1998.
33. Zanjani E, Almeida-Porada G, Livingston A, et al: Human bone marrow CD34− cells engraft in vivo and undergo multilineage expression that includes giving rise to CD34+ cells. Exp Hematol 26:353, 1998.
34. Osawa M, Hanada K, Hamada H, et al: Long-term lymphohematopoietic reconstitution by single CD34-low/negative hematopoietic stem cell. Science 273:242, 1996.
35. Goddel M, Brose K, Paradis G, et al: Isolation and functional properties of murine hematopoietic stem cells that are replicating in vitro. J Exp Med 183:1797, 1996.
36. Goodell M, Rosenzweig M, Kim H, et al: Dye efflux studies suggest that hematopoietic stem cells expressing low or undetectable levels of CD34 antigen exist in multiple species. Nature Med 3:1337, 1997.
37. Bhatia M, Bonnet D, Murdoch B, et al: A newly discovered class of human hematopoietic cells with SCID-repopulating activity. Nature Med 4:1038, 1998.
38. Zanjani E, Almeida-Porada G, Livingston A, et al: Long term engrafting capabilities of CD34-negative adult marrow cells. Blood 92(Suppl 1):504a, 1998.
39. Nakauchi H: Hematopoietic stem cells: are they CD34-positive or CD34-negative? Nature Med 4:1009, 1998.
40. Donnelly DS, Zelterman D, Sharkis S, Krause DS: Functional activity of murine CD34+ and CD34− hematopoietic stem cell populations. Exp Hematol 27:788, 1999.
41. Surgrue MW, Hutchinson CE, Fisk DD, et al: The effect of overnight storage of leukapheresis stem cell products on cell viability, recovery, and cost. J Hematother 7:431, 1998.
42. Preti RA, Razis E, Ciavarella D, et al: Clinical and laboratory comparison study of refrigerated and cryopreserved bone marrow for transplantation. Bone Marrow Transplant 13:253, 1994.
43. Pettengell R, Woll PJ, O'Connor DA, et al: Viability of hemapoietic progenitors from whole blood, bone marrow and leukapheresis product: effects of storage media, temperature and time. Bone Marrow Transplant 14:991, 1994.
44. Lane TA, Young D, Mullen M, et al: Effect of storage on engraftment of mobilized peripheral blood cells (PBPC) [Abstract 4229]. Blood 90(Suppl 1):329b, 1997.
45. Jestice HK, Scott MA, Ager S, et al: Liquid storage of peripheral blood progenitor cells for transplantation. Bone Marrow Transplant 14:991, 1994.
46. Hechler G, Weide R, Heymanns J, et al: Storage of noncryopreserved peripheral blood stem cells for transplantation. Ann Hematol 72:303, 1996.
47. Ahmed T, Wuest D, Ciavararella D, et al: Marrow storage techniques: a clinical comparison of refrigerated versus cryopreservation. Acta Haemotol 85:173, 1991.
48. Koppler H, Pfluger KH, Havemann K: Hematopoietic reconstitution after high dose chemotherapy and autologous nonfrozen bone marrow rescue. Ann Hematol 63:253, 1991.
49. Mazur P: Cryobiology: the freezing of biological systems. Science 168:939, 1970.
50. Meryman HT, Williams R: Mechanisms of freezing injury, natural tolerance, and principles of artificial cryoprotection. In Withers LA, Williams JT (eds): Crop Genetics Resources: The Conservation of Difficult Material, Paris, International Union of Biological Sciences Press, 1980, pp 5–37.
51. Meryman HT, Williams RJ, Douglas M: Freezing injury from "solution effects" and its prevention by natural and artificial cryopreservation. Cryobiology 14:287, 1977.
52. Schwartz GJ, Diller KR: Osmotic response of individual cells during freezing: I. Experimental volume measurements. Cryobiology 20:61, 1983.
53. Takahashi T, Inada S, Pommier CG, et al: Osmotic stress and the freeze-thaw cycle cause shedding of Fc and C3b receptors by human polymorphonuclear leukocytes. J Immunol 134:4062, 1985.
54. Mazur P: The role of intracellular freezing in the death of cells cooled at supraoptimal rates. Cryobiology 14:251, 1977.
55. Meryman HT, Hornblower M: A method for freezing and washing red blood cells using a high glycerol concentration. Transfusion 12:145, 1972.
56. Mazur P, Miller RH: Permeability of human erythrocytes to glycerol in 1 and 2 M solutions at 0 or 20°C. Cryobiology 13:507, 1976.
57. Cicoria AD, Hempling HG: Osmotic properties of differentiating bone marrow precursor cells: membrane permeability to non-electrolytes. J Cell Physiol 105(1):129, 1980.
58. Hempling HG, White S: Permeability of cultured megakaryocytopoietic cells of the rat to dimethyl sulfoxide. Cryobiology 21(2):133, 1984.
59. Mazur P, Rall WF, Leibo SP: Kinetics of water loss and the likelihood of intracellular freezing in mouse ova: influence of the method of calculating the temperature dependence of water permeability. Cell Biophys 6(3):197, 1984.
60. Harvey B, Kelley RN, Ashwood-Smith MJ: Permeability of intact and dechorionated zebra fish embryos to glycerol and dimethyl sulfoxide. Cryobiology 20(4):432, 1983.
61. Mironescu S: Hyperosmotic injury in mammalian cells: volume and alkali cation alterations of CHO cells in unprotected and DMSO-treated cultures. Cryobiology 15(2):178, 1978.
62. Leibo SP, Farrant J, Mazur P, et al: Effects of freezing on marrow stem cell suspensions: interactions of cooling and warming rates in the presence of PVP, sucrose or glycerol. Cryobiology 6:315, 1970.
63. Takahashi T, Hirsh A, Erbe E, Williams RJ: Mechanisms of cryoprotection by extracellular polymeric solutes. Biophys J 54:509, 1988.
64. Law P, Meryman HT: Cryopreservation of human bone marrow grafts. In Gee AP (ed): Bone Marrow Processing and Purging: A Practical Guide. Boca Raton, FL, CRC Press, 1991, pp 332–340.
65. Buckner CD, Rudolph RJ, Fejes A, et al: High dose cyclophosphamide therapy for malignant disease: toxicity, tumor response and the effect of stored autologous marrow. Cancer 29:357, 1972.
66. Rowley SD, Bensinger WI, Gooley TA, Buckner CD: Effect of cell concentration on bone marrow and peripheral blood stem cell cryopreservation. Blood 83:2731, 1994.
67. Stiff PJ, Murgo AJ, Zaroulis CG, et al: Unfractionated marrow cell cryopreservation of myeloid stem cells from human bone marrow. Cryobiology 20:17, 1983.
68. Stiff PJ, Dvorak K, Schulz W: A simplified bone marrow cryopreservation method. Blood 72:1102, 1988.
69. Fountain D, Ralston M, Higgins N, et al: Liquid nitrogen freezers: a potential source of microbial contamination of hematopoietic stem cell components. Transfusion 37(6):585, 1997.
70. Tedder RS, Zuckerman MA, Goldstone AH, et al: Hepatitis B transmission from contaminated cryopreservation tank. Lancet 346(8968):137, 1995.
71. Carroll WE, Pinnick HA, Ellis ML: Viruses, skin lesions, and liquid nitrogen [Letter] [see comments]. Lancet 345(8954):929, 1995.
72. Jones SK, Darville JM, Burton JL: Viruses, skin lesions, and liquid nitrogen [Letter; comment]. Lancet 345(8961):1369, 1995.
73. Douay L, Gorin NC, David R, et al: Study of granulocyte-macrophage progenitor (CFUc) preservation after slow freezing of bone marrow in the gas phase of liquid nitrogen. Exp Hematol 10:360, 1982.
74. Gorin NC: Collection: manipulation and freezing of hematopoietic stem cells. Clin Haematol 15:19, 1986.

75. Smith DM, Weisenburger DD, Bierman P, et al: Acute renal failure associated with autologous bone marrow transplantation. Bone Marrow Transplant 2:195, 1987.

76. Davis JM, Rowley SD, Braine HG, et al: Clinical toxicity of cryopreserved bone marrow graft infusion. Blood 70:974, 1987.

77. Stroncek DF, Fautsch SK, Lasky LC, et al: Adverse reactions in patients transfused with cryopreserved marrow. Transfusion 31:521, 1991.

78. Areman EM, Rhodes PL, Mazumder A, Meehan KP: Differential effects of IL-2 incubation of hematopoietic potential of autologous bone marrow and mobilized PBSC from patients with hematological malignancies. J Hemather 8:39, 1999.

79. Meehan KR, Badros A, Frankel SR, et al: A pilot study evaluating interleukin-2-activated hematopoietic stem cell transplantation for hematologic malignancies. J Hematother 6:457, 1997.

80. Areman EM, Mazumder A, Kotula P, et al: Hematopoietic potential of IL-2-cultured peripheral blood stem cells from breast cancer patients. Bone Marrow Transplant 18:521, 1996.

81. Bender JG, To LB, Williams S, et al: Defining a therapeutic dose of peripheral blood stem cells. J Hematother 1:329, 1992.

82. Johnsen HE, Knudsen L: Nordic flow cytometry standards for CD34+ cell enumeration in blood and leukapheresis products: report from the second Nordic Workshop: Nordic Stem Cell Laboratory Group (NSCL-G). J Hematother 5:237, 1996.

83. Sutherland DR: Assessment of peripheral blood stem cell grafts by CD34+ cell enumeration: toward a standardized flow cytometric approach. J Hematother 5:209, 1996.

84. Law P, Traylor L, Recktenwald D: Cell analysis for hematopoietic stem/progenitor cell transplantation. Cytometry 38(2):47, 1999.

85. Bashey A, Lane TA, Mullen M, et al: Value of percentage of CD34 positive cells in leukapheresis product as a predictor of platelet engraftment in autologous transplants. Blood 90(10)(Suppl 1):1997.

86. Gratama JW, Kraan J, Levering W, et al: Analysis of variation results of CD34+ hematopoietic progenitor cell enumeration in a multicenter study. Cytometry 30:109, 1997.

87. Verwer BJH, Ward DM: An automated classification algorithm for ProCOUNT™ flow cytometric acquisition and analysis. J Hematother 6:169, 1997.

88. Terstappen LW, Gandour D, Huang S, et al: Assessment of hematopoietic cell differentiation by multidimensional flow cytometry. J Hematother 2(3):431, 1993.

89. Terstappen LW, Hollander Z, Meiners H, Loken MR: Quantitative comparison of myeloid antigens on five lineages of mature peripheral blood cells. J Leukocyte Biol 48(2):138, 1990.

90. Terstappen LW, Buescher S, Nguyen M, Reading C: Differentiation and maturation of growth factor expanded human hematopoietic progenitors assessed by multidimensional flow cytometry. Leukemia 6(10):1001, 1992.

91. Huang S, Terstappen LW: Lymphoid and myeloid differentiation of single human CD34+, HLA-DR+, CD38− hematopoietic stem cells. Blood 83(6):1515, 1994.

92. Terstappen LW, Huang S: Analysis of bone marrow stem cell. Blood Cells 20(1):45, 1994.

93. Pecora AL, Preti RA, Gleim GW, et al: CD34+CD33− cells influence days to engraftment and transfusion requirements in autologous blood stem-cell recipients. J Clin Oncol 16(6):2093, 1998.

94. Rowley SD, Zuchlsdorf M, Braine HG, et al: CFU-GM content of bone marrow graft correlates with time to hematologic reconstitution following autologous bone marrow transplantation with 4-hydroperoxycyclophosphamide-purged marrow. Blood 70:271, 1987.

95. Janssen WE, Lee C: Transportation of bone marrow for in vitro processing and storage. In Gee AP (ed): Bone Marrow Processing and Purging: A Practical Guide. Boca Raton, FL, CRC Press, 1991, pp 39–51.

96. Strauss LC, Trischmann TM, Rowley SD, et al: Selection of normal human hematopoietic stem cells for bone marrow transplantation using immunomagnetic microspheres and CD34 antibody. Am J Pediatric Hematol Oncol 13:217, 1991.

97. Civin CI, Trischman T, Kadan KS, et al: Highly purified CD34+ cells reconstitute hematopoiesis. J Clin Oncol 14:2224, 1996.

98. Hardwick RA, Kulcinski D, Mansour V, et al: Design of large-scale separation systems for positive and negative immunomagnetic selection of cells using super-paramagnetic microspheres. J Hematother 1:379, 1992.

99. Radbruch A, Mechtold B, Thiel A, et al: High-gradient magnetic cell sorting. Methods Cell Biol 42(Part B):387, 1994.

100. Miltenyi S, Müller W, Weichel W, Radbruch A: High gradient magnetic cell separation with MACS. Cytometry 11:231, 1990.

101. Fraser JK, Cairo MS, Wagner EL, et al: Co Transplantation Study (COBLT): cord blood bank standard operating procedures. J Hematother 6:521, 1998.

102. Schumm M, Lang P, Taylor G, et al: Isolation of highly purified autologous and allogeneic peripheral CD34+ cells using the CliniMACS device. J Hematother 8:200, 1999.

103. Goodell MA: CD34+ or CD34−: Does it really matter? Blood 94:2545, 1999.

104. Sato T, Laver JH, Ogawa M: Reversible expression of CD34 by murine hematopoietic stem cells. Blood 94:2548, 1999.

CHAPTER TWENTY-NINE

Purging of Contaminating Tumor Cells

Davood Vafai, M.D., James J. Vredenburgh, M.D., and Edward D. Ball, M.D.

High-dose chemotherapy with autologous peripheral blood or marrow hematopoietic cell support is an effective therapy for a number of malignancies. Patients with diseases such as acute myeloid leukemia (AML), acute lymphoblastic leukemia (ALL), non-Hodgkin lymphoma (NHL), Hodgkin disease, breast cancer, and multiple myeloma are potential candidates for this treatment. Prolonged disease-free survival (DFS) can be achieved for a substantial portion of patients. A major cause of treatment failure is disease relapse, which can result from resistant residual malignant cells in vivo or the infusion of contaminating tumor cells collected with the hematopoietic stem cells (HSC). In a landmark study, Brenner et al. demonstrated that autologous marrow cells marked with the neomycin-resistant gene from children with leukemia and neuroblastoma can contribute to relapse after autologous transplantation.[1] The marker gene was detected in the blasts of the two patients in relapse. Since then, infused tumor cells have been implicated as contributing to relapse in other diseases.[2-4] Treatment strategies to overcome resistance and eliminate residual malignant cells in vivo are discussed in Chapters 34 and 35. We focus on the incidence of contaminating tumor cells, the prognostic significance of malignant cells in the harvested hematopoietic cells from marrow or peripheral blood progenitor cells (PBPC) products, and techniques to eliminate the contaminating malignant cells.

Clinical results that correlated the level of purging to increased treatment efficacy (in terms of decrease in relapse or increase in DFS) can be interpreted in alternative ways. The marrow or PBPC that remained positive after purging might contain increased numbers of malignant cells as a result of greater tumor bulk. The inability to eliminate all tumor cells in vitro might identify patients with more-resistant disease. Residual tumor cells after purging might represent clonogenic cells capable of growth upon infusion. Although the exact mechanism is not always clear, there are apparent clinical benefits in using purged marrow or PBPC in certain diseases.

HISTORY AND BACKGROUND

The first experimental evidence for purging was reported from the bone marrow transplantation program of the Johns Hopkins Oncology Center in the 1980s. In the study, normal marrow and AML cells, both from rats, were mixed and incubated with graded doses of 4-hydroperoxycyclophosphamide (4-HC). The cell suspensions were then in-

fused into lethally irradiated rats. Only animals receiving cell suspensions incubated with higher doses of 4-HC survived without the appearance of leukemia, indicating that tumor cells were eliminated from marrow cells without completely destroying the pluripotent HSC.[5] In 1982, Krolick et al. reported selective killing of leukemia cells by antibody-toxin conjugates.[6] Results of a phase I study in 1985 showed that hematopoietic engraftment was achieved after infusion of 4-HC–treated autologous marrow in patients with leukemia and lymphoma.[7] One year later, Chang et al. reported a patient with AML receiving autologous marrow after long-term culture which was employed as a method of purging.[8] In a phase II study, Yeager et al. summarized results from 25 patients with AML in second and third remission (CR2 and CR3) who underwent transplantation with marrow purged by 4-HC.[9] Neutrophil and platelet engraftment ($\geq 500/mm^3$ and $50,000/mm^3$, respectively) were attained at median intervals of 29 and 57 days, respectively. Of the 25 patients, 11 remained in remission at a median of over 400 days. After this report, several centers conducted phase II trials using different purging methods. These trials have demonstrated different and at times conflicting results. Information regarding the efficacy of purging in different diseases is reviewed separately.

DETECTION OF MINIMAL RESIDUAL DISEASE

Autologous peripheral blood or marrow HSC support is usually performed when the patient is in complete remission and the marrow is free of malignant cells by histology. Unfortunately, the sensitivity of histologic detection of tumor cells is about 1 in 10^3 cells. A variety of different techniques have been developed to detect and quantify minimal residual disease (Table 29–1).[10-16] The most commonly used technique is immunocytochemistry (ICC). This method is applicable to tumors that can be identified with monoclonal antibodies (mAb) and allows the detection of one malignant cell in 10^5 normal cells from marrow or PBPC. The quality of this technique depends on the reactivity of the mAb with the targeted markers. False-positive results can arise from specific or nonspecific binding of the mAb to normal cells. Counterstaining and microscopic visualization by experienced personnel can eliminate some of these events. False-negative results can occur when the target antigens are altered by prior treatment to the patient or during the staining procedures.

TABLE 29–1. METHODS FOR DETECTING MINIMAL RESIDUAL DISEASES

TABLE 29–1. METHODS FOR DETECTING MINIMAL RESIDUAL DISEASES

METHOD	SENSITIVITY
Morphology	1 in 10^2
Immunocytochemistry	1 in 10^4–10^6
Polymerase chain reaction (DNA or RNA)	1 in 10^5–10^6
Clonogenic assays	1 in 10^4–10^6
Flow cytometry	1 in 10^3–10^4
Southern blot	1 in 10^2
Fluorescence in situ hybridization	1 in 10^2

Flow cytometry has been used for detection of tumor cells.[17–19] Marrow cells or PBPC are stained with fluorochrome-labeled mAb, and the proportions of fluorescent cells are measured together with the light-scattering properties of the cells. The accuracy of this technique depends on the experience of the operator and the quality of the mAb.[20] Automated gating and three- or four-color analysis (in which tumor cells and normal cells are stained with different mAb) have helped to improve the consistency in gating and analysis, leading to higher sensitivity of the procedure. The level of detection depends on the tumor and the mAb, and generally ranges from one tumor cell in 10^4–10^5 cells. The main advantages of flow cytometry are the speed of data acquisition and the number of events (can be $> 10^5$ compared with 10^3–10^4 in immunocytochemistry) collected by the cytometers.

Detection of gene rearrangements can be performed using polymerase chain reaction (PCR) to amplify the specific DNA sequences of disease markers.[21] The procedure is routinely used as a diagnostic tool for AML, chronic myelogenous leukemia, and NHL that contains genetic rearrangements. The method has been applied to detecting residual tumor cells before and after purging (see discussion of NHL). Reverse transcriptase-PCR (RT-PCR) amplifies specific sequences of messenger RNA (mRNA). The mRNA can be transcribed from rearranged DNA sequences or from genes that are normally inactive in nonmalignant cells. The specificity of RT-PCR depends on the availability of primers specific for the target tumor cells.[15, 22] PCR and RT-PCR can detect 1 tumor cell in 10^6 cells. Despite its high sensitivity, the potential for false-positive results is high because counterstaining and visual observation is not possible. The technique is unable to differentiate between viable clonogenic cells and nonviable cells. Quantifying the number of tumor cells in a specimen requires tedious calibration and control.[15, 21, 22]

In vitro culture of clonogenic tumor cells has been reported.[16] The existence of such clones in marrow or PBPC has been correlated with relapse and DFS. The procedure requires long culture duration, typically 14 days or more, and has not gained wide acceptance in clinical practice.

PURGING TECHNIQUES

Table 29–2 summarizes the most common methods of purging malignant cells from marrow or PBPC. Of those, pharmacologic and immunologic procedures are most popular. Each technique has advantages and disadvantages, which are listed in Table 29–3. The efficacy of purging can be evaluated by the same detection methods as mentioned earlier and is expressed as the log reduction of tumor cells in the HSC collections. Changes to the HSC (CD34+ cells, colony-forming units–granulocyte-macrophage [CFU-GM], and burst-forming units—erythroid [BFU-E]) are always measured to evaluate possible damage to the grafts.

PHARMACOLOGIC METHODS

Pharmacologic purging of autografts in patients with AML primarily utilizes metabolites of cyclophosphamide such as 4-HC or mafosfamide.[5, 23, 24] Both agents were more toxic to differentiated myeloid progenitors than to primitive HSC in animals and in humans. 4-HC is primarily used in the United States, mafosfamide primarily in Europe. Pharmacologic methods are relatively easy to perform and are inexpensive, but they are associated with delayed engraftment and the possibility of selecting drug-resistant tumor-cell clones. Toxicity to hematopoietic progenitor cells is the major cause of delayed engraftment. There are also variations in the dose response of tumor cells and CFU-GM among patients and HSC collections.[25, 26] Killing of tumor cells and CFU-GM by 4-HC and mafosfamide is modulated by the presence of aldehyde dehydrogenase in contaminating erythrocytes.[27] Removing erythrocytes and other mature blood cells via density gradient separation produces more-uniform results.[25]

Normal hematopoetic progenitor cells can be protected

TABLE 29–2. TUMOR CELL PURGING TECHNIQUES

1. Pharmacologic
   4-Hydroperoxycyclophosphamide
   Mafosfamide
2. Immunologic
   Negative removal of tumor cells
      Unconjugated monoclonal antibody(ies) + complement
      Unconjugated monoclonal antibody(ies) + paramagnetic microspheres
         Similar antibodies + beads (Dynal or equivalent) coated with secondary antimouse antibody(ies)
      Monoclonal antibody(ies) conjugated to
         Chemotherapeutic agents
         Toxic substance(s) such as ricin-A chain (immunotoxins)
         Paramagnetic beads (Dynal or equivalent)
         Radionuclide
   Positive selection of CD34+ cells
      CellPro: Indirect binding of biotinylated antibody (12.8, IgM), captured by avidin column and release by mechanical disruption
      Nexell: Indirect binding of anti-CD34 antibody (9C5, IgG), captured by paramagnetic beads, and release by competitive displacement
      Miltenyi: Direct binding anti-CD34 antibody (QBend-10, IgG) coated microbeads, captured with high gradient magnetic field, no release
3. Physical separation
   Counter flow elutriation (Size)
   Density gradient centrifugation
4. Cytokine activation of immune effector cells
5. Genetic and molecular manipulation
6. Binding to lectins and/or other synthetic molecules

TABLE 29-3. COMPARISON OF PURGING TECHNIQUES

METHODS	ADVANTAGES	DISADVANTAGES
1. Pharmacologic	1. Relatively inexpensive 2. Standardized procedure(s)	1. Possibility of resistant clones 2. Associated with delayed engraftment 3. Variable tumor sensitivity to agents among patients
2. Antibody- and complement-mediated lysis	1. Simple technique requiring no specialized equipment 2. 2–3 log depletion	1. Dependent on the type of antibody 2. Time-consuming, needing multiple rounds of treatment 3. Evaluation of each complement lot for toxicity and efficacy 4. Possibility of resistant clones
3. Immunomagnetic beads	1. Relatively rapid 2. 5–6 log depletion	1. Expensive (cost of beads) 2. Nonspecific cell loss
4. Immunotoxin	1. Standardized procedure(s) 2. 5–6 log depletion	1. Requirement of internalization of complex 2. Availability of suitable antigens 3. Nonspecific toxicity 4. Development of resistant clones

from the toxic effect of 4-HC or mafosfamide by pretreatment with amifostine (W-2721).[28–30] Originally designed as a protective agent for ionizing radiation,[31, 32] this phosphorylated sulfhydryl compound has been used to protect normal tissues against the toxic side effects of antineoplastic drugs.[33, 34] Early clinical results from pharmacologic purging of marrow pretreated with amifostine showed that the period of delayed engraftment was shortened.[29, 30] Survival and relapse data are not yet available. The combined use of this reagent and pharmacologic purging of PBPC remain to be investigated.

IMMUNOLOGIC METHODS

Murine mAb against tumor cell surface markers have been used for purging.[35–40] Most targeted markers represent differentiation antigens and are present on both normal and malignant cells. A majority of AML blasts expresses at least one of the myeloid antigens CD14, CD15, CD33, or p124. mAb to CD10, CD19, and/or CD20 had been used for purging of lymphoma cells, and mAb to cytokeratine has been used in breast cancer purging. An ideal marker for purging is one that is (1) expressed only on clonogenic tumor cells, sparing the normal HSC, (2) expressed on target cells in high density without heterogeneity, and (3) stable enough for manipulations necessary in the treatment steps. Despite initial enthusiasm, no unique tumor-specific surface marker has been identified, with the exception of the unique idiotype of the surface immunoglobulin expressed by a B cell neoplasm.

mAb are usually not toxic by themselves and need to be combined with other agents to eliminate the target cells. Common techniques include complement-mediated lysis, immunomagnetic beads coated with secondary antibody directed against the murine mAb (e.g., sheep or goat anti-mouse immunoglobulin G [IgG]) together with magnetic field, and linkage to cytotoxic chemicals (immunotoxins). A single cycle of mAb and complement treatment can reduce the tumor burden by 3 logs.[35, 36] Adding more mAb (against different tumor cell markers) can augment this effect (i.e., using three antibodies and complement can remove up to 6 logs of the tumor cells).[39, 40] Multiple cycles of mAb and complement treatment are more efficient than

a single treatment.[41] The advantages of complement are that it is a simple technology requiring no specialty device or machinery and is relatively inexpensive. Disadvantages include the necessity to screen each complement lot for efficacy of lysing and for potential toxicity to normal HSC; the lengthiness of treatment time, because of the multiple cycles of mAb and complement; production of cell lysis debris that can cause nonspecific clumping of nontarget cells; and the fact that not all mAb can fix complement.[39, 42]

Immunomagnetic beads can also be used with mAb for purging. The biologic variability between different complement lots is avoided. Marrow or PBPC products are first sensitized with mAb. After the excess mAb is removed by washing, paramagnetic microspheres coated with anti-mouse antibodies are added. Sensitized target cells are rosetted with the magnetic beads, and the rosettes are then captured using a magnetic field. Tumor cell depletion of 4–6 logs can be achieved.[43, 44] Advantages of the method are no cell lysis debris, the effectiveness of a single treatment cycle, and the relative small loss in the normal HSC.[43] Disadvantages include the expense of clinically approved microspheres, the need for sophisticated magnetic systems or devices for capturing the target cell/bead rosettes, nonspecific cell trapping by the beads, and the infusion of residual beads into patients.

Immunotoxin-based purging technology can also cause 5- to 6-log depletion of the tumor cells. The mAb is typically conjugated to toxins such as ricin-A chain, but other components such as saporin 6 have been used.[6, 45–50] The procedure is relatively simple in that the marrow or PBPC are mixed and incubated with the immunotoxins with no requirement for special equipment. Application of this procedure is limited by the concern for residual ricin toxicity,[48–50] the difficulty in finding appropriate target antigens,[49] and the conjugation of a sufficient quantity of potent toxins to the mAb.[49]

POSITIVE SELECTION

HSC are identified by the CD34 surface marker. The CD34+ stem/progenitor cells can be sensitized using anti-CD34 mAb (with or without biotinylation), captured on solid substrates such as immunomagnetic beads or avidin-coated column, and released using specific and nonspecific means (see Chapters 28 and 30). Selection of CD34+ cells can decrease tumor-cell contamination by 2–3 logs.[42, 51]

POSITIVE-NEGATIVE SELECTION

The hematopoietic stem/progenitor cells are first selected using the CD34 marker, and the enriched cell suspension is further depleted of tumor cells by an immunologic procedure using mAb directed against tumor markers.[52, 53] This technique can eliminate tumor cells by more than 5 logs. Positive-negative selection has been used in diseases such as lymphoma, myeloma, breast cancer, and AML. Reasons for the combined positive-negative approach include reduction of purging cell volume, especially for PBPC collections, leading to smaller consumption of antibodies[52]; no cross-reactivity between solid tumor markers and the CD34+ cells, leading to higher power of tumor-cell reduction[53]; and release reagent specifically designed for CD34+ cells, leading to the possibility of combining both procedures into a single step.[54]

RESULTS OF CLINICAL TRIALS

ACUTE MYELOGENOUS LEUKEMIA

Several clinical trials with pharmacologic agents and mAb have been performed. Most studies are phase I or phase II nonrandomized trials. Miller et al. reported 295 patients who received autologous 4-HC–purged or –unpurged bone marrow.[55, 56] Patients underwent transplantation within 6 months of achieving CR1 or CR2. Results showed that 4-HC purging decreased late treatment failures without increasing early mortality. The relative risk of relapse for patients receiving purged autologous marrow after 12 months is 0.37 versus those receiving unpurged cells (P = .007).[55, 56]

Sixty-nine patients underwent transplantation while in CR1 with autologous marrow purged with mafosfamide at one of 34 centers in the European Bone Marrow Transplant (EBMT) group.[57] For patients with standard risk using a conditioning regimen based on total body irradiation (TBI), the leukemia-free survival rate was higher (63% vs. 34%, P = .05) and the probability of relapse was lower in recipients of purged than unpurged marrow (23% vs. 55%; relative risk = 0.34, $P \le$ .05). Patients who underwent transplantation within 6 months of achieving CR benefited the most from purging. The investigators concluded that marrow purging with mafosfamide can be valuable for patients receiving autografts in CR1.

Chao et al. reported a retrospective single-center study using 4-HC–purged marrow in patients receiving busulfan and etoposide.[58] Results were compared with historical controls who received the same conditioning regimen but nonpurged marrow.[58] Patients underwent transplantation while in CR1 (34 patients), in CR2 (12 patients), or in relapse (4 patients). Neutrophil and platelet engraftment for patients infused with unpurged marrow occurred at 23

days (absolute neutrophil count [ANC] $\ge$ 500/mm³) and 56 days (platelet count $\ge$ 20,000/mm³), versus 31 days and 73 days, respectively, for those infused with purged marrow. Follow-up of survivors ranged from 6 to 66 months (median, 31 months). Patients receiving purged marrow experienced an actuarial DFS of 57% with a relapse rate of 28% compared with 32% and 62%, respectively, for patients receiving unpurged marrow.[58]

Ball et al. reported results of purging in different prognostic categories.[35, 52, 59, 60] Between August 1984 and February 1995, 131 patients underwent autologous bone marrow transplantation using antibody + complement purging: 108 patients were in complete remission (CR1: 24, CR 2/3: 84) and 23 patients were in first relapse (R1). Marrow was purged with two mAb (PM-81 for CD15 and AML-2-23 for CD14) and complement. Conditioning regimens included busulfan/cyclophosphamide, cyclophosphamide/TBI, and busulfan/etoposide (VP-16). Median 2-year survival for patients undergoing transplantation in CR1 was 71% with CY/TBI and 58% with BU/VP-16. In patients in CR2/3, the median survival with BU/CY was 50% and 33% with CY/TBI. For patients in R1 who received BU/CY, survival was 37%. Patients in CR2/3 or R1 were examined for the possible effect of cytogenetic subgroup, history of extramedullary disease, history of myelodysplastic syndrome, or therapy-related AML for impact on survival, and no statistically significant correlation between any of the parameters to DFS or overall survival was identified. Results of other trials are summarized in Table 29–4.

In summary, DFS for patients with AML who received purged marrow varies between 41% and 61% (see Table 29–4). Engraftment appeared to be similar among those receiving purged versus unpurged marrow except for pharmacologic purging. Single-center and multicenter studies have reported improvement of DFS and decrease of relapse rates, although a randomized trial has not been performed. It is interesting that the DFS reported with unpurged marrow varies from 35% to 51% and from 35% to 42% with unpurged PBPC, which overlaps substantially with the values for those receiving purged grafts.[24] It is possible that PBPC have fewer contaminating tumor cells in AML than with other malignancies.[16, 64, 65] Given the increased use of PBPC to replace marrow in autologous transplantation, the efficacy of purging should be evaluated independently.

NON-HODGKIN LYMPHOMA

Gribben et al. demonstrated that the level of purging of translocation t(14;18) containing lymphoma cells from marrow correlates with DFS.[36] In this study, 114 patients with B-cell lymphoma received autologous marrow after mAb + complement purging using three mAb. Three-log to 6-log reduction of tumor cells was achieved after purging, and no residual lymphoma cells could be detected in the marrow of 57 patients using PCR for t(14;18). Only 4 of 57 patients (7%) whose marrow became PCR-negative experienced relapse compared with 26 of 57 patients (46%) receiving PCR-positive marrow.

Horning et al. performed transplantation in 37 patients with advanced-stage follicular lymphoma who were in CR or PR with marrow purged by mAb and complement.[66]

TABLE 29–4. AML: PURGED BONE MARROW TRIALS

INVESTIGATORS	NO. OF PATIENTS	MEDIAN AGE (YR)	DISEASE STATUS	CONDITIONING REGIMEN	RELAPSE RATE (%)	DFS (%)	COMMENTS
Yeager et al.[9]	48	25	CR2, CR3	BU/CY	49	41	4-HC, patients with poor prognosis
Linker et al.[61]	50	Up to 60	CR1	BU/VP-16	27	70	4-HC
	25		CR2, CR3	BU/VP-16	35	52	4-HC
Chao et al.[58]	20	40	CR1, CR2, CR3, R	BU/VP-16	62	32	Unpurged marrow
	28		CR1, CR2, CR3, R		28	57	4-HC purged marrow
Körbling et al.[62]	22	35	CR1	CY/TBI	36	61	Mafosfamide
Selvaggi et al.[59]	56	36	CR2, CR3, R	CY/TBI	58	21	mAb + C'
			CR2, CR3, R	BU/CY	39	48	mAb + C'
Cassileth et al.[63]	35	36	CR1	BU/CY	33	54	4-HC
Laporte et al.[23]	60	33	CR1	CY/TBI	25	58	Mafosfamide
	24		CR2	CY/TBI	48	34	Mafosfamide

CR, complete remission; R, relapse, BU, busulfan; CY, cyclophosphamide; 4-HC, 4-hydroperoxycyclophosphamide; TBI, total body irradiation; mAb + C', monoclonal antibody + complement; VP-16, etoposide.

The conditioning regimen consisted of fractionated TBI, etoposide, and cyclophosphamide. With median follow-up of 4.5 years, the actuarial survival rate at 5 years was 87% and the progression-free survival (PFS) rate was 73%. PCR measurement for t(14;18) was performed in 25 patients, 15 of whom achieved PCR-negative status after purging. One of three patients receiving PCR-positive marrow experienced relapse compared with 5 of 22 patients receiving PCR-negative marrow.

In a study by Freedman et al., 83 untreated patients with advanced follicular lymphoma received six to eight cycles of induction CHOP (cyclophosphamide, hydroxydaunomycin, Oncovin, prednisone) therapy. Their bone marrow was purged with mAb (CD10 and CD20) and complement.[67] The initial CR rate after CHOP was 36% compared with 70% reported in other studies,[68] indicating that the patient population was skewed toward poor prognostic features. Marrow after purging was evaluated for tumor contamination using PCR for bcl-2: 77 patients underwent bone marrow harvest, and 71 were PCR-positive. After purging, grafts from 30 patients (43%) became PCR-negative. Among the 30 patients, 5 experienced relapse after autologous transplantation compared with 21 relapses among the 40 patients who received PCR-positive marrow. The 3-year freedom-from-relapse rate for the PCR-negative patients is 88% compared with 51% for those receiving PCR-positive grafts. It should be noted that median time for PFS in patients receiving conventional treatment is 2 years.[68] The study showed that patients receiving marrow without PCR-detectable lymphoma cells remain in clinical and molecular CR much longer than patients whose marrow remains PCR-positive, and that such treatment compares favorably to conventional treatment.

In 1997, Freedman et al. published the updated results of 153 patients who received purged marrow in CR2 or higher using the same mAb and complement purging from their previous report. Seventy percent of patients were alive at a median time of 12 years after diagnosis, which is superior to the median survival time of 10–12 years for patients receiving conventional therapy or for the matched controls of those receiving unpurged marrow.[69]

High-grade lymphoma, such as Burkitt and lymphoblastic lymphoma, often involves the bone marrow. Improving the result of autologous transplantation with purging may be important in these patients. Currently, few studies have been reported, and the number of enrolled patients is small, yielding no conclusion on the efficacy of purging.[70, 71]

Purging of bone marrow in NHL has been evaluated by the EBMT Lymphoma Registry.[72] By July 1, 1994, results from 1726 patients receiving autologous bone marrow transplantation were reported to the registry. Of these, 270 received marrow purged with different techniques such as 4-HC or mafosfamide, mAb and complement, and selection for CD34+ cells. Complete information from 224 patients was submitted to EBMT and was matched with information from 224 patients who received unpurged marrow within the European registry. All histologic data, including low-grade, intermediate-grade, and high-grade lymphomas (Burkitt, lymphoblastic, and others), were included. Patients were evaluated according to stage at diagnosis (stage I/II vs. III/IV), marrow involvement at diagnosis and transplantation, disease status at transplantation (CR1 vs. CR2/3, primary refractory, sensitive relapse vs. resistant relapse, untreated relapse), and conditioning regimens (chemotherapy vs. TBI-based). No difference in PFS was found between the purged and the unpurged groups. The 5-year survival rate in the purged group was 44.3% compared with 44.6% in the unpurged group. Even in patients with marrow involvement, in whom a potential benefit was likely, the data from the purged versus the unpurged group revealed no difference: 17.3% of patients with previous marrow involvement in the purged group experienced relapse compared with 18.3% in the unpurged group. Patients with low-grade lymphoma appeared to derive some benefit from purging. Although PFS was not different, the overall 5-year survival rate in 50 purged patients was 83.9% compared with 47.6% in the 50 unpurged patients. Increased use of TBI in the unpurged patients might have contributed to this observation. Other causes could include experience among bone marrow transplant centers: 42 of the purged patients were treated in centers that had transplanted more than 10 low-grade lymphoma transplantation patients previously, as compared to 12 in the unpurged patient group.

In summary, there is some evidence that purging may be beneficial in low-grade lymphoma, especially during CR. Analysis by the EBMT and single-center studies showed that the overall 5-year survival rate in patients receiving purged marrow in CR1 was 80–85%. Most published reports had a median follow-up of 4–5 years, but a longer time is needed to confirm the efficacy because by nature low-grade lymphoma have an indolent course. One interesting summary is that DFS in these patients receiving purged or unpurged marrow in CR1 has increased significantly with time. It is possible that the level of purging may be used as a prognostic marker such that patients whose marrow can be purged to PCR-negative status may have biologically different tumor cells than otherwise, such that the disease is more chemotherapy-responsive, leading to lower tumor burden after treatment. The DFS rate in patients with relapsed low-grade lymphoma who have received purged marrow in CR2 or higher varies but is comparable to the DFS for those receiving unpurged marrow; still, there might an advantage in overall survival with purging.[73]

ACUTE LYMPHOBLASTIC LEUKEMIA

Simonsson et al. performed transplantation in 54 adult patients (21 in CR1, 29 in CR2, 3 in CR3, and 1 in relapse) with marrow purged with mAb and complement.[37] Safety of the purged marrow was not compromised because neutrophil and platelet engraftment (ANC $\geq$ 500/mm^3 and platelet count $\geq$ 50,000/mm^3) was 24 and 40 days, respectively. Six of 21 patients in CR1 experienced relapse and the actuarial DFS rate was 65% (median follow-up, 16 months). Eighteen of 32 patients in CR2/3 experienced relapse, and the DFS rate was 31%.

Doney et al. reported results from 89 patients receiving marrow purged by immunologic or pharmacologic (4-HC) techniques.[74] Ten patients were in CR1, 52 in CR2 or greater, and 27 in relapse. Median age was 18.4 years. The DFS rate at 1 year was 50% for patients in CR1, 27% for patients in CR2 or greater, and 8% for patients in relapse. Neutrophil and platelet engraftment ranged from 19 to 24 days and from 27 to 35 days, respectively. Some patients received post-transplantation immunotherapy with interferon ($n = 10$), interleukin-1 ($n = 2$), or GM-CSF ($n = 6$). Factors associated with improved survival were transplantation in CR1 and self-sustained platelet count of more than 20,000/mm^3 in a short period of time. The use of post-transplantation immunotherapy made it difficult to compare these results with other studies.

Soiffer et al. performed transplantation in 22 patients (median age 28 years) with B-lineage disease using marrow purged with mAb (CD10 and CD19) and complement.[75] Five of 22 patients were alive and disease-free at a median of 6.5 years (range, 2.5–7.5), and the estimated DFS rate for all patients was 20%. For the evaluable patients, the 5 younger ones (<28 years old) had an estimated DFS rate of 45%; in sharp contrast, none of the older 12 patients (>28 years old) survived. The result compared favorably

with allogeneic transplantation in a similar group of patients.

Blaise et al. treated 47 high-risk patients with autologous or allogeneic marrow.[76] The autografts were purged with immunologic and pharmacologic methods. Eight patients were younger than 15 years old, an arbitrary analysis parameter chosen by the investigators. There was no difference in engraftment between autografts and allografts. The probability of relapse was 9% for patients who had received allografts and 52% for autografts (P <.01). The DFS rate was 71% for allogeneic transplants and 40% for autologous transplants (statistical significance was not provided).

Poweles et al. reported the result of autologous transplantation in 50 adult patients in CR1.[77] Only 7 patients received purged marrow, and 12 patients received unpurged PBPC. All patients received weekly maintenance chemotherapy with methotrexate and 6-mercaptopurine after hematologic recovery. The actuarial 5-year overall survival rate was 56.2%. The authors concluded that maintenance chemotherapy after autologous transplantation reduces the relapse rate. Evaluation of purging efficacy is complicated by maintenance therapy.

Gilmore et al. performed transplantation in 27 adults in CR1 using marrow purged with mAb and complement.[78] Retrospective analysis of 19 purged grafts by immunophenotyping and immunoglobulin gene rearrangement demonstrated no evidence of tumor cells. The actuarial DFS rate was 32%, and the primary cause of treatment failure was disease recurrence. Purging appeared to have no effect on treatment outcome.

In summary, the results of purging in ALL appeared more variable than in AML or NHL because the studies included children and adults, making interpretation of results difficult (treatment responses of pediatric and adult ALL are different). The use of different forms of post-transplantation therapy applied to both purged and unpurged marrow also contributed to the difficulties in interpretation.

NEUROBLASTOMA

Tumor-cell infiltration in marrow can be as high as 86% in stage 4 disease. Typically, patients initially receive three to four cycles of induction therapy to reduce the tumor bulk in the marrow. The rate of tumor cell contaminating marrow dropped to 35%.[79] Evidence suggests the potential efficacy for purging. Some patients who received unpurged marrow experienced diffuse lung infiltration, possibly from tumor embolization.[80, 81] A study using neomycin resistance gene transduction of autologous marrow showed that tumor cells found at relapse carried the molecular marker.[1, 80, 82]

Evidence against the utility of purging relies on the fact that most patients experience relapse in the areas of previous disease.[83] Matthay et al. argued that aggressive early surgery, more-effective conditioning regimens, and post-transplantation therapy could have a stronger impact on the overall survival of these patients compared with purging.[84]

Garaventa et al. reported the results of a large cooperative experience with 135 children with metastatic disease.[38] Unpurged marrow was given to 117 patients; others received unpurged autologous PBPC ($n = 13$) or allogeneic marrow ($n = 5$). The 8-year DFS rate was 34.6% for patients undergoing transplantation in CR1, 36.4% for patients in CR2 or higher, 23.6% for patients in PR1, and 8% for patients experiencing progression or with advanced disease. The result is comparable to those reported from the International Bone Marrow Transplant Registry (IBMTR), EBMT, Children's Cancer Group (CCG), and Pediatric Oncology Group (POG).[85] The probability of 2-year survival in all patients (including purged and unpurged) is 39 ± 7%.[38] The DFS rate at 2 years and 4–5 years in 500 patients enrolled by the EBMT was 52% and 29%, respectively for purged and unpurged marrow. The CCG and POG used only purged marrow, and the DFS rate at 2 years was 51% and 40%, respectively, and at 4–5 years, 40% and 32%, respectively.[85]

In summary, there is substantial overlap in DFS between autologous transplantation using purged and unpurged marrow. Given the facts that purging did not adversely affect the course or post-transplantation recovery and that genetically marked tumor cells were detected at relapse, most transplant centers have continued to employ purged marrow grafts for patients with neuroblastoma.

BREAST CANCER

Given the current controversy surrounding autologous transplantation for patients with breast cancer (see Chapter 10), a more-detailed discussion on this subject will be provided.

Tumor-Cell Contamination

Malignant cells contaminating the marrow at the time of the initial diagnosis are not uncommon.[86–89] The presence of marrow tumor cells portends a higher likelihood of relapse and a decreased survival.[86, 87] In the largest series, Diel et al. found that the presence of marrow micrometastatic disease is a more important determinant of survival than axillary lymph node involvement.[86] The bone marrow microenvironment is a likely sanctuary for metastatic breast carcinoma. Using predominately ICC techniques, 30–100% of women with metastatic breast cancer were found to have malignant cells in marrow.[90–93] The incidence of marrow micrometastases is higher in women with bone metastases compared with other foci.[90]

Even after aggressive induction chemotherapy, many patients treated with high-dose chemotherapy and HSC support have residual tumor cells in the marrow or PBPC.[94–96] Table 29–5 summarizes a number of studies that examined the incidence of tumor-cell contamination in marrow or PBPC and possible correlation with survival. Although it is unclear whether the breast cancer cell contamination of PBPC had any bearing on post-transplantation survival, most studies show that PBPC contain fewer tumor cells than marrow does. Utilizing a sensitive ICC assay, Vredenburgh et al. showed that of 57 patients who received high-dose chemotherapy with HSC support for high-risk primary breast carcinoma, tumor cells were detected in only two (4%).[64] Statistical correlation to survival was not possible. In a large series from a number of centers, Moss et al. reported that tumor cells in the PBPC were predictive of decreased survival.[95] In a later publication, however, Cooper et al. found that patients receiving PBPC contaminated with occult tumor cells experienced a similar survival rate and time to progression as did those whose PBPC were not contaminated.[97] At least one report showed that the regimen for mobilization might influence tumor-cell contamination in PBPC products.[98]

It is clear from Table 29–5 that when marrow is the source of autologous HSC, contamination by breast cancer cells is predictive of a worse outcome. Vredenburgh et al. reported on a phase II study of high-dose chemotherapy with HSC support for patients with 10 or more positive axillary lymph nodes at the time of initial diagnosis.[99] The patients received four cycles of CAF (cyclophosphamide-Adriamycin-fluorouracil) induction followed by marrow harvest after either the third or the fourth cycle. Two thirds of the patients also received cytokine-primed PBPC. The presence of tumor cells in the harvested marrow and PBPC was detected by ICC in 31 of 83 patients (37%). Those 31 patients experienced a decreased survival compared with patients whose tumor cells were not detected. In addition, multivariate analysis showed that the number of tumor cells was also statistically associated with decreased survival. Survival is similarly decreased in patients with metastatic disease receiving high-dose chemotherapy and HSC support if the marrow is contaminated with tumor cells.[100] Patients with multiple bone metastases tend to experience a higher incidence of contamination in the marrow grafts. Over 90% of cases of metastatic breast cancer and contaminated marrow recurred within 2 years of autologous transplantation.[100]

TABLE 29–5. DETECTION OF BREAST CANCER IN MARROW OR PBPC COLLECTION: POSSIBLE CORRELATION WITH SURVIVAL IN AUTOLOGOUS TRANSPLANTATION

INVESTIGATORS	N	STAGING	% MARROW POSITIVE	% PBPC POSITIVE	CORRELATION WITH SURVIVAL
Ross et al.[113]	48	II-IV	66.7	19	NS
Shpall et al.[105]	44	IV	34	50	NS
Umiel et al.[114]	144	II/III	18	NA	$P < .001$
Vredenburgh et al.[99]	85	II	36	4	$P < .04$
Vredenburgh et al.[100]	147	IV	80	28	NS
Moss et al.[95]	130	IV	NA	29	$P < .001$

NA, not available; NS, not significant.

With PBPC, it is less clear whether occult tumor cells negatively affect relapse rate and/or DFS. It is equally unclear whether the malignant cells in marrow or PBPC are responsible for relapse or just a marker of tumor burden or resistance to chemotherapy.

Different Purging Technologies

Pharmacologic

4-HC has been the most commonly used agent. A laboratory study showed that 1–2 logs of tumor cell purging can be achieved with acceptable loss of CFU-GM.[71] In a phase I/II clinical study for patients with metastatic disease, Shpall et al. found that increasing the purging dose of 4-HC led to delayed neutrophil and platelet engraftment,[25] as shown in Table 29–6. 4-HC purging was performed on marrow mononuclear cells after density gradient separation (see Chapter 28). Conditioning regimen consisted of cyclophosphamide, cisplatin, and carmustine (BCNU). With a minimum of 10 years' follow-up, 2 of the 27 patients were alive and progression-free. Administration of G-CSF immediately after infusion marrow purged with 4-HC had shortened the time to neutrophil engraftment, leading to a decreased number of febrile days, but did not alter platelet recovery.[101] Other growth factors had been used with a similar effect.[102] Kennedy et al. treated buffy coat preparations from marrow with 4-HC (at 100 $\mu g/mm^3$, because of presence of red blood cells—see earlier) for 30 patients.[26] Cyclophosphamide and thiotepa were used for conditioning. With a median follow-up of 27 months, 4 of 30 patients (13%) were alive and progression-free. The 3-year DFS rate for similar patients treated with the same regimen by unpurged marrow was 10–15%.[26] Because both studies were not randomized trials, the contribution of 4-HC purging could not be evaluated. Currently, 4-HC is not under any clinical trials for FDA approval. The lack of availability of the drug and the delayed engraftment make a randomized study for breast cancer unlikely.

Immunologic

A number of mAb have been developed that react to breast cancer tumor cells but not to normal HSC. The procedure of mAb + complement was not successful because the tumor cells were relatively resistant to lysis. Laboratory results, however, showed that immunomagnetic procedures could remove 4–5 logs of breast cancer cells from the bone

TABLE 29–6. DOSE OF 4-HC ON ENGRAFTMENT OF PATIENTS WITH BREAST CANCER RECEIVING PURGED MARROW

4-HC ($\mu g/mL$)	NO. OF PATIENTS	ANC ≥500 (DAYS)	PLATELETS >20,000 (DAYS)
20	4	17	22
40	4	20	21
60	8	19	25
80	9	28	33

4-HC, 4-hydroperoxycyclophosphamide; ANC, absolute neutrophil count.

TABLE 29–7. MONOCLONAL ANTIBODIES REACTIVE WITH BREAST CANCER CELLS

IDENTIFICATION	REACTIVE EPITOPE
113F1	73-kDa glycoprotein
260F9	58-kDa glycoprotein
317G5	42-kDa glycoprotein
520C9	185-kDa glycoprotein (Her-2-neu receptor)
2G3	High-molecular-weight mucin

marrow or PBPC.[39, 40] In a trial enrolling 13 patients with metastatic disease, Vredenburgh et al. used a panel of five mAb (Table 29–7) for immunomagnetic purging of marrow; neutrophil and platelet engraftment were similar to historical controls.[103]

PBPC offers the advantage of early engraftment, but the quantity of cells to be treated in purging is 1–2 logs more than that in a marrow graft. Nevertheless, immunomagnetic purging was performed by Tyer et al. in PBPC collections.[40] Only three of the original five mAb were used (260F9, 317G5, and 520C9—see Table 29–7) because laboratory study results showed that the new combination was as effective as the original panel.[40] Twenty-three patients underwent transplantation with purged PBPC using a conditioning regimen of cyclophosphamide, cisplatin, and BCNU. Kinetics of neutrophil and platelet engraftment was similar to those in historical control patients receiving unpurged PBPC. ICC determination showed that 6 of 23 had tumor cells in PBPC but none after purging.[40]

Combined Pharmacologic and Immunologic Purging

Clinical results for transplanting purged marrow or PBPC do not reveal a satisfactory outcome, as discussed earlier. Because pharmacologic and immunologic methods use different mechanisms for eliminating tumor cells, it is likely that a combination may provide more depletion than either technique alone. Laboratory experiments have confirmed the possibility.[104] In a phase I study wherein marrow was first treated with 4-HC before additional purging with immunomagnetic procedures, engraftment was markedly delayed (ANC ≥ 500/mm³ on day 38, platelet count ≥ 20,000/mm³ on day 50), with kinetics similar to those reported with 4-HC purging alone.[40] As summarized in Table 29–8, subsequent patients were given IL-3, GM-CSF, or both; a slight improvement in ANC engraftment was achieved, but platelet engraftment was still delayed. The DFS rate and relapse rate have not been reported.

Selection of CD34+ Cells

Breast cancer cells do not express the surface CD34 marker found on the primitive and committed hematopoietic stem/progenitor cells.[105, 106] Enrichment for the CD34+ cells can be used for passive purging. In experiments wherein breast cancer cells were spiked into marrow or PBPC, selection of CD34+ cells removed 1.5–4.0 logs of tumor cells and the final product contained 60–90% CD34+ cells with a yield of cells of 40–80%.[102] Although the CellPro system using biotinylated antibody and avidin column was the first sys-

TABLE 29–8. ENGRAFTMENT IN PATIENTS WITH ADVANCED METASTATIC BREAST CANCER TREATED WITH HIGH-DOSE CHEMOTHERAPY AND MARROW PURGED WITH COMBINED 4-HC AND IMMUNOMAGNETIC PURGING

GROUP	NO. OF PATIENTS	CYTOKINE	ANC ≥500 (DAYS)	PLATELET COUNT ≥20,000 (DAYS)
Control	9	None	36	38
1	11	IL-3	27	31
2	8	GM-CSF	28	40
3	12	IL-3 + GM-CSF	24	52

ANC, absolute neutrophil count; GM-CSF, granulocyte-macrophage colony-stimulating factor; IL-3, interleukin-3; 4-HC, 4-hydroperoxycyclophosphamide.

tem to be approved for clinical application, comparison experiments showed that the purity and recovery of CD34+ cells, and hence the level of purging, was inferior to that achieved with other, newer systems (see Chapter 28).[106]

Shpall et al. conducted a phase II trial of high-dose chemotherapy and transplantation of CD34+ cells enriched using the CellPro system.[105] A total of 44 patients was enrolled. The first cohort was supported with CD34+ marrow cells, the second with CD34+ cells from bone marrow and PBPC, and the third with CD34+ PBPC. Except for the first 7 patients, GM-CSF or G-CSF was administered after transplantation. Engraftment kinetics of the three cohorts is shown in Table 29–9 and were not different from those in similar patients receiving unmanipulated marrow or PBPC. Tumor-cell contamination was determined by ICC in 54 marrow or PBPC products (some patients received both marrow and PBPC) before and after enrichment and was reduced by over 2 logs.

Sixty-seven women with metastatic breast cancer and positive bone marrow biopsies or more than 3 bone metastases underwent transplantation by Vredenburgh et al.[102] PBPC were collected after mobilization with G-CSF or cyclophosphamide plus docetaxel followed by G-CSF. CD34+ cells were enriched with the Nexell ISOLEX system. According to a sensitive two-color immunofluores-

TABLE 29–9. ENGRAFTMENT IN PATIENTS WITH BREAST CANCER RECEIVING HIGH-DOSE CHEMOTHERAPY AND ENRICHED CD34+ CELLS

COHORT	N	SOURCE OF STEM CELLS/CYTOKINE SUPPORT	ANC ≥500 (DAYS)	PLATELET COUNT >20,000 (DAYS)
1	7	Bone marrow/no cytokine	22	22
	11	Bone marrow/G-CSF	11	20
	8	Bone marrow/GM-CSF	17	33
2	11	Bone marrow + PBPC/GM-CSF	11	14
3	7	PBPC alone/G-CSF	11	17

ANC, absolute neutrophil count; G-CSF, granulocyte colony-stimulating factor; GM-CSF, granulocyte-macrophage colony-stimulating factor; PBPC, peripheral blood progenitor cell.

cence technique, 13 of the patients had tumor cells in PBPC before selection and only 1 after selection. All patients experienced rapid engraftment.

Combining positive selection and negative purging was studied in the laboratory setting.[53] Especially with the Nexell immunomagnetic procedure in which CD34+ cells are released by a competitive displacement reagent specific for the antibody, it may be possible to combine both procedures into a single step.[54] Initial laboratory results have appeared promising.

Other Methods

Soybean agglutinin has been used for T-cell depletion (see Chapter 30). Ben-Yosef et al. attempted to purge breast cancer cells from 13 patients (with high-risk and metastatic diseases) before infusion of autologous cells.[107] Compared with 35 similar patients receiving unpurged products, engraftment was significantly delayed and no advantage in DFS, overall survival, or relapse rate was found. The authors concluded that soybean agglutination is not an effective method for purging in breast cancer.

IL-2 had been used to activate lymphocytes into tumor killing cells.[108, 109] It is possible to incubate marrow or PBPC directly in IL-2 to promote in vitro activation of lymphocytes to kill breast cancer cells without toxicity to the hematopoietic progenitors[109] or to preactivate lymphocytes from peripheral blood in vitro before mixing with marrow or PBPC.[108] Clinical trials are currently underway (see Chapter 31).

Long-term marrow culture had been used for purging in AML.[8] The procedure has been incorporated into an automated clinical device (see Chapter 32). When marrow mononuclear cells harvested from patients with breast cancer—cells that were intended for transplantation but not used clinically—were thawed and cultured, complete removal of tumor cells was detected in 7 of 10 samples and the level of contamination was reduced in the other 3.[110] The possibility of clinical trials was suggested.

In 1999, a replication deficient adenovirus containing the tumor suppressing p53 gene was developed.[111] Experiments incubating PBPC spiked with tumor cells and the construct showed that complete removal of malignant cells could be achieved. Other approaches to gene-mediated purging are possible. Chen et al. showed that integrin-mediated update of a replication-defective adenoviral vector in breast cancer cells was five orders of magnitude stronger than that from blood, marrow, or CD34+ cells.[112] This difference in transduction could be exploited for selective killing of tumor cells using vectors containing the HSV-tk gene and incubation with ganciclovir in a purging procedure.

Summary

Breast cancer cells can be effectively removed from marrow or PBPC using a variety of techniques of positive selection or purging. Although delayed engraftment is associated with pharmacologic procedures, immunologically purged grafts provided comparable engraftment when compared with unmanipulated products. Survival and relapse rates were similar in patients receiving purged versus unpurged products in early studies; however, improved techniques of tumor cell detection combined with the latest purging and/or positive selection methods, leading to accurate assessment of higher levels of tumor cell reduction, may provide clinical benefits not achievable by the earlier studies. In view of the poor outcome of patients with breast cancer and the controversies surrounding the application of autologous transplantation in this disease, randomized trials of purging versus no purging are sorely needed.

CONCLUSION

A variety of techniques have been developed for removing tumor cells from marrow and PBPC. The levels of tumor cell reduction have ranged from 1–5 logs using different methods for detection. Results from clinical trials using autologous purged marrow and/or PBPC showed that pharmacologic procedures using 4-HC or mafosfamide led to delayed engraftment because of damage to committed progenitor cells, although administration of cytokine(s) after transplantation had shortened the duration for neutropenia. Protective agent(s) may be added to the procedure without compromising tumor-cell killing by the cytotoxic agents.

The actual clinical benefit of purging is unclear. Some centers have demonstrated advantages in DFS and relapse rates in patients undergoing transplantation with purged marrow. Other studies, however, have sometimes shown comparable DFS rates in similar patient populations using unpurged marrow. Comparisons and interpretations of results are complicated by differences in patient selection criteria, disease status at transplantation, prior treatment history, purging procedures, and conditioning regimens. Registry data (EBMT and ABMTR) have suggested that purging may be beneficial in selected patients (e.g., neuroblastoma, low-grade lymphoma in CR, and AML in remission).

Most clinical data on purging were obtained using marrow for autografting. PBPC typically contain more cells (10-fold to 100-fold) than marrow and are collected on multiple days, thus adding logistical hurdles to the purging procedure. PBPC can be stored overnight and pooled with subsequent collections before processing. The purging procedure has to be modified from that used for marrow to account for the increased cell number and differences in components (e.g., the level of red blood cell contamination). The level of tumor-cell contamination in PBPC is reported to be lower than that of marrow for most diseases. Given the relative lack of data with purged PBPC, the necessity of purging PBPC is unknown.

Multicenter randomized trials comparing purged and nonpurged marrow or PBPC are not likely any time soon. Despite the need for conclusive clinical data, the number of patients and the cost of such a trial in any disease is prohibitive. The expected differences in DFS rate and relapse rate are relatively small (~10–20%), though clinically significant. Patients on each arm of a particular disease study must be stratified to address a multitude of related questions (e.g., age, disease status, prior treatments). Because long follow-up (5–10 years) is necessary before the randomized trials would be considered intrepretable, new

and improved therapies might render the test modalities less relevant, even if improved outcome benefits can be confirmed.

Despite the conflicting results in DFS and overall survival in patients receiving purged cells, it is possible that purging can be used as a prognostic factor for autologous transplantation. Many studies suggest that the absence of tumor cells after purging correlates with the incidence of relapse. For patients whose marrow or PBPC cannot be completely purged of cancer cells, post-transplantation therapy may be initiated early to prevent the higher relapse rate. Because patients would have received high-dose chemotherapy for the transplantation, other forms of therapeutic modalities, such as vaccine or cell-based immunotherapy (see Chapters 31 and 58), might be employed. For those patients whose marrow or PBPC are purged free of tumor, improved conditioning therapies and adjunctive immunotherapies may ultimately lead to the goal of greater cure rates for a variety of diseases. It seems obvious that it is better to infuse a tumor-free product than one contaminated with cancer cells. At present, the difficulty in demonstrating a clinical benefit of purging relates to obstacles in eradicating tumor cells from the patient more so than the graft.

REFERENCES

1. Brenner MK, Rill DR, Moen RC, et al: Gene-marking to trace origin of relapse after autologous bone-marrow transplantation. Lancet 341:85–86, 1993.
2. Deisseroth AB, Zu Z, Claxton D, et al: Genetic marking shows that Ph + cells present in autologous transplants of chronic myelogenous leukemia (CML) contribute to relapse after autologous bone marrow in CML. Blood 83(10):3068–3076, 1994.
3. Rill DR, Santana VM, Roberts WM, et al: Direct demonstration that autologous bone marrow transplantation for solid tumors can return a multiplicity of tumorigenic cells. Blood 84(2):380–383, 1994.
4. Heslop HE, Brenner MK, Krance RA, et al: Use of double marking with retroviral vectors to determine rate of reconstitution of untreated and cytokine expanded CD34 + selected marrow cells in patients undergoing autologous bone marrow transplantation. Hum Gene Ther 7(5):655–667, 1996.
5. Sharkis SJ, Santos GW, Calvin M: Elimination of acute myelogenous leukemia cells from marrow and tumor suspensions in rat with 4-hydroperoxycyclophosphamide. Blood 55:521–523, 1980.
6. Krolick KA, Uhr JW, Vitetta ES: Selective killing of leukemic cells by antibody-toxin conjugates: implication for autologous bone marrow transplantation. Nature 295:604–605, 1982.
7. Kaizer H, Stuart RK, Brookmyer R, et al: Autologous bone marrow transplantation in leukemia: a phase I study of in vitro treatment of marrow with 4-hydroperoxycyclophosphamide to purge tumor cells. Blood 65:1504–1510, 1985.
8. Chang J, Morgenstern G, Deakin D, et al: Reconstitution of hematopoietic system with autologous marrow taken during relapse of acute myeloblastic leukemia and grown in long-term culture. Lancet 1:294–295, 1986.
9. Yeager AM, Kaizer H, Santos GW, et al: Autologous bone marrow transplantation in patients with acute nonlymphocytic leukemia, using ex vivo marrow treatment with 4-hydroperoxycyclophosphamide. N Engl J Med 315:141–147, 1986.
10. Vredenburgh JJ, Silva O, Tyer CL, et al: A comparison of immunohistochemistry, two-color immunofluorescence and flow cytometry with cell sorting for the detection of micrometastatic breast cancer in the bone marrow. J Hematother 5:57–62, 1996.
11. Cote RJ, Rosen PP, Hakes TB, et al: Monoclonal antibodies detect occult breast carcinoma metastases in the bone marrow of patients with early stage disease. Am J Surg Pathol 12:333–340, 1988.
12. Schlimok G, Funke I, Holzmann B, et al: Micrometastatic cancer cells in bone marrow: in vitro detection with anti-cytokeratin and in vivo labeling with anti-17–1A monoclonal antibodies. Proc Natl Acad Sci U S A 84:8672–8676, 1987.

13. Berger U, Bettelheim R, Mansi JL, et al: The relationship between micrometastases in the bone marrow, histopathologic features of the primary tumor in breast cancer and prognosis. Am J Clin Pathol 90:1–6, 1988.

14. Mansi JL, Berger U, McDonnell T, et al: The fate of bone marrow micrometastases in patients with primary breast cancer. J Clin Oncol 7:445–449, 1989.

15. Datta YH, Adams PT, Drobyski WR, et al: Sensitive detection of occult breast cancer by the reverse-transcriptase polymerase chain reaction. J Clin Oncol 12:475–482, 1994.

16. Sharp JG, Joshi SS, Armitage JO, et al: Significance of detection of occult non-Hodgkin's lymphoma in histologically uninvolved bone marrow by a culture technique. Blood 79(4):1074–1080, 1992.

17. Wells DA, Hall MC, Shulman HM, Loken MR: Occult B cell malignancies can be detected by three-color flow cytometry in patients with cytopenias. Leukemia 12(12):2015–2023, 1998.

18. Wells DA, Sale GE, Shulman HM, et al: Multidimensional flow cytometry of marrow can differentiate leukemic from normal lymphoblasts and myeloblasts after chemotherapy and bone marrow transplantation. Am J Clin Pathol 110(1):84–94, 1998.

19. Sievers EL, Loken MR: Detection of minimal residual disease in acute myelogenous leukemia. J Pediatr Hematol/Oncol 17(2):123–133, 1995.

20. Stewart CC, Behm FG, Carey JL, et al: U.S.-Canadian Consensus recommendations on the immunophenotypic analysis of hematologic neoplasia by flow cytometry: selection of antibody combinations. Cytometry 30(5):231–235, 1997.

21. Lee MS, Chang KS, Calabanillas E, et al: Detection of minimal residual disease cells carrying t(14:18) by DNA sequence amplification. Science 237:175–178, 1987.

22. Radich JP, Slovak ML: The laboratory evaluation of minimal residual disease. In Thomas ED, Blume K, Forman SJ (eds): Hematopoietic Stem Cell Transplantation. Malden, MA, Blackwell, 1999, pp 235–247.

23. Laporte JP, Douay L, Lopez M, et al: One hundred twenty-five adult patients with primary acute leukemia autografted with marrow purged by mafosfamide: a 10-year single institution experience. Blood 84(11):3810–3818, 1994.

24. Stein AS, Forman SJ: Autologous hematopoietic cell transplantation for acute myeloid leukemia. In Thomas ED, Blume K (eds): Hematopoietic Stem Cell Transplantation. Malden, MA, Blackwell, 1999, pp 963–977.

25. Shpall EJ, Jones RB, Bast RC Jr, et al: 4-Hydroperoxycyclophosphamide purging of breast cancer from the mononuclear cell fraction of bone marrow in patients receiving high dose chemotherapy and autologous marrow support: a phase I trial. J Clin Oncol 9:85–93, 1991.

26. Kennedy MJ, Beveridge RA, Rowley SD, et al: High-dose chemotherapy with reinfusion of purged autologous bone marrow following dose-intense induction as initial therapy for metastatic breast cancer. J Natl Cancer Inst 83:920–926, 1991.

27. Kohn FR, Landkammer GJ, Manthey CL, et al: Effect of aldehyde dehydrogenase inhibitors on the ex vivo sensitivity of human multipotent and committed hematopoietic progenitor cells and malignant blood cells to oxazophosphorines. Cancer Res 47:3180–3185, 1987.

28. Balzarotti M, Grisanti S, Granzow K, et al: Ex vivo manipulation of hematopoietic stem cells for transplantation: the potential role of amifostine. Semin Oncol 26:66–71, 1999.

29. Cagnoni PJ, Jones RB, Bearman SI, et al: Use of amifostine in bone marrow purging. Semin Oncol 23:44–48, 1996.

30. Gorin NC: The potential of amifostine (Ethyol) in haematological malignancies. Eur J Cancer 32A (Suppl 4):S31–39, 1996.

31. Castiglione F, Dalla Mola A, Porcile G: Protection of normal tissues from radiation and cytotoxic therapy: the development of amifostine. Tumori 85(2):85–91, 1999.

32. Wasserman T: Radioprotective effects of amifostine. Semin Oncol 26 (2 Suppl 7):89–94, 1999.

33. List AF: Use of amifostine in hematologic malignancies, myelodysplastic syndrome, and acute leukemia. Semin Oncol 26 (2 Suppl 7):61–65, 1999.

34. Links M, Lewis C: Chemoprotectants: a review of their clinical pharmacology and therapeutic efficacy. Drugs 57(3):293–308, 1999.

35. Ball ED, Phelps V, Wilson J: Bone marrow transplantation for acute leukemia in remission or first relapse using monoclonal antibody-purged marrow. Blood 88:485a, 1996.

36. Gribben JG, Freedman AS, Neuberg D, et al: Immunological purging of marrow assessed by PCR before autologous bone marrow transplantation for B-Cell lymphoma. N Engl J Med 325:1525–1533, 1991.

37. Simonsson B, Burnett AK, Prentice HG, et al: Autologous bone marrow transplantation with monoclonal antibody purged marrow for high risk acute lymphoblastic leukemia. Leukemia 9:631–636, 1989.

38. Garaventa A, Rondelli R, Lanino E, et al: Myeloablative therapy and bone marrow rescue in advanced neuroblastoma: report from the Italian Bone Marrow Transplant Registry. Bone Marrow Transplant 18:125–130, 1996.

39. Vredenburgh JJ, Simpson W, Memoli VA, Ball ED: Reactivity of anti-CD15 monoclonal antibody PM-81 with breast cancer and elimination of breast cancer cells from human bone marrow by PM-81 and immunomagnetic beads. Cancer Res 51:2451–2455, 1991.

40. Tyer CL, Vredenburgh JJ, Heimer M, et al: Breast cancer cells are effectively purged from peripheral blood progenitor cells using an immunomagnetic technique. Clin Cancer Res 2:81–86, 1996.

41. Kamani NR: Autotransplants for neuroblastoma. Bone Marrow Transplant 17:301–304, 1996.

42. Gribben JG, Nadler LM: Bone marrow purging for autologous bone marrow transplantation. Leuk Lymph 11 (Suppl 2):141–148, 1993.

43. Moss TJ, Xu ZJ, Mansour VH, et al: Quantitation of tumor cell removal from bone marrow: a preclinical model. J Hematother 1:65–74, 1992.

44. Hardwick RA, Kulcinski D, Mansour V, et al: Design of large-scale separation systems for positive and negative immunomagnetic selection of cells using super-paramagnetic microspheres. J Hematother 1:379–386, 1992.

45. Gobbi M, Tazzari PL, Cavo M, et al: Autologous bone marrow transplantation with immunotoxin purged marrow for multiple myeloma: long term results in 14 patients with advanced disease. Bone Marrow Transplant 7 (Suppl 2):30, 1991.

46. Preijers FW, De Witte T, Wessels JM, et al: Autologous transplantation of bone marrow purged in vitro with anti-CD7-(WT1-) ricin A immunotoxin in T-cell lymphoblastic leukemia and lymphoma. Blood 74(3):1152–1158, 1989.

47. Gorin NC, Douay L, Laporte JP, et al: Autologous bone marrow transplantation with marrow decontaminated by immunotoxin T 101 in the treatment of leukemia and lymphoma: first clinical observations. Cancer Treat Rep 69(9):953–959, 1985.

48. Roy DC, Ouellet S, Le Houillier C, et al: Elimination of neuroblastoma and small-cell lung cancer cells with an anti-neural cell adhesion molecule immunotoxin. J Natl Cancer Inst 88(16):1136–1145, 1996.

49. Roy DC, Perreault C, Bélanger R, et al: Elimination of B-lineage leukemia and lymphoma cells from bone marrow grafts using anti-B4-blocked-ricin immunotoxin. J Clin Immunol 15(1):51–57, 1995.

50. Barbieri L, Dinota A, Gobbi M, et al: Immunotoxins containing saporin 6 and monoclonal antibodies recognizing plasma cell-associated antigens: effects on target cells and on normal myeloid precursors (CFU-GM). Eur J Haematol 42(3):238–245, 1989.

51. Civin C, Trischmann T, Kadan NS, et al: Highly purified CD34+ cells reconstitute hematopoiesis. J Clin Oncol 14(8):2224–2233, 1996.

52. Nimgaonkar M, Kemp A, Lancia J, Ball ED: A combination of CD34 selection and complement-mediated immunopurging (anti-CD15 monoclonal antibody) eliminates tumor cells while sparing normal progenitor cells. J Hematother 5(1):39–48, 1996.

53. Bertolini F, Thomas T, Battaglia M, et al: A new "two step" procedure for 4.5 log depletion of T and B cells in allogeneic transplantation and of neoplastic cells in autologous transplantation. Bone Marrow Transplant 19(6):615–619, 1997.

54. Tseng-Law J, Szalay P, Guillermo R, et al: Identification of a peptide directed against the anti-CD34 antibody, 9C5, by phage display and its use in hematopoietic stem cell selection. Exp Hematol 27(5):936–945, 1999.

55. Miller CB, Rowlings PA, Jones RJ, et al: Autotransplants for acute myelogenous leukemia (AML) effects of purging with 4-hydroperoxycyclophosphamide (4-HC) [Abstract]. Blood 100a, 1996.

56. Miller CB, Rowlings PA, Jones RJ, et al: Autotransplants for acute myelogenous leukemia (AML) effects of purging with 4-hydroperoxycyclophosphamide (4-HC). Proc Am Soc Clin Oncol 15:338, 1996.

57. Gorin NC, Aegerter P, Auvert B, et al: Autologous bone marrow

transplantation for acute myelocytic leukemia in first remission: a European Survey of the role of marrow purging. Blood 75:1606–1614, 1990.

58. Chao NJ, Stein AS, Long GD, et al: Busulfan/etoposide initial experience with a new preparatory regimen for autologous bone marrow transplantation in patients with acute nonlymphocytic leukemia. Blood 81:319–323, 1993.

59. Selvaggi KJ, Wilson JW, Mills LE, et al: Improved outcome for high-risk acute myeloid leukemia patients usiing autologous bone marrow transplantation and monoclonal antibody-purged bone marrow. Blood 83:1698–1705, 1994.

60. Hammert LC, Ball ED: Purging of autologous bone marrow with monoclonal antibodies for transplantation in acute myelogenous leukemia. Blood Rev 11:1–11, 1997.

61. Linker CA, Ries CA, Damon LE, et al: Autologous bone marrow transplantation for acute myeloid leukemia using 4-hydroperoxy-cyclophosphamide-purged bone marrow and the busulfan/etoposide preparative regimen: a follow-up report. Bone Marrow Transplant 22(9):865–872, 1998.

62. Körbling M, Fliedner TM, Holle R, et al: Autologous blood stem cell (ABSCT) versus purged bone marrow transplantation (pABMT) in standard risk AML: influence of source and cell composition of the autograft on hemopoietic reconstitution and disease-free survival. Bone Marrow Transplant 7(5):343–349, 1991.

63. Cassileth PA, Andersen J, Lazarus HM, et al: Autologous bone marrow transplant in acute myeloid leukemia in first remission. J Clin Oncol 11(2):314–319, 1993.

64. Vredenburgh JJ, Peters WP, Rosner G, et al: Detection of tumor cells in the bone marrow of stage IV breast cancer patients receiving high dose chemotherapy: the role of induction chemotherapy. Bone Marrow Transplant 16:815–821, 1995.

65. Weaver CH, Moss T, Schwartzberg LS, et al: High-dose chemotherapy in patients with breast cancer: evaluation of infusing peripheral blood stem cells containing occult tumor cells. Bone Marrow Transplant 21(11):1117–1124, 1998.

66. Horning SJ, Chao NJ, Negrin RS, et al: High-dose therapy and autologous hematopoietic progenitor cell transplantation for recurrent or refractory Hodgkin's disease: analysis of the Stanford University results and prognostic indices. Blood 89:801–813, 1997.

67. Freedman A, Gribben J, Neuberg D, et al: High dose therapy and autologous bone marrow transplantation in patients with follicular lymphoma during first remission. Blood 88:2780–2786, 1996.

68. Lister TA: Follicular lymphoma: grounds for optimism. Ann Oncol 8(suppl 1):89–92, 1997.

69. Freedman A, Gribben J, Neuberg D, et al: Long term prolongation of disease free survival and overall survival following autologous bone marrow transplantation in patients with advanced relapsed follicular lymphoma. Proc Am Soc Clin Oncol 89 (abstract 304), 1997.

70. Preijers FW, De Witte T, Wessels JM, et al: Autologous transplantation of bone marrow purged in vitro with anti-CD7-(WT1-) ricin. An immunotoxin in T-cell lymphoblastic lymphoma. Blood 74:1152–1158, 1989.

71. Santini G, Coser P, Chiesi T, et al: Autologous bone marrow transplantation for advanced stage adult lymphoblastic lymphoma in first complete remission. Ann Oncol 2:181–185, 1991.

72. Williams CD, Goldstone AH, Pearce RM, et al: Purging of bone marrow in autologous bone marrow transplantation for non-Hodgkin's lymphoma: a case-matched comparison with unpurged cases by the European Blood and Marrow Transplant Lymphoma Registry. J Clin Oncol 14:2454–2464, 1996.

73. Bierman PJ, Vose JM, Anderson JR, et al: High-dose therapy with autologous hematopoietic rescue for follicular low-grade non-Hodgkin's lymphoma. J Clin Oncol 15:445–450, 1997.

74. Doney K, Buckner CD, Fisher L, et al: Autologous bone marrow transplantation for acute lymphoblastic leukemia. Bone Marrow Transplant 12:315–321, 1993.

75. Soiffer RJ, Roy DC, Gonin R, et al: Monoclonal antibody purged autologous bone marrow transplantation in adults with acute lymphoblastic leukemia at high risk of relapse. Bone Marrow Transplant 12:243–251, 1993.

76. Blaise D, Gaspard MH, Stoppa AM, et al: Allogeneic or autologous bone marrow transplantation for acute lymphoblastic leukemia in first remission. Bone Marrow Transplant 5:7–12, 1990.

77. Poweles R, Mehta J, Singhal S, et al: Autologous bone marrow or

peripheral blood stem cell transplantation followed by maintenance chemotherapy for adult acute lymphoblastic leukemia in first remission: 50 cases from a single center. Bone Marrow Transplant 16:241–247, 1995.

78. Gilmore M, Hamon MD, Prentice HG, et al: Failure of purged autologous bone marrow transplantation in high-risk acute lymphoblastic leukaemia in first complete remission. Bone Marrow Transplant 8:19–26, 1991.

79. Seeger RC, Reynolds CP: Hematopoietic cell transplantation for neuroblastoma. In Thomas ED, Blume K, Forman SJ (eds): Hematopoietic Cell Transplantation. Malden, MA, Blackwell, 1999, pp 1071–1083.

80. Medencia RD, Nava EF, Freeman AL: Diffuse pulmonary infiltration of neuroblastoma following autologous bone marrow transplantation [Abstract]. Blood 66:261a, 1985.

81. Glorieux P, Bouffet E, Phillip I, et al: Metastatic interstitial pneumonitis after autologous bone marrow transplantation: a consequence of reinjection of malignant cells? Cancer 58:2136–2139, 1986.

82. Treleaven J, Gibson F, Udelstad J: Removal of neuroblastoma cells from bone marrow with monoclonal antibodies conjugated to magnetic microspheres. Lancet 2:70–76, 1984.

83. Matthay KK, Atkinson JB, Stram DO, et al: Patterns of relapse after autologous purged bone marrow transplantation for neuroblastoma: a Children's Cancer Group Pilot study. J Clin Oncol 11:2226–2233, 1993.

84. Matthay KK, Reynolds CP, Stram DO, Seeger RC: Quantitative tumor cell content of bone marrow and blood as an early predictor of response in high risk neuroblastomas: a Children's Cancer Group study [Abstract]. Proc Am Soc Clin Oncol 16:512, 1997.

85. Kamani NR: Autotransplants for neuroblastoma. Bone Marrow Transplant 17:301–304, 1996.

86. Diel I, Kaufmann M, Goerner R, et al: Detection of tumor cells in bone marrow of patients with primary breast cancer: a prognostic factor for distant metastasis. J Clin Oncol 10:1534–1539, 1992.

87. Osborne M, Wong G, Cote R, et al: Bone marrow micrometastasis detected by monoclonal antibodies predicts early relapse in patients with breast cancer. Breast Cancer Res Treat 23:136, 1992.

88. Mansi J, Easton D, Berger U, et al: Bone marrow micrometastases in primary breast cancer: prognostic significance after 6 years' follow-up. Eur J Cancer 27:1552–1555, 1991.

89. Coombes R, Berger U, Mansi J, et al: Prognostic significance of micrometastases in bone marrow in patients with primary breast cancer. Natl Cancer Inst Monogr 1:51–53, 1986.

90. Vredenburgh J, Tyer C, Broadwater G, et al: The incidence of significance of tumor cell contamination of the hematopoietic chemotherapy. Proc Am Soc Clin Oncol 16:338, 1997.

91. Berger U, Bettelheim R, Mansi JL, et al: The relationship between micrometastases in the bone marrow, histopathologic features of the primary tumor in breast cancer and prognosis. Am J Clin Pathol 90:1, 1988.

92. Passos-Coelho J, Ross AA, Davis JM, et al: Bone marrow micrometastases in chemotherapy-responsive advanced breast cancer: effect of ex vivo purging with 4-hydroperoxycyclophosphamide. Cancer Res 54:2366–2371, 1994.

93. Rill DR, Santana VM, Roberts M, et al: Direct demonstration that autologous bone marrow transplantation for solid tumors can return a multiplicity of tumorigenic cells. Blood 2:380–383, 1994.

94. Pecora AL, Lazarus HM, Cooper B, et al: Breast cancer contamination in peripheral blood stem cell (PBSC) collections associated with bone marrow disease and type of mobilization. Blood 90:99a, 1997.

95. Moss TJ, Umiel T, Herzig RM, et al: The presence of clonogenic breast cancer cells in peripheral blood stem cell (PBSC) products correlates with an extremely poor prognosis for patients with stage IV disease. Proc Am Soc Clin Oncol 17:106a, 1998.

96. Umiel T, Moss TJ, Cooper B, et al: The prognostic value of bone marrow (BM) micrometastases in stage II/III breast cancer patients undergoing autologous transplant (AMBT) therapy. Proc Am Soc Clin Oncol 17:79a, 1998.

97. Cooper BW, Moss TJ, Ross AA, et al: Occult tumor contamination of hematopoietic stem-cell products does not affect clinical outcome of autologous transplantation in patients with metastatic breast cancer. J Clin Oncol 16(11):3509–3517, 1998.

98. Brugger W, Bross KJ, Glatt M, et al: Mobilization of tumor cells and hematopoietic progenitor cells into peripheral blood of patients with solid tumors. Blood 83(3):636–640, 1994.

99. Vredenburgh JJ, Silva O, Broadwater G, et al: The significance of tumor contamination in the bone marrow from high-risk primary breast cancer patients treated with high dose chemotherapy and hematopoietic support. Biol Blood Marrow Transplant 3:91–97, 1997.

100. Fields KK, Elfenbein GJ, Trudeau WL, et al: Clinical significance of bone marrow metastases as detected using the polymerase chain reaction in patients with breast cancer undergoing high dose chemotherapy and autologous bone marrow transplantation. J Clin Oncol 14:1868–1876, 1996.

101. Kennedy MJ, Davis J, Passos-Coelho J, et al: Administration of human recombinant granulocyte colony-stimulating factor (filgrastim) accelerates granulocyte recovery following high-dose chemotherapy and autologous marrow transplantation with 4-hydroperoxy-cyclophosphamide-purged marrow in women with metastatic breast cancer. Cancer Res 53(22):5424–5428, 1993.

102. Vredenburgh JJ, Long GD, Rizzieri D, et al: High dose chemotherapy (HDC) with CD34 cellular support for women with poor prognosis metastatic breast cancer (MBC). Proc Am Soc Clin Oncol 18:49a, 1999.

103. Vredenburgh J, Shpall EJ, Ross M, et al: Immunopharmacologic bone marrow purging and high-dose chemotherapy with autologous bone marrow support (ABMS) for patients with metastatic breast cancer. Proc Am Soc Clin Oncol 11:58, 1992.

104. Anderson I, Shpall EJ, Leslie D, et al: Elimination of malignant clonogenic breast cancer cells from human bone marrow. Cancer Res 49:4659–4664, 1989.

105. Shpall EJ, Jones RB, Bearman SI, et al: Transplantation of enriched CD34-positive autologous marrow into breast cancer patients following high-dose chemotherapy: influence of CD34-positive peripheral-blood progenitors and growth factors on engraftment. J Clin Oncol 12(1):28–36, 1994.

106. Kruger W, Gruber M, Henning S, et al: Purging and haemopoietic progenitor cell selection by CD34+ cell separation. Bone Marrow Transplant 21:665–671, 1998.

107. Ben-Yosef R, Or R, Naparstek E, et al: Should soybean agglutinin purging be performed in breast cancer patients undergoing autologous transplantation? A retrospective analysis of 48 patients. Am J Clin Oncol 20:419–423, 1997.

108. Margolin KA, Wright C, Forman SJ: Autologous bone marrow purging by IL-2 activation of endogenous killer cells. Leukemia 11:723–728, 1997.

109. Meehan KR, Verma UN, Rajogopal C, et al: Stem cell transplantation with chemoradiotherapy myeloablation and interleukin-2. J Infusion Chemother 6:28–32, 1996.

110. Lundell BI, Vredenburgh JJ, Tyer C, et al: Ex vivo expansion of bone marrow from breast cancer patients: reduction of tumor cell content through passive purging. Bone Marrow Transplant 22:153–159, 1998.

111. Hirai M, Kelsey LS, Maneval DC, et al: Adenovirus p53 purging for human breast cancer stem cell products. Acta Haematol 101:97–105, 1999.

112. Chen L, Pulsipher M, Chen D, et al: Selective transgene expression for detection and elimination of contaminating carcinoma cells in hematopoietic cell sources. J Clin Invest 98:2539–2548, 1996.

113. Ross AA, Cooper BW, Lazarus HM, et al: Detection and viability of tumor cells in peripheral blood stem cell collections from breast cancer patients using immunocytochemical and clonogenic assay techniques [see comments]. Blood 82:2605–2610, 1993.

114. Umiel T, Moss TJ, Cooper B, et al: The prognostic value of bone marrow (BM) metastases in stage II/III breast cancer patients undergoing autologous transplant (ABMT) therapy. Proc Am Soc Clin Oncol 17:79a, 1998.

CHAPTER THIRTY

T-Cell Depletion and Allograft Engineering

Albert D. Donnenberg, Ph.D.

Unmanipulated aspirated bone marrow was the first source of hematopoietic stem cells (HSC) to be used in clinical allotransplantation. Recently, peripheral blood progenitor cells (PBPC) obtained by leukapheresis after cytokine mobilization gained acceptance as a source of HSC for allogeneic transplantation. Both marrow and PBPC are most frequently used without further modification or cell selection.

The first attempts to modify bone marrow aspirates to meet specific clinical requirements took place in the early 1980s. Clinical T-cell depletion was performed using soybean lectin agglutination followed by rosetting with sheep red blood cells to remove T cells from the marrow graft. This procedure permitted transplantation of paternal bone marrow to a human leukocyte antigen (HLA)-A, -B, and -DR nonidentical child.[1] Techniques to deplete erythrocytes were developed at about the same time, allowing transplantation in the setting of major ABO incompatibility.[2] There are still cogent reasons for allograft engineering in general and T-cell depletion in particular. This chapter concentrates on the biology of T-cell depletion, its indications, and the consequences of its use.

METHODS OF T-CELL DEPLETION

Among the most widely used methods for T-cell depletion are monoclonal antibody–based negative selection techniques, separation based on lectin-mediated agglutination, and physical separation by size and density. More recently, positive selection of CD34+ cells has been used to eliminate T cells. Similar success in eliminating acute graft-versus-host disease (GVHD) has been reported for all of these processes, providing that they achieved a T-cell reduction of about 2 orders of magnitude (logs) or greater.

MONOCLONAL ANTIBODIES

Monoclonal antibodies are an important tool for graft processing. Their advantages include specificity, homogeneity, and virtually unlimited supply. Several different monoclonal antibody–based technologies are available for T-cell depletion. These include incubation with complement or with antiglobulin-conjugated magnetic beads, conjugation to immunotoxins, and conjugation to other solid phase substrates. Most of these methods, when optimally applied, yield a depletion of 2–3 logs and thus are sufficient to

prevent GVHD in a majority of HLA-matched transplants. Monoclonal antibodies directed against surface antigens found on T cells or T-cell subsets have been used alone and in combination in clinical trials. These include OKT-3 (anti-CD3)[3]; Campath-1 (anti-CD52)[4]; CT2 (anti-CD2)[5]; anti-CD6 plus anti-CD8[6]; anti-CD2, anti-CD5, plus anti-CD7[7]; TA-1, UCHT-1 (anti-CD3), and T101 (anti-CD5)[8]; anti-CD8 alone[9]; and anti-CD6 alone[10] and T10B9 (anti-α/β T-cell receptor).[11] It is uncertain whether any of these antibodies or combinations of antibodies offers a clear advantage.

Another promising antibody-mediated T-cell depletion technique was originally developed for CD34+ cell selection in autologous HSC transplantation (HSCT). The CellPro CEPRATE SC, which has been used in clinical protocols to select for CD34+ cells, depletes T cells incidental to CD34+ cell purification. The extent of T-cell depletion (approximately 3 orders of magnitude) is comparable to that of many techniques expressly developed for T-cell depletion.[12, 13] Even greater T-cell depletion has been reported using positive immunomagnetic selection of CD34+ cells.[14] Future software developments for the Nexell Isolex 300i system, which also uses immunomagnetic selection and includes an integrated cell washer, may permit one-step positive/negative selection wherein CD34+ cells are positively selected and T cells are negatively selected in a single run. Such developments hold the promise of virtually quantitative elimination of T cells.

SOY BEAN AGGLUTININ AND E ROSETTE DEPLETION

Preclinical experiments revealed that the plant lectin soy bean agglutinin (SBA) could be used to agglutinate and deplete a wide variety of lineage-committed marrow cells, including lymphocytes. The majority of hematopoietic progenitor cells do not bind SBA. Addition of a second T cell–specific round of depletion using treated sheep red blood cells or monoclonal antibody–based methods resulted in up to 3 logs of T-cell depletion. The first clinical implementation of HSCT with lymphocyte-depleted marrow was performed using this technique.[1] Reisner et al., at Memorial Sloan-Kettering Cancer Center, also successfully applied lectin separation to parental haplo-mismatched HSCT for severe combined immune deficiency syndrome (SCID).[15] Since its implementation, this technique has been refined considerably, permitting more-rapid processing of the larger marrow volumes needed for adult transplantation. Typically, a 2.4-log T-cell depletion is achieved, with about 6% recovery of harvested leukocytes and 38% recovery of granulocyte monocyte colony-forming units (CFU-GM). The SBA-positive fraction is irradiated (3000 cGy) and infused with the T-depleted SBA-negative/E rosette–negative fraction (about 5×10^7 cells/kg).

ELUTRIATION

Counterflow centrifugal elutriation is a rapid, nondestructive, and reproducible method of large-scale cell manipulation. Elutriation separates cell populations on the basis of their sedimentation coefficients. Cells suspended in medium are pumped into a spinning chamber in a direction opposing the centrifugal field. By loading cells into the chamber at a counterflow rate that balances the centrifugal force, cells remain in suspension and align themselves with respect to their sedimentation velocities. In clinical applications, lymphocyte depletion of bone marrow has been effected either by increasing the medium flow rate[16] or by decreasing the centrifugation speed.[17] With both procedures, smaller, slower sedimenting cells are eluted first, followed by larger cells with faster sedimentation coefficients. The former population contains the majority of lymphocytes, whereas the latter is enriched myeloid cells, including a modest enrichment for CD34+ cells.

Two major systems are in use for clinical elutriation—the Beckman 5.0 rotor (Beckman Instruments, Palo Alto, CA), equipped with a high capacity $10 \times$ chamber, and the MCCC system supplied by Dijkstra, Amsterdam, Netherlands. Both systems offer rapid separation, viable cell recovery exceeding 90% and the capability to further manipulate lymphocyte-enriched fractions.

The elutriation protocol at the University of Pittsburgh Cancer Institute starts with a granulocyte-depleted leukapheresis bone marrow buffy coat that has been adjusted to contain a fixed number of erythrocytes (1.5×10^{11}) in a standardized volume of autologous plasma (175 mL). Three fractions are collected at increasing flow rates while centrifugation speed is held constant. Cells remaining in the chamber compose the final fraction, designated "rotor off" (R/O), which is collected by stopping the rotor while maintaining fluid flow. In a single elutriation procedure, cell recovery in the R/O fraction is 34 ± 4% for nucleated cells, 33 ± 11% for CFU-GM cells, and 28 ± 13% for lineage-negative CD34+ cells (mean ± SD) compared with the input product. T-cell depletion in this fraction is greater than 2.5 logs. The lymphocyte-rich elutriation fractions are pooled, brought to the volume and erythrocyte concentration of the original product, and subjected to a second round of lymphocyte depletion by elutriation. Patients are given the lymphocyte-depleted R/O fractions from the first and second elutriations plus a volume of the lymphocyte-rich fraction from the second elutriation sufficient to bring the total T-cell dose to 0.5×10^6/kg. The total lineage-negative CD34+ cell dose in the graft product averages $1.6 \pm 0.6 \times 10^6$/kg (mean ± SEM)—a 1.8-fold increase over the dose that would have been attained with a single elutriation.[18]

HETEROGENEITY OF THE UNMANIPULATED GRAFT PRODUCT

Surrogate markers such as the proportion of nucleated cells expressing CD34 or forming hematopoietic colonies in vitro are routinely used to measure graft progenitor cell content. The hematopoietic progenitor cell content of a graft is usually expressed relative to recipient body weight (ideal or actual). Hematopoietic progenitor cells make up a very small minority of cells in aspirated bone marrow (Table 30–1) or PBPC products prepared by leukapheresis (Table 30–2). Pluripotential HSC, the subset of progenitor cells capable of giving rise to sustained multilineage engraftment, account for an even smaller fraction: 0.05% of nucleated cells at most.[20]

The mechanical process of bone marrow aspiration ensures that the unmanipulated bone marrow graft consists of a relatively small volume of bone marrow suspended in a large volume of peripheral blood. As a result, mature T cells, which can mediate both beneficial and detrimental effects, outnumber CD34+, lineage-negative cells by approximately 13 to 1. In PBPC products, circulating mononuclear cells predominate and the T-cell dose is approxi-

TABLE 30–1. VARIABILITY IN THE COMPOSITION OF BONE MARROW HARVESTED FOR USE IN ALLOGENEIC TRANSPLANTATION

PARAMETER	MEAN	SD
Volume (mL)	1567	519
BFU-E/10^5 nucleated cells	35.6	20.8
GM/10^5 nucleated cells	83.2	54.2
GEMM/10^5 nucleated cells	3.2	3.2
Lineage negative CD34+ (%)	0.71	0.36
CD3+ (%)	9.27	3.48
CD3+/CD56+ (%)	1.32	0.82
CD3+/CD4+ (%)	5.90	2.58
CD3+/CD8+ (%)	4.33	1.84
CD4/CD8 ratio	1.50	0.70
Total nucleated cells	2.78×10^{10}	9.83×10^9
Total erythrocytes	4.37×10^{12}	2.42×10^{12}
Total BFU-E	1.46×10^7	1.05×10^7
Total GM	6.35×10^6	3.96×10^6
Total GEMM	5.67×10^5	5.74×10^5
Total lineage negative CD34+	1.94×10^8	1.36×10^8
Total CD3+	2.55×10^9	1.47×10^9
Total CD3+ CD56+	3.36×10^8	2.17×10^8
Total CD4+	1.78×10^9	9.57×10^8
Total CD8+	1.31×10^9	7.23×10^8
Nucleated cells/kg of recipient weight	6.93×10^8	4.07×10^8
BFU-E/kg of recipient weight	4.35×10^5	5.33×10^5
GM/kg of recipient weight	1.81×10^5	2.03×10^5
GEMM/kg of recipient weight	1.19×10^4	1.01×10^4
Lin neg. CD34+/kg of recipient weight	4.78×10^6	4.09×10^6
CD3+/kg of recipient weight	6.30×10^7	4.62×10^7
CD56+/kg of recipient weight	9.62×10^6	1.06×10^7
CD4+/kg of recipient weight	3.21×10^7	2.77×10^7
CD8+/kg of recipient weight	2.64×10^7	2.66×10^7

The results are from 31 donors harvested at the University of Pittsburgh Cancer Institute. BFU-E, erythroid burst forming units; GM, granulocyte/monocyte colony forming units; GEMM, granulocyte/erythroid/monocyte/megakaryocyte colony forming units. CD34+, lineage negative cells were defined by a cocktail consisting of antibodies to lymphoid cells (anti-CD3, anti-CD11b, anti-CD19), erythroid cells (anti-glycophorin A), and myeloid cells (anti-CD14 and anti-CD15).

TABLE 30–2. VARIABILITY IN THE COMPOSITION OF MOBILIZED NORMAL DONOR LEUKAPHERESIS PRODUCTS USED FOR ALLOTRANSPLANTATION

PARAMETER	MEAN	SD
CD34+ CD45^{dim} (%)	0.90	0.38
CD3+ (%)	23.73	3.01
CD3+/CD56+ (%)	3.84	1.90
CD3+/CD4+ (%)	14.85	2.12
CD3+/CD8+ (%)	8.31	1.77
CD19+ (%)	6.54	2.59
Total nucleated cells	1.14×10^{11}	6.29×10^{10}
Total CD34+ CD45^{dim}	8.58×10^{8}	2.97×10^{8}
Total CD3+	2.61×10^{10}	1.34×10^{10}
Total CD3+ CD56+	3.89×10^{9}	2.30×10^{9}
Total CD4+	1.65×10^{10}	8.92×10^{9}
Total CD8+	9.04×10^{9}	4.80×10^{9}
Total CD19+	7.07×10^{9}	5.03×10^{9}
Nucleated cells/kg of recipient weight	1.70×10^{9}	8.98×10^{8}
CD34+/kg of recipient weight	1.25×10^{7}	3.01×10^{6}
CD3+/kg of recipient weight	3.95×10^{8}	2.05×10^{8}
CD3+ CD56+/kg of recipient weight	5.72×10^{7}	2.89×10^{7}
CD4+/kg of recipient weight	2.49×10^{8}	1.32×10^{8}
CD8+/kg of recipient weight	1.37×10^{8}	7.65×10^{7}
CD19+/kg of recipient weight	1.03×10^{8}	6.44×10^{7}

The results are from 12 donors harvested at the University of Pittsburgh Cancer Institute. Donors received recombinant human-GCSF at 16 μg/kg (ideal body weight) per day subcutaneously for 4 days prior to the initiation of apheresis. CD34+ CD45^{dim} cells were quantified according to the method of Sutherland et al.[19]

mately tenfold higher than that of a marrow graft (see Table 30–2). The number, and hence dose, of progenitor cells varies considerably from product to product. In bone marrow, the standard deviations for CD34+ cell doses and CFU doses are almost as great as the respective mean values (see Table 30–1). The large variance in progenitor dose is attributable to the variability of the volume of blood relative to marrow aspirated and of the recipient's weight. PBPC products harvested from normal donors tend to have less subject-to-subject variability than bone marrow (see Table 30–2).

In the autologous transplant setting, CD34+ cell dose is highly correlated with speed of engraftment. In a detailed study examining parameters affecting speed of engraftment in a large cohort of autograft recipients, the CD34+ cell dose ranged from 0.5 to 112.6×10^{6} cells/kg.[21] In this series, days to neutrophil engraftment (absolute neutrophil count [ANC] > 500 cells/mm^3) ranged from 5 to 38 days; platelet engraftment (platelet count > 20,000/mm^3) ranged from 4 to 53+ days. Multivariate analysis revealed CD34+ cell dose to be the single greatest factor affecting time to neutrophil and platelet engraftment. Studies comparing engraftment of autologous PBPC grafts with CD34-enriched PBPC grafts indicate that in the autologous setting, CD34– cells do not demonstrably affect the tempo of engraftment.[22]

T-CELL AND HEMATOPOIETIC STEM CELL CONTENT AFFECT ENGRAFTMENT IN ALLOTRANSPLANTATION

In contrast with autologous transplantation, allogeneic transplants are characterized by the two-way immunologic recognition of major and minor histocompatibility disparities between donor and host. Thus, graft lymphocytes, and perhaps accessory cells, can affect the tempo and even the ultimate outcome of engraftment. Despite the immunoablative properties of dose-intensive conditioning regimens, residual host immunity, though short lived, can oppose engraftment. When T-replete grafts from major histocompatibility complex (MHC)-matched sibling donors are used, the two-way reaction of graft and host immune cells strongly favors the graft and rejection is rare. Depletion of graft T-cells can tip this balance in favor of host immunity, increasing the likelihood of graft rejection, a complication that is usually fatal. The incidence of graft rejection has ranged from 5% to 60%, depending on the depletion technique, marrow ablative regimen, immunosuppressive regimen, donor sex, and donor and patient age.[23]

A study of 39 consecutive patients treated for acute myeloid leukemia (AML) with T-depleted matched sibling donor grafts reported no cases of immune mediated graft rejection.[24] In this study, patients considered at risk for immune-mediated graft rejection received antithymocyte globulin (ATG) and methylprednisolone in the peritransplantation period. The incidence of rejection is even higher when alternative donors (matched unrelated or partially matched related) are used. For example, in the setting of MHC-matched sibling donor transplantation, the combined incidence of graft rejection in two published series using counterflow centrifugal elutriation as a method of T-depletion was approximately 5%.[25] Application of the same procedure in the matched unrelated donor setting resulted in four graft failures in the first six transplants.[26] When the procedure was modified by the use of a more-immunosuppressive conditioning regimen including ATG, the incidence of graft failure was decreased to 17% in the published series and 13% at the University of Pittsburgh Cancer Institute. It has been postulated that graft T cells, and perhaps other lymphoid populations, oppose rejection that is actively mediated by residual host-derived cells or directly promote engraftment by as yet uncharacterized mechanisms.[27] Irrespective of the mechanism, the T-cell content of an allograft positively affects its engraftment potential. This effect is most pronounced when the allograft is obtained from an alternative donor.

As in autotransplantation, HSC dose appears to exert a strong effect on the pace of engraftment in allotransplantation. Although the number of pluripotential HSC required for engraftment is arguably small, the lower engraftable limit of HSC dose is not known. In murine models, as few as 100 primitive HSC, defined by surface marker expression, can rescue a lethally irradiated animal and provide durable multilineage engraftment.[28] In a series of T cell–depleted, matched unrelated donor transplantations performed at the University of Pittsburgh Cancer Institute, the lowest cell dose that gave rise to successful multilineage long-term engraftment was 1×10^{5} lineage-negative CD34+ cells/kg. This represents about 2% of the dose achieved with the average unmanipulated bone marrow graft (see Table 30–1). Engraftment (ANC >500 cells/mm^3) occurred on day 28. It is probable that even lower HSC doses could provide durable engraftment providing the graft does not meet with immunologic resistance from residual host immunity.

On the opposite end of the dose spectrum, animal studies show that transplantation with very high HSC doses can overcome immunologically mediated graft rejection, even in sublethally irradiated recipients MHC disparate to the stem cell donor.[29] This observation has been extended to human studies with encouraging results in terms of engraftment. Haplo-mismatched PBPC were first depleted of T cells by rosetting with sheep red blood cells and then positively selected for CD34+ cells using the CellPro CEPRATE SC column. The average CD34+ cell dose was $10.6 \pm 5.4 \times 10^6$/kg of recipient weight, with an average T-cell dose of $3.5 \pm 4.2 \times 10^4$/kg. This represented a 4.3-log T-depletion with a 69.8% recovery of CD34+ cells. Forty-one of 43 patients studied experienced durable engraftment, with neutrophil counts greater than 1000/mm³ at a median of 11 days and platelet counts greater than 50,000/mm³ at a median of 29 days. None of the patients experienced acute or chronic GVHD. The limiting toxicity of this procedure appears to be related to a sustained and severe immunocompromised state after transplantation. CD4+ T-cell counts were below 200 cells/mm³ at 16 months post transplantation, and infection was the major cause of death other than leukemia. Actuarial probability of relapse at 18 months post transplantation was $85 \pm 13\%$ for patients receiving transplants for acute lymphocytic leukemia (ALL) in relapse, $44 \pm 17\%$ for patients receiving transplants for ALL in remission, and $13 \pm 8\%$ for patients receiving transplants for AML.[30]

In addition to HSC dose, it is important to consider progenitor cell heterogeneity and the relative contributions of progenitor cells that give rise to short- and long-term engraftment. Surface marker expression (CD38[31], HLA-DR[32]), and functional markers, such as the ability to actively exclude dyes such as Hoecsht 33342[33] and rhodamine 123,[34] can be used to define hematopoietic progenitor cell subsets that give rise to short-term and long-term reconstitution, respectively.[20] Lineage-committed progenitor cells almost certainly give rise to the first wave of graft-derived mature myeloid cells because expansion of donor neutrophils has been documented as early as 48 hours after graft infusion.[35] Quantification of the most primitive HSC has been complicated by the observation that in the mouse, and probably in humans as well, a subpopulation of primitive engraftable cells does not express CD34. This population is recognized by the ability to exclude dyes that are substrates of the multiple drug resistance pump MDR-1.[33] These cells do not directly give rise to hematopoietic colonies in vitro but, when cultured on stromal cells, become CD34+ and are highly enriched for long-term culture initiating cells. They are almost certainly excluded from grafts that have been highly enriched for CD34+ cells by affinity column or magnetic bead separation and thus do not appear to be essential for durable engraftment. It is not known to what extent such cells contribute to hematopoietic progenitor *reserve*, the capacity for hematopoietic regeneration after injury.

LOSS OF HEMATOPOIETIC PROGENITOR CELLS DURING T-CELL DEPLETION

Despite the advantages of maximal HSC dose, most T-cell depletion techniques result in a loss of about half of the CD34+ cells present in the harvested product. Antibody and complement-based methods such as using Campath-1 and T10B9 have a yield of ~50% CD34+ cells.[36] Mechanical methods such as elutriation may recover as few as 25% of the CD34+ cells in the T cell–depleted fraction, depending on the precise separation conditions employed. Fortunately, because elutriation is nondestructive, a significant portion of CD34+ cells can be recovered from the lymphocyte-rich fractions either by an additional round of elutriation[18] or with the aid of an immunoaffinity column.[37]

An issue unique to elutriation is due to the fact that this procedure separates cells on the basis of size and density. The lymphocyte-depleted fraction, by definition, consists of cells that are larger and/or denser than lymphocytes. Thus it is reasonable to ask whether the CD34+ cells isolated in the lymphocyte-depleted fraction are more differentiated and therefore less capable of maintaining sustained engraftment than those that co-separate with lymphocytes.[38] Small-scale elutriation has, in fact, been used to enrich CD34+ cells into small lineage-negative and larger lineage-positive CD34+ fractions.[39] Fortunately, late graft failure has not been observed despite extensive clinical experience with this procedure, indicating that sufficient long-term engrafting cells are present in the elutriated product. This conundrum raises an important issue concerning the limitations of extrapolation from small-scale pilot experiments to large-scale clinical applications.

In the case of elutriation, such extrapolations are particularly difficult because varying proportions of CD34+ cells co-purify with lymphocytes, depending on the elutriation conditions. Factors such as the total number of cells loaded, the ratio of red blood cells to white blood cells, and even the size and density distribution of the input population as a whole can affect the resolution of the separation. The finding that the most primitive HSC are the smallest in diameter[39] does not necessarily preclude their separation from small T cells in a clinical-scale procedure. Stokes' law, which has been used to predict the elutriation characteristics of cells, describes the sedimentation rate of a cell in terms of volume and density, the density and viscosity of the separation medium, and the force applied to the cell. In elutriation, cell density is often a critical parameter. For example, under the conditions of clinical elutriation, small dense nucleated red blood cells co-purify with the largest of myeloid cells. In order to quantify lineage-uncommitted CD34+ cells in elutriated grafts, the bone marrow processing laboratory at the University of Pittsburgh Cancer Institute reports the dose of lineage-negative CD34+ cells[26] (see Table 30–1) rather than total CD34+ cells. These are defined as CD34+ cells that fail to express CD3, CD11b, CD19, glycophorin A, CD14, or CD15.

Although it is clear from this discussion that lineage-committed CD34+ cells may play an essential role in early engraftment, it is important to note that the most prevalent lineage-committed CD34+ cell in bone marrow is an early B cell progenitor (CD34+ CD19+). Although CD34+ B cells account for approximately 25% of all bone marrow CD34+ cells, they do not contribute to myeloid, erythroid, or platelet engraftment. In unmanipulated bone marrow, CD34+ CD19− progenitor cells have higher forward light scatter than their CD34+ CD19+ counterparts. This indicates that early B cells are physically smaller than the majority of CD34+ progenitor cells. The elutriated graft fraction (rotor off) is relatively depleted of CD34+ CD19+ cells. Thus, at least part of the loss of CD34+ "progenitor cells" observed after elutriation represents the selective depletion of early B cells rather than HSC.

HSC loss is also a problem in positive selection techiques for CD34+ cells, which in the allogeneic setting have been proposed for T-cell depletion. These methods result in the loss of 20–68% of the CD34+ cells present in the initial product (Table 30–3). This is the case for both the avidin-biotin affinity column–based CellPro CEPRATE SC and the immunomagnetic-based Nexell Isolex system. Recovery and purity are highly correlated with the CD34 content and quality of initial product. Products with high CD34+ cell content, high viability, and little cellular debris yield greater CD34 purity and recovery after separation. Preclinical reports on the performance of a cell-selection device developed by Miltenyi Biotec, which is also immunomagnetic based, indicate a mean CD34 recovery of 81.7% ± 6% (median, 78%). It will be important to confirm these results in the clinical setting. Recent patent and licensure issues have given Baxter-Nexell exclusive rights in the United States for sales of clinical devices that enrich CD34+ cells. The disposables and reagents for the CEPRATE system are no longer available at this time.

Another promising methodology for T-cell depletion, being developed by Eligix (Boston), involves the use of dense nickel particles conjugated either to an antiglobulin or to specific monoclonal antibodies.[40] Dense beads are admixed with cells, agitated for a short period of time, and then allowed to quickly settle to the bottom of the vessel. The supernatant, depleted of the targeted cell population, is decanted. This rapid procedure can be repeated for multiple rounds, with very low nonspecific cell loss. Although still in the early phases of clincal trials, the simplicity and rapidity of the procedure make it an attractive emerging technology. Discussion of comparative aspects of CD34+ cell enrichment can be found in Chapter 28.

Although most current methods of T-depletion result in progenitor cell loss, it is clearly desirable to provide as large an HSC dose as possible.[53] In the allogeneic setting, not only does an increased HSC dose appear to overcome barriers to engraftment, but hastened engraftment translates into shorter periods of transfusion dependence, decreased risk of infections associated with neutropenia, and shorter hospital stays.

OTHER BENEFICIAL FUNCTIONS OF GRAFT T CELLS

The preceding discussion of the role of graft T cells focused on their ability to promote engraftment in the allogeneic transplant setting. Although an exegesis is beyond the scope of this chapter, it should be mentioned that graft T cells play an important and sometimes critical role in the therapeutic efficacy of allogeneic HSCT, especially in the context of matched sibling donor transplantation. The most dramatic example is in chronic myeloid leukemia (CML), where graft T-cell depletion dramatically increases the post-transplantation relapse rate[54] and therapeutic donor lymphocyte infusion can be used to induce remission in transplant recipients experiencing relapse.[55] Application of donor lymphocytic infusion in CML after allogeneic HSCT can be found in Chapter 4. T-cell depletion, however, does not invariably lead to an increased relapse rate. In patients with AML treated in first remission with T cell–depleted matched sibling bone marrow, the actuarial relapse rate at 4 years can be as low as 3%.[24] T-cell depletion, which in practice is not complete, does not appear to ablate the graft-versus-leukemia effect in the matched unrelated donor setting, even in the treatment of CML.[56]

In addition to mediating graft-versus-leukemia effects, mature lymphocytes present in the graft can also mediate

TABLE 30–3. PURITY AND RECOVERY OF CD34+ CELLS ISOLATED BY POSITIVE SELECTION METHODS

PRODUCT	METHOD	PURITY	RECOVERY	AUTHORS
Auto PBPC	Isolex 300i positive/negative	98.5% (range, 96–99.8%)	32%	Paulus et al, 1997[41]
Auto PBPC	Isolex 50	85.9% (range, 69.8–92.9%)	48.1% (range, 21.0–85.2%)	Roots-Weiss et al, 1997[42]
Auto PBPC	Isolex 300 SA	95% (range, 82–99%)	80% (range, 27–132%)	Hohaus et al, 1997[43]
Auto PBPC	Isolex 300	Not available	71%	Farley et al, 1997[44]
Auto PBPC	Isolex 300	97% (range, 94.7–99.7%)	54% (35–68%)	Kvalheim et al, 1996[45]
Auto PBPC	CellPro	42 ± 20%	36 ± 20%	Handgretinger et al, 1997[46]
Auto PBPC	CellPro	61 ± 11%	68 ± 12%	Bertolini et al, 1997[47]
Allo bone marrow	CellPro	44.6% (range, 13–91%)	42%	Hassan et al, 1996[48]
Allo PBPC	CellPro	50.4% (range, 15–77%)	79%	
Auto PBPC	CellPro	49% (range, 18.4–98%)	31.4% (range, 21–37.8%)	Johnson et al, 1996[49]
Auto PBPC	CellPro	92 ± 2.3%	71 ± 10.7%	Bohbot et al, 1995[50]
Auto PBPC	MACS	74.1%	60.3%	Papadimitriou et al, 1995[51]
Auto PBPC	Isolex	83.3%	43.4%	
Allo PBPC	Campath-1	1.7%	56%	Dreger et al, 1995[36]
Allo PBPC	Isolex	94%	36	
Allo PBPC	CellPro	65%	27%	
Allo PBPC (G-CSF)	Isolex	81% ± 11%	48% ± 12%	Lane et al, 1995[52]
Allo PBPC (GM-CSF)	Isolex	77% ± 21%	51% ± 15%	

Purity is expressed as percent CD34+ cells in the product. Recovery (percent) is the number of CD34+ cells after separation divided by the number of CD34+ cells before separation × 100. Auto, autologous; Allo, allogeneic; PBPC, peripheral blood progenitor cell.

adoptive transfer of immunity from donor to recipient. When successful, adoptive transfer provides a shortcut to the generation of immune memory cells; de novo memory cell production generally does not occur until the second year after transplantation. The success of this strategy depends largely on three factors: the frequency of antigen-specific lymphocytes in the graft, the presence of antigen in the recipient at the time of transplantation, and the agents used for prophylaxis of GVHD.[57] In T-replete allo-transplantation, immunization of the donor 1 week prior to transplantation and of the recipient at the time of transplantation can facilitate transfer of cell-mediated and antibody responses to antigens such as tetanus and diphtheria toxoids. Natural exposure to endogenous viral antigens can also result in transfer of donor immunity to herpesviruses and BK virus.[58]

Not surprisingly, T-depletion of the graft ablates adoptive transfer of donor T-cell responses,[57] although antibody responses may be transferred given appropriate immunization in the peritransplantation period.[59] Long-term immune reconstitution involves the de novo generation of memory cells and takes months to years to accomplish in both T cell–replete and T cell–depleted HSCT. Although the most widely used methods of T-depletion do not demonstrably retard this process,[60, 61] it is possible that more-stringent T-depletion may delay the kinetics of immune reconstitution.[30] Similarly, although the incidence of infectious complications has not been increased in most series, removal of virus-specific donor memory cells may leave the host more susceptible to secondary lymphoproliferative disorders induced by Epstein-Barr virus.[62]

DETRIMENTAL EFFECTS OF GRAFT T CELLS: ACUTE GRAFT-VERSUS-HOST DISEASE

Studies in human and animal models clearly identify T lymphocytes as the causative agent of GVHD.[63] Thus, the presence of mature allogeneic lymphocytes ($3–5 \times 10^9$ in the average marrow graft, up to tenfold more in a PBPC graft) provide the rationale for T-depletion. Despite chemo-prophylactic regimens, clinically significant GVHD (clinical stage 2 or higher) occurs in 45% of recipients of HLA-identical sibling marrow and 75% of recipients of HLA-mismatched grafts.[64] GVHD ranks above infection and leukemia relapse as the leading cause of treatment failure. Elimination of T cells from the graft has markedly reduced the incidence and severity of acute and chronic GVHD. Reviews of the international literature have estimated that the incidence of acute GVHD has been reduced to 10–11% in recipients of T cell–depleted HLA-matched marrow grafts.[64, 65] Significant reductions have also occurred in matched unrelated transplants, especially when molecular HLA disparities not detectable by serology were present.[66] Discussions of GVHD can be found in Chapters 39, 45, and 54.

EFFECT OF LYMPHOCYTE DOSE ON GRAFT-VERSUS-HOST DISEASE

In its modern form, the clonal selection theory posits that the generation of T-cell antigen specificity occurs at random

through rearrangement of the genes encoding the T-cell receptor (TCR). Selective clonal expansion occurs when T cells with a useful specificity (i.e., an antigen receptor that recognizes foreign peptide in the context of self-MHC) encounters its cognate antigen and simultaneously receives costimulation by specialized antigen-presenting cells. Through this mechanism, a T cell bearing unique receptor specificity is clonally expanded such that its progeny constitute a detectable proportion of circulating T cells. Because alloreactive cells are present at relatively high frequency even in unprimed persons and because these cells proliferate on contact with antigen, it is not surprising that a steep dose-response relationship exists between the number of graft T cells and the incidence and severity of GVHD.

Studies performed using elutriation for T-cell depletion permitted T cells to be added back to the graft at a known dose. T-cell depletion to 1.0×10^6 lymphocytes/kg (approximately 8×10^5 T cells/kg)[67] resulted in acute GVHD (all stages) in 19 of 39 evaluable patients (49%); 5 (13%) experienced organ GVHD ($\geq$stage 2) and 8 experienced chronic GVHD. A further 50% reduction in lymphocyte dose to 0.5×10^6/kg[25] resulted in a remarkable decrease in the incidence and severity of GVHD (15% for all stages). No patients died from acute GVHD or experienced organ (stage 2 or higher) or chronic GVHD.

Application of the same technique in the matched unrelated donor setting resulted in a much higher incidence of acute GVHD (3 of 10 stage 2 or higher).[26] In patients who received matched unrelated donor grafts T-cell depleted with the monoclonal antibody T10B9 plus complement, both the frequency and dose of host-specific cytotoxic lymphocyte precursors (CTLp) were associated with severe acute GVHD and chronic GVHD. Even after adjustment for covariates such as known HLA disparity, CTLp frequency remained associated with survival, and the frequency of host-specific helper T-lymphocyte precursors was associated with the incidence of chronic GVHD.[68] T-cell depletion followed by CD34+ cell selection offers 4 logs or greater of T-depletion (with total T-cell doses in the range of a million or less). Although available data were scarce, the results of Aversa et al. indicate that this level of depletion may completely eliminate GVHD, even in haplo-mismatched transplantation.[30]

At the opposite end of the dose-response spectrum, greatly increased T-cell dose, such as that obtained with T-replete HLA-matched allogeneic PBPC grafts, does not appear to greatly increase the incidence or severity of acute GVHD over that observed with T-replete bone marrow grafts. This has been demonstrated both in animal models[69] and in human models.[70] Thus, the dose-response relationship for acute GVHD appears to rise sharply at low T-cell doses and plateau at higher doses. In contrast with acute GVHD, follow-up studies reveal a distinct increase in the incidence of chronic GVHD in recipients of allogeneic PBPC grafts.[71–73] Thus, it appears likely that T-cell depletion, quantitative or partial, may come to play a role in allogeneic PBPC transplants if they are to be used to their full potential.

In addition to major and minor histocompatibility disparities, two additional factors that appear to influence the T cell–GVHD dose-response relationship are (1) acute tissue damage and cytokine release associated with the conditioning regimen and (2) the short-term persistence of host immune cells and antigen-presenting cells. In a dose-escalation trial performed in patients with CML in relapse after allogeneic HSCT, GVHD developed in only one of eight patients who received an infusion of 10×10^6 donor T cells/kg. In contrast, 8 of 11 patients who received a T-cell dose of at least 50×10^6 T cells/kg experienced GVHD.[74] This indicates that the T cell–acute GVHD dose-response curve may be shifted by as much as an order of magnitude after the acute injuries incident to transplantation have resolved.

RISK VS. BENEFIT

The present generation of T cell–depletion methods has surpassed regimens relying on chemoprophylaxis alone in its ability to eliminate acute GVHD as a cause of transplant mortality in the matched sibling setting. Further, it has succeeded where other approaches have failed in significantly reducing the incidence and severity of chronic GVHD, a prominent cause of late treatment failure. Reduction of these complications through allograft T-cell depletion should, in theory, significantly improve the success rate of allogeneic HSCT and expand the donor pool. Unfortunately, clinical experience with T-cell depletion has demonstrated the positive roles played by graft T cells in facilitation of engraftment, elimination of residual leukemia, and transfer of donor immune memory. In many trials conducted to date, the loss of these beneficial effects has offset the advantages of GVHD ablation to the extent that, in the aggregate, disease-free survival in T cell–depleted and T cell–replete allogeneic HSCT has been similar.[65]

Despite this apparent stalemate, there appear to be particular indications for which T-cell depletion can provide a significant advantage. For example, the risk of severe GVHD is particularly high in unrelated donor marrow transplantation.[75] Recognizing this, the National Heart, Lung, and Blood Institute has sponsored a multicenter randomized trial to determine whether "a reduction in GVHD can be achieved without a counterbalancing increase in graft failure and relapse of leukemia in patients receiving an unrelated-donor marrow transplant."[76]

Patients enrolled in this study are randomized to receive T cell–depleted or unmanipulated marrow. Two methods of T-cell depletion, elutriation with CD34+ cell add-back and treatment with the monoclonal antibody T10B9 (anti–T cell receptor α/β) plus complement, are being evaluated. Enrollment is projected at 560 patients with a median follow-up time of 3 years. Study end-points include disease-free survival, incidence and severity of acute and chronic GVHD, infection, graft failure, and relapse. In addition to these clinical end-points, extensive laboratory data, including studies of graft composition, chimerism, and immune reconstitution, are being collected. Although results are not yet available, the completion of this trial should provide a definitive answer concerning the advisability of T-cell depletion in the unrelated-donor setting.

The use of parental haploidentical donors has long been recognized as another potentially important indication for T-depletion. Finally, in diseases wherein the graft-versus-

leukemia effect appears to be less prominent, such as AML treated with HSCT in remission, T-depletion may provide a net benefit even in the setting of HLA-matched sibling transplantation.

THE FUTURE OF T-CELL DEPLETION: ACHIEVING A BALANCE

Most trials performed to date have eliminated T cells *en masse* without regard to functional characteristics, maturational stage, or antigen specificity. In the first generation of trials, the degree of T-depletion was limited by the available technology. The most recent studies show that virtually absolute T-cell depletion may be obtained while maintaining relatively high CD34+ cell dose. A second generation of trials attempted to surmount T-cell depletion–related complications by reintroducing a fixed T-cell dose to the graft or by excluding specific lymphocyte subsets.[9] Although the ability to substantially overcome the obstacles of GVHD and graft rejection are important accomplishments, currently available methods are an approximation of the ultimate goal, which is to formulate a product that reliably and rapidly engrafts, demonstrates enhanced antitumor and antimicrobial activity, and is tolerant of the host.

It is clear that successful allograft engineering requires that the HSC dose be maximized. This approach promises to hasten engraftment and reduce the incidence of rejection. It may also obviate the need for more-radical forms of peritransplantation immunosuppression, such as total lymphoid irradiation and administration of antithymocyte globulin. Although HSC may be increased in the future through ex vivo expansion (see Chapter 32), the use of PBPC in preference to bone marrow can increase the progenitor cell dose in T-depleted grafts by as much as an order of magnitude. Regarding the optimal degree of T-cell depletion, it has also become increasingly evident that the question is no longer how many logs of T cells should be removed, but how many of which types of T cells should be given back, and when. Once engraftment has been achieved without GVHD, the goal is to prevent relapse and viral and fungal infections by hastening T-cell and B-cell reconstitution.

The premise of T-cell add-back requires quantitative T-depletion as a starting point; the technology is now available to routinely obtain in excess of 4 logs of depletion. T cells for add-back could then be selected on the basis of surface marker expression, antigen specificity as detected by peptide-MHC tetramer binding capacity,[77] or ex vivo expansion after exposure to specific antigens.[78] In terms of infusing polyclonal T cells or T-cell subsets, the literature on donor lymphocyte infusion is instructive and indicates that donor T cells are better tolerated after the patient has healed from cytoreductive therapy. Timing of the infusion may be less critical when antigen-specific T-cell clones are selectively expanded and infused. The first success of such a strategy was achieved in the context of T-replete allogeneic HSCT when infusion of cytomegalovirus-specific donor-derived T cells were shown to transfer cytomegalovirus-specific cell-mediated immunity to the graft recipient.[79] In addition to transferring donor-derived antimicrobial responses, donor T cells specific for tumor antigens such as bcr-abl,[80] lymphoma idiotype,[81] or Epstein-Berr virus antigens expressed on Reed-Sternberg cells[82] could be given as adjunctive therapy after transplantation with a T-depleted graft. Similarly, T cells reactive to minor histocompatibility determinants present on host-derived hematopoietic cells, but not other tissues, may mediate the graft-vs.-leukemia effect without accompanying GVHD.[83]

The tools and procedures for successful allograft engineering are largely in place. The key will be to find more practical and cost-effective means for their implementation so that GVHD can be eliminated, engraftment and immune reconstitution can be hastened, and the donor pool can be expanded.

CONCLUSION

Mature T lymphocytes can be successfully removed from allogeneic bone marrow or PBPC grafts. Active T cell depletion methods include separation using size and density differences (elutriation) or surface characteristics (agglutination and rosetting) and immunologic identification (monoclonal antibody directed against T cell markers together with solid substrate or complement-mediated lysis). T lymphocytes can also be passively depleted by selecting for CD34+ HSC. Various commercial systems are available or in different stages of clinical development for CD34+ cell selection. The level of T cell depletion in the active and passive methods is adequate to reduce GVHD. However, the poor yield of HSC (generally ~50%) is a major concern for the manipulation. Newer selection systems may decrease the loss of HSC. Although the incidence and severity of GVHD is reduced, patients receiving T cell–depleted HSCT are at higher risk for graft failure and disease relapse. In the future, with more advanced cell selection procedures, it may be possible to engineer allografts such that patients will initially receive a sufficient quantity of HSC and T cells (or subpopulation) to achieve engraftment with donor cells without severe GVHD. Infusions of donor lymphocytes (or subpopulations of lymphocytes, with or without activation) can be administered later to enhance antitumor effects and to prevent rejection.

REFERENCES

1. Reisner Y, Kapoor N, Kirkpatrick D, et al: Transplantation for acute leukemia with HLA-A and B nonidentical parental marrow cells fractionated with soybean agglutinin and sheep red blood cells. Lancet 2:327–331, 1981.
2. Braine HG, Sensenbrenner LL, Wright SK, et al: Bone marrow transplantation with major ABO blood group incompatibility using erythrocyte depletion of marrow prior to infusion. Blood 60:420–425, 1982.
3. Filipovich AH, McGlave PB, Ramsay NK, et al: Pretreatment of donor bone marrow with monoclonal antibody OKT3 for prevention of acute graft-versus-host disease in allogeneic histocompatible bone-marrow transplantation. Lancet 1:1266–1269, 1982.
4. Hale G, Bright S, Chumbley G, et al: Removal of T cells from bone marrow for transplantation: a monoclonal antilymphocyte antibody that fixes human complement. Blood 62:873–882, 1983.
5. Mitsuyasu RT, Champlin RE, Gale RP, et al: Treatment of donor bone marrow with monoclonal anti-T-cell antibody and complement for the prevention of graft-versus-host disease: a prospective, randomized, double-blind trial. Ann Intern Med 105:20–26, 1986.
6. Patterson J, Prentice HG, Brenner MK, et al: Graft rejection following

   HLA matched T-lymphocyte depleted bone marrow transplantation. Br J Haematol 63:221–230, 1986.
7. Racadot E, Herve P, Beaujean F, et al: Prevention of graft-versus-host disease in HLA-matched bone marrow transplantation for malignant diseases: a multicentric study of 62 patients using 3-pan-T monoclonal antibodies and rabbit complement. J Clin Oncol 5:426–435, 1987.
8. Filipovich AH, Vallera DA, Youle RJ, et al: Graft-versus-host disease prevention in allogeneic bone marrow transplantation from histocompatible siblings: a pilot study using immunotoxins for T cell depletion of donor bone marrow. Transplantation 44:62–69, 1987.
9. Champlin R, Ho W, Gajewski J, et al: Selective depletion of CD8+ T lymphocytes for prevention of graft-versus-host disease after allogeneic bone marrow transplantation. Blood 76:418–423, 1990.
10. Soiffer RJ, Ritz J: Selective T cell depletion of donor allogeneic marrow with anti-CD6 monoclonal antibody: rationale and results. Bone Marrow Transplant 12(Suppl 3):S7–S10, 1993.
11. Drobyski WR, Ash RC, Casper JT, et al: Effect of T-cell depletion as graft-versus-host disease prophylaxis on engraftment, relapse, and disease-free survival in unrelated marrow transplantation for chronic myelogenous leukemia. Blood 83:1980–1987, 1994.
12. Cottler-Fox M, Cipolone K, Yu M, et al: Positive selection of CD34+ hematopoietic cells using an immunoaffinity column results in T cell-depletion equivalent to elutriation. Exp Hematol 23:320–322, 1995.
13. Colter M, Jones M, Heimfeld S: CD34+ progenitor cell selection: clinical transplantation, tumor cell purging, gene therapy, ex vivo expansion, and cord blood processing. J Hematother 5:179–184, 1996.
14. Fujimori Y, Kanamaru A, Hashimoto N, et al: Second transplantation with CD34+ bone marrow cells selected from a two-loci HLA-mismatched sibling for a patient with chronic myeloid leukaemia. Br J Haematol 94:123–125, 1996.
15. Reisner Y, Kapoor N, Kirkpatrick D, et al: Transplantation for severe combined immunodeficiency with HLA-A, B, D, DR incompatible parental marrow cells fractionated by soy bean agglutinin and sheep red blood cells. Blood 61:341–348, 1983.
16. Gao IK, Noga SJ, Wagner JE, et al: Implementation of a semiclosed large scale counterflow centrifugal elutriation system. J Clin Apheresis 3:154–160, 1987.
17. de Witte T, Hoogenhout J, de Pauw B, et al: Depletion of donor lymphocytes by counterflow centrifugation successfully prevents acute graft-versus-host disease in matched allogeneic marrow transplantation. Blood 67:1302–1308, 1986.
18. Donnenberg AD, Neudorf SML, Pople M, et al: Sequential elutriation enhances CD34 yield of T-depleted bone marrow. Blood 90(Suppl 1):350b, 1997.
19. Sutherland DR, Anderson L, Keeney M, et al: The ISHAGE guidelines for CD34+ cell determination by flow cytometry. International Society of Hematotherapy and Graft Engineering. J Hematother 5:213–226, 1996.
20. Morrison SJ, Uchida N, Weissman IL: The biology of hematopoietic stem cells. Ann Rev Cell Dev Biol 11:35–71, 1995.
21. Weaver CH, Hazelton B, Birch R, et al: An analysis of engraftment kinetics as a function of the CD34 content of peripheral blood progenitor cell collections in 692 patients after the administration of myeloablative chemotherapy. Blood 86:3961–3969, 1995.
22. Watts MJ, Jones HM, Sullivan AM, et al: Accessory cells do not contribute to G-CSF or IL-6 production nor to rapid haematological recovery following peripheral blood stem cell transplantation. Br J Haematol 91:767–772, 1995.
23. Kernan NA, Bordignon C, Heller G, et al: Graft failure after T-cell-depleted human leukocyte antigen identical marrow transplants for leukemia: I. Analysis of risk factors and results of secondary transplants. Blood 74:2227–2236, 1989.
24. Papadopoulos EB, Carabasi MH, Castro-Malaspina H, et al: T-cell-depleted allogeneic bone marrow transplantation as postremission therapy for acute myelogenous leukemia: freedom from relapse in the absence of graft-versus-host disease. Blood 91:1083–1090, 1998.
25. Wagner JE, Donnenberg AD, Noga SJ, et al: Lymphocyte depletion of donor bone marrow by counterflow centrifugal elutriation: results of a phase I clinical trial. Blood 72:1168–1176, 1988.
26. Neudorf SM, Rybka W, Ball E, et al: The use of counterflow centrifugal elutriation for the depletion of T cells from unrelated donor bone marrow. J Hematother 6:351–359, 1997.
27. Gaines BA, Colson YL, Kaufman CL, Ildstad S: Facilitating cells enable

engraftment of purified fetal liver stem cells in allogeneic recipients. Exp Hematol 24:902–913, 1996.

28. Uchida N, Aguila HL, Fleming WH, et al: Rapid and sustained hematopoietic recovery in lethally irradiated mice transplanted with purified Thy-1.1lo Lin-Sca-1+ hematopoietic stem cells. Blood 83:3758–3779, 1994.

29. Bachar-Lustig E, Rachamim N, Li HW, et al: Megadose of T cell-depleted bone marrow overcomes MHC barriers in sublethally irradiated mice. Nature Med 1:1268–1273, 1995.

30. Aversa F, Tabilio A, Velardi A, et al: Treatment of high-risk acute leukemia with T-cell-depleted stem cells from related donors with one fully mismatched HLA haplotype. N Engl J Med 339:1186–1193, 1998.

31. Lansdorp PM: Stem cell biology for the transfusionist. Vox Sanguin 74 (Suppl 2):91–94, 1998.

32. Messner HA: Assessment and characterization of hemopoietic stem cells. Stem Cells 13(Suppl 3):13–18, 1995.

33. Goodell MA, Rosenzweig M, Kim H, et al: Dye efflux studies suggest that hematopoietic stem cells expressing low or undetectable levels of CD34 antigen exist in multiple species. Nature Med 3:1337–1345, 1997.

34. Uchida N, Combs J, Chen S, et al: Primitive human hematopoietic cells displaying differential efflux of the rhodamine 123 dye have distinct biological activities. Blood 88:1297–1305, 1996.

35. Lapointe C, Forest L, Lussier P, et al: Sequential analysis of early hematopoietic reconstitution following allogeneic bone marrow transplantation with fluorescence in situ hybridization (FISH). Bone Marrow Transplant 17:1143–1148, 1996.

36. Dreger P, Viehmann K, Steinmann J, et al: G-CSF-mobilized peripheral blood progenitor cells for allogeneic transplantation: comparison of T cell depletion strategies using different CD34+ selection systems or CAMPATH-1. Exp Hematol 23:147–154, 1995.

37. Noga SJ, Vogelsang GB, Seber A, et al: CD34+ stem cell augmentation of allogeneic, elutriated marrow grafts improves engraftment but cyclosporine A is still required to reduce GVHD and morbidity. Transplant Proc 29:728–732, 1997.

38. Chang Q, Harvey K, Akard L, et al: Counterflow centrifugal elutriation as a method of T cell depletion may cause loss of immature CD34+ cells. Bone Marrow Transplant 19:1145–1150, 1997.

39. Wagner JE, Collins D, Fuller S, et al: Isolation of small, primitive human hematopoietic stem cells: distribution of cell surface cytokine receptors and growth in SCID-Hu mice. Blood 86:512–523, 1995.

40. Zwemer RK, Schmittling RJ, Russell TR: A simple and rapid method for removal of specific cell populations from whole blood. J Immunol Method 198:199–202, 1996.

41. Paulus U, Schmitz N, Viehmann K, et al: Combined positive/negative selection for highly effective purging of PBPC grafts: towards clinical application in patients with B-CLL. Bone Marrow Transplant 20:415–420, 1997.

42. Roots-Weiss A, Papadimitriou C, Serve H, et al: The efficiency of tumor cell purging using immunomagnetic CD34+ cell separation systems. Bone Marrow Transplant 19:1239–1246, 1997.

43. Hohaus S, Pforsich M, Murea S, et al: Immunomagnetic selection of CD34+ peripheral blood stem cells for autografting in patients with breast cancer. Br J Haematol 97:881–888, 1997.

44. Farley TJ, Ahmed T, Fitzgerald M, Preti RA: Optimization of CD34+ cell selection using immunomagnetic beads: implications for use in cryopreserved peripheral blood stem cell collections. J Hematother 6:53–60, 1997.

45. Kvalheim G, Pharo A, Holte H, et al: High-dose therapy of cancer with CD34 positive cells as stem cell support. Tidsskrift for Den Norske Laegeforening 116:2542–2546, 1996.

46. Handgretinger R, Greil J, Schurmann U, et al: Positive selection and transplantation of peripheral CD34+ progenitor cells: feasibility and purging efficacy in pediatric patients with neuroblastoma. J Hematother 6:235–242, 1997.

47. Bertolini F, Thomas T, Battaglia M, et al: A new "two step" procedure for 4.5 log depletion of T and B cells in allogeneic transplantation and of neoplastic cells autologous transplantation. Bone Marrow Transplant 19:615–619, 1997.

48. Hassan HT, Zeller W, Stockschlader M, et al: Comparison between bone marrow and G-CSF-mobilized peripheral blood allografts undergoing clinical scale CD34+ cell selection. Stem Cells 14:419–429, 1996.

49. Johnson RJ, Owen RG, Smith GM, et al: Peripheral blood stem cell transplantation in myeloma using CD34 selected cells. Bone Marrow Transplant 17:723–727, 1996.

50. Bohbot A, Feugeas O, Cuillerot JM, et al: Peripheral blood CD34+ cells: method of purification and ex vivo expansion. Nouv Rev Francaise Hematol 37:359–365, 1995.

51. Papadimitriou CA, Roots A, Koenigsmann M, et al: Immunomagnetic selection of CD34+ cells from fresh peripheral blood mononuclear cell preparations using two different separation techniques. J Hematother 4:539–544, 1995.

52. Lane TA, Law P, Maruyama M, et al: Harvesting and enrichment of hematopoietic progenitor cells mobilized into the peripheral blood of normal donors by granulocyte-macrophage colony-stimulating factor (GM-CSF) or G-CSF: potential role in allogeneic marrow transplantation. Blood 85:275–282, 1995.

53. Reisner Y, Martelli MF: Bone marrow transplantation across HLA barriers by increasing the number of transplanted cells. Immunol Today 16:437–440, 1995.

54. Marks DI, Hughes TP, Szydlo R, et al: HLA-identical sibling donor bone marrow transplantation for chronic myeloid leukaemia in first chronic phase: influence of GVHD prophylaxis on outcome. Br J Haematol 81:383–390, 1992.

55. Kolb HJ, Holler E: Adoptive immunotherapy with donor lymphocyte transfusions. Curr Opin Oncol 9:139–145, 1997.

56. Hessner MJ, Endean DJ, Casper JT, et al: Use of unrelated marrow grafts compensates for reduced graft-versus-leukemia reactivity after T-cell-depleted allogeneic marrow transplantation for chronic myelogenous leukemia. Blood 86:3987–3996, 1995.

57. Donnenberg AD, Hess AD, Duff SC, et al: Regeneration of genetically restricted immune functions following human marrow transplantation: influence of four different strategies for graft-versus-host disease (GVHD) prophylaxis. Transplant Proc 19(Suppl. 7):144–152, 1987.

58. Drummond JE, Shah KV, Saral R, et al: BK virus specific humoral and cell mediated immunity in allogeneic bone marrow transplant (BMT) recipients. J Med Virol 23:331–344, 1987.

59. Wimperis JZ, Brenner MK, Prentice HG, et al: Transfer of a functioning humoral immune system in transplantation of T-lymphocyte-depleted bone marrow. Lancet 1:339–343, 1986.

60. Keever CA, Small TN, Flomenberg N, et al: Immune reconstitution following bone marrow transplantation: comparison of recipients of T-cell depleted marrow with recipients of conventional marrow grafts. Blood 73:1340–1350, 1989.

61. Bär BMAM, Santos GW, Donnenberg AD: Reconstitution of antibody response following allogeneic BMT: effect of lymphocyte depletion by counterflow centrifugal elutriation (CCE) on the expression of hemagglutinins. Blood 76:1410–1418, 1990.

62. Zutter MM, Martin PJ, Sale GE, et al: Epstein-Barr virus lymphoproliferation after bone marrow transplantation. Blood 72:520–529, 1988.

63. Billingham RE: The biology of graft-versus-host reactions. In The Harvey Lectures, vol 62. New York, Academic Press, 1966, pp 21–78.

64. Butturini A, Gale RP: T cell depletion in bone marrow transplantation for leukemia: current results and future directions. Bone Marrow Transplant 3:185–192, 1988.

65. Poynton CH: T cell depletion in bone marrow transplantation. Bone Marrow Transplant 3:265–279, 1988.

66. Gajewski J, Gjertson D, Cecka M, et al: The impact of T-cell depletion on the effects of HLA DR beta 1 and DQ beta allele matching in HLA serologically identical unrelated donor bone marrow transplantation. Biol Blood Marrow Transplant 3:76–82, 1997.

67. Wagner JE, Donnenberg AD, Noga SJ, et al: Lymphocyte depletion of bone marrow by counterflow centrifugal elutriation: results of a phase I clinical trial. Blood 72:1168–1176, 1988.

68. Keever-Taylor CA, Passweg J, Kawanishi Y, et al: Association of donor-derived host-reactive cytolytic and helper T cells with outcome following alternative donor T cell-depleted bone marrow transplantation. Bone Marrow Transplant 19:1001–1009, 1997.

69. Glass B, Uharek L, Zeis M, et al: Allogeneic peripheral blood progenitor cell transplantation in a murine model: evidence for an improved graft-versus-leukemia effect. Blood 90:1694–1700, 1997.

70. Bensinger WI, Clift R, Martin P, et al: Allogeneic peripheral blood stem cell transplantation in patients with advanced hematologic malignancies: a retrospective comparison with marrow transplantation. Blood 88:2794–2800, 1996.

71. Storek J, Gooley T, Siadak M, et al: Allogeneic peripheral blood stem cell transplantation may be associated with a high risk of chronic graft-versus-host disease. Blood 90:4705–4709, 1997.

72. Scott MA, Gandhi MK, Jestice HK, et al: A trend towards an increased incidence of chronic graft-versus-host disease following allogeneic peripheral blood progenitor cell transplantation: a case controlled study. Bone Marrow Transplant 22:273–276, 1998.

73. Harada M, Shinagawa K, Kawano T, et al: Allogeneic peripheral blood stem cell transplantation for standard-risk leukemia: a multicenter pilot study: Japanese experience. Japan Blood Cell Transplantation Study Group. Bone Marrow Transplant 21(Suppl 3):S54–S56, 1998.

74. Mackinnon S, Papadopoulos EB, Carabasi MH, et al: Adoptive immunotherapy evaluating escalating doses of donor leukocytes for relapse of chronic myeloid leukemia after bone marrow transplantation: separation of graft-versus-leukemia responses from graft-versus-host disease. Blood 86:1261–1268, 1995.

75. Kernan NA, Bartsch G, Ash RC, et al: Analysis of 462 transplantations from unrelated donors facilitated by the National Marrow Donor Program. N Engl J Med 328:593–602, 1993.

76. Howe C, Wagner J, Kernan N, et al: T-cell depletion in unrelated-donor marrow transplantation. Blood 86(Suppl 1):391a, 1995.

77. Altman JD, Moss PAH, Goulder PJR, et al: Phenotypic analysis of antigen-specific T lymphocytes. Science 274:94–96, 1996.

78. Yee C, Riddell SR, Greenberg PD: Prospects for adoptive T cell therapy. Curr Opin Immunol 9:702–708, 1997.

79. Walter EA, Greenberg PD, Gilbert MJ, et al: Reconstitution of cellular immunity against cytomegalovirus in recipients of allogeneic bone marrow by transfer of T-cell clones from the donor. N Engl J Med 333:1038–1044, 1995.

80. Chen W, Qin H, Reese VA, Cheever MA: CTLs specific for bcr-abl joining region segment peptides fail to lyse leukemia cells expressing p210 bcr-abl protein. J Immunother 21:257–268, 1998.

81. Casper CB, Levy S, Levy R: Idiotype vaccines for non-Hodgkin's lymphoma induce polyclonal immune responses that cover mutated tumor idiotypes: comparison of different vaccine formulations. Blood 90:3699–3706, 1997.

82. Sing AP, Ambinder RF, Hong DJ, et al: Isolation of Epstein-Barr virus (EBV)-specific cytotoxic T lymphocytes that lyse Reed-Sternberg cells: implications for immune-mediated therapy of EBV+ Hodgkin's disease. Blood 89:1978–1986, 1997.

83. Warren EH, Greenberg PD, Riddell SR: Cytotoxic T-lymphocyte–defined human minor histocompatibility antigens with a restricted tissue distribution. Blood 91:2197–2207, 1998.

CHAPTER THIRTY-ONE

Immunomodulation After Transplantation

Kenneth R. Meehan, M.D., Udit N. Verma, M.D., and Amitabha Mazumder, M.D.

The graft-versus-tumor (GVT) effect following allogeneic hematopoietic stem cell transplantation (HSCT) suggests that immune mechanisms are important for eradication of residual disease in the recipient.[1–3] Graft-versus-host disease (GVHD) contributes to a GVT effect and reduces relapse rates compared with the situation in patients receiving autologous HSCT (autoHSCT).[1] The lack of a GVT effect after autoBMT, along with reinfusion of clonogenic tumor cells within the autologous graft, may contribute to the increased relapse rate.[4] Because of the nonhematologic dose-limiting toxicity of current autoHSCT preparative regimens, innovative therapeutic modalities are needed. Post-transplantation immunotherapy is an attractive strategy.

Both tumor-*specific* and -*nonspecific* immunotherapeutic approaches to cancer therapy have been evaluated in experimental models and clinical trials. Definition of oncogenes and their products and the discovery of antigenic molecules on tumor cells that are either aberrantly expressed or products of mutated genes have paved the way for differentiating the malignant cell from "self."[5–9] These discoveries have renewed interest in tumor-specific immunotherapy.

This chapter reviews laboratory and clinical immunotherapy for solid tumors and hematologic malignancies in the HSCT setting.

NONSPECIFIC IMMUNOTHERAPY

Immune defense mechanisms involve cells and cytokines. The critical cells involved in the body's innate defense mechanism include macrophages, non–major histocompatibility complex (MHC)-restricted killer cells of either natural killer (NK) cell or T-cell origin, and activated NK or lymphokine-activated killer (LAK) cells. In addition, cytokines secreted by these cells, including interferon-γ (IFN-γ) and tumor necrosis factor (TNF), demonstrate potent antitumor activity. Manipulations of the cellular or cytokine immune mechanisms have been attempted, including (1) in vitro activation of lymphoid cells with cytokines, antibodies, or lectins; (2) in vivo administration of cytokines to generate antitumor effector cells; and (3) a combination of these two approaches.[10–16] Because results were encouraging in the nontransplant setting in patients with melanoma and renal cell carcinoma, these approaches are being evaluated for use in the period that follows both allogeneic and autologous HSCT.[17]

GVHD and GVT effects are caused by immunocompetent cells contained in the graft that recognize major or minor histocompatibility antigens on recipient cells.[18–21] Although the mechanism of GVHD is uncertain, clinical trials have been designed to generate GVT activity by infusing various cytokines (interleukin-2 [IL-2], IFN) or cells (donor-specific leukocytes) after autologous or allogeneic HSCT (as is discussed later).[3, 22] It is conceivable that the induction of autologous GVHD after autoHSCT may lead to preferential lysis of tumor cells and a GVT effect.[23–25]

Most clinical trials of the post-HSCT period have focused on nonspecific immunotherapy and are discussed in the following paragraphs.

INTERLEUKIN-2 WITH OR WITHOUT LYMPHOKINE-ACTIVATED KILLER CELLS

Human IL-2 is primarily secreted by T cells and acts via a specific IL-2 receptor consisting of α, β, and γ subunits.[26, 27] In addition to T-cell proliferation, IL-2 leads to activation and proliferation of NK cells and increases their tumoricidal activity and augments B-cell growth and immunoglobulin production.[28] IL-2 also enhances IFN-γ and TNF-β production from T cells, IL-6 production by monocytes, modulation of histamine release by basophils, and enhanced expression of the IL-2 receptor.

The antitumor activity of IL-2 may be due to the induction of endogenous LAK activity and elaboration of tumor inhibitory cytokines such as IFN-γ and TNF.[32] LAK cells, generated when peripheral blood mononuclear cells are incubated with IL-2, lyse a variety of tumor cells both in vitro and in vivo in an MHC-unrestricted manner.[28, 29] LAK cell activity resides in activated NK cells, with variable contributions from T cells and other cell types.[30] Administration of LAK cells has demonstrated efficacy in several experimental models and clinical trials, particularly in patients with renal cell carcinoma and melanoma.[31] The administration of IL-2 with or without LAK cell infusion is being evaluated in autologous and allogeneic transplantation (results are summarized later). Murine studies suggest that IL-2 therapy is most effective in a situation of low tumor burden.[33] Because minimal residual disease status follows transplantation, HSCT offers an attractive setting for evaluation of IL-2 therapy.

Autologous Hematopoietic Stem Cell Transplantation

IL-2 administration improves immunologic function directly by the induction of cellular changes and indirectly by stimulating the release of cytokines.[34, 35] Normally, after HSCT, endogenous NK cells appear in 4–6 weeks. These cells are highly responsive to IL-2 both in vitro and in vivo.[36] During IL-2 therapy, circulating lymphocytes exhibit increased spontaneous activity against NK-sensitive and NK-resistant tumor targets and inhibit autologous leukemic blast growth in vitro.[37] IL-2 incubation of lymphocytes collected after IL-2 administration has resulted in the generation of potent antitumor effector cells.[38] In addition to inducing changes in the cellular immune compartment, IL-2 results in the secretion of cytokines, most importantly IFN-γ and TNF, both possessing antitumor effects.[39] The administration of IL-2 to patients undergoing autoHSCT induces the expression of messenger RNA (mRNA) for granulocyte macrophage colony-stimulating factor, IL-3, IL-4, and IL-6 in mononuclear cells, which could result in proliferation of myeloid precursors.[40]

IL-2 alters the reactivity of the autologous lymphocytes regenerating after autoHSCT. The administration of IL-2 and LAK cells after autoHSCT resulted in infiltration of T cells in the skin with histologic changes consistent with cutaneous GVHD.[41] It is possible that this reaction in the autoHSCT setting reflects the induction of a GVT phenomenon.

Clinical trials using IL-2 after autoHSCT have reported similar hematologic effects, including a modest drop in hemoglobin levels, a dose-related increase in circulating neutrophils, and, occasionally, eosinophilia.[37, 38, 42–44] A slight fall in circulating lymphocytes occurs, followed by a significant rise persisting above baseline levels for several days to weeks after discontinuation of IL-2.[37, 38] Some studies have shown an increase in both CD4+ and CD8+ lymphocytes, whereas others have observed a greater increase in CD8+ than in CD4+ lymphocyte populations.[42] Prolonged infusion of low-dose IL-2 can significantly increase the number of circulating NK cells with no significant effect on the numbers of CD3 cells.[43–45]

Early reports suggested that IL-2 alone administered after autoHSCT induced responses in patients with advanced malignancies.[46] Since then, results from several phase I/II clinical trials have been published.[37–43] Although the dose and schedule of IL-2 therapy in these trials varied, results suggest that low doses of IL-2 therapy were well tolerated. At moderate to high dosages, toxicity was common but manageable, with similar side effects observed in the nontransplant settings. There was initial concern that IL-2 after HSCT would delay engraftment because bone marrow progenitor cell activity can be suppressed by LAK cells in vitro.[47] Subsequently, the absence of harmful effects of IL-2 and LAK cells on bone marrow growth has been confirmed.[48, 49] Most clinical trials, however, have employed IL-2 therapy after the engraftment following transplantation.

Gottlieb et al. administered IL-2 to patients with acute myeloid leukemia or multiple myeloma in a phase I dose-escalation study.[37] IL-2 was started at 1.5×10^6 IU/m²/day, with doubling of the dose every 48 hours, until the maximum tolerated dose was reached. When IL-2 therapy was started immediately after HSCT, severe toxicity resulted, requiring cessation of treatment. In subsequent patients, IL-2 infusion was initiated after neutrophil engraftment. Mild to moderate toxicity was observed, with hypotension being the dose-limiting toxicity. Blaise et al. administered IL-2 to 10 patients undergoing autoHSCT for various hematologic malignancies and solid tumors.[38] IL-2 was administered at 18×10^6 IU/m²/day (3×10^6 Cetus units/m²/day) as a continuous infusion for 6 days, beginning 79 days (median) after HSCT. Moderate toxicity occurred in all patients and involved the skin, gastrointestinal tract, and liver but was well tolerated. Changes in hemodynamic parameters necessitated cessation of treatment on a few occasions, yet 91% of the planned dosage are administered with no toxic deaths. Although this was a small study with limited follow-up, five patients were in continuous complete response (CR) at 8–10 months after HSCT.

Higuchi et al. examined immunologic changes induced by IL-2 in 16 patients undergoing autoHSCT for hematologic malignancy.[42] IL-2 was administered at a dose of 0.3×10^6 to 4.5×10^6 Hoffman La Roche Units (RU) (specific activity, 1.2–1.5 units/mg protein)/m²/day as a continuous infusion for 5 days beginning 33 days (median) posttransplant. After 5 days of rest, a 10-day maintenance course (0.3×10^6 RU/m²/day) was administered. Most patients experienced mild to moderate dose-related toxicity, including fever, rash, nausea, diarrhea, dyspnea, and weight gain with rapid reversal after completion of treatment. There were no treatment-related deaths, and all patients received the prescribed IL-2 maintenance therapy. Nine of the 16 patients were in continuous CR 7–23 months after HSCT.

Soiffer et al. have examined immunologic changes with prolonged infusion of low-dose IL-2 with the aim of producing a GVT effect after autoHSCT for various hematologic and solid tumor malignancies.[43] IL-2 was initiated several months after HSCT at a dose of 2×10^5 RU/m²/day as a continuous intravenous infusion for 90 days. Toxicity was mild and included rash, dyspnea, weight gain, and hypothyroidism. Sixty-nine percent of the patients completed the full course of therapy, and most experienced immunologic changes suggestive of a GVT effect in vitro. Weisdorf et al. evaluated IL-2 instituted immediately after autoHSCT in 14 patients with acute lymphoblastic leukemia (ALL).[44] IL-2 was started as a continuous IV infusion (0.5–2.0×10^6 RU/m²/day) for 4 days each week for 3 weeks. Ten patients received IL-2 therapy as planned; 4 were removed because of fever or respiratory distress. Overall, patients treated with IL-2 experienced a shorter hospital stay (median, 38 days) compared with a control group of similar patients not receiving IL-2 (median, 63 days). Two of 14 patients died of toxicity attributed to IL-2 therapy, however.

The combination of IL-2 and LAK cell therapy has also been evaluated. Some laboratory and clinical studies demonstrate a greater antitumor response when IL-2 and LAK cells are combined.[31, 45, 50] Significant endogenous LAK cell activity can be generated only when *high doses* of parenteral IL-2 are administered. Unfortunately, these doses are toxic and poorly tolerated. Animal studies confirm that the increase in cure rate achieved by high-dose IL-2 therapy (attempting to generate in vivo LAK activity) is offset by increased toxic mortality.[50] In the transplant setting, animal models show that a combination of IL-2 and LAK cells may suppress engraftment and induces a GVT effect in a syngeneic model of HSCT for acute myeloid leukemia.[33] Thus, treatment with a combination of IL-2 and LAK cells may be effective in eradicating minimal residual disease and reducing relapse rates after autoHSCT.

Sixteen patients with malignant lymphoma undergoing autoHSCT received IL-2 with or without LAK cells.[15, 42] IL-2 was administered 51 days (median) after transplantation. Five of 16 patients underwent leukapheresis on days 6–8 after initial IL-2 therapy (3×10^6 RU/m²/day for 5 days). Lymphocytes were incubated with IL-2 for 5 days to generate LAK cells. A median of 136×10^9 LAK cells were infused into patients on days 12–14, and low-dose IL-2 (3×10^5 RU/m²/day) was administered on days 12–21. LAK cell infusions were well tolerated with transient fever, rigors, and dyspnea. Eleven patients remained in CR up to 21 months after HSCT. Another study evaluated the feasibility of IL-2 alone or in combination with LAK cells after autoHSCT for patients with acute myeloid leukemia.[13] Toxicities were comparable to those of previous trials.[15, 42] Of the 14 patients treated in this trial, 10 remained in continuous CR for 13–48 months. This trial also analyzed the results of IL-2 alone or with LAK cells after autoHSCT in 14 patients with acute myeloid leukemia.[13] One patient died during IL-2 therapy, but 10 patients remained in CR at 34 months (median). The actuarial probability of relapse was 23% and the probability of survival was 71%, far superior to the rates with historical control patients undergoing autoHSCT without IL-2.

Allogeneic Hematopoietic Stem Cell Transplantation

Administration of IL-2 after alloHSCT can lead to exacerbation of GVHD by expansion and maintenance of allosensitized T cells and possibly NK cells. In experimental models, *delayed* institution of IL-2 treatment after alloHSCT potentiates GVHD.[51, 52] *Early* institution (on the day of transplantation) nullifies GVHD, possibly by preventing sensitization of unprimed alloreactive T cells.[53, 54] Although the mechanisms responsible for modulation of GVHD by IL-2 are poorly understood, the induction of veto cell activity in the host may be responsible. Veto cells suppress the generation of cytotoxic T lymphocytes in an MHC-specific manner with MHC specificity determined by the antigens expressed on the surface of veto cells. LAK cells can mediate veto activity and thus can potentially reduce the incidence and severity of GVHD in alloHSCT.[55] IL-2 therapy after transplantation with T cell–depleted allogeneic bone marrow enhances veto activity in a mouse model.[56] Interestingly, this reduction in GVHD by post-transplant IL-2 therapy is not associated with a reduction in GVT effect induced by allogeneic T cells.[53, 54, 57]

Delayed administration of IL-2 (4 months after alloHSCT) in a patient with neuroblastoma led to reactivation of GVHD. Cessation of IL-2 therapy and treatment with corticosteroids resulted in rapid resolution of GVHD.[46] More recently, low doses of IL-2 after alloHSCT with T cell–depleted bone marrow were administered to patients with hematologic malignancies.[43, 58] IL-2 was initiated after engraftment and continued over 3 months by continuous intravenous infusion. Toxicity was mild and consisted of fever, hypotension, nausea, vomiting, and weight gain. No patient experienced GVHD. The increase in the lymphocyte

population was due to an increase in NK cell number from 15% to 70% during therapy. These cells exhibited potent activity against both NK-sensitive and NK-resistant tumor targets. The antitumor activity of these cells rapidly fell to baseline levels after cessation of IL-2 therapy. Relapse and disease-free survival rates were determined in the 25 patients who completed at least 4 weeks of IL-2 treatment. Compared with historical control patients who did not have a history of GVHD, the patients treated with IL-2 had a lower risk of relapse (hazard ratio, 0.34; range, 0.14–0.82) and superior disease-free survival rates (hazard ratio, 0.39; range, 0.18–0.87).[58] These observations suggest a possible benefit of IL-2 therapy after alloHSCT.

IL-2 WITH IL-2–ACTIVATED BONE MARROW OR PERIPHERAL BLOOD PROGENITOR CELL GRAFTS

The autograft lacks the GVT effect that plays a critical role in eradication of minimum residual disease or in maintaining tumor dormancy in alloHSCT.[4, 59–61] The importance of the GVHD and its associated GVT effects is corroborated by the fact that patients experiencing allogeneic GVHD have a lower probability of relapse, possibly from a "heightened" immune system.[62]

Autologous grafts do not have the immune capabilities of allogeneic bone marrow. Therefore, innovative strategies aimed at inducing a GVT effect are needed. Our group has demonstrated that when autologous bone marrow is incubated with IL-2 in vitro, significant antitumor activity results.[33, 63] This IL-2 "activation" of marrow results in a purging effect of the marrow and generates cytotoxic effector cells, which may mediate a GVT effect in vivo.[49] Thus, IL-2 incubation of the bone marrow is a potential approach to therapy that might decrease relapse rates after autoHSCT.

When murine and human bone marrow are incubated with IL-2, potent cytotoxic effector T cells are generated.[49, 63–66] These effector cells, like LAK cells, lyse a wide variety of both NK-sensitive and NK-resistant tumor cell targets in an MHC-unrestricted manner. The cytolytic activity of these cells was found to be superior to LAK cells and was maintained for longer periods of time.[63, 66] The in vivo antitumor efficacy of activated bone marrow was evident in a murine melanoma model when IL-2-incubated bone marrow infusion followed by IL-2 treatment led to regression of pulmonary metastasis of chemoradiotherapy-resistant melanoma (B16) and methylcholanthrene (MCA) tumors in mice.[63, 66] Subsequently, similar observations were made in murine acute myeloid leukemia models.[33, 64] These studies demonstrated that transplantation with IL-2-activated bone marrow combined with post-transplant IL-2 treatment was associated with significant antitumor responses. Results were inferior with the administration of IL-2 after transplantation with unmanipulated fresh bone marrow or with transplantation with IL-2-activated bone marrow alone without post-transplant IL-2.

In a comparable set of in vivo experiments, splenic LAK cells demonstrated far less antitumor efficacy than did IL-2–activated bone marrow cells.[67] Further studies suggested that tumor eradication was obtained when IL-2 was instituted immediately post transplant in a state of minimum residual disease.[64] The superior antitumor effects with IL-2–activated marrow and post-transplant administration of IL-2 may be due to effectors primed in vitro with a high dose of IL-2. These "effector cells" can maintain their cytotoxic potential in vivo with low serum levels of IL-2, which can be achieved without undue toxicity.[68] The combination of IL-2–activated bone marrow infusion and low-dose IL-2 after autologous transplantation has the advantage of mediating antitumor responses immediately after transplantation in a condition of low tumor burden.[69, 70] The early institution of IL-2 may be necessary for in vivo survival and expansion of these antitumor effector T cells.

In addition to the generation of cytotoxic effector cells that may mediate a GVT effect in vivo, the eradication of contaminating tumor cells in the graft and the maintenance of hematopoietic reconstitution ability are critically important for successful application of this strategy. Both of these parameters were evaluated using human and murine bone marrow. Short-term culture of bone marrow with IL-2 was associated with significant clearing of contaminating leukemic cells without loss of hematopoietic precursors.[49]

We have shown that cytotoxic effector cells generated by IL-2 in long-term culture (1–3 weeks) lyse a variety of tumor cell lines in vitro.[71] Prolonging the duration of IL-2 exposure in culture leads to a progressive increase in cytotoxicity. The number of hematopoietic precursors declines after 7 days, however, with the number of normal hematopoietic clonogenic cells highest at 7 days. These results indicated that marrow cultured for 7 days with IL-2 can be successfully used for transplantation. In a model of in vitro purging, IL-2 incubation in long-term culture successfully purged marrow of 10% of contaminating tumor cells. Studies using bone marrow from patients with chronic myelogenous leukemia indicate that such long-term culture with IL-2 leads to eradication of Philadelphia chromosome positive (Ph+) metaphases.[71] The feasibility of long-term culture of bone marrow autografts with IL-2 with the aim of achieving purging and generation of cytotoxic effectors has also been demonstrated by Klingemann et al.[72, 73] Earlier, several groups demonstrated that LAK cells preferentially lyse contaminating neoplastic cells present in bone marrow and that these LAK cells can be used for in vitro purging.[48, 74] IL-2 activation of marrow provides a possible advantage over LAK cell purging because it is a single-step procedure and leads to generation of effector cells that may mediate in vivo reactivity against tumor in the presence of low-dose IL-2.

Because autologous peripheral blood progenitor cell (PBPC) transplantation results in faster hematopoietic recovery and may reduce the risk of contamination by tumor cells compared with marrow, we evaluated IL-2 activation of PBPC.[75–77] We examined the capacity of chemotherapy and growth factor–mobilized PBPC to generate antitumor cytotoxic effector cells when cultured with IL-2 in vitro.[78, 79] IL-2 activation of mobilized PBPC from patients with different neoplastic disorders led to the generation of potent cytotoxic effector cells without loss of hematopoietic progenitors. Further experiments showed that the cytotoxicity achieved using growth factor–mobilized PBPC was equal to or higher than that achieved using bone marrow.

Based on our preclinical studies, phase I/II clinical trials are in progress at our center in patients with hematologic malignancies and solid tumors to evaluate the feasibility of administering IL-2–activated autografts after high-dose chemoradiotherapy.

Sixty-one patients with breast cancer have undergone transplantation with PBPC mobilized with rhG-colony-stimulating factor and chemotherapy (either cyclophosphamide or paclitaxel).[24, 25] The patient population consisted of patients with high-risk stage 2 (n = 20), stage 3 (n = 16), and stage 4 disease (n = 25). Ten of 61 patients had resistant disease at the time of transplantation, with the remaining patients demonstrating responsive disease. After high-dose chemotherapy with carboplatin and cyclophosphamide, PBPC incubated for 24 hours with IL-2 were reinfused. IL-2 administration was initiated on the day of transplantation (day 0) at escalating doses and increasing duration. The initial five patients received only IL-2–activated PBPC, whereas subsequent patients received IL-2 initially at a starting dose of 6×10^5 IU/m²/day beginning on day 0.

Rapid hematopoietic reconstitution occurred in all patients, with 11.5 days (mean) required for the absolute neutrophil count to reach 0.5×10^9/L for 3 days and 11.7 days (mean) for the platelet count to be maintained at 20×10^9/L for 3 days.

The combination of IL-2–activated PBPC transplantation with systemic IL-2 therapy was associated with prevalent but tolerable side effects. Not all of the toxic effects could be attributed to IL-2 alone and may have resulted from the combination of chemotherapy and IL-2.[80] One patient died during hospitalization from a nontraumatic cerebral bleed. In general, the prevalence and severity of toxicity was associated with increasing doses and duration of IL-2.[81] The maximal tolerated dose was 6×10^5 IU/m²/day administered for 5 of 7 days each week for 4 weeks.

A unique and interesting phenomenon included skin findings suggestive of autologous GVHD. Although these data are being evaluated, findings suggestive of autologous skin GVHD manifesting as a diffuse erythematous rash were observed (stage 2 GVHD) and documented pathologically. The rash improved within days of discontinuing the IL-2, and no patient required therapy.

Follow-up is too short to determine the possible impact of IL-2-activated PBPC transplantation on relapse and survival in these patients. The clinical outcomes, including overall and disease-free survival for the various stages of breast cancer, are comparable to the results in the literature. Two patients with refractory disease, one patient with stage 3A disease and one patient with stage 4 disease, were disease free at 38 + and 14 + months after transplantation, respectively. Additional interesting findings include clinical and histologic findings suggestive of autologous GVHD, successful hematopoietic reconstitution, and tolerable toxicity. These results suggest successful alteration of immune status with this regimen. It remains to be determined whether these immunologic effects will translate into clinical benefit due to a possible associated autologous GVT effect. These initial results with IL-2–activated PBPC, however, clearly demonstrate the feasibility of such an approach. Similar studies are currently evaluating this therapy in patients with hematologic malignancies.

INTERFERONS AFTER TRANSPLANTATION

In addition to a direct cytotoxic effect on tumor cells, INF act through cytokine mediators.[82] For example, cell surface expression on tumor cells, including integrins and MHC molecules, is regulated by IFN-γ.[83, 84] IFN-α and IFN-γ act either alone or with IL-2 as potent inducers of cytolytic activity of NK cells. Enhanced expression of MHC antigens results in increased immunogenicity of tumor cells, possibly mediated by improved antigen presentation by tumor cells. Unfortunately, IFN inhibit hematopoietic progenitor cell proliferation.[85] Therefore, in most of transplantation trials, IFN therapy is instituted after engraftment.[86]

Autologous Transplantation

Several small, nonrandomized studies using IFN-α after autoHSCT have been performed in patients with hematologic malignancies.[87–93] The dose of IFN varied from 1 to 3 × 10[6] U/day for 3–7 days each week starting at hematologic reconstitution. Mild constitutional symptoms and occasional thrombocytopenia occurred. Neloni et al. reported their results with use of IFN-α in 34 patients with chronic myelogenous leukemia (CML) who underwent transplantation during chronic phase.[94] After a median follow-up of 13 months, 12 of 12 patients who previously received IFN and 19 of 22 previously untreated patients were in CR. In another study, 13 patients with CML in chronic phase and 2 patients in accelerated phase or blast crisis were treated with IFN-α after autoHSCT.[91] Five of eight patients in first chronic phase were in complete hematologic remission after 8–19 months, whereas two of seven patients in second chronic phase or accelerated/blastic phase were in complete hematologic remission after more than 16 months. Ascensao et al. reported results of IFN-α therapy in 58 patients with non-Hodgkin lymphoma or Hodgkin disease.[95] After minimal follow-up of 19 months, the overall survival rate was 83% with event-free survival at 64%. Attal et al. reported a progression-free survival rate of 53% at 33 months post HSCT in patients with multiple myeloma treated with IFN.[93]

These results indicate that IFN-α can be used safely after autoHSCT. In the absence of large controlled randomized trials, however, valid conclusions regarding the efficacy of treatment cannot be reached.

Allogeneic Transplantation

In allogeneic HSCT, IFN-α therapy has been used in patients with CML in combination with donor lymphocyte infusion (discussed later). Meyers et al. evaluated IFN-α in patients with acute lymphoblastic leukemia.[96] Treatment was instituted after engraftment and continued for 80 days after transplantation. This led to a significant reduction in relapse rate at 4 years.

CYCLOSPORIN-INDUCED AUTOLOGOUS GVHD

Glazier et al. described the development of syngeneic GVHD after syngeneic or autologous transplantation in rats after a brief course of cyclosporin.[97] This autologous-immune phenomenon of cyclosporin-induced GVHD has been studied extensively. Cytotoxic lymphocytes circulating in these animals with GVHD lyse tumor cells expressing the Ia[+] antigens.[98] Various tumor cells express class II MHC antigens. In some malignancies, MHC expression can be induced by the administration of IFN. Tumor cells expressing class II MHC molecules can thus be susceptible to lysis by autoreactive lymphocytes induced by post-transplant cyclosporin therapy.[98, 99] This technique of inducing GVHD is being evaluated in clinical trials in an attempt to obtain GVHD and GVT effects after autoHSCT.[100, 101] Cyclosporin has been evaluated in phase I/II trials in patients with metastatic breast cancer, lymphoma, CML, and acute non-lymphocytic leukemia in dosages of 1–3.75 mg/kg/day from day 0 to day 28. Most of the patients treated with cyclosporin had evidence of grade I–II cutaneous GVHD without visceral GVHD. Decreased relapse and improved disease-free survival rates have been reported in a study of 14 patients with non-Hodgkin lymphoma compared with historical controls.[102] It is difficult to draw conclusions about the antitumor effect of this mode of therapy, although preliminary results appear promising.

DONOR LYMPHOCYTE INFUSION

The GVL effect of alloHSCT is dependent on mature T cells contained within allogeneic grafts. In an effort to induce GVHD and thus augment the GVL effect in patients experiencing relapse after transplantation, researchers have infused peripheral blood mononuclear cells from the original donors into patients experiencing relapsed CML with promising results.[103] Helg et al. reported successful reinduction of complete hematologic, cytogenetic, and molecular remission in two patients experiencing relapse who were in chronic stable phase at initiation of leukocyte infusions and IFN-α therapy.[104] A third patient was treated in accelerated phase and died with bone marrow aplasia after donor lymphocyte infusion (DLI). Similar results were reported by others.[3]

In a limited number of clinical trials in patients with hematologic malignancies other than CML, results with DLI have not been as impressive. These results have been confirmed in a multicenter trial in patients with CML, acute myeloid leukemia (AML), polycythemia vera, myelodysplastic syndrome (MDS) (myelodysplasia), and ALL.[103] The best results occurred in patients with CML when DLI was administered in early cytogenetic or hematologic relapse. Of the evaluable 67 patients with CML, 53 patients achieved complete remission. Results were poor if DLI was started in the accelerated or transformed stage of the disease. No remissions were induced in 22 patients with ALL; CR was observed in 29% of patients with AML (n = 17) and 25% of patients with MDS (n = 4). Considerable toxicity was associated with DLI, the most common being GVHD and bone marrow aplasia. In this study, 59% of all patients receiving DLI experienced GVHD. Myelosuppression was a common side effect, and 50% of patients with CML who were in hematologic relapse with mixed chimerism experienced myelosuppression. In contrast, patients with cytogenetic relapses or with chemotherapy-induced remission were less prone to this effect. This suggests that myelosuppression in these patients may be the result of suppression of recipient-derived hematopoiesis. Six deaths were attributable to myelosuppression, and four other patients died of combined myelosuppression and GVHD. In most patients, myelosuppression reversed spontaneously or after a boost with donor marrow. Other studies have reported similar side effects. It remains to be determined whether the infusion of donor cells and the resultant immune response selectively suppress the neoplastic clone or whether recipient-derived hematopoietic cells are indiscriminately eliminated.

TUMOR-SPECIFIC IMMUNOTHERAPY

Tumor-specific immunotherapy has been attempted by several investigators.[105–110] Vaccines consisting of irradiated autologous or allogeneic tumor cells, tumor cell lysates, or purified tumor antigens in combination with immunologic adjuvants have been used in tumor-specific immunotherapy in the nontransplant setting with encouraging results in patients with melanoma, colon cancer, and lung cancer.[5, 111–114]

Preclinical data and anecdotal clinical reports indicate that some tumors are immunogenic and that systemic antitumor immunity plays a role in eradication or control of the tumor growth or metastasis. Cancer patients may have B and T cells that recognize antigens expressed by autologous tumor cells, including products of mutated oncogenes and various differentiation antigens.[115] Although most of these antigens are expressed on normal cells, aberrant expression on tumor tissues, due to either quantitative or qualitative alterations, makes these tumors immunogenic.[111] Despite a detectable immune response against autologous tumor cells, progression of the malignancy can be explained by inherently weak immunogenicity of tumor antigens.[111] Studies in experimental models, however, suggest that even weakly immunogenic cancers can be rejected by the host's immune response after effective immunization.[116, 117]

Several methods can enhance the immunogenicity of tumor cells, including culturing tumor cells with IFN-γ to up-regulate MHC molecules and transfecting malignant cells with genes of co-stimulatory molecules and various cytokines, including IL-2 and IFN-γ.[84, 108, 113, 117–119] All of these strategies have resulted in enhancement of tumor cells' immunogenic potential. One encouraging finding has been that antitumor immunity induced by modified tumor cells extends to wild-type tumors as well.[120] Host factors may be important determinants of the outcome of immunization, especially in the context of immunotherapy. Immunosuppression in tumor-bearing hosts can be the result of several known factors, such as a defective CD3 complex in T cells, elaboration of cytokines such as transforming growth factor (TGF)-β, and other undefined factors.[121, 122] Because the magnitude of immunosuppression parallels the tumor burden, the chances of success with immunotherapy are improved if applied in a state of minimum residual disease, such as after transplantation.[123] Several other variables associated with transplantation may enhance the success of immunotherapy, including elimination of suppressor cells and disruption of architectural integrity of residual tumor by the conditioning regimen, thus making tumor cells more susceptible to damage by immune effector mech-

anisms. The phenomenon of general immune suppression associated with HSCT may be a potential concern, however. In most of the studies addressing immune status after autologous transplantation, nonspecific functions of T and B cells have been evaluated that are likely to be influenced by the overwhelming majority of de novo differentiating lymphocytes.[124, 125] In contrast, there are reports of successful transfer of immunity to different viral and bacterial antigens by transplantation, suggesting "carryover" memory cells.[126, 127] Furthermore, immunity can be boosted by post-transplant immunization.[128] Interestingly, when antitumor immunity is evaluated, animals that received lethal irradiation demonstrate higher resistance to tumor after transplantation than do normal mice.[129] In addition, the occurrence of a GVT effect with GVHD suggests that, despite immunosuppression associated with HSCT, effective antitumor immune mechanisms are operative.

Kwak et al. demonstrated the transfer of humoral anti-idiotypic response with resultant protective immunity to a murine B cell tumor.[130] Our results in B16 murine melanoma suggest that antitumor immunity can be successfully transferred by HSCT. Mice undergoing transplantation with immune-stimulated bone marrow reject fresh tumor, and in tumor-bearing animals this leads to a potent antitumor effect. Our preliminary results in the same model suggest that bone marrow from animals that are not fully immune to the tumor elicit more potent immunity in secondary recipients after HSCT. Thus, HSCT may present an ideal situation for the application of tumor-specific immunotherapy. In addition, there is the possibility of in vitro manipulation of bone marrow before reinfusion into the host to augment induced immune responses by procedures such as in vitro sensitization.

Despite these possible advantages associated with application of immunotherapeutic strategies after transplantation, efforts have been limited. Currently, no published results evaluate tumor-specific immunotherapy with autoHSCT. In 1992, Kwak et al. reported successful transfer of myeloma idiotype-specific immunity from an actively immunized bone marrow donor.[131] A normal sibling bone marrow donor was immunized with two doses of myeloma immunoglobulin G (idiotype) conjugated to keyhole limpet hemocyanin (KLH) and emulsified in an adjuvant. Tumor-specific immunity in the form of lymphoproliferative responses was noted in the recipient at 30 and 60 days after transplantation. A CD4 + cell line of donor origin was developed from the recipient's peripheral blood mononuclear cells, and this cell line proliferated in response to immunizing antigen. The patient was clinically well with a stable M component 2 years after transplantation. The report suggests that it may be possible to transfer tumor-specific immunity by HSCT. These results, in conjunction with earlier work in experimental models, should provide the basis for future evaluation of this strategy in large clinical trials.

REFERENCES

1. Barrett AJ, Horowitz MM, Gale RP, et al: Marrow transplantation for acute lymphoblastic leukemia: factors affecting relapse and survival. Blood 74:862–871, 1989.
2. Champlin R: Graft-versus-leukemia without graft-versus-host dis-

ease: an elusive goal of bone marrow transplantation. Semin Hematol 29:46–52, 1992.

3. Porter DL, Roth MS, McGarigle C, et al: Induction of graft-versus-host disease as immunotherapy for relapsed chronic myeloid leukemia. N Engl J Med 330:100–106, 1994.

4. Brenner MK, Rill DR, Moen RC, et al: Gene-marking to trace origin of relapse after autologous bone-marrow transplantation. Lancet 341:85–86, 1993.

5. Quan WD Jr, Mitchell MS: Immunology and immunotherapy of melanoma. Cancer Treat Res 65:257–277, 1993.

6. Morton DL: Active immunotherapy against cancer: present status. Semin Oncol 13:180–185, 1986.

7. Wang RF, Robbins PF, Kawakami Y, et al: Identification of a gene encoding a melanoma tumor antigen recognized by HLA-A31-restricted tumor-infiltrating lymphocytes. J Exp Med 181:799–804, 1995.

8. Bernhard H, Karbach J, Wolfel T, et al: Cellular immune response to human renal-cell carcinomas: definition of a common antigen recognized by HLA-A2-restricted cytotoxic T-lymphocyte (CTL) clones. Int J Cancer 59:837–842, 1994.

9. Van der Bruggen P, Bastin J, Gajewski T, et al: A peptide encoded by human gene mage-3 and presented by HLA-A2 induces cytolytic T lymphocytes that recognize tumor cells expressing MAGE-3. Eur J Immunol 24:3038–3043, 1994.

10. Whittington R, Faulds D: Interleukin-2: a review of its pharmacological properties and therapeutic use in patients with cancer. Drugs 46:446–514, 1993.

11. Ghosh AK, Cerny T, Wagstaff J, et al: Effect of in vivo administration of interferon gamma on expression of MHC products and tumor associated antigens in patients with metastatic melanoma. Eur J Cancer Clin Oncol 1989, 25:1637–1643, 1989.

12. Hirte HW, Clark DA, O'Connell G, et al: Reversal of suppression of lymphokine-activated killer cells by transforming growth factor-beta in ovarian carcinoma ascitic fluid requires interleukin-2 combined with anti-CD3 antibody. Cell Immunol 142:207–216, 1992.

13. Benyunes MC, Massumoto C, York A, et al: Interleukin-2 with or without lymphokine-activated killer cells as consolidative immunotherapy after autologous bone marrow transplantation for acute myelogenous leukemia. Bone Marrow Transplant 12:159–163, 1993.

14. Simpson C, Seipp CA, Rosenberg SA: The current status and future applications of interleukin-2 and adoptive immunotherapy in cancer treatment. Semin Oncol Nurs 4:132–141, 1988.

15. Fefer A, Benyunes M, Higuchi C, et al: Interleukin-2 ± -lymphocytes as consolidative immunotherapy after autologous bone marrow transplantation for hematologic malignancies. Acta Haematol 89(Suppl 1):2–7, 1993.

16. Pavletic Z, Benyunes MC, Thompson JA, et al: Induction by interleukin-7 of lymphokine-activated killer activity in lymphocytes from autologous and syngeneic marrow transplant recipients before and after systemic interleukin-2 therapy. Exp Hematol 21:1371–1378, 1993.

17. Rosenberg SA: Immunotherapy of cancer using interleukin 2: current status and future prospects. Immunol Today 9:58–62, 1988.

18. Champlin R: T-cell depletion for allogeneic bone marrow transplantation: impact on graft-versus-host disease, engraftment, and graft-versus-leukemia. J Hematother 2:27–42, 1993.

19. Bron D: Graft-versus-host disease. Curr Opin Oncol 6:358–364, 1994.

20. Noga SJ, Hess AD: Lymphocyte depletion in bone marrow transplantation: will modulation of graft-versus-host disease prove to be superior to prevention? Semin Oncol 20:28–33, 1993.

21. Champlin R: Immunobiology of bone marrow transplantation as treatment for hematologic malignancies. Transplant Proc 23:2123–2127, 1991.

22. Boiron JM, Cony-Makhoul P, Mahon FX, et al: Treatment of hematological malignancies relapsing after allogeneic bone marrow transplantation. Blood Rev 8:234–240, 1994.

23. Kennedy MJ, Vogelsang GB, Jones RJ, et al: Phase I trial of interferon gamma to potentiate cyclosporine-induced graft-versus-host disease in women undergoing autologous bone marrow transplantation for breast cancer. J Clin Oncol 12:249–257, 1994.

24. Meehan KR, Rajagopal C, Verma UN, et al: Biological and clinical correlates of interleukin-2 administration in peripheral blood stem cell transplantation for breast cancer. Blood 86:389a, 1995.

25. Meehan KR, Verma UN, Rajagopal C, et al: Stem cell transplantation

with high dose chemoradiotherapy and interleukin-2. J Infus Chemother 6:28–32, 1995.

26. Smith KA: Interleukin-2: inception, impact, and implications. Science 240:1169–1176, 1988.

27. Waldmann TA, Pastan IH, Gansow OA, Junghans RP: The multichain interleukin-2 receptor: a target for immunotherapy. Ann Intern Med 116:148–160, 1992.

28. Grimm EA, Mazumder A, Zhang HZ, Rosenberg SA: Lymphokine-activated killer cell phenomenon: lysis of natural killer–resistant fresh solid tumor cells by interleukin 2–activated autologous human peripheral blood lymphocytes. J Exp Med 155:1823–1841, 1982.

29. Lotze MT, Grimm EA, Mazumder A, et al: Lysis of fresh and cultured autologous tumor by human lymphocytes cultured in T-cell growth factor. Cancer Res 41:4420–4425, 1986.

30. Chadwick BS, Miller RG: Heterogeneity of the lymphokine-activated killer cell phenotype. Cell Immunol 132:168–176, 1991.

31. Rosenberg SA, Lotze MT, Yang JC, et al: Experience with the use of high-dose interleukin-2 in the treatment of 652 cancer patients. Ann Surg 210:474–484, 1989.

32. Rosenberg SA: Karnofsky memorial lecture: the immunotherapy and gene therapy of cancer. J Clin Oncol 10:180–199, 1992.

33. Charak BS, Brynes RK, Groshen S, et al: Bone marrow transplantation with interleukin-2-activated bone marrow followed by interleukin-2 therapy for acute myeloid leukemia in mice. Blood 76:2187–2190, 1990.

34. Bosly AE, Staquet PJ, Doyen CM, et al: Recombinant human interleukin-2 restores in vitro T-cell colony formation by peripheral blood mononuclear cells after autologous bone marrow transplantation. Exp Hematol 15:1048–1054, 1987.

35. Borradori L, Hirt A, Baumgartner C, Morell A: Influence of exogenous interleukin-2 on the proliferation of lymphocytes from normal donors and from patients after autologous bone marrow transplantation. Acta Haematol 77:129–134, 1987.

36. Reittie JE, Gottlieb D, Heslop HE, et al: Endogenously generated killer cells circulate after autologous and allogeneic bone marrow transplantation but not after chemotherapy. Blood 73:1341–1358, 1989.

37. Gottlieb DJ, Brenner MK, Heslop HE, et al: A phase I clinical trial of recombinant interleukin 2 following high dose chemo-radiotherapy for haematological malignancy: applicability to the elimination of minimal residual disease. Br J Cancer 60:610–615, 1989.

38. Blaise D, Olive D, Stoppa AM, et al: Hematologic and immunologic effects of the systemic administration of recombinant interleukin-2 after autologous bone marrow transplantation. Blood 76:1092–1097, 1990.

39. Heslop HE, Gottlieb DJ, Bianchi ACM, et al: In vivo induction of γ interferon and tumor necrosis factor by interleukin-2 infusion following intensive chemotherapy or autologous bone marrow transplantation. Blood 74:1374–1380, 1989.

40. Heslop HE, Bello-Fernandez C, Reittie JE, et al: Interleukin 2 infusion after autologous bone marrow transplantation or chemotherapy enhances hematopoietic regeneration [Abstract]. Blood 76(Suppl 1):544a, 1990.

41. Massumoto C, Sale G, Benyunes M, et al: Cutaneous GVHD associated with IL-2 + LAK therapy after autologous bone marrow transplantation (ABMT) for hematologic malignancies [Abstract]. Proc Am Soc Clin Oncol 11:825a, 1992.

42. Higuchi CM, Thompson JA, Petersen FB, et al: Toxicity and immunomodulatory effects of interleukin-2 after autologous bone marrow transplantation for hematologic malignancies. Blood 77:2561–2568, 1991.

43. Soiffer RJ, Murray C, Cochran K, et al: Clinical and immunologic effects of prolonged infusion of low-dose recombinant interleukin-2 after autologous and T-cell-depleted allogeneic bone marrow transplantation. Blood 79:517–526, 1992.

44. Weisdorf DJ, Anderson PM, Blazar BR, et al: Interleukin 2 immediately after autologous bone marrow transplantation for acute lymphoblastic leukemia-a phase I study. Transplantation 55:61–66, 1993.

45. Papa MZ, Mule JJ, Rosenberg SA: Antitumor efficacy of lymphokine-activated killer cells and recombinant interleukin 2 in vivo: successful immunotherapy of established pulmonary metastases from weakly immunogenic and nonimmunogenic murine tumors of three district histological types. Cancer Res 46:4973–4978, 1986.

46. Favrot MC, Floret D, Negrier S, et al: Systemic interleukin-2 therapy in children with progressive neuroblastoma after high dose chemo-

therapy and bone marrow transplantation. Bone Marrow Transplant 4:499–503, 1989.

47. Fujimori Y, Hara H, Nagai K: Effect of lymphokine activated killer cell fraction on the development of human hematopoietic progenitor cells. Cancer Res 48:534–538, 1987.

48. van den Brink MRM, Voogt PJ, Marijt WAF, et al: Lymphokine activated killer cells selectively kill tumor cells in bone marrow without compromising bone marrow stem cell function in vitro. Blood 74:354–560, 1989.

49. Charak BS, Malloy B, Agah R, Mazumder A: A novel approach to purging of leukemia by activation of bone marrow with interleukin-2. Bone Marrow Transplant 6:193–198, 1990.

50. Peace DJ, Cheever MA: Toxicity and therapeutic efficacy of high-dose interleukin 2: in vivo infusion of antibody to NK-1.1 attenuates toxicity without compromising efficacy against murine leukemia. J Exp Med 169:161–173, 1989.

51. Sprent J, Schaefer M, Gao EK, Korngold R: Role of T cell subsets in lethal graft-versus-host disease (GVHD) directed to class I versus class II H-2 differences: I. L3T4+ cells can either augment or retard GVHD elicited by Lyt-2+ cells in class I different hosts. J Exp Med 167:556–569, 1988.

52. Malkovsky M, Brenner MK, Hunt R, et al: T-cell depletion of allogeneic bone marrow prevents acceleration of graft-versus-host disease induced by exogenous interleukin 2. Cell Immunol 103:476–480, 1986.

53. Sykes M, Abraham BS, Harty MW, Pearson DA: IL-2 reduces graft-versus-host disease and preserves a graft-versus-leukemia effect by selectively inhibiting CD4+ T cell activity. J Immunol 150:197–205, 1993.

54. Sykes M, Harty MW, Szot GL, Pearson DA: Interleukin-2 inhibits graft versus host disease promoting activity of CD4+ cells while preserving CD4− and CD8− mediated graft versus leukemia effects. Blood 83:2560–2569, 1994.

55. Azuma E, Kaplan J: Role of lymphokine-activated killer cells as mediators of veto and natural suppression. J Immunol 141:2601–2606, 1988.

56. Nakamura H, Gress RE: Interleukin-2 enhancement of veto suppressor cell function in T-cell-depleted bone marrow in vitro and in vivo. Transplantation 49:931–937, 1990.

57. Sykes M, Romick ML, Sachs DH: Interleukin-2 prevents graft-versus-host disease while preserving the graft-versus-leukemia effect of allogeneic T cells. Proc Natl Acad Sci U S A 87:5633–5637, 1990.

58. Soiffer RJ, Murray C, Gonin R, Ritz J: Effect of low-dose interleukin-2 on disease relapse after T-cell-depleted allogeneic bone marrow transplantation. Blood 84:964–971, 1994.

59. Gribben JG, Freedman AS, Neuberg D, et al: Immunological purging of marrow assessed by PCR before autologous bone marrow transplantation for B cell lymphoma. N Engl J Med 325:1525–1533, 1991.

60. Ringden O, Horowitz MM: Graft-versus-leukemia reactions in humans: the Advisory Committee of the International Bone Marrow Transplant Registry. Transplant Proc 21:2989–2992, 1989.

61. Truitt RL, Horowitz MM, Atasoylu AA, et al: Graft-versus-leukemia effect of allogeneic bone marrow transplantation: clinical and experimental aspects of late leukemia relapse. In Stewart THM, Wheelock EF (eds): Cellular Immune Mechanisms and Tumor Dormancy. Boca Raton, FL, CRC Press, 1992, pp 111–128.

62. Horowitz MM, Gale RP, Sondel PM, et al: Graft-versus-leukemia reactions after bone marrow transplantation. Blood 75:555–562, 1990.

63. Agah R, Malloy B, Kerner M, Mazumder A: Generation and characterization of IL-2 activated bone marrow cells as a potent graft versus tumor effector in transplantation. J Immunol 143:3039–3099, 1989.

64. Charak BS, Brynes RK, Katsuda S, et al: Induction of graft versus leukemia effect in bone marrow transplantation: dosage and time schedule dependency of interleukin 2 therapy. Cancer Res 51:2015–2020, 1991.

65. Charak BS, Agah R, Gray D, Mazumder A: Interaction of various cytokines with interleukin-2 in the generation of killer cells from human bone marrow: application in purging of leukemia. Leuk Res 15:801–810, 1991.

66. Keever CA, Pekle K, Gazzola MV, et al: NK and LAK activities from human bone marrow progenitors: I. The effects of interleukin-2 and interleukin-1. Cell Immunol 126:211–226, 1990.

67. Agah R, Malloy B, Kerner M, et al: Potent graft antitumor effect in natural killer–resistant disseminated tumors by transplantation of interleukin-2-activated syngeneic bone marrow in mice. Cancer Res 49:5959–5963, 1989.

68. Lotze MT, Matory YL, Ettinghausen SE, et al: In vivo administration of purified human interleukin-2: half life, immunologic effects, and expansion of peripheral lymphoid cells in vivo with recombinant IL-2. J Immunol 135:2865–2875, 1985.

69. Kedar E, Klein E: Cancer Immunotherapy: are the results discouraging? can they be improved? Adv Cancer Res 59:245–322, 1992.

70. Mitchell MS: Combining chemotherapy with biological response modifiers in the treatment of cancer. J Natl Cancer Inst 80:1445–1450, 1988.

71. Verma UN, Bagg A, Brown E, Mazumder A: Interleukin-2 activation of human bone marrow in long term cultures: an effective strategy for purging and generation of anti-tumor cytotoxic effectors. Bone Marrow Transplant 13:115–123, 1994.

72. Klingemann HG, Deal H, Reid D, Eaves CJ: Pre-clinical evaluation of a bone marrow autograft culture procedure for generating lymphokine-activated killer cells in vitro. Can J Infect Dis 3:123B–127B, 1992.

73. Klingemann HG, Deal H, Reid D, Eaves CJ: Design and validation of a clinically applicable culture procedure for the generation of interleukin-2 activated natural killer cells in human bone marrow autografts. Exp Hematol 21:1263–1270, 1993.

74. Long GS, Cramer DV, Harnaha JB, Hiserodt JC: Lymphokine-activated killer (LAK) cell purging of leukemic bone marrow: range of activity against different hematopoietic neoplasms. Bone Marrow Transplant 6:169–177, 1990.

75. Chao N, Schriber J, Grimes K, et al: Granulocyte colony-stimulating factor "mobilized" peripheral blood progenitor cells accelerate granulocyte and platelet recovery after high dose chemotherapy. Blood 81:2031–2035, 1993.

76. Kessinger A, Armitage JO: The evolving role of autologous peripheral stem cell transplantation following high-dose therapy for malignancies. Blood 77:211–213, 1991.

77. Kessinger A, Bierman P, Vose J, Armitage JO: High-dose cyclophosphamide, carmustine, and etoposide followed by autologous peripheral stem cell transplantation for patients with relapsed Hodgkin's disease. Blood 77:2322–2325, 1991.

78. Verma UN, Areman E, Dickerson SA, et al: Interleukin-2 activation of chemotherapy and growth factor mobilized peripheral blood stem cells for generation of cytotoxic effectors. Bone Marrow Transplant 15:199–206, 1995.

79. Areman EM, Mazumder A, Kotula P, et al: Hematopoietic potential of IL-2 cultured peripheral blood stem cells from breast cancer patients. Bone Marrow Transplant 18:521–525, 1996.

80. Spitzer TR, Cirenza E, McAfee S, et al: Phase I–II trial of high dose cyclophosphamide, carboplatin and autologous bone marrow or peripheral blood stem cell rescue. Bone Marrow Transplant 15:537–542, 1995.

81. Meehan KR, Verma UN, Cahill R, et al: Interleukin-2-activated hematopoietic stem cell transplantation for breast cancer: investigation of dose level with clinical correlates. Bone Marrow Transplant 20:643–651, 1997.

82. Price G, Brenner MK, Prentice HG, et al: Cytotoxic effects of tumor necrosis factor and gamma interferon on acute myeloid leukemia blast cells. Br J Cancer 55:287–290, 1987.

83. Guadagni F, Schlom J, Johnston WW, et al: Selective interferon-induced enhancement of tumor-associated antigens on a spectrum of freshly isolated human adenocarcinoma cells. J Natl Cancer Inst 81:502–512, 1989.

84. Jabrane-Ferrat N, Faille A, Loiseau P, et al: Effect of gamma interferon on HLA class-I and -II transcription and protein expression in human breast adenocarcinoma cell lines. Int J Cancer 45:1169–1176, 1990.

85. Carlo Stella C, Cazzola M: Interferons as biologic modulators of hematopoietic cell proliferation and differentiation. Haematologica 73:225–237, 1988.

86. Bilgrami S, Silva M, Cardoso A, et al: Immunotherapy with autologous bone-marrow transplantation: rationale and results. Exp Hematol 22:1030 1050, 1994.

87. Winston DJ, Ho WG, Schroff RW, et al: Safety and tolerance of recombinant leukocyte α-interferon in bone marrow transplant recipients. Antimicrob Agents Chemother 23:846–851, 1983.

88. McGlave PB, Arthur D, Miller WJ, et al: Autologous transplantation

for CML using marrow treated ex vivo with recombinant human interferon gamma. Bone Marrow Transplant 6:115–120, 1990.

89. Lo Coco F, Mandelli F, Diverio D, et al: Therapy-induced Ph1 suppression in chronic myeloid leukemia: molecular and cytogenetic studies in patients treated with alpha-2b IFN, high-dose chemotherapy and autologous stem cell infusion. Bone Marrow Transplant 6:253–258, 1990.

90. Higuchi W, Moriyama Y, Kishi K, et al: Hematopoietic recovery in a patient with acute lymphoblastic leukemia after an autologous marrow graft purged by combined hyperthermia and interferon in vitro. Bone Marrow Transplant 7:163–166, 1991.

91. Kantarjian HM, Talpaz M, Le Maistre CF, et al: Intensive combination chemotherapy and autologous bone marrow transplantation leads to the reappearance of philadelphia chromosome–negative cells in chronic myelogenous leukemia. Cancer 67:2959–2965, 1991.

92. Klingemann HG, Grigg AP, Wilkie-Boyd K, et al: Treatment with recombinant interferon (alpha-2b) early after bone marrow transplantation in patients at high risk for relapse. Blood 78:3306–3311, 1991.

93. Attal M, Huguet F, Schlaifer D, et al: Intensive combined therapy for previously untreated aggressive myeloma. Blood 79:1130–1136, 1992.

94. Neloni G, De Fabritiis P, Alimena G, et al: Autologous bone marrow or pheripheral blood stem cell transplantation for patients with chronic myeloid leukemia in chronic phase. Bone Marrow Transplant 4(Suppl 4):92, 1989.

95. Ascensao JL, Miller KB, Tuck D, et al: Immunotherapy with interferon-alpha-2b (IFN) following autologous bone marrow transplantation (ABMT) for lymphomas: an update [Abstract]. Proc Am Soc Clin Oncol 12:380, 1993.

96. Meyers JD, Flournoy N, Sanders JE, et al: Prophylactic use of human leukocyte interferon after allogeneic marrow transplantation. Ann Intern Med 107:809–816, 1987.

97. Glazier AD, Tutschka PJ, Farmer ER, Santos GW: Graft-versus-host disease in cyclosporine A treated rats following syngeneic and autologous bone marrow reconstitution. J Exp Med 158:1–8, 1983.

98. Hess AD, Horwitz L, Beschorner WE, Santos GW: Development of graft-verses-host disease–like syndrome in cyclosporine-treated rats after syngeneic bone marrow transplantation: I. Development of cytotoxic T lymphocytes with apparent polyclonal anti-Ia specificity, including autoreactivity. J Exp Med 161:718–730, 1985.

99. Hess AD, Jones RC, Santos GW: Autologous graft-versus-host disease: mechanism and potential therapeutic effect. Bone marrow transplant 12(Suppl 3):S65, 1993.

100. Jones RJ, Vogelsang GB, Hess AD, et al: Induction of graft versus host disease after autologous bone marrow transplantation. Lancet 1:754–757, 1989.

101. Yeager AM, Vogelsang GB, Jones RJ, et al: Induction of cutaneous graft-versus-host reaction by administration of cyclosporine to patients undergoing autologous bone marrow transplantation for acute myeloid leukemia. Blood 79:3031–3035, 1992.

102. Santos GW: Autologous graft vs host disease [Abstract]. Exp Hematol 19:463, 1991.

103. Kolb HJ, Schattenberg A, Goldman JM, et al: Graft-versus-leukemia effect of donor lymphocyte transfusions in marrow grafted patients. Blood 86:2041–2050, 1995.

104. Helg C, Roux E, Beris P, et al: Adoptive immunotherapy for recurrent CML after BMT. Bone Marrow Transplant 12:125–129, 1993.

105. Mitchell MS, Harel W, Kan-Mitchell J, et al: Active specific immunotherapy of melanoma with allogeneic cell lysates: rationale, results, and possible mechanisms of action. Ann N Y Acad Sci 690:153–166, 1993.

106. Berd D, Maguire HC Jr, McCue P, Mastrangelo MJ: Treatment of metastatic melanoma with an autologous tumor-cell vaccine: clinical and immunologic results in 64 patients. J Clin Oncol 8:1858–1867, 1990.

107. Hanna MG Jr, Ransom JH, Pomato N, et al: Active specific immunotherapy of human colorectal carcinoma with an autologous tumor cell/Bacillus Calmette-Guerin vaccine. Ann N Y Acad Sci 690:135–146, 1993.

108. Gilboa E, Lyerly HK, Vieweg J, Saito S: Immunotherapy of cancer using cytokine gene-modified tumor vaccines. Semin Cancer Biol 5:409–417, 1994.

109. Barth A, Hoon DS, Foshag LJ, et al: Polyvalent melanoma cell vaccine induces delayed-type hypersensitivity and in vitro cellular immune response. Cancer Res 54:3342–3345, 1994.

110. Plaksin D, Porgador A, Vadai E, et al: Effective anti-metastatic melanoma vaccination with tumor cells transfected with MHC genes and/or infected with newcastle disease virus (NDV). Int J Cancer 59:796–801, 1994.

111. Finn OJ: Tumor-specific immune responses and opportunities for tumor vaccines. Clin Immunol Immunopathol 71:260–262, 1994.

112. Mastrangelo MJ, Schultz S, Kane M, Berd D: Newer immunologic approaches to the treatment of patients with melanoma. Semin Oncol 15:589–594, 1988.

113. Pardoll DM: Cancer vaccines. Trends Pharmacol Sci 14:202–208, 1993.

114. Golumbek P, Levitsky H, Jaffee L, Pardoll DM: The antitumor immune response as a problem of self-nonself discrimination: implications for immunotherapy. Immunol Res 12:183–192, 1993.

115. Houghton AN: Cancer antigens: immune recognition of self and altered self. J Exp Med 180:1–4, 1994.

116. Johnston D, Bystryn JC: Immunogenicity and tumor protective activity of B16 melanoma vaccines. Mol Biother 1:218–222, 1989.

117. Sainouchi R, Terata N, Kodama M: The induction of enhanced antitumor effect against a nonimmunogenic tumor by highly immunogenic variants obtained by mutagen treatment. Jpn J Cancer Res 79:1247–1253, 1988.

118. Guadagni F, Roselli M, Schlom J, Greiner JW: In vitro and in vivo regulation of human tumor antigen expression by human recombinant interferons: a review. Int J Biol Markers 9:53–60, 1994.

119. Pardoll DM: New strategies for enhancing the immunogenicity of tumors. Curr Opin Immunol 5:719–725, 1993.

120. Vanky F, Stuber G, Rotstein S, Klein E: Auto-tumor recognition following in vitro induction of MHC antigen expression on solid human tumors: stimulation of lymphocytes and generation of cytotoxicity against the original MHC-antigen-negative tumor cells. Cancer Immunol Immunother 28:17–21, 1989.

121. Mizoguchi H, O'Shea JJ, Longo DL, et al: Alterations in signal transduction molecules in T lymphocytes from tumor-bearing mice. Science 258:1795–1798, 1992.

122. Sulitzeanu D: Immunosuppressive factors in human cancer. Adv Cancer Res 60:247–267, 1993.

123. Deckers PJ, Davis RC, Parker GA, Mannick JA: The effect of tumor size on concomitant immunity. Cancer Response 33:33–39, 1973.

124. Verma UN, Mazumder A: Immune reconstitution following bone marrow transplantation. Cancer Immunol Immunother 37:351–360, 1993.

125. Roberts MM, To LB, Gillis D, et al: Immune reconstitution following peripheral blood stem cell transplantation, autologous bone marrow transplantation and allogeneic bone marrow transplantation. Bone Marrow Transplant 12:469–471, 1993.

126. Ilan Y, Nagler A, Shouval D, et al: Development of antibodies to hepatitis B virus surface antigen in bone marrow transplant recipient following treatment with peripheral blood lymphocytes from immunized donors. Clin Exp Immunol 97:299–302, 1994.

127. Ljungman P, Lewensohn-Fuchs I, Hammarstrom V, et al: Long-term immunity to measles, mumps, and rubella after allogeneic bone marrow transplantation. Blood 84:657–663, 1994.

128. Hammarstrom V, Pauksen K, Azinge J, et al: Pneumococcal immunity and response to immunization with pneumococcal vaccine in bone marrow transplant patients: the influence of graft versus host reaction. Support Care Cancer 1:195–199, 1993.

129. Kwak LW, Grand LC, Williams RM: Radiation-induced augmentation of host resistance to histocompatible tumor in mice: detection of a graft antitumor effect of syngeneic bone marrow transplantation. Transplantation 51:1244–1248, 1991.

130. Kwak LW, Campbell M, Levy R: Idiotype vaccination post-bone marrow transplantation for B-cell lymphoma: initial studies in a murine model. Cancer Detect Prev 15:323–325, 1991.

131. Kwak LW, Campbell MJ, Czerwinski DK, et al: Induction of immune responses in patients with B-cell lymphoma against the surface-immunoglobulin idiotype expressed by their tumors. N Engl J Med 327:1209–1215, 1992.

CHAPTER THIRTY-TWO

Ex Vivo Stem Cell Expansion
Yago Nieto, M.D., and Elizabeth J. Shpall, M.D.

Hematopoietic stem cell transplantation (HSCT) is presently considered a potentially curative therapy for a variety of malignant and inherited bone marrow diseases. It also provides hematopoietic support to patients receiving myeloablative treatment for solid tumors. The broad application of HSCT, however, is limited by several features. The acquisition of enough stem cells for clinical use requires either a bone marrow harvest under general anesthesia or peripheral blood leukapheresis; both are expensive and potentially morbid procedures. Next, grafts contain only a limited number of useful hematopoietic progenitors. Additionally, the kinetics of short-term stem cell engraftment are such that for the first 1–3 weeks after infusion, these cells offer little hematopoietic support, and therefore the recipients remain profoundly myelosuppressed.

Umbilical cord blood is increasingly used as a source of hematopoietic stem cells for unrelated allogeneic transplantation. To date, the procedure has been limited almost exclusively to the pediatric patients because cord blood might not provide sufficient numbers of progenitors to allow reconstitution in an adult.

In recent years, these limitations of HSCT have been addressed by attempts to increase the number of primitive and committed hematopoietic progenitors by ex vivo cultures prior to transplantation. These progenitor cell cultures have been technically developed to the stage at which they merit clinical testing. Clinical trials are under way in a number of different clinical settings. Potential applications of ex vivo stem cell expansion include the following:

- Supplementing stem cell grafts with more mature precursors to shorten or potentially prevent pancytopenia
- Increasing the number of primitive progenitors to ensure hematopoietic support for multiple cycles of high-dose therapy
- Obtaining a sufficient number of stem cells from a single marrow aspirate or pheresis procedure, thus reducing the need for large-scale harvesting of marrow or multiple leukaphereses
- Generating sufficient cells from a single cord-blood unit to allow reconstitution in an adult after high-dose chemotherapy
- Purging stem cell products of contaminating tumor cells
- Generating large volumes of immunologically active cells with antitumor activity to be used in immunotherapeutic regimens
- Increasing the pool of stem cells that could be targets for the delivery of gene therapy

HEMATOPOIETIC CELL ASSAYS

In vitro hematopoietic cell assays are based on the clonal growth of cell colonies in the presence of marrow stromal support and/or cytokine combinations.

SHORT-TERM COLONY-FORMING ASSAY

In the 1960s, Bradley and Metcalf introduced the short-term colony-forming assay.[1] This semisolid culture system allowed the investigators to identify committed hematopoietic cells in vitro and characterize the kinetics of their growth and differentiation. Hematopoiesis in such colony assays lasts only 2–4 weeks, even with nutrient and cytokine support, at which point the physiologic connection between hematopoietic progenitors and, presumably, the supportive marrow and/or stromal cells is perturbed.

LONG-TERM COLONY-FORMING ASSAYS

In the late 1970s, Dexter et al.[2] developed the liquid *long-term bone marrow culture* (LTBMC) assay, in which human hematopoietic cells closely interact with an adherent feeder layer of marrow stroma. This system tries to recapitulate the tridimensional stromal meshwork of normal bone marrow. When very primitive hematopoietic cells are cocultured with stroma, they are selectively retained in the adherent layer[3] while continuously releasing their maturing granulopoietic progeny (granulocyte-macrophage colony–forming units [CFU-GM]) into the nonadherent fraction.[4] Unlike similar long-term murine bone marrow cultures, however, human pluripotent stem cells have a limited lifespan in the Dexter LTBMC.

The LTBMC system does not provide any information about the numbers of primitive progenitor cells that are responsible for the production of CFU-GM. Sutherland et al. developed the quantitative *long-term culture-initiating cell* (LTC-IC) assay.[5] LTC-IC are identified on the basis of their ability to give rise to clonogenic progeny in the presence of irradiated layers of marrow stroma. These investigators demonstrated a linear relationship between the numbers of cells that were inoculated onto the preformed stroma and the numbers of CFU-GM released into the supernatant 5 weeks later, identified in methylcellulose-based short-term tissue culture assays. Therefore, LTC-IC are defined as primitive progenitors that are able to reinitiate secondary stromal cultures. The cloning efficiency of LTC-IC is typically one to two per 10^4 normal marrow cells; LTC-IC constitute 1–2% of the CD34+ cell population.[6]

The number of LTC-IC starts to decrease by 1 week in LTBMC,[7] and 70–80% of them are lost over a culture period of 5–8 weeks.[8] Although the relationship between LTC-IC and totipotent human hematopoietic stem cells capable of reconstituting hematopoiesis in vivo has not been definitely established, the LTC-IC likely represents a more primitive hematopoietic progenitor than the CFU-GM represented in the short-term assay.[9]

EX VIVO CULTURE SYSTEMS

STROMA-FREE LIQUID SUSPENSION CULTURES

Incubation of hematopoietic cells with combinations of hematopoietic growth factor (HGF) in stroma-free static liquid cultures has been the most commonly studied ex vivo culture technique.[10–15] A major finding in the vast majority of those studies is that CD34 selection is necessary prior to culture initiation, if optimal progenitor cell expansion is desired. This requirement is demonstrated in Figure 32–1, which shows how Purdy et al. produced a 5- and 17-fold expansion of marrow progenitors when buffy coat and mononuclear cell fraction, respectively, were cultured for 10 days in media plus stem cell factor (SCF), interleukin-3 (IL-3), IL-6, and granulocyte colony-stimulating factor (G-CSF), compared with a 189-fold CFU-GM expansion obtained when CD34-selected marrow was cultured.[10]

Haylock et al.[11] reported that mobilized CD34 + peripheral blood progenitor cells could be stimulated to proliferate when a combination of interleukins (IL-1β, IL-3, IL-6), G-CSF, granulocyte-macrophage colony–stimulating factor (GM-CSF), and SCF were added to the liquid suspension culture. Under these conditions, the CFU-GM pool expanded a median of 66-times over 14 days and more mature nucleated progenitors were generated at an exponential rate. Other investigators have reproduced these results with different HGF combinations, some of which included erythropoietin (Epo) and/or Flt-3 ligand, in addition to those already mentioned.[12–14] These static culture systems all employ multiple HGF and CD34-enriched progenitor cells. In these studies, CD34 selection is performed prior to culture initiation using a solid-phase immunoselection device[10] or fluorescent activated cell sorting.[11]

A closed liquid culture system that uses gas-permeable teflon-coated bags instead of flasks, without exchange of media or HGF, has been designed for clinical use. Different investigators have reported advantages of such bags, including their capacity to expand larger volumes of progenitors and the low likelihood of contamination and/or technical processing errors.[10, 15]

Although expansion protocols differ with respect to the specific combination of HGF used, the common conclusion is that a single HGF generates minimal hematopoietic cell growth, whereas when combined, HGF synergistically expand the myeloid progenitor cell compartment.

Although the CFU-GM or colony-forming cells are often expanded substantially in these cultures, the number of CD34 + cells and LTC-IC seldom increases yet often declines. In contrast, published data suggest that such cultured grafts retain sufficient primitive stem cells capable of long-term engraftment.[16, 17] Absent a good assay, it is difficult to assess the clinical impact of these cultures on the primitive human hematopoietic stem cell. For some therapeutic applications, expansion of the primitive stem cell may not be required. For instance, patients receiving high-dose nonmyeloablative therapy retain substantial numbers of endogenous stem cells contributing to the long-term stable production of blood cells.[18] In these cases, transplantation of large numbers of intermediately differentiated progenitors could hasten short-term peripheral blood count recovery.

STROMAL NONCONTACT CULTURES

Stroma-Progenitor Interaction in Bone Marrow Cultures

Verfaillie et al. compared three different types of culture conditions, both with and without exogenous HGF: nonstromal, "stroma-contact," and "stroma-noncontact" in which stromal and hematopoietic cells were separated by a 0.45-μm microporous cell-impermeable membrane.[19] In the studies in which no HGF were added, no primitive progenitors were detectable in the stroma-free cultures after 8 weeks. This confirmed that in the absence of exogenous HGF, stroma was necessary for ex vivo hematopoiesis. Comparison of the stroma-noncontact and stroma-contact cul-

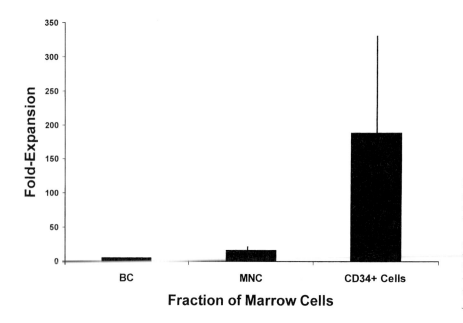

FIGURE 32–1. Effect of CD34 + cell selection on CFU-GM expansion. Bone marrow buffy coat (BC), mononuclear (MNC), or CD34 + cells were cultured in G-CSF, SCF, IL-3, and IL-6, at 10 ng/mL, in X-Vivo 10 medium with 10% autologous plasma. Each culture was initiated with 1 × 10⁶ cells in 50 mL of medium. (Data from Purdy MH, Hogan CJ, Hami L, et al: Large volume ex vivo expansion of CD34-positive hematopoietic progenitor cells for transplantation. J Hematother 4:515–525, 1995.)

tures showed that in the former system, a greater percentage of input LTC-IC was recovered (50%) and a larger number of CFU-GM was produced at the expense of other committed progenitors. These results suggested that, essential as it may seem for the regulated production of all lineages, direct stroma–progenitor cell contact is not required for conservation or differentiation of primitive progenitors.

Subsequent experiments used both stroma-noncontact and stroma-free cultures, with and without an HGF combination of IL-3, G-CSF, SCF, and leukemia-inhibitory factor.[20] The stromal layers produced soluble factors that synergistically induced maturation and proliferation of LTC-IC in combination with the exogenous HGF. These factors also prevented the terminal differentiation of the LTC-IC. None of the HGF added to the cultures, either alone or in combination, were able to expand the LTC-IC population after 5 weeks. Loss of LTC-IC from ex vivo long-term cultures may be the result of excessive stimulation of the otherwise quiescent primitive hematopoietic compartment, resulting in their irreversible terminal differentiation.

Stroma-Produced Soluble Factors

Further research was aimed at a better definition of these putative stromal soluble factors. Macrophage inflammatory protein-1α (MIP-1α), originally described as "stem cell inhibitor," inhibits in vitro and in vivo proliferation of colony-forming units/granulocyte-ethythrocyte-macrophage-megakaryocyte (CFU-GEMM) progenitors.[21, 22] Verfaillie et al.[23] reported that the addition of either MIP-1α or IL-3 to stroma-noncontact cultures did not increase the number of LTC-IC and therefore did not seem to prevent LTC-IC differentiation. After the concurrent addition of MIP-1α and IL-3, however, LTC-IC recovery after 8 weeks of culture was 100% of input. MIP-1α + IL-3 + SCF, however, failed to maintain LTC-IC in stroma-free cultures at 5–8 weeks, which seems to confirm the essential role of these unidentified diffusible stroma-derived factors. Only with a combination of MIP-1α, IL-3, and stromal factors was it possible to maintain LTC-IC in vitro for at least 2 months.

Stroma-Containing Continuous-Perfusion Cultures

Continuous-perfusion cultures of hematopoietic cell populations attempt to mimic the normal human bone marrow milieu, in which the proliferation and regulated differentiation of the hematopoietic stem cell is directed by the surrounding stromal cells. Marrow stroma constitutes a complex meshwork of cells and extracellular matrix that secretes HGF and provides the necessary adhesive microenvironment for the maintenance of high local HGF concentrations and cell-to-cell contact. Early studies showed that long-term bone marrow cultures are not feasible without the stroma.[24, 25]

RATIONALE FOR RAPID MEDIUM EXCHANGE SYSTEMS

An important observation from the liquid culture experience is that secreted products of mature granulocytes and macrophages are toxic to progenitors.[26] Removal of maturing myeloid cells allowed the growth of erythroid and megakaryocytic cells in vitro, which would not otherwise occur. Macrophages arising in liquid cultures have been shown to directly damage cultured stroma and hematopoietic progenitors.[27] Therefore, a continuous perfusion of culture medium that removed mature cells as they lose their stromal adhesion receptors could protect the cultured cells from toxic byproducts, such as lactate or ammonium.

The calculated in vivo human vascular perfusion rate to the bone marrow is approximately 0.1 mL of serum/mL of marrow per minute (0.23 mL serum per 10^6 cells per day),[28] seven times higher than the standard single weekly exchange typically employed for static liquid cultures. A continuous medium and oxygen exchange stimulates stromal cell metabolism and a local supply of certain proliferative and differentiative CSF, such as GM-CSF[29, 30] or IL-3.[27] Schwarz et al.[31] showed that the addition of IL-3, GM-CSF, and Epo to a rapid culture medium exchange enhanced the expansion of progenitors and increased survival of cultured stem cells.

In cultures targeting the expansion of the most primitive hematopoietic progenitor cells (LTC-IC), continuous perfusion is critical for both stimulating stroma and removing the metabolic byproducts produced by maturing progenitors.

DEVELOPMENT OF BIOREACTORS

Flat-Plate Bioreactors

A clinical-scale bioreactor device with a continuously perfused culture system has been developed by Aastrom Biosciences Inc.[32] that is based on a prior small-scale culture chamber designed by Palsson et al.[33] Using the medium perfused flat-plate Aastrom device, Koller et al. reported, for the first time, a significant expansion of LTC-IC.[35] Marrow mononuclear cells were cultured for 14 days with low doses of SCF, IL-3, GM-CSF, and Epo. The total number of cells was increased ten-fold, marrow mononuclear cells and CFU-GM were expanded 10- to 20-fold, and LTC-IC were a expanded a median of 7.5-fold (range, 4- to 9.8-fold).

The issue of the optimal degree of cell purification prior to its culture under perfusion conditions was studied by different investigators. Sandstrom et al.[34] compared marrow mononuclear cell cultures, with and without CD34 selection, in both static suspension and continuously perfused systems containing IL-3, IL-6, G-CSF, and SCF. Both types of cultures yielded similar expansion of total cells and CFU-GM for both marrow mononuclear cells and CD34+ cell cultures, although samples that performed poorly in static cultures expanded at normal levels when continuously perfused. Within perfusion systems, CD34+ cell cultures gave a higher total cell, similar CFU-GM, and lower LTC-IC output than cultures initiated with marrow mononuclear cells.

Koller et al.[35] cultured CD34-selected cells with HGF in perfusion systems that were either stroma-free or contained preformed stroma. Stroma-free culturing of CD34-selected cells resulted in a 50% reduction of LTC-IC regardless of the specific HGF combination added. When CD34-enriched cells were cultured with preformed stroma, the net result was a maintenance, but not an expansion, of LTC-IC. A third step showed that as the purity of CD34+ cells decreases in cultures, the output of total cells, CFU-GM, and LTC-IC increases by three to five times. The authors concluded that the lack of LTC-IC expansion with CD34 selection was likely related to the removal of important CD34– nonstromal accessory cells normally present in the marrow mononuclear cell compartment.

Stirred Suspension Bioreactors

An experimental suspension system in stirred flask bioreactors described by Sardonini et al.[36] is an alternative approach to the flat-based bioreactor. As opposed to the adherent flat-based bioreactors, these bioreactors employ a stirred suspension perfusion culture wherein the medium and growth factor environment is easier to measure and optimize. The system offers the advantages of a greater homogeneity and lack of dependance on the formation and maintenance of an adherent layer. Zandstra et al.[37] reported 7- and 22-fold expansion of LTC-IC and colony-forming cells, respectively, with this system.

SOURCES OF HEMATOPOIETIC CELLS FOR EXPANSION

BONE MARROW

Bone marrow has been the primary hematopoietic cell source in cultures that employ perfusion systems. The known content of primitive hematopoietic progenitors, as well as the stromal mesenchymal and nonstromal accessory cells required for optimal expansion of colony-forming cells and LTC-IC in bioreactors,[33] is responsible for the selection of marrow over peripheral blood progenitor cells (PBPC) or cord blood when expansion in continuously perfused devices is desired.

MOBILIZED PERIPHERAL BLOOD

Preclinical studies of mobilized PBPC have reported high levels of committed progenitor cell expansion, often exceeding 50-fold.[10–15] A potential concern is the long-term durability of cultured PBPC grafts in patients who have undergone myoablation. It has been shown that although there may be higher numbers of LTC-IC in mobilized PBPC than in marrow, the potential of PBPC-derived LTC-IC to expand ex vivo seems more limited than with marrow-derived LTC-IC.[38] Ongoing clinical trials will address this issue.

UMBILICAL CORD BLOOD

Observations in the 1980s showed that murine fetal stem cells had a competitive repopulating advantage over adult stem cells.[39] Similarly, human umbilical cord blood contained much higher numbers of clonogenic progenitor cells

(one to five per 1000 mononuclear cells) than adult peripheral blood (one to five per 20,000 mononuclear cells).[40] Moreover, the progenitor-derived colonies observed were very large, often macroscopic, and multifocal.[41, 42] These studies suggest that cord blood contains progenitors that are similar to the primitive progenitors in the fetal liver. Other investigators later confirmed these results.[43] Subsequent studies demonstrated a higher proliferative capacity and a higher capacity of self-renewal of cord blood stem cells over adult marrow or PBPC.[44, 45] CD34+ cord blood cells can generate several thousand more mature cord blood cells in culture without reducing the number of CD34+ cells with which the cultures were inoculated. This is in contrast with cultures of adult bone marrow, in which CD34+ cells decline quickly.[46, 47]

These studies suggest that cord blood progenitors may have an increased capacity to support self-renewal and the production of more mature cells in culture when compared with marrow and PBPC and that cord blood might be a superior source of expanded stem and progenitor cells for clinical transplantation.

CLINICAL STUDIES INVOLVING STEM CELLS CULTURED EX VIVO

Both stroma-free liquid suspension cultures and the Aastrom bioreactor have been used in clinical studies.

EXPANDED CD34+ CELL REINFUSION AFTER NON-MYELOABLATIVE AND MYELOABLATIVE CHEMOTHERAPY

Brugger et al.[48] conducted a pilot trial with a PBPC product consisting of expanded CD34+ PBPC in patients treated with ifosfamide (12 g/m^2), carboplatin (750 mg/m^2), etoposide (1.5 g/m^2), and epirubicin (150 mg/m^2). Autologous PBPC were mobilized with chemotherapy plus G-CSF, collected in a single apheresis procedure, CD34-selected, and cultured ex vivo for 12 days in static liquid cultures containing serum-free media plus SCF, IL-1β, IL-3, IL-6, and Epo. Engraftment rates were identical to those of historical control patients who received the same conditioning regimen and uncultured CD34+ PBPC. In another study using myeloablative chemotherapies (total body irradiation)/cyclophosphamide and busulfan/melphalan, all four patients failed to experience sustained engraftment and required infusion of unmanipulated back-up PBPC.[49]

REINFUSION OF BOTH UNMANIPULATED AND CULTURED STEM CELLS AFTER MYELOABLATIVE CHEMOTHERAPY

Several pilot trials have tested the combination of expanded progenitors with unmanipulated marrow or PBPC after myeloablative chemotherapy. Naparstek et al.[50] reinfused 20 leukemic patients with allogeneic cells, a third of which had been incubated in a static device with IL-3 and GM-CSF for 4 days. The patients who received the cultured cells experienced more-rapid platelet engraftment and a reduced hospital stay compared with historical controls who received only unmanipulated marrow.

Champlin et al.[51] cultured marrow from nine patients with breast cancer in the Aastrom bioreactor for 12 days, with an input number of 2.25×10^8 mononuclear cells. After high-dose cyclophosphamide (6 g/m²), thiotepa (720 mg/m²), and BCNU (1,3-bis(2-chloroethyl)-1-nitrosourea; carmustine) (450 mg/m²), patients were reinfused with both their cryopreserved unmanipulated bone marrow and the cultured fractions. Granulocytes and platelets engrafted on days 11 (10–13) and 16 (13–21), respectively. These engraftment rates compared favorably to those of historical controls who received the same chemotherapy regimen with only unmanipulated marrow support.

Alcorn et al.[52] reported the safe clinical use of expanded PBPC that were cryopreserved before their culture. These frozen cells were thawed, CD34-selected, and cultured in a static system. The cultured cells and unmanipulated PBPC were subsequently reinfused in 10 patients with myeloma, breast cancer, or non-Hodgkin lymphoma after a variety of myeloablative conditioning regimens. No difference was found in neutrophil or platelet engraftment rates in patients after high-dose therapy compared with their historical controls. The same authors also reported on two subsequent patients who were reinfused with cultured cells alone.[53] The CFU-GM content of the grafts in these two patients was lower than that in their earlier patients who received both unmanipulated and expanded PBPC. The first patient, who received 6×10^4 CFU-GM/kg, did not experience engraftment by day +14, at which point an unmanipulated PBPC back-up fraction was infused; the patient subsequently experienced engraftment. The second patient, with her second stem cell transplants, received 1.033×10^7 CFU-GM/kg, and her neutrophil engraftment rate was normal by day +15.

Zimmerman et al.[54] cultured PBPC from 11 patients with breast cancer in a static device that contained serum-free media supplemented with PIXY321 (a fusion protein: IL-3/GM-CSF). Patients were reinfused the cultured PBPC and an unmanipulated PBPC fraction after high-dose cyclophosphamide (6 g/m²), thiotepa (600 mg/m²), and carboplatin (800 mg/m²). Time to engraftment was normal in all patients. The reinfused number of CD34+ cells in both the cultured and the unmanipulated PBPC products inversely correlated with the depth and duration of neutropenia. A subsequent study from the same group showed that a substantial portion of the expanded cells were accumulated by the reticuloendothelial system.[55]

CULTURED CELLS AS SOLE HEMATOPOIETIC SUPPORT AFTER MYELOABLATIVE CHEMOTHERAPY

Stiff et al.[56] reported results from the first trial that used cultured marrow as the sole source of hematopoietic support after high-dose chemotherapy. Small 40-mL bone marrow aliquots were aspirated and cultured in an Aastrom bioreactor; the cultured cells were subsequently infused into six patients with breast cancer who had received high-dose cyclophosphamide (6 g/m²), thiotepa (500 mg/m²),

and carboplatin (800 mg/m²). Times to neutrophil and platelet engraftment were 18 days (range, 13–22) and 22 days (range, 19–27), respectively. A subsequent study confirmed this observation.[57] In 1998, marrow cells expanded with the Aastrom system were infused in addition to PBPC after Solid Tumor Autologous Marrow Program V (STAMP V) chemotherapy. Accelerated neutrophil and placement engraftment time was reported.[58] These results are similar to results with historical controls who received a standard unmanipulated bone marrow autograft.

OTHER PROMISING CLINICAL APPLICATIONS OF EX VIVO STEM CELL CULTURES

EX VIVO EXPANSION OF CORD BLOOD–DERIVED PROGENITORS

Preliminary data suggest that umbilical cord blood contains eightfold higher numbers of early hematopoietic progenitors than does adult marrow.[59] Cord blood transplantations have been performed in recent years, primarily in pediatric patients. A major concern with respect to cord blood transplantation in adults is the relatively small number of hematopoietic progenitors in cord blood units, which may not allow for rapid engraftment. Cord blood–derived progenitors have shown an enhanced proliferative potential when cultured ex vivo compared with marrow-derived progenitors.[60, 61]

Clinical trials are under way to evaluate the efficacy of expanded cord blood progenitors in adult patients receiving high-dose chemotherapy. Preliminary results using expanded and unmanipulated cord blood progenitors together in the same patients showed that infusion of such grafts was safe and did not compromise engraftment.[62]

IMMUNOTHERAPY WITH CULTURED HEMATOPOIETIC PROGENITORS

Production of lineage-restricted progenitors and differentiated populations can be manipulated by varying the HGF combinations. For instance, lymphoid progenitors can be obtained and then driven to differentiate into cells with a critical role in the antitumor immune response, such as dendritic cells,[63] or those with a potent cytotoxic capacity, such as natural killer cells.[64]

Generation of Dendritic Cells

Dendritic cells are "professional" antigen-presenting cells, considered to be among the most-effective stimulators of T-cell immunity. They are found in many nonlymphoid tissues, such as skin (Langerhans cells) and mucosa, and they migrate after antigen capture through the afferent lymphatic system or bloodstream to lymphoid organs, where they present the antigen to the T cells.

Dendritic-cell progenitors have been identified in the CD34+ hematopoietic fraction, from which they can be isolated.[63, 65] Dendritic cells from bone marrow, cord blood, and PBPC have been expanded ex vivo with different cytokine combinations. The specific cytokines vary according to the source of the progenitors. GM-CSF and tumor necrosis factor α (TNFα) are effective for marrow[66]; cord blood,[67] G-CSF–mobilized PBPC,[68] and IL-4 + GM-CSF are effective for steady-state peripheral blood.[68] The addition of stem-cell targeted cytokines, SCF,[66, 69] Flt-3 ligand,[70] and transforming growth factor β (TGFβ)[71] further augment the effect of these combinations. The dendritic cells cultured with these cytokines possess normal antigen-presenting capability.[72]

By retrovirally transducing the human breast cancer antigen MUC-1 into dendritic cells, Henderson et al. from the University of Pittsburgh obtained a population with stable, high-level MUC-1 expression. MUC-1 + dendritic cells displayed a more-potent allostimulation of CD4 + T cells compared with MUC-1 − dendritic cells.[73]

Ongoing clinical studies with cultured dendritic cells will determine their capacity to generate therapeutic T-cell responses to tumor antigens in patients with cancer.

Production of Natural Killer Cells

Natural killer (NK) cells are a small population of peripheral blood lymphocytes with the capacity to kill foreign cells in a human leukocyte antigen (HLA)-unrestricted manner. Several groups are investigating the use of NK cells that are expanded ex vivo and then used for immunotherapy after autologous bone marrow transplantation.

Miller et al.[64] showed that NK cells could be generated by culturing CD34 + /HLA-DR − marrow mononuclear cells, in stroma-containing media, in the presence of IL-2 and human serum. Eighty-five percent of the cultured cells expressed the characteristic CD56 + /CD3 − NK phenotype. NK cells generated in the cultures were Philadelphia chromosome–negative, or Ph − .[74] In a second step, the NK cells, when incubated with IL-2 in stroma-noncontact cultures, were shown to expand, in the presence of monocytes. This method yielded NK cell production at a large scale adequate for its use in vivo.[75] In a subsequent study, in vitro–generated and IL-2-activated NK cells suppressed chronic myelogenous leukemia LTC-IC while sparing normal LTC-IC, proving that non–HLA-restricted NK cytotoxic activity suppressed malignant hematopoiesis. This effect did not depend on soluble factors but on direct cell-to-cell contact.[76]

TUMOR PURGING ROLE FOR EX VIVO CULTURES OF STEM CELL PRODUCTS

Chronic Myelogenous Leukemia

Chronic myelogenous leukemia (CML) is characterized by the Philadelphia chromosome (Ph), in which a translocation of chromosomes 9 and 22 [t(9;22)] produces a molecular rearrangement of the bcr-abl gene. Malignant CML progenitors exhibit an altered function of various adhesion receptors and a reduced adherence to normal stroma.[77, 78] The stroma does not, therefore, exert its usual inhibitory effect on stem cell proliferation and differentiation.[79] It has been shown that marrow stromal macrophages are Ph + and bcr-abl + ,[80] as opposed to stromal fibroblasts, which

have long been known to be Ph(−).[81, 82] As a result of both the abnormalities in CML malignant progenitors themselves and the impaired interactions between these progenitors and marrow stroma, a global picture of abnormal hematopoiesis becomes apparent in these patients.

This abnormal in vivo hematopoiesis translates into a survival advantage for the benign progenitors compared with the CML progenitors in ex vivo cultures.[83, 84] These data allow for the possibility that the malignant clone could be eradicated by culturing the marrow of patients with CML.

Long-term culture of CML marrow in early studies did not result in the elimination of disease in most patients.[85, 86] Refinement of these early culture techniques will be necessary for complete eradication of the malignant clone.

Verfaillie et al.[87] demonstrated that when CML marrow cells expressing the CD34 + /HLA-DR − phenotype were cultured ex vivo, they did not exhibit the Philadelphia chromosome or the corresponding bcr/abl mRNA. Conversely, when the CD34 + /HLA-DR + population was cultured ex vivo, the cells remained Ph(+) and bcr/abl mRNA(+). In 1996, the same investigators showed that selection of benign progenitors was only possible when marrow from patients in early chronic phase (within their first year from initial diagnosis) was cultured.[88] These studies have led to plans for clinical evaluation of marrow harvesting and CD34 selection followed by fluorescent-activated cell sorting to isolate the CD34 + /HLA-DR − /bcr-abl(−) fraction for ex vivo culturing. If this strategy proves to be effective in future clinical studies, autologous transplantation could become an attractive option for those patients with CML who are not candidates for allogeneic transplantation.

Other Tumors

The presence of the t(14;18) translocation, identified by the rearrangement of the bcl-2 gene in most cases of follicular non-Hodgkin lymphoma, offers an opportunity for molecular monitoring by polymerase chain reaction (PCR) for subclinical disease and the efficacy of in vitro purging. Both immunologic purging[89] and CD34-selection procedures[90, 91] have been explored, but an insufficient purging capacity has been reported for both techniques. Widmer et al.[92] reported the results from CD34-selecting and then expanding nine samples from patients with non-Hodgkin lymphoma positive by PCR for the t(14;18) translocation. Seven samples remained bcl-2 + by PCR after CD34 selection with an immunoadsorption column. After a 14-day incubation with HGF in a suspension culture, six of the seven samples became PCR-negative for bcl-2. The authors hypothesized that ex vivo culture resulted in a predominant myelomonocytic differentiation, whereas lymphoma B cells did not proliferate and became undetectable.

Reported results from studies of acute myeloid leukemia cell lines show a preferential differentiation and inhibition of the growth of malignant cells, when cultured in the presence of vitamin D and analogues, relative to normal progenitors.[93]

Preliminary data show that breast cancer[94] and myeloma[95] tumor cells do not appear to expand in liquid cultures. On the contrary, these studies suggest that malignant cells that contaminate the stem cell products might have a growth disadvantage with respect to CD34+ progenitors under these conditions. Additional studies are needed to confirm these data.

GENE THERAPY

Gaucher disease is a congenital metabolic storage disease characterized by deficient activity of the glucocerebrosidase enzyme involved in lipid metabolism. In 1992, retroviral vectors were first reported to efficiently transfer the glucocerebrosidase gene into bone marrow hematopoietic progenitor cells of patients with this disease. This resulted in normal levels of glucocerebrosidase enzyme activity.[96] CD34 selection is initially performed to increase the retrovirus/cell ratio because retroviral infection of stem cells has low efficiency and high titers of the appropriate retrovirus cannot yet be obtained. CD34+ PBPC have produced higher transfection rates than CD34+ marrow cells.[97, 98] Subsequent culture of the CD34+ retrovirally transfected stem cell population can provide a sufficient number of primitive progenitors that express normal levels of the enzyme. An ongoing clinical trial at the University of Pittsburgh is testing this therapeutic approach to Gaucher disease.[99]

Patients with other diseases caused by a bone marrow–derived gene deficiency, such as Fanconi anemia,[100] chronic granulomatous disease,[101] or X-linked severe combined immunodeficiency syndrome,[102] may someday benefit from this promising therapy.

CONCLUSION

It is possible to expand hematopoietic progenitor cells in stroma-containing or nonstromal systems. While the effect on primitive hematopoietic stem cells cannot be determined for lack of an assay, expansion systems have been shown to be capable of increases in CFU-GM of more than 100-fold. Enrichment of CD34+ cells is required before expansion in nonstromal cultures but may not be necessary in stroma-containing systems. Early results of clinical trials are encouraging and demonstrate that the engraftment potential of the expanded hematopoietic cells is not compromised by culture. Expansion of cord blood–derived hematopoietic cells is especially important because of the limited number of cells that can be collected. Successful expansion of primitive and committed hematopoietic cells from cord blood will allow more extensive use in clinical transplantation, particularly in adult patients. Other possible applications of stem cell expansion include purging of tumor cells; production of immune-competent cells, such as dendritic cells and NK cells; and gene therapy.

REFERENCES

1. Bradley TR, Metcalf D: The growth of mouse bone marrow cells in vitro. Aust J Exp Biol Med Sci 44:287, 1966.
2. Dexter TM, Allen TD, Lajtha LG: Conditions controlling the proliferation of hemopoietic stem cells in vitro. J Cell Physiol 91:335, 1977.
3. Coulumbel L, Eaves AC, Eaves CJ: Enzymatic treatment of long-term human marrow cultures reveals the preferential location of primitive hematopoietic progenitors in the adherent layer. Blood 62:291–297, 1983.
4. Slovick FT, Abboud CN, Brennan JK, Lichtman MA: Survival of granulocytic progenitors in the nonadherent and adherent compartments of human long-term marrow cultures. Exp Hematol 12:327–338, 1984.
5. Sutherland HJ, Eaves CJ, Eaves AC, et al: Characterization and partial purification of human marrow cells capable of initiating long-term hematopoiesis in vitro. Blood 74:1563–1570, 1989.
6. Sutherland HK, Lansdorp PM, Hemkelman DH, et al: Functional characterization of individual hematopoietic stem cells cultured at limiting dilution on supportive marrow stromal layers. Proc Natl Acad Sci U S A 87:3584–3588, 1990.
7. Sutherland HJ, Hogge DE, Cook D, Eaves CJ: Alternative mechanisms with and without steel factor support primitive human hematopoiesis. Blood 81:1465, 1993.
8. Sutherland HJ, Eaves CJ, Lansdorp PM, et al: Differential regulation of primitive human hematopoietic cells in long-term cultures maintained on genetically engineered murine stromal cells. Blood 78:666, 1991.
9. Eaves CJ, Sutherland HJ, Udomsakdi C, et al: The human hematopoietic stem cell in vitro and in vivo. Blood Cells 18:301–307, 1992.
10. Purdy MH, Hogan CJ, Hami L, et al: Large volume ex vivo expansion of CD34-positive hematopoietic progenitor cells for transplantation. J Hematother 4:515–525, 1995.
11. Haylock DN, To LB, Dowse TL, et al: Ex vivo expansion and maturation of peripheral blood CD34+ cells into the myeloid lineage. Blood 80:1405–1412, 1992.
12. Srour EG, Brandt JE, Briddell RA, et al: Long-term generation and expansion of human primitive hematopoietic progenitor cells in vitro. Blood 81:661, 1993.
13. Coutinho LH, Will A, Radford J, et al: Effects of recombinant human granulocyte colony-stimulating factor (G-CSF), human granulocyte-macrophage colony stimulating factor (GM-CSF), and gibbon interleukin-3 on hematopoiesis in human long-term bone marrow culture. Blood 75:2118, 1990.
14. Brugger W, Mocklin W, Heimfeld S, et al: Ex vivo expansion of enriched peripheral blood CD34+ progenitor cells by stem cell factor, interleukin-β (IL-1β), IL-6, IL-3, interferon-γ, and erythropoietin. Blood 81:2579–2584, 1993.
15. Shapiro F, Yao T-J, Raptis G, et al: Optimization of conditions for ex vivo expansion of CD34+ cells from patients with stage IV breast cancer. Blood 84:3567–3574, 1994.
16. Muench MO, Firpo MY, Moore MA: Bone marrow transplantation with interleukin-1 plus kit-ligand ex vivo expanded bone marrow accelerates hematopoietic reconstitution in mice without the loss of stem cell lineage and proliferative potential. Blood 81:3463–3473, 1993.
17. Henschler R, Brugger W, Luft T, et al: Maintenance of transplantation potential in ex vivo expanded CD34+-selected human peripheral blood progenitor cells. Blood 84:2898–2903, 1994.
18. Petz LD, Yam P, Wallace RB, et al: Mixed hematopoietic chimerism following bone marrow transplantation for hematologic malignancies. Blood 70:1331–1337, 1987.
19. Verfaillie CM: Direct contact between human primitive hematopoietic progenitors and bone marrow stroma is not required for long-term in vitro hematopoiesis. Blood 79:2821–2826, 1992.
20. Verfaillie CM: Soluble factor(s) produced by human bone marrow stroma increase cytokine-induced proliferation and maturation of primitive hematopoietic progenitors while preventing their terminal differentiation. Blood 82:2045–2053, 1993.
21. Graham GJ, Wright EG, Hewick R, et al: Identification and characterization of an inhibitor of hemopoietic stem cell proliferation: Nature 344:442, 1990.
22. Lord BI, Dexter TM, Clements JM, et al: Macrophage-inflammatory protein protects multipotent hematopoietic cells from the cytotoxic effects of hydroxyurea in vivo. Blood 79:2605, 1992.
23. Verfaillie CM, Catanzarro PM, Li W: Macrophage inflammatory protein 1α, interleukin 3 and diffusible marrow stromal factors maintain human hematopoietic stem cells for at least eight weeks in vitro. J Exp Med 179:643–649, 1994.
24. Dexter TM, Allen TD, Lajtha LG: Conditions controlling the proliferation of hemopoietic stem cells in vitro. J Cell Physiol 91:335–344, 1977.
25. Chamberlain W, Barone J, Kedo A, Fried W: Lack of recovery of

murine hematopoietic stromal cells after irradiation-induced damage. Blood 44:385–392, 1974.

26. Tsai S, Emerson SG, Sieff SA, Nathan DG: Isolation of a human stromal cell strain secreting hemopoietic growth factors. J Cell Physiol 127:137–145, 1986.

27. Meagher RC, Salvado AJ, Wright DJ: An analysis of the multi lineage production of human hematopoietic progenitors in long-term bone marrow culture: evidence that reactive oxygen intermediates derived from mature phagocytic cells have a role in limiting progenitor cell self-renewal. Blood 72:273–281, 1988.

28. Martiat PH, Ferrant A, Cogneau M, et al: Assessment of bone marrow blood flow using positron emission tomography: no relationship with bone cellularity. Br J Haematol 66:307–310, 1987.

29. Caldwell J, Palsson BO, Locey B, Emerson SG: Culture perfusion schedules influence the metabolic activity and granulocyte-macrophage colony stimulating factor production rates of human bone marrow stromal cells. J Cell Physiol 147:344–353, 1991.

30. Guba SC, Sartor CI, Gottschalk LR, et al: Bone marrow stromal fibroblasts secrete interleukin-6 and granulocyte-macrophage colony-stimulating factor in the absence of inflammatory stimulation: demonstration by serum-free bioassay, enzyme-linked immunosorbent assay, and reverse transcriptase polymerase chain reaction. Blood 80:1190–1198, 1992.

31. Schwartz RM, Emerson SG, Clarke MF, Palsson BO: In vitro myelopoiesis stimulated by rapid medium exchange and supplementation with hematopoietic growth factors. Blood 78:3155–3161, 1991.

32. Koller MR, Emerson SG, Palsson BO: Large-scale expansion of human hematopoietic stem and progenitor cells from bone marrow mononuclear cells in continuous perfusion culture. Blood 82:378–384, 1993.

33. Palsson BO, Paek SH, Schwartz RM, et al: Expansion of human bone marrow progenitor cells in a high cell density continuous perfusion system. Biotechnology 11:368, 1993.

34. Sandstrom CE, Bender JG, Papoutsakis ET, Miller WM: Effects of CD34+ cell selection and perfusion on ex vivo expansion of peripheral blood mononuclear cells. Blood 86:958–970, 1995.

35. Koller MR, Palsson MA, Manchel I, Palsson BO: Long-term culture-initiating cell expansion is dependent on frequent medium exchange combined with stroma and other accessory cell effects. Blood 86:1784–1793, 1995.

36. Sardonini CA, Wu Y-J: Expansion and differentiation of human hematopoietic cells from static cultures from small-scale bioreactors. Biotechnol Prog 9:131–137, 1993.

37. Zandstra PW, Eaves CJ, Piret JM: Expansion of hematopoietic progenitor cell populations in stirred suspension bioreactors of normal human bone marrow cells. Bio Technol 12:909–914, 1994.

38. Srour EF, Bregni M, Traycoff CM, et al: Long-term hematopoietic culture-initiating cells are more abundant in mobilized peripheral blood grafts than in bone marrow but have a more limited ex vivo expansion potential. Blood Cells Mol Dis 22:68–81, 1996.

39. Fleischman RA, Mintz B: Development of adult bone marrow stem cells in H-2-compatible and -incompatible mouse fetuses. J Exp Med 159:731, 1984.

40. Broxmeyer HE, Douglas GW, Hangoc G, et al: Human umbilical cord blood as a potential source of transplantable hematopoietic stem/progenitor cells. Proc Natl Acad Sci USA 86:3828, 1989.

41. Broxmeyer HE, Hangoc G, Cooper S, et al: Growth characteristics and expansion of human umbilical cord blood and estimation of its potential for transplantation in adults. Proc Natl Acad Sci U S A 89:4109, 1992.

42. Broxmeyer HE, Kutzberg J, Gluckman E, et al: Umbilical cord blood hematopoietic stem and repopulating cells in human clinical transplantation. Blood Cells 17:313, 1991.

43. Traycoff C, Abboud M, Laver J, et al: Evaluation of the in vitro behavior of phenotypically defined populations of umbilical cord blood hematopoietic progenitor cells. Exp Hematol 22:215–222, 1994.

44. Lu L, Xiao M, Shen RN, et al: Enrichment, characterization, and responsiveness of single primitive CD34+++ human umbilical cord blood hematopoietic progenitors with high proliferative and repleating potential. Blood 81:41–48, 1993.

45. Carow CE, Hangoc G, Broxmeyer HE: Human multipotential progenitor cells (CFU-GEMM) have extensive repleating capacity for secondary CFU-GEMM: an effect enhanced by cord blood plasma. Blood 81:942–949, 1993.

46. Lansdorp PM, Dragowska W, Mayani H: Ontogeny-related changes in proliferative potential of human hematopoietic cells. J Exp Med 178:787, 1993.

47. Mayani H, Lansdorp PM: Thy-1 expression is linked to functional properties of primitive hematopoietic progenitor cells from human umbilical cord blood. Blood 83:2410, 1994.

48. Brugger W, Heimfeld S, Berenson RJ, et al: Reconstitution of hematopoiesis after high-dose chemotherapy by autologous progenitor cells generated ex vivo. N Engl J Med 333:283–287, 1995.

49. Holyoake TL, Alcorn MJ, Richmond L, et al: CD34 positive PBPC expanded ex vivo may not provide durable engraftment following myeloablative chemoradiotherapy regimens. Bone Marrow Transplant 19:1095–1101, 1997.

50. Naparstek E, Hardan Y, Ben-Shahar M, et al: Enhanced marrow recovery by short preincubation of marrow allografts with human recombinant interleukin-3 and granulocyte-macrophage colony stimulating factor. Blood 80:1673–1678, 1992.

51. Champlin R, Mehra R, Gajewski J, et al: Ex vivo expanded progenitor cell transplantation in patients with breast cancer. Blood 86:295a, 1995.

52. Alcorn MJ, Holyoake TL, Richmond L, et al: CD34-positive cells isolated from cryopreserved peripheral-blood progenitor cells can be expanded ex vivo and used for transplantation with little or no toxicity. J Clin Oncol 14:1839–1847, 1996.

53. Holyoake TL, Alcorn MJ, Richmond L, et al: A phase I study to evaluate the safety of reinfusing CD34 expanded ex vivo as part or all of PBPC transplant procedure. Blood 86:294a, 1995.

54. Zimmerman TM, Bender JG, Lee WJ, et al: Impact of ex vivo expanded myeloid progenitors on neutropenia after high-dose chemotherapy. Blood 88:605a, 1996.

55. Zimmerman TM, Bender G, Lee WJ, et al: Infusion and localization of ex vivo expanded myeloid progenitors after high-dose chemotherapy in patient with metastatic breast cancer. Blood 88:605a, 1996.

56. Stiff P, Oldenberg D, Hsi E, et al: Successful hematopoietic engraftment following high dose chemotherapy using only ex-vivo expanded bone marrow grown in Aastrom (stromal-based) bioreactors. Proc ASCO 16:88a, 1997.

57. Pecora A, Preti R, Jennis A, et al: Aastrom Replicell™ system expanded bone marrow enhances hematopoietic recovery in patients receiving low doses of G-CSF primed blood stem cells. Blood 92:132a, 1998.

58. Stiff P, Parthasarathy M, Chen B, et al: A single apheresis combined with ex vivo expanded bone marrow cells from a small starting aliquot leaps to rapid hematopoietic engraftment following autotransplantation. Blood 92:132a, 1998.

59. Traycoff C, Abboud M, Laver J, et al: Evaluation of the in vitro behavior of phenotypically defined populations of umbilical cord blood hematopoietic progenitor cells. Exp Hematol 22:215–222, 1994.

60. Traycoff C, Abboud MR, Laver J, et al: Human umbilical cord blood hematopoietic progenitor cells: are they the same as their adult bone marrow counterparts? Blood Cells 20:382–390, 1994.

61. Moore MA, Hoskins T: Ex vivo expansion of cord blood-derived stem cells and progenitors. Blood Cells 20:468–479, 1994.

62. Jaroscak J, Martin P, Waters-Pick B, et al: A phase I trial of augmentation of unrelated umbilical cord blood transplantation with ex vivo expanded cells. Blood 92:646a, 1998.

63. Caux C, Dezutter-Dambuyant C, Schmitt D, Bancherau J: GM-CSF and TNF-α cooperate in the generation of dendritic Langerhans cells. Nature 360:258–261, 1992.

64. Miller JS, Verfaillie CM, McGlave PM: The generation of human natural killer cells from CD34+/DR− primitive progenitors in long-term bone marrow culture. Blood 80:2182–2187, 1992.

65. Reid CD, Stackpoole A, Meager A, Tikerpae J: Interactions of tumor necrosis factor with granulocyte-macrophage colony-stimulating factor and other cytokines in the regulation of dendritic cell growth in vitro from early bipotent CD34+ progenitors in human bone marrow. J Immunol 149:2681–2688, 1992.

66. Young JW, Skabolcs P, Moore MA: Identification of dendritic cell colony-forming units among normal human CD34+ progenitors that are expanded by c kit ligand and yield pure dendritic cell colonies in the presence of GM-CSF and TNF-α. J Exp Med 182:1111–1119, 1995.

67. Caux C, Vanbervliet B, Massacrier C, et al: CD34+ hematopoietic progenitors form human cord blood differentiate along two indepen-

dent dendritic cell pathways in response to GM-CSF + TNF-alpha. J Exp Med 184:695–706, 1996.

68. Romani N, Gruner S, Brang D, et al: Proliferating dendritic cell progenitors in human blood. J Exp Med 180:83–93, 1994.

69. Santiago-Schwarz F, Rappa DA, Laky K, Carsons SE: Stem cell factor augments TNF/GM-CSF-mediated dendritic cell hematopoiesis. Stem Cells 13:186–197, 1995.

70. Siena S, Di Nicola M, Bregni M, et al: Massive ex vivo generation of functional dendritic cells from mobilized CD34 + blood progenitors from anticancer therapy. Exp Hematol 23:1463–1471, 1995.

71. Strobl H, Riedl E, Scheinecker C, et al: TGF-beta 1 promotes in vitro development of dendritic cells from CD34 + hemopoietic progenitors. J Immunol 157:1499–1507, 1996.

72. Bernhard H, Disis ML, Heimfeld S, et al: Generation of immunostimulatory dendritic cells from human CD34 + hematopoietic progenitor cells of the bone marrow and peripheral blood. Cancer Res 55:1099–1104, 1995.

73. Henderson RA, Nimgaonkar MT, Watkins SC, et al: Human dendritic cells genetically engineered to express high levels of the human epithelial tumor antigen (MUC-1). Cancer Res 56:3763–3670, 1996.

74. Miller JS, Verfaillie CM, McGlave PM: Expansion and activation of human natural killer cells for autologous therapy. J Hematother 3:71–74, 1994.

75. Miller JS, Klingsporn S, Lund J, et al: Large scale ex vivo expansion and activation of human natural killer cells for autologous therapy. Bone Marrow Transplant 14:555–562, 1994.

76. Cervantes F, Pierson BA, McGlave PB, et al: Autologous activated natural killer cells suppress primitive chronic myelogenous leukemia progenitors in long-term culture. Blood 87:2476–2485, 1996.

77. Gordon MY, Dowding CR, Riley GP, et al: Altered adhesive interactions with marrow stroma of hematopoietic progenitor cells in chronic myelogenous leukemia. Nature 328:342, 1984.

78. Verfaillie CM, McCarthy JB, McGlave PB: Mechanisms underlying abnormal trafficking of malignant progenitors in chronic myelogenous leukemia: decreased adhesion to stroma and fibronectin but increased adhesion to the basement membrane components laminin and collagen type IV. J Clin Invest 90:1232, 1992.

79. Eaves AC, Cashman JD, Gaboury LA, et al: Unregulated proliferation of primitive chronic myelogenous leukemia progenitors in the presence of normal marrow adherent cells. Proc Natl Acad Sci U S A 83:5306, 1986.

80. Bhatia R, McGlave PB, Dewald GW, et al: Abnormal function of the bone marrow microenvironment in chronic myelogenous leukemia: role of malignant stromal macrophages. Blood 85:3636–3645, 1995.

81. Greenberg BR, Wilson FD, Woo L, Henks HM: Cytogenetics of fibroblastic colonies in Ph 1 positive chronic myelogenous leukemia. Blood 51:1039, 1978.

82. O'Brien S, Kantarjian H, Shtalrid M, et al: Lack of breakpoint cluster region rearrangement in marrow fibroblasts of patients with Philadelphia chromosome–positive chronic myelogenous leukemia. Hematol Pathol 2:25, 1988.

83. Eaves CJ, Barnett MJ, Eaves AC: In vitro culture of bone marrow cells for autografting in CML. Leukemia 7 (Suppl 2):126–129, 1993.

84. Spencer A, Yan XH, Chase A, et al: BCR-ABL-positive lymphoblastoid cells display limited proliferative capacity under in vitro culture conditions. Br J Heaematol 94:654–658, 1996.

85. Deisseroth AB, Zhifei Z, Claxton D, et al: Genetic marking shows that Ph + cells present in autologous marrow of chronic myelogenous leukemia (CML) contribute to relapse after autologous bone marrow transplant in CML. Blood 83:3068, 1994.

86. Coutinho LH, Testa NG, Chang J, et al: The use of cultured bone marrow cells in autologous transplantation. Prog Clin Biol Res 333:415, 1989.

87. Verfaillie CM, Miller WJ, Boylan K, McGlave PB: Selection of benign primitive hematopoietic progenitors in chronic myelogenous leukemia on the basis of HLA-DR antigen expression. Blood 79:1003–1010, 1992.

88. Verfaillie CM, Bhatia R, Miller W, et al: BCR/ABL-negative primitive progenitors suitable for transplantation can be selected from the marrow of most early-chronic phase but not accelerated-phase chronic myelogenous leukemia patients. Blood 87:4770–4779, 1996.

89. Gribben JG, Freedman AS, Neuberg D, et al: Immunologic purging of marrow assessed by PCR before autologous bone marrow transplantation for B-cell lymphoma. N Engl J Med 325:1525–1533, 1991.

90. Gorin NC, Lopez M, Laporte JP, et al: Preparation and successful engraftment of purified CD34 + bone marrow progenitor cells in patients with non-Hodgkin's lymphoma. Blood 85:1647–1654, 1995.

91. Mahe B, Milpied N, Hermouet S, et al: G-CSF alone mobilizes sufficient peripheral blood CD34 + cells for positive selection in newly diagnosed patients with myeloma and lymphoma. Br J Haematol 92:263–268, 1996.

92. Widmer L, Pichert G, Jost LM, Stahel RA: Fate of contaminating t(14;18)+ lymphoma cells during ex vivo expansion of CD34-selected hematopoietic progenitor cells. Blood 88:3166–3175, 1996.

93. Pettengel R, Shido K, Kanz L, et al: Preferential expansion of hematopoietic versus acute myeloid leukemia cells ex vivo. Blood 86:145a, 1995.

94. Vogel W, Behringer D, Scheding S, et al: Ex vivo expansion of CD34 + peripheral blood progenitor cells: implications for the expansion of contaminating epithelial tumor cells. Blood 88:2707–2713, 1996.

95. Van Riet I, Schots R, Juge N, et al: Cytokine-mediated generation of myeloid progenitors in stroma-free cultures of mobilized CD34 + blood cells: no evidence for tumor cell expansion in multiple myeloma [Abstract]. Blood 86(Suppl 1):62a, 1995.

96. Nolta JA, Yu XJ, Bahner I, Kohn DB: Retroviral-mediated transfer of the human glucocerebrosidase gene into cultured Gaucher bone marrow. J Clin Invest 90:342–348, 1992.

97. Bregni M, Magni M, Siena S, et al: Human peripheral blood hematopoietic progenitors are optimal targets of retroviral-mediated gene transfer. Blood 80:1418–1422, 1992.

98. Dunbar CE, Cottler-Fox M, O'Shaughnessy JA, et al: Retrovirally marked CD34-enriched peripheral blood and bone marrow cells contribute to long-term engraftment after autologous transplantation. Blood 85:3048–3057, 1995.

99. Nimgaokar M, Mierski J, Beeler M, et al: Cytokine mobilization of peripheral blood stem cells in patients with Gaucher disease with a view to gene therapy. Exp Hematol 23:1633–1641, 1995.

100. Walsh CE, Grompe M, Vanin E, et al: A functionally active retrovirus vector for gene therapy in Fanconi anemia group C. Blood 84:453–459, 1994.

101. Malech HL, Horwitz ME, Linton GF, et al: Extended production of oxidase normal neutrophils in ex-linked chronic granulomatous disease (CGD) following gene therapy with gp91p^{hox} transduced CD34 + cells. Blood 92:690a, 1998.

102. Qazilbash MH, Walsh CE, Russell SM, et al: Retroviral vector for gene therapy of X-linked severe combined immunodeficiency syndrome. J Hematother 4:91–98, 1995.

CHAPTER THIRTY-THREE

Hematopoietic Stem Cells as Targets for Gene Therapy

Alfred B. Bahnson, Ph.D., and Edward D. Ball, M.D.

The importance of hematopoietic stem cells (HSC) as targets for gene therapy can hardly be overemphasized. Their ready availability from autologous sources, including peripheral blood and cord blood at birth; the proven effectiveness of cryopreservation; the ease of transplantability by simple infusion; their ability to be manipulated in vitro, their proliferative potential; their quiescent protection from acquired disease, from radiation, and from senescence; their ability to yield progeny that circulate and infiltrate organs and tissues throughout the body; and their position as the source of a renewable immune system and as upstream somatic carriers of mutations, which, when expressed in their progeny, result in a wide variety of common and rare human diseases are all compelling reasons for approaches to gene therapy.

A wealth of animal studies have guided and encouraged the entry into initial clinical trials.[1-3] The remarkable studies of Lemishka et al. using retroviral marking of murine bone marrow cells transplanted into lethally irradiated recipients confirmed the stability of retroviral vectors in HSC cells and accented the expansion and self-renewal capacities of gene-marked pluripotent stem cells. In time-dependent patterns of hematopoietic reconstitution, over the course of several months the condition of most animals stabilized with hematopoietic systems that showed oligoclonal and monoclonal patterns of vector integration.[4] Furthermore, when these primary recipients were used as bone marrow donors, multiple secondary recipients were fully reconstituted with the same gene-marked clones observed in the donors.[5] Such impressive self-renewal capacities cannot currently be achieved in vitro, despite much effort (see Chapter 17), but evidence is emerging for long-lasting engraftment of gene-modified progenitors in humans. Discovery of crucial factors involved in cell cycling and maintenance of pluripotency is anticipated by investigators seeking methods to enhance gene delivery and to preserve or expand primitive cells in vitro. Much of what follows reflects the active and inconclusive nature of this search.

GENE TRANSFER METHODS

With very few exceptions, clinical trials using gene transfer into HSC have relied on retrovirus-mediated gene transfer methods. Retroviruses fill the need for stable and relatively efficient integration of engineered genetic elements into the chromosomes of the target T cells. Other viral vector systems currently available, such as adenovirus or adenovirus-associated viral vectors, or transfection methods, such as lipofection, electroporation, calcium phosphate precipitation, or bioballistics, lack efficiency for long-term expression of the transgenes in dividing HSC. This is because the vectors do not enter the cells in sufficient numbers without cytotoxicity and/or they do not integrate stably into the chromosomes with useful efficiency. In dividing cells, unintegrated DNA is diluted and lost. Adenoviral vectors are also highly immunogenic.

Currently, retroviral vectors are preferred by investigators in transducing HSC. We are exploiting a gene transfer system naturally optimized through untold millions of years of selection and evolution. It is likely that progressive improvements in recombinant vector design and packaging systems will further increase the efficiency of retroviral vectors for achieving clinical goals. Among numerous developments, the recent promise shown by vectors derived from lentivirus, of which the human immunodeficiency virus (HIV) is a member, for integration of therapeutic genes into nondividing cells[6] is noteworthy. Vectors based on type C retroviruses, of which the Moloney murine leukemia virus (MMLV) has been most extensively employed, require that the target cell be in cycle in order for integration to occur.[7] Inducing the normally quiescent HSC[8] to divide in vitro, however, is commonly associated with loss of engraftment potential and/or pluripotency.[9]

In the murine model, several steps contribute to a solution to this problem using MMLV-based vectors. First, donor mice are pretreated with 5-fluorouracil to stimulate recruitment of HSC into cycle. An additional benefit of this pretreatment is the reduction in number of mature cells with consequent reductions in culture volumes. Second, extracted donor bone marrow cells are further stimulated in vitro with cytokine "cocktails" that commonly include interleukin-3 (IL-3), IL-6, and stem cell factor. Finally, the stimulated cells are transduced by direct coculture with cells that produce murine vector, which provide high-efficiency gene transfer and which likely supply extracellular matrix factors associated with maintenance of stem cell engraftment potential and pluripotency.[10]

Elements of each of these steps have been incorporated into most human clinical protocols for transduction of HSC (Table 33–1). For studies aimed at autologous HSC targets in adults, pretreatment of the patient/donor with granulocyte-colony stimulating factor (G-CSF) is used to mobilize HSC into the peripheral blood (peripheral blood progenitor cells, or PBPC). After harvest of sufficient numbers of PBPC or bone marrow cells, various enrichment methods for

	TARGET CELL	TRANSDUCTION METHOD	CYTOKINES	TRANSGENE LEVELS IN VIVO
ADA-SCID				
Blaese[24]	PBL	Supernatant 3–5 times over initial 72 hr of 9–12 day expansion	IL-2 and OKT3	PB: <0.01, 0.3 copy/cell (6 yr)
Kohn[19, 20]	CB CD34+	Supernatant 3 times over 3 days	IL-3, IL-6, SCF (20, 50, 100 ng/ml)	BM: 4–6% CFU-C (G418R), PB: 0.00001–0.003 copy/cell (PCR)—rising after PEG-ADA reduction (1 yr)
Bordignon[21]	PBL, BM,	BM—supernatant 3 days on stroma; PBL—6–7 day coculture with producer cells	BM: none; PBL: IL-2	PBL: 2–5% CFU-C, BM: 17–25% CFU-C (G418R) (1.5 yr)
Huggerbrugge[40]	BM CD34+	Coculture 80 hr	IL-3 (50 ng/mL)	PB&BM ± detection up to 6.5 mo, not thereafter
GAUCHER DISEASE				
Karlsson[50]	PB, BM CD34+	Supernatant 3 days, stroma optional	Optional IL-1, 3, 6, SCF (50 ng/mL)	<0.02% in PB at 1–2 mo.
Schuening[49]	PB CD34+	Supernatant 5 days on autologous stroma		Nondetectable in PB
Barranger[58]	PB CD34+	16-hr prestimulation, 4-hr centrifugation	IL-3, 6, SCF (10 ng/mL)	0.1–1% PCR+ PB cells up to 1 yr
CHRONIC GRANULOMATOUS DISEASE				
Malech[61]	PB CD34+	3 times over 3 days	PIXY, G-CSF	Peak 0.07% in PB, nondetectable after 6 mo
CANCER				
Rosenberg[66]	TIL	Supernatant 2 hr 2 times (1/3–1/2 of infusion)	IL-2	Marked PB all 5 pts up to 22 d, one pt out to 60 d; 1–2%-marked TIL in tumor at 64 d, expanded, reinfused, detected in PB at 189 d
Brenner[69]	ABMT	Supernatant 6 hr (30% of cells), cryopreserve		Up to 15% G418R BM CFU-C (18 mo), marked B and T cells (18 mo)
Cornetta[81]	BM	Supernatant 4 hr 1 time	None	365d PCR + 1 pt, 4 pts negative, (NOTE: variable bkg G418R colonies at 1000 μg/mL)
Deisseroth[80]	BM CD34+	Supernatant 6 hr (30% of cells), cryopreserve	None	Marked leukemic (up to 18%) and normal cells detected up to 280 d
Dunbar[79]	BM/PB CD34+	Supernatant 3 times over 3 days (same supernatant source as Bremner)	IL-3, 6 (brca only), SCF (20, 50, 100 ng/mL)	0.02–1% PB and/or BM PCR+ at 20d, intermittent PCR+ up to 2 yr, not detectable in brca at relapse
Stewart[78]	ABMT (LTMC)	Supernatant 3 times over 3 wk on stroma	None	19% G418R CFU, 17% in situ PCR+ BM cells (12 mo, 2 pts), up to
Bordignon[127]	Allogenic-PBL	Coculture >48 hr	IL-2, PHA	13% total PB and 5.3% BM (FACS)
AIDS				
Riddell[45]	HIV-specific CD8+ clones	Supernatant (HyTK) 2 times, days 3 & 5	IL-2	0.03–0.1% after two infusions, 4/5 pts <0.003% after third infusion

PBL, peripheral blood leukocytes; CB, cord blood; BM, bone marrow; TIL, tumor infiltrating lymphocytes; ABMT, autologous bone marrow transplant; LTMC, long-term marrow culture; IL, interleukin; SCF, stem cell factor; PIXY, IL-3/GM-CSF fusion protein; CFU-C, colony-forming units in culture; G418R, resistance to the antibiotic G418; PCR, polymerase chain reaction; PEG-ADA, polyethylene glycol–adenosine deaminase replacement therapy; FACS, fluorescence-activated cell sorting.

CD34+ cells can reduce the number of mature cells being handled by 2 logs with associated reductions in volume of cultures and costs of expensive recombinant cytokines during ex vivo procedures. In several European studies, direct coculture of HSC with murine producer cells has been used for the gene transduction step, whereas in the United States, because the coculture method poses safety concerns to the Food and Drug Administration (FDA), transduction with filtered supernatants is more common, often in the presence of an autologous stromal cell layer.

The choice of an ex vivo transduction method is currently a matter of considerable study and debate, made all the more difficult by the fact that there is no proven in vitro assay for human pluripotent HSC. Even if such an assay did exist, the ultimate decision as to what will and will not work in the clinic must be made in the clinic. Progress will surely accelerate in light of clinical trials that show therapeutic benefit and provide unique opportunities for insight into human hematopoiesis and hematology. Accordingly, this chapter outlines results from these pioneering trials, highlights the methods used, and provides practical information regarding FDA regulatory and safety concerns.

PIONEERING CLINICAL TRIALS

GENETIC DISORDERS

The urge to advance medicine early in the development of mammalian gene transfer technology led to a 1980 attempt to transfer the β-globin gene into bone marrow from two patients with β-thalassemia.[11] The protocol made use of calcium phosphate precipitation of a recombinant plasmid containing the herpes simplex virus thymidine kinase (TK) gene and human β-globin cDNA. This experiment succeeded in awakening the scientific community to the need for meeting defined criteria prior to initiation of gene therapy clinical trials in the United States. In 1983, the National Institutes of Health Recombinant DNA Advisory Committee (NIH-RAC) set up the Human Gene Therapy Subcommittee to provide a public forum for this purpose, and in 1985 the first draft of "Points to Consider" was published in the Federal Register. It was 3 years before the first proposal was evaluated and 4 more before two potentially therapeutic protocols were approved. The RAC Gene Therapy Subcommittee minutes and proceedings, published in *Human Gene Therapy,* provide insight into the continuing public discussion of the ethics and science of human gene therapy.

ADENOSINE DEAMINASE DEFICIENCY

In the period immediately following this β-globin gene therapy experiment, it became clear that hemaglobinopathies would pose a long-term challenge, not a starting point, for gene therapy. Instead, a rare severe combined immune disorder (SCID) resulting from genetic deficiency of adenosine deaminase (ADA) provided the focus for the first feasible gene therapy clinical trial for genetic disease. The development of retroviral packaging cell lines[12, 13] and helper virus-free vector preparations that could efficiently transfer and express the ADA cDNA in human peripheral blood lymphocytes (PBL) under in vitro stimulation provided the means to target the pathobiologically relevant T-cell progenitors.[14] Gene expression could range widely without harm and with probable benefit. A SCID mouse model was used to demonstrate correction of the ADA deficiency in human immune cells by retrovirus-mediated gene transfer.[15] Finally, in 1990 and 1991, under Blaese et al. at the National Institutes of Health (NIH), the first two patients with ADA-SCID were begun on a series of treatments that marked the beginning of human gene therapy.

The emerging use of enriched CD34+ cells for transplantation[16] and for retrovirus-mediated gene transfer[17, 18] encouraged protocol modifications aimed at a more durable source of ADA-expressing T cells than expected from the initial PBL transduction protocol in patients with SCID. In 1993, primitive HSC were targeted using CD34+ enrichment of umbilical cord blood from three ADA-deficient newborns at Children's Hospital, Los Angeles in a collaborative effort by Kohn et al., including NIH colleagues.[19, 20] Concurrent trials were initiated in Italy using a combination of PBL and bone marrow[21] and in the Netherlands using density gradient purified bone marrow stem cells.[22, 23] These and similar clinical trials introduced methods, successes, and problems associated with gene transfer into HSC.

NATIONAL INSTITUTES OF HEALTH

The murine retroviral vector used by Blaese et al. is designated *LASN* to denote an *LTR*-driven *ADA* gene with an internal *SV40*-driven *neomycin* resistance gene (neo). The "LTR," or long terminal repeat, is a multifunctional component of retroviruses containing strong enhancer and promoter elements (Fig. 33–1). The neo gene confers resistance to the toxic antibiotic, G418, which is used in some cases as an in vitro selective agent. Similar vectors expressing both the normal human ADA gene and the bacterial neo gene were used in the other ADA trials. Development of these vectors, and the packaging cells that "produce" them, involved scientists too numerous to mention here.

The patient T-cell transduction procedure involved exposure of PBL to filtered retroviral vector-containing supernatant three to five times over the initial 72 hours of a 9- to 12-day ex vivo T-cell expansion period using IL-2 and OKT3 stimulation. At the times of infusion at the end of each ex vivo transduction procedure, gene transfer efficiency varied between 1–10% and 0.1–1% for the first and second patients with ADA-SCID, respectively, at the NIH. The tenfold or lower transduction efficiency for the second patient in comparison with the first was consistent over the course of more than 10 transduction/infusion cycles for each patient.

Although various T-cell functional parameters (e.g., delayed-type hypersensitivity skin test reactivity, IL-2 production, cytolytic reactivity) indicate clinical benefit, evaluation of the therapeutic contribution from ADA gene replacement in the patients with SCID is obscured by concurrent polyethlyene glycol (PEG)–ADA enzyme therapy.[19–21, 24] An analogous problem complicates evaluation of gene therapy for Gaucher disease, a prototype disorder discussed later, because patients generally respond clinically to alglucerase (a

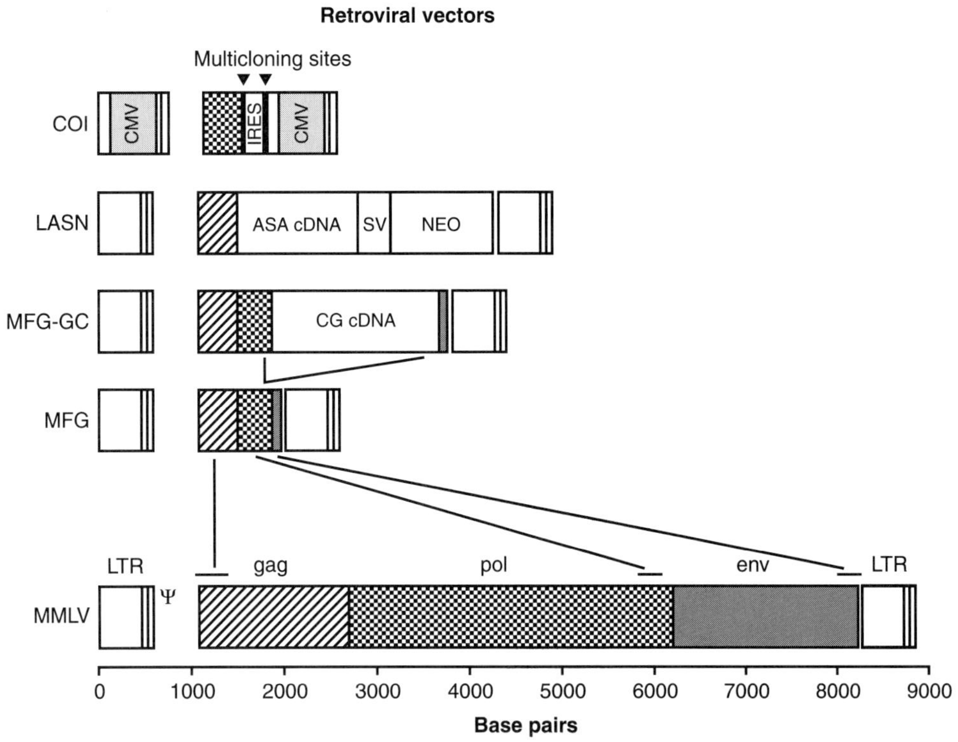

Retroviral vectors

FIGURE 33-1. Retroviral vectors derived from Moloney murine leukemia virus (MMLV). The MFG vector backbone is essentially derived through recombination of three fragments. The first fragment includes the 5' long terminal repeat (LTR—*three-segmented box*) continuing through the untranslated region (*solid line* including the "Ψ" region) and into approximately 420 base pairs of the 5' coding region for the gag polypeptide (*cross-hatched box*). The untranslated region contains a splice donor site; the "Ψ" region indicates sequences required for efficient packaging of RNA transcripts into virions. The first fragment is joined to a second fragment obtained from the 3' end of the polymerase coding region (pol—*dotted pattern*). This fragment contains a splice acceptor site and ends precisely at the adenine-thymine-guanine (ATG) start site of the following envelope gene (env—*checkerboard box*). Finally, the third fragment consists of the 3' end of the env gene connected by a short untranslated segment to the 3' LTR. The MFG-GC vector illustrates insertion of the cDNA for normal human glucocerebrosidase (GC) into the vector backbone so that the ATG start site coincides with that of the deleted env gene. The LASN vector illustrates one member of a family of vectors developed by Miller and colleagues (Hock et al., 1989[14]). These vectors lack the pol splice acceptor site and portion of the env gene included in the MFG vector; many contain an internal promoter such as the SV40 promoter (SV) for driving transcription of a selectable marker gene such as neo (NEO). The COI vector was developed from the MFG backbone by deletion of gag and env coding regions and through replacement of a portion of the LTR with promoter/enhancer sequences from cytomegalovirus (CMV). Multicloning sites provide for convenient insertion of desired genes at two locations, and an internal ribosome entry site (IRES) enables efficient translation of the second inserted gene. In vitro studies have shown that this vector expresses as efficiently or better than the original MFG (Kim et al., 1998[106]), and it should be safer because it provides less homology for possible recombination leading to replication competent retrovirus.

modified glucocerebrosidase) enzyme replacement therapy. Nevertheless, results for transgene persistence and expression are highly informative and set the stage for further progress toward definitive therapy.

Unexpectedly, patients receiving multiple infusions of transduced and expanded peripheral blood T cells have maintained circulating gene-modified cells at constant levels now for over 6 years of follow-up since the last infusion, and levels of ADA transgene expression remain without evidence of silencing over this period (RM Blaese: Personal communication). Analyses approximately 2 years after the last infusions indicated that vector frequencies of greater than 0.3 and less than or equal to 0.01 copies per cell had been achieved for the first and second patients, respectively, with Southern blot confirmation of approximately one vector copy per cell in the first patient's PBL.[24]

In ADA-deficient patients, expression of the ADA transgene may contribute a selective advantage favoring survival of transduced T cells. The long-term carriage and sustained expression of the transgene in these patients, however, go beyond expected survival of mature T cells. Sustained in vivo expansion, perhaps "self-renewal," of

transduced immature T-cell progenitors is implied. A concept that includes durable self-renewal of progenitors in vivo would enhance prospects for therapeutic benefit from many gene therapy protocols that fail to achieve transduction of primitive pluripotent HSC. The predominant problem is that the most primitive HSC are normally quiescent, and at this stage they apparently lack sufficient retroviral receptors.[25–28] Because cell cycling is a requirement for retroviral vector integration,[7] efforts have been directed toward stimulation of stem cell cycling without induction of differentiation during the ex vivo transduction procedures. This is a greater challenge than transduction of early cycling progenitors. Nonetheless, the results from Blaese et al. at the NIH support the possibility that therapeutic goals may be achieved over still undefined long-term intervals using conditions that favor expansion and transduction of committed progenitors.

MILAN, ITALY

Results using a combination of transduced PBL and bone marrow by Bordignon et al. in Italy corroborate the findings at the NIH of long-term gene carriage with likely selection for ADA expression.[21] Sixteen months after the last infusions, clonal assays indicated that 2–5% of the PBL progenitors and 17–25% of clonable bone marrow progenitors from two patients expressed the neo marker genes present in the vectors (based on colony resistance to G418). ADA enzyme activity ranged between 5% and 18% of normal in total peripheral blood nucleated cells from both patients and was near or higher than normal in G418-resistant bone marrow colony-forming cells and in patient T cells transplanted into SCID mice.

The Milan protocol further enabled an informative comparison of the relative contribution to engraftment from transduced PBL versus bone marrow progenitor cells. Different distinguishable vectors were used to permit this analysis. Initially, proviral DNA analysis indicated that circulating gene-modified lymphocytes arose from transduced PBL, whereas circulating gene-modified granulocytes arose from transduced bone marrow cells. One year after the last infusions, clonable circulating T cells shifted to the bone marrow–derived vector type. Patient numbers are too small to generalize these results.

The transduction protocol used by Bordignon et al. for bone marrow cells involved addition of vector-containing supernatants over the first 3 days of culture in a long-term culture system with adherent monolayers and without added cytokines. The presence of stromal/adherent T cells appears to foster preservation and transduction of early HSC,[1, 2, 29–35] and the culture system has been shown to be effective for maintenance of hematopoietic reconstituting cells.[36] Transduction efficiencies averaged from 30–40% according to G418 resistance of colony-forming progenitor cells expressing the neo transgene.

PBL were transduced by coculture with murine retroviral vector producer cells using a low IL-2 concentration and 6- to 7-day total incubation times. This PBL coculture transduction protocol has been shown to preserve immune repertoire (pre T-cell receptor-β germline rearrangement) and in vivo proliferative potential of transduced PBL.[37, 38] Transduction efficiencies increased from less than or equal to 2.5–40% with PBL-producer coculture and the introduction of a new vector packaging line partway through this study.

CHILDREN'S HOSPITAL, LOS ANGELES

For the three ADA-deficient newborns, CD34+ enriched cord blood cells were transduced by daily exposure over 3 days to vector-containing supernatant in the presence of IL-3 (20 ng/mL), IL-6 (50 ng/mL), and stem cell factor (100 ng/mL). Estimated transduction efficiencies at the time of infusion ranged from 12.5–21.5%. Significant engraftment was indicated in bone marrow biopsies taken after 12 months based on vector neo gene expression conferring G418 resistance in 4–6% of the granulocyte-macrophage–colony-forming units (CFU-GM), whereas vector frequencies in circulating cells were much lower at this time: 0.00001–0.0003 copies per cell.[19] This apparent imbalance between vector frequencies in bone marrow progenitors and circulating cells compares with the similar apparent imbalance reported by Bordignon et al. (discussed earlier). This imbalance implies progenitor expansion within the marrow compartment and blockage to maturation and/or fenestration. Kohn et al. caution that the apparent failure to complete maturation may be due to interference of normal cellular biochemistry by expression of the bacterial neomycin resistance gene or by overexpression of ADA.[19]

PEG-ADA replacement enzyme dosages were reduced after the babies reached 18 months of age, and the vector frequency in circulating cells rose to as high as 0.003 copies per cell, with 0.01–0.1 copies per cell among fluorescence-activated cell sorting (FACS)-sorted CD3+ cells.[20] The differential steps in gene frequencies with PEG-ADA withdrawal and with T-cell enrichment are clearly indicative of selective pressure for ADA-expressing transduced cells. More recently, when PEG-ADA was stopped completely in the patient with the highest gene marking level, absolute numbers of B lymphocytes and natural killer cells dropped by over 100 times and CD3+ and CD4+ T lymphocytes decreased by 50%, but the fraction of peripheral blood T lymphocytes containing the transgene increased to 30–100%. PEG-ADA therapy was resumed after oral thrush and upper respiratory infection developed.[20, 39]

THE NETHERLANDS

No advantage was apparent using irradiated vector producer cells for direct coculture of CD34+ enriched bone marrow cells from three patients with ADA-SCID in a study by Hoogerbrugge et al.[40] Transduction efficiency was 6–12% according to ADA expression in CFU-GM, and detection of the gene in patient peripheral blood cells was intermittent by polymerase chain reaction (PCR) up to a maximum of 6 months after treatment.[40] Expression of the transgene was not evident.

EXPRESSION AND IMMUNE REACTION TO GENE THERAPY PRODUCTS

Expression of the ADA transgene in T cells appears to correlate with levels of vector frequency, based on ADA activity in peripheral blood lymphocytes,[24] in cultured T lymphocytes selected in G418[19] or in total PBL and bone marrow cells.[21] Persistent expression of retroviral transgenes in humans in these and other trials appears to reduce long-held concerns about in vivo "down-regulation" of the transgene, for which there is much evidence in mice.[41–44] The lack of any evidence for silencing of the normal ADA and the bacterial neomycin resistance genes also indicates an absence of strong immune rejection against the cells expressing new gene products, both of which are foreign molecules to these patients. The deficient immune status of these and other patients may play a role in tolerance to transgene products. As discussed later, immune rejection of transgene-expressing cells has been reported in other human trials[15, 16] and is a serious concern with gene therapy. In addition, some patients have antibodies to bovine serum proteins used as culture supplements during ex vivo T-cell transduction and expansion, despite extensive washing of cells prior to patient infusion.[45, 47, 48]

GAUCHER DISEASE

Clinical trials for Gaucher disease have exhibited widely varying results, possibly because of differing transduction protocols for CD34+ enriched cells from peripheral blood of G-CSF stimulated patients and, in one case, from bone marrow. Schuening et al.[49] used a 5-day transduction of enriched peripheral blood CD34+ cells with vector-containing supernatant and cytokines (50 ng/mL IL-1, IL-3, IL-6, and stem cell factor) on a pre-established autologous stromal layer. Karlsson et al.[50] have maintained options to use or not to use cytokines and stroma during a 3-day supernatant transduction period for peripheral blood or bone marrow cells. Both of these protocols incorporated only a single infusion of cells for each patient. In the protocol of Barranger et al. (Fig. 33–2), transduction is performed using centrifugation for 4 hours at room temperature following overnight prestimulation in low-concentration cytokine-containing medium (10 ng/mL each of IL-3, IL-6, and stem cell factor). Centrifugation at 2400g with

retroviral vector-containing supernatant enhances the transduction process.[51, 52] Two patients have received four or more cycles of treatment over 3-month intervals, each cycle consisting of two infusions of transduced cells. A third patient was discontinued after two cycles because of G-CSF induced thrombocytopenia. None of the Gaucher or ADA cases involved myeloablation prior to reinfusion of transduced cells.

Schuening et al. reported transduction efficiencies in the range of 0.01–0.1% prior to infusion for their initial three patients, with enzyme elevation in treated cells at least twofold above the deficient low levels in nontreated patient control cells.[53] No detectable evidence of vector carriage has been found in peripheral blood cells after infusion, however. Karlsson et al. observed somewhat higher transduction efficiencies for peripheral blood CD34+ enriched cells prior to infusion into two patients (up to 10%) and for CD34+ bone marrow cells infused into one patient (up to 2.5%). Vector sequences were detected at minimum levels (< 0.02%) in two patients at 1–3 months post infusion.[54, 55]

Preliminary results of Barranger et al. for treatment of Gaucher disease at the University of Pittsburgh are more encouraging. Transduction efficiency prior to cell infusion

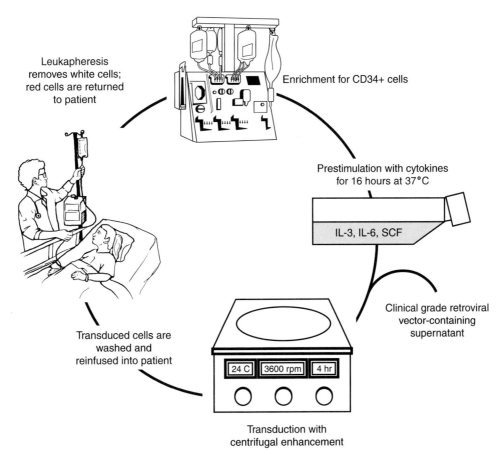

Leukapheresis removes white cells; red cells are returned to patient

Enrichment for CD34+ cells

Prestimulation with cytokines for 16 hours at 37°C

IL-3, IL-6, SCF

Transduced cells are washed and reinfused into patient

Clinical grade retroviral vector-containing supernatant

24 C   3600 rpm   4 hr

Transduction with centrifugal enhancement

FIGURE 33–2. Gene therapy clinical trial for Gaucher disease. Leukapheresis is performed on 2 successive days following granulocyte colony-stimulating factor mobilization of peripheral blood stem cells. Each leukapheresis product is enriched for CD34+ cells by immunoaffinity column separation (CellPro, Bothell, Washington). As the CellPro system is no longer commercially available, the Nexell-300 system, an FDA-approved device, is illustrated. The cells are then prestimulated for 16 hours in a mixture of cytokines (IL-3, IL-6, and stem cell factor at 10 ng/mL) in culture medium. Stimulated cells are mixed with FDA-approved retroviral vector–containing supernatant in the presence of protamine sulfate (8 μg/mL) and are centrifuged in blood bags for 4 hours at 2400 g. After centrifugation, the cells are washed and reinfused into the patient shortly after the second leukapheresis product is obtained and the cycle is repeated.

has varied between 5% and 30% for CFU-GM colonies, with an average of 9.4 ± 3.5% (n = 10) for high proliferative potential-colony forming cells (HPP-CFC).[56] The numbers of HPP-CFC did not differ between infected and non-infected cells, but infected cells were less actively cycling compared with prestimulated noncentrifuged cells according to ^{3}H-thymidine suicide assay. The latter finding suggests that conditions imposed by centrifugation with retrovirus may counteract the cycling induced by cytokine prestimulation, possibly reversing an engraftment defect observed after ex vivo transduction.[57] Glucocerebrosidase enzyme activity of bulk transduced cells after expansion in culture indicated levels up to 20 times those of the non-treated control cells of patients with Gaucher disease.

The transgene is consistently present in peripheral blood leukocytes in all of these patients with Gaucher disease; it has persisted in one patient now over 1 year since the last infusion at levels as high as 1% in circulating cells according to semiquantitative polymerase chain reaction (PCR). Glucocerebrosidase enzyme elevation in peripheral blood leukocytes is evident in all three patients, in one of whom levels have approached those of heterozygote carriers.[58] In this patient, replacement enzyme therapy was gradually reduced and finally discontinued without signs of clinical reversal. The possibility of a selective advantage for enzyme expressing monocyte/macrophages in this patient may become more evident after complete discontinuation of alglucerase enzyme replacement therapy. Transgene expression has apparently compensated for enzyme withdrawal, and persistence of the transgene in circulating cells suggests that early progenitors have been transduced and have engrafted.

Several contributing factors may account for these results. Multiple cycles of treatment may boost patient response and compensate for less than optimal conditions in some cycles of the highly variable transduction procedures. The MFG-based vector has been shown to provide superior transgene expression,[59, 60] which could account for the observed near-normal average glucocerebrosidase activity among circulating nucleated cells in the patient with vector frequencies up to 1%. Finally, centrifugation allows use of a significantly shortened transduction period. Combined with the use of a minimal (16-hour) prestimulating incubation time, these conditions may favor vector transfer into minimally differentiated CD34+ cells capable of re-engraftment. One could speculate that many of the cells carry unintegrated vector intermediates at the time of reinfusion, and if a single round of cell division were part of the engraftment process, integration could occur at this point in vivo.

If substantiated, the results of Barranger et al. provide encouragement for other protocols envisioned to involve transduction of CD34+ cells from G-CSF stimulated adult patients followed by reinfusion without myeloablative conditioning. As with the ADA trial results described earlier, in vivo expression from the retroviral vector remains high, countering down-regulation of transcription or immune elimination of transgene-expressing cells. Discussion of gene therapy in Gaucher disease can be found in Chapter 17.

OTHER GENETIC DISEASE GENE THERAPY TRIALS

Other genetic disorders currently under investigation in clinical gene therapy trials using HSC include chronic gran-ulomatous disease, Fanconi anemia, Fabry disease, and mild Hunter syndrome (mucopolysaccharidosis type III). Results have been reported for five patients with p47phox-deficient chronic granulomatous disease who were treated with a single round of two infusions of transduced G-CSF mobilized peripheral blood CD34+ enriched cells.[61] The centrifugation-enhanced transduction with a p47phox ret-rovirus-containing supernatant in the 3-day presence of PIXY321 (GM-CSF/IL-3 fusion protein) and G-CSF yielded transduction efficiencies of 10–30%. At 3–7 weeks post treatment, oxidase-positive neutrophils peaked at levels of 0.004–0.05% among total peripheral blood neutrophils and declined thereafter to nondetectible levels over 3–6 months. Correction of oxidase activity to normal levels in individual neutrophils was evident in all patients by flow cytometry, and gene-modified cells were detected in an empyema from one patient who had pneumonia 3 weeks after gene therapy. A protocol leading to higher accumulation and more-durable engraftment of transduced cells would likely benefit these patients.

Three patients with group C Fanconi anemia received three or four cycles of infusion of retrovirally transduced autologous HSC carrying the corrective complementation group C gene.[62] Transient detection of the transgene in peripheral blood coincided with increased numbers of colony-forming cells and transient improvement in bone marrow cellularity. Liu et al. plan to use gene-modified autologous HSC in patients who have undergone mye-loablation in whom allogeneic transplantation has failed. No patients have yet been enrolled in the trial proposing to use retroviral vector-mediated transfer of the iduonate-2-sulfatase gene into lymphocytes for treatment of mild Hunter syndrome[63]; the likelihood of intercellular cross-correction by transduced patient T cells has been demonstrated.[64]

These are bold studies, particularly in light of the fact that some of the patients with genetic disorders have access to alternative treatments and they are likely to lead full lives. The latter expectation is not so true with many of the advanced cancer and HIV-infected patients described later. These studies were performed in a comparatively nonab-lated hematopoietic environment, in contrast with the environment of cancer patients who have endured chemotherapy and often radiotherapy and surgery. The clear signs of progenitor cell engraftment without myeloablation are extremely encouraging and might not have been predicted on the basis of large-animal data.[9] Even with the handful of patients treated so far, results show probable benefit and hint at the broad information to be gathered about human HSC biology.

GENE MARKING AND GENE THERAPY FOR MALIGNANCY

Brenner makes a strong case for the value of gene marking in hematopoietic cell transplantation and ultimately in studies of other self-renewing tissues.[65] Information about trafficking patterns of activated lymphocytes, mechanisms of relapse after autologous HSCT for malignancy, evaluation of purging technologies, contributions to engraftment from peripheral blood versus bone marrow HSC, comparative effectiveness of methods for in vivo donor cell mobilization, HSC enrichment and sorting, and ex vivo maintenance and expansion—these are some of the issues that may be approached for the first time with integrating vectors, even without insertion of "therapeutic" genes.

Accordingly, the first approved gene transfer clinical trial was a marking study designed to evaluate persistence and trafficking of tumor infiltrating lymphocytes (TIL) in patients with advanced melanoma. Ex vivo expansion and reinfusion of TIL with high-dose IL-2 administration had shown promise for enhanced immune rejection of tumor cells,[66] and gene marking permitted evaluation of the longevity and reinfiltration of these cells.[67] Although T cells are rarely found in the blood, gene-marked TIL were detected in the bloodstream of all five patients at levels as high as 0.003 vector copies per cell within 3 days of infusion, declining thereafter with discontinuation of IL-2 administration to less than or equal to 0.0001 vector copies per cell detectible for as long as 95 days post infusion in one patient. Gene-marked TIL were detected in tumor biopsies from three of five patients, in one case for as long as 9 weeks (reviewed in reference 68).

At St. Jude's Children's Research Hospital in Memphis, long-term marking of normal marrow progenitor cells, peripheral blood mononuclear cells (MNC), B cells, and T cells was demonstrated for at least 15 months after autologous HSCT for neuroblastoma and acute myelogenous leukemia.[69] Persistence and expression of the transgene in mature progeny has continued for up to 4 years in some patients.[65] As in the studies involving ADA-deficient patients, bone marrow from the cancer patients appeared to harbor higher frequencies of gene-modified progenitors (five times higher) than is reflected by gene frequencies in peripheral blood.[70] Brenner, like Kohn et al., suggests that the neo transgene product may retard progenitor cell growth and differentiation in vivo or that a weak immune response against mature neo-expressing cells could play a role in the apparently imbalanced steady-state equilibrium between marked progenitors and mature progeny. Selection against neo-expressing hematopoietic cells was not observed, however, in a murine competitive repopulation study using neo transgenic mice as donors.[71] Additionally, frequencies vary among lineages in the mature circulating cells of cancer patients, with marked myeloid cells outnumbering marked B lymphocytes.[65] Preferential transduction of myeloid versus B-lymphoid progenitors is being supported by in vitro studies.[72]

In the earlier-described study of acute myelogenous leukemia and neuroblastoma, marrow was harvested 2–6 weeks after intensive chemotherapy, a time of hyperactive HSC cycling. One third of the harvested marrow MNC were transduced using retroviral supernatant for 6 hours without cytokines prior to cryopreservation. Patients were conditioned with chemotherapy, and both transduced (one third) and nontransduced (two thirds) cells were returned. The contribution of reinfused cells to resurgent malignancy was demonstrated in two patients with acute myelogenous leukemia who experienced relapse 67 and 180 days after transplantation.[73] Approximately 2% of the malignant blast T cells were marked with the neo transgene based on G418 resistance and PCR of colonies from malignant-immuno-

type sorted cells. The same colonies were positive by reverse PCR for the fusion transcript resulting from the (8;21) translocation in one patient. In three patients with neuroblastoma who experienced relapse, marker-gene positive cells constituted 0.1–1% of the malignant T-cell population.[74] The technique of inverse PCR[75] was used to enumerate two or four different vector integration sites among malignant T-cell clones from two patients. These data, combined with transduction efficiencies (2–9%) in the one-third portion of marked cells, enable an estimate of approximately 100–1000 tumorigenic cells contributing to relapse.

Contribution to relapse from reinfused gene-modified cells has also been demonstrated after autologous HSCT with intensive chemotherapy for chronic myeloid leukemia[76] and in a different study involving neuroblastoma.[77] Additional studies have been attempted or are in progress to assess this issue in multiple myeloma,[78, 79] chronic lymphoid leukemia,[80] acute lymphcytic leukemia,[81] and breast cancer.[79, 82]

Because recurrence is the major cause of autologous HSCT treatment failure for malignant disease, the demonstrations that marked tumor cells contribute to relapse have intensified efforts to achieve more-effective ex vivo purging. Gene marking provides a powerful tool for evaluation. Through the use of two different markers, two different purging techniques can be compared on different portions of the autologous HSCT in the same patient. At least two trials are under way.[65] An interesting early finding is the evidence for long-term gene marking of normal progenitors, "even when 4-hydroperoxycyclophosphamide (4HC) purging had rendered the HSC preparation entirely free of colony-forming cells," confirming "that measurement of gene transfer into committed progenitor cells is an inappropriate surrogate for assessing gene transfer into pluripotent progenitor cells."[65] Marked cells have persisted for more than 3 years after 4HC purging. In contrast, IL-2 purging yielded only transiently detectable marked cells.[70] Lack of an appropriate surrogate assay for pluripotent HSC limits the extent of useful information that can be obtained from preclinical in vitro studies, raising the importance of these and other clinical trials involving gene transfer into HSC. Discussion of purging and autologous HSCT can be found in Chapter 29.

A study using two distinguishable marking vectors for comparing the reconstituting effectiveness of peripheral blood versus bone marrow CD34+ enriched cells for autologous HSCT in patients with myeloma and breast cancer showed that both sources contributed to marked peripheral blood cells in one patient with myeloma, whereas two other patients showed only peripheral blood marked cells more than 1 year after transplantation.[79] Similar studies are currently underway for lymphoma and chronic lymphoid leukemia[83] and for pediatric solid tumors.[84]

Dual gene-marking studies can take many forms. For example, comparison between engraftment potential of cytokine stimulated/expanded and nonstimulated CD34+ enriched cells is being evaluated by Brenner et al.[65] Results from this study should show whether ex vivo cytokine stimulation and expansion result in faster initial engraftment and whether this leads to commitment to differentiation with loss of long-term reconstituting potential. Generally, cytokine stimulation enhances transduction efficiency based on surrogate assays. However, Brenner et al. note that pre-transplantation gene frequencies were much higher in the study of Dunbar et al. using a 3-day ex vivo transduction protocol with cytokine stimulation,[79] but long-term post-transplantation gene frequencies were higher using a 6-hour ex vivo transduction period without cytokines.[74] Again, this result points to the irrelevance of progenitor cell assays for predicting gene transfer rates in long-term engrafting cells. Given the variety of transduction protocols, we might anticipate that dual gene marking studies, in which patients act as their own controls, will play an increasing role in evaluating these techniques as well as for comparison of the relative efficacy of expansion, purging, enrichment, and depletion technologies for treatment of malignancies.

Deisseroth et al. reported findings from a trial designed to explore the potential for transgene enhancement of hematopoietic recovery from post-transplantation taxol chemotherapy in patients with advanced carcinomas of the breast or ovary.[83] Retrovirus-mediated transduction of the multidrug resistance gene (MDR-1) into CD34+ enriched peripheral blood or bone marrow cells is being compared using a 4-hour transduction without cytokines or a 2-day transduction on stromal monolayers with IL-3 and IL-6. Although surrogate assays indicated no difference in transduction efficiency between the two transduction procedures, post-transplantation gene marking frequencies of up to 3–7% were detected by in situ PCR in five of eight patients when stromal layers were used, whereas none of the 10 patients treated with cells transduced in suspension showed detectable levels of gene transfer. The shortened transduction protocol was apparently too inefficient for transduction of engrafting progenitors or stem cells. Several other trials have been approved for MDR resistance gene transfer into hematopoietic cells.[86]

Adoptive transfer of donor-derived Epstein-Barr virus (EBV)-specific cytotoxic T lymphocytes (CTL) has been shown to be effective in treatment of EBV lymphoma, a common complication that occurs after allogeneic HSCT using T cell–depleted marrow. Heslop et al. used neo gene marking to track levels of EBV-specific CTL in 14 bone marrow transplant recipients. Marked cells were detected in peripheral blood from 11 patients at levels of 0.002–0.02%, suggesting a 2- to 3-log expansion 1 month after infusion, based on a median transduction efficiency of 2% and the small numbers of CTL infused (2×10^7 to 1.2×10^8) relative to the total lymphocyte population in vivo.[87] Therapeutic benefit was demonstrated by rapid reduction in titers of EBV DNA coincident with increased frequencies of gene marked cells. Vector marked cell frequency fell to below detection levels in all patients at 4–5 months after infusion but reappeared in one patient after 18 months simultaneously with reactivation of EBV. More recently, marked cells have been shown to accumulate and expand at tumor sites with erradication of tumor cells.[88] Trafficking of gene-marked EBV-specific CTL is also being studied in EBV-positive Hodgkin disease.[89]

A rapidly expanding technology is illustrated by the use of the "suicide" gene, herpes simplex–thymidine kinase (HS-tk), in transduced T cells. Cells expressing HS-tk in vivo are killed by administration of ganciclovir. This system allows for elimination of transduced cells within the patient. Trials employing this system have been initiated for allogeneic marrow transplant recipients at risk for graft-versus-host disease (GVHD). In one study, T cell–depleted allogeneic marrow is being combined with infusion of G418-selected gene-modified primary allogeneic T cells (2×10^5/kg) to favor killing of residual tumor cells after intensive chemotherapy and total body irradiation.[90] The retroviral vector contains both the HS-tk gene and the neo G418 resistance gene. Two of three treated patients experienced grade II and III GVHD, and both responded completely to treatment with ganciclovir. One patient who experienced EBV lymphoma was successfully treated with an additional infusion of transduced allogeneic T cells (2×10^6/kg).

In a similar study, a nonfunctional form of the low-affinity nerve growth factor receptor gene, ΔLNGFR, was incorporated into the HS-tk vector to permit flow cytometry sorting of transduced T cells prior to infusion and for analysis post infusion.[46] As many as 13.4% of circulating PBL expressed the transgenes after infusion with escalating doses of 1×10^5 to 4×10^7 transduced donor PBL/kg. Three of eight treated patients experienced acute GVHD that responded in all cases to near resolution with ganciclovir treatment. Immunity against the HS-tk transgene, however, was observed in one patient, with sharp reduction of transduced cells.

Most of the studies are ongoing, and more definitive results are forthcoming. Nevertheless, it is already clear that important contributions have been made, and the use of gene-modified HSC is becoming a valuable, if not indispensable, tool for understanding and enhancing successful clinical outcomes in the field of HSCT for malignant diseases.

GENE THERAPY FOR INFECTIOUS DISEASE

Induction of immunity against transgene-expressing cells has decidedly complicated the gene therapy approach used by Riddell et al. for HIV-infected patients.[45] Based on previous successful results for reconstitution of cellular immunity against cytomegalovirus in allogeneic transplant recipients by infusion of cytomegalovirus-specific donor CTL,[91] a protocol was initiated in six HIV-seropositive patients using genetically modified HIV-specific autologous CTL. Retrovirus-mediated transfer of an HyTK fusion gene resulted in expression of hygromycin phosphotransferase (Hy), which enabled positive selection of transduced cells in hygromycin B–containing medium prior to infusion into the patients. In case toxicity occurred, HS-tk provided for ablation of gene-modified cells with ganciclovir.

Four escalating doses of transgene-expressing cells, ranging from 1×10^8 to 3.3×10^9 cells/m^2, were infused into each patient. In all of the patients, circulating gene-modified cells were detected after the first two infusions at frequencies up to one marked cell per 1000 peripheral blood MNC. In five of the six patients, however, rapid elimination of infused cells was evident after the third and fourth infusions. Strong cytolytic reactivity specific for HyTK-transduced target T cells was demonstrated in MNC cultures prepared 1 week after the fourth infusion from these five patients, whereas pretreatment cultures were not reactive nor were cultures from the sixth patient, who exhibited detectable gene-modified cells in peripheral blood after all four infusions. More rigorous analysis of CTL precursor clones indicated that epitopes derived from both the TK and Hy domains of the expressed protein contributed to induction of cytolytic reactivity. These findings once again underscore the potential for immune reaction against novel transgene products in gene therapy.

A similar CTL-mediated response has been observed against the neo transgene product in four HIV-infected patients involved in a gene marking study (Blaese RM: Personal communication). These patients have received three cycles of treatment, given at 6-week intervals, with expanded syngeneic T lymphocytes from HIV-seronegative identical twins. The donor apheresis products were separated into CD4+ and CD8+ cell enriched fractions, which were transduced with distinctive retroviral neo-containing vectors and expanded 10- to 1000-fold over approximately 2 weeks of culture with anti-CD3 and IL-2 stimulation prior to infusion.[92] The finding of CTL-mediated immunity against the neo transgene product in this case may have implications for the ADA-deficient patients and cancer patients in whom neo-containing vectors were used.

Several additional clinical trials involving gene transfer into HSC have been approved and/or submitted for HIV-infected patients. In one trial using HIV-specific autologous CTL and in another using CTL from twins, cells were transduced with vectors containing a CD4-zeta-chain fusion protein.[86] This chimeric universal T-cell receptor is expected to enhance killing of HIV-infected cells.

In a trial by Kohn et al., autologous CD34+ cells will be transduced with retroviral vectors carrying HIV Rev-responsive element (RRE) sequences.[94] Transcripts derived from these sequences are called *RRE decoys* because they bind with the HIV Rev protein and interfere with the normal Rev-RRE interaction required for export of viral RNA from the nucleus to the cytoplasm of infected cells. Preclinical studies indicate up to 99.9% inhibition of HIV-1 replication in myelomonocytic progeny of transduced progenitor cells.[93] Bone marrow CD34+ cells from four HIV-1–infected pediatric subjects were transduced with RRE decoy genes, and then were reinfused without adverse effects. However, the level of transgene-containing leukocytes was extremely low at 1 year after infusion.[94]

Nabel et al. conducted a clinical trial involving transduction of autologous CD4+ T cells with a transdominant negative mutant form of the Rev M10 protein.[95] A unique feature of this study is the use of gold particle–mediated gene delivery of plasmid DNA in addition to retroviral vector–mediated gene transfer. The former method produced a fourfold to fivefold survival advantage for Rev M10–transfected cells in comparison with cells transfected with δ-Rev M10, a frameshift control vector, in four HIV-infected patients.[96] The duration of engraftment was short-lived, however: up to 2 months in one patient but not detectable after 2 weeks in two other patients. More recently, T cells transduced with a retroviral vector expressing Rev M10 exhibited a survival advantage over control transduced cells for 4 months in three HIV-infected patients and for 9 months in one patient.[97]

Morgan and Walker are using genes for transdominant

Rev and/or antisense RNA, which inhibits transactivation of the HIV-1 LTR by the transactivator protein (tat) by hybridizing to sequence within the *cis*-acting transactivation response (TAR) element or the overlapping tat/rev genes.[98] Vectors are transduced into CD4+ lymphocytes from identical twins of HIV-1-infected patients using a centrifugation-enhanced protocol. A unique feature of this transduction protocol is the incorporation of phosphate-depleted media, which up-regulates the phosphate symporter molecules that serve as receptors for amphotropic and gibbon ape leukemia virus vector pseudotypes.[99] Preliminary results for eight patients indicate transduction efficiencies up to 40% and transgene frequencies up to 2% in MNC immediately after infusion. Transient increases in CD4+ cell counts have persisted up to 28 weeks.[100] A study in rhesus macaques, published in 1998, showed significant reduction in viral load, sustained CD4+ cell numbers, and reduced lymph node pathology for three animals receiving challenge infection with SIV mac239 after multiple infusions of tat/rev antisense vector-transduced CD4 lymphocytes.[101]

Two protocols propose the use of retroviral vectors encoding anti-HIV ribozymes for inhibition of HIV replication in transduced T cells or progeny of transduced CD34+ progenitors from HIV-infected patients.[86] Ribozymes are RNA molecules that recognize specific target sequences within RNA transcripts and inactivate the target molecules by cleavage. Finally, Marasco proposes to use a new class of therapeutic molecules known as intracellular antibodies or "intrabodies" consisting of human single-chain antibodies that remain within the cytoplasm.[102] One such intrabody against the HIV envelope glycoprotein, gp120, blocks processing and production of infectious HIV particles in infected cells. Retroviral vectors carrying the gene for this intrabody will be transduced into autologous T cells for reinfusion into patients. Prolonged survival of transduced CD4+ T cells is anticipated.

Because HIV integrates into the genome of infected cells, some of which form a quiescent reservoir,[103, 104] and because mosaicism of expression is a feature of retroviral vectors, even if true latency is not, it seems unlikely that HIV infection will ever be permanently curable. But numerous approaches have been designed to augment T-cell numbers, to inhibit virus spread, to suppress virus activity, and to protect uninfected cells from infection. The use of HIV-based vectors may become a particularly useful approach for CD4+ T-cells.[105]

RETROVIRAL VECTORS

Although a set of detailed protocols for transduction of human HSC has been published,[2] the review of current clinical trials makes evident many unresolved issues regarding clinical transduction procedures for HSC using retroviruses.[65] Differences between multiple variables—different vectors, different packaging lines, producer cells and supernatant products of widely varying titer, different cytokine concentrations, different transduction schedules, even different gravitational field strengths—complicate comparisons between the results of one group and another (see Table 33–1). In many cases, intellectual property ties shape the picture. Moreover, the variety of vectors, packaging cell types, and transduction techniques will likely increase in the clinical setting for some time.

Development of a retrovirus-mediated gene transfer system making use of existing technology can be summarized as follows. The therapeutic gene, usually in the form of cDNA, is inserted into the vector of choice. Inclusion of multicloning site(s) facilitates this step.[106] Two or three genes can be expressed from a single RNA transcript using internal ribosome entry sites, thereby avoiding interference problems associated with use of internal heterologous promoters within a single vector (see Fig. 33–1). The vector construct in plasmid form is cloned and amplified in a large-scale bacterial preparation. Purified plasmid is then transfected into packaging cells. A variety of packaging cells are available;[107] the most commonly used in clinical trials are PA317, ψCRIP, GP + AM12, and GP13. Generation of stable retroviral vector-producing cells may be achieved by cotransfection with a selectible plasmid vector such as pSV2neo, followed by selection in G418,[108] and screening of clones for vector activity in target T cells. Alternatively, the plasmid can be transiently expressed in highly transfectable packaging cells[109] or cotransfected with vectors providing packaging functions to obtain small quantities of vector-containing supernatant. Because cell receptors differ for ecotropic versus amphotropic forms of retrovirus envelope in the packaging system, ecotropic vector particles can cross-infect amphotropic packaging cells. Multiple cross-infections can generate nearly 100% infection in the producer cell population, from which clones are obtained by limiting dilution and are screened directly for vector activity (Fig. 33–3). The fidelity and stability of integrated vectors is generally better with retroviral *transduction* in comparison with *transfection* with plasmid DNA, and evidence indicates that expression is on the average more efficient from transduced genes.[110]

A tremendous advantage with retroviral vectors is that once a stable producer cell is generated, it can be expanded without limit. Retroviral vector production has no cytotoxic effect in the producer cells unless the transgene product itself is toxic. The cells are grown to confluence, and vector-containing supernatant can be collected daily with feeding of fresh medium to the monolayer. With ψCRIP cells, we have found that titer maximizes about 4 days after confluence and remains on a plateau thereafter as long as the cells remain healthy.[111] On the other hand, PA317 monolayers appear to peel off after approximately 1 week (unpublished data). Alternative vectors, such as adenovirus, adeno-associated virus, herpesvirus, or vesicular stomatitis virus G protein (VSV-G) pseudotype retrovirus, involve cytotoxic events in their production, which complicates large-scale production.

All of the retroviral vector systems used to date have been based on modifications of murine leukemia virus.

Cross-infection strategy for generating amphotropic producers

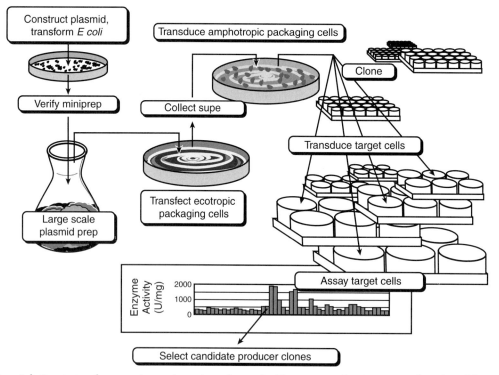

FIGURE 33–3. Cross-infection strategy for generating amphotropic producer cells. The vector provirus is constructed in plasmid form, cloned, verified, and prepared in quantity. The purified DNA is used to transfect a highly transfectible cell line such as 293 cells. Packaging functions can be provided by stable incorporation of gag, pol, and env genes such as in BOSC 23 cells,[109] or these genes can be cotransfected into the cells along with the vector DNA. Transient production of vector particles occurs. If these particles contain the ecotropic envelope, the supernatant (supe) may be used to transduce a stable amphotropic packaging line such as PA317 or ΨCRIP. Multiple transduction may be performed to increase the copy number and probability of obtaining amphotropic producing clones, which express high titers of vector. These clones are evaluated by transduction and analysis of transgene expression in target cells.

Only in a few cases have properly controlled direct comparisons been made between vector expression levels, although vector design is associated with wide variation in expression levels. The "MFG" family of vectors (see Fig. 33–1), initially generated at the Massachusetts Institute of Technology and further developed at many sites, including the University of Pittsburgh under the direction of Paul Robbins, has consistently yielded expression superior to that of other vectors.[59, 60, 112] Even so, conjectures about the reasons for superior expression of MFG vectors, including the need for 5' partial gag sequences and coincidence of the translation start site of the inserted gene with that of the deleted envelope gene (env), have not been supported by further study.[106] Deletion of unnecessary gag and env sequences should yield vectors less prone to recombination with packaging elements contained in the producer cells, reducing the risk of generating a replication-competent retrovirus.

Remarkably, Kim et al. have shown that almost all of the native untranslated U3 region of the long terminal repeat (LTR) can be deleted and replaced with human cytomegalovirus enhancer sequences to provide equivalent or better expression and at the same time provide reduced genetic homology for undesirable recombination in the murine packaging cells.[106] Similar enhancer replacement modifications using eukaryotic erythroid-specific promoters inserted into the U3 region have shown promise for targeting expression of retroviral constructs to specific cell lineages.[113]

Cell type–specific control of expression presents a major challenge, if hemoglobinopathies are to be treated using retroviruses. Genes involved in metabolic genetic disorders are frequently expressed constitutively. Partial correction may provide therapeutic benefit, and inappropriate expression or overexpression does not present problems. For most applications, however, control of expression would be advantageous if not necessary. The tetracycline and doxorubicin systems have shown value for in vitro control of expression,[114] but methods for in vivo control are still lacking. Within the size limit imposed by retroviral vectors of about 5 kb of payload sequence, numerous additional possibilities exist for molecular control of expression. Examples involve inclusion of a scaffold attachment region[115] or construction of novel chimeric signal transduction proteins.[116]

ENHANCEMENT OF TRANSDUCTION

Currently, low transduction efficiency is a major impediment to clinical success. Ideally 100% of the target cells would be transduced prior to reinfusion into patients. Instead, fewer than 50%, and in many cases fewer than 10%, of the treated progenitor cells are transduced. In preliminary studies, it is often assumed that the measured transduction efficiency of progenitors (CFU-GM, HPP-CFC, or LTC-IC) correlates with transduction efficiency of self-renewing cells that can engraft in patients. Most likely, the opposite is true: conditions evidently yielding higher transduction of progenitors could associate with differentiation and loss of primitive HSC, particularly when cytokine stimulation continues for periods of several days. Thus, conclusions regarding which method is "better" must be viewed with caution when transduction efficiency is expressed in terms of commonly employed progenitor cell assays. Enhancement methods can improve transduction efficiency. Polycation (e.g., polybrene) is almost universally used. Additional methods include the use of fibronectin,[117] cationic lipids,[118] flow-through transduction,[119] and calcium phosphate concentration.[120] Pseudotyping of retroviral vectors with VSV-G protein has allowed concentration of vectors by ultracentrifugation.[121]

With continued development of better vectors and higher-titer production techniques, we might anticipate the future capability of vector insertion in target cells to whatever extent we will. In cultured cells, 50 or more copies may be introduced per cell without apparent harmful effects, although the growth rate may lag at higher multiplicities of infection (unpublished observation). Immortalized cells tell little about the leukemogenicity of these integration events, however. The downside of superefficient transduction may be the occurrence of leukemia or other undesirable effects resulting from non–replication-competent retrovirus "insertional mutagenesis," not yet a known factor in the risk/benefit analysis.

SAFETY AND REGULATORY ISSUES

All of the retrovirus-mediated gene therapy trials have demonstrated a major phase I objective (i.e., safety). There have been few reported adverse reactions. The cell infusions have been well tolerated and, in fact, uneventful. The ADA-deficient patients each received a total of approximately 5×10^9 transduced cells arising from some 10^8 vector integrations during the initial ex vivo transduction periods. In the case of multiply treated patients with Gaucher disease, 20% transduction of the target cell dose of 2×10^6 CD34 + cells/kg for four treatment cycles represents, once again, about 10^8 vector integrations per patient. Except in association with their disease, all patients have not undergone myeloablation, as dictated by the Recombinant DNA Advisory Committee and the desire to reduce risks, including the risk of retroviremia, should a replication-competent retrovirus (RCR) arise from recombination with endogenous genes in the murine vector packaging system or with retroviral elements in the human cells.

Two early studies indicated lack of acute pathogenicity or malignancy from amphotropic RCR in immunosuppressed and myeloablated primates.[122, 123] However, in a subsequent study with transplantation of transduced CD34 + enriched bone marrow cells into myeloablated monkeys, it was found that malignant disease could be transmitted. Three of eight lethally irradiated rhesus monkeys experienced lymphoma after treatment using supernatants known to contain RCR at levels of 10^3–10^4 particles/mL.[124] Integrated proviral RCR containing the amphotropic envelope gene were present in the tumor cells at 10–50 copies per cell. This study underscored the importance of rigid testing of supernatants and, in most cases, of transduced cells for RCR prior to reinfusion. Even with replication-defective vectors and/or immunocompetent hosts, however, the risks of insertional mutagenesis leading to neoplasia are finite, though very small.[125]

The FDA's approach to regulation of gene therapy trials has been evolving in response to the rapid growth in this area. Definitions and statements concerning the manner in which the FDA's statutory authorities govern somatic cell therapy and gene therapy products were issued in October 1993 as *Application of Current Statutory Authorities to Human Somatic Cell Therapy Products and Gene Therapy Products* (58 FR 53248). Human research experiments involving use of recombinant DNA (i.e., human gene therapy experiments) are reviewed and approved by the NIH through submission to the Office of Recombinant DNA Activities (ORDA) of relevant information as described in *Points to Consider in the Design and Submission of Protocols for the Transfer of Recombinant DNA Molecules into One or More Human Subjects* (Jan 1997), Appendix M of the ORDA document, *Guidelines for Recombinant DNA Activities*. Prior to submission to Federal agencies, the experiments must be approved by the local institutional review board (IRB) and the institutional biosafety committee (IBC). Changes have recently been or are currently being implemented in the requirements of this process as well as in the makeup of the Recombinant DNA Advisory Committee (RAC) committee itself, which has traditionally reviewed and recommended approval of such protocols to the NIH director. Since 1995, some categories of protocols determined not to represent a novel gene therapy delivery strategy or target disease are processed by consolidated review by the RAC and are forwarded directly to the FDA for approval.

Guidelines and "Points to Consider" documents prepared by the RAC and the FDA concerning use of recombinant DNA for therapeutic purposes should be consulted during the planning stages and undertaking of preliminary gene-modification experiments. These include the *Points to Consider in Human Somatic Cell Therapy and Gene Therapy* (August 1991) and a *1/96 Draft Addendum* to this document, providing background information needed for investigational new drug applications for gene therapy experiments along with current regulatory concerns for production, testing, and administration of recombinant vectors for gene therapy. Other pertinent documents include *Points to Consider in the Production and Testing of New Drugs and Biologicals Produced by Recombinant DNA Technology* (1985) and *Points to Consider in the Characterization of Cell Lines Used to Produce Biologicals* (1993) for the construction of gene therapy vectors and preparation of other biologic products by recombinant DNA technology. The documents set standards for clinical trials that are likely to be required for FDA and RAC approval. These documents are readily available through the Internet at http://www.fda.gov.cber (U.S. FDA Center for Biologic Evaluation and Research) or through the FDA fax: (888-223-7329). Current status and issues in the regulation of HSCT are discussed in Chapter 65.

Different vector systems are associated with different safety concerns and testing requirements. The costs for these tests can become a major consideration (Table 33-2). For viral vectors, testing includes certification of the producer cell bank(s) for adventitious agents (inappropriate viruses), *Mycoplasma,* sterility, and replication-competent viruses of the vector type (e.g., RCR for retroviral vectors and replication-competent adenoviruses for adenoviral vectors); certification of the vector sequence and, if applicable, the seed stock; certification of each lot of final product for similar contaminants and for general safety (in vivo test); and finally, periodic monitoring of the patient for RCR.

TABLE 33–2. SAFETY TESTING AND ASSOCIATED COSTS FOR RETROVIRUS-MEDIATED GENE THERAPY*

	COST
Vector	
DNA sequence	Depends on base pair
Preliminary testing of candidate producer cell	
Sterility	$500
Mycoplasma	$1,200
RCR by S+/L− focus assay	$1,300
Total for preliminary testing	*$3,000*
Master cell bank	
Sterility	$500
Isoenzymes	$1,400
Mycoplasma	$1,200
Extended XC plaque	$1,200
RCR: cocultivation of producer cells with Mus dunni cells	$3,200
RCR: supernatant amplification on Mus dunni cells	$4,000
Mouse antibody production (MAP)	$1,500
In vitro assay for adventitious viral contaminants	$11,000
In vivo assay for adventitious viral contaminants	$11,000
Total for master cell bank production	*$35,000*
Bulk unfiltered supernatant	
Bulk product sterility	$700
Mycoplasma	$1,200
RCR: supernatant amplification on Mus dunni cells	$5,300
Filtered supernatant product	
Endotoxin	$600
General safety	$800
Bacteriostasis/fungistasis	$900
Final product GMP sterility	$2,200
End-of-production cells	
RCR: cocultivation with Mus dunni cells	$6,300
Total for supernatant production per lot	*$11,700*
Testing of ex-vivo transduced cells	
Sterility	$500
Mycoplasma	$1,200
RCR: cocultivation with Mus dunni cells	$3,200
RCR: supernatant amplification on Mus dunni cells	$4,200
Total for ex-vivo transduced cells	*$9,100*
Grand Total	**$58,800**

*Tests are from current recommendations based on FDA guidelines. Costs are approximated from current pricing from two independent contract testing laboratories.

GMP, good manufacturing practice; RCR, replication-competent retrovirus.

Validated testing may be performed by the sponsoring institution in compliance with Good Laboratory Practices, but the investment in personnel time for small numbers of samples may not be cost effective.

Testing requirements and costs should be born in mind when pursuing plans for protocols involving gene transfer. Generally, regulations have taken the form of "guidelines" rather than strict legal codes in order to allow flexibility in light of the evolving science. It may be helpful to maintain contact with the relevant offices throughout the course of proposed investigations and, when possible, to participate in and provide input to public conferences and meetings related to Center for Biologic Evaluation and Research (CBER) activities.

In 1994, the NIH established a program for support of gene therapy clinical trials through an interactive group of academic production laboratories known as the National Gene Vector Laboratories (NGVL). Investigators may apply for assistance in the production of cell bank(s) and clinical grade vector-containing materials through a peer-review process based on scientific merit, feasibility, and availability of NGVL resources. Application may be made through the Coordinating Center at the Indiana University School of Medicine (317-274-0448), with submission deadlines in March and September of each year. In addition, it may be possible to obtain material through collaborative agreement with centers such as the University of Pittsburgh Human Gene Therapy Applications Laboratory and elsewhere where good manufacturing practice (GMP) facilities have been successfully established.

CONCLUSION

Numerous disorders, including leukemias and other cancers, infectious diseases, and a broad list of genetic diseases, of which ADA deficiency and Gaucher disease are prototypes, may be responsive to gene alteration of HSC and their progeny. We are clearly approaching the threshold of a new era in medical treatment. Our understanding of what works and what doesn't work is still largely based on a process of trial and error. This process will become more predictable with increased understanding of the factors involved in normal gene regulation. The 1998 report of Yuh et al.[126] demonstrates the potential for detailed functional analysis of cis-regulatory elements leading to quantitative predictions for gene expression. Retroviral vectors are providing stable integration into target progenitor cells, and except in some instances of immune rejection of foreign transgene products, adequate in vivo expression can be maintained over long-term periods.

Currently, one of the greatest hurdles is less-than-adequate transduction efficiency using retroviruses for gene transfer into primitive HSC and progenitor cells. This hurdle is likely to be overcome through advances in recombinant vector design and through various methods of concentration and/or technologies for enhancement of transduction. These technologies are in their infancy, and there is every reason to be optimistic about improvements in gene transfer efficiency and about incorporating new and more-refined mechanisms into vectors for control of transgene expression. In parallel with these advances, we may anticipate progress toward a more-complete understanding of factors involved in normal hematopoiesis and toward improvements in technologies for HSC maintenance and expansion in vitro.

REFERENCES

1. Nolta JA, Kohn DB: Haematopoietic stem cells for gene therapy. *In* Potten C (ed): Stem Cells. London, Academic Press, 1997, p 447.
2. Nolta JA, Kohn DB: Human hematopoietic cell culture, transduction, and analyses. *In* Dracopoli NC, Haines JL, Korf BR, et al (eds): Current Protocols in Human Genetics, Suppl. 14. John Wiley & Sons, New York, 1998.
3. Havenga M, Hoogerbrugge P, Valerio D, van Es HHG: Retroviral stem cell gene therapy. Stem Cells 15:162–179, 1997.
4. Lemischka IR, Raulet DH, Mulligan RC: Developmental potential of pluripotent hematopoietic stem cells. Cell 45:917–927, 1986.
5. Jordon CT, Lemischka IR: Clonal and systemic analysis of long-term hematopoiesis in the mouse. Genes Dev 4:220, 1990.
6. Naldini L, Blomer U, Gally P, et al: In vivo gene delivery and stable transduction of nondividing cells by a lentiviral vector. Science 272:263, 1996.
7. Miller DG, Adam MA, Miller AD: Gene transfer by retrovirus vectors occurs only in cells that are actively replicating at the time of infection. Mol Cell Biol 10:4239, 1990.
8. Abkowitz JL, Persik M, Shelton G, et al: Behaviour of hematopoietic stem cells in a large animal. Proc Natl Acad Sci U S A 92:2031, 1995.
9. Stewart FM, Crittenden RB, Lowry PA, et al: Long-term engraftment of normal and post-5-fluorouracil murine marrow into normal non-myeloablated mice. Blood 81:2544, 1993.
10. Roberts RA, Spoonser E, Parkinson EK, et al: Metabolically inactive 3T3 cells can substitute for marrow stromal cells to promote the proliferation and development of multipotent haematopoietic stem cells. J Cell Physiol 132(2):203, 1987.
11. Thompson L: The risks of progress. *In* Correcting the Code. New York, Simon & Schuster, 1994, p 189.
12. Miller AD, Jolly DJ, Friedman T, Verma IM: A transmissible retrovirus expressing human hypoxanthine phosphoribosyltransferase(HPRT): gene transfer into cells obtained from humans deficient in HPRT. Proc Natl Acad Sci U S A 80:4709, 1983.
13. Miller AD, Buttimore C: Redesign of retrovirus packaging cell lines to avoid recombination leading to helper virus production. Mol Cell Biol 6:2895, 1986.
14. Hock RA, Miller AD, Osborne WRA: Expression of human adenosine deaminase from various strong promoters after gene transfer into human hematopoietic cell lines. Blood 74:876, 1989.
15. Ferrari G, Rossini S, Giavazzi R, et al: An in vivo model of somatic cell gene therapy for human severe combined immunodeficiency. Science 251:1363, 1991.
16. Berenson RJ: Transplantation of CD34+ hematopoietic precursors: clinical rationale. Transplant Proc 24:3032, 1992.
17. Cassel A, Cottler-Fox M, Doren S, Dunbar CE: Retroviral-mediated gene trasfer into CD34+-enriched human peripheral blood stem cells. Exp Heme 21:585, 1993.
18. Bregni M, Magni M, Sienna S, et al: Human peripheral blood hematopoietic progenitors are optimal targets of retroviral-mediated gene transfer. Blood 80:1418, 1992.
19. Kohn DB, Weinberg KI, Nolta JA, et al: Engraftment of gene-modified umbilical cord blood cells in neonates with adenosine deaminase deficiency. Nature Med 1(10):1017, 1995.
20. Kohn DB, Hershfield MS, Carbonaro D, et al: T lymphocytes with a normal ADA gene accumulate after transplantation of transduced autologous umbilical cord blood CD34+ cells in ADA-deficient SCID neonates. Nature Med 4:775–780, 1998.
21. Bordignon C, Motarangelo LD, Nobili N, et al: Gene therapy in peripheral blood lymphocytes and bone marrow for ADA-immuno-deficient patients. Science 270:470, 1995.
22. Hoogerbrugge PM, van Beusechem VW, Vossen JMJJ, Valerio D: Treatment of patients with severe combined immunodeficiency due to adenosine deaminase (ADA) deficiency by autologous transplantation of genetically modified bone marrow cells. Hum Gene Ther 3:553, 1992.
23. Hoogerbrugge PM, van Beusechem VW, Kaptein LCM, et al: Gene therapy for adenosine deaminase deficiency. Br Med Bull 51:72, 1995.
24. Blaese RM, Culver KW, Miller AD, et al: T lymphocyte–directed gene therapy for ADA-SCID: initial trial results after 4 years. Science 270:475, 1995.
25. Crooks GM, Kohn DB: Growth factors increase amphotropic retrovirus binding to human CD34+ bone marrow progenitor cells. Blood 82:3290, 1993.
26. Orlic D, Girard LJ, Jordan CT, et al: The level of mRNA encoding the amphotropic retrovirus receptor in mouse and human hematopoietic stem cells is low and correlates with the efficiency of retrovirus transduction. PNAS93:11097, 1996.
27. MacDonald C, Corney C, Watts M, et al: Receptor binding is a limiting factor in the transduction of CD34+ hematopoietic cell with amphotropic retroviral vectors [Abstract 507]. Blood 90(10):116a, 1997.
28. Horwitz M, Malech HL, Anderson SM, et al: G-CSF mobilized peripheral blood CD34+ CD38− cells are target cell for high efficiency retrovirus gene transfer [Abstract 2669]. Blood 90(10):601a, 1997.

29. Moore KA, Deisseroth AB, Reading CL, et al: Stromal support enhances cell-free retroviral vector transduction of human bone marrow long-term culture-initiating cells. Blood 79:1393, 1992.

30. Bodine DM, Moritz T, Donahue RE, et al: Long-term expression of a murine adenosine deaminase (ADA) gene in rhesus hematopoietic cells of multiple lineages following retroviral mediated gene transfer into CD34+ bone marrow cells. Blood 82:1975, 1993.

31. Chertkov JL, Jiang S, Lutton JD, et al: The hematopoietic stromal microenvironment promotes retrovirus-mediated gene transfer into hematopoietic stem cells. Stem Cells 11: 218, 1993.

32. Bienzle D, Abrams-Ogg ACG, Kruth SA, et al: Gene transfer into hematopoietic stem cells: long-term maintenance of in vitro activated progenitors without marrow ablation. Proc Natl Acad Sci U S A 91:350, 1994.

33. Wells S, Malik P, Pensiero M, et al: The presence of an autologous marrow stromal cell layer increases glucocerebrosidase gene transduction of long-term culture initiating cells (LTCICs) from the bone marrow of a patient with Gaucher disease. Gene Ther 2:512, 1995.

34. Dube ID, Kruth S, Abrams-Ogg A, et al: Preclinical assessment of human hematopoietic progenitor cell transduction in long-term marrow cultures. Hum Gene Ther 7:2089, 1996.

35. Takiyama N, Mohney T, Swaney W, et al: Comparison of methods for retroviral mediated transfer of glucocerebrosidase gene to CD34+ hematopoietic progenitor cells. Eur J Haematol 61:1–6, 1998.

36. Barnett MJ, Eaves CJ, Phillips GL, et al: Autografting with cultured marrow in chronic myeloid leukemia: results of a pilot study. Blood 84:724, 1994.

37. Ferrari G, Rossini S, Nobili N, et al: Transfer of the ADA gene into human ADA-deficient T lymphocytes reconstitutes specific immune functions. Blood 80:1120, 1992.

38. Mavilio F, Ferrari F, Rossini S, et al: Peripheral blood lymphocytes as target cells of retroviral vector-mediated gene transfer. Blood 83:1988, 1994.

39. Kohn DB, Weinberg KI, Shigeoka A, et al: PEG-ADA reduction in recipients of ADA gene-transduced autologous umbilical cord blood CD34+ cells [Abstract 1798]. Blood 90(10): 404a, 1997.

40. Hoogerbrugge PM, van Veusechem VW, Fischer A, et al: Bone marrow gene transfer in three patients with adenosine deaminase deficiency. Gene Ther 3:179, 1996.

41. Williams DA, Orkin SH, Mulligan RCL: Retrovirus-mediated transfer of human adenosine deaminase gene sequences into cells in culture and into murine hematopoietic cells in vivo. Proc Natl Acad Sci U S A 83:2566, 1985.

42. Moore KA, Fletcher RA, Villalon DK, et al: Human adenosine deaminase expression in mice. Blood 75:1393, 1990.

43. Challita PM, Kohn DB: Lack of expression from a retroviral vector after transduction of murine hematopoietic stem cells is associated with methylation in vivo. Proc Natl Acad Sci U S A 91:2567, 1994.

44. Lange C, Blankenstein T: Loss of retroviral gene expression in bone marrow reconstituted mice correlates with down-regulation of gene expression in long-term culture initiating cells. Gene Ther 4:303, 1997.

45. Riddell SR, Elliott M, Lewinsohn DA, et al: T-cell mediated rejection of gene-modified HIV-specific cytotoxic T lymphocytes in HIV-infected patients. Nature Med 2:216, 1996.

46. Bonini C, Ferrari G, Verzeletti S, et al: HSV-TK gene transfer into donor lymphocytes for control of allogeneic graft-versus-leukemia. Science 276:1719, 1997.

47. Selvaggi TA, Walker RE, Fleisher TA: Development of antibodies to fetal calf serum with arthus-like reactions in human immunodeficiency virus-infected patients given syngeneic lymphocyte infusions. Blood 89:776, 1997.

48. Bunnell BA, Metzger M, Bytne E, et al: Efficient in vivo marking of primary CD4+ T lymphocytes in nonhuman primates using a gibbon ape leukemia virus-derived retroviral vector. Blood 89:1987, 1997.

49. Schuening F, Sanders J, Scott CR, et al: Retrovirus-mediated transfer of the cDNA for human glucocerebrosidase into peripheral blood repopulating cells of patients with Gaucher's disease. Human Gene Transfer Protocol 9312-061. Bethesda, MD, Office of Recombinant DNA Activities, NIH, 1993.

50. Karlsson S, Dunbar C, Kohn DB: Retroviral mediated transfer of the cDNA for human glucocerebrosidase into hematopoietic stem cells of patients with Gaucher disease. Hum Gene Ther 7:231, 1996.

51. Bahnson AB, Dunigan JT, Baysal BE, et al: Centrifugal enhancement of retroviral mediated gene transfer. J Virol Method 54:131, 1995.

52. Nimgaonkar MT, Bahnson A, Kemp A, et al: Long term expression of the glucocerebrosidase gene in mouse and human hematopoietic progenitors. Leukemia 9(Suppl 1):38, 1995.

53. Schuening F, Longo WL, Atkinson ME, et al: Retrovirus-mediated transfer of the cDNA for human glucocerebrosidase into peripheral blood repopulating cells of patients with Gaucher's disease. Hum Gene Ther 8:2143–2160, 1997.

54. Kohn DB, Schuening F, Dunbar C, et al: Early trials of gene transfer for Gaucher disease. In Desnick RJ (ed): Advances in Jewish Genetic Diseases. New York, Oxford University Press, 1997, p 1.

55. Dunbar CE, Kohn DB, Schiffmann R, et al: Retroviral transfer of the glucocerebrosidase gene into CD34+ cells from patients with Gaucher disease: in vivo detection of transduced cells without myeloablation. Hum Gene Ther 9:2629–2640, 1998.

56. Becker PS, Riel GJ, Debatis ME, et al: Transfer of the glucocerebrosidase gene to CD34+ cells results in marking of HPP-CFC [Abstract 1043]. Blood 90:237a, 1997.

57. Kittler EL, Peters SO, Crittenden RB, et al: Cytokine-facilitated transduction leads to low-level engraftment in nonablated hosts. Blood 90:865, 1997.

58. Barranger JA, Rice E, Sansieri C, et al: Transfer of the glucocerebrosidase gene to CD34 cells and their autologous transplantation in patients with Gaucher disease [Abstract 1802]. Blood 90(10):405a, 1997.

59. Krall WJ, Skelton DC, Yu X-J, et al: Increased levels of spliced RNA account for augmented expression from the MFG retroviral vector in hematopoietic cells. Gene Ther 3:37, 1996.

60. Byun J, Kim SH, Kim JM, et al: Analysis of the relative level of gene expression from different retroviral vectors used for gene therapy. Gene Ther 3:780, 1996.

61. Malech HL, Maples PB, Whiting-Theobald N, et al: Prolonged production of NADPH oxidase-corrected granulocytes after gene therapy of chronic granulomatous disease. Proc Natl Acad Sci U S A 94:12133, 1997.

62. Liu JM, Kim S, Read EJ, et al: Engraftment of hematopoietic progenitor cells transduced with the Fanconi anemia group C gene (FANCC). Hum Gene Ther 10:2337–2346, 1999.

63. Whitley CB, McIvor RS, Aronovich EL, et al: Retroviral-mediated transfer of the iduronate-2-sulfatase gene into lymphocytes for treatment of mild Hunter syndrome. Hum Gene Ther 7:537, 1996.

64. Braun SE, Pan D, Aronovich EL, et al: Preclinical studies of lymphocyte gene therapy for mild Hunter syndrome (mucopolysaccharidosis type II). Hum Gene Ther 7:283, 1996.

65. Brenner M: Gene marking. Hum Gene Ther 7:1927, 1996.

66. Rosenberg SA, Packard BS, Aebersold PM, et al: Use of tumor-infiltrating lymphocytes and interleukin-2 in the immunotherapy of patients with metastatic melanoma: a preliminary report. N Engl J Med 319:1676, 1988.

67. Rosenberg SA, Aebersold P, Cornetta K, et al: Gene transfer into humans—immunotherapy of patients with advanced melanoma, using tumor-infiltrating lymphocytes modified by retroviral gene transduction. N Engl J Med 323:570, 1990.

68. Rosenberg SA: The gene therapy of cancer. Prev Med 23:624, 1994.

69. Brenner MK, Rill DR, Holladay MS, et al: Gene marking to determine whether autologous marrow infusion restores long-term haemopoiesis in cancer patients. Lancet 342:1134, 1993.

70. Rill DR, Holliday M, Heslop HE, et al: Long term transgene expression by human hemopoietic cells in vivo [Abstract 1799]. Blood 90(10):405a, 1997.

71. Wu T, Bloom ML, Yu JM, et al: Murine bone marrow stem cells expressing the neomycin resistance gene have no competitive disadvantage assessed in vivo [Abstract 512]. Blood 90(10):118a, 1997.

72. Hao Q-L, Peterson D, Thiemann FT, et al: Primary human progenitors with B lymphoid potential are resistant to retroviral marking [Abstract 1155]. Blood 90(10):263a, 1997.

73. Brenner MK, Rill DR, Moen RC, et al: Gene-marking to trace origin of relapse after autologous bone-marrow transplantation. Lancet 341:85, 1993.

74. Brenner MK, Cunningham JM, Sorrentino B, et al: Gene transfer into human hemopoietic progenitor cells. Br Med Bull 51:167, 1995.

75. Ochman HA, Gerber S, Hart DL: Genetic application of an inverse polymerase chain reaction. Genetics 120:621, 1988.

76. Deisseroth AB, Zu S, Claxton D, et al: Genetic marking shows that Ph+ cells present in autologous transplants of chronic myelogenous leukemia (CML) contribute to relapse after autologous bone marrow in CML. Blood 83:3068, 1994.

77. Rill DR, Santana VM, Roberts WM, et al: Direct demonstration that autologous bone marrow transplantation for solid tumors can return a multiplicity of tumorigenic cells. Blood 84:380, 1994.

78. Stewart AK, Sutherland DR, Nanji S, et al: Engraftment of gene-marked hematopoietic progenitors in myeloma patients after transplant of autologous long-term marrow cultures. Hum Gene Ther 10:1953–1964, 1999.

79. Dunbar CE, Cottler-Fox M, O'Shaughnessy JA, et al: Retrovirally marked CD34-enriched peripheral blood and bone marrow cells contribute to long-term engraftment after autologous transplantation. Blood 85:3048, 1995.

80. Deisseroth AB: Use of retroviral markers to identify efficacy of purging and origin of relapse following autologous bone marrow and peripheral blood cells transplantation in indolent B cell neoplasms (follicular non-Hodgkins's lymphoma or chronic lymphocytic leukemia (CLL) patients. Hum Gene Ther 4:821, 1993.

81. Cornetta K, Srour EF, Moore A, et al: Retroviral gene transfer in autologous bone marrow transplantation for adult acute leukemia. Hum Gene Ther 7:1323, 1996.

82. O'Schaughnessy JA, Cowan KH, Nienhuis AW, et al: Retroviral mediated transfer of the human multidrug resistance gene (MDR-1) into hematopoietic stem cells during autologous transplantation after intensive chemotherapy for metastatic breast cancer. Hum Gene Ther 5:891, 1994.

83. Deisseroth AB, Kantarjian H, Talpaz M, et al: Use of two retroviral markers to test relative contribution of marrow and peripheral blood autologous cells to recovery after preparative therapy. Hum Gene Ther 4:71, 1993.

84. Santana VM, Brenner MK, Ihle J, et al: A phase I trial of high-dose carboplatin and etoposide with autologous marrow support for treatment of stage D neuroblastoma in first remission: use of marker genes to investigate the biology of marrow reconstitution and the mechanism of relapse. Hum Gene Ther 2:257, 1991.

85. Rahman Z, Kavanagh J, Champlin R, et al: Chemotherapy immediately following autologous stem-cell transplantation in patients with advanced breast cancer. Clin Cancer Res 4:2717–2721, 1998.

86. Marcel T, Grausz JD: The TMC worldwide gene therapy enrollment report (June 1996). Hum Gene Ther 7:2025, 1996.

87. Heslop HE, Ng CYC, Li C, et al: Long-term restoration of immunity against Epstein-Barr virus infection by adoptive transfer of gene-modified virus-specific T lympocytes. Nature Med 2:551, 1996.

88. Rooney CM, Smith CA, Ng CY, et al: Infusion of cytotoxic T cells for the prevention and treatment of Epstein-Barr virus-induced lymphoma in allogeneic transplant recipients. Blood 92:1549–1555, 1998.

89. Roskrow MA, Suzuki N, Heslop HE, et al: Genetically modified EBV-specific cytotoxic T cells for adoptive transfer to patients with EBV-positive Hodgkin disease [Abstract 2679]. Blood 88(Suppl 1):673a, 1996.

90. Tiberghien P, Cahn JY, Brion A, et al: Use of donor T-lymphocytes expressing herpes-simplex thymidine kinase in allogeneic bone marrow transplantation: a phase I-II study. Hum Gene Ther 8:615–624, 1997.

91. Walter EA, Greenberg PD, Gilbert MJ, et al: Reconsitution of cellular immunity against cytomegalovirus in recipients of allogeneic bone marrow by transfer of T-cell clones from the donor. N Engl J Med 333:1038–1044, 1995.

92. Walker R, Blaese RM, Carter CS, et al: A study of the safety and survival of the adoptive transfer of genetically marked syngeneic lymphocytes in HIV-infected identical twins. Hum Gene Ther 4(5):659, 1993.

93. Bahner I, Kearns K, Hao QL, et al: Transduction of human CD34+ hematopoietic progenitor cells by a retroviral vector expressing an RRE decoy inhibits human immunodeficiency virus type 1 replication in myelomonocytic cells produced in long-term culture. J Virol 70(7):4352, 1996.

94. Kohn DB, Bauer G, Rice CR, et al: A clinical trial of retroviral-mediated transfer of a rev-responsive element decoy gene into CD34+ cells from the bone marrow of human immunodeficiency virus–1-infected children. Blood 94:368, 1999.

95. Nabel GJ, Fox BA, Post L, et al: A molecular genetic intervention for AIDS—effects of a transdominant negative form of Rev. Hum Gene Ther 5:79, 1994.

96. Woffendin C, Ranga U, Yang Z, et al: Regulation of human retroviral latency by the NF-kappa B/I kappa B family: inhibition of human immunodeficiency virus replication by I kappa B through a Rev-dependent mechanism. Proc Natl Acad Sci U S A 93:2889, 1996.

97. Ranga U, Woffendin C, Verma S, et al: Enhanced T cell engraftment after retroviral delivery of an antiviral gene in HIV-infected individuals. Proc Natl Acad Sci U S A 95:1201, 1998.

98. Morgan RA, Walker R: Gene therapy for AIDS using retroviral mediated gene transfer to deliver HIV-1 antisense TAR and trans dominant Rev protein genes to syngeneic lymphocytes in HIV-1 infected identical twins. Hum Gene Ther 7:1281, 1996.

99. Bunnell BA, Muul LM, Donahue RE, et al: High-efficiency retroviral-mediated gene transfer into human and nonhuman primate peripheral blood lymphocytes. Proc Natl Acad Sci U S A 92:7739–7743, 1995.

100. Morgan RA, Bunnell B, Walker R, et al: An AIDS gene therapy trial in HIV-1 discordant identical twins [Abstract 1803]. Blood 90:405a, 1997.

101. Donahue RE, Bunnell BA, Zink MC, et al: Reduction in SIV replication in rhesus macaques infused with autologous lymphocytes engineered with antiviral genes. Nature Med 4(2):181, 1998.

102. Marasco WA: Intrabodies turning the humoral immune system outside in for intracellular immunization. Gene Ther 4:11, 1997.

103. Wong JK, Hezareh M, Gunthard HF, et al: Recovery of replication-competent HIV despite prolonged suppression of plasma viremia. Science 278:1291, 1997.

104. Finzi D, Hermankova M, Pierson T, et al: Identification of a reservoir for HIV-1 in patients on highly active antiretroviral therapy. Science 278:1295, 1997.

105. Corbeau P, Kraus G, Wong-Staal F: Efficient gene transfer by a human immunodeficiency virus type 1 (HIV-1)-derived vector utilizing a stable HIV packaging cell line. Proc Natl Aca Sci U S A 93:14070, 1996.

106. Kim SH, Yu SS, Park JS, et al: Construction of retroviral vectors with improved safety, gene expressioin and versatility. J Virol 72:994, 1998.

107. Miller AD: Production of retoviral vectors. In Dracopoli NC, Haines JL, Korf BR, et al (eds): Current Protocols in Human Genetics, Suppl. 11. New York, John Wiley & Sons, 1996.

108. Southern PJ, Berg P: Transformation of mammalian cells to antibiotic resistance with a bacterial gene under control of the SV40 early region promoter. J Mol Appl Genet 1:327, 1982.

109. Pear WS, Nolan GP, Scott ML, Baltimore D: Production of high-titer helper-free retroviruses by transient transfection. Proc Natl Acad Sci U S A 90:8392, 1993.

110. Hwang L-HS, Gilboa E: Expression of genes introduced into cells by retroviral infection if more efficient than that of genes introduced into cells by DNA transfection. J Virol 50:417, 1984.

111. Bahnson AB, Nimagonkar M, Fei Y, et al: Transduction of CD34+ enriched cord blood and Gaucher bone marrow cells by a retroviral vector carrying the glucocerebrosidase gene. Gene Ther 1:176, 1994.

112. Ohashi TS, Boggs S, Robbins PD, et al: Efficient transfer and sustained high expression of the human glucocerebrosidase gene in mice and their functional macrophages following transplantation of bone marrow transduced by a retroviral vector. Proc Natl Acad Sci U S A 89, 11332, 1992.

113. Grande A, Piovani B, Aiuti A, et al: Transcriptional targeting of retroviral vectors to the erythropoietic progeny of transduced hematopoietic stem cells. Blood 93:3276–3285, 1999.

114. Iida A, Chen ST, Friedmann T, Yee JK: Inducible gene expression by retrovirus-mediated transfer of a modified tetracycline-regulated system. J Virol 70(9):6054, 1996.

115. Plavec I, Agarwal M, Chen J, Bohnlein E: Scaffold attachment region-mediated enhancement of trangene expression in quiescent primary T cells: implication for gene therapy of HIV disease [Abstract 2671]. Blood 90(10):601a, 1997.

116. Kume A, Ueda Y, Ito K, et al: G-CSF receptor-gyrase B chimera: a new type of selective amplifier gene for expansion of the genetically engineered hematopoietic cells. Blood 2474:5562, 1997.

117. Moritz T, Patel VP, Williams DA: Bone marrow extracellular matrix molecules improve gene transfer into human hematopoietic cells via retroviral vectors. J Clin Invest 93:1451, 1994.

118. Swaney WP, Sorgi FL, Bahnson AB, Barranger JA: The effect of cationic liposome pretreatment and centrifugation on retrovirus-mediated gene transfer. Gene Ther 4:1379, 1997.

119. Chuck AS, Palsson BO: Consistent and high rates of gene transfer can be obtained using flow-through transduction over a wide range of retroviral titers. Hum Gene Ther 7:743, 1996.

120. Morling FJ, Russell SJ: Enhanced transduction efficiency of retroviral vectors coprecipitated with calcium phosphate. Gene Ther 2:504, 1995.

121. Burns JC, Friedmann T, Driever W, et al: Vesicular stomatitis virus G glycoprotein pseudotyped retroviral vectors: concentration to very high titer and efficient gene transfer into mammalian and non-mammalian cells. Proc Natl Acad Sci U S A 90:8033, 1993.

122. Cornetta K, Moen RC, Culver K, et al: Amphotropic murine leukemia retrovirus is not an acute pathogen for primates. Hum Gene Ther 1:13, 1990.

123. Cornetta K, Morgan RA, Gillio A, et al: No retroviremia or pathology in long-term follow-up of monkeys exposed to a murine amphotropic retrovirus. Hum Gene Ther 2:215, 1991.

124. Donahue RE, Kessler SW, Bodine D, et al: Helper virus induced T cell lymphoma in nonhuman primates after retroviral mediated gene transfer. J Exp Med 176:1125, 1992.

125. Anderson WF: What about those monkeys that got T-cell lymphoma? Hum Gene Ther 4:1, 1993.

126. Yuh CH, Bolouri H, Davidson EH: Genomic cis-regulatory logic: experimental and computational analysis of a sea urchin gene. Science 279:1896, 1998.

127. Bordignon C, Bonini C, Verzeletti S, et al: Transfer of the HSV-tk gene into donor peripheral blood lymphocytes for in vivo modulation of donor anti-tumor immunity after allogeneic bone marrow transplantation. Hum Gene Ther 6:813–819, 1995.

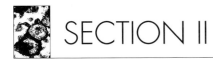 SECTION II

Issues Relevant to The Immediate Transplant Period

Treatment Regimens

CHAPTER THIRTY-FOUR

High-Dose Chemotherapy Conditioning Regimens for Autologous or Allogeneic Hematopoietic Stem Cell Transplantation

Pablo J. Cagnoni, M.D., Yago Nieto, M.D., and Roy B. Jones, M.D., Ph.D.

Several potential goals must be defined prior to the design of a high-dose chemotherapy regimen. The first is whether the regimen will be used in allogeneic or autologous transplantation. Although in autologous transplantation the antitumor effect is of singular importance, in the allogeneic setting equally important goals are to achieve myeloablation and immunosuppression. Another consideration is the pattern of chemosensitivity of the targeted disease.

In this chapter we first describe some pharmacologic studies of the drugs used in conditioning regimens; we then describe the most commonly used high-dose therapy regimens that have been developed in recent decades. Unfortunately, as the reader will recognize, more often than not high-dose chemotherapy regimens are simple ad hoc combinations of the most effective agents for a particular disease given at high doses. We emphasize that a firm pharmacodynamic rationale for a particular drug combination, followed by a well-designed phase I study with thorough pharmacokinetic evaluation, strengthens the design and understanding of high-dose chemotherapy regimens.

PHARMACOLOGIC STUDIES IN HIGH-DOSE CHEMOTHERAPY

The study of pharmacokinetic/pharmacodynamic correlations is potentially of great importance in high-dose chemotherapy. If toxicities produced by a regimen can be correlated with particular pharmacokinetic parameters, directed dose adjustments are possible. Also, if the response rate or disease-free survival produced by a particular regimen can be correlated with the drug exposure for a particular drug within the combination, this information may prove valuable in planning future studies. To date, few reports of pharmacokinetic/pharmacodynamic correlations have been published.[1] We summarize several of the most relevant ones.

BUSULFAN

The disposition of busulfan has wide inter- and intra-patient variability—numerous studies have shown both in children and adults.[2–4] Considering the well-described correlation between busulfan's area under the time-concentration curve (AUC) and veno-occlusive disease (VOD) of the liver, it is easy to understand the importance of this variability.[5, 6] Part of this variability is probably due to the fact that busulfan is routinely given with the anticonvulsant phenytoin to prevent seizures produced by busulfan.[7] Phenytoin is a well-known inducer of the P450 system, which is responsible for the metabolism of busulfan. An alternative would be to use a different anticonvulsant. Diazepam has been shown by Hassan et al. to have much less effect on busulfan's pharmacokinetics than phenytoin in a group of 17 patients.[8] In addition, busulfan is routinely combined with cyclophosphamide, which also modifies P450 activity. Cyclophosphamide is known to induce its own metabolism, and therefore it could potentially modify busulfan disposition as well.[9]

An additional variable is the difference in busulfan clearance between adults and children.[10] Vassal et al. found that children below the age of 3 years have a busulfan clearance twice that of adults and 50% higher than that of older children.[11, 12] Yeager et al. conducted a dose-escalation study of busulfan based on body surface area in children, targeting the AUC observed in adults given busulfan/cyclophosphamide.[13] They showed that the median dose of busulfan to achieve the desired AUC was 26.4 mg/kg, which is a 60% increase over the traditional 16 mg/kg given when the dose is based on body weight. These data suggest that a significant number of children who receive 16 mg/kg of busulfan are being underdosed compared with adults.

An important example of a pharmacokinetics/pharmacodynamics correlation in patients who receive high-dose chemotherapy, and one that has resulted in the only dose-adjustment trial in high-dose chemotherapy, is found in the data published by Grochow et al. evaluating the correlation between AUC and VOD.[5] They showed that in patients who receive the busulfan/cyclophosphamide regimen, the AUC of busulfan correlates with the risk of VOD, a potentially fatal complication of this regimen.[5] Other investigators confirmed these observations.[6] Grochow conducted a trial testing the possibility of busulfan dose adjustment.[12]

The AUC was calculated after the first dose of busulfan, and doses 5–16 were adjusted if the initial AUC was more than one standard deviation above or below the median. Of 27 patients in whom the dose was adjusted because of high AUC, only 18% (5 of 27 patients) experienced VOD and 3 died of VOD. This compared favorably with eight patients with similar AUC in whom the dose was not adjusted. Seven of these eight patients experienced VOD, and four of them died.

A study in patients who received different busulfan/cyclophosphamide variants as conditioning prior to receiving related or partially matched unrelated allogeneic transplants found that minimal steady-state concentrations of busulfan of 200 ng/mL and 600 ng/mL, respectively, were required to avoid marrow graft rejection.[14] Moreover, in a multivariate analysis that included, among other variables, the dose of cyclophosphamide, only the steady-state concentration of busulfan was a significant determinant of marrow graft rejection.

Until very recently, busulfan existed only in the form of tablets for oral administration. Oral administration of the drug introduces another factor that can produce interdose and interpatient variability in drug exposure as a result of different bioavailability. The recent development of an intravenous formulation of busulfan should permit more-accurate dosing and better dose adjustment.[15]

BCNU

Jones et al. showed that the AUC of high-dose bis-chloro-ethyl-nitrosourea (BCNU, or carmustine) correlates with the risk of drug-induced lung injury in patients who receive high-dose cyclophosphamide, cisplatin, and BCNU.[16] Unfortunately, the use of a single dose of BCNU in this regimen precludes dose adjustment. Additionally, another factor that can influence the toxicity due to BCNU is the wide interpatient variability of BCNU's AUC when the drug is given in combination. Jones et al. showed in animal studies that both cyclophosphamide and cisplatin can significantly alter the pharmacokinetics of BCNU.[17] In rats, the AUC of BCNU is increased by more than 75% when cyclophosphamide, compared with placebo, is administered in three daily doses prior to BCNU. This pharmacokinetic variability can be reflected in pharmacodynamic differences such as increased incidence of lung injury.[17]

CYCLOPHOSPHAMIDE

Ayash et al. studied the pharmacokinetics of cyclophosphamide in a group of patients with breast cancer treated with high-dose cyclophosphamide, thiotepa, and carboplatin (see later discussion of STAMP V). They found that patients with a lower cyclophosphamide AUC had a higher incidence of cardiac toxicity and longer duration of response than patients with a higher AUC.[18] This was the first time that drug exposure was correlated with treatment efficacy in high-dose chemotherapy. The authors postulated that because cyclophosphamide has to be metabolized by the liver to originate both the active (phosphoramide mustard) and toxic (acrolein) metabolites, an increase in cyclophos-

phamide activation with a correspondingly lower cyclophosphamide AUC was responsible for the differences observed. These conclusions assume an inverse relationship between parent drug and its active and toxic metabolites.

Such a relationship was confirmed by Slattery et al. when they studied cyclophosphamide in patients who received cyclophosphamide/total body irradiation (TBI) and busulfan/cyclophosphamide.[19] They found an inverse relationship between the AUC for hydroxycyclophosphamide and cyclophosphamide. Importantly, Chen et al. showed that the pharmacokinetics of high-dose cyclophosphamide are nonlinear, with saturable elimination when high doses of the drug are given over a short period of time.[20] The same investigators studied cyclophosphamide and its metabolites (4-hydroxycyclophosphamide [4-HC] and aldophosphamide) by mass spectrometry in a similar group of patients.[21] In this study, the magnitude of change for the metabolite was less than that for the parent drug and in the opposite direction. Anderson et al. also observed a nonproportional increase in the cyclophosphamide AUC from the first course (cyclophosphamide alone) to the second course (cyclophosphamide and thiotepa), whereas the AUC for 4-HC was higher after the first course. They postulated a possible, but not confirmed, interaction of cyclophosphamide with thiotepa. Additionally, Slattery et al. showed that in patients who receive cyclophosphamide/TBI, exposure to hydroxycyclophosphamide is greater than in patients given busulfan/cyclophosphamide, possibly because the prior exposure to busulfan and/or phenytoin affects the rate of metabolic activation of cyclophosphamide.[19]

PACLITAXEL

In 1996, the group from the University of Colorado demonstrated that the AUC and maximum clearance (Cmax) of high-dose paclitaxel correlate with the severity of the polyneuropathy and mucositis produced by a regimen containing cyclophosphamide, cisplatin, and paclitaxel.[22]

THIOTEPA

In 1987, Egorin et al. studied the pharmacokinetics of thiotepa in 14 patients who received either single-agent thiotepa or different combinations.[23] The dose of thiotepa ranged from 70 to 475 mg/m². They described linear disposition of thiotepa with nonsaturable kinetics. A study by O'Dwyer et al. of the pharmakokinetics of conventional dose thiotepa, however, found evidence consistent with a saturable step in the conversion of thiotepa into triethylenephosphoramide (TEPA).[24] The author's interpretation for this difference was that in the latter study, blood sampling continued after 4 hours and therefore Egorin et al. may have underestimated the AUC of TEPA. Animal studies performed by the same group appear to support this hypothesis.[25] When studying the pharmacokinetics of thiotepa in patients who received cyclophosphamide, busulfan, and thiotepa, Przepiorka et al. found a correlation between the regimen-related toxicity and both TEPA peak concentrations and combined thiotepa and TEPA AUC.[26]

DRUG-DRUG INTERACTIONS IN HIGH-DOSE CHEMOTHERAPY

These correlations between certain pharmacokinetic parameters and outcome, toxicity, or antitumor effect stress the potential importance of drug-drug interactions among the chemotherapy agents that might alter exposure to these agents or alter pharmacodynamic effects. For example, we and others have reported the differences in the pharmacokinetics of high-dose cyclophosphamide and cisplatin, depending on the antiemetics used.[27, 28] Also, as discussed earlier, the type of anticonvulsant prophylaxis can affect the pharmacokinetics of busulfan[8] or cyclophosphamide.[19]

In the following discussion, we discuss details of specific regimens, describing whenever possible the pharmacokinetic/pharmacodynamic data underlying their design and use.

BUSULFAN/CYCLOPHOSPHAMIDE AND RELATED COMBINATIONS FOR HEMATOLOGIC MALIGNANCIES

BUSULFAN/CYCLOPHOSPHAMIDE

Rationale

Soon after the initial results using a TBI-containing regimen (cyclophosphamide/TBI) (Fig. 34–1) in allogeneic transplantation became available, it became clear that a non–TBI-containing regimen was necessary. The reason for this was the lack of availability of adequate radiation oncology equipment needed to deliver TBI at many institutions[29] and the substantial number of patients with prior radiation exposure who required intensive treatment. With this in mind, Santos and Tutschka developed a non–TBI-containing regimen for use in allogeneic transplantation.[29, 30] Busulfan was thought to be an ideal drug for such a regimen because of its myeloablative properties and potent antileukemic effects.[29, 30] A regimen suitable for allogeneic transplantation, however, must also be immunosuppressive,

and an animal model by Santos and Tutschka had suggested that busulfan had only a weak immunosuppressive effect.[31]

Cyclophosphamide, a potent immunosuppressor, was then tested first in the same animal model and finally combined with busulfan, laying the foundations for the busulfan/cyclophosphamide regimen and its subsequent variants.[32] The initial busulfan/cyclophosphamide regimen, now called *big busulfan/cyclophosphamide* or *busulfan/cyclophosphamide 4*, delivers busulfan, 1 mg/kg every 6 hours PO for 4 days, followed by cyclophosphamide, 50 mg/kg/day intravenously for 4 days (Fig. 34–2). The busulfan/cyclophosphamide regimen thus combines the three important properties that are desirable in a regimen for allogeneic transplantation in hematologic malignancies: antitumor (antileukemic) effect, myeloablation, and immunosuppression. Initial results using this regimen in patients with acute leukemia were encouraging, with a disease-free survival rate of more than 60% in adults with acute myelogenous leukemia (AML).[33]

It soon became apparent that the two main toxicities of this regimen were mucositis and liver toxicity. Twenty to 30% of patients experienced VOD that was fatal in 50% of those affected.[34] For this reason, attempts were made to develop a less toxic and equally effective regimen. With the concept that the main role of cyclophosphamide in the busulfan/cyclophosphamide regimen was immunosuppression, Tutschka et al. developed what its now called *little busulfan/cyclophosphamide* or *busulfan/cyclophosphamide 2*, a variant with a reduced dose of cyclophosphamide.[35] The dose of cyclophosphamide was reduced to 120 mg/kg over 2 days (Fig. 34–3). As a result, the incidence of VOD was reduced to approximately 10–15%, fatal in only 5% of all the patients treated.[36]

Efficacy and Toxicity

One of the main questions regarding busulfan/cyclophosphamide is whether it is as effective as TBI-containing regimens. A randomized trial in patients with AML in first remission who underwent allogeneic transplantation compared busulfan/cyclophosphamide 2 with cyclo-

Day	-8	-7	-6	-5	-4	-3	-2	-1	0
Cy	X	X							
TBI 200 cGy/d			X	X	X	X	X	X	
HSC									X

FIGURE 34–1. Cyclophosphamide-TBI. IV, intravenous; HSC, hematopoietic stem cells; cGy, centiGray; TBI, total body irradiation; Cy, cyclophosphamide.

Day	-9	-8	-7	-6	-5	-4	-3	-2	-1	0
Bu 4 mg/kg/d PO	X	X	X	X						
Cy 50 mg/kg/d IV					X	X	X	X		
HSC										X

FIGURE 34–2. BuCy4. PO, oral; IV, intravenous; Cy, cyclophosphamide; Bu, busulfan; HSC, hematopoietic stem cells.

phosphamide/TBI. Patients treated with the latter experienced better survival and disease-free survival.[37] A similar study in patients with chronic myeloid leukemia showed no differences in the 3-year probability of survival or on the event-free survival.[38] The Nordic Bone Marrow Transplantation Group published another randomized comparison of these two regimens in patients with adult and pediatric leukemia (acute and chronic). The 3-year actuarial survival was significantly worse in patients who received busulfan, and a multivariate analysis identified busulfan treatment as one of the factors associated with poor survival.[39]

Dusenbery et al. performed a randomized trial in patients with AML in first or subsequent complete remission. Autologous bone marrow that had been purged with 4-HC was the source of the graft. Importantly, this is the only randomized comparison of busulfan/cyclophosphamide 4 with cyclophosphamide/TBI, and it showed no difference in disease-free survival for patients with AML in first complete remission but a trend toward superior disease-free survival in patients with more advanced disease who received the TBI-containing regimen.[40] A retrospective comparison of patients with acute leukemia from the European Bone Marrow Transplant Registry database who underwent allogeneic or autologous transplantation was published in 1996. The only subgroup with a benefit for the TBI-containing regi-

Day	-7	-6	-5	-4	-3	-2	-1	0
Bu 4 mg/kg/d PO	X	X	X	X				
Cy 60 mg/kg/d IV					X	X		
HSC								X

FIGURE 34–3. BuCy2. PO, oral; IV, intravenous; Cy, cyclophosphamide; Bu, busulfan; HSC, hematopoietic stem cells.

men was patients with acute lymphoblastic leukemia in intermediate stages who went more than 2 years from diagnosis to transplantation.[41] The Southwest Oncology Group conducted a randomized study comparing busulfan/cyclophosphamide with TBI/etoposide in patients with leukemia "not in first remission."[42] The study found no differences in either disease-free survival or overall survival.

In summary, the current evidence suggests that busulfan/cyclophosphamide 2 and cyclophosphamide/TBI with allogeneic transplantation are equivalent in the chronic phase of chronic myeloid leukemia. In patients with AML undergoing allogeneic transplantation, cyclophosphamide/TBI appears to be superior to busulfan/cyclophosphamide 2, although it might be equivalent to busulfan/cyclophosphamide 4 in the autologous setting; one must, however, remember that the only available randomized trial is small. For all other indications, cyclophosphamide/TBI remains the standard against which new regimens should be compared.

As discussed earlier, one of the potential advantages of busulfan/cyclophosphamide is the possibility of using it in patients who have been previously irradiated. Thirty-seven patients with prior chest radiation therapy were treated with busulfan/cyclophosphamide 2 for hematologic malignancies prior to autologous transplantation.[43] Their incidence of fatal interstitial pneumonitis was 5%, compared with 32% for historical controls treated with a TBI-containing regimen.

Another potential advantage of busulfan-containing regimens over TBI-containing regimens is the apparent lack of impairment in development and growth in children who undergo bone marrow transplantation,[44, 45] although not all published studies have shown such an advantage.[46] The effects of both cyclophosphamide/TBI and busulfan/cyclophosphamide on fertility have also been reported. Sanders et al. reviewed more than 1500 records of patients treated with cyclophosphamide alone, cyclophosphamide/TBI, or busulfan/cyclophosphamide.[47] They concluded that all

pregnancies among female marrow transplant recipients should be considered high risk because women who received TBI had an increased risk of spontaneous abortion and women who received high-dose cyclophosphamide had an increased risk of preterm labor and delivery of low-birth-weight babies. The incidence of congenital anomalies was not increased, however.

BUSULFAN/CYCLOPHOSPHAMIDE VARIANTS

Attempts have been made to improve the busulfan/cyclophosphamide regimen by adding other drugs with known antileukemic effect. Several studies are described here. When reading these reports, one should keep in mind that many of them represent phase I trials, which traditionally include patients with advanced disease and who are more heavily pretreated. For these and other reasons, toxicity tends to be higher in initial phase I reports of new regimens.

Etoposide-Busulfan/Cyclophosphamide 2

Vaughan et al. published the results of a study that incorporated etoposide into busulfan/cyclophosphamide 2.[48] Twenty-four patients with advanced hematologic malignancies who underwent allogeneic transplantation were treated. The authors used a dose of etoposide of 60 mg/kg (Fig. 34–4). The transplant-related mortality rate was 46%, with 40% of the patients alive and free of disease at the time of report. The authors concluded that the therapeutic efficacy appeared better than that obtained with a TBI-containing regimen for 12 historical controls with similar risk of disease, but the high toxicity is obviously of concern. In 1996, Vaughan et al. presented their results in using this regimen in 11 patients with non-Hodgkin lymphoma prior to autologous hematopoietic stem cell support.[49] All patients expe-

Day	-8	-7	-6	-5	-4	-3	-2	-1	0
Bu 4 mg/kg/d PO	X	X	X	X					
Cy 60 mg/kg/d IV					X	X			
VP16 60 mg/kg/d IV					X				
HSC									X

FIGURE 34–4. BuCy-VP16. PO, oral; IV, intravenous; Cy, cyclophosphamide; Bu, busulfan; VP16, etoposide; HSC, hematopoietic stem cells.

Day	-10	-9	-8	-7	-6	-5	-4	-3	-2	-1	0
Bu 4 mg/kg/d PO	X	X	X	X							
Cy 60 mg/kg/d IV					X	X					
Ara C 1-1.5 g/m²/48 hs IV CI								▬▬▬▬▬▬▬▬▬▬			
HSC											X

FIGURE 34–5. BuCy-Ara C. PO, oral; IV, intravenous; CI, continuous infusion; Cy, cyclophosphamide; Bu, busulfan; HSC, hematopoietic stem cells.

rienced skin rash, mucositis, and hyperbilirubinemia, but no patient experienced VOD.

Cytosine Arabinoside–Busulfan/Cyclophosphamide 2

Two studies have evaluated incorporating cytosine arabinoside into busulfan/cyclophosphamide 2. Geller et al. published the results of a phase I study of 17 patients with refractory or relapsed leukemia or lymphoma who were given busulfan/cyclophosphamide 2 plus escalated doses of cytosine arabinoside given as a 48-hour continuous infusion (Fig. 34–5).[50] The maximum tolerated dose for cytosine arabinoside was 1500 mg/m², and the dose-limiting

toxicity was lung injury. The other study added cytosine arabinoside at a dose of 2 g/m² every 12 hours for a total of four doses in 21 patients with AML who underwent allogeneic bone marrow transplantation (Fig. 34–6).[51] Ten percent of the patients experienced fatal VOD, and the event-free survival rate was 52% with a median follow-up of 18.3 months.

Busulfan/Cyclophosphamide–TBI

Peterson et al. at the Fred Hutchinson Cancer Research Center combined busulfan/cyclophosphamide with TBI in a phase I study (Fig. 34–7). The maximum tolerated dose for this regimen was busulfan, 6.9 mg/kg for 6 days; cyclo-

Day	-9	-8	-7	-6	-5	-4	-3	-2	-1	0
Bu 4 mg/kg/d PO	X	X	X	X						
Cy 60 mg/kg/d IV							X	X		
Ara C 2 g/m²/12 hs IV					X	X				
HSC										X

FIGURE 34–6. BuCy-Ara C. PO, oral; IV, intravenous; Cy, cyclophosphamide; Bu, busulfan; HSC, hematopoietic stem cells.

Day	-12	-11	-10	-9	-8	-7	-6	-5	-4	-3	-2	-1	0
Bu 8.7 mg/kg PO	X	X	X	X									
Cy 47 mg/kg IV					X	X							
FTBI 12 Gy								X	X	X	X	X	
HSC													X

FIGURE 34–7. BuCy-FTBI. PO, oral; IV, intravenous; Cy, cyclophosphamide; Bu, busulfan; FTBI, fractionated total body irradiation; HSC, hematopoietic stem cells.

phosphamide, 47 mg/kg; and TBI, 200 cGy/day for 6 days. The dose-limiting toxicities for this regimen were VOD and interstitial pneumonitis. A total of 36 patients with different diagnoses were treated, and at the maximum tolerated dose, the death rate from drug toxicity was zero.[52] When this regimen was evaluated in a subsequent phase II study in patients with acute and chronic myeloid leukemia, no improvement over historical controls treated with busulfan/ cyclophosphamide or cyclophosphamide/TBI was noted.[53] Because of the high variability of busulfan's pharmacokinetics in these patients, the same investigators conducted a new phase I study with the same doses of cyclophosphamide and TBI but with a pharmacologically guided dose

escalation of busulfan.[54] They demonstrated that it was feasible to reduce the interpatient variability of busulfan's pharmacokinetics, but the overall results were similar to those of the previous phase II study.

Cyclophosphamide/Thiotepa

In 1996, Bacigalupo et al. published their results with the use of a non-TBI, non–busulfan-containing regimen in allogeneic transplantation.[55] They treated 31 patients with hematologic malignancies with thiotepa, 15 mg/kg, and cyclophosphamide, 120–150 mg/kg, followed by allogeneic peripheral blood progenitor cell transplantation (Fig. 34–

Day	-7	-6	-5	-4	-3	-2	-1	0
TT 5 mg/kg x 3 IV	X	X						
Cy 60 mg/kg/d IV					X	X		
HSC								X

FIGURE 34–8. Cy-thiotepa. Cy, cyclophosphamide; IV, intravenous; TT, thiotepa; HSC, hematopoietic stem cells.

Day	-9	-8	-7	-6	-5	-4	-3	-2	-1	0
TT 250 mg/m²/d IV	X	X	X							
Bu 1.0 mg/kg x 10 PO				X	X	X				
Cy 60 mg/kg/d IV							X	X		
HSC										X

FIGURE 34–9. BuCy-thiotepa. Bu, busulfan; Cy, cyclophosphamide; IV, intravenous; TT, thiotepa; HSC, hematopoietic stem cells.

8). Twenty-nine of 30 evaluable patients experienced prompt engraftment with a transplant-related mortality rate of 29%, mostly due to graft-versus-host disease, sepsis, and infection.

Busulfan/Cyclophosphamide/Thiotepa

Dimopoulos et al. showed that it is feasible to incorporate thiotepa into busulfan/cyclophosphamide 2 with reduced doses of busulfan.[56] Forty patients with multiple myeloma were treated with busulfan (10 mg/kg), cyclophosphamide (120 mg/kg), and thiotepa (750 mg/m²) (Fig. 34–9). There were five toxic deaths, one due to VOD and another one due to diffuse alveolar hemorrhage.

HIGH-DOSE CHEMOTHERAPY REGIMENS FOR HODGKIN DISEASE AND NON-HODGKIN LYMPHOMA

CBV

Undoubtedly, the most popular treatment for these diseases remains the CBV (cyclophosphamide, BCNU, and etoposide) regimen developed at the M.D. Anderson Cancer Center.[57, 58] This regimen has a number of variants, mainly modifying the dose and schedule of BCNU, whereas the dose and schedule of cyclophosphamide and etoposide have remained relatively stable (Figs. 34–10, 34–11).[59–64] Investigators have reported important differences in both

Day	-6	-5	-4	-3	-2	-1	0
Cy 1,500 mg/m²/d IV	X	X	X	X			
BCNU 300 mg/m² IV	X						
VP16 50-75 mg/kg/12 hs IV	X	X	X				
HSC							X

FIGURE 34–10. Standard CBV. Cy, cyclophosphamide; VP16, etoposide; HSC, hematopoietic stem cells; IV, intravenous.

Day	-6	-5	-4	-3	-2	-1	0
Cy 1,800 mg/m²/d IV	X	X	X	X			
BCNU 600 mg/m² IV				X			
VP16 400 mg/m²/12 hs IV	X	X	X				
HSC							X

FIGURE 34–11. Augmented CBV. Cy, cyclophosphamide; VP16, etoposide; HSC, hematopoietic stem cells; IV, intravenous.

antitumor response and toxicity with the different CBV variants (Table 34–1). These differences might be attributed to patient selection, to the different doses of BCNU used in each protocol or, as described earlier, to drug-drug interactions produced by the different schedules. Animal data cited earlier suggest that the BCNU AUC of 600 mg/m² administered after three daily cyclophosphamide doses might be equivalent to the AUC of a much higher BCNU dose administered prior to cyclophosphamide.[17] Even though the response rate appears to be superior in the "augmented CBV" variants, their toxic death rate is also higher, and therefore the ultimate value of these regimens is not clear.

At least three groups have reported on the use of CBV prior to allogeneic transplantation, confirming reliable engraftment.[65–67] The doses of the three drugs were different in each of the reports: cyclophosphamide, 6.0–7.2 g/m²; BCNU, 300–600 mg/m²; and etoposide, 600–2400 mg/m².

TABLE 34–1. COMPARISON OF DIFFERENT REGIMENS USED FOR HODGKIN DISEASE AND NON-HODGKIN LYMPHOMA

	CBV		BEAC	BEAM
	Standard	**Augmented**		
Doses (mg/m²)				
CPA	6000	7200	6000	300
BCNU	300	450–600	300	800
Etoposide	600–900	2000–2400	800	1600
Cytosine arabinoside			800	140
Melphalan				
Main grade 3–4 toxicities	Mucositis (27%)	Mucositis (76%) Pneumonitis (15%)	Mucositis (15–20%) Pneumonitis (5%) Renal (9%) Liver (7%)	Mucositis (15%) Pneumonitis (7%)
Toxic deaths	4–11%	17–21%	5%	5–10%
Salvage therapy for HD				
CR in refractory HD	47–59%	43–79%		51%
Long-term DFS	24–40%	47%		50%
Salvage therapy for NHL				
Long-term DFS			46%	35%
Long-term OS			55%	41%

BCNU, bis-chloroethyl-nitrosourea; BEAC, cyclophosphamide, BCNU, etoposide, cytosine arabinoside; BEAM, melphalan, BCNU, etoposide, cytosine arabinoside; CBV, cyclophosphamide, BCNU, etoposide; CPA, cyclophosphamide; CR, complete remission; DFS, disease-free survival; HD, Hodgkin disease; NHL, non-Hodgkin lymphoma; OS, overall survival.

BEAC

A regimen very similar to CBV is BEAC, in which cytosine arabinoside is added and the schedule slightly modified. BEAC is composed of BCNU, 300 mg/m²/day × 1; etoposide, 200 mg/m²/day × 4 days; cytosine arabinoside, 200 mg/m²/day × 4 days; and cyclophosphamide, 1500 mg/m²/day × 4 days (Fig. 34–12; see Table 34–1).

BEAC was the high-dose regimen chosen for Multicenter European trial, also known as The Parma study, the only randomized trial published so far in the setting of high-grade non-Hodgkin lymphomas in sensitive relapse. After two courses of second-line conventional chemotherapy with DHAP (dexamethasone, cisplatin, and cytosine arabinoside), responding patients were randomized to receive four additional courses of DHAP plus radiotherapy or BEAC with autologous bone marrow transplantation followed by radiotherapy. At 5 years of follow-up, the high-dose arm had significantly better disease-free survival (46% versus 12%, P = .001) and overall survival (53% versus 32%, P = .038) than the conventional chemotherapy arm.[68] The main nonhematologic toxicities of BEAC that have been reported are hepatic toxicity 7%, interstitial pneumonitis 5%, renal toxicity 9%, and grade 3–4 mucositis 17%, with an overall toxic death rate of 5%.

BEAM

Another major chemotherapy combination used in Hodgkin disease and non-Hodgkin lymphoma is the BEAM regimen, in which melphalan is substituted for cyclophosphamide. Melphalan is an attractive agent to use in this setting because it is not part of first-line conventional regimens (e.g., MOPP, ABVD, CHOP) and has been shown to be effective as a single agent in high doses in Hodgkin disease.[69] Additionally, it is not believed to undergo metabo-lism, thus decreasing the likelihood of unpredictable drug-drug interactions with other chemotherapeutic agents.

The BEAM regimen was originally developed by Linch et al. at University College in Great Britain, and it includes BCNU (300 mg/m²), etoposide (800 mg/m²), cytosine arabinoside (1600 mg/m²), and melphalan (140 mg/m²) (Fig. 34–13). Complete remission rates in excess of 50% have been reported in refractory Hodgkin disease with a low (5–10%) death rate from drug toxicity.[70, 71] The main toxicity of this regimen is interstitial pneumonitis (7%), with mucositis also being prominent.

Importantly, BEAM has been used in the only published randomized trial of high-dose versus conventional chemotherapy in refractory Hodgkin disease. This English study, which was closed prematurely because of patient refusal to be randomized, showed a significant benefit in terms of disease-free survival for the high-dose arm.[72] In patients with refractory high-grade non-Hodgkin lymphoma as salvage treatment after a single cycle of conventional second-line chemotherapy, BEAM produced 5-year disease-free and overall survival rates of 35% and 41%, respectively.[73]

FRACTIONATED TBI–ETOPOSIDE/ CYCLOPHOSPHAMIDE

The use of fractionated TBI in combination with etoposide (60 mg/kg) and cyclophosphamide (100 mg/kg) has been extensively evaluated in the treatment of non-Hodgkin lymphoma and Hodgkin disease (Fig. 34–14).[74, 75] Two different groups obtained similar 2- to 3-year disease-free survival rates (55–59%), and the toxic mortality rate was less than 10%. A retrospective comparison of this regimen with CBV in a large number of patients with non-Hodgkin lymphoma found no significant differences in outcome.[76]

Day	-6	-5	-4	-3	-2	-1	0
Cy 35 mg/kg/d IV		X	X	X	X		
BCNU 300 mg/m² IV	X						
VP16 100 mg/m²/12 hs IV		X	X	X	X		
Ara C 100 mg/m²/12 hs IV		X	X	X	X		
HSC							X

FIGURE 34–12. BEAC (BCNV, etoposide, Ara-C, cyclophosphamide). Cy, cyclophosphamide; VP16, etoposide; HSC, hematopoietic stem cells; IV, intravenous.

Day	-6	-5	-4	-3	-2	-1	0
L-PAM 140 mg/m² IV						X	
BCNU 300 mg/m² IV	X						
VP16 100 mg/m²/12 hs IV		X	X	X	X		
Ara C 200 mg/m²/12 hs IV		X	X	X	X		
HSC							X

FIGURE 34–13. BEAM (BCNU, etoposide, Ara-C, melphalan). Cy, cyclophosphamide; VP16, etoposide; L-PAM, melphalan; HSC, hematopoietic stem cells; IV, intravenous.

BCHE

This regimen is a CBV variant with the addition of hydroxyurea (oral hydroxyurea, 1.5 g/m²/6 hours PO × 12 doses or IV hydroxyurea, 12 g/m² in 72-hour continuous infusion) (Fig. 34–15).[77] These two hydroxyurea-containing regimens were developed by Vaughan et al. at the University of Nebraska in primary refractory or refractory relapsed non-Hodgkin lymphoma.[77] IV BCHE showed more activity (57% versus 29% complete remission) and less toxicity (4% versus 29% toxic deaths) than oral BCHE. In this extremely poor-prognosis patient population, IV BCHE of-fered a 33% disease-free survival rate at 4 years and a 12% rate for oral BCHE. Mucositis was the major nonhematologic toxicity associated with oral and IV BCHE: 100% of patients at the maximum tolerated dose of hydroxyurea in the IV BCHE regimen experienced severe mucositis.

HIGH-DOSE CHEMOTHERAPY REGIMENS FOR BREAST CANCER

RATIONALE

In the mid-1980s, the Solid Tumor Autologous Marrow Program (STAMP) at the Dana-Farber Cancer Institute, un-

Day	-8	-7	-6	-5	-4	-3	-2	-1	0
FTBI 12 Gy	X	X	X	X					
VP 60 mg/kg IV					X				
Cy 100 mg/kg IV							X		
HSC									X

FIGURE 34–14. Cy-VP-FTBI. IV, intravenous; Cy, cyclophosphamide; VP, etoposide; FTBI, fractionated total body irradiation; HSC, hematopoietic stem cells.

Day	-8	-7	-6	-5	-4	-3	-2	-1	0
BCNU 300 mg/m² IV	X								
Cy 2.5 g/m²/d IV	X	X							
VP16 150 mg/m²/ 1–2 hs IV				X	X	X			
HU 10 g/m² IV CI				▬▬▬▬▬▬▬▬					
HSC							X		

FIGURE 34–15. BCHE (BCNU, cyclophosphamides hydroxyurea, etoposide). Cy, cyclophosphamide; HU, hydroxyurea; VP16, etoposide; HSC, hematopoietic stem cells; IV, intravenous; CI, continuous infusion.

der the direction of Emil Frei III, began a series of clinical trials testing different high-dose alkylating agent combinations with autologous hematopoietic stem cell support. The evidence of a dose-response effect together with lack of cross-resistance among different alkylating agents and the potential for synergism formed the scientific basis for these trials.[78–80]

RESULTS AND TOXICITY

In 1986, Peters et al. published the results from a phase I study that showed that cyclophosphamide, cisplatin, and BCNU (STAMP I) could be combined at high doses (Fig. 34–16).[81] When this regimen was tested in the treatment of metastatic breast cancer, 54% of patients obtained a complete response, a result unprecedented in this disease.[82] Five of 22 patients treated died as a result of toxicity, but 14% of the patients continued free of disease at more than 10 years of follow-up.[83] Subsequent studies have shown a much lower mortality rate with the use of peripheral blood progenitor cells, growth factors, and hyperhydration during chemotherapy.[84] Elias et al. described a modification of this regimen (dose of BCNU reduced to 480 mg/m² and a schedule modification) in patients with small cell lung cancer.[85]

Day	-6	-5	-4	-3	-2	-1	0
Cy 1,875 mg/m²/d IV	X	X	X				
Cis 165 mg/m² IV CI	▬▬▬▬▬▬▬▬						
BCNU 600 mg/m² IV				X			
HSC							X

FIGURE 34–16. STAMP I. STAMP, Solid Tumor Autologous Marrow Program; Cy, cyclophosphamide; Cis, cisplatin; IV, intravenous; CI, continuous infusion; HSC, hematopoietic stem cells.

In 1990, Jones et al. attempted to replace cisplatin with carboplatin in STAMP I.[86] Unfortunately, despite the relatively low dose of carboplatin (450 mg/m²), three of four patients experienced VOD, which was fatal in two of them, and so this modification was discarded. This small study stresses the fact that it is difficult to predict the toxicities of a regimen when high-dose combination chemotherapy is used.

In an attempt to reduce the high mortality encountered during the initial phase I/II studies with STAMP I, Eder et al. conducted a new phase I/II study that combined cyclophosphamide, carboplatin, and thiotepa given as a continuous infusion (Fig. 34–17).[87] In breast cancer, the overall response rate to this regimen, called STAMP V, was 81%, and this regimen conferred a mortality rate of only 7%.

Williams et al. conducted a phase I study of high-dose thiotepa and cyclophosphamide and reached the following a maximum tolerated dose: cyclophosphamide, 7.5 g/m² and thiotepa, 700 mg/m², both given over 3 days (Fig. 34–18).[88] The toxic death rate in that study was 25%. A subsequent phase II study confirmed the value of this regimen in patients with chemotherapy-responsive metastatic breast cancer.[89] Kennedy et al. used a similar regimen, but giving both drugs as a continuous infusion they had a comparable response rate without toxic fatalities in 30 patients (Fig. 34–19).[90] Dunphy et al. published the results of a phase I/II study using two sequential cycles of high-dose cyclophosphamide (4.5–5.25 g/m²), cisplatin (120–180 mg/m²), and etoposide (750–1200 mg/m²)[91] (Fig. 34–20). The toxic mortality rate in this study was only 6%, and 18% of patients with breast cancer and metastatic disease were alive and progression free at the time of the last report.[92] Somlo et al. used a similar regimen, but they divided the total dose of both cisplatin and etoposide in half and they administered them 7 days apart in an attempt to reduce the nephrotoxicity and neurotoxicity (Fig. 34–

21).[93] Only two of 30 patients died as a result of toxicity, and the maximum tolerated dose was cisplatin, 125 mg/m² × 2; etoposide, 30 mg/kg × 2; and cyclophosphamide, 100 mg/kg. Fields et al. performed a phase I study of ifosfamide, carboplatin, and etoposide in patients with poor-prognosis malignancies (99 of 154 had breast cancer).[94] The maximum tolerated dose for this combination was ifosfamide, 20,100 mg/m²; carboplatin, 1800 mg/m²; and etoposide, 3000 mg/m², all given in divided doses over 6 days (Fig. 34–22). The dose-limiting toxicities for the combination were central nervous system toxicity and acute renal failure. In a subsequent analysis of this study, the authors suggested that patients with anthracycline-responsive breast cancer treated at the higher dose levels experienced a higher response rate than those treated at the lower doses.[95]

One possible way to improve the results in patients with metastatic breast cancer is the incorporation of drugs with different mechanisms of action. In a 1996 phase I study, Cagnoni et al. demonstrated the feasibility of incorporation of paclitaxel in a high-dose chemotherapy regimen.[100] The rationale for this study was the promising antitumor activity of paclitaxel in breast cancer, the lack of life-threatening extrahematologic toxicity of conventional dose paclitaxel, the preclinical evidence for a dose-response effect with paclitaxel, and the in vitro synergism exhibited when paclitaxel and cisplatin are combined.[96–99] The maximum tolerated dose for this regimen was paclitaxel, 775 mg/m², infused over 24 hours; cyclophosphamide, 5625 mg/m² in three daily doses; and cisplatin, 165 mg/m² IV given by continuous infusion over 72 hours followed by AHPCS (Fig. 34–23). It is too early to determine whether this regimen will be an improvement over the currently available high-dose regimens for the treatment of breast cancer, but the fact that it incorporates a drug with very high activity in breast cancer, together with the ability to dose-escalate this drug almost fourfold above standard doses, makes this approach attractive.

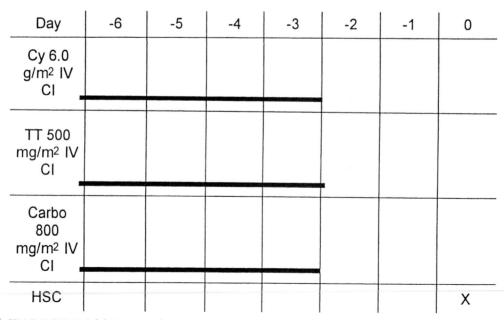

FIGURE 34–17. STAMP V. STAMP, Solid Tumor Autologous Marrow Program; Cy, cyclophosphamide; TT, thiotepa; Carbo, carboplatin; IV, intravenous; CI, continuous infusion; HSC, hematopoietic stem cells.

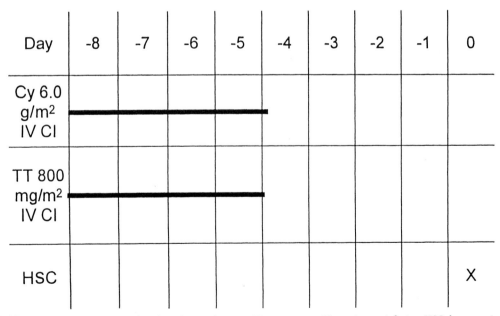

Day	-6	-5	-4	-3	-2	-1	0
Cy 2.5 g/m²/d IV	X		X		X		
TT 225 mg/m²/d IV	X		X		X		
HSC							X

FIGURE 34–18. Cy-thiotepa. Cy, cyclophosphamide; TT, thiotepa; IV, intravenous; HSC, hematopoietic stem cells.

Day	-8	-7	-6	-5	-4	-3	-2	-1	0
Cy 6.0 g/m² IV CI	━━━━━━━━━━━━━━━━								
TT 800 mg/m² IV CI	━━━━━━━━━━━━━━━━								
HSC									X

FIGURE 34–19. Cy-thiotepa CI. Cy, cyclophosphamide; TT, thiotepa; IV, intravenous; CI, continuous infusion; HSC, hematopoietic stem cells.

Day	-6	-5	-4	-3	-2	-1	0
Cy 1.5-1.75 g/m²/d IV	X	X	X				
VP16 250-400 mg/m²/d IV	X	X	X				
Cis 40-60 mg/m²/dl V	X	X	X				
HSC							X

FIGURE 34–20. Cy-VP16-Cisplatin. Cy, cyclophosphamide; VP16, etoposide; Cis, cisplatin; IV, intravenous; HSC, hematopoietic stem cells.

Day	-12	-11	-10	-9	-8	-7	-6	-5	-4	-3	-2	-1	0
Cis 125 mg/m² IV	X							X					
VP 30 mg/kg IV	X							X					
Cy 100 mg/kg IV										X			
HSC													X

FIGURE 34–21. Cy-VP16-Cisplatin. Cy, cyclophosphamide; VP16, etoposide; Cis, cisplatin; IV, intravenous; HSC, hematopoietic stem cells.

Day	-8	-7	-6	-5	-4	-3	-2	-1	0
Ifo 20.1 g/m² IV	X	X	X	X					
VP 3.0 g/m² IV	X	X	X	X					
Carbo 3.0 g/m² IV	X	X	X	X					
HSC									X

FIGURE 34–22. ICE (ifosfamide, carboplatin, etoposide). IFO, ifosfamide; Carbo, carboplatin; VP, etoposide; IV, intravenous; HSC, hematopoietic stem cells.

After the completion of this phase I study, a follow-up study was started that attempts to incorporate BCNU into this high-dose, paclitaxel-based regimen.[100] Somlo et al. conducted a phase I study of etoposide (60 mg/kg) and cyclophosphamide (100 mg/kg) with escalated doses of doxorubicin (Adriamycin) given as a continuous infusion over 96 hours (Fig. 34–24).[101] The maximum tolerated dose for doxorubicin in this combination was determined to be 165 mg/m², and no toxic fatalities occurred. At least two groups have tested the value of busulfan/cyclophosphamide in patients with breast cancer. Klumpp et al. treated 15 patients with breast cancer with busulfan, 16 mg/kg, and cyclophosphamide; 6.0 g/m², and obtained a median progression-free survival time of 164 days.[102] Using busulfan/cyclophosphamide 2, Kalaycioglu et al. treated 21 patients with chemosensitive breast cancer and observed only one toxic fatality, and the estimated 2-year disease-free survival rate was 25% at the time of report.[103]

Discussion of hematopoietic stem cell transplantation in breast cancer can be found in Chapter 10.

HIGH-DOSE CHEMOTHERAPY REGIMENS USED FOR OVARIAN CARCINOMA

The two main regimens used for this disease are usually referred to by the name of the institution at which they

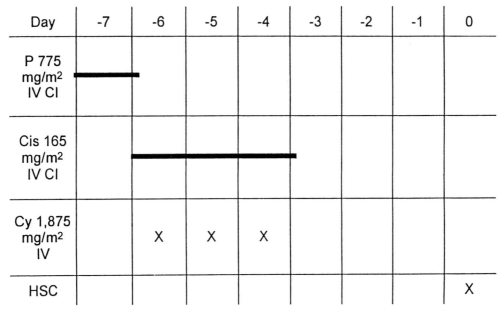

Day	-7	-6	-5	-4	-3	-2	-1	0
P 775 mg/m² IV CI	▬▬▬							
Cis 165 mg/m² IV CI		▬▬▬▬▬▬						
Cy 1,875 mg/m² IV		X	X	X				
HSC								X

FIGURE 34–23. PCC (paclitaxel, cisplatin, cyclophosphamide). P, paclitaxel; Cis, cisplatin; Cy, cyclophosphamide; IV, intravenous; CI, continuous infusion; HSC, hematopoietic stem cells.

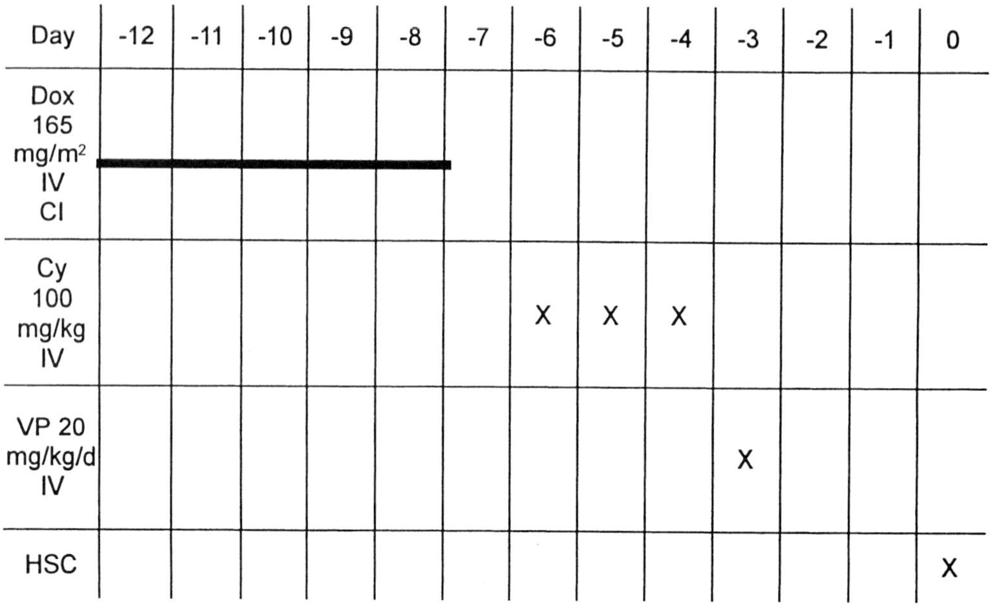

Day	-12	-11	-10	-9	-8	-7	-6	-5	-4	-3	-2	-1	0
Dox 165 mg/m² IV CI	▬▬▬▬▬▬▬▬▬▬▬▬▬												
Cy 100 mg/kg IV							X	X	X				
VP 20 mg/kg/d IV										X			
HSC													X

FIGURE 34–24. Dox, doxorubicin; VP, etoposide; Cy, cyclophosphamide; IV, intravenous; CI, continuous infusion; HSC, hematopoietic stem cells.

were developed: the Duke/Colorado regimen and the Loyola regimen.

DUKE/COLORADO REGIMEN

Using preclinical data showing synergism of different alkylating agents against ovarian cancer cell lines,[104] Shpall et al. developed a regimen containing three alkylating agents at the following doses: cyclophosphamide (5.6 g/m²), cisplatin (165 mg/m²), and thiotepa (600 mg/m²) (Fig. 34–25).[105] The response rate to this regimen in heavily pretreated patients was 60%.[106]

LOYOLA REGIMEN

Preclinical data supported the inclusion of mitoxantrone in a dose-intensive regimen for patients with ovarian cancer. In vitro studies showed that both alkylating agents and mitoxantrone have a dose-response effect against ovarian cancer cell lines.[107] These data prompted Stiff et al. to explore a combination of mitoxantrone combined with two alkylating agents, carboplatin and cyclophosphamide, at the following doses[108, 109]: cyclophosphamide (120 mg/kg), mitoxantrone (30–75 mg/m²), and carboplatin (1500 mg/m²) (Fig. 34–26). The dose-limiting toxicities were mucositis and diarrhea, and the response rate in 30 patients was 89%.

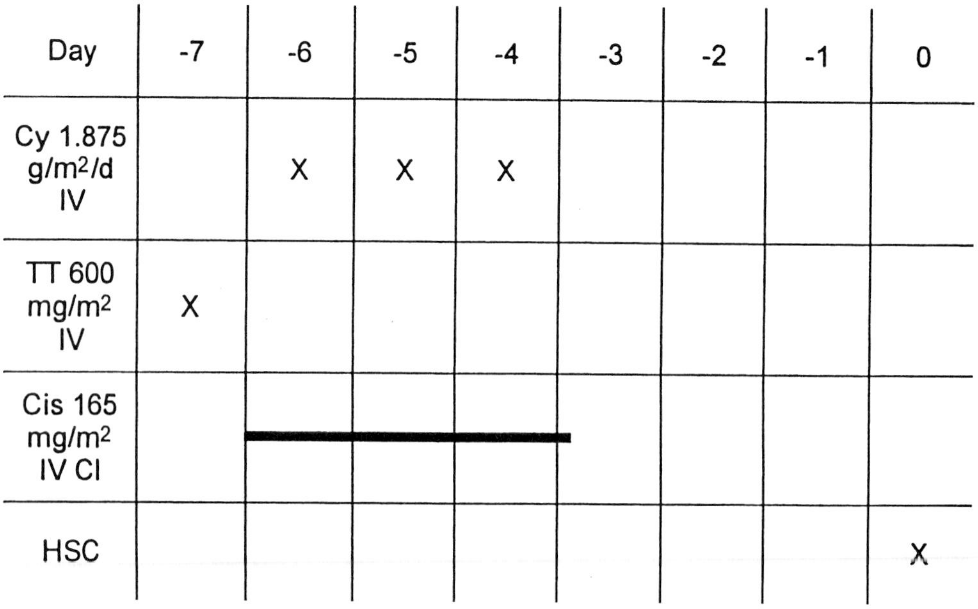

Day	-7	-6	-5	-4	-3	-2	-1	0
Cy 1.875 g/m²/d IV		X	X	X				
TT 600 mg/m² IV	X							
Cis 165 mg/m² IV CI		▬▬▬▬▬▬▬▬▬▬						
HSC								X

FIGURE 34–25. Duke/Colorado regimen. Cy, cyclophosphamide; TT, thiotepa; Cis, cisplatin; IV, intravenous; CI, continuous infusion; HSC, hematopoietic stem cells.

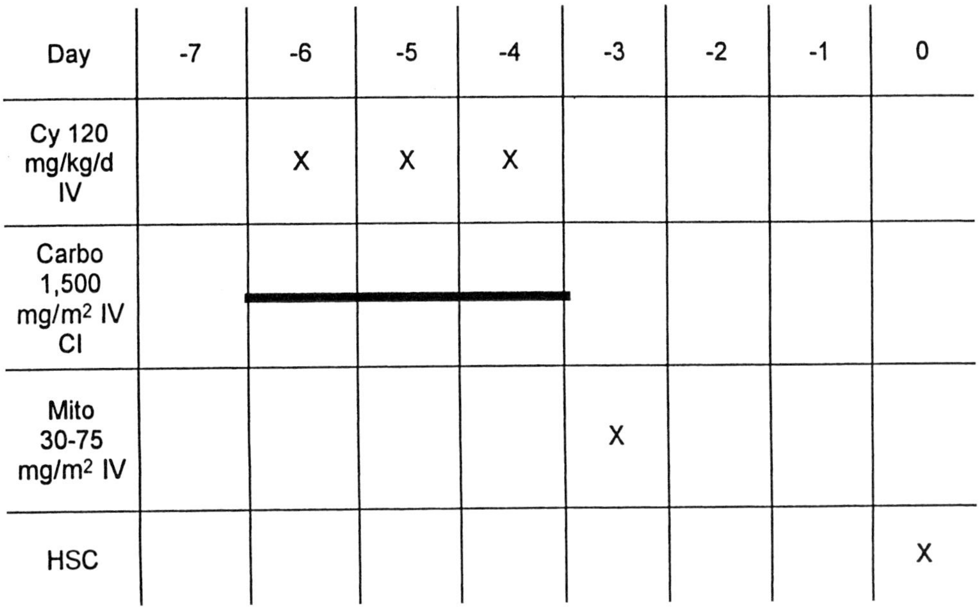

Day	-7	-6	-5	-4	-3	-2	-1	0
Cy 120 mg/kg/d IV		X	X	X				
Carbo 1,500 mg/m² IV CI		▬▬▬▬▬▬▬▬▬▬						
Mito 30-75 mg/m² IV					X			
HSC								X

FIGURE 34–26. Loyola regimen. Cy, cyclophosphamide; Mito, mitoxantrone; Carbo, carboplatin; IV, intravenous; CI, continuous infusion; HSC, hematopoietic stem cells.

CONCLUSION

In recent decades, many high-dose chemotherapy regimens have been developed. If we expect to continue to make progress in this field, future regimens must be designed more rationally. To date, randomized comparison of high-dose regimens has been limited to the busulfan/cyclophosphamide versus cyclophosphamide/TBI trials in patients with leukemia. These trials will continue to be difficult to perform. Maximal information must be obtained from phase I–II studies of newer regimens to optimize the potential outcome of patients after high-dose chemotherapy. Pharmacokinetic monitoring is an indispensable component of such studies so that we can, among other things, better understand how drugs can be combined, which drugs are more important in a regimen, and whether dose adjustment of a particular drug is feasible and necessary. A critical question that remains is whether a particular regimen is optimal for each indication. Although some doubt remains that outcome will be improved with newer regimens, precedents from trials of cancer treatment regimens used in conventional doses suggest that this view is incorrect. The only way to answer this and other questions is to enroll patients in well-designed clinical studies that ask clinically relevant questions about maximally effective regimens.

REFERENCES

1. Jones RB, Cagnoni PJ, Bearman SI, Shpall EJ: Pharmacology of high-dose therapy with bone marrow transplantation. *In* Carella AM (ed): Autologous Stem Cell Transplantation: Biological and Clinical Results in Malignancies. Newark, Gordon & Breach, 1997, pp 81–88.
2. Henner WD, Furlong EA, Flaherty MD, et al: Measurement of busulfan in plasma by high-performance liquid chromatography. J Chromatogr 416:426–432, 1987.
3. Hassan M, Ehrsson H, Smedmyr B, et al: Cerebrospinal fluid and plasma concentrations of busulfan during high-dose therapy. Bone Marrow Transplant 4:113–114, 1989.
4. Vassal G, Gouyette A, Hartmann O, et al: Pharmacokinetics of high-dose busulfan in children. Cancer Chemother Pharmacol 24:386–390, 1989.
5. Grochow LB, Jones RJ, Brundrett RB, et al: Pharmacokinetics of busulfan: correlation with veno-occlusive disease in patients undergoing bone marrow transplantation. Cancer Chemother Pharmacol 25:55–61, 1989.
6. Dix SP, Wingard JR, Mullins RE, et al: Association of busulfan area under the curve with veno-occlusive disease following BMT. Bone Marrow Transplant 17:225–230, 1996.
7. Sureda A, Perez de Oteyza J, Garcia Larana J, et al: High-dose busulfan and seizures. Ann Intern Med 111:543–544, 1989.
8. Hassan M, Oberg G, Bjorkholm M, et al: Influence of prophylactic anticonvulsant therapy on high-dose busulfan kinetics. Cancer Chemother Pharmacol 33:181–186, 1993.
9. Moore MJ, Hardy RW, Thiessen JJ, et al: Rapid development of enhanced clearance after high-dose cyclophosphamide. Clin Pharmacol Ther 44:622, 1988.
10. Grochow LB, Krivit W, Whitley CB, et al: Busulfan disposition in children. Blood 75:1723–1727, 1990.
11. Vassal G, Fischer A, Challine D, et al: Busulfan disposition below the age of three: alterations in children with lysosomal storage disease. Blood 82:1030–1034, 1993.
12. Grochow LB: Busulfan disposition: the role of therapeutic monitoring in bone marrow transplantation induction regimens. Semin Oncol 20:18–25, 1993.
13. Yeager AW, Wagner JE, Graham ML, et al: Optimization of busulfan dosage in children undergoing bone marrow transplantation: a pharmacokinetic study of dose escalation. Blood 80:2425–2428, 1992.
14. Slattery JT, Sanders JE, Buckner CD, et al: Graft-rejection and toxicity following bone marrow transplantation in relation to busulfan pharmacokinetics. Bone Marrow Transplant 16:31–42, 1995.
15. Bhagwatwar HP, Phadubgpojna S, Chow DS-L, et al: Formulation and stability of busulfan for intravenous administration in high-dose chemotherapy. Cancer Chemother Pharmacol 37:401–408, 1996.
16. Jones RB, Matthes S, Shpall EJ, et al: Acute lung injury following treatment with high-dose cyclophosphamide, cisplatin and carmustine: pharmacodynamic evaluation of carmustine. J Natl Cancer Inst 85:640–647, 1993.
17. Jones RB, Matthes S, Kemme D, et al: Cyclophosphamide, cisplatin, and carmustine: pharmacokinetics of carmustine following multiple alkylating-agent interactions. Cancer Chemother Pharmacol 35:59–63, 1994.
18. Ayash LJ, Wright JE, Tretyakov O, et al: Cyclophosphamide pharma-

cokinetics: correlation with cardiac toxicity and tumor response. J Clin Oncol 10:995–1000, 1992.

19. Slattery JT, Kalhorn TF, McDonald GB, et al: Conditioning regimen-dependent disposition of cyclophosphamide and hydroxycyclophosphamide in human marrow transplantation patients. J Clin Oncol 14:1484–1494, 1996.

20. Chen T-L, Passos-Coelho JL, Noe DA, et al: Nonlinear pharmacokinetics of cyclophosphamide in patients with metastatic breast cancer receiving high-dose chemotherapy followed by autologous bone marrow transplantation. Cancer Res 55:810–816, 1995.

21. Anderson LW, Chen L-T, Colivin OM, et al: Cyclophosphamide and 4-hydroxycyclophosphamide/aldophosphamide kinetics in patients receiving high-dose cyclophosphamide chemotherapy. Clin Cancer Res 2:1481–1487, 1996.

22. Stemmer SM, Cagnoni PJ, Shpall EJ, et al: High-dose paclitaxel, cyclophosphamide, and cisplatin with autologous hematopoietic progenitor cell support: a phase I trial. J Clin Oncol 14:1463–1472, 1996.

23. Egorin MJ, Cohen BE, Herzig RH, et al: Human plasma pharmacokinetics and urinary excretion of thiotepa and its metabolites in patients receiving high-dose thiotepa therapy. In Herzig GP (ed): High-Dose Thiotepa and Autologous Marrow Transplantation. New York, Park Row, 1987, pp 3–8.

24. O'Dwyer PJ, LaCreta F, Engstrom PF, et al: Phase I/pharmacokinetic reevaluation of thiotepa. Cancer Res 51:3171–3176, 1991.

25. LaCreta FP, Tinsley PW, O'Dwyer PJ: Dose dependent elimination of thiotepa by the isolated perfused rat liver. Proc Am Assoc Cancer Res 31:386, 1990.

26. Przepiorka D, Madden T, Ippoliti C, et al: Dosing of thiotepa for myeloablative therapy. Cancer Chemother Pharmacol 37:155–160, 1995.

27. Cagnoni PJ, Matthes S, Dufton C, et al: Ondansetron significantly reduces the area under the curve of cyclophosphamide and cisplatin. Proc Am Soc Clin Oncol 14:462a, 1995.

28. Gilbert CJ, Petros WP, Cavanaugh C, et al: Influence of ondansetron on the pharmacokinetics of high-dose cyclophosphamide. Proc Am Soc Clin Oncol 14:316a, 1995.

29. Santos GW: The development of busulfan/cyclophosphamide preparative regimens. Semin Oncol 20:12–16, 1993.

30. Santos GW, Tutschka PJ: Marrow transplantation in the busulfan treated rat—pre-clinical models of aplastic anemia. J Natl Cancer Inst 53:1781–1785, 1974.

31. Santos GW, Tutschka PJ: Effect of busulfan on antibody production and skin allograft survival in the rat. J Natl Cancer Inst 53:1775–1780, 1974.

32. Tutschka PJ, Santos GW: Marrow transplantation in the busulfan treated rat: I. Effect of cyclophosphamide and rabbit anti-rat thymocyte serum as immunosuppression. Transplantation 20:101–106, 1975.

33. Santos GW, Tutschka PJ, Brookmeyer R, et al: Marrow transplantation for acute nonlymphocytic leukemia after treatment with busulfan and cyclophosphamide. N Engl J Med 309:1347–1353, 1983.

34. Jones RJ, Lee KSK, Beschorner WE, et al: Venoocclusive disease of the liver following bone marrow transplantation. Transplantation 44:778–783, 1987.

35. Tutschka PJ, Copelan EA, Klein JP: Bone marrow transplantation for leukemia following a new busulfan and cyclophosphamide regimen. Blood 70:1382–1388, 1987.

36. Copelan EA, Biggs JC, Thompson JM, et al: Treatment of acute myelocytic leukemia with allogeneic bone marrow transplantation following preparation with BuCy2. Blood 78:838–843, 1991.

37. Blaise D, Maraninchi D, Archimbaud E, et al: Allogeneic bone marrow transplantation for acute myeloid leukemia in first remission: a randomized trial of a busulfan-cytoxan versus cytoxan-total body irradiation as preparative regimen: a report from the Groupe d'Etudes de la Greffe de Moelle Osseuse. Blood 79:2578–2582, 1992.

38. Clift RA, Buckner CD, Thomas ED, et al: Marrow transplantation for chronic myeloid leukemia: a randomized study comparing cyclophosphamide and total body irradiation with busulfan and cyclophosphamide. Blood 84:2036–2043, 1994.

39. Ringden O, Ruutu T, Remberger M, et al: A randomized trial comparing busulfan with total body irradiation as conditioning in allogeneic marrow transplant recipients with leukemia: a report from the Nordic Bone Marrow Transplantation Group. Blood 83:2723–2730, 1994.

40. Dusenbery KE, Daniels KA, McClure JS, et al: Randomized comparison of cyclophosphamide-total body irradiation versus busulfan-cyclophosphamide conditioning in autologous bone marrow transplantation for acute myeloid leukemia. Int J Radiat Oncol Biol Phys 31:119–128, 1995.

41. Ringden O, Labopin M, Tura S, et al: A comparison of busulfan versus total body irradiation combined with cyclophosphamide as conditioning for autograft or allograft bone marrow transplantation in patients with acute leukemia. Br J Hematol 93:637–645, 1996.

42. Blume KG, Kopecky KJ, Henslee-Downey JP, et al: A prospective randomized comparison of total body irradiation-etoposide versus busulfan-cyclophosphamide as preparatory regimens for bone marrow transplantation in patients with leukemia who were not in first remission: a Southwest Oncology Group Study. Blood 81:2187–2193, 1993.

43. Van der Jagt FR, Appelbaum FR, Petersen FB, et al: Busulfan and cyclophosphamide as a preparative regimen for bone marrow transplantation in patients with prior chest radiotherapy. Bone Marrow Transplant 8:211–215, 1991.

44. Giorgiani G, Bozzola M, Locatelli F, et al: Role of busulfan and total body irradiation on growth of prepubertal children receiving bone marrow transplantation and results of treatment with recombinant human growth hormone. Blood 86:825–831, 1995.

45. Urban C, Schwingshandl J, Slavc I, et al: Endocrine function after bone marrow transplantation without the use of preparative total body irradiation. Bone Marrow Transplant 3:291, 1988.

46. Wingard JR, Plotnick LP, Freemer CS, et al: Growth in children after bone marrow transplantation: busulfan plus cyclophosphamide versus cyclophosphamide plus total body irradiation. Blood 79:1068–1073, 1992.

47. Sanders JE, Hawley J, Levy W, et al: Pregnancies following high-dose cyclophosphamide with or without high-dose busulfan or total-body irradiation and bone marrow transplantation. Blood 87:3045–3052, 1996.

48. Vaughan WP, Dennison JD, Reed EC, et al: Improved results of allogeneic bone marrow transplantation for advanced hematologic malignancy using busulfan, cyclophosphamide and etoposide as cytoreductive and immunosuppressive therapy. Bone Marrow Transplant 8:489–495, 1991.

49. Vaughan WP, Briggs AD, Salzman DE, et al: High dose busulfan, cytoxan, etoposide supported by autologous peripheral stem cell rescue for intermediate grade non-Hodgkin lymphoma at high risk of relapse. Presented at the Second Annual Scientific Meeting of the American Society for Blood and Marrow Transplantation, San Diego, October 2–6, 1996, p 39.

50. Geller RB, Myers S, Devine S, et al: Phase I study of busulfan, cyclophosphamide and timed sequential escalating doses of cytarabine followed by bone marrow transplantation. Bone Marrow Transplant 9:41–47, 1992.

51. Ratanatharathorn V, Karanes C, Lum LG, et al: Allogeneic bone marrow transplantation in high-risk myeloid disorders using busulfan, cytosine arabinoside and cyclophosphamide. Bone Marrow Transplant 9:49–55, 1992.

52. Petersen FB, Buckner CD, Appelbaum FR, et al: Busulfan, cyclophosphamide and fractionated total body irradiation as a preparatory regimen for marrow transplantation in patients with advanced hematological malignancies: a phase I study. Bone Marrow Transplant 4:617–623, 1989.

53. Lynch MHE, Petersen FB, Appelbaum FR, et al: Phase II study of busulfan, cyclophosphamide and fractionated total body irradiation as a preparatory regimen for allogeneic bone marrow transplantation in patients with advanced myeloid malignacies. Bone Marrow Transplant 15:59–64, 1995.

54. Demirer T, Buckner CD, Appelbaum FR, et al: Busulfan, cyclophosphamide and fractionated total body irradiation for allogeneic marrow transplantation in advanced acute and chronic myelogenous leukemia: a phase I dose escalation of busulfan based on targeted plasma levels. Bone Marrow Transplant 17:341–346, 1996.

55. Bacigalupo A, Van Lint MT, Valbonesi M, et al: Thiotepa cyclophosphamide followed by granulocyte colony-stimulating factor mobilized allogeneic peripheral blood cells in adults with advanced leukemia. Blood 88:353–357, 1996.

56. Dimopoulos MA, Alexanian R, Przepiorka D, et al: Thiotepa, busulfan, and cyclophosphamide: a new preparative regimen for autologous marrow or blood stem cell transplantation in high-risk multiple myeloma. Blood 82:2324–2328, 1993.

57. Spitzer G, Dicke KA, Litam J, et al: High-dose combination chemotherapy with autologous bone marrow transplantation in adult solid tumors. Cancer 45:3075, 1980.

58. Jagannath S, Dicke K, Armitage JO, et al: High-dose cyclophosphamide, carmustine, and etoposide and autologous bone marrow transplantation for relapsed Hodgkin's disease. Ann Intern Med 104:163–168, 1986.

59. Jagannath S, Armitage JO, Dicke KA, et al: Prognostic factors for response and survival after high-dose cyclophosphamide, carmustine and etoposide (CBV) with autologous bone marrow transplantation for relapsed Hodgkin's Disease. J Clin Oncol 7:179–185, 1989.

60. Armitage JO, Bierman PJ, Vose JM, et al: Autologous bone marrow transplantation for patients with relapsed Hodgkin's disease. Am J Med 91:605, 1991.

61. Carella A, Congiu AM, Gaozza E, et al: High-dose chemotherapy with autologous bone marrow transplantation in 50 advanced resistant Hodgkin's disease patients: an Italian Study Group Report. J Clin Oncol 6:1411–1416, 1988.

62. Reece DE, Connors JM, Spinelli JJ, et al: Intensive therapy with cyclophosphamide, carmustine, etoposide ± cisplatin, and autologous bone marrow transplantation for Hodgkin's disease in first relapse after combination chemotherapy. Blood 83:1193–1199, 1994.

63. Wheeler C, Antin JH, Churchill WH, et al: Cyclophosphamide, carmustine and etoposide with autologous bone marrow transplantation in refractory Hodgkin's disease and non-Hodgkin's lymphoma: a dose-finding study. J Clin Oncol 8:648–656, 1990.

64. Reece DE, Barnett MJ, Connors JM, et al: Intensive chemotherapy with cyclophosphamide, carmustine, and etoposide followed by autologous bone marrow transplant for relapsed Hodgkin's disease. J Clin Oncol 10:1871–1879, 1991.

65. Demirer T, Weaver CH, Buckner CD, et al: High-dose cyclophosphamide, carmustine and etoposide followed by allogeneic bone marrow transplantation in patients with lymphoid malignancies who had received prior dose-limiting radiation therapy. J Clin Oncol 13:596–602, 1995.

66. Zander AR, Culbert S, Jagannath S, et al: High dose cyclophosphamide, BCNU and VP-16 (CBV) as a conditioning regimen for allogeneic bone marrow transplantation for patients with acute leukemia. Cancer 59:1083–1086, 1987.

67. Ratanatharathorn V, Uberti J, Karanes C, et al: Prospective comparative trial of autologous versus allogeneic bone marrow transplantation in patients with non-Hodgkin's lymphoma. Blood 84:1050–1055, 1994.

68. Philip T, Guglielmo C, Hagenbeek A, et al: Autologous bone marrow transplantation as compared with salvage chemotherapy in relapses of chemotherapy-sensitive non-Hodgkin's lymphoma. N Engl J Med 333:1540–1545, 1995.

69. Russell JA, Selby PJ, Ruether BA, et al: Treatment of advanced Hodgkin's disease with high dose melphalan and autologous bone marrow transplantation. Bone Marrow Transplant 4:425–429, 1989.

70. Gribben JG, Linch DC, Singer CRJ, et al: Successful treatment of refractory Hodgkin's disease by high-dose combination chemotherapy and autologous bone marrow transplantation. Blood 73:340–344, 1989.

71. Chopra R, McMillan AK, Linch DC, et al: The place of high-dose BEAM therapy and autologous bone marrow transplantation in poor-risk Hodgkin's disease: a single-center eight-year study of 155 patients. Blood 81:1137–1145, 1993.

72. Linch DC, Winfield D, Goldstone AH, et al: Dose intensification with autologous bone-marrow transplantation in relapsed and resistant Hodgkin's disease: results of a BNLI randomized trial. Lancet 341:1051–1054, 1993.

73. Mills W, Chopra R, McMillan A, et al: BEAM chemotherapy and autologous bone marrow transplantation for patients with relapsed or refractory non-Hodgkin's lymphoma. J Clin Oncol 13:588–595, 1995.

74. Nademanee A, Sniecinski I, Schmidt GM, et al: High-dose therapy followed by autologous peripheral blood stem cell transplantation for patients with Hodgkin's disease and non-Hodgkin's lymphoma using unprimed and granulocyte colony-stimulating factor-mobilized peripheral blood stem cells. J Clin Oncol 12:2176–2186, 1994.

75. Horning SJ, Negrin RS, Chao NJ, et al: Fractionated total-body irradiation, etoposide, and cyclophosphamide plus autografting in Hodgkin's disease and non-Hodgkin's lymphoma. J Clin Oncol 12:2552–2558, 1994.

76. Stockerl-Goldstein KE, Horning SJ, Negrin RS, et al: Influence of preparatory regimen and source of hematopoietic cells on outcome of autotransplantation for non-Hodgkin's lymphoma. Biol Blood Bone Marrow Transplant 2:76–85, 1996.

77. Vaughan WP, Kris E, Vose J, et al: Phase I/II study incorporating intravenous hydroxyurea into high-dose chemotherapy for patients with primary refractory or relapsed and refractory intermediate-grade and high-grade malignant lymphoma. J Clin Oncol 13:1089–1095, 1995.

78. Schabel FM: Animal models as predictive systems. In Cancer Chemotherapy—Fundamental Concepts and Recent Advances. Chicago, Yearbook Medical, 1975, pp 323–355.

79. Frei E III, Cucchi CA, Rosowsky A, et al: Alkylating agent resistance: in vitro studies with human cell lines. Proc Natl Acad Sci U S A 82:2158–2162, 1985.

80. Schabel F, Trader M, Laster W, et al: Patterns of resistance and therapeutic synergy among alkylating agents. Antibiot Chemother 23:200–215, 1978.

81. Peters WP, Eder JP, Henner WD, et al: High-dose combination alkylating agents with autologous bone marrow support: a phase I trial. J Clin Oncol 4:646–654, 1986.

82. Peters WP, Shpall EJ, Jones RB, et al: High-dose alkylating agents with bone marrow support as initial treatment for metastatic breast cancer. J Clin Oncol 6:1368–1376, 1988.

83. Peters WP: Personal communication, 1996.

84. Peters WP, Ross M, Vredenburgh JJ, et al: High-dose chemotherapy and autologous bone marrow support as consolidation after standard-dose adjuvant therapy for high-risk primary breast cancer. J Clin Oncol 11:1132–1143, 1993.

85. Elias AD, Ayash L, Frei E III, et al: Intensive combined modality therapy for limited stage small cell lung cancer. J Natl Cancer Inst 85:559–566, 1993.

86. Jones RB, Shpall EJ, Ross M, et al: High-dose carboplatin, cyclophosphamide, and BCNU with autologous bone marrow support: excessive hepatic toxicity. Cancer Chemother Pharmacol 26:155–156, 1990.

87. Eder JP, Elias A, Shea TC, et al: A phase I–II study of cyclophosphamide, thiotepa, and carboplatin with autologous bone marrow transplantation in solid tumor patients. J Clin Oncol 8:1239–1245, 1990.

88. Williams SF, Bitran JD, Kaminer L, et al: A phase I–II study of bialkylator chemotherapy, high-dose thiotepa, and cyclophosphamide with autologous bone marrow reinfusion in patients with advanced cancer. J Clin Oncol 5:260–265, 1987.

89. Williams SF, Mick R, Desser R, et al: High-dose consolidation therapy with autologous stem cell rescue in stage IV breast cancer. J Clin Oncol 7:1824–1830, 1989.

90. Kennedy MJ, Beveridge RA, Rowley SD, et al: High-dose chemotherapy with reinfusion of purged autologous bone marrow following dose-intense induction as initial therapy for metastatic breast cancer. J Natl Cancer Inst 83:920–926, 1991.

91. Dunphy FR, Spitzer G, Buzdar AU, et al: Treatment of estrogen receptor-negative or hormonally refractory breast cancer with double high-dose chemotherapy intensification and bone marrow support. J Clin Oncol 8:1207–1216, 1990.

92. Dunphy FR, Spitzer G: Use of very high-dose chemotherapy with autologous bone marrow transplantation in treatment of breast cancer. J Natl Cancer Inst 84:128–129, 1992.

93. Somlo G, Doroshow JH, Forman SJ, et al: High-dose cisplatin, etoposide, and cyclophosphamide with autologous stem cell reinfusion in patients with responsive metastatic or high-risk breast cancer. Cancer 73:125–134, 1994.

94. Fields KK, Elfenbein GJ, Lazarus HM, et al: Maximum-tolerated doses of ifosfamide, carboplatin and etoposide given over 6 days followed by autologous stem-cell rescue: toxicity profile. J Clin Oncol 13:323–332, 1995.

95. Perkins JB, Fields KK, Elfenbein GJ: Ifosfamide/carboplatin/etoposide chemotherapy for metastatic breast cancer with or without autologous hematopoietic stem cell transplantation: evaluation of dose-response relationships. Semin Oncol 22:5–8, 1995.

96. Rowinsky EK, Citardi MJ, Noe DA, et al: Sequence-dependent cytotoxic effects due to combinations of cisplatin and the antimicrotubule agents taxol and vincristine. J Cancer Res Clin Oncol 119:727–733, 1993.

97. Rowinsky EK, Donehower RC, Jones RJ, et al: Microtubule changes and cytotoxicity in leukemic cell lines treated with Taxol. Cancer Res 48:4093–4100, 1988.

98. Milas L, Hunter NR, Kurdoglu B, et al: Kinetics of mitotic arrest and apoptosis in murine mammary and ovarian tumors treated with Taxol. Cancer Chemother Pharmacol 35:297–303, 1995.

99. McCloskey DE, Davidson NE: Paclitaxel-induced programmed cell death in human breast cancer cells [Abstract]. Proc Am Assoc Cancer Res 36:416, 1995.

100. Cagnoni PJ, Shpall EJ, Bearman SI, et al: Paclitaxel-containing high-dose chemotherapy: the University of Colorado experience. Semin Oncol 23:43–48, 1996.

101. Somlo G, Doroshow JH, Forman SJ, et al: High-dose doxorubicin, etoposide, and cyclophosphamide with stem cell reinfusion in patients with metastatic or high-risk primary breast cancer. Cancer 73:1678–1685, 1994.

102. Klumpp TR, Mangan KF, Glenn LD, et al: Phase II pilot study of high-dose busulfan and CY followed by autologous BM or peripheral blood stem cell transplantation in patients with advanced chemosensitive breast cancer. Bone Marrow Transplant 11:337–339, 1993.

103. Kalaycioglu ME, Lichtin AE, Andresen SW, et al: High-dose busulfan and cyclophosphamide followed by autologous bone marrow transplantation and/or peripheral blood progenitor cell rescue for metastatic breast cancer. Am J Clin Oncol 18:491–494, 1995.

104. Lidor YJ, Shpall EJ, Peters WP, et al: Synergistic toxicity of different alkylating agents for epithelial ovarian cancer. Int J Cancer 49:704–707, 1991.

105. Shpall EJ, Jones RB, Bearman SI, et al: Future strategies for the treatment of advanced epithelial ovarian cancer using high-dose chemotherapy and autologous bone marrow support. Gynecol Oncol 54:357–361, 1994.

106. Shpall EJ, Clark-Pearson D, Soper JT, et al: High-dose alkylating agent chemotherapy with autologous bone marrow support in patients with stage III/IV epithelial ovarian cancer. Gynecol Oncol 38:386–391, 1990.

107. Alberts DS, Young L, Mason N, et al: In vitro evaluation of anticancer drugs against ovarian cancer at concentrations achievable by intraperitoneal administration. Semin Oncol 12:38–42, 1985.

108. Stiff PJ, McKenzie RS, Alberts DA, et al: Phase I clinical and pharmacokinetic study high-dose mitoxantrone, carboplatin, and cyclophosphamide and autologous bone marrow rescue: high response rate for refractory ovarian carcinoma. J Clin Oncol 12:176–183, 1994.

109. Stiff PJ, Bayer R, Camarda M, et al: A phase II trial of high-dose mitoxantrone, carboplatin, and cyclophosphamide with autologous bone marrow rescue for recurrent epithelial ovarian carcinoma: analysis of risk factors for clinical outcome. Gynecol Oncol 57:278–285, 1995.

CHAPTER THIRTY-FIVE

Choice of Conditioning Regimens

Kenneth F. Mangan, M.D.

When selecting a regimen to prepare a patient for peripheral blood progenitor cell (PBPC) or bone marrow transplantation, the transplant physician is faced with a wide variety of options. Regimens with multiple chemotherapy drugs and immunobiologic agents are employed alone or in various combinations with or without radiation. The types of chemotherapeutic drugs, doses, schedules, and techniques for administering the drugs or radiotherapy are not standardized and vary from institution to institution. In general, most conditioning regimens are classified into four major types: (1) pure high-dose chemotherapy regimens, (2) total body irradiation (TBI) regimens, (3) regimens containing both high-dose chemotherapy and TBI, and (4) innovative regimens that target marrow or lymphoid tissue with radioimmune conjugates. Unfortunately, very few controlled data have been published that directly compare the toxicity and efficacy of different conditioning regimens. Therefore, the transplant physician must consider several factors before selecting a regimen for a specific patient.

CRITERIA FOR AN IDEAL CONDITIONING REGIMEN

The primary biologic goals of the conditioning regimen are to (1) create space in the host marrow microenvironment to allow engraftment of donor cells, (2) provide enough immunosuppression to allow immunologically diverse donor cells to engraft, and (3) eliminate any residual malignancy or nonmalignant disease. These goals should be considered when choosing a conditioning regimen. In addition to these three major biologic goals, the ideal regimen should be relatively nontoxic to the patient's vital organs and be inexpensive and easy to administer. Seven major factors that affect the selection of an appropriate conditioning regimen for any given patient are discussed in the following.

FACTORS TO CONSIDER WHEN SELECTING A CONDITIONING REGIMEN

ABLATIVE POTENCY

The first goal of any conditioning regimen is to create space for donor hematopoietic stem cells (HSC) to engraft in host recipient marrow. Current understanding of the engraftment process suggests that multipotential HSC home to marrow niches supported by stromal cells in the microenvironment.[1] The stromal cells and other accessory cells provide important growth factors that sustain and proliferate HSC. Only a small proportion of HSC are dividing (i.e., are in cell cycle) at any given time. The remainder are resting (i.e., in stage G_o of the cell cycle). Therefore, it is difficult to completely eliminate every host HSC. Sufficient numbers of HSC must be eliminated to allow any new autologous or allogeneic HSC to engraft, however.

When selecting a conditioning regimen, it is important to consider whether it is necessary to completely ablate residual marrow. Supralethal myeloablative conditioning regimens consistently result in severe life-threatening aplasia by damaging HSC. These aggressive regimens may also cause severe damage to the microenvironment. For truly ablative regimens, marrow HSC rescue is absolutely necessary to avoid aplastic deaths in nearly 100% of patients. In contrast, for many conditioning regimens, although severe pancytopenias may result, damage to HSC compartments and/or the microenvironment is sublethal.

For sublethal regimens, theoretically speaking, excellent supportive care could allow autologous recovery to take place *without* marrow rescue. The inclusion of busulfan, melphalan, nitrosureas (carmusfine [BCNU], lomustine [CCNU]), and TBI in conditioning regimens ensures maximum toxicity to multipotential HSC and the microenvironment.[2-5] These agents are therefore most useful in preparing patients with hematologic malignancies such as leukemia, myeloma, and lymphoma wherein the disease process is primarily confined to HSC compartments of the bone marrow.

In contrast, for patients with nonhematologic malignancies, use of a supralethal myeloablative conditioning regimen may not be necessary. Agents that can be dose escalated by over 100 times, such as cyclophosphamide and etoposide, may be administered at "transplant doses" even without marrow or HSC rescue if one is willing to support the patient for up to 5–6 weeks.[6] These agents are particularly effective in eliminating the progenitor cell compartments in the bone marrow but spare multipotential and pluripotential HSC compartments and cause minimal damage to the microenvironment, in contrast with busulfan, nitrosureas, and TBI. Therefore, agents that are nontoxic to HSC are ideal for inclusion in conditioning regimens supported by PBPC, especially in malignant diseases in which the activity of these agents is high.

The administration of PBPC that are enriched in progenitor cells provides the patient with a primary wave of engraftment as early as 9 days after transplantation.[7] After

30 days, autologous multipotential HSC that survive the nonmyeloablative therapy may provide a secondary wave of long-term engraftment if agents nontoxic to HSC (such as cyclophosphamide and etoposide) are employed.[8]

For autologous transplants, there is little need for an ablative regimen toxic to HSC unless a multipotential or pluripotential HSC is involved as part of the malignant disease. In autologous transplant recipients, the primary focus should be on selecting agents that are effective for ablating the malignancy; however, for autologous transplantation in HSC malignancies, such as acute and chronic leukemias, agents toxic to HSC such as busulfan or TBI are necessary.

For allogeneic transplants, removal of residual recipient HSC to create space for donor cells is essential. The goal for most allogeneic transplant recipients treated for malignancies is to achieve full chimerism because mixed chimerism often correlates with relapse.[9] Thus, in general, the need to use a more myeloablative regimen is greater in most allogeneic transplant settings than in autologous transplant settings (see the discussion of non myeloablative or reduced-dose-intensity regimens, later).

IMMUNOSUPPRESSIVE POTENCY

Conditioning regimens vary greatly in their effects on the immune system. Therefore, the immunosuppressive potency of a regimen is a primary concern in selecting a conditioning regimen. For autologous transplants, the ideal conditioning regimen would have little or no effect on the lymphoid (immune) system because there is no requirement to suppress host immune response to prevent graft rejection. In contrast, for allogeneic marrow transplant recipients, suppression of host immune response is an absolute requirement for success. For autologous transplants, the goal should be to employ a regimen that induces as little immunosuppression as possible and allows for rapid recovery of the immune system. Regimens that employ TBI, massive doses of cyclophosphamide or anti–T cell agents such as antithymocyte globulin, or purine analogues such as cladribine or fludarabine invariably result in delayed immune recovery post transplantation and may increase the risk of opportunistic infections such as *Pneumocystis carinii,* cytomegalovirus, and fungal infections.[10] High doses of etoposide, carboplatin, cisplatin, BCNU, and busulfan are much less immunosuppressive than the aforementioned agents and therefore are frequently incorporated into regimens used for autografting. Unfortunately, because some agents are particularly useful in ablating the malignant clone, it may not be possible to completely avoid some degree of immunosuppression in autografting.

For allografting, the issue is not whether one needs immunosuppression but how much should be used. The risk of graft rejection increases with the degree of human leukocyte antigen (HLA) disparity across major HLA-A,-B,-C,-D loci barriers and with increasing minor antigen disparity.[11] The risk of graft rejection is increased in patients undergoing unrelated versus related marrow transplants in general and in those receiving T cell–depleted grafts.[12, 13] Transfusion-sensitized aplastic recipients are also at high

risk for graft rejection.[14] In all such instances, the immunosuppressive strength of the conditioning regimen should be increased if consistent engraftment is the goal. For patients receiving TBI, one may need to increase total dose or adjust the fractionation schedule to increase immunosuppressive potency.[15] Addition of agents specific for T cells or natural killer cells such as antibodies against these cells have been used to suppress host immune cells that may survive aggressive doses of TBI and participate in graft rejection.[16] Use of cyclophosphamide, 2-deoxycoformycin, total lymphoid irradiation, cyclosporin, FK-506, and other T cell–specific agents have been employed to suppress host immune cells and enhance engraftment.[17] An alternative approach to enhance engraftment is to infuse massive numbers of PBPC, which may supplement T cell–depleted marrows.[18] This approach is a relatively nontoxic way to enhance the immunosuppressive effects of conditioning regimens required to cross major HLA barriers.

An entirely unique approach to allograft focuses on providing enough immunosuppressive potency but abandoning the use of toxic myeloablative regimens. This approach has recently been employed by Khouri et al in elderly patients with chronic lymphocytic leukemia. These investigators employ fludarabine as a lymphoid toxic and immunosuppressive agent to enhance engraftment of allogeneic HSC without massive myelablation.[19] The goal is to utilize the natural antileukemia potency of a graft-versus-leukemia effect to eliminate residual leukemia rather than rely on an ablative regimen. This concept is discussed in detail later.

DISEASE-RELATED FACTORS

One must consider several disease-related factors when selecting a conditioning regimen. They include (1) whether the patient is undergoing transplantation for malignant or for nonmalignant disease, (2) whether the patient has bulky disease at transplantation or minimal residual disease, (3) whether one is anticipating a graft-versus-tumor or graft-versus-leukemia effect, (4) the degree of tumor resistance at the time of transplantation, (5) whether there is medullary or extramedullary disease, (6) the presence of any potential sanctuary sites such as central nervous system (CNS) disease, and (7) whether the patient will require any post-transplant therapy or a second transplant. All of these disease-related factors may influence the choice of a conditioning regimen.

Malignant Versus Nonmalignant Disease

For patients undergoing transplantation for a malignancy, the selection of a conditioning regimen is greatly influenced by the sensitivity of the tumor to various agents included in the regimen. In contrast, for patients who undergo transplantation for marrow failure such as aplastic anemia, or an immunodeficiency such as severe combined immunodeficiency disease, or congenital diseases such as sickle cell anemia or thalassemia, the primary concern of the conditioning regimen is to create space by removing nonmalignant but abnormal clones.[20] The immunosuppressive effects of autologous and allogeneic transplantation, rather than their myeloablative effects, are gaining importance as transplant therapies have been increasingly employed to treat patients with autoimmune disease such as rheumatoid arthritis or multiple sclerosis.[21, 22]

Treatment of Bulky Versus Minimal Residual Disease

Most patients undergoing transplantation for a malignancy present to the transplant center with a tumor load of 10^8–10^{12} tumor cells. Conditioning regimens may escalate chemotherapeutic drug doses up to 100 times. Very few, if any, current conditioning regimens can reliably and permanently eliminate massive tumor bulk, however. For autologous transplants, the conditioning regimen should best be viewed as a means to eliminate minimal residual disease because high doses of single agents or TBI can rarely be expected to eliminate more than 3–4 logs of tumor.[23] Combinations of agents, however, may do considerably better (i.e., 6–10 logs).[24, 25]

Nonetheless, conditioning regimens rarely, if ever, cure bulky disease. Cure rates are highest in patients who present to the transplant center with chemosensitive disease, who are in complete or near-complete remission, and who have undergone a minimum of pretransplant therapy to prevent induction of tumor resistance.[26] Patients with bulky disease (defined as tumor masses >5 cm) or in full leukemic relapse should either undergo pretransplant therapy or be considered for post-transplant consolidation therapy if one hopes to achieve a prolonged disease-free survival or possible cure.

These observations dictate that conditioning regimens as much as possible employ agents that are not only useful in a given malignancy but are not cross-resistant to previous pretransplant therapy and are compatible with planned post-transplant therapy. This requires close coordination between referring oncologists and transplant centers. For example, it is particularly useful to employ a dose-escalated etoposide-based regimen in a patient with non-Hodgkin lymphoma who has been previously treated with the cyclophosphamide, hydroxydaunomycin, Oncovin, prednisone (CHOP) protocol. If this is combined with TBI, the patient with lymphoma is treated with two modalities that have not yet been used in this patient. The likelihood of greater response is thus increased. Post-transplant consolidative irradiation therapy can be safely administered to areas of bulk disease even in patients receiving TBI if excessive radiation has not been used before transplantation.

Presence or Absence of Graft-Versus-Tumor Effect

For patients receiving allogeneic transplants with unmanipulated marrow, it is widely acknowledged that for many malignancies, especially chronic and acute myelogenous leukemia, a potent antileukemia effect called graft-versus-leukemia (GVL) or graft-versus-tumor (GVT) effect is an important mechanism for removing minimal residual disease.[27–29] In the allogeneic setting, it is therefore not necessary that the conditioning regimen eliminate every last tumor cell.[19] If, however, donor marrow is manipulated to reduce T cells in an attempt to eliminate graft-versus-host disease, the beneficial effects of the GVL effect may be lost,

putting more burden on the conditioning regimen to reduce the abnormal clone.[30] The observation that the immune system may play a primary role in the allogeneic bone marrow transplant setting has prompted some investigators to modify conditioning regimens to reduce toxicity or build immunomodulating therapy into the transplantation process to enhance the GVL or GVT effect.

Thus, in chronic myelogenous leukemia, in which GVL is potent, reduction of the dose-intensive conditioning regimen may become more common as post-transplantation donor lymphocyte therapy takes precedence.[31] Similarly, in autologous bone marrow transplantation, administration of post-transplant immunomodulators such as interferon-α, interleukin-2, or roquinimex (Linomide) may allow one to consider a less aggressive conditioning regimen and rely more on GVL effects.[32, 33] The value of the GVL or GVT effect is more established in hematologic malignances but is largely unknown for solid tumors such as breast cancer.[29] Further work in the solid tumors is needed before heavy emphasis can be placed on immunomodulatory therapy rather than intensive chemoradiotherapy regimens.

Drug Resistance

Drug resistance is often a major reason for a referral for transplantation in hopes that dose-intensive therapy will overcome resistance and allow elimination of refactory malignancy. Although the value of dose-intensive transplant therapy is well established for most hematologic malignancies, the role of this approach in solid tumors is still controversial.[34] For many chemotherapeutic agents, the maximum tolerated dose has been established. The limits of tolerance for TBI are also widely known.[35] Approaches that use targeted single-dose therapy or multiple-hit high-dose therapy provide novel ways to overcome tumor resistance and increase cure rates.[36–39] Sequential dose-intensive chemotherapy is made possible by the wide application of the PBPC transplants.[38, 39] Targeted radiotherapy allows one to concentrate the radiation in the desired area with limited systemic effects.[36, 37] Future conditioning regimens may involve use of radiosensitizers or chemosensitizers that protect normal tissue and increase tumor cell kill, providing a wider therapeutic index.[40, 41]

Medullary Versus Extramedullary Disease

The selection of appropriate agents for inclusion in a conditioning regimen is influenced by the primary site of the tumor. For patients with hematologic malignancies, potent HSC toxins such as busulfan, BCNU, and radiation are most appropriate because disease may arise in the multipotential or pluripotential HSC. In contrast, it is not necessary to use HSC toxins for tumors that arise outside the marrow unless the agent has a high degree of activity against the tumor. For example, in the treatment of breast cancer, busulfan and TBI—agents commonly employed in leukemia—are rarely used and probably add little except toxicity to conditioning regimens for the treatment of this disease. The transplanter must consider the potential for excessive toxicity due to delayed engraftment with HSC toxins when selecting agents for treatment of solid tumors.

Sanctuary Sites

Disease sanctuary sites may influence the choice of transplant therapy. In general, patients with CNS disease are excluded from transplantation because no transplant regimen can reliably cure established CNS disease. Some regimens, however—namely those with TBI and CNS-penetrating chemotherapy agents such as nitrosureas, cytosine arabinoside, and high-dose methotrexate—may prove useful in preventing future CNS disease or in eliminating occult CNS disease. In allogeneic transplant recipients, the GVT effect may not be as active in eliminating disease in the CNS.[42] Patients with disease in traditional sanctuary sites such as the CNS, testes, or ovaries should undergo additional therapy specifically directed at these sites rather than rely on the conditioning regimen. The conditioning regimen, however, may influence the choice of therapy for prophylaxis at these sites.

Post-Transplantation Therapy and Second Transplants

Whether a patient will require post-transplant therapy or even a second transplant may influence the decision for selecting a conditioning regimen for the first transplant. As noted earlier, patients with large tumor cell masses are rarely cured with transplant therapy alone. Therefore, it is highly likely that some form of post-transplant consolidative therapy or radiotherapy will be required to "burn out" potential sites of relapse. The use of post-transplant radiotherapy may limit the use of TBI or influence the decision to use an ablative regimen because stable long-term engraftment may be difficult to achieve if post-transplant radiotherapy is applied immediately after transplantation. In some patients, a lower-risk autologous transplant may be used first, often at the patient's request. Later, after relapse, the patient may be more willing to accept a higher-risk allogeneic transplant. It is not possible for a patient to receive TBI twice, although patients have successfully undergone retransplantation with non-TBI regimens if the first transplant conditioning regimen was TBI based.[43, 44] Clearly, the condition of the patient at the time of second transplantation dictates the type of conditioning regimen that can be used safely.

PATIENT-RELATED FACTORS

The ideal conditioning regimen would have negligble toxicity in all patients, allowing the transplant physician to weigh the other factors discussed earlier in deciding on the conditioning regimen. Unfortunately, no conditioning regimen is completely free of potentially life-threatening toxicity (Table 35–1). Careful pretransplant testing is done primarily to determine the patient's ability to tolerate agents with known extramedullary toxicity. Patients who come to transplantation with serious pre-existing cardiac disease, for example, should generally avoid high-dose cyclophosphamide, which may lead to irreversible cardiomyopathy.[45] Patients with pre-existing lung disease are particularly vulnerable to BCNU, busulfan, and TBI.[46] Patients with borderline renal function may not be able to tolerate car-

TABLE 35–1. MAJOR EXTRAMEDULLARY TOXICITIES OF SOME PREPARATIVE REGIMEN AGENTS

AGENT	TOXICITIES
Antithymocyte globulin	Serum sickness, thrombocytopenia, renal insufficiency
BCNU (carmustine)	Pneumonitis, hepatic veno-occlusive disease (VOD), renal insufficiency, CNS encephalopathy
Busulfan	Interstitial pneumonitis, hepatic VOD, seizures, skin rashes
Cyclophosphamide	Hemorrhagic cystitis, cardiomyopathy, intersititial pneumonitis
Cytarabine (Ara-C)	Mucositis, cerebellar ataxia, hepatitis, skin rashes
Carboplatin	Renal insufficiency, ototoxicity, peripheral neuropathy
Cisplatin	Renal insufficiency, ototoxicity, peripheral neuropathy
Etoposide	Mucositis, hemorrhagic cystitis, hepatitis
Ifosfamide	Hemorrhagic cystitis, CNS encephalopathy, renal insufficiency
Melphalan	Mucositis, hepatitis
Mitoxantone	Cardiomyopathy, mucositis
Paclitaxel (Taxol)	Mucositis, peripheral neuropathy, anaphylaxis, cardiac arrhythmias
Thiotepa	Mucositis, skin rash
Total body irradiation	Interstitial pneumonitis, hepatic VOD, mucositis, diarrhea

boplatin or cisplatin. Pre-existing liver disease is a risk factor for hepatic veno-occlusive disease, a serious complication of most high-dose therapy regimens, particularly those including busulfan.[47]

Although it may be impossible to avoid any toxicity by appropriate selection of regimens, it is possible to reduce the risk of regimen-related toxicity without sacrificing overall response rates. For example, substitution of etoposide for BCNU in a cyclophosphamide/cisplatin combination may not only reduce serious lung toxicity but may synergize and increase activity against certain tumors.[48]

The pretransplant therapy that a patient has experienced may influence the choice of conditioning regimen. First, patients may already have experienced significant decrements in major organ function because of conventional chemotherapy and may not be able to tolerate some high-dose chemotherapy agents. Second, the patient's tumor may already be resistant to certain classes of agents. There may be little reason to hope that dose escalation can overcome significant resistance, and a non-cross-reactive drug would be a better choice. Third, extensive pretransplant therapy may damage marrow HSC or stromal cells to the extent that further use of myeloablative regimens toxic to HSC may prove too risky in an autologous transplant setting, leading to the risk of failed, delayed, or weak engraftment. Finally, patients who have undergone prior involved field or local irradiation may have already reached tissue tolerance for TBI, effectively eliminating TBI-based options. For all these reasons, referring oncologists are urged to consult transplant centers well before referral of transplant candidates to discuss the most compatible pretransplant therapy.

INFLUENCE OF STEM CELL PRODUCTS

The source and quality of the HSC product and whether it has been purged or manipulated may influence the design of the conditioning regimen. HSC may be derived from the PBPC marrow or cord blood. They may be enriched by CD34+ cell selection or purged through removal of T cells or tumor cells. The subsequent HSC product may possess variable engraftment characteristics. For products that have been purged by some agents, such as 4-hydroperoxycyclophosphamide, one can anticipate slow engraftment characteristics in the setting of heavily myeloablative regimens such as busulfan, cyclophosphamide, or cyclophosphamide/TBI.[49] There is less concern when using purged products if submyeloablative regimens are employed because autologous HSC recovery is more likely. For T cell–depleted allogeneic HSC products, it is mandatory that one use highly immunosuppressive conditioning regimens. For sequential double autografts, HSC are preferable to marrow to ensure rapid engraftment.[39] In some patients with functionally poor HSC due to extensive heavy exposure to multiple agents toxic to HSC before coming to transplantation, it may not be desirable to employ a maximally ablative conditioning regimen in which autologous HSC recovery is further diminished. In sum, one should always consider the quality and source of the HSC product one intends to use before choosing a particular conditioning regimen.

PHARMACOLOGIC AND RADIOBIOLOGIC CONSIDERATIONS

The toxicities of chemotherapeutic agents administered at high doses may be profoundly influenced by pharmacokinetics and drug-drug interactions. For example, the lung toxicity of BCNU, the cardiac toxicity of cyclophosphamide, and the hepatic toxicity of busulfan and carboplatin have been correlated with the area under the curve (AUC) for plasma drug elimination.[50] It is now well known that simultaneous administration of cisplatin may result in wide variability of BCNU/AUC, explaining why the maximum tolerated dose of BCNU administered with cisplatin and cyclophosphamide must be reduced by approximately 50% for safety reasons.[51] For busulfan, metabolism varies widely between children and adults such that children may be underdosed and adults easily overdosed, resulting in an increased risk of hepatic veno-occlusive disease.[52, 53] Alkylating agents such as cyclophosphamide or ifosfamide require metabolic activation in the liver, forming reactive intermediates that may induce liver or bladder toxicity.[50, 53, 54]

Most conditioning regimens involve two or three combinations of drugs administered in high doses. Single doses of drugs can be expected to kill no more than 4 logs of tumor, and one may have to eliminate 8–12 logs in order to achieve extended survival. Ideally, combinations of chemotherapeutic agents should produce synergistic cytotoxicity in tumor cells but not damage normal tissue and still allow substantial dose escalation.[55] If one must reduce an active drug to add a second or third drug, antitumor efficacy ultimately becomes compromised. The mode of administration as well as the sequence of administration of high-dose therapy may also effect the outcome. For example, prolonged etoposide levels are more tumoricidal than short exposure to high doses.[56, 57] Concomitant administration of cisplatin or cyclophosphamide may further enhance

etoposide's antitumor effect.[58] Cyclophosphamide is more cytotoxic when preceded by administration of busulfan or thiotepa.[58] These observations suggest that the design of the conditioning regimen may profoundly affect toxicity and antitumor efficacy.

TBI-containing conditioning regimens may vary tremendously in their antitumor effects and toxicities. Total dose, dose rate and schedule, and simultaneous use of chemotherapeutic agents must be considered. Single-dose TBI delivered at high-dose rates (4–7 cGy per minute) is more toxic to lung, gastrointestinal, and normal renal tissue compared with fractionated TBI.[59] Fractionated schedules of 200–225 cGy, twice per day for 3 days, are often employed. Fractionation of three times per day has also been employed. As the fractionation schedule increases, the chance for recovery of normal HSC and normal tissue increases, and this allows one to escalate a total dose from 1000 cGy up to 1575 cGy.[60] At higher doses, risk of leukemia relapse decreases. Because fractionation may spare normal HSC, higher total doses may be required to ensure engraftment when rejection is likely to be a concern, particularly with T cell–depleted transplants and HLA-nonidentical transplants. Engraftment, on the other hand, is enhanced by administration of cyclophosphamide within 24 hours of TBI but not if given 72 hours before TBI.[61] In sum, the design of the conditioning regimen, whether using multiple chemotherapeutic agents or TBI, must be considered during selection of a conditioning regimen for any given patient.

PRACTICAL CONSIDERATIONS—OUTPATIENT CONDITIONING REGIMENS

Although choice of conditioning regimen should be primarily influenced by the clinical and biologic factors reviewed earlier, increasingly, the transplant physician must consider other factors that primarily deal with resources and cost. As high-dose therapy is moved into an outpatient setting in response to cost-containment measures, it becomes clear that certain chemotherapeutic regimens are more suitable to outpatient protocols. High-dose melphalan, cyclophosphamide, and paclitaxel can be administered as single agents over short periods, making these agents attractive for outpatient protocols. In some instances, oral busulfan and TBI can be administered in a closely monitored outpatient setting. In contrast, agents that require continuous 24-hour infusions (such as etoposide or carboplatin) and that are associated with severe nausea, vomiting, and mucositis may be more difficult to manage in an outpatient setting. Furthermore, because TBI requires specialized equipment and dosimetry, TBI may not always be available at all transplant centers. Chemotherapeutic agents administered at high doses are expensive. If there is no difference in toxicity or survival between one conditioning regimen and another, some transplant centers may be pressured to use less-expensive agents in their regimen.

COMMON CONDITIONING REGIMENS

Because there is no perfect candidate regimen that provides optimal space and immunosuppression and completely ablates the tumor and is relatively nontoxic to the patient, no universal recommendation can be made regarding conditioning regimens. Two regimens that have withstood the test of time and have been widely used are (1) cyclophosphamide, 120 mg/kg, with TBI of 1000–1440 cGy and (2) busulfan, 16 mg/kg, with cyclophosphamide, 120–200 mg/kg. These regimens are generally well tolerated and useful as supralethal myeloablative regimens for treatment of hematologic malignancies, especially leukemias. Randomized controlled studies in of chronic myelogenous leukemia comparing these two regimens in the allogeneic setting have shown no differences in overall or disease-free survival.[62, 63] The busulfan/cyclophosphamide regimen, however, may be better tolerated.[63] Given that both are equally effective regimens, the transplanter may choose one over the other because of the specific patient-related factors noted earlier. A randomized trial in acute leukemia comparing the two regimens reported a survival advantage for cyclophosphamide/TBI.[64] In contrast, Blume et al. reported no differences in survival between busulfan/cyclophosphamide and a VP-16/TBI regimen in high-risk leukemia.[65]

For patients with multiple myeloma, melphalan-TBI conditioning regimens appear ideal because melphalan is highly active in myeloma and myeloma is sensitive to radiation.[66] Finally, if patients are given pretransplant vincristine, doxorubicin, dexamethasone therapy, melphalan may be used for the first time in a dose-escalated fashion, which may overcome tumor resistance. Busulfan/cyclophosphamide with or without thiotepa is also a useful regimen for myeloma autografts.[67, 68] In Hodgkin disease and non-Hodgkin lymphoma, most patients have already had extensive prior exposure to alkylating agents and anthracycline-based regimens such as mechlorethamine, Oncovin, procarbazine, prednisone (MOPP), Adriamycin, bleomycin, vinblastine, dacarbazine (ABVD), and CHOP. Etoposide, BCNU, and platinum compounds are attractive agents for lymphoma because they have excellent activity and may synergize in a non-cross-resistant way to most induction therapies for lymphomas.[69, 70] Cyclophosphamide/TBI or VP-16/TBI regimens are also used in the lymphomas, particularly if patients have not received prior radiation therapy.

There is no consensus for the best conditioning regimen for most solid tumors. Cyclophosphamide, BCNU, and cisplatin and cyclophosphamide, thiotepa, and carboplatin have been widely employed with excellent activity in patients with breast cancer.[71, 72] Paclitaxel melphalan, and thiotepa are also active as single agents and can be dose escalated for treatment of breast cancer.[73] Current evidence suggests that up to 60% of chemosensitive breast cancers may enter complete remission after these therapies but only 25–30% of these remissions will be durable, indicating that the optimal conditioning regimen for treatment of breast cancer has not yet been designed. Popular conditioning regimens for common transplant indications are summarized in Table 35–2.

NONMYELOABLATIVE OR REDUCED-DOSE-INTENSITY CONDITIONING REGIMENS FOR ALLOGENEIC HSC TRANSPLANTATION

Since the 1960s, transplant physicians based the design of conditioning regimens on the notion that maximum dose intensity was required to create space for the seeding of new donor HSC and to provide optimal immunosuppression of the host to allow engraftment. It was thought that high-dose regimens were necessary to ablate every last malignant or nonmalignant clone. The high-dose chemoradiotherapy approach was always problematic because massive doses of chemoradiotherapy, no matter how modified, exposed vital organs to considerable toxicity. Furthermore, this approach led to excessive compromise of host defenses with increased risk of infection. A reduction in dose intensity of the conditioning regimen would be desirable but could compromise engraftment and/or relapse rates.

In recent years, increasing evidence from preclinical animal models and pilot studies in humans has shown that a full myeloablative conditioning regimen is not necessary to establish an allogeneic graft in the recipient.[90, 91] There is now ample evidence to suggest that if the host is given enough immunosuppression and large doses of HLA-identical PBPC or marrow HSC, donor cells can create their own space and engraft in the recipient.[18, 90–94] After receiving such transplants, most patients experience "mixed chimerism," indicating that there are varying proportions of donor and recipient cells reconstituting the host's lymphohematopoietic system. Mixed chimerism is usually assessed by the use of genetic markers that indicate the proportion of cells in the blood or marrow sample derived from the donor or recipient. In sex-mismatched transplants, fluorescence-in-situ-hybridization (FISH) with X and Y probes provides a convenient way to quantify mixed chimerism. For same-sex transplants, DNA analysis using variable N terminal repeat (VNTR) analysis is required. Full donor chimerism is generally complete when the lymphohematopoietic system is greater than 97% donor. In the mixed chimera, graft-versus-host disease (GVHD) may be mild or absent. As the recipient expresses a greater proportion of donor cells, GVHD may occur.

A GVT or GVL effect may also accompany a GVHD.[27–29] A GVL effect is responsible for the cure of most patients with chronic myelogenous leukemia in chronic phase and may be particularly useful in patients with chronic lymphoid leukemias, follicular non-Hodgkin lymphoma, and multiple myeloma.[31, 32, 94–96] GVL effect may be present but is generally less potent in patients with chronic myelogenous leukemia in blast crisis, acute myelogenous or lymphoblastic leukemia, or aggressive large cell lymphomas.[94, 95] There is a potential for GVT effect in patients with breast cancer, renal cell carcinoma, and malignant melanoma or other tumors that may respond to the immunotherapeutic effects of donor T or natural killer cells.[97–99] These observations are firmly based on the fact that malignant clones disappear in the allogeneic transplant setting after infusion of HLA-identical donor lymphocytes in patients who have experienced relapse after allogeneic transplantation. These potent immunotherapeutic affects, presumably mediated by T lymphocytes and natural killer cells, have encouraged marrow transplanters to develop conditioning regimens that rely more on the ability of the donor cells to generate GVL or GVT effect than on the high-dose chemotherapeutic regimen. This strategy, if done in a stepwise manner, relies on the initial establishment of mixed chimerism followed by the subsequent titration of donor lymphocytes. With this approach, it may be possible

TABLE 35–2. POPULAR PREPARATIVE REGIMENS FOR COMMON TRANSPLANT INDICATIONS

ACRONYM	AGENTS	USUAL TOTAL DOSES	USUAL DISEASE INDICATIONS	REFERENCES
Cy/TBI	Cyclophosphamide	120–200 mg/kg	AML, ALL, CML, MDS, HD, NHL, SAA, MM, CLL	59, 60, 62, 88
	Total body irradiation	1000–1440 cGy		
VP/TBI	Etoposide (VP-16)	60 mg/kg	AML, ALL, NHL, HD	65, 74
	Total body irradiation	1320 cGy		
Bu/Cy	Busulfan	16 mg/kg	AML, CML, MDS	75, 76
	Cyclophosphamide	120–200 mg/kg	MM, Thal, NHL	20, 68
Cy	Cyclophosphamide	200 mg/kg	SAA	77
Cy/ATG	Cyclophosphamide	200 mg/kg	SAA	78
	Antithymocyte globulin	90 mg/kg		
Cy/TLI	Cyclophosphamide	200 mg/kg	SAA	79
	Total lymphoid irradiation	750 cGy		
Mel/TBI	Melphalan	140 mg/m^2	MM	66
	Total body irradiation	1200 cGy		
Mel	Melphalan	200 mg/m^2	MM, breast cancer	89
CBC	Cyclophosphamide	5.625 g/m^2	Breast cancer	80
	Carmustine (BCNU)	600 mg/m^2		
	Cisplatin	165 mg/m^2		
CTCb	Cyclophosphamide	6 g/m^2	Breast cancer	72
	Thiotepa	500 mg/m^2		
	Carboplatin	800 mg/m^2		
ICE	Ifosfamide	16 g/m^2	Breast cancer, NHL, testicular cancer	81
	Carboplatin	1.8 g/m^2		
	Etoposide	1.5 g/m^2		
CEC	Cyclophosphamide	6 g/m^2	Breast cancer	82
	Etoposide	2.4 g/m^2		
	Carboplatin	1.2 g/m^2		
CEP	Cyclophosphamide	6 g/m^2	Breast cancer, NHL, HD	48, 83
	Etoposide	1.2–2.4 g/m^2		
	Cisplatin	150 mg/m^2		
CT	Cyclophosphamide	6 g/m^2	Breast cancer	84
	Thiotepa	500 mg/m^2		
CBV	Cyclophosphamide	6 g/m^2	NHL, HD	69
	Carmustine	300–600 mg/m^2		
	Etoposide	600–1200 mg/m^2		
BEAM	Carmustine	300 mg/m^2	NHL, HD	85
	Etoposide	800 mg/m^2		
	Cytarabine	800 mg/m^2		
	Melphalan	140 mg/m^2		
BACT	Carmustine	200 mg/m^2	NHL	86
	Cytarabine	800 mg/m^2		
	Cyclophosphamide	200 mg/kg		
	6-Thioguanine	800 mg/m^2		
MCC	Mitoxantrone	75 mg/m^2	Ovarian cancer	87
	Carboplatin	1.5 g/m^2		
	Cyclophosphamide	120 mg/m^2		

AMI, acute myelogenous leukemia; ALL, acute lymphoblastic leukemia; CML, chronic myelogenous leukemia; MDS, myelodysplastic syndrome; HD, Hodgkin disease; NHL, non-Hodgkin lymphoma; MM, multiple myeloma; SAA, severe aplastic anemia; Thal, thalassemia major.

to avert aggressive acute GVHD and the toxicity of high-dose conditioning regimens while taking advantage of the potent GVL or GVT effects of the allogeneic graft.

In a series of careful studies in a canine model, Storb et al. showed that the dose of TBI could be reduced to a submyeloablative level of 200 cGy if cyclosporin and mycophenolate mofetil were employed to provide additional immunosuppression.[91] Only one of 11 dogs experienced rejection of its donor leukocyte antigen–identical allograft. The remaining 10 achieved stable mixed chimerism consisting of donor cells in the range of 45–85%. Further reduction of TBI dose in the dogs treated with cyclosporin and mycophenolate mofetil resulted in graft rejection in all animals. This could be partially averted, however, by use of granulocyte colony-stimulating factor

mobilized PBPC rather than bone marrow in over half of the animals. Collectively, these studies suggest that a full myeloablative TBI dose is not required to create space for donor cells and that donor cells may engraft at submyeloablative doses if supplemented with additional immunosuppression, such as cyclosporin and mycophenolate mofetil. These studies also suggest that PBPC may have a more potent engrafting potential than marrow HSC, which may assist in establishment of the graft. This is attractive because it is possible to collect larger numbers of PBPC with current mobilization procedures than can be harvested from bone marrow under general anesthesia.

Armed with the knowledge that allogeneic grafts with mixed chimerism could be established with submyeloablative regimens and that HLA-identical donor lymphocytes

TABLE 35–3. NONMYELOABLATIVE OR REDUCED-DOSE-INTENSITY PREPARATIVE REGIMENS FOR ALLOGENEIC STEM CELL TRANSPLANTS

INSTITUTION	PREPARATIVE REGIMEN (TOTAL DOSES)	POST-TRANSPLANT IMMUNOSUPPRESSION	REFERENCE
Fred Hutchinson Cancer Research Center	200 cGy TBI	CyA/MMF[2]	100
Jerusalem	Fludarabine (180 mg/m²) Busulfan (8 mg/kg) ATG (40 mg/kg)	CyA	101
M.D. Anderson*	Fludarabine (90–120 mg/m²) Cyclophosphamide (900–2000 mg/m²) *or* Melphalan (140 mg/m²)	Tacrolimus/MTX	102 104
M.D. Anderson†	Fludarabine (90–120 mg/m²) Idarubicin (36 mg/m²) Cytarabine (8 g/m²)	Tacrolimus/MTX	103
NIH	Fludarabine (125 mg/m²) Cyclophosphamide (120 mg/kg)	CyA	105

CyA, cyclosporine; MMF, mycophenolate mofetil; MTX, methotrexate; TBI, total body irradiation.
*For lymphoid/plasma cell malignancies.
†For myeloid malignancies.

could mediate potent GVL or GVT effect, several groups have begun clinical pilot trials in patients with hematologic malignancies and selected solid tumors to determine the efficacy and toxicity of this submyeloablative or reduced-dose-intensity approach, sometimes called a *minitransplant*. In 1998, McSweeney et al. at Fred Hutchinson Cancer Research Center reported results of a submyeloablative regimen (based on their canine studies) using just 200 cGy of TBI in humans with daily mycophenolate mofetil and cyclosporin.[100] Donor lymphocytes were administered after day 65 if there was no evidence of GVHD and there was residual disease with varying degrees of mixed chimerism. They demonstrated that all patients were able to achieve mixed chimerism. One patient with chronic lymphocytic leukemia who was treated with this approach was able to experience clearance of malignant lymphocytes and full donor chimerism by day 150 with only mild, grade II GVHD, which responded to corticosteroids. No donor lymphocytes were needed to supplement the graft. This case demonstrated that in some patients it may be possible to deliver submyeloablative regimens on an outpatient basis and perform the transplantation with minimal leukopenia and risk of infection. This approach may also reduce the need for platelet and red blood cell transfusion support. In addition, toxic symptoms such as mucositis and other typical side effects that occur in full myeloablative regimens may be completely averted.

Several groups of investigators have omitted the TBI in conditioning regimens altogether and exploited the immunosuppressive effects of fludarabine in low-intensity regimens (Table 35–3). Fludarabine is a potent T cell–lytic purine synthesis inhibitor that can be combined with reduced doses of alkylating agents to assist in engraftment of HLA-identical HSC. Although considered submyeloablative, some of these regimens are probably best described as "reduced-dose-intensity regimens." Slavin et al. reduced the busulfan dose from 16 mg/kg to 8 mg/kg in 26 patients

with acute and chronic myelogenous leukemia and other hematologic malignancies.[101] These patients were rescued with HLA-identical granulocyte colony-stimulating factor mobilized PBPC. Host immunosuppression was provided by administering 30 mg/m² of fludarabine over 6 days (total dose, 180/m²) supplemented with antithymocyte globulin (ATG) over 4 days at a dose of 10 mg/mg/day. Using this protocol, they observed stable mixed chimerism and reduced incidence of acute GVHD in all 26 patients. In three patients who experienced relapse, infusion of donor lymphocytes successfully induced complete remission. Eighty-one percent of the patients were disease-free after 1 year, and 85% were alive. This group has also shown that the fludarabine/ATG/busulfan regimen may allow engraftment in a matched unrelated donor setting.

Investigators from M.D. Anderson Cancer Center combined fludarabine with either cyclophosphamide or melphalan with or without cisplatin and/or cytarabine for lymphoid malignancies.[102–104] Fludarabine (total dose, 125 mg/m²) plus idarubicin or cytarabine was given for myeloid malignancies in the matched related or unrelated donor setting. No ATG or TBI was included. Thirteen to 15 patients with myeloid malignancies and 11 of 15 patients with lymphoid malignancies experienced engraftment. Those patients who did not experience engraftment recovered autologous hematopoiesis. Complete remissions were observed with both chemosensitive and refractory disease. Although preliminary, these studies show that fludarabine-based regimens may result in durable engraftment and complete remissions in patients with hematologic malignancies. Childs et al. at National Heart, Lung and Blood Institute of NIH combined fludarabine with cyclophosphamide (120 mg/kg) in patients with hematologic malignancies and in selected solid tumors, including breast, kidney, and melanoma cancers.[105] In some patients, thymic radiation was also administered. Full engraftment was achieved, and clinical response of malignancy was observed.

In summary, preclinical studies and early clinical pilot studies allow the following conclusions to be drawn regarding use of submyeloablative or reduced-dose-intensity conditioning regimens:

1. Engraftment can be achieved using closely matched HLA-identical related or HLA-identical unrelated donors.
2. Peritransplant morbidity and mortality with a conditioning regimen is markedly reduced, and sometimes such regimens allow transplantation in the outpatient setting.
3. Acute and chronic GVHD are still observed but their incidence and severity may be markedly reduced.
4. Achievement of stable mixed chimerism has allowed a platform for the use of donor lymphocytes to exploit a useful GVT or GVL effect in many patients.
5. In nonmalignant disease, stable mixed donor chimerism may be curative without risking full donor chimerism in GVHD with donor lymphocytes.[106]

Thus, for some patients with hematologic disorders such as thalassemia, stable mixed donor chimerism may be curative without risking GVHD.

Ultimately, randomized controlled studies with much longer follow-up are needed to confirm the encouraging results of these early phase I and II studies and to determine whether this approach is truly more effective and less toxic than a full myeloablative regimen.

CONCLUSION

The large variety of conditioning regimens and the lack of randomized controlled data comparing one regimen with another dictate that the transplant physician must consider a number of biologic, clinical, and practical factors before selecting a particular conditioning regimen for any given transplant candidate. Important biologic factors that must be considered are the requirement for space and the need for using a supralethal myeloablative conditioning regimen versus a less-intensive regimen. The requirement for immunosuppression and the anticipated source and quality of the HSC product must be considered. Multiple disease- and patient-related factors should be carefully considered in choosing a particular conditioning regimen. Finally, practical considerations, including the ability to administer a particular regimen and cost, are also important factors that need to be considered before a conditioning regimen is chosen. Further controlled studies are required to ultimately determine the value of one conditioning regimen over another in specific clinical settings.

REFERENCES

1. Quesenberry PJ: Hemopoietic stem cells, progenitor cells, and growth factors. *In* Williams WJ, et al (eds): Hematology, 4th ed. New York, McGraw Hill, 1990, pp 129–147.
2. Tutschka PJ, Santos GW: Bone marrow transplantation in the busulfan treated rat III: in relationship between myelosuppression and immunosuppression for conditioning bone marrow recipients. Transplantation 24:52–62, 1992.
3. Vriesendorp HM: Radiobiological speculation on therapeutic total body irradiation. Crit Rev Hematol Oncol 10:211–224, 1990.
4. Henner WD, Peters WP, Eder JP, et al: Pharmacokinetics and imme-diate effects of high dose carmustine in man. Cancer Treat Rep 70:877–880, 1986.
5. Samules BL, Bitran JD: High dose intravenous melphalan: a review. J Clin Oncol 13:1786–1799, 1995.
6. Brown RA, Herzig RH, Wolff SN, et al: High dose etoposide and cyclophosphamide without bone marrow transplantation for resistant-hematologic malignancy. Blood 76:473–479, 1990.
7. Kessinger A, Armitage J, Landmark J: Reconstitution of human hematopoietic function with autologous cryopreserved circulating stem cells. Exp Hematol 14:192–196, 1986.
8. Jones RJ, Celano P, Sharkes SJ, Sensenbrenner LL: Two phases of engraftment established by serial bone marrow transplantation in mice. Blood 73:397–401, 1989.
9. Petz LD: Documentation of engraftment and characteristics of chimerism following marrow transplantation. In Forman SJ, Blume KG, Thomas ED (eds): Bone Marrow Transplantation. London, Blackwell Scientific, 1994, p 141.
10. Lum LG: The kinetics of immune reconstitution after human bone marrow transplantation. Blood 69:369–380, 1987.
11. Beatty PG, Clift RA, Mickelson EM, et al: Marrow transplantation from related donors other than HLA identical siblings. N Engl J Med 313:765–771, 1985.
12. Kernan NA, Bartsch G, Ash RC: Retrospective analysis of 462 unrelated marrow transplants facilitated by the National Marrow Donor Program (NMDP) for treatment of acquired and congenital disorders of the lymphohematopoietic system and congenital metholic diseases. N Engl J Med 328:593–602, 1993.
13. Kernan NA, Flomenberg N, Dupont B, O'Reilly RJ: Graft rejection in recipients of T-cell depleted HLA non identical marrow transplants for leukemia. Transplantation 43:842–847, 1987.
14. Storb R, Prentice RL, Thomas ED: Marrow transplantation for treatment of aplastic anemia: an analysis of factors associated with graft rejection. N Engl J Med 296:61–66, 1977.
15. Down JD, Tarbele NJ, Thames HD, March PM: Syngeneic and allogeneic bone marrow engraftment after total body irradiation: dependence on dose, dose rate, and fractionation. Blood 77:661–669, 1991.
16. Butturini A, Saeger RC, Gale RP: Recipient immune competent T lymphocytes can survive intensive conditioning for bone marrow transplantation. Blood 68:954–956, 1986.
17. Vogelsang G: Pharmacology and use of immunosuppressive agent after bone marrow transplantation. *In* Forman S, Blume RG, Thomas ED (eds): Bone Marrow Transplantation. London, Blackwell Scientific, 1994, pp 114–123.
18. Aversa F, Tabilio A, Velandi A, et al: Treatment of high-risk acute leukemia with T-cell depleted stem cells from related donors with one fully mismatched HLA haplotype. N Engl J Med 339:1186–1193, 1998.
19. Khouri I, Keating M, Przepiorka D, et al: Engraftment and induction of GVL with fludarabine based non-ablative preparative regimen in patients with chronic lymphocytic leukemia and lymphoma. Blood 88(Suppl 1):301a, 1996.
20. Lucarelli G, Galimberti M, Polch P, et al: Bone marrow transplantation in patients with thalassemia. N Engl J Med 332:417–421, 1990.
21. Ikhara S, Good RA, Nakamora T, et al: Rationale for bone marrow transplantation in the treatment of autoimmune diseases. Proc Natl Acad Sc U S A 82:2483–2487, 1985.
22. Liu Yin JA: Resolution of immune mediated diseases following bone marrow transplants for leukemia. Bone Marrow Transplant 9:31–33, 1992.
23. Vriesendorp HM: Radiobiological speculations on therapeutic total body irradiation. Hematol Oncol 10:211–244, 1990.
24. Skipper HE: Criteria associated with destruction of leukemia and solid tumor cells in animals. Cancer Res 27:2636–2645, 1967.
25. Skipper HE: Combination therapy: some concepts and results. Cancer Chemother Rep 4:137–145, 1974.
26. Armitage JO: Bone marrow transplantation for treatment of patients with lymphoma. Blood 73:1749–1758, 1989.
27. Weiden PL, Sullivan KM, Flournoy N, et al: Antileukemia effect of chronic graft vs. host disease: contribution to improved survival after allogeneic bone marrow transplantation. N Engl J Med 304:1529–1533, 1981.
28. Horowitz MM, Gale RP, Sondel P, et al: Graft versus leukemia reaction after bone marrow transplantation. Blood 75:555–562, 1990.

29. Kennedy MJ, Vogelsang GB, Beveridge R, et al: Phase I trial of intravenous cyclosporine to induce graft versus host disease in women undergoing autologous bone marrow transplantation for breast cancer. J Clin Oncol 11:478–484, 1993.

30. Marmont AM, Horowitz MM, Gale RP: T cell depletion of HLA identical transplants in leukemia. Blood 78:2120–2130, 1991.

31. Kolb JH, Mittermuller J, Clemin C, et al: Donor leukocyte transfusions for treatment of recurrent chronic myelogenous leukemia in marrow transplant patients. Blood 76:2462–2465, 1990.

32. Rowe J, Ryan D, Dipersio J, et al: Autografting in chronic myelogenous leukemia followed by immunotherapy. Stem Cells 11(Suppl 3):34–42, 1993.

33. Rowe JM, Nilsson BI, Simonsson B: Treatment of minimal residual disease in myeloid leukemia: the immuno therapeutic options with emphasis on linomide. Leuk Lymphoma 11:321–329, 1993.

34. Kennedy MJ: High dose chemotherapy of breast cancer: "Is the question answered?" J Clin Oncol 13:2472–2479, 1995.

35. Shank B: Radiotherapeutic principles of bone marrow transplantation. In Forman SJ, Blume KG, Thomas ED (eds): Bone Marrow Transplantation. London, Blackwell Scientific, 1994, pp 98–100.

36. Appelbaum F, Brown PA, Sandmaier BM, et al: Specific marrow ablation before marrow transplantation using an aminophosphic acid conjugate, 166 HOEDTMP. Blood 80:1608–1613, 1992.

37. Press OW, Eary JF, Badget CC: Treatment of refractory non-Hodgkin's lymphoma with radiolabelled MB-1 anti CD37 antibody. J Clin Oncol 7:1027–1038, 1989.

38. Tepler I, Cannistra SA, Frei E III, et al: Use of peripheral blood progenitor cells abrogates the myelotoxicity of repetitive outpatient high dose carboplatin and cyclophosphamide chemotherapy. J Clin Oncol 11:1583–1591, 1993.

39. Shea TC, Mason JR, Storniolo AM, et al: Sequential cycles of high dose carboplatin administered with recombinant human granulocyte-macrophage colony stimulating factor and repeated infusions of autologous peripheral blood progenitor cells: a novel and effective method for delivering multiple courses of dose intensive therapy. J Clin Oncol 10:464–473, 1992.

40. Coia L, Krigel R, Haskins G, et al: A phase I study of WR2721 in combination with total body irradiation in patients with refractory lymphoid malignancies. Int J Radiat Oncol Biol Phys 22:791–794, 1992.

41. Dore MJ, Bedarich G, Kallman RF: Protection of interleukin-1 against lung toxicity caused by cyclophosphamide and irradiation. Radiat Res 128:316–319, 1991.

42. Goldberg SL, Mangan KF, Klumpp TR, et al: Lack of graft vs. leukemia effect in an immunologically privileged sanctuary site. Bone Marrow Transplant 14:180–181, 1994.

43. Champlin RE, Ho HG, Leuarsky C, et al: Successful second bone marrow transplants for treatment of acute myelogenous or acute lymphoblastic leukemia. Transplant Proc 17:496–499, 1985.

44. Sanders JE, Buckner CD, Clift RA: Second marrow transplant in patients with leukemia who relapse after allogeneic marrow transplantation. Bone Marrow Transplant 3:11–19, 1988.

45. Goldberg MA, Antin J, Guinan EC, Rappaport JM: Cyclophosphamide cardiotoxicity: an analysis of dosing as a risk factor. Blood 68:1114–1118, 1986.

46. Smith AL, Boyd MR: Preferential effects of 1.3 bis (2 chloroethyl)-1 nitrosurea (carmustine) on pulmonary glutathione reductase and glutathione/cylotathione disulfide ratios: possible implication for lung toxicity. J Pharmacol Exp Ther 229:658–663, 1984.

47. Morgan M, Dodds A, Atkinson K, et al: The toxicity of busulfan and cyclophosphamide as a preparative regimen for bone marrow transplantation. Br J Haematol 77:529–534, 1991.

48. Klumpp TR, Mangan KF, Glenn LD, et al: A phase I/II study of high dose cyclophosphamide, cisplatin, and etoposide followed by autologous bone marrow or peripheral blood stem cell transplantation in patients with poor prognosis Hodgkin's or non-Hodgkin's lymphoma. Bone Marrow Transplant 13:337–345, 1993.

49. Yeager AM, Kaizer H, Santos G, et al: Autologous bone marrow transplantation in patients with acute non lymphocytic leukemia using ex vivo marrow treatment with 4-hydroperoxy cyclophosphamide. N Engl J Med 315:141–147, 1986.

50. Jones RB: The pharmacology of alkalating agents. Marrow Transplant Rev 4:9–12, 1994.

51. Peters WP, Eder JD, Henry WD, et al: High dose combination alkalating agents with autologous bone marrow support: a phase I trial. J Clin Oncol 4:646–654, 1986.

52. Groshow LB, Brundett NB, et al: Pharmacokinetic of busulfan: correlation with venoocclusive disease in patients undergoing bone marrow transplantation. Cancer Chemother Pharmacol 25:55–61, 1989.

53. Hassen M, Ljungmai P, Bolme P, et al: Busulfan bioavailability. Blood 84:2144–2150, 1994.

54. Allen LN, Creaven PJ: Effect of microsomal activation on interaction between ifosfamide and DNA. J Pharm Sci 61:2009–2011, 1972.

55. Frei E: Pharmacologic strategies for high dose chemotherapy. In Armitage JO, Antman KH (eds): High Dose Cancer Therapy, 2nd ed. Baltimore, William & Wilkins, 1995, pp 3–16.

56. Herzig R: High dose etoposide and marrow transplantation. Cancer 67(Suppl 1):292–298, 1991.

57. Mross K, Bewermeie P: Pharmacokinetics of high dose VP-16: 6 hour infusion versus 39 hour infusion. Bone Marrow Transplant 13:423–430, 1991.

58. Teicher BA, Holden SA, Jones SM, et al: Influence of scheduling in two drug combination of alkalating agents in vivo. Cancer Chemother Pharmacol 25:161–166, 1989.

59. Thomas ED, Clift R, Herman J, et al: Marrow transplantation for acute non lymphoblastic leukemia in first remission using fractionated or single dose irradiation. Int J Radiat Oncol Biol Phys 8:817–821, 1982.

60. Buckner C, Clift R, Appelbaum F, Thomas E: A randomized trial of 12 or 15.75 cGy of total body irradiation in patient with ANLL and CML followed by marrow transplantation. Exp Hematol 17:522, 1989.

61. Down J, March P: The effect of combining cyclophosphamide with total body irradiation on donor bone marrow engraftment. Transplantation 51:1309–1311, 1991.

62. Devergie A, Blaise D, Ahai M, et al: Allogeneic bone marrow transplantation for chronic myeloid leukemia in first chronic phase: a randomized trial of busulfan-cyclophosphamide versus cytoxan-total body irradiation as preparative regimen a report for the French Society of Bone Marrow Graft. Blood 85:2263–2268, 1995.

63. Clift RA, Buckner CD, Thomas ED: Marrow transplantation for chronic myeloid leukemia: a randomized study comparing cyclophosphamide total body irradiation with busulfan and cyclophosphamide. Blood 84:2036–2043, 1994.

64. Ringden O, Ruuta T, Renberger M, et al: A randomized trial comparing busulfan with total body irradiation as conditioning in allogeneic bone marrow transplant recipients with leukemia: a report from the Nordic Bone Marrow Transplant Corporation. Blood 83:2723–2730, 1994.

65. Blume KG, Kopeckey K, Downey JP, et al: A prospective randomized comparison of total body irradiation-etoposide versus busulfan-cyclophosphamide as preparative regimens for bone marrow transplantation in patients with leukemia who were not in first remission: a Southwest Oncology Group Study. Blood 81:2187–2193, 1993.

66. Barlogie B, Alexanian R, Dicke K, et al: High dose chemoradiotherapy and autologous bone marrow transplant for resistant multiple myeloma. Blood 70:869–872, 1987.

67. Bensinger WI, Buckner CD, Clift RA, et al: Phase I study of busulfan and cyclophosphamide in preparation for allogeneic marrow transplants for patients with multiple myeloma. J Clin Oncol 10:1492–1497, 1992.

68. Dimopoulos M, Alexanian R, Przepiorka D, et al: Thiotepa, busulfan, and cyclophosphamide: a new preparative regimen for autologous marrow or blood stem cell transplantation in high risk myeloma. Blood 82:2324–2328, 1993.

69. Jagannath S, Dicke K, Armitage JO, et al: High dose cyclophosphamide, carmustine, and etoposide and autologous bone marrow transplantation for relapsed Hodgkin's disease. Ann Intern Med 104:163–168, 1986.

70. Crilley P, Lazarus H, Topolsky D, et al: Comparison of preparative transplantation regimens using carmustine/etoposide/cisplatin or busulfan/etoposide/cyclophosphamide in lymphoid malignancies. Semin Oncol 20:50–54, 1993.

71. Peters WP, Shpall EJ, Jones RB, et al: High dose combination alkalating agents with bone marrow support as initial treatment for metastatic breast cancer. J Clin Oncol 6:1368–1376, 1988.

72. Antman K, Ayash L, Elias A, et al: A phase II study of high dose cyclophosphamide, thiotepa, and carboplatin with advanced autologous marrow support in women with measurable advanced breast cancer responding to standard dose therapy. J Clin Oncol 10:102–110, 1992.

73. Antman K, Gale RP: Advanced breast cancer high dose chemotherapy and bone marrow transplants. Ann Intern Med 108:570–579, 1988.

74. Blume KG, Forman SJ, O'Donnell MR, et al: Total body irradiation and high dose etoposide: a new preparatory regimen for bone marrow transplantation in patients with advanced hematologic malignancies. Blood 69:1015–1020, 1987.

75. Santos GW, Tutschka PI, Brookmeyer R, et al: Marrow transplantation for acute nonlymphocytic leukemia after treatment with busulfan and cyclophosphamide. N Engl J Med 309:1347–1353, 1983.

76. Tutschka PJ, Copelan EA, Klein JP: Bone marrow transplantation for leukemia following a new buslufan and cyclophosphamide regimen. Blood 70:1382–1388, 1987.

77. Storb R, Thomas EP, Buckner CD, et al: Marrow transplantation in thirty untransfused patients with severe aplastic anemia. Ann Intern Med 92:30–36, 1980.

78. Storb R, Etzini R, Anasetti C, et al: Cyclophosphamide combined with antithymocyte globulin in preparation for allogeneic marrow transplant in patients with aplastic anemia. Blood 84:941–949, 1994.

79. McGlave P, Haake R, Miller W, et al: Therapy of severe aplastic anemia in young adults and children with allogeneic bone marrow transplantation. Blood 90:1325–1330, 1981.

80. Peters WP, Eden JP, Henner WD, et al: High dose combination agents with autologous bone marrow support: a phase I trial. J Clin Oncol 4:646–654, 1986.

81. Siegert W, Beyer T, Storbscheer I, et al: High dose treatment with carboplatin, etoposide, and ifosamide followed by autologous stme cell transplantation in relapsed and refractory germ cell cancer: a phase I/II study. J Clin Oncol 12:1223–1231, 1994.

82. Klumpp TR, Goldberg SL, Magdalinski AJ, Mangan KF: A phase II study of high dose cyclophosphamide, etoposide, and carboplatin (CEC) followed by autologous hematopoietic stem cell rescue in women with metastatic or high risk non metastatic breast cancer. Bone Marrow Transplant 20:277–281, 1997.

83. Dunphy FR, Spitzer G, Buzda AU, et al: Treatment of estrogen receptor negative or hormonally refractory breast cancer with double dose high dose chemotherapy intensification and bone marrow support. J Clin Oncol 8:1207–1216, 1990.

84. Williams S, Gilewski T, Mick R, Bitran J: High dose consolidation therapy with autologous stem cell rescue in stage IV breast cancer: follow up report. J Clin Oncol 10:1743–1747, 1992.

85. Gribben JL, Linch DC, Singer CA: Successful treatment of refractory Hodgkin's disease by high dose combination chemotherapy and autologous bone marrow transplantation. Blood 73:340, 1989.

86. Philip T, Birm P, Maraninch D, et al: Massive chemotherapy with autologous bone marrow transplantation in 50 cases of bad prognosis non-Hodgkin's lymphoma. Br J Haematol 60:599–609, 1985.

87. Stiff PS, McKenzie E, Alberts PS, et al: Phase I clinical and pharmacokinetic study of high dose mitoxantrone, combined with carboplatin, cyclophosphamide, and autologous bone marrow rescue: high repair rate for refractory ovarian carcinoma. J Clin Oncol 12:176–183, 1994.

88. Phillips GC, Wolff SN, Sterzy WH, et al: Treatment of progressive Hodgkin's disease with intensive chemotherapy and autologous bone marrow transplantation. Blood 73:2086, 1989.

89. Ayash CJ, Elias A, Wheeler C, et al: Double dose intensive chemotherapy with autologous marrow and peripheral blood progenitor cell support for metastatic breast cancer: a feasibility study. J Clin Oncol 12:37–44, 1994.

90. Yu L, Storb M, Mathey B, et al: DLA identical bone marrow grafts after low dose total body irradiation effects of high corticosteroids and cyclosporin on engraftment. Blood 86:4376, 1995.

91. Storb R, Yu L, Wagner JL, et al: Stable mixed hematopoietic chimerism in DLA-identical litter mates given sublethal total body irradiation before and pharmacological immunosuppressives after marrow transplantation. Blood 89:3048, 1997.

92. Rao SS, Peters SO, Crittendon RB, et al: Stem cell transplantation in the normal nonmyeloablative host: relationship between cell dose, schedule, and engraftment. Exp Hematol 25:114, 1997.

93. Slavin S, Naparstek E, Nagler A, et al: Allogeneic cell therapy with donor peripheral blood cells and recombinant interleukin-2 to treat leukemia relapse after allogeneic bone marrow transplantation. Blood 87:2195–2204, 1996.

94. Johnson BD, Drobyski WR, Truitt RL: Delayed infusion of normal donor cells after MHC-matched bone marrow transplants provides an anti-leukemia reaction without graft vs. host disease. Bone Marrow Transplant 11:329–336, 1993.

95. Collins RH, Shiplberg W, Drobask W, et al: Donor leukocyte infusion in 140 patients with relapsed malignancy after allogeneic bone marrow transplantation. J Clin Oncol 15:433–444, 1997.

96. Lokhorst H, Schattenberg A, Cornelisser J, et al: Donor leukocyte infusions are effective in relapsed multiple myeloma after allogeneic bone marrow transplantation. Blood 90:4205–4211, 1997.

97. Rosenberg SA, Packard BS, Aebersold PN, et al: Tumor-infiltrating lymphocytes and interleukin-2 in the immunotherapy of patients with metastatic melanoma. J Clin Oncol 7:250–261, 1989.

98. Bellgrun A, Muul L, Rosenberg S: Interleukin-2 expanded tumor in infiltrating lymphocytes in human renal cell cancer: isolation, characterization and antitumor activity. Cancer Res 48:206–214, 1988.

99. Eibl B, Schwaighofer H, Nachbauer D, et al: Evidence for a graft versus tumor effect in a patient treated with marrow ablative chemotherapy and allogeneic bone marrow transplantation for breast cancer. Blood 88:1501–1508, 1996.

100. McSweeney PA, Wagner JL, Maloney DG, et al: Outpatient peripheral blood stem cell allograft using immunosuppression with low dose TBI before and cyclosporine and mycophenolate mofetil after transplant. Blood 92(Suppl 1):519a, 1998.

101. Slavin S, Nagler A, Naparstek E, et al: Nonmyeloablative stem cell transplantation and cell therapy as an alternative to conventional bone marrow transplantation with lethal cytoreduction for the treatment of malignant and non malignant hematologic diseases. Blood 91:756–763, 1988.

102. Khouri I, Keating M, Korbling M, et al: Transplant-lite: induction of graft vs malignancy using fludarabine based nonablative chemotherapy and allogeneic blood progenitor cell transplantation as treatment for lymphoid malignancies. J Clin Oncol 16:2817–2824, 1998.

103. Giralt S, Estey E, Albiter M, et al: Engraftment of allogeneic hematopoietic progenitor cells with purine analog-containing chemotherapy: harnessing graft-versus-leukemia without myeloablative therapy. Blood 89:4531–4536, 1997.

104. Giralt S, Cohen A, Claxton N, et al: Fludarabine/melphalan as a less intense preparative regimen for unrelated donor transplants in patients with hematologic malignancies. Blood 92(Suppl 1):289a, 1998.

105. Childs R, Clave E, Contentin N, et al: Engraftment kinetics after nonmyeloablative allogeneic peripheral stem cell transplantation: full donor T-cell chimerism precedes alloimmune reponses. Blood 94:3234–3241, 1999.

106. Andreani M, Manna M, Lucarelli G, et al: Persistence of mixed chimerism in patients transplanted for the treatment of thalassemia. Blood 87:3494–3499, 1996.

Infection Prophylaxis

CHAPTER THIRTY-SIX

Viral Infections

Per Ljungman, M.D., Ph.D.

Viral infection is an important cause of morbidity and mortality after autologous and allogeneic hematopoietic stem cell (HSC) transplantation (HSCT). Because T cell–mediated immune response is the primary defense for controlling viruses in an immunocompetent person, the state of immunocompromise induced by the conditioning regimen (autologous and allogeneic HSCT) and the treatment for graft-vs.-host disease (GVHD) (allogeneic HSCT) depress all cell-mediated immune functions (cytotoxic T lymphocyte, helper T lymphocyte, and B lymphocyte). The cytotoxic T cells are important in the control of primary viral infections such as influenza as well as latent viruses that can reactivate in immunocompromised persons. Antibodies are important for preventing reinfections with exogenous viruses. Thus, the gradual loss of specific antibodies occurring in many patients undergoing allogeneic HSCT with time will increase the risk for reinfections with viruses previously encountered in life. T-helper cell defects are important for recruitment of both B cells and cytotoxic T cells as a response to viral challenges. The main focus of this chapter is prevention of virus infection. Therapy options are addressed in Chapter 43.

The main techniques for diagnosis of viral infections in immunocompetent individuals are detection of specific antibodies (seroconversion, immunoglobulin M [IgM] production), virus isolation, and antigen detection. In transplant recipients, the capacity for specific antibody production in response to viral infection is frequently severely depressed, making seroconversion and IgM production unreliable tools. Virus isolation can be used but takes a few days to several weeks to complete. In transplant recipients, rapid diagnosis of infections is crucial to quickly initiate specific therapies. Thus, in many viral infections, antigen detection by immunocytochemistry is preferred. Molecular biology techniques such as polymerase chain reaction (PCR) for detection of either DNA or, more rarely, RNA and DNA hybridization are increasingly being used. The selected technique depends on the material obtained for diagnostic purposes (e.g., blood, biopsy material) and the virus suspected of causing the infection.

HERPESVIRUS

The most common viral infections after HSCT are due to herpesviruses. The group consists currently of eight different members, six of which have been implicated as important pathogens in transplant recipients. These viruses share characteristics crucial for the understanding of their

importance: The viruses are ubiquitous, infecting between 50% and 95% of the population, usually early in life. After primary infection, they remain in the individual for life, able to reactivate and replicate many years after the primary infection. Finally, cytotoxic T cells appear to be the most important mode of control of these viruses after the primary infection.

During recent decades, development of antiviral agents has resulted in a number of drugs being considered for prevention or therapy in transplant patients. Such drugs include acyclovir and its prodrug valacyclovir, penciclovir with its prodrug famciclovir, ganciclovir, cidofovir, and foscarnet. All except for foscarnet are nucleoside or nucleotide analogues and require phosphorylation by viral or cellular enzymes to become activated. Acyclovir, valacyclovir, ganciclovir, and foscarnet have been used in controlled trials for prevention of herpesvirus disease in transplant recipients. Famciclovir has been used extensively in non-immunocompromised hosts, and cidofovir has been used as therapy of cytomegalovirus retinitis in HIV-infected patients.

HERPES SIMPLEX VIRUS

EPIDEMIOLOGY AND CLINICAL MANIFESTATIONS

Herpes simplex virus (HSV) types 1 and 2 establish latency in ganglia after the primary infection and reactivate in a large proportion of infected persons. For immunocompetent individuals, the infections are usually self-limiting, although severe complications, such as encephalitis, can occur. Many different external influences are associated with reactivations, such as sunlight, other infections, and stress. In transplant recipients, reactivations are common, occurring in more than 60% of pretransplantation seropositive patients. Primary infections are rare but can be severe, and nosocomial transmission from family members and staff is the main route.

The disease caused by HSV reactivation in transplant recipients is usually local in the orofacial or urogenital area, although disseminated fatal infections can occur.[1] Symptoms are frequently uncharacteristic and difficult to differentiate from the toxicity caused by chemotherapeutic agents and/or radiation therapy in the conditioning regimens. HSV reactivations are frequently undiagnosed unless specific procedures are used. HSV reactivations are frequently painful and can interfere with the patient's ability to eat or drink. Furthermore, it has been documented in patients with acute leukemia that HSV ulcerations are associated with an increased risk of bacteremias.[2] Thus, prevention of HSV reactivations is important in the transplant recipient.

PREVENTION

Antiviral prophylaxis with acyclovir is effective in preventing HSV reactivations. Several randomized, controlled trials of acyclovir prophylaxis in transplant recipients have been published.[3–5] It is important to consider drug absorption, particularly early after transplantation and in patients who are vomiting or have diarrhea, because breakthroughs can occur.[6–8] In these patients, intravenous acyclovir should be considered. The duration of antiviral prophylaxis should be individually adapted but should at least last through the aplastic phase in both allogeneic and autologous transplant recipients. In allogeneic cases, longer duration of prophylaxis should be considered in patients with GVHD. It is important to realize that HSV reactivations frequently occur quickly after prophylaxis is stopped and might require therapy.[3, 4, 8, 9] Long-term prophylaxis studies with acyclovir have been performed, and the results show that the frequency of reactivations has been lower after stopping prophylaxis. Long-term prophylaxis, however, is rarely indicated because reactivations occurring after the aplastic phase usually are mild.[5, 10] Therapy of established HSV disease can be given either orally or intravenously. The most commonly used drug is acyclovir.

The most frequently used agents for HSV prophylaxis and therapy (acyclovir, famciclovir, valacyclovir) all require the viral enzyme thymidine kinase for activation. Resistant virus, usually a mutant lacking this enzyme, can develop. Although acyclovir has been widely administered for years, there has only been a moderate increase in detection rate of acyclovir-resistant strains.[11–13] These HSV mutants are usually less virulent than wild-type virus. Most breakthroughs or failures of therapy are caused by poor absorption of the agent. If reactivation is documented in patients receiving adequate prophylaxis or in patients not responding to therapy, however, a resistant strain should be suspected. Resistance can be confirmed by different techniques. If a resistant virus is documented or strongly suspected, therapy should be changed to foscarnet in a dose of 60 mg/kg three times daily adjusted for renal function.[14] Ganciclovir is not effective for therapy of thymidine kinase–deficient HSV. There is no indication for HSV prophylaxis with foscarnet in transplant recipients, however.

VARICELLA-ZOSTER VIRUS

EPIDEMIOLOGY AND CLINICAL MANIFESTATIONS

Varicella-zoster virus (VZV) infections occur frequently in both allogeneic and autologous transplant recipients. Most adult patients and older children are seropositive against VZV, and primary infections are rare during the early post-transplantation period. During long-term follow-up, however, patients, especially those with chronic GVHD, may lose specific antibodies to VZV, rendering them vulnerable to external reinfection with VZV. It has been well documented that such patients can experience an infection similar to primary varicella infection (chickenpox). Obviously, those patients who are seronegative before transplantation can also become infected. With these exceptions, however, the most common manifestation in transplant recipients is VZV reactivation—herpes zoster.

PREVENTION

One frequently asked clinical question is what to do with a seronegative patient who has been exposed to VZV (in school or in the hospital). It is frequently difficult to adequately assess the quality of the exposure. If a patient is likely to have been exposed to varicella, however, preventive measures are indicated. The recommended prophylaxis is to use zoster-immune globulin, which has been shown to be effective if given within 3 days of exposure. Another option, if immune globulin cannot be given within the recommended period, would be antiviral chemoprophylaxis, but there are no published data regarding the efficacy of such treatment. VZV vaccine has been used safely in children with leukemia in remission, but there are no reported studies in transplant recipients about safety or efficacy.

Primary VZV infection is a severe complication to both HSC and organ transplant recipients. Because of the epidemiologic pattern of infection, the risk is highest in children.

In contrast with HSV, which reactivates rapidly and causes disease during the first few weeks after transplantation, the peak risk of herpes zoster infection is between 3 and 6 months after HSCT. Thus, the duration of antiviral prophylaxis must be long to prevent reactivated VZV disease. Two randomized, controlled studies have been performed comparing 6 months of prophylactic acyclovir with placebo.[5, 15] Both studies showed that acyclovir was effective in reducing the risk of herpes zoster during the 6 months of therapy, but at 12 months there was no longer any difference. Thus, there is no obvious advantage of acyclovir as prophylaxis against reactivated VZV disease in allogeneic transplant recipients, although it could be argued that it might be beneficial to postpone the reactivation to a time when the patients are less immunosuppressed and therefore less likely to experience severe complications. This assumption has not been proven, however. Valacyclovir has not been studied for VZV prophylaxis, but the rate of VZV disease was reduced when the agent was compared with acyclovir as cytomegalovirus prophylaxis (Ljungman et al., unpublished data).

CYTOMEGALOVIRUS

EPIDEMIOLOGY AND CLINICAL MANIFESTATIONS

Cytomegalovirus (CMV) has been one of the most feared infectious complications in allogeneic HSCT. Several risk factors for CMV disease have been identified, including CMV seropositivity of the patient, CMV-seronegative patients receiving cells from seropositive donors, the use of total body irradiation, increasing age, and GVHD. Reactivation of CMV occurs in approximately 80% of seropositive (before HSCT) patients, whereas about one third of seronegative patients with seropositive donors experience primary CMV infection.

Before the introduction of specific prophylaxis, the risk for CMV disease was reported to be 20–30%. CMV can cause multiorgan disease after HSCT, including pneumonia, hepatitis, gastroenteritis, retinitis, and encephalitis. It is also the most likely cause of fever of unknown origin early after HSCT. CMV has also been implicated as a cause of pancytopenia after HSCT. CMV isolation, particularly CMV viremia, has been shown to be a strong predictor for CMV disease, but simultaneous detection of viremia and development of disease occur infrequently. Recent developments have shown that antigenemia or polymerase chain reaction for CMV DNA has higher sensitivity than CMV viremia for diagnostic purposes. The positive predictive value, however, is low for both these techniques.

The role of CMV as a pathogen after autologous HSCT is less obvious than after allogeneic transplantation. Several studies show that the incidence of CMV pneumonia after autologous transplantation ranges from 1% to 5%.[16–18] Furthermore, the outcome of CMV pneumonia after autologous HSCT has been similar to the outcome after allogeneic transplantation. Other types of CMV disease have been rarely reported after autologous HSCT. There has been some controversy in the published literature regarding the influence of CMV on engraftment. No data exist regarding CMV and engraftment after autologous HSCT using peripheral blood progenitor cells.

PREVENTING INFECTION

If possible, CMV-seronegative patients should undergo HSCT using a CMV-negative donor.[19] This is often not possible because only a limited number of donors are available and the time to find a donor is frequently critical. In patients with chronic myelogenous leukemia undergoing HSCT from a matched unrelated donor, CMV status should be included as a donor selection criterion. The risk for CMV transmission is mainly through blood products in a seronegative patient receiving HSC from a seronegative donor. Two options exist for reducing this risk of CMV transmission: using only blood products from CMV-seronegative donors and using blood products after leukodepletion filters. These two options were tested in a randomized trial and shown to be comparable.[20] The latter is preferred in view of the cost in procuring CMV-negative blood products.

If a CMV-seropositive HSCT donor has to be used for a seronegative patient, the risk of transmission to the recipient is approximately 35%. Immune globulin is not effective in preventing primary infection.[21, 22] These patients should be considered to be at risk for CMV disease, and preventive strategies similar to those used in CMV-seropositive patients should be considered.

PREVENTING CMV DISEASE

CMV-seropositive patients have a risk of reactivating CMV of approximately 75%, and if no preventive measures are taken, approximately 20–30% of patients risk CMV disease. Because the prognosis of therapy of established CMV disease is still poor (see later), preventive measures are important. These can be divided into either prevention of reactivation (prophylaxis) or prevention of developing disease when reactivation has occurred (pre-emptive therapy).

Prophylaxis

For allogeneic HSCT, the first studied preventive measure was the use of intravenous immune globulin (IVIG). Several randomized trials have been performed, giving diverging results. Bass et al. summarized these trials in a meta-analysis, showing a slight but significant reduction in CMV disease and pneumonia.[23] Because of the expense of high-dose IVIG and the modest effect, it has been replaced in most transplant centers by prophylactic strategies through antiviral agents. These can be divided into low-potency and high-potency prophylaxis. Drugs of low potency include acyclovir and valacyclovir, with only modest effects in vitro and in vivo on CMV replication. High-potency drugs, such as ganciclovir and foscarnet, effectively inhibit CMV replication. Two large studies of acyclovir prophylaxis have been performed, and both show a reduction of CMV infection and an improvement in survival.[24–26] The survival benefit of these studies is probably not only mediated through a reduction in CMV disease, however, and breakthroughs of CMV disease are not infrequent. If these agents are to be used as CMV prophylaxis, they must be combined with a strategy of pre-emptive therapy (see later).

Ganciclovir has been tested in two randomized trials, both showing a strong reduction in CMV disease but no effect on survival.[27, 28] There are two possible reasons for the lack of survival benefit. First, these studies were performed before the widespread use of growth factors such as granulocyte colony-stimulating factor (G-CSF), and gancyclovir-induced neutropenia was a problem in both studies. Second, ganciclovir prophylaxis has been associated with delayed immune reconstitution to CMV, thereby potentially causing the development of late CMV disease.[29, 30]

Foscarnet has been used in three small trials. Although it inhibits CMV replication effectively and its major side effect, renal toxicity, can be reduced with careful monitoring and hydration, no data on survival have been presented.[31–33]

The risk of CMV disease after autologous HSCT is low; however, the prognosis, particularly pneumonia when it occurs, is poor. The benefit of prophylaxis in autologous transplant recipients is small, and no controlled trials have been performed. In a retrospective analysis, Boeckh et al. showed that high-dose acyclovir did not influence the risk of CMV disease.[34] It could be logical, however, to try to prevent primary infections in autologous transplant recipients. This strategy has not been tested.

Pre-Emptive Therapy

An alternative to giving prophylaxis to all patients with varying risks of CMV disease is the use of early or pre-emptive therapy based on detection of CMV. The advantage is that only patients at risk receive treatment, thus reducing the risk of side effects to all patients and potentially the cost. The disadvantage is that some patients might experience CMV disease before the indicator technique yields positive results.

The requirements for the use of a preemptive strategy are as follows:

1. Availability of a fast and reliable diagnostic technique to measure early infection
2. Close surveillance
3. Procurement of the adequate samples

Several studies have shown that CMV viremia is predictive for the development of CMV disease.[35-37] Even so, the earlier techniques such as rapid or standard isolation were not sensitive enough to allow diagnosis of CMV soon enough to initiate antiviral therapy before the disease had developed in a significant proportion of patients. This was shown in a study by Goodrich et al., who showed that although the risk of CMV disease was significantly reduced in the pre-emptive therapy group, 12% of patients experienced CMV disease before antiviral therapy was initiated.[38] Schmidt et al. used rapid isolation to analyze bronchoalveolar lavage fluid obtained from asymptomatic patients at day 35 after HSCT and showed that pre-emptive therapy reduced the risk of progression to CMV pneumonia.[37] In the same study, however, the technique failed to identify 12% of patients who experienced CMV pneumonia. More sensitive techniques are currently available, and two of the most common ones are discussed in the following paragraphs.

Polymerase Chain Reaction. Einsele et al. showed recently in a randomized trial that the use of a polymerase chain reaction (PCR)-based diagnostic technique reduced the incidence of CMV disease and CMV-associated mortality compared with rapid isolation.[39] Ljungman et al. compared PCR-based diagnosis with historical control patients followed with rapid isolation and found that PCR allowed significantly earlier initiation of therapy and reduced the risk of CMV disease. Furthermore, when the PCR-positive samples were analyzed semiquantitatively, a higher amount of CMV DNA was associated with an increased risk of CMV disease.[40] This finding indicates that the pre-emptive therapy strategy can be developed even further and that the proportion of patients needing antiviral therapy might be reduced without increasing the risk of breakthrough CMV disease.

Antigenemia. In a randomized study, Boeckh et al. showed that antigenemia-based pre-emptive therapy could be used in preventing CMV disease with the same efficacy as ganciclovir prophylaxis.[30] Ganciclovir prophylaxis was more effective in preventing CMV disease during the time it was given (the first 100 days after HSCT), whereas the risk of late CMV disease was higher in the ganciclovir prophylaxis group, equalizing the risk of CMV disease and survival at 180 days after transplantation.

Either ganciclovir or foscarnet is efficacious for pre-emptive therapy. Ganciclovir has been used in most published studies so far. In a small study by Moretti et al., no difference was reported between foscarnet therapy and ganciclovir therapy.[41] A larger randomized trial by the European Group for Blood and Marrow Transplantation (EBMT),

presented in abstract form in 1999, found no difference in efficacy and no difference in renal toxicity, but there was less neutropenia in the foscarnet arm.[42] The combination of ganciclovir and foscarnet has been used with high efficacy in patients with high-level antigenemia, and no additional toxicity was reported.[43]

The duration of pre-emptive therapy has varied greatly in published studies. In the earliest studies by Goodrich et al. and Schmidt et al., ganciclovir continued until day 100 after HSCT, translating to therapy duration of 6–8 weeks in most patients. More recently, shorter periods of therapy have been used.[39, 44] The disadvantage of shorter courses is that treatment might have to be reinstituted, but the advantages are lower cost and less risk of side effects, and, potentially, the short duration therapy allows a better reconstitution of the specific immune response to CMV.

NEW STRATEGIES AND NEW DRUGS

Despite major advances in CMV management, several problems still exist. Prophylaxis and pre-emptive therapy can produce an increased incidence of CMV disease with delayed onset. Lack of specific immunity to CMV from both cytotoxic T cells and helper T cells has been associated with a high risk of CMV disease. A series of landmark studies by Riddell et al. at the Fred Hutchinson Cancer Research Center in Seattle have shown that specific cytotoxic T cells can be cloned in vitro, can be safely given to the patient, and have their activity detected during follow-up.[45-47] Preliminary data indicate that these cells decrease the risk of CMV disease, but further studies are ongoing.

Both foscarnet and ganciclovir have disadvantages associated with significant side effects, and until recently only intravenous formulations were available. An oral formulation of ganciclovir was shown to be effective for maintenance therapy of CMV retinitis in patients with AIDS, and studies are ongoing in HSCT patients. Cidofovir is a new compound that is highly effective against CMV and only needs to be given once weekly. It is associated with significant renal toxicity, however. Preliminary experience presented at meetings showed good effectiveness but a risk of renal toxicity in approximately 20% of patients (Ljungman et al., unpublished observation). Further studies are needed to define the role of cidofovir in allogeneic HSCT.

EPSTEIN-BARR VIRUS

EPIDEMIOLOGY AND CLINICAL MANIFESTATIONS

Despite the fact that Epstein-Barr virus (EBV) is frequent in the general population and that a majority of adults have been infected, little is known about its importance after allogeneic HSCT and none after autologous transplantation. A few published studies indicate that it is of minor importance. EBV can be detected in oropharynx after HSCT. In a study by Wang et al., a majority of allogeneic transplant recipients were reported to have detectable EBV DNA in circulating blood cells, but the observation has not been associated with clinical symptoms.[48] Rare case reports exist in the literature regarding pneumonia and meningoencephalitis. Lymphoproliferative disorders after HSCT are discussed in more detail in Chapter 57.

EBV LYMPHOPROLIFERATION

The most important clinical manifestation of EBV infection is post-transplantation lymphoproliferative disease. This usually monoclonal disease occurs in less than 1% of patients after allogeneic HSCT. The frequency can be much higher in mismatched and unrelated transplants, however, particularly if the grafts are T cell–depleted. In a series from the University of Minnesota, the frequency was 24% in mismatched, T cell–depleted transplants.[49]

The lymphoproliferative syndromes occur in two phases. The early phase during the first 2–3 months after HSCT is almost always of donor origin and is thought to be caused by a lack of specific T-cell control of the EBV-driven B-cell proliferation. This group usually shows a rapid progressive course. The late phase frequently starts more than a year after HSCT and is usually of recipient origin. Therapeutic attempts have usually been unsuccessful. Two groups have used adoptive T-cell therapy with encouraging results. Rooney et al. at St. Jude Medical Center have used cloned EBV-specific donor T cells,[50] whereas Papadopoulus et al. at the Memorial Sloan-Kettering Cancer Center employed nonspecific donor lymphocyte infusions.[51] Both strategies were effective with regression of the tumor masses, but the use of nonspecific donor lymphocyte infusions was associated with an increased risk of severe acute GVHD. EBV-specific T-cell infusions have also been used prophylactically to prevent EBV lymphoproliferative disorders after HSCT.[50] Lower EBV viral load was reported.[52]

HUMAN HERPESVIRUS TYPE 6

EPIDEMIOLOGY AND CLINICAL MANIFESTATIONS

Human herpesvirus type 6 (HHV-6) exists in two subtypes that differ from each other in 4–8% of the DNA. Subtype B is the cause of exanthem subitum in childhood and is the most common cause of admission to hospital in infants below 1 year of age. It has also been linked to febrile seizures in childhood. It is unclear what disease is caused by subtype A. Because this infection is common early in life, the rate of seropositivity in adults is more than 95%.

HHV-6 has been associated with interstitial pneumonia, encephalitis, hepatitis, and bone marrow suppression after HSCT. Carrigan et al. described two cases of interstitial pneumonia in which HHV-6 could be isolated from respiratory specimens and in one case also from lung tissue.[53] Furthermore, in a study by Cone et al., HHV-6 DNA could be found in much higher amounts in lung tissue from patients with "early idiopathic interstitial pneumonia" compared with patients who had pneumonia of other origin.[54] HHV-6 has been implicated as a cause of meningoencephalitis in healthy children and seems to have a propensity for the central nervous system. In 1999, Wang et al. reported HHV-6 as the cause of a large proportion of encephalitis of

"unknown origin" in HSCT cases.[55] Carrigan et al. showed a correlation between post-transplantation late marrow suppression and presence of HHV-6 in the bone marrow and a correlation between HHV-6 and rejection of marrow graft.[56] Finally, Wang et al. demonstrated a correlation between levels of HHV-6 DNA in peripheral blood leukocytes and delayed engraftment.[48] The role of HHV-6 as a potential pathogen in autologous HSCT is still unknown.

DIAGNOSIS

Because seropositivity is so common after infancy, serology has little or no use in diagnosing HHV-6 disease. Virus isolation can be performed, but several studies indicate that presence of HHV-6 in leukocytes after HSCT is common and that its predictive value is limited. Detection of HHV-6 DNA by PCR can be performed on cerebrospinal fluid and appears to be both sensitive and specific for the diagnosis of HHV-6 central nervous system disease in immunocompromised patients.[55, 57]

PREVENTION AND THERAPY

There is no published study on the use of antiviral prophylaxis against HHV-6. In an epidemiologic study, Wang et al. showed that patients who received high-dose acyclovir had lower HHV-6 DNA levels and were less likely to suffer from delayed marrow engraftment.[48] In vitro studies show that both ganciclovir and foscarnet should be effective against HHV-6. At present, there is no controlled study of antiviral prophylaxis or therapy against HHV-6 with either agent.

RESPIRATORY VIRUSES

Respiratory viruses such as respiratory syncytial virus (RSV), parainfluenza viruses, and influenza A and B are widespread in the community with major seasonal variations. Although these viruses are so common, it is only during recent years that their role as pathogens in immunocompromised patients has started to be appreciated. Additional discussion of these viral infections can be found in Chapter 48.

Rapid diagnosis of respiratory virus infections is possible. The most common technique is immunofluorescence using monoclonal antibodies. Virus isolation is more sensitive but takes longer to complete. If routine investigations for respiratory viruses are performed, the frequency of infected patients is substantial. At Huddinge University Hospital, investigations of respiratory viruses have been routine in patients with upper or lower respiratory symptoms since 1989, and the frequency of respiratory virus infections is approximately 6%.[58] Even higher frequency has been found in a study from the M.D. Anderson Cancer Center.[59]

An important aspect of respiratory viruses is that these infections can easily be spread nosocomially through immuncompetent staff and patient relatives. The infections can be spread through the air by droplets but more commonly are spread through hand contact. Thus, infection-control measures are of major importance.

RESPIRATORY SYNCYTIAL VIRUS

EPIDEMIOLOGY AND CLINICAL MANIFESTATIONS

RSV is a paramyxovirus with single-stranded RNA. The incubation period is short, between 1 and 4 days. RSV is the most common cause of severe respiratory infections in healthy infants during the first 6 months of life and causes bronchiolitis and pneumonia. Reinfection is common in older immunocompetent children and adults, and it usually causes mild upper respiratory symptoms and acute bronchitis. RSV is highly contagious and is spread through direct contact, but it can also be spread through droplets expelled after sneezing or coughing. Thus, nosocomial transmission from family members and staff to the patient undergoing HSCT is a major concern.

RSV pneumonia is associated with a high mortality. Harrington et al. described an outbreak at the Fred Hutchinson Cancer Research Center in which 31 cases of RSV infection were documented, and the overall mortality rate was 45%.[60] Eighteen patients experienced pneumonia, and the mortality rate in patients with pneumonia was 78%. Whimbey et al. reported on 33 patients, with an overall mortality rate of 37%.[61]

PREVENTION AND THERAPY

A few small phase II studies have been performed. In the series by Harrington et al., 13 patients with pneumonia were treated with aerosolized ribavirin and four patients survived.[60] Whimbey et al. combined aerosolized ribavirin with high-titer anti-RSV immune globulin and showed that patients who were treated with the combination before respiratory failure developed experienced a mortality rate of 31%.[62] Patients in whom therapy was instituted when ventilatory support was necessary, however, experienced a mortality rate of 100%. Sparrelid et al. used the combination of aerosolized and intravenous ribavirin in a small number of patients with some early promising results.[63] Controlled studies are necessary to assess the relative efficacy of the different treatment options.

PARAINFLUENZA VIRUSES

EPIDEMIOLOGY AND CLINICAL MANIFESTATIONS

There are four different parainfluenza subtypes. The most common manifestation of parainfluenza viruses is upper respiratory infection. Other symptoms, however—such as parotitis and pneumonia—have been documented. There may be differences in virulence between the subtypes, and parainfluenza virus type 3 appears to be more virulent in that pneumonia is more common. Ljungman et al. de-

scribed 11 cases after HSCT with no mortality. In this series, two patients had parainfluenza 3 and both experienced pneumonia but survived, whereas nine patients had parainfluenza 1 and all had mild and self-limiting infections. Wendt et al. described 27 cases of parainfluenza virus infections with a 22% mortality rate.[64] Nineteen of 27 patients had parainfluenza type 3. The frequency of pneumonia was 70%, and of patients with pneumonia the mortality rate was 32%. In a study published in 1996 from the M.D. Anderson Cancer Center, Lewis et al. described 61 cases during a 3½ year period, representing 5.2% of HSCT cases. Twenty-seven of these patients experienced pneumonia, and 10 patients died. Thus, the overall mortality rate was 16% and the mortality rate in patients with pneumonia was 37%. Allogeneic transplant recipients who experienced parainfluenza virus before day 100 had a higher frequency of pneumonia (61%) compared with autologous recipients (42%), with a similar trend in parainfluenza-associated mortality (55% vs. 30%). In this series, all but three patients had parainfluenza 3. In an EBMT survey, 2 of 13 infected patients (15%) died.[58]

PREVENTION AND THERAPY

The usefulness of antiviral therapy remains to be determined. The available antiviral agent is ribavirin. In a study by Wendt et al., there was no clear effect of ribavirin therapy.[64] At the Huddinge University Hospital, two patients experienced severe pneumonia and needed ventilator support. Both were treated with a combination of intravenous and aerosolized ribavirin and survived. In the study by Lewis et al., five patients were treated with aerosolized ribavirin. Three were treated before respiratory failure developed and survived, whereas two patients required ventilator support and both died.[65]

INFLUENZA VIRUSES

EPIDEMIOLOGY AND CLINICAL MANIFESTATIONS

Despite the fact that influenza virus infections are common in the community, few cases of severe infections after HSCT have been described in the literature. Ljungman et al. described a prospective study over 2 years in which seven patients had influenza A infection and one experienced fatal pneumonia.[66] In a later report, this experience was extended and two of 14 patients experienced fatal pneumonia (14%).[58] Aschan et al. described four patients with influenza B infections, of which one was fatal.[67] Although significant, this experience contradicts the data of Whimbey et al. from the M.D. Anderson Cancer Center in which most patients with influenza experienced pneumonia; the mortality rate with pneumonia was 78%.[68] The reason for this difference is unknown but can be due to patient and virus factors because influenza strains differ in pathogenicity from year to year.

PREVENTION

No controlled study has been performed regarding either prevention or therapy of influenza in patients undergoing

HSCT. The possibilities for prevention include amantadin/rimantadin and immunization. Amantadin/rimantadin has been effective in elderly patients, but the rate of developing resistance is rapid. Although anecdotal reports exist, these case reports do not allow assessment of whether the therapy is useful. Immunization was shown to be ineffective in eliciting a protective antibody response if given earlier than 6 months after allogeneic and autologous HSCT.[69] Pauksen et al. performed a randomized trial studying the addition of granulocyte macrophage (GM)-CSF to influenza vaccine and found a slight but significant advantage to the addition, in particular regarding the response against influenza B.[70]

HEPATITIS B VIRUS

EPIDEMIOLOGY AND CLINICAL MANIFESTATIONS

Hepatitis B (HBV) infections are common in some parts of the world, and therefore patients and/or their donors might be positive for HBV antibody or antigen before HSCT. Patients who are infected with HBV and who are hepatitis B surface antigen (HBsAg)-positive at the time of transplantation rarely experience severe hepatitis during the early post-transplantation phase.[71] After reconstitution of the immune system, however, severe and sometimes fatal acute hepatitis can develop, particularly at the time of discontinued immunosuppressive therapy. Patients who are antibody-positive at the time of transplantation can become HBsAg and HBV-DNA positive during long-term follow-up as a consequence of loss of specific antibodies to HBV. Additional discussions on hepatitis viruses and post-HSCT liver complications are found in Chapter 46.

The HBV status of the donor appears to be more important than the status of the patient. If the donor is antibody-positive but HBsAg-negative, the risk of transmission to the patient appear to be negligible. If the donor is HBsAg-positive, however, the likelihood of transfer to the patient is high. Furthermore, it was shown in a study by Locasciulli et al. that the use of an HBsAg-positive donor increased the risk of severe liver complications after transplantation, especially if the patient was antibody-negative.[72] Furthermore, in patients who are infected by HBV, it has been shown that the use of either marrow or lymphocytes from HBV-immune donors, either from natural infection or immunization, can clear the HBV infection in the patient.[73, 74]

PREVENTION AND THERAPY

In a seronegative recipient, the use of an HBsAg-positive donor should be avoided. If that is not possible, different strategies can be considered, although none has been tested in a controlled clinical trial. Vaccination of the patient before HSCT seems logical because Locasciulli et al. showed that patients who are antibody-positive before transplantation were less likely to experience severe liver complications.[72] There is, however, frequently not enough time for a vaccination schedule to be carried out. If the patient's clinical status allows a delay of the transplantation, however, vaccination could be considered.

HBV-specific immune globulin was given to some patients before HSCT in the study by Locasciulli et al.[72] The number of patients was too low to draw any conclusions regarding the effectiveness of this strategy, however. It has been shown that famciclovir has anti-HBV efficacy. Because many patients need anti-HSV prophylaxis (see earlier), the use of famciclovir could be considered with the aim of both preventing HSV reactivation and potentially reducing the risk of HBV transmission. Unpublished data from Huddinge Unversity Hospital showed that famciclovir could be safely given through the HSCT procedure. The effect on HBV, however, cannot be assessed because the number of treated patients is small. Another antiviral agent, lamivudine, with more potent anti-HBV activity, has been licensed. No studies have been performed with this agent in transplant recipients, however.

In antibody-positive patients, no specific preventive measures seem to be indicated before HSCT.

In patients who are HBsAg-positive before HSCT, the risk of severe liver complications after transplantation appears not to be increased.[71, 72] The numbers of patients in these two studies were small, however, and pretransplantation abnormal liver function has been shown to be an independent risk factor for VOD in several studies. Thus, it is unclear whether any preventive measure in patients with pretransplantation HBV infection who have abnormal liver function would be helpful.

HEPATITIS C VIRUS

EPIDEMIOLOGY AND CLINICAL MANIFESTATIONS

Hepatitis C virus (HCV) is an RNA virus and is the major agent causing non-A, non-B hepatitis. It is mainly spread through blood transfusions and plasma-derived products, although other modes of transmission such as sexual contact occur. Today, the risk of transmission from blood products has been greatly reduced through testing of blood donors. Thus, the number of HCV-positive patients coming to HSCT during the forthcoming years is likely to be limited. IVIG has also been shown to transmit HCV. Many manufacturers have introduced new virus inactivation methods, as well as methods of screening the plasma sources and final product, that probably will reduce the risk for transmission. If the donor is HCV RNA–positive, the risk of transmission to the patient is very high. In a study by Shuhart et al., however, the clinical course of the patients was mild.[85]

Several studies have investigated the risk of severe liver complications such as VOD in patients who are HCV RNA–positive before HSCT. The results have been divergent, but most large series indicate that the risk of VOD is probably not substantially increased over noninfected patients.[75–78] The situation might be different in HCV-infected patients, however, who have biochemical signs of liver dysfunction compared with patients with normal liver function. A liver biopsy is indicated in potential allogeneic HSCT recipients with HCV infection.[79] Later, after transplantation, severe and sometimes fatal acute hepatitis can develop, especially at the time of discontinued immunosuppressive therapy. The long-term effects of HCV in patients undergoing HSCT appear not to be more severe than in immunocompetent persons. Data from the Fred Hutchinson Cancer Research Center suggest that patients surviving more than 20 years after allogeneic bone marrow transplantation who have HCV infection are at a high risk for liver cirrhosis.[79] Ljungman et al. showed a low incidence of chronic active hepatitis in a study with shorter median follow-up.[80] Further studies with longer follow-up are needed.

Because of the immunodeficiency of the patient both before and after HSCT, serology might be unreliable, and PCR for HCV RNA should be used.

PREVENTION AND TREATMENT

It is unclear whether any specific preventive measures are needed in patients who are HCV RNA–positive before HSCT. In a small series, Ljungman et al. showed that ribavirin given orally can probably be given through the transplant procedure without severe side effects.[81] Furthermore, three of three long-term survivors became free from HCV during extended follow-up. Further studies are needed.

Because the severity of long-term effects of HCV is currently unclear, the need for other interventions is also unclear. It is logical to avoid the use of an HCV-positive donor if an alternative exists. Whether antiviral prophylaxis in the patient would reduce the risk for transmission is unknown. Interferon-α with the addition of ribavirin is the treatment of choice in immunocompetent persons. Anecdotal experience with long-term survivors after HSCT suggests that interferon-α can be given safely and that HCV negativity can be maintained.[80, 82] Whether the therapy would change the long-term outcome and reduce the risk for late complications is currently unknown, however.

ADENOVIRUSES

EPIDEMIOLOGY AND CLINICAL MANIFESTATIONS

Adenoviruses are DNA viruses that are common causes of infections in immunocompetent persons, especially children under the age of 5 years. Because of the epidemiology of these viruses in the community, patients can be primarily infected from nosocomial and other sources. Because adenovirus can cause latent infections, reactivations are possible. Chronic shedding has been described in immunocompetent persons. Adenoviruses exist in more than 40 antigenically separate serotypes, and the different subtypes cause different symptoms, such as upper respiratory symptoms, conjunctivitis, and gastroenteritis, most commonly in children and young adults. More severe infections can also develop in normal children, including hepatitis and hemorrhagic cystitis.

Adenovirus can be a cause of severe disseminated infections in transplant recipients. Shields et al. showed a frequency of adenovirus infections of 5%.[83] Approximately one third of those (1.7% of all recipients) had severe infections, and the total mortality rate was 0.4%. Flomenberg et al. documented an adenovirus infection frequency of 20.8% and adenovirus disease in one third of these

patients.[84] There was a higher incidence of adenovirus infections in pediatric patients than in adults, and the time of onset of adenovirus infection after HSCT was earlier in pediatric patients than in older patients. The data indicate that most infections are mild, and acute GVHD has been associated with development of adenovirus disease. As in immunocompetent persons, the most severe disease manifestations are pneumonia, encephalitis, and fulminant hepatitis, but hemorrhagic cystitis and gastroenteritis are also frequent.

Adenovirus infections can be diagnosed by several techniques, including isolation, antigen detection, and histopathology with immunohistochemistry. PCR is also under development for diagnosis of adenovirus infections.

PREVENTION AND THERAPY

Currently, there is no established effective prophylaxis or therapy for adenovirus infections in transplant recipients. Anecdotal cases of the use of IVIG have been published.[84] Ribavirin has been used with reported success in some patients. Because spontaneous recovery is not unusual, however, these reports are difficult to evaluate. An interesting possibility is the use of adoptive immunotherapy with lymphocytes as in CMV and EBV infections. Cidofovir might have effect against adenovirus infection, but no controlled studies have been performed in stem cell transplant recipients.

CONCLUSION

Viral infections are an important factor contributing to post-HSCT mortality and morbidity. Preventive measures for some of the more-common viruses, such as HSV, VZV, and CMV, are available (Table 36–1). For other viruses, such as EBV or respiratory viruses, fortunately with a relatively low incidence, no satisfactory pharmacologic prophylactic measures are available. New pharmacologic agents

TABLE 36–1. RECOMMENDED PREVENTION MEASURES FOR SELECTED VIRUSES AFTER HEMATOPOIETIC STEM CELL TRANSPLANTATION

VIRUS	AGENT(S)	COMMENTS
HSV	Acyclovir	Development of resistant strains can occur
VZV	Zoster-immune globulin	Indicated in seronegative patients after exposure to VZV
	Acyclovir, valacyclovir, famciclovir	Long-term use necessary to prevent herpes zoster
CMV prophylactic treatment	Acyclovir, valacyclovir, ganciclovir	Must be combined with pre-emptive therapy; risk for side effects, increased rate of late CMV disease
CMV pre-emptive therapy	Ganciclovir, foscarnet	Fast and reliable diagnostic techniques must be used (pp65, PCR)

CMV, cytomegalovirus; HSV, herpes simplex virus; PCR, polymerase chain reaction; VZV, varicella-zoster virus.

and biologic approaches are under study and will undoubtably add to our ability to decrease the morbidity and mortality of viral infections in the future.

REFERENCES

1. Ramsay P, Fife K, Hackman R, et al: Herpes simplex virus pneumonia. Ann Intern Med 97:813–820, 1982.

2. Lönnqvist B, Palmblad J, Ljungman P, et al: Oral acyclovir as prophylaxis for bacterial infections during induction therapy for acute leukaemia in adults: the Leukemia Group of Middle Sweden. Support Care Cancer 1(3):139–44, 1993.

3. Hann IM, Prentice HG, Blacklock HA, et al: Acyclovir prophylaxis against herpes virus infections in severely immunocompromised patients: randomised double blind trial. Br Med J 287(6389):384–388, 1983.

4. Saral R, Burns WH, Laskin OL. et al: Acyclovir prophylaxis of herpes-simplex-virus infections. N Engl J Med 305(2):63–67, 1981.

5. Ljungman P, Wilczek H, Gahrton G, et al: Long-term acyclovir prophylaxis in bone marrow transplant recipients and lymphocyte proliferation responses to herpes virus antigens in vitro. Bone Marrow Transplant 1(2): 185–192, 1986.

6. Engelhard D, Morag A, Or R, et al: Prevention of herpes simplex virus (HSV) infection in recipients of HLA-matched T-lymphocyte-depleted bone marrow allografts. Isr J Med Sci 24(3):145–150, 1988.

7. Gluckman E, Lotsberg J, Devergie A, et al: Prophylaxis of herpes infections after bone-marrow transplantation by oral acyclovir. Lancet 2(8352):706–708, 1983.

8. Wade JC, Newton B, Flournoy N, Meyers JD: Oral acyclovir for prevention of herpes simplex virus reactivation after marrow transplantation. Ann Intern Med 100(6):823–828, 1984.

9. Wade JC, Day LM, Crowley JJ, Meyers JD: Recurrent infection with herpes simplex virus after marrow transplantation: role of the specific immune response and acyclovir treatment. J Infect Dis 149(5):750–756, 1984.

10. Shepp DH, Dandliker PS, Flournoy N, Meyers JD: Sequential intravenous and twice-daily oral acyclovir for extended prophylaxis of herpes simplex virus infection in marrow transplant patients. Transplantation 43(5):654–658, 1987.

11. Wade JC, McLaren C, Meyers JD: Frequency and significance of acyclovir-resistant herpes simplex virus isolated from marrow transplant patients receiving multiple courses of treatment with acyclovir. J Infect Dis 148(6):1077–1082, 1983.

12. Englund JA, Zimmerman ME, Swierkosz EM, et al: Herpes simplex virus resistant to acyclovir: a study in a tertiary care center. Ann Intern Med 112(6):416–422, 1990.

13. Reusser P, Cordonnier C. Einsele H, et al: European survey of herpesvirus resistance to antiviral drugs in bone marrow transplant recipients: Infectious Diseases Working Party of the European Group for Blood and Marrow Transplantation (EBMT). Bone Marrow Transplant 17(5):813–817, 1996.

14. Safrin S, Assaykeen T, Follansbee S, Mills J: Foscarnet therapy for acyclovir-resistant mucocutaneous herpes simplex virus infection in 26 AIDS patients: preliminary data. J Infect Dis 161(6):1078–1084, 1990.

15. Selby PJ, Powles RL, Easton D, et al: The prophylactic role of intravenous and long-term oral acyclovir after allogeneic bone marrow transplantation. Br J Cancer 59(3):434–438, 1989.

16. Ljungman P, Biron P, Bosi A, et al: Cytomegalovirus interstitial pneumonia in autologous bone marrow transplant recipients. Bone Marrow Transplant 13:209–212, 1994.

17. Reusser P, Fisher LD, Buckner CD, et al: Cytomegalovirus infection after autologous bone marrow transplantation: occurrence of cytomegalovirus disease and effect on engraftment. Blood 75(9): 1888–1894, 1990.

18. Wingard JR, Chen DY, Burns WH, et al: Cytomegalovirus infection after autologous bone marrow transplantation with comparison to infection after allogeneic bone marrow transplantation. Blood 71(5):1432–1437, 1988.

19. Bowden RA, Slichter SJ, Sayers MH, et al: Use of leukocyte-depleted platelets and cytomegalovirus-seronegative red blood cells for prevention of primary cytomegalovirus infection after marrow transplant. Blood 78(1):246–250, 1991.

20. Bowden R, Cays M, Schoch G, et al: Comparison of filtered blood (FB) to seronegative blood products (SB) for prevention of cytomegalovirus (CMV) infection after marrow transplant. Blood 86:3598–3603, 1995.

21. Ruutu T, Ljungman P, Brinch L, et al: No prevention of cytomegalovirus infection by anti-cytomegalovirus hyperimmune globulin in seronegative bone marrow transplant recipients: the Nordic BMT Group. Bone Marrow Transplant 19(3):233–236, 1997.

22. Bowden RA. Fisher LD, Rogers K, et al: Cytomegalovirus (CMV)-specific intravenous immunoglobulin for the prevention of primary CMV infection and disease after marrow transplant. J Infect Dis 164(3):483–487, 1991.

23. Bass E, Powe N, Goodman S, et al: Efficacy of immune globulin in preventing complications of bone marrow transplantation: a meta-analysis. Bone Marrow Transplant 12:179–183, 1993.

24. Meyers JD, Reed EC, Shepp DH, et al: Acyclovir for prevention of cytomegalovirus infection and disease after allogeneic marrow transplantation. N Engl J Med 318(2):70–75; 1988.

25. Prentice HG, Gluckman E, Powles RL, et al: Impact of long-term acyclovir on cytomegalovirus infection and survival after allogeneic bone marrow transplantation: European Acyclovir for CMV Prophylaxis Study Group. Lancet 343(8900):749–753, 1994.

26. Prentice HG, Gluckman E, Powles RL, et al: Long-term survival in allogeneic bone marrow transplant recipients following acyclovir prophylaxis for CMV infection: the European Acyclovir for CMV Prophylaxis Study Group. Bone Marrow Transplant 19(2):129–133, 1997.

27. Goodrich J, Bowden R, Fisher L, et al: Ganciclovir prophylaxis to prevent cytomegalovirus disease after allogeneic marrow transplant. Ann Intern Med 118:173–178, 1993.

28. Winston DJ, Ho WG, Bartoni K, et al: Ganciclovir prophylaxis of cytomegalovirus infection and disease in allogeneic bone marrow transplant recipients: results of a placebo-controlled, double-blind trial. Ann Intern Med 118(3):179–184, 1993.

29. Li CR, Greenberg PD, Gilbert MJ, et al: Recovery of HLA-restricted cytomegalovirus (CMV)-specific T-cell responses after allogeneic bone marrow transplant: correlation with CMV disease and effect of ganciclovir prophylaxis. Blood 83(7):1971–1979, 1994.

30. Boeckh M, Gooley TA, Myerson D, et al: Cytomegalovirus pp65 antigenemia-guided early treatment with ganciclovir versus ganciclovir at engraftment after allogeneic marrow transplantation: a randomized double-blind study. Blood 88(10):4063–4071, 1996.

31. Bacigalupo A, Tedone E, Van Lint MT, et al: CMV prophylaxis with foscarnet in allogeneic bone marrow transplant recipients at high risk of developing CMV infections. Bone Marrow Transplant 13(6):783–788, 1994.

32. Ringdén O, Lönnqvist B, Aschan J, Sundberg B: Foscarnet prophylaxis in marrow transplant recipients [Letter]. Bone Marrow Transplant 4(6), 1989.

33. Reusser P, Gambertoglio JG, Lilleby K, Meyers JD: Phase I–II trial of foscarnet for prevention of cytomegalovirus infection in autologous and allogeneic marrow transplant recipients [see comments]. J Infect Dis 166(3):473–479, 1992.

34. Boeckh M, Gooley TA, Reusser P, et al: Failure of high-dose acyclovir to prevent cytomegalovirus disease after autologous marrow transplantation. J Infect Dis 172(4):939–943, 1995.

35. Meyers JD, Ljungman P, Fisher LD: Cytomegalovirus excretion as a predictor of cytomegalovirus disease after marrow transplantation: importance of cytomegalovirus viremia. J Infect Dis 162(2):373–380, 1990.

36. Ljungman P, Aschan J, Azinge JN, et al: Cytomegalovirus viraemia and specific T-helper cell responses as predictors of disease after allogeneic marrow transplantation. Br J Haematol 83(1):118–124, 1993.

37. Schmidt GM, Horak DA, Niland JC, et al: A randomized, controlled trial of prophylactic ganciclovir for cytomegalovirus pulmonary infection in recipients of allogeneic bone marrow transplants: the City of Hope-Stanford-Syntex CMV Study Group. N Engl J Med 324(15):1005–1011, 1991.

38. Goodrich JM, Mori M, Gleaves CA, et al: Early treatment with ganciclovir to prevent cytomegalovirus disease after allogeneic bone marrow transplantation. N Engl J Med 325(23):1601–1607, 1991.

39. Einsele H, Ehninger G, Hebart H, et al: Polymerase chain reaction monitoring reduces the incidence of cytomegalovirus disease and the duration and side effects of antiviral therapy after bone marrow transplantation. Blood 86(7):2815–2820, 1995.

40. Ljungman P, Loré K, Aschan J, et al: Use of a semi-quantitative PCR for cytomegalovirus DNA as basis for preemptive therapy in allogeneic bone marrow transplant recipients. Bone Marrow Transplant 17:583–587, 1996.

41. Moretti S, Zikos P, Van Lint MT, et al: Foscarnet vs ganciclovir for

cytomegalovirus (CMV) antigenemia after allogeneic hemopoietic stem cell transplantation (HSCT): a randomised study. Bone Marrow Transplant 22(2):175–180, 1998.

42. Reusser P, Einsele H, Lee J, et al: Randomized, multicenter, open-label trial of foscarnet versus ganciclovir for preemptive therapy of cytomegalovirus infection after allogeneic stem cell transplantation. In Interscience Conference on Antimicrobial Agents and Chemotherapy, 1999, San Francisco, 1999 [Abstract].

43. Bacigalupo A, van Lint M, Tedone E, et al: Combined foscarnet + ganciclovir treatment of CMV infections after allogeneic BMT. Bone Marrow Transplant 15(Suppl 2):S128, 1995.

44. Ljungman P, Lore K, Aschan J, et al: Use of a semi-quantitative PCR for cytomegalovirus DNA as a basis for pre-emptive antiviral therapy in allogeneic bone marrow transplant patients. Bone Marrow Transplant 17(4):583–587, 1996.

45. Reusser P, Riddell SR, Meyers JD, Greenberg PD: Cytotoxic T-lymphocyte response to cytomegalovirus after human allogeneic bone marrow transplantation: pattern of recovery and correlation with cytomegalovirus infection and disease. Blood 78(5):1373–1380, 1991.

46. Riddell SR, Watanabe KS, Goodrich JM, et al: Restoration of viral immunity in immunodeficient humans by the adoptive transfer of T cell clones. Science 257(5067):238–241, 1992.

47. Walter EA, Greenberg PD, Gilbert MJ, et al: Reconstitution of cellular immunity against cytomegalovirus in recipients of allogeneic bone marrow by transfer of T-cell clones from the donor [see comments]. N Engl J Med 333(16):1038–1044, 1995.

48. Wang FZ, Dahl H, Linde A, et al: Lymphotropic herpesviruses in allogeneic bone marrow transplantation. Blood 88(9):3615–3620, 1996.

49. Shapiro RS, McClain K, Frizzera G, et al: Epstein-Barr virus associated B cell lymphoproliferative disorders following bone marrow transplantation. Blood 71(5):1234–1243, 1988.

50. Rooney CM, Smith CA, Ng CY, et al: Use of gene-modified virus-specific T lymphocytes to control Epstein-Barr-virus–related lymphoproliferation. Lancet 345(8941):9–13, 1995.

51. Papadopoulos EB, Ladanyi M, Emanuel D, et al: Infusions of donor leukocytes to treat Epstein-Barr virus–associated lymphoproliferative disorders after allogeneic bone marrow transplantation. N Engl J Med 330(17):1185–1191, 1994.

52. Gustafsson Å, Levitsky V, Zou J-Z, et al: Epstein-Barr virus (EBV) load in bone marrow transplant recipients at risk to develop post-transplant lymphoproliferative disease: prophylactic infusion of EBV-specific cytotoxic T-cells. Blood 95:807–814, 2000.

53. Carrigan DR, Drobyski WR, Russler SK, et al: Interstitial pneumonitis associated with human herpesvirus-6 infection after marrow transplantation. Lancet 338(8760):147–149, 1991.

54. Cone RW, Hackman RC, Huang ML, et al: Human herpesvirus 6 in lung tissue from patients with pneumonitis after bone marrow transplantation. N Eng I J Med 329(3):156–161, 1993.

55. Wang FZ, Linde A, Hägglund H, et al: Human herpesvirus 6 DNA in cerebrospinal fluid specimens from allogeneic bone marrow transplant patients: does it have clinical significance? Clin Infect Dis 28(3):562–568, 1999.

56. Carrigan DR, Knox KK: Bone marrow suppression by human herpesvirus-6: comparison of the A and B variants of the virus [Letter]. Blood 86(2):835–836, 1995.

57. Cinque P, Vago L, Dahl H, et al: Polymerase chain reaction on cerebrospinal fluid for diagnosis of virus-associated opportunistic diseases of the central nervous system in HIV-infected patients. AIDS 10:951–958, 1996.

58. Ljungman P: Respiratory virus infections in bone marrow transplant recipients: the European perspective. Am J Med 102(Suppl 3A), 1997.

59. Whimbey E, Englund J, Couch R: Community respiratory virus infections in immunocompromised patients with cancer. Am J Med 102(3A):10–18, 1997.

60. Harrington R, Hooton T, Hackman R, et al: An outbreak of respiratory syncytial virus in a bone marrow transplant center. J Infect Dis 165:987–993, 1992.

61. Whimbey E, Champlin RE, Couch RB, et al: Community respiratory virus infections among hospitalized adult bone marrow transplant recipients. Clin Infect Dis 22(5):778–782, 1996.

62. Whimbey E, Champlin R, Englund J, et al: Combination therapy with aerosolized ribavirin and intravenous immunoglobulin for respiratory syncytial virus disease in adult bone marrow transplant recipients. Bone Marrow Transplant 16:393–399, 1995.

63. Sparrelid E, Ljungman P, Ekelof-Andstrom E, et al: Ribavirin therapy in bone marrow transplant recipients with viral respiratory tract infections. Bone Marrow Transplant 19(9):905–908, 1997.

64. Wendt C, Weisdorf D, Jordan M, et al: Parainfluenza virus respiratory infection after bone marrow transplantation. N Engl J Med 326:921–926, 1992.

65. Lewis V, Champlin R, Englund J, et al: Respiratory disease due to parainfluenza virus in adult bone marrow transplant recipients. Clin Infect Dis 23:1033–1037, 1996.

66. Ljungman P, Andersson J, Aschan J, et al: Influenza A in immunocompromised patients. Clin Infect Dis 17(2):244–247, 1993.

67. Aschan J, Ringden O, Ljungman P, et al: Influenza B in transplant patients. Scand J Infect Dis 21(3):349–350, 1989.

68. Whimbey E, Elting LS, Couch RB, et al: Influenza A virus infections among hospitalized adult bone marrow transplant recipients. Bone Marrow Transplant 13(4):437–440, 1994.

69. Engelhard D, Nagler A, Hardan I, et al: Antibody response to a two-dose regimen of influenza vaccine in allogeneic T cell–depleted and autologous BMT recipients. Bone Marrow Transplant 11(1):1–5, 1993.

70. Pauksen K, Hammarström V, Linde A, et al: Granulocyte macrophage-colony-stimulating factor (GM-CSF) as immunomodulating factor together with influenza vaccination in stem cell transplant patients. Clin Infect Dis 30:342–348, 2000.

71. Reed E, Myerson D, Corey L, Meyers J: Allogeneic marrow transplantation in patients positive for hepatitis B surface antigen. Blood 77:195–200, 1991.

72. Locasciulli A, Alberti A, Bandini G, et al: Allogeneic bone marrow transplantation from HBsAg+ donors: a multicenter study from the Gruppo Italiano Trapianto di Midollo Osseo (GITMO). Blood 86(8):3236–3240, 1995.

73. Ilan Y, Nagler A, Adler R, et al: Adoptive transfer of immunity to hepatitis B virus after T cell–depleted allogeneic bone marrow transplantation. Hepatology 18(2):246–252, 1993.

74. Ilan Y, Nagler A, Adler R, et al: Ablation of persistent hepatitis B by bone marrow transplantation from a hepatitis B–immune donor. Gastroenterology 104(6):1818–1821, 1993.

75. Frickhofen N, Wiesneth M, Jainta C, et al: Hepatitis C virus infection is a risk factor for liver failure from veno-occlusive disease after bone marrow transplantation. Blood 83:1998–2004, 1994.

76. Locasciulli A, Alberti A, de Bock R, et al: Impact of liver disease and hepatitis infections on allogeneic bone marrow transplantation in Europe: a survey from the European Bone Marrow Transplantation (EBMT) Group—Infectious Diseases Working Party. Bone Marrow Transplant 14(5):833–837, 1994.

77. Locasciulli A, Bacigalupo A, VanLint MT, et al: Hepatitis C virus infection and liver failure in patients undergoing allogeneic bone marrow transplantation. Bone Marrow Transplant 16(3):407–411, 1995.

78. Locasciulli A, Testa M, Pontissi P, et al: Hepatitis C virus genotypes and liver disease in patients undergoing allogeneic bone marrow transplantation. Bone Marrow Transplant 18:237–240, 1997.

79. Strasser S, McDonald G: Hepatitis viruses and hematopoietic cell transplantation: a guide to patient and donor management. Blood 93:1127–1136, 1999.

80. Ljungman P, Johansson N, Aschan J, et al: Long-term effects of hepatitis C virus infection in allogeneic bone marrow transplant recipients. Blood 86(4):1614–1618, 1995.

81. Ljungman P, Andersson J, Aschan J, et al: Oral ribavirin for prevention of severe liver disease caused by hepatitis C virus during allogeneic bone marrow transplantation. Clin Infect Dis 23(1):167–169, 1996.

82. Giardini C, Galimberti M. Lucarelli G, et al: Alpha-interferon treatment of chronic hepatitis C after bone marrow transplantation for homozygous beta-thalassemia. Bone Marrow Transplant 20:767–772, 1997.

83. Shields A, Hackman R, Fife K, et al: Adenovirus infections in patients undergoing bone marrow transplantation. N Engl J Med 312:529–533, 1985.

84. Flomenberg P, Babbitt J, Drobyski W, et al: Increasing incidence of adenoviruss disease in bone marrow transplant recipients. J Infect Dis 169:775–781, 1994.

85. Shuhart MC, Myerson D, Spurgeon CL, et al: Hepatitis C virus (HCV) infection in bone marrow transplant patients after transfusions from anti–HCV-positive blood donors. Bone Marrow Transplant 17:601–606, 1996.

CHAPTER THIRTY-SEVEN

Bacteria

Edward J. Wing, M.D., and Richard B. Hart II, M.D.

Hematopoietic stem cell transplantation (HSCT) is now widely accepted as therapy for selected malignant and genetic disorders. HSCT, however, is associated with morbidity and mortality from infectious complications.[1] The incidence of infection in this patient population is difficult to assess because studies have not used a standard definition of infection or defined evaluation periods during the HSCT process. Fever or documented infection is common during HSCT. Almost 100% of patients undergoing HSCT experience fever shortly after receiving a graft.[2, 3] More importantly 10–59% of these patients experience bacteremia at some point during their course.[4] The incidence of these complications may be decreased by peripheral blood progenitor cell transplantation with its associated shortened engraftment time.

Fever is almost universal among patients undergoing HSCT, yet it remains an important indicator of infection because approximately 60% of febrile episodes are associated with significant infection.[5] This sign of infection was stressed in a study investigating 344 infections in patients with granulocytopenic cancer. Infectious processes involving the respiratory tract, gastrointestinal tract, and soft tissue were evaluated. There was a marked reduction in the classic signs and symptoms of infection such as exudates, fluctuance, ulceration, fissures, cutaneous hyperthermia, adenopathy, and swelling; only local tenderness and erythema correlated with infection.[6] The atypical clinical findings hamper the physician's ability to diagnose and initiate early therapy. Furthermore, the advanced nature of the infection when treatment is initiated may contribute to a poorer outcome. Thus, the ability to prevent infection during HSCT becomes of paramount importance.

During HSCT many factors interact to create a complex environment that predisposes the patient to infection. Prior to HSCT, T-cell depletion and other pretransplantation processing of the graft can be employed to reduce the incidence of graft vs. host disease (GVHD). This processing causes a profound defect of cellular immunity. High-dose myeloablative therapy results in severe granulocytopenia and can cause extensive mucosal ulceration. These host defense deficits result in a marked susceptibility to infection. After the granulocytopenia and mucositis resolve, significant functional defects in the cellular and humoral host defense systems persist, which may slowly recover over a period of months to years. The kinetics of the immune system's reconstitution can be further inhibited by GVHD and the immunosuppressive therapy given to treat or prevent this complication. Furthermore, factors including prolonged central venous catheterization, mismatched transplants, increasing age of the patient, changing nosocomial

pathogens, antibiotic susceptibility patterns, and immunosuppressive therapy all play important roles in the patient's predisposition to infection.[7–13]

Interventions that favor the patient's natural defenses may reduce or prevent infectious complications. Preventive measures, however, may also have a negative effect on the patient's susceptibility to infection, which may or may not be known prior to institution. Examples in which there are both positive and negative effects of a preventive measure include (1) titration of immunosuppressive therapy to a point of balance between GVHD prevention and increased risks of infection, (2) graft T-cell depletion to reduce GVHD versus engraftment failure, delayed normalization of T-cell function, or relapse of the initial disease state, (3) prolonged central venous catheterization with the concomitant increased risk of infection, and (4) antibiotic prophylaxis, which may result in increased cost, side effects, and antibiotic resistance.

This chapter reviews the risk of bacterial infection associated with HSCT. In addition, the various prophylactic and preventive strategies used to prevent bacterial infections are discussed. Many of these practices remain highly controversial.

CHRONOLOGIC RISK OF INFECTION

Host defense deficits vary predictably over time in the HSCT process. There is a well-defined chronologic order of infectious complications, which can be divided into three parts: first, a pre-engraftment phase lasting from approximately day zero to day 30; second, the early postengraftment phase, encompassing day 30 to day 100; and last, the late postengraftment phase, after day 100 and forward. Each of these periods has characteristic host defense deficits, types of infectious complications, and microbiologic pathogens.

PRE-ENGRAFTMENT PHASE

This period's host defense defects are characterized by postmyeloablative granulocytopenia, which typically resolves within a period of 10–30 days, and damage to mucosal barriers by cytoreductive conditioning regimens. Additionally, prolonged central venous catheterization and invasive procedures place the patient at risk by breaching natural barriers.

Bacterial pathogens that typically cause infection during this period include those that colonize the patient's skin and gastrointestinal tract. It is not surprising that central venous catheter sites and damaged gastrointestinal mucosa commonly serve as sources of pathogenic bacteria. These pathogens include gram-negative bacteria such as *Pseudomonas aeruginosa*, members of the Enterobacteriaceae family, and gram-positive bacteria including *Staphylococcus aureus, Staphylococcus epidermidis, Streptococcus viridans, Bacillus* species, and *Corynebacterium* species. Figure 37–1 illustrates the incidence of infection and the most common bacterial pathogens for not only the pre-engraftment period but also the early and late postengraftment periods. Specific types of infection during this period include bacteremia[4, 14] and soft tissue and sinus infections. The incidence of documented nosocomial bacterial pneumonia has been shown to be unexpectedly low during this period. A study evaluating the incidence of pneumonia in patients undergoing HSCT showed that 55 of 275 consecutive patients experienced this complication. The etiology was determined in 67% of patients, but only 11% had documented bacterial pneumonia.[15]

EARLY POSTENGRAFTMENT PHASE

This period, day 30 through day 100, is characterized by a return of the neutrophil count; however, the immunologic deficits due to lymphocyte dysfunction become increasingly apparent. The impaired cell-mediated immunity is characterized by decreased T-helper lymphocyte counts, increased T-cytotoxic-suppressor lymphocyte counts, and impaired natural killer or T-cell cytotoxicity. The degree and duration of the cellular immune dysfunction is influenced by multiple factors, including the type of HSCT (allogeneic vs. autologous), human leukocyte antigen (HLA) matching of donor and recipient, and methods used to manipulate the graft.[9, 13] The humoral arm of the immune system is also dysfunctional during this period. Characteristic deficits include a decrease in the number of B lymphocytes and impaired production of antibody to various antigenic stimuli.[11, 12]

Additionally, acute GVHD occurs and can interrupt immunologic repair, and the immunosuppressive therapy for GVHD inhibits immunologic reconstitution. This period's profound lymphocytic deficits increase the susceptibility to fungal and viral infection. In addition, as with the pre-engraftment phase, patients frequently have central venous catheters in place and undergo invasive procedures. This period mimics characteristics of the pre-engraftment phase with regard to bacterial pathogens, type of infection, and site of the infectious process, although at a reduced rate (see Fig. 37–1).

LATE POSTENGRAFTMENT PERIOD

The late post-engraftment phase begins after day 100 and continues indefinitely. This period is characterized by slow reconstitution of the cellular and humoral arms of the immune system.[9, 13] Immunologic repair proceeds over years and is associated with a continually decreasing risk of infection. An important feature during this time is the presence or absence of chronic GVHD. Chronic GVHD involves multiple organ systems, particularly the skin, gastrointestinal tract, and respiratory tract. Not only do the chronic GVHD and resulting immunosuppressive therapy significantly delay lymphopoietic reconstitution, but chronic GVHD increases the adherence and colonization of mucosal surfaces by bacteria.[9, 16–17] Further immunologic dysfunction is characterized by decreased serum opsonizing activity, immunoglobulin G levels, and reticuloendothelial function of the liver and spleen.[18, 19] Many patients require chronic central venous catheters and periodic invasive procedures, which continue to place them at risk for infectious complications.

Bacterial pathogens during the late postengraftment phase are most commonly encapsulated bacteria such as *Streptococcus pneumoniae, Haemophilus influenzae,* and *Neisseria meningitidis.* Less commonly, infections can continue to be caused by gram-negative bacteria and staphylococcal

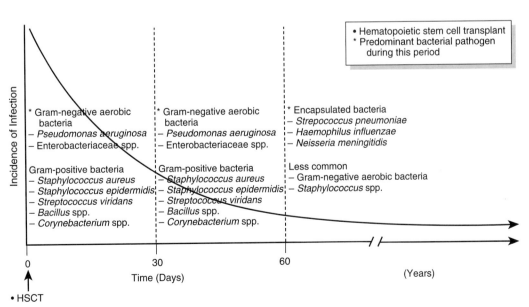

FIGURE 37–1. Incidence and type of bacterial pathogen after HSCT.

species. It is important to emphasize that cellular and humoral immunity during this period continue to slowly reconstitute, resulting in a steadily diminishing risk of infection. As with the previous two phases of HSCT, late infectious complications involve characteristic sites. During the late postengraftment phase, blood stream and upper and lower respiratory tract infections are most common.[16, 17]

PREVENTION

Once the chronology of the immunologic dysfunction and repair, the host defense deficits, and the microbiology of bacterial infections were understood, investigators began to design a strategy to prevent bacterial infections in patients undergoing HSCT. Numerous studies evaluated the effect of antibiotics on the incidence of infection in such patients. Different methods of antibiotic use, such as absorbable systemic antibiotic delivery, nonabsorbable gastrointestinal decontamination protocols, and periprocedure antibiotic delivery, were investigated. Other trials have evaluated the effects of growth factors, intravenous immunoglobulin, and immunization on immunologic recovery and reduction of infection during at-risk periods. Additional studies have investigated laminar air flow systems, patient isolation, antibacterial mouthwash, nursing barrier techniques, and sterilized food to determine if these reduce infectious complications. In addition, total parenteral nutrition was evaluated for its possible effect at reducing the risk of infection in patients undergoing HSCT. Last, hospital surveillance for infectious trends and changing bacterial resistance patterns has been shown to be invaluable.

Even with the significant morbidity and mortality caused by infection in the patient undergoing HSCT and the tremendous effort in studying preventive measures, there are no universally accepted prophylactic methods. This lack of proof of the efficacy of preventive measures results from problems with study design and, in some cases, no statistically significant benefit to the patient.

Clinical HSCT is an extremely complex procedure. The clinical investigator must contend with multiple variables that are difficult to control when one is designing studies and interpreting data. Many trials evaluating prophylactic measures in patients undergoing HSCT involve multiple centers. Therefore, nosocomial infections that develop in this population may have center-dependent characteristics that make interpretation of data difficult.

With more extensive prophylactic measures, the number of drugs ingested daily by the patient undergoing HSCT also increases. Pharmaceutical agents have multiple interactions, and the exact nature of these drug-drug interactions is often unknown. It is possible that a prophylactic measure that has been shown to be of benefit in a clinical trial may actually have a detrimental effect when incorporated into multidrug prophylaxis. In any event, these potential interactions add to the complexity of interpreting data on the effectiveness of a particular prophylactic method. Lastly, cost-benefit considerations have placed constraints on the universal acceptance of some prophylactic measures, especially when no long-term benefit has been demonstrated.[7]

SPECIFIC PREVENTIVE MEASURES

Because of the significant morbidity and mortality associated with bacterial infections in patients undergoing HSCT, numerous studies have evaluated the effects of prophylactic antibiotic regimens on the incidence of infection. The characteristics of the "ideal" prophylactic agent include a spectrum of activity targeted toward typical pathogens, a long half-life, complete absorption, parenteral and oral forms, low cost, minimal drug-drug interaction, and minimal drug toxicity. Goals of the "ideal" prophylactic agent include prevention of frequent infections associated with morbidity and mortality during periods of high risk, improved survival, low superinfection rate, minimal induction of resistant bacterial pathogens, and a decrease in documented infection.[20] Specific antibiotic classes are discussed in the order of their general acceptance as prophylactic agents rather than by historical evaluation and use. Selected studies are cited to present the current data on each prophylactic agent.

FLUOROQUINOLONE PROPHYLAXIS

The fluoroquinolone class of antibiotics has undergone extensive evaluation as a source of prophylactic agents in the prevention of bacterial infections in the HSCT setting. This class of antibiotic was chosen because of its excellent activity against gram-negative bacterial pathogens, which cause life-threatening sepsis early in HSCT.[21] Multiple studies have documented the effectiveness of fluoroquinolones (norfloxacin, ciprofloxacin, and ofloxacin) in reducing the incidence of gram-negative bacterial infections in HSCT. These studies have also shown the fluoroquinolones to be safe and well tolerated.[22–32]

Ciprofloxacin has been evaluated in multiple studies, which have included HSCT and other neutropenic cases, and has consistently reduced the incidence of serious gram-negative bacterial infections.[3, 22–25] Lew et al.[22] conducted a prospective, randomized, double-blind, placebo-controlled trial evaluating the effectiveness of ciprofloxacin versus placebo in reducing bacterial infections in patients with hematologic malignancy and HSCT. Patients treated with ciprofloxacin had no episodes of gram-negative bacterial sepsis, whereas those given placebo experienced a 27% incidence. Additionally, ciprofloxacin increased the time to first neutropenic fever and decreased the time in which patients received intravenous antibiotics.

DePauw et al.[3] prospectively assessed ciprofloxacin's ability to prevent infection in allogeneic HSCT. Ciprofloxacin completely prevented the development of gram-negative bacterial sepsis. Gilbert et al.[23] showed that ciprofloxacin plus rifampin reduced the incidence of gram-negative aerobic bacterial sepsis from 17% in the historical control group to 3% in the treatment group. Additionally, this study showed that ciprofloxacin plus rifampin decreased the time that patients received systemic antibiotics, decreased total days of fever, and increased the time to first neutropenic fever.

Norfloxacin has also been evaluated for its ability to prevent gram-negative bacterial infections.[2, 26, 27] Menichetti et al.[2] showed that norfloxacin prevented documentable gram-negative bacterial infections in 44 consecutive patients who underwent allogeneic HSCT. Another study conducted by Karp et al.[26] compared norfloxacin and placebo in a randomized, double-blind, placebo-controlled trial of neutropenic acute leukemic patients. In this study, only 11% of the norfloxacin-treated patients experienced gram-negative bacterial infection compared with 39% of the placebo-treated patients. The norfloxacin group also experienced an increased time to first neutropenic fever, decreased days of fever, and a decrease in total days treated with systemic antibiotics.

The last fluoroquinolone to be evaluated for its ability to prevent infection, ofloxacin, has also shown efficacy.[28–30] Winston et al.[28] compared ofloxacin with oral vancomycin and polymyxin in patients undergoing HSCT. The ofloxacin group experienced no gram-negative sepsis events, whereas the incidence in the vancomycin/polymyxin group was 16%. In this trial, there was no statistical difference in time to first neutropenic fever, total days of fever, or total time treated with systemic antibiotics. In another study, Schmeiser et al.[29] evaluated ofloxacin's ability to prevent infection in patients undergoing HSCT. In this open, noncomparative trial, only 1 of 101 patients experienced gram-negative bacterial sepsis.

Bow et al. compared norfloxacin, ofloxacin, and ofloxacin plus rifampin in neutropenic patients undergoing cytotoxic therapy for acute leukemia or bone marrow autografting. Microbiologically documented infection rates for norfloxacin, ofloxacin, and ofloxacin plus rifampin were 47%, 24%, and 9%, respectively. Ofloxacin plus rifampin was particularly effective in reducing documented gram-positive infections. Despite differences in the overall documented infection rate, the incidence of febrile episodes was not different between the groups.

Several fluoroquinolones have been shown to be effective in prevention of aerobic gram-negative bacterial infections, but it is not clear which agent is the most effective. The Gruppo Italiano Malattie Ematologiche Maligne dell'Adulto (GIMEMA) Infection Program[25] conducted a randomized, multicenter trial comparing norfloxacin with ciprofloxacin. The incidence of gram-negative bacterial sepsis was 4% in the ciprofloxacin group and 9% in the norfloxacin group, a statistically significant difference. Ciprofloxacin prophylaxis, when compared with norfloxacin, did result in an increase in time to first neutropenic fever and a decrease in both total febrile days and systemic antibiotic use. There was no difference in the incidence of gram-positive infections or infection-related mortality. An additional advantage of ciprofloxacin was illustrated by a study by Imrie et al.[31] that compared oral ciprofloxacin with co-trimoxazole in neutropenic patients undergoing autologous HSCT. Ciprofloxacin was associated with a significantly shorter period of neutropenia than the co-trimoxazole group, 16 days versus 22, respectively.

The advantages of fluoroquinolone prophylaxis in neutropenic patients must be weighed against its potential negative effects. Problems include the development of resistant bacteria, an increase in infections caused by bacterial pathogens unaffected by fluoroquinolone prophylaxis, the inability to consistently show clinical benefit in patients undergoing fluoroquinolone prophylaxis, and cost.

A major obstacle to universal acceptance of fluoroquino-lone prophylaxis is that no study has ever shown a reduction in infection-related mortality. In a meta-analysis of studies evaluating fluoroquinolone prophylaxis, Cruciani et al.[32] found a statistically significant reduction in gram-negative bacteremia when fluoroquinolone prophylaxis was compared with control group regimens (co-trimoxazole, oral nonabsorbable antibiotics, or placebo). No significant reduction in gram-positive bacteremia, fever-related morbidity, or infection-related mortality was demonstrated, however.

Fluoroquinolone resistance in both gram-negative[33] and gram-positive[3] pathogens has been documented in patients treated prophylactically. Gram-positive bacterial resistance to fluoroquinolones was illustrated in a study by DePauw et al. evaluating ciprofloxacin prophylaxis after HSCT. Fever evaluations led to 42 positive blood cultures, in which 35 isolates were identified as *Streptococcus viridans*. All but one isolate displayed reduced sensitivity to ciprofloxacin. Newer fluoroquinolones such as levofloxacin allow once-a-day dosing with improved gram-positive coverage. Systematic evaluation in patients undergoing HSCT, however, is not available.

GRAM-POSITIVE PROPHYLAXIS

In the 1970s gram-negative bacteria were the primary cause of serious infections in patients undergoing HSCT. In the 1980s, however, this trend reversed itself, and in many studies gram-positive bacteria had become the primary pathogens. For example, the European Organization for Research and Treatment of Cancer (EORTC)[34] showed that 65% of bacteremias were caused by gram-positive pathogens. Other studies have documented the increase of gram-positive pathogens in neutropenic cancer patients.[35–37] and in patients undergoing HSCT.[14, 38, 39] The increasing incidence of gram-positive bacterial infections in neutropenic patients is likely multifactorial, resulting from more intensive chemoradiotherapy, the increased use and the chronicity of central venous canulation, and the use of prophylactic agents directed at patients' gram-negative microflora.[38] Additionally, gram-positive bacterial infections in neutropenic patients have been shown to be associated with serious complications, such as adult respiratory distress syndrome (ARDS) and septic shock, resulting in significant morbidity and mortality.[38, 40–41]

Kern et al.[37] evaluated 55 cases of streptococcal bacteremia in neutropenic patients with acute leukemia. *Streptococcus viridans* was the most frequently isolated gram-positive pathogen, accounting for 82% of isolates. The spectrum of clinical infection included soft tissue infections, lower respiratory infections, and sepsis; clinical features ranged from fever to ARDS and septic shock. Of special note, the 40 patients in whom streptococci constituted the only pathogen isolated from the blood were compared with 36 patients who had aerobic gram-negative bacteremia. Patients who developed streptococcal bacteremia were more likely to have received fluoroquinolone prophylaxis than patients who developed aerobic gram-negative bacteremia (75% vs. 22%, respectively). Mortality for patients with streptococcal bacteremia was 18% compared with 17% for patients with gram-negative bacteremia. These mortality data indicate that both pathogens carry a potential for a poor outcome. Analysis of data related to the increase in gram-positive infections in neutropenic patients leads to two conclusions. First, there is a marked increase in gram-positive infections in patients who receive fluoroquinolones prophylactically. Second, these infections are associated with complications resulting in morbidity and mortality comparable to the gram-negative bacterial infections.

Because gram-positive pathogens were causing an increased frequency of serious infections in granulocytopenic patients in the 1980s, clinical researchers began to evaluate the addition of gram-positive bacteria prophylaxis to existing regimens. Multiple antibiotics with gram-positive antibacterial activity were studied in a prophylactic role in several different patient populations.[38, 42–46] In 1994, a prospective, randomized, double-blind, placebo-controlled trial conducted by the EORTC[38] evaluated penicillin or placebo plus pefloxacin for prophylaxis in granulocytopenic patients; 95% had undergone HSCT. The two primary end-points were fever and gram-positive bacteremia. In the penicillin arm, 71% of patients had fever and 14% had gram-positive bacteremia. In the placebo group, 80% of patients had fever and 22% had gram-positive bacteremia. Both of these end-points were statistically significant. The authors concluded that penicillin G plus pefloxacin decreased the incidence of gram-positive bacteremia and fever in granulocytopenic patients. Fourteen patients, however, experienced streptococcal bacteremia in the penicillin arm of the study; 11 isolates were available for testing and 46% were resistant to penicillin G. In addition, there was no statistical difference in infection-related mortality. Two studies have evaluated the effectiveness of roxithromycin in combination with a fluoroquinolone for the prophylaxis of gram-positive bacteremia.[42, 43] Both studies showed a decreased incidence of streptococcal bacteremia with the use of prophylactic roxithromycin but no decrease in mortality.

The effect of oral vancomycin on the incidence of gram-positive infections in neutropenic patients has also been evaluated.[39, 44] Classen et al.[39] evaluated 21 consecutive HSCT recipients assigned to either norfloxacin or the combination of oral vancomycin, tobramycin, and polymixin as prophylaxis for streptococcal bacteremia. *Streptococcus mitis* bacteremia occurred in 8% of patients receiving the oral vancomycin regimen and in 55% of patients receiving norfloxacin, a statistically significant finding. Similarly, Archimbiaud et al.[44] demonstrated that in neutropenic patients, pefloxacin plus oral vancomycin resulted in a decreased incidence of gram-positive as well as gram-negative bacterial infections when compared with colistin (polymixin E) and gentamicin prophylaxis.

Vancomycin given intravenously has also been evaluated for the prophylaxis of gram-positive infections. Attal et al.[45] conducted a prospective randomized trial in patients undergoing HSCT to evaluate the effect of prophylactic intravenous vancomycin on the incidence of gram-positive infections. No patient in the vancomycin group experienced a gram-positive infection, whereas 37% of patients in the control group suffered gram-positive infections. There were also fewer days of fever and empirical antibiotic therapy in the vancomycin group compared with the placebo group. Intravenous prophylactic vancomycin has also been studied

to evaluate whether it reduces the incidence of catheter-related sepsis when given before and after insertion. The data on this issue are conflicting.[46, 47]

A meta-analysis was performed to determine whether the addition of gram-positive bacteria prophylaxis (penicillin, macrolide, or vancomycin) to fluoroquinolone reduced the incidence of clinically significant end-points.[32] The combined prophylactic regimen significantly reduced the incidence of gram-positive bacteremia compared with fluoroquinolone or nonabsorbable antibiotics alone but did not decrease fever-related morbidity or infection-related mortality.

Trimethoprim-sulfamethoxazole (TMP-SMX) is another antibiotic that has been used for years as prophylaxis against bacterial infections in granulocytopenic patients. The effectiveness in reducing microbiologically documented infections using TMP-SMX has been shown in several studies.[48–50] The use of TMP-SMX, however, has diminished because of bacterial resistance, fungal overgrowth resulting in superinfection, inactivity against *Pseudomonas aeruginosa,* patient intolerance, myleosuppressive effects on engraftment, and drug toxicity.[49–52]

BOWEL DECONTAMINATION

Another prophylactic antibiotic method that has been studied for its ability to reduce infection is selective and total bowel decontamination. Both gram-positive and gram-negative bacteria colonize the patient's skin and mucosal surfaces before becoming invasive. Specifically, in the pre-engraftment phase of HSCT, mucosal barrier disruption and granulocytopenia predispose to systemic infection caused by gastrointestinal colonizing bacteria. Various nonabsorbable antibiotics have been used to decrease (selective bowel decontamination; SBD) or eliminate (total bowel decontamination; TBD) colonizing bowel flora. Examples of these antibiotics include gentamicin, neomycin, colistin, tobramycin, vancomycin, and framycetin.

SBD is a process by which nonabsorbable antibiotics are administered to eliminate aerobic gram-negative bacteria from the gastrointestinal tract. This allows the remaining anaerobic bacteria to proliferate and inhibit the regrowth of the aerobic gram-negative bacteria, a phenomenon that has been called *colonization resistance.*[20] SBD has been studied most extensively in the intensive care setting.[53–59] Others have also evaluated this practice in immunocompromised patients.[60, 61] Many of these studies demonstrated a decreased incidence of infection, but end-points such as length of stay in the intensive care unit, days of systemic antibiotics, and rates of colonization with resistant bacteria vary widely among the studies. Most importantly, no consistent, statistically significant decrease in mortality has been shown with SBD procedures. TBD differs in that the nonabsorbable antibiotics are directed toward both the aerobic and anaerobic alimentary tract bacteria. Studies evaluating TBD have shown results similar to those using SBD. Interestingly, when TBD regimens are compared with SBD, GVHD is decreased in both animal and human studies.[62, 63]

The practice of using nonabsorbable antibiotics for bowel decontamination has not gained wide acceptance among

HSCT centers for several reasons. These include patient intolerance, increased incidence of gram-positive infection, induction of multiantibiotic-resistant bacteria, cost, compliance issues, and unproved benefit to the patient. Additionally, with the advent of fluoroquinolone prophylaxis, the incidence of infection with alimentary tract bacterial pathogens (i.e., gram-negative bacteria) has decreased.

LATE POST-TRANSPLANTATION PROPHYLAXIS

When a patient reaches the late post-transplantation phase of HSCT, the predominant bacterial pathogens and consequently the focus of antibacterial prophylaxis change. The predominant bacterial pathogens include encapsulated bacteria as discussed previously (see Fig. 37–1). Predisposition to infection during this phase includes the presence of GVHD, lack of lymphopoietic reconstitution, and type of HSCT. The overall incidence of infection decreases markedly, although patients with GVHD who have undergone HSCT remain at risk. The potential magnitude of the increased risk of infection was highlighted by reports of pneumococcal infection rates as high as 27% in long-term survivors.[64]

Antibacterial prophylaxis during this phase of HSCT has centered around the use of oral penicillin or TMP-SMX. Even though no controlled studies have evaluated this practice, prophylaxis directed at reducing the incidence of infection with encapsulated organisms in patients with chronic GVHD during the late post-HSCT phase is generally accepted. Antibacterial prophylaxis during this phase is also beset with many of the problems associated with other prophylactic regimens, however, including the appearance of antibiotic resistance, "breakthrough" pathogens,[20, 65] and lack of data supporting a reduction in fever-related morbidity or infection-related mortality.

Thus, even though antibacterial prophylaxis is used in the late post-HSCT period, issues related to the development of resistance and the absence of data supporting clinical benefit have prevented universal acceptance. There are special cases in which prophylaxis should be instituted, such as patients who have undergone splenectomy and patients who have survived a documented preventable infection. In these cases, the prophylactic antibacterial agent should be continued during the patient's entire immunocompromised state.

HEMATOPOIETIC GROWTH FACTORS

To date, two hematopoietic growth factors have been extensively studied and used in clinical HSCT: granulocyte colony-stimulating factor (G-CSF) and granulocyte macrophage colony-stimulating factor (GM-CSF). The role of growth factors in clinical HSCT has centered around their ability to induce hematopoietic reconstitution and decrease the duration of neutropenia, possibly reducing the incidence of infection. Multiple studies have demonstrated a statistically significant relationship between prolonged neutropenia and an increased incidence of infection.[66, 67] In an observational retrospective study of 219 patients who

underwent autologous HSCT, Mossad et al.[67] found that the incidence of infection varied directly with time. In patients who experienced engraftment in less than 10 days, the incidence of infection was 14%; in patients in whom engraftment took 11–16 days, the risk of infection increased to 46%.

The use of growth factors has gained wide acceptance in HSCT; however, the available research evaluating the effect of growth factors has yielded mixed results. These studies have included patients with a variety of indications for HSCT who underwent both autologous and allogeneic HSCT. Growth factors have been consistently shown to enhance neutrophil recovery and decrease the time in which the patient is neutropenic independent of the type of HSCT. Data, however, are conflicting on the ability of these growth factors to reduce infection rates, total days of antibiotics, total hospitalization days, and mortality.[68–76] Until further trials are carried out, it is difficult to definitively recommend the use of growth factors in HSCT for reduction of infection.

IMMUNIZATION

Most patients who undergo allogeneic HSCT with a history of pre-HSCT immunization revert to seronegative status shortly after transplantation,[77] and both allogeneic and autologous procedures yield suboptimal response to vaccination against polysaccharide encapsulated organisms after HSCT.[19, 77–80] Factors that contribute to both a diminished and an increased response to vaccination have been identified, including the vaccine's biochemical composition, timing of administration, donor and recipient immunization status before and after HSCT, and patient characteristics.

Polysaccharide-conjugate vaccines, such as *Haemophilus influenzae* type B (HIB), appear to induce an antibody response in a higher percentage of patients than do vaccines that are pure polysaccharides, such as the pneumococcal vaccine. Molrine et al.[78] demonstrated this point with a study of 65 patients undergoing allogeneic HSCT in terms of antibody response to HIB and to the 23-valent pneumococcal vaccine. The HIB-conjugate vaccine was given at 3, 6, 12, and 24 months after HSCT; the 23-valent pneumococcal vaccine was given at 12 and 24 months posttransplantation. Additionally, 32 patients received bone marrow grafts from donors who had been immunized prior to transplantation, and 33 patients received bone marrow grafts from donors who had not been immunized. In the donor HIB vaccination group, protective antibody levels at 3 months were 97% and at 24 months were 92%. In recipients of bone marrow grafts from unimmunized donors, protective antibody levels were noted to be 55% and 47% at 3 and 24 months, respectively. In the 23-valent polysaccharide pneumococcal vaccine group, there was no statistically significant increase in antibody concentrations in the immunized donor and unimmunized donor groups after HSCT.

Additional studies have documented the response to the HIB-conjugate vaccine[79] and the lack of response to the polysaccharide pneumococcal vaccine.[77, 79, 81] Winston et al.[80] noted a poor response to the 14-valent pneumococcal vaccine when studying 39 patients who underwent allogeneic HSCT. In this study, additional markers for poor response were early vaccination post transplantation, corticosteroid therapy for GVHD, male sex, and other illnesses. Of note, toxicity and intolerance to immunization were virtually nonexistent in these patients.

It has been difficult to draw conclusions regarding the true effectiveness of immunization on patients undergoing HSCT because most reports have had few patients, lacked studies with clinical infection rates, had varying times of immunization, had limited evaluation of immunized serotypes, and had prophylactic antiobiotic regimens. Furthermore, new studies are needed to determine the effect of donor immunization, repetitive early immunization, and whether polysaccharide-conjugate vaccines other than HIB provoke a stronger, longer-lasting immunologic response.

INTRAVENOUS IMMUNOGLOBULIN

The role of intravenous immunoglobulin (IVIG) preparations in HSCT remains unclear despite multiple trials evaluating their impact in reducing the incidence of infection. Wolff et al.[81] performed a randomized, stratified, nonblinded study of 170 patients undergoing HSCT to compare weekly IVIG to no intervention. Clinical infection and bacteremia occurred in 43% and 35%, respectively, of the IVIG-treated group and in 44% and 34%, respectively, in the control group. Infection-related mortality occurred in 4.9% of the IVIG-treated group and in 2.3% of the control group. There was no statistically significant difference between the two groups in gram-negative or gram-positive bacteremia or in infection-related mortality. There was, however, a significant increase in the mortality in the treatment group that was accounted for by a higher incidence of toxicity related to the myeloablative chemotherapy. On the other hand, Sullivan et al.[82] showed that patients undergoing HSCT who received IVIG exhibited a reduced incidence of local infection and gram-negative bacteremia.

Studies evaluating IVIG and its effects have indicated that the type and preparation of immunoglobulin may affect the incidence of infection and toxicity.[83, 84] The dosing of IVIG has been evaluated for its ability to prevent infection in patients undergoing HSCT. Spitzer et al.[85] compared continuous IVIG with weekly IVIG using historical controls. In patients who survived longer than 3 weeks post transplantation, the incidence of documented infection in the continuous IVIG group was 19% compared with 57% in the weekly dosing group. IVIG has been shown in multiple studies[82, 86] to reduce the incidence of GVHD, and because GVHD is a risk factor for infection, IVIG use may translate into a reduction of infection in patients undergoing HSCT. Nonetheless, we do not recommend the use of IVIG in light of the conflicting data and its extraordinary cost. Further prospective, randomized, double-blind, placebo-controlled trials are necessary to determine the efficacy, optimal dosing regimen, duration of treatment, and clinical effectiveness of different IVIG preparations.

MISCELLANEOUS PREVENTIVE MEASURES

Protective isolation has been used as a preventive measure in HSCT since its origin. Techniques that filter the air for potential pathogens, such as laminar air flow (LAF) and high-efficiency particulate air (HEPA) filters, have been studied for their potential in reducing the incidence of infection in patients undergoing HSCT. Additional efforts, including various heat, gas, and chemical methods of sterilization, have been used to decontaminate all objects that are in or enter the patient's room. Levine et al.[86] showed that in neutropenic acute leukemic patients, the employment of isolation and LAF plus a prophylactic antibiotic regimen decreased severe infections by 50% and life-threatening infections by 25% compared with patients who received oral nonabsorbable antibiotics only and patients who received care on a conventional ward with no prophylactic antibiotics or isolation. In a prospective, randomized trial of patients undergoing HSCT, Buckner et al.[88] found that LAF plus decontamination procedures reduced the incidence of sepsis and major local infections compared with controls. There was no statistically significant difference in mortality. The problem in drawing conclusions from studies evaluating isolation and decontamination procedures is determining the specific contribution of each intervention to the decreased incidence of infection observed. Because of the cost, tremendous demands on supportive personnel in maintaining the protective environment, and the lack of data supporting reduction in mortality, we do not recommend strict isolation for the prevention of bacterial infections.

Surveillance cultures in patients undergoing HSCT and neutropenic patients with cancer is another area in which no firm consensus has been reached. Results of clinical trials have shown a benefit in detecting patients colonized with antibiotic-resistant organisms[89] but no benefit in predicting infection with nasal, vaginal, urine, and throat surveillance cultures.[90] Oral flora contribute significantly to the pathogenesis of systemic infection in neutropenic patients during periods in which myeloablative chemoradiotherapy-induced oromucositis is present. For this reason, various mouthwashes with antibacterial properties have been evaluated in reducing the incidence of infection. The results of these studies are conflicting, with both reduction of bacteremia[91] and no effect on bacteremia[92, 93] demonstrated.

Total parental nutrition (TPN) has also been evaluated for its potential protective role in patients undergoing HSCT. Ziegler et al.[94] conducted a double-blind, randomized, controlled clinical trial to determine whether glutamine-supplemented TPN reduced the incidence of infection. This study showed a reduced incidence of clinical infection, improved nitrogen balance, decreased microbial colonization, and a shorter hospital stay in patients receiving glutamine-supplemented TPN. Of interest, however, was the lack of a statistically significant difference in fever, antibiotic requirement, or time of neutropenia.

CONCLUSION

Since its initiation as a therapeutic modality, HSCT has been associated with significant infection-related morbidity and mortality. Antibiotic prophylaxis has been the major focus in the prevention of bacterial infections. The term *prophylaxis,* as used in HSCT, is flawed. Prophylaxis is a meaningful concept only when a specific offending bacterial pathogen and antimicrobial agent are targeted for a focused preventive effort. In HSCT, the targeting of patients' skin and gastrointestinal flora for prophylaxis has resulted in multiantibiotic-resistant bacteria, the selection of novel pathogens, and the emergence of fungal pathogens. Additionally, prophylactic agents are costly and they increase the potential for drug-drug interactions and toxicity. Finally, and most important, no prophylactic antibiotic regimen has been shown to decrease infection-related mortality or even consistently reduce infection-related morbidity. For these reasons, none of the currently available prophylactic antibiotic methods can be recommended with absolute certainty. Changing this recommendation can occur only after a prophylactic regimen justifies its existence by reducing infection-related morbidity and mortality while minimizing cost, intolerance, toxicity, drug-drug interactions, superinfections, and resistance.

Three other preventive methods used extensively are growth factors, IVIG, and immunization. Growth factors have gained widespread acceptance and have been proven to reduce the duration of neutropenia during the pre-engraftment phase of HSCT. Studies evaluating their effectiveness on infection-related morbidity and mortality, however, have yielded conflicting data. Thus, from the standpoint of prevention of bacterial infections, growth factors cannot be recommended. IVIG studies have also provided inconsistent results, requiring further investigation to prove clinical benefit prior to its recommendation. The role of immunization has not been completely defined. Many questions regarding host response, efficacy, vaccine composition, and timing of immunization remain to be answered. In light of the minimal cost and the apparent lack of toxicity, however, immunization should continue pending further definitive studies.

Many other preventive measures have been studied, but general acceptance has not occurred because consistent clinically significant benefits have been difficult to document. Ongoing clinical research will better define the exact role of each preventive strategy in HSCT. Until this occurs, most of the prophylactic and preventative measures studied to date cannot be recommended with confidence.

REFERENCES

1. van der Meer JWM, Guiot HFL, van den Broek PJ, van Furth R: Infections in bone marrow transplant recipients. Semin Hematol 2:123–136, 1984.
2. Menichetti F, Felicine R, Bucaneve G, et al: Norfloxacin in prophylaxis for neutropenic patients undergoing bone marrow transplantation. Bone Marrow Transplant 4:489–492, 1989.
3. DePauw BE, Donnelly JP, DeWitte T, et al: Options and limitations of long-term oral ciprofloxacin as antibacterial prophylaxis in allogeneic bone marrow transplant recipients. Bone Marrow Transplant 5:179–182, 1990.
4. Donnelly JP: Bacterial complications of transplantation: diagnosis and treatment. J Antimicrob Chemother 36(Suppl B):59–72, 1995.
5. Walter EA, Bowden RA: Infection in the bone marrow transplant recipient. In Rubin RH (ed): Infectious Disease Clinics of North America. Philadelphia, W.B. Saunders, 1995, pp 823–848.
6. Sickles EA, Greene WH, Wiernik PH: Clinical presentation of infection in granulocytopenic patients. Arch Intern Med 135:715–719, 1975.
7. Schuler U, Ehninger G: New approaches to the prophylaxis and treatment of bacterial and fungal infections in allogeneic marrow transplant recipients. Bone Marrow Transplant 14(Suppl 4):S61–S65, 1994.
8. Storb R, Prentice RL, Buckner CD, et al: Graft-versus-host disease and survival in patients with aplastic anemia treated by marrow grafts from HLA-identical siblings. N Engl J Med 6:302–307, 1983.
9. Lunn LG: The kinetics of immune reconstitution after human marrow transplantation. Blood 69:369–380, 1987.
10. van Leeuwen JEM, van Tol MJD, Joosten AM, et al: Relationship between patterns of engraftment in peripheral blood and immune reconstitution after allogeneic bone marrow transplantation for (severe) combined immunodeficiency. Blood 11:3936–3947, 1994.
11. Witherspoon RP, Storg R, Ochs HD, et al: Recovery of antibody production in human allogeneic marrow graft recipients: influence of time post-transplantation, the presence or absence of chronic graft-versus-host disease, and antithymocyte globulin treatment. Blood 2:360–367, 1981.
12. Storek J, Saxon A: Reconstitution of B cell immunity following bone marrow transplantation. Bone Marrow Transplant 9:395–408, 1992.
13. Roberts MM, To LB, Gillis D, et al: Immune reconstitution following peripheral blood stem cell transplantation, autologous bone marrow transplantation and allogeneic bone marrow transplantation. Bone Marrow Transplant 12:469–475, 1993.
14. Villablanca JG, Steiner M, Kersey J, et al: The clinical spectrum of infections with viridians streptococci in bone marrow transplant patients. Bone Marrow Transplant 6:387–393, 1990.
15. Pannuti CS, Gingrich RD, Pfaller MA, Wenzel RP: Nosocomial pneumonia in adult patients undergoing bone marrow transplantation: a 9-year study: J Clin Oncol 1:77–84, 1991.
16. Atkinson K, Farewell V, Storb R, et al: Analysis of late infections after human bone marrow transplantation: role of genotypic nonidentify between marrow donor and recipient and of nonspecific suppresser cells in patients with chronic graft-versus-host disease. Blood 3:714–720, 1982.
17. Sullivan KM, Agura E, Anasetti C, et al: Chronic graft-versus-host disease and other late complication of bone marrow transplantation. Semin Hematol 3:250–259, 1991.
18. Atkinson K: Chronic graft-versus-host disease. Bone Marrow Transplant 5:69–82, 1990.
19. Giebink GC, Warkentin PI, Ramsay NKC, Kersey JH: Titers of antibody to pneumococci in allogeneic bone marrow transplant recipients before and after vaccination with pneumococcal vaccine. J Infect Dis 4:590–596, 1986.
20. Momin F, Chandrasekar PH: Antimicrobial prophylaxis in bone marrow transplantation. Ann Intern Med 123:205–215, 1995.
21. Wolfson JS, Hooper DC: Norfloxacin: a new targeted fluoroquinolone antimicrobial agent. Ann Intern Med 108:238–251, 1988.
22. Lew MA, Kehoe K, Ritz J, et al: Prophylaxis of bacterial infections with ciprofloxacin in patients undergoing bone marrow transplantation. Transplantation 51:630–636, 1991.
23. Gilbert C, Meisenberg B, Vredenburg J, et al: Sequential prophylactic oral and empiric once-daily parenteral antibiotics for neutropenia and fever after high-dose chemotherapy and autologous bone marrow support. J Clin Oncol 12:1005–1011, 1994.
24. Dekker AW, Rozenberg-Arska M, Verhoef J: Infection prophylaxis in acute leukemia: a comparison of ciprofloxacin with trimethroprim-sulfamethoxazole and colistin. Ann Intern Med 106:7–11, 1987.
25. GIMEMA: Prevention of bacterial infection in neutropenic patients with hematologic malignancies: a randomized, multicenter trial comparing norfloxacin with ciprofloxacin. GIMEMA Infection Program Ann Intern Med 115:7–12, 1991.
26. Karp JE, Merz WG, Hendricksen C, et al: Oral norfloxacin for prevention of gram-negative bacterial infections in patients with acute leukemia and granulocytopenia. Ann Intern Med 106:1–7, 1987.
27. Winston DJ, Ho WG, Nakao SL, et al: Norfloxacin versus vancomycin/polymyxin for prevention of infections in granulocytopenic patients. Am J Med 80:884–888, 1986.
28. Winston DJ, Ho WG, Bruckner DA, et al: Ofloxacin versus vancomycin/polymyxin for prevention of infections in granulocytopenic patients. Am J Med 88:36–41, 1990.
29. Schmeiser T, Kern WV, Hay B, et al: Single-drug oral antibacterial prophylaxis with ofloxacin in BMT recipients. Bone Marrow Transplant 12:57–63, 1993.
30. Bow EJ, Mandell LA, Louie TJ, et al: Quinolone-based antibacterial chemoprophylaxis in neutropenic patients: effect of augmented gram-positive activity on infectious morbidity. Ann Intern Med 125:183–190, 1996.
31. Imrie KR, Prince HM, Couture F, et al: Effect of antimicrobial prophy-

laxis on hematopoietic recovery following autologous bone marrow transplantation: ciprofloxacin versus co-trimoxazole. Bone Marrow Transplant 15:267–270, 1995.

32. Cruciani M, Rampazzo R, Malena M, et al: Prophylaxis with fluoroquinolones for bacterial infections in neutropenic patients: a meta-analysis. Clin Infect Dis 23:795–805, 1996.

33. Cometta A, Calandra T, Bille J, Glauser MP: *Escherichia coli* resistant to fluoroquinolones in patients with cancer and neutropenia [Letter]. N Engl J Med 330:1240–1241, 1994.

34. International Antimicrobial Therapy Cooperative Group of the European Organization for Research and Treatment of Cancer: Efficacy and toxicity of single daily doses of amikacin and ceftriaxone versus multiple daily doses of amikacin and ceftazidime for infection in patients with cancer and granulocytopenia. Ann Intern Med 119:584–593, 1993.

35. Karp JE, Dick JD, Angelopulous C, et al: Empiric use of vancomycin during prolonged treatment-induced granulocytopenia: randomized, double-blind, placebo-controlled clinical trial in patients with acute leukemia. Am J Med 81:237–2421, 1986.

36. Rubin M, Hathorn JW, Marshall D, et al: Gram-positive infections and the use of vancomycin in 550 episodes of fever and neutropenia. Ann Intern Med 108:30–35, 1988.

37. Kern W, Kurrle E, Schmeiser T: Streptococcal bacteremia in adult patients with leukemia undergoing aggressive chemotherapy: a review of 55 cases. Infection 18:138–143, 1990.

38. International Antimicrobial Therapy Cooperative Group of the European Organization for Research and Treatment of Cancer: Reduction of fever and streptococcal bacteremia in granulocytopenic patients with cancer: a trial of oral penicillin V or placebo combined with pefloxacin. JAMA 272:1183–1189, 1994.

39. Classen DC, Burke JP, Ford CD, et al: *Streptcococcus mitis* sepsis in bone marrow transplant patients receiving oral antimicrobial prophylaxis. Am J Med 89:441–446, 1990.

40. Martino R, Nomdedeu J, Sureda A, et al: Acute rhabdomyolysis complicating viridians streptococcal shock syndrome. Acta Haematol 92:140–141, 1994.

41. Awada A, van der Auwera P, Meunier F, et al: Streptococcal and enterococcal bacteremia in patients with cancer. Clin Infect Dis 15:33–48, 1992.

42. Rozenberg-Arska M, Dekker A, Verdonck L, Verhoef L: Prevention of bacteremia caused by α-hemolytic streptococci by roxithromycin (RU-28 965) in granulocytopenic patients receiving ciprofloxacin. Infection 17:240–244, 1989.

43. Kern WV, Hay B, Kern P, et al: A randomized trial of roxithromycin in patients with acute leukemia and bone marrow transplant recipients receiving fluoroquinolone prophylaxis. Antimicrob Agents Chemother 38:465–472, 1994.

44. Archimbaud E, Guyotat D, Maupas J, et al: Pefloxacin and vancomycin versus gentamicin, colistin sulphate and vancomycin for prevention of infections in granulocytopenic patients: a randomized double-blind study. Eur J Cancer 27:174–178, 1991.

45. Attal M, Schlaifer D, Rubie H, et al: Prevention of gram-positive infections after bone marrow transplantation by systemic vancomycin: a prospective, randomized trial. J Clin Oncol 9:865–870, 1991.

46. Rangoon MR, Oppenheim BA, Jackson A, et al: Double-blind placebo controlled study of vancomycin prophylaxis for central venous catheter insertion in cancer patients. J Hosp Infect 15:95–102, 1990.

47. Vassilomanolakis M, Plataniotis G, Koumakis G, et al: Central venous catheter-related infections after bone marrow transplantation in patients with malignancies: a prospective study with short-course vancomycin prophylaxis. Bone Marrow Transplant 15:77–80, 1995.

48. Gurwith MJ, Brunton JL, Lank BA, et al: A prospective controlled investigation of prophylactic trimethoprim/sulfamethoxazole in hospitalized granulocytopenic patients. Am J Med 66:248–256, 1979.

49. Gualtieri RJ, Donowitz GR, Kaiser DL, et al: Double-blind randomized study of prophylactic trimethoprim/sulfamethoxazole in granulocytopenic patients with hematologic malignancies. Am J Med 74:934–940, 1983.

50. Gurwith M, Truog K, Hinthorn D, Liu C: Trimethoprim-sulfamethoxazole and trimethoprim alone for prophylaxis of infection in granulocytopenic patients. Rev Infect Dis 4:593–601, 1982.

51. Wilson JM, Guiney DG: Failure of oral trimethoprim-sulfamethoxazole prophylaxis in acute leukemia. N Engl J Med 306:16–20, 1982.

52. Murray BE, Rensimer ER, DuPont HL: Emergence of high-level trimethoprim resistance in fecal *Escherichia coli* during oral administra-

tion of trimethoprim or trimethoprim-sulfamethoxazole. N Engl J Med 306:130–135, 1982.

53. Craven DE: Use of selective decontamination of the digestive tract: is the light at the end of the tunnel red or green? [Editorial]. Ann Intern Med 117:609–611, 1992.

54. European Society for Intensive Care Medicine: Selective digestive decontamination in intensive care unit patients. Intensive Care Med 18:182–188, 1992.

55. Fink MP: Selective digestive decontamination: a gut issue for the nineties [Editorial]. Crit Care Med 20:559–562, 1992.

56. Flaherty J, Nathan C, Kabins SA, Weinstein RA: Pilot trial of selective decontamination for prevention of bacterial infection in an intensive care unit. J Infect Dis 162:1393–1397, 1990.

57. Cockerill FR, Muller SR, Anhalt JP, et al: Prevention of infection in critically ill patients by selective decontamination of the digestive tract. Ann Intern Med 117:545–553, 1992.

58. Selective Decontamination of the Digestive Tract Trialists' Collaborative Group: Meta-analysis of randomized controlled trials of selective decontamination of the digestive tract. Bone Marrow J 307:525–532, 1993.

59. Verhoef J, Verhage EAE, Visser MR: A decade of experience with selective decontamination of the digestive tract as prophylaxis for infections in patients in the intensive care unit: what have we learned? Clin Infect Dis 17:1047–1054, 1993.

60. Guiot HFL, van den Broek PJ, van der Meer JWM, van Furth R: Selective antimicrobial modulation of the intestinal flora of patients with acute nonlymphocytic leukemia: a double-blind, placebo-controlled study. J Infect Dis 147:615–623, 1983.

61. Guiot HFL, van der Meer JWM, van Furth R: Selective antimicrobial modulation of human microbial flora: infection prevention in patients with decreased host defense mechanisms by selective elimination of potentially pathogenic bacteria. J Infect Dis 143:644–654, 1981.

62. Beelen DW, Haralambie E, Brandt H, et al: Evidence that sustained growth suppression of intestinal anaerobic bacteria reduces the risk of acute graft-versus-host disease after sibling marrow transplantation. Blood 80:2668–2676, 1992.

63. Heidt PJ, Vossen JM: Experimental and clinical antibiotics: influence of the microflora on graft-versus-host disease after allogeneic bone marrow transplantation. J Med 23:161–173, 1992.

64. Winston DJ, Schiffman G, Wang DC, et al: Pneumococcal infections after human bone marrow transplantation. Ann Intern Med 91:835–841, 1979.

65. D'Antonio D, DiBartolomeo P, Iacone A, et al: Meningitis due to penicillin-resistant *Streptococcus pneumoniae* in patients with chronic graft-versus-host disease. Bone Marrow Transplant 9:299–300, 1992.

66. Nosanchuk JD, Sepkowitz KA, Pearse RN, et al: Infectious complications of autologous bone marrow and peripheral stem cell transplantation for refractory leukemia and lymphoma. Bone Marrow Transplant 18:355–359, 1996.

67. Mossad SB, Longworth DL, Goormastic M, et al: Early infectious complications in autologous bone marrow transplantation: a review of 219 patients. Bone Marrow Transplant 18:265–271, 1996.

68. Appelbaum FR: The use of colony stimulating factors in marrow transplantation. Cancer Suppl 72:3387–3392, 1993.

69. Rabinowe SN, Neuberg D, Bierman PJ, et al: Long-term follow-up of a phase III study of recombinant human granulocyte-macrophage colony-stimulating factor after autologous bone marrow transplantation for lymphoid malignancies. Blood 81:1903–1908, 1993.

70. Gulati SC, Bennett CL: Granulocyte-macrophage colony-stimulating factor (GM-CSF) as adjunct therapy in relapsed Hodgkin disease. Ann Intern Med 116:117–182, 1992.

71. Link H, Boogaerts MA, Carella AM, et al: A controlled trial of recombinant human granulocyte-macrophage colony-stimulating factor after total body irradiation, high-dose chemotherapy, and autologous bone marrow transplantation for acute lymphoblastic leukemia or malignant lymphoma. Blood 80:2188–2195, 1992.

72. Gisselbrecht C, Prentice HG, Bacigalupo A, et al: Placebo-controlled phase III trial of lenograstim in bone marrow transplantation. Lancet 343:696–700, 1994.

73. Stahel RA, Jost LM, Cerny T, et al: Randomized study of recombinant human granulocyte colony-stimulating factor after high-dose chemotherapy and autologous bone marrow transplantation for high-risk lymphoid malignancies. J Clin Oncol 12:1931–1938, 1994.

74. Linch DC, Scarffe H, Proctor S, et al: Randomized vehicle-controlled dose-finding study of glycosylated recombinant human granulocyte

colony-stimulating factor after bone marrow transplantation. Bone Marrow Transplant 11:307–311, 1993.

75. DeWitte T, Gratwohl A, van der Lely N, et al: Recombinant human granulocyte-macrophage colony-stimulating factor accelerates neutrophil and monocyte recovery after allogeneic T-cell-depleted bone marrow transplantation. Blood 5:1359–1365, 1992.

76. Powels R, Treleaven J, Millar J, et al: Human recombinant GM-CSF in allogeneic bone marrow transplantation for leukemia: double-blind placebo controlled trial. Bone Marrow Transplant 7(Suppl 7):85–86, 1991.

77. Somani J, Larson RA: Reimmunization after allogeneic bone marrow transplantation. Am J Med 98:389–398, 1995.

78. Molrine DC, Guinan EC, Antin JH, et al: Donor immunization with *Haemophilus influenza* type b (HIB)-conjugate vaccine in allogeneic bone marrow transplantation. Blood 87:3012–3018, 1996.

79. Guinan EC, Molrine DC, Antin JH, et al: Polysaccharide conjugate vaccine responses in bone marrow transplant patients. Transplantation 57:677–684, 1994.

80. Winston DJ, Ho WG, Schiffman G, et al: Pneumococcal vaccination of recipients of bone marrow transplants. Arch Intern Med 143:1735–1737, 1983.

81. Wolff SN, Fay JW, Herzig RH, et al: High-dose weekly intravenous immunoglobulin to prevent infections in patients undergoing autologous bone marrow transplantation or severe myelosuppresive therapy. Ann Intern Med 118:937–942, 1993.

82. Sullivan KM, Kopecky KJ, Jocom J, et al: Immunomodulatory and antimicrobial efficacy of intravenous immunoglobulin in bone marrow transplantation. N Engl J Med 323:705–712, 1990.

83. Peltier MKH, Filipovich AH, Bechtel M, et al: Randomized double-blind comparison of three intravenous immunoglobulin products in bone marrow transplantation. Semin Hematol 29:112–115, 1992.

84. Poynton CH, Jackson S, Fegan C, et al: Use of IgM enriched intravenous immunoglobulin (pentaglobin) in bone marrow transplantation. Bone Marrow Transplant 9:451–457, 1992.

85. Spitzer TR, Cottler-Fox M, Sullivan P, et al: Continuous infusion intravenous immunoglobulin is associated with a reduced incidence of infection and achieves higher serum immunoglobulin G levels than intermittent infusion following bone marrow transplantation. Semin Hematol 29(Suppl 2):123–126, 1992.

86. Guglielmo BJ, Wong-Beringer A, Linker CA: Immune globulin therapy in allogeneic bone marrow transplant: a critical review. Bone Marrow Transplant 13:499–510, 1994.

87. Levine AS, Siegel SE, Schreiber AD, et al: Protective environments and prophylactic antibiotics: a prospective controlled study of their utility in the therapy of acute leukemia. N Engl J Med 288:477–483, 1973.

88. Buckner CD, Clift RA, Sanders JE, et al: Protective environment for marrow transplant recipients. Ann Intern Med 89:893–901, 1978.

89. Wingard JR, Dick J, Charache P, Saral R: Antibiotic-resistant bacteria in surveillance stool cultures of patients with prolonged neutropenia. Antimicrob Agents Chemother 30:435–439, 1986.

90. Riley DK, Pavia AT, Beatty PG, et al: Surveillance cultures in bone marrow transplant recipients: worthwhile or wasteful? Bone Marrow Transplant 15:469–473, 1995.

91. Ferretti GA, Ash RC, Brown AT, et al: Control of oral mucositis and candidiasis in marrow transplantation: a prospective double-blind trial of chlorhexidine digluconate oral rinse. Bone Marrow Transplant 3:483–493, 1988.

92. Weisdorf DJ, Bostrom B, Raether D, et al: Oropharyangeal mucositis complicating bone marrow transplantation: prognostic factors and the effect of chlorhexidine mouth rinse. Bone Marrow Transplant 4:89–95, 1989.

93. Epstein JB, Vickars L, Spinelli J, Reece D: Efficacy of chlorhexidine and nystatin rinses in prevention of oral complications in leukemia and bone marrow transplantation. Oral Surg Oral Med Oral Pathol 73:682–689, 1992.

94. Ziegler TR, Young LS, Benfell K, et al: Clinical and metabolic efficacy of glutamine-supplemented parenteral nutrition after bone marrow transplantation. Ann Intern Med 116:821–828, 1992.

CHAPTER THIRTY-EIGHT

Fungi and Other Organisms

Han Myint, M.B.B.S., M.R.C.Path.

Invasive fungal infection has been increasingly recognized as one of the important causes of morbidity and mortality in patients receiving immunosuppressive chemotherapy for hematologic malignancy and in hematopoietic stem cell transplantation (HSCT) recipients. The typical invasive mold infections are caused by members of the *Aspergillus* species. Likewise, the typical yeast infections are caused by *Candida*. These are the most common fungal pathogens in patients undergoing HSCT[1]; however, increasingly recognized invasive fungal infections caused by uncommon organisms such as species of *Fusarium, Mucorales* or *Zygomycetes, Scedosporium, Paecilomyces,* and *Trichosporon* are often unresponsive to currently available antifungal therapy[2] (Table 38–1).

YEAST INFECTIONS

Candida can cause acute or chronic deep-seated infection in recipients of HSCT and in immunocompromised hosts. They are more often associated with superficial infection in immunocompetent hosts. *C. albicans* is the most important cause of superficial (mucosal, cutaneous, and nail) and deep-seated fungal infection.

COLONIZATION

Candida organisms are normal fungal inhabitants of the gastrointestinal tract, but colonization was lower in healthy persons (median, 6%) than in hospital patients of any kind (median, 47%) in nine studies.[3] Yeast can be isolated from the genital tract in 20% of normal women. *C. albicans* is the most common isolate (60–80% from the mouth and 80–90% from the genital tract). *Candida* species rarely colonize normal skin unless there are breaks that promote colonization. Air samples are consistently negative for *Candida* species.

CANDIDA INFECTIONS

Both humoral and cell-mediated immunity prevent the colonizing organism from establishing an infection. Even trivial impairment of immune function, however, is often sufficient to allow *C. albicans* to establish a superficial infection. More serious impairment of the host can lead to life-threatening, deep-seated infection.

C. albicans is the most commonly isolated *Candida* species from the blood and deep tissue of immunocompromised patients. The three non-*albicans* species considered to be the most important nosocomial pathogens are *C. tropicalis, C. glabrata,* and *C. parapsilosis.* Two other less common non-*albicans Candida* species are *C. krusei* and *C. lusitaniae,* the latter being associated with resistance to antifungal agents including amphotericin B. The recently described *Candida dubliniensis* has been recovered primarily

TABLE 38–1. FUNGAL PATHOGENS AND THE SITE OF INFECTION

SITE OF DISEASE	CLINICAL FEATURES		LIKELY ORGANISMS
Pulmonary	Cough Pleuritic pain Hemoptysis Infiltrates	⟷	*Aspergillus* *Mucorales* *Scedosporium* *Paecilomyces*
Sinus, nose, face	Sinusitis Epistaxis Facial swelling	⟷	*Aspergillus flavus* *Fusarium* *Mucorales*
Brain	Stroke Epilepsy Rhinocerebral mucormycosis	⟷	*Aspergillus* *Scedosporium apiospermum*

Liver, spleen
Skin
	Rising liver enzyme levels
	Maculopapular rashes
	    Necrotic
	    Macronodular
		⟷	*Mucorales (Rhizopus* spp.)
			Candida
			Fusarium
			Aspergillus
			Mucorales, Acremonium
			Candida spp.

Nonspecific	Neutropenic fever unresponsive to broad-spectrum antibiotics		All organisms

From Working Party of the British Society for Antimicrobial Chemotherapy: Therapy of deep infection in haemotological malignancy. J Antimicrob Chemother 40:779, 1997.

from superficial oral candidiasis in patients infected with human immunodeficiency virus (HIV).[4] Three cases of candidemia due to *Candida dubliniensis*, however, were described in recipients of HSCT and patients with chemotherapy-induced neutropenia.[5]

Candida infections are usually acquired by endogenous activation; however, exogenous acquisition from food, environment, and hospital staff may also occur. Because colonization of the gut and indwelling catheters by *Candida* is common, mucosal disruption by chemotherapy and/or radiotherapy and the use of broad-spectrum antibiotics may facilitate the overgrowth and the translocation of *Candida* organisms, allowing them to enter the bloodstream and to disseminate throughout the body. The most common *Candida* infection during the pre-engraftment period is oral thrush, although chronic disseminated candidiasis (hepatosplenic candidiasis) usually is first recognized after engraftment.[6]

When *Candida* infection develops, it is associated with high mortality in recipients of HSCT.[7] The mortality rate is 39% in fungemia without tissue involvement, but it increases to 90% with tissue involvement.

MOLD INFECTIONS

The infectious molds are divided into three groups:

- *Mucormycosis*—Nonseptate hyphae in tissue (e.g., *Mucorales* or *Zygomycetes* species)
- *Hyalohyphomycosis*—Colorless septate hyphae in tissue (*Aspergillus, Fusarium, Scedosporium,* and *Paecilomyces* species)
- *Phaehyphomycosis*—Pigmented septate hyphae in tissue (*Alternaria, Bipolaris,* and *Curvularia* species)

ASPERGILLUS INFECTIONS

The most common mold-causing organism is *Aspergillus*, which is responsible for 70% of non-*Candida* fungal infections in recipients of HSCT.[8] *A. fumigatus* is the most common *Aspergillus* species that causes pulmonary infection, followed by *A. flavus*, causing a disproportionate number of sinus and nasal infections.

The most common presentation of invasive pulmonary fungal infection is dry cough with fever unresponsive to broad-spectrum antibiotics and a pulmonary infiltrate. Chest pain is common and usually mild but may be pleuritic. Hemoptysis and dyspnea are uncommon symptoms. High-resolution computed tomography (CT) is very sensitive for detecting "halo sign" and "crescent sign," which are virtually characteristic of invasive pulmonary fungal infection.[9–11]

Cerebral invasive aspergillosis occurs in 10% of invasive aspergillosis cases and has a particularly poor outcome.[12] A stroke-like syndrome with fever is the most common presentation, but seizures and altered mental status are also common. Cerebral involvement is usually associated with pulmonary fungal infection, but it may also spread from *Aspergillus* infections of the sinuses or from the ears. Multiple or single hypodense areas due to embolic infarction or

multiple ring-enhancing lesions due to abscesses are visible on CT or magnetic resonance imaging (MRI). Many fungal infections are diagnosed only at autopsy because currently available diagnostic tools are inadequate. The introduction of the polymerase chain reaction (PCR) assay to detect fungal DNA has yet to have an impact on the early diagnosis of invasive fungal infection. The optimal prophylactic strategy is not defined, but patients would benefit from early detection.

FUSARIOSIS

Fusariosis has been increasingly recognized as one of the emerging fungal pathogens in HSCT.[13–15] *Fusarium solani* is the most common pathogen in immunocompromised patients that causes disseminated invasive infection, but other species such as *F. oxysporum, F. proliferatum,* and *F. moniliforme* have been incriminated.[16, 17] Infection is characterized by erythematous papulonodular skin lesions, myalgias, fungemia, and multiorgan involvement. Facial or periorbital cellulitis are common in patients with fusarial sinusitis.[18, 19]

Although *Fusarium* shares features with *Aspergillus* in morphology and in the propensity for invasion of blood vessels leading to tissue infarction, there are three important differences.[15] First, blood cultures are positive in 70% of patients with fusariosis, whereas blood cultures are rarely positive in *Aspergillus* infections. Second, fusariosis is characteristically associated with disseminated skin lesions. Pulmonary lesions, however, are identical to those of *Aspergillus* infection. Third, a single-center experience from M.D. Anderson Cancer Center has shown that *Fusarium* is usually resistant to treatment and associated with high mortality.[15] The response rate is about 30–40%, and response is associated with neutrophil recovery. Relapse frequently occurs with subsequent myelosuppressive therapy.

MUCORALES

Rhizopus arrhizus, Rhizomucor pusillus, and *Absidia corymbifera* are the most common organisms of mucormycosis. Infection usually follows inhalation. The two most common presentations are rhinocerebral and pulmonary mucormycoses. Rhinocerebral mucormycosis begins as a nasal or paranasal sinus infection and invades through bone to involve the orbit or brain. The usual presenting symptoms and signs are unilateral facial swelling, proptosis, and ophthalmoplegia with a serosanguineous nasal discharge and characteristic black intranasal or palatal eschars.[20] Because of mucormycosis' aggressiveness, prompt diagnosis is essential for a successful outcome, including CT of the sinuses and biopsy and débridement of necrotic tissue.[21] Primary mucormycosis of the lung is less common, but terminal widespread dissemination is common in neutropenic patients with involvement of brain, lung, heart, and spleen.

OTHER RARE FUNGI

Scedosporium has been associated with invasive fungal infections in recipients of HSCT. Disseminated infection due to

Scedosporium apiospermum[22, 23] (previously named *Pseudallescheria boydii*) is resistant to amphotericin B and *S. prolificans* (previously known as *S. inflatum*) is resistant to all known antifungal agents.[24] It may occasionally respond to granulocyte infusion.[25]

Trichosporon beigelii (formerly known as *T. cutaneum*), which is a yeast organism, has been established as a cause of disseminated invasive fungal infection in immunocompromised patients.[26–29] It presents with neutropenic fever unresponsive to antibiotics with widespread involvement of liver, spleen, and lungs and multiple, erythematous, maculopapular skin lesions. Blood culture is positive in 50% of cases, although trichosporonosis is usually diagnosed at autopsy.[30] Most of the strains are resistant to therapy, but occasional long-term survivors after HSCT have been reported.[31]

Paecilomyces lilacinus, a colorless mold, has been associated with an outbreak of invasive fungal infection transmitted from a contaminated skin lotion[32] to recipients of HSCT. Skin involvement is common, with papular, pustular, and necrotic skin eruptions. Direct cutaneous invasion was thought to be the mode of entry. These infections are often resistant to amphotericin B. Other rare fungal infections have been reported in bone marrow transplant recipients, including *Phialophora verrucosa*,[33] *Neosartorya fischeri*,[34] *Hansenula anomala*,[35, 36] *Cokeromyces recurvatus*,[37] *Cladophialophora bantiana*,[38] and *Scopulariopsis brevicaulis*.[39, 40]

RISK FACTORS FOR INVASIVE FUNGAL INFECTION

Fungi are rarely as invasive or pathogenic as many bacteria or viruses, so certain risk factors must be present in the seriously ill immunosuppressed patient to allow infection with these fungi as opportunistic fungal pathogens (Table 38–2).

Prolonged neutropenia is one of the risk factors for invasive fungal infection. Furthermore, the duration of neutropenia is directly correlated with an increase in the incidence of invasive aspergillosis. For example, the rate of invasive pulmonary aspergillosis increases progressively after the 6th day of neutropenia at a rate of 1% per day. The rate increases to 4.5% per day between the 24th and 36th days of neutropenia, reaching 70% after 30 days of neutropenia.[41] Likewise, oropharyngeal candidiasis developed after 6 days of neutropenia and rose to 65% after 12 days of neutropenia in patients without prophylaxis.[42]

Corticosteroid therapy is another risk factor for invasive

fungal infection because it suppresses the monocyte-macrophage system, resulting in impaired killing of fungal spores by macrophages and impaired mobilization of neutrophils around the fungus.

Other risk factors for fungal infection in immunocompromised patients include indwelling catheters, broad-spectrum antibiotics, high-dose cytosine arabinoside, previous fungal infection, cytomegalovirus infection, graft-versus-host disease (GVHD), and environmental exposure. A well-established risk factor for the acquisition of *Aspergillus* infections, especially in HSCT units, is construction work in the hospital environment.

HSCT recipients are at risk for invasive fungal infection because of their underlying disease, the type of transplant and the conditioning regimen, and the type of immunosuppressive therapy administered. By and large, patients undergoing autologous peripheral blood progenitor cell transplantation are at less risk of invasive fungal infection because the duration of neutropenia is shorter than that in allogeneic HSCT recipients. Post-transplantation immunotherapy after autologous HSCT further increases the risk of an invasive fungal infection.[43] In contrast, recipients of unrelated donor or mismatched donor bone marrow are at the greatest risk of invasive fungal infection. During the pre-engraftment period, the risk is increased by disruption of the mucosal barrier, T-cell depletion, prolonged neutropenia, and immunosuppression with steroid and methotrexate. In the immediate postengraftment period the risk is increased by acute GVHD, causing further damage to the mucosal barrier, therapy of acute GVHD with immunosuppression using agents such as cyclosporine and steroids and in the late engraftment period by chronic GVHD and immunosuppression related to its treatment.

PREVENTION OF FUNGAL INFECTION IN HEMATOPOIETIC STEM CELL TRANSPLANTATION

REDUCTION OF ENVIRONMENTAL EXPOSURE

Because the major routes of fungal acquisition are contact, food, water, and air supply, physical measures play a major role in minimizing the risk of contracting invasive fungal infection. They include reverse barrier nursing, careful handwashing, removal of plants, avoidance of food with fungal contamination, housing recipients of HSCT in rooms with either high-efficiency particulate air (HEPA) or laminar airflow (LAF) ventilation, and sealing of nearby construction areas (Table 38–3).

Strict attention to hand hygiene, including careful washing followed by decontamination with alcoholic chlorhexidine of the hands before contacting neutropenic patients, avoids nosocomial infection because there is a high frequency of yeast carriage on hands of hospital personnel.[44]

Candida species are recovered from various food products including vegetables, salads, cereals, fruits, and fruit juice. In general, all juices packaged and sealed with foil wraps are contaminated, whereas canned and bottled juices are free of fungi. Therefore, serving patients a neutropenic diet (e.g., avoidance of salads, uncooked vegetables, unpasteur-

TABLE 38–2. RISK FACTORS FOR INVASIVE FUNGAL INFECTION

Prolonged neutropenia	Steroids
Impaired cell-mediated immunity	Indwelling catheters
Fungal colonization	Environmental exposure
Immunosuppressive agents	Plants
Cytomegalovirus infection	Contaminated food
Graft-versus-host disease	Building work
High-dose cytosine arabinoside	

TABLE 38–3. REMOVAL OF ENVIRONMENTAL FACTORS

Reverse barrier nursing
Careful hand washing
Removal of plants
Avoidance of fungus-contaminated food
High-efficiency particulate air (HEPA) filter
Laminar airflow
Sealing of nearby construction area

ized milk and fruit juices, fresh fruits, and ground pepper[45]) is also an important part of preventing invasive fungal infection.

The use of HEPA filters or LAF is the most effective means of keeping *Aspergillus* from a patient's environment. Sherertz et al. showed in 1987 that there was no case of fungal infection among the 39 allogeneic HSCT recipients who were housed in isolation rooms with whole-wall HEPA filtration units with horizontal laminar flow compared with 14 cases of invasive fungal infection in 74 patients who were housed elsewhere in the hospital.[46] Furthermore, air sampling showed a significantly reduced number of *Aspergillus* spores in the filtered rooms compared with all other areas of the hospital. Barnes and Rogers showed that 6 out of 19 children undergoing HSCT died of invasive pulmonary aspergillosis in the adjacent ward during the construction of a new bone marrow transplantation unit when air sampling confirmed heavy fungal spore contamination.[47] The introduction of LAF isolation terminated the outbreak with no subsequent cases of invasive pulmonary aspergillosis in 19 patients who underwent transplantation in the rooms with LAF. A large retrospective cohort study of 2496 recipients of HSCT, however, showed that the LAF environment protects against early *Aspergillus* infection (onset before day +40 of transplantation) but not late (onset after day +40 of transplantation) infection.[48] Furthermore, the protection is lost when patients are removed from the protected environment (e.g., transportation to the radiology department for CT or chest radiography). In addition, regular engineering maintenance of the air supply system must be performed to achieve the best outcome. This should include changing the air filters, air sampling, and smoke tests to ensure effective ventilation. The rooms should be cleaned regularly when vacated by immunocompromised patients.

MEDICAL PROPHYLAXIS

Because establishing the diagnosis of fungal infection is problematic and once established is associated with high mortality, the two paradigms for the prevention of invasive fungal infection are medical prophylaxis and empirical therapy. The agents most frequently used are amphotericin B, fluconazole, and itraconazole. For the prevention of fungal infection, the azoles have been used for some time. The first azole employed was clotrimazole, which could not be given intravenously and was poorly absorbed with oral administration. Miconazole also had a very poor absorption, but the topical preparation has been successfully used for superficial mycoses. Ketoconazole is well absorbed after

oral administration and has a wide spectrum of antifungal therapy. Its wide variety of side effects, however—including hepatotoxicty and endocrine abnormalities—led to its replacement by the newer triazoles, fluconazole and itraconazole.

Fluconazole

A summary of prophylactic fluconazole administration to patients undergoing HSCT is presented in Table 38–4. Goodman et al. performed a double-blind, randomized, multicenter trial in which patients undergoing HSCT were randomly assigned to receive placebo or fluconazole (400 mg daily).[49] Either fluconazole or placebo was assigned as prophylaxis from the start of the conditioning regimen until the neutrophil count returned to 1000/mm^3, toxicity was suspected, or a systemic fungal infection was suspected or proved. One hundred seventy-seven patients were assigned to receive placebo, of whom 67% had a positive fungal culture from specimens from any site as compared with 30% of the 179 patients assigned to fluconazole. Superficial infections were diagnosed in 33% of patients who received placebo and in 8% of the patients who received fluconazole ($P < .001$). Systemic fungal infections occurred in 28 (16%) in the placebo arm compared with 5 (3%) in the fluconazole arm ($P < .001$). During the trial period, colonization increased to 78% and 32% in the placebo and fluconazole groups, respectively. Fluconazole prevented infection with all species of *Candida* except *C. krusei*. There were fewer deaths in the group who received fluconazole due to acute systemic fungal infection than in the group who received placebo (1 of 179 vs. 10 of 177, $P < .001$). The authors concluded that fluconazole prophylaxis reduces not only the frequency of candidiasis but also the number of deaths from fungal infection.

In another prospective, randomized, double-blind, placebo-controlled study, the efficacy of prophylactic fluconazole, 400 mg once daily, was assessed in the prevention of fungal infections during the first 75 days after marrow transplantation.[50] Among the 152 fluconazole-treated patients, proven systemic fungal infections occurred in 10 (7%) compared with 26 (18%) of 148 placebo-treated patients ($P = .004$). There were no *C. albicans* infections in fluconazole recipients compared with 18 in placebo recipients ($P < .001$). The occurrence of other non-*albicans* infections and *C. glabrata* were not significantly increased in the two study arms. Prophylactic fluconazole also significantly reduced the incidence of superficial fungal infection ($P < .001$), fungal colonization ($P = .037$), and empirical amphotericin B use ($P = .005$) Mortality at the end of the study was not significantly different. The probability of dying up to day 110 after transplantation, however, was reduced in the fluconazole arm compared with placebo recipients (31 vs. 52, $P = .004$). The authors concluded that the prophylactic use of fluconazole is safe and significantly reduces systemic fungal infection with other benefits, including improved survival at day 110 after marrow transplantation.

In another double-blind, multicenter trial, 257 patients undergoing chemotherapy for acute leukemia were randomly assigned to receive either fluconazole, 400 mg daily, or placebo.[51] The study drug was started at the initiation

TABLE 38–4. SUMMARY OF PROPHYLACTIC FLUCONAZOLE STUDIES IN HEMATOPOIETIC STEM CELL TRANSPLANTATION RECIPIENTS AND LEUKEMIC PATIENTS

STUDY	RANDOMIZED DOUBLE-BLIND PLACEBO-CONTROLLED?	FLUCONAZOLE VS. PLACEBO	DOSAGE	FUNGAL COLONIZATION	SYSTEMIC FUNGAL INFECTION	SUPERFICIAL FUNGAL INFECTION	EMPIRIC AMPHOTERICIN B USE	MORTALITY
Goodman et al.[49]	Yes	179 vs. 177 (BMT)	400 mg	↓	↓	↓	Not addressed	↓
Slavin et al.[50]	Yes	152 vs. 148 (BMT)	400 mg	↓	↓	↓	↓	↔
Winston et al.[51]	Yes	119 vs. 122 (BMT)	400 mg	↓	↔	↓	↔	↔
Alangaden et al.[119]	No (compared with historical control of patients with no prophylaxis)	112 (BMT)	100–200 mg	↓ C. albicans but ↑ C. glabrata	↓	Not addressed	↓	Not addressed

BMT, Bone marrow transplantation.

of chemotherapy and continued until recovery of the neutrophil count, development of proven or suspected invasive fungal infection, or the occurrence of a drug-related toxicity. Fungal colonization was decreased in the study group (34 of 119 [29%]) compared with the placebo group (83 of 122 [68%]) ($P < .001$). Fewer patients had proven fungal infections in the fluconazole group (9%) than in the placebo group (21%, $P = .02$). The occurrence of superficial fungal infections was also less in the fluconazole arm (6% vs. 15%, $P = .01$). There was no difference, however, in the development of invasive fungal infection (4% vs. 8%, $P = .3$). The incidence of *Aspergillus* infection was no different between the two arms (three cases each). The authors concluded that prophylactic fluconazole prevents colonization and superficial infection by *Candida* species other than *C. krusei* in patients undergoing chemotherapy for acute leukemia. In addition, fluconazole could not be clearly shown to be effective for preventing invasive fungal infection, reducing the use of amphotericin B, or decreasing the number of deaths.

Fluconazole has become the prophylactic agent of choice in patients with neutropenia due to either chemotherapy or HSCT. Its use, however, is associated with an increase in the incidence of non-*albicans* species such as *C. krusei*[52] and *C. glabrata*,[53] and the emergence of drug resistance has been reported.[54] Furthermore, an autopsy study of 355 HSCT recipients showed an increase in the incidence of *Aspergillus* infections, although *Candida* infections appeared to be significantly lower in patients who had received fluconazole prophylaxis.[55] Despite the extensive use of prophylactic fluconazole in recipients of HSCT, systemic fungal infections caused by *Aspergillus*, *Mucorales*, and *Fusarium* remain a problem because the drug is ineffective, regardless of the dose, against *Aspergillus* species and other fungal pathogens. Therefore, there is a clear need for better antifungal prophylaxis.

Itraconazole

Itraconazole is a triazole compound with a broad spectrum of in vitro activity against fungi, including *Aspergillus* and non-*albicans Candida*. An important limitation of itraconazole, however, is its erratic absorption, especially in patients who have sustained damage to the intestinal epithelium

due to radiation or chemotherapy. It is no surprise that so little information is available from well-designed, placebo-controlled, randomized studies in HSCT recipients because the drug was only available in capsule form until recently. This view may change—first because of the introduction of the new oral formulation of itraconazole suspended in cyclodextrin solution, which appears to have overcome the problem of erratic absorption, and second because of the arrival of the new intravenous formulation, which has recently been approved by the FDA.

In a randomized study, the efficacy and safety of itraconazole in capsule form was studied for the prevention of fungal infection in neutropenic patients given cytotoxic chemotherapy for hematologic malignancy.[56] Patients were randomly allocated to receive either an itraconazole capsule, 200 mg BID (n = 46), or placebo (n = 46). In addition, oral amphotericin B was given until either fungal infection developed or antileukemic treatment was complete. There was no difference in the development of fungal infection: 9 in the itraconazole group, of which 4 cases were histologically or microbiologically proven, and 15 in the placebo group, of which 8 were proven ($P < .12$)—and they were treated with intravenous amphotericin B. Although the incidence of *C. albicans* infections appeared to be lower in the itraconazole group, the authors concluded that there was no measurable improvement in the prevention of fungal infection or mortality by itraconazole.

Tricot et al. reported the preliminary results of a single-center experience on the comparison of two consecutive, nonrandomized studies of ketoconazole, 200 mg BID (n = 52), and itraconazole, 200 mg BID (n = 45), in patients with hematologic malignancies other than HSCT recipients with severe neutropenia.[57] The incidence of fatal fungal infection was significantly higher in patients who received ketoconazole than in those who received itraconazole. Drug levels were measured in 42 of 45 patients, of whom half had an inadequate serum itraconazole level (<250 ng/mL for at least 7 consecutive days). Proven or suspected fungal infection developed in 11 of 21 patients with inadequate serum itraconazole levels, in contrast with 4 of 21 patients with adequate serum levels. In another study, the same group suggested that a relationship exists between serum itraconazole levels and its prophylactic efficacy, although a precise determination of the optimal serum itraconazole level has not been established.[58]

Because the itraconazole molecule is virtually insoluble, the liquid is prepared by addition of hydroxypropyl-β-cyclodextrin. In an open study, the pharmacokinetics of itraconazole oral solution was studied in seven patients who received high-dose chemotherapy followed by autologous HSCT.[59] Itraconazole was given at 5 mg/kg/day as either a once- or twice-daily dose. Drug concentrations reached steady state by day 15 in both groups. The mean predose itraconazole serum concentration at hour 0, day 8 was 385 ng/mL in the once-a-day group and 394 ng/mL in the BID group, rising to 762 and 845 ng/mL, respectively, by day 15. The authors concluded that serum concentrations of itraconazole suitable for antifungal prophylaxis can be attained within a week in neutropenic patients. This finding led to further randomized studies of itraconazole oral solution in patients with hematologic malignancy, including recipients of HSCT (Table 38–5).

Menichetti et al. conducted a study in 405 neutropenic patients with hematologic malignancy, the majority being acute leukemia.[60] In this double-blind, multicenter study, patients were randomly assigned to prophylactic itraconazole, 2.5 mg/kg BID (201 patients), or placebo (204 patients). Both groups received oral nystatin. There were 37 patients who underwent autologous HSCT in each arm of the study. Recipients of allogeneic HSCT or high-dose cytosine arabinoside were excluded from the study. Serum itraconazole concentration was greater than 250 ng/mL in 86–100% of the treatment group after day 12 of therapy. Itraconazole significantly reduced the incidence of proven and suspected deep fungal infection, which occurred in 24% of the itraconazole group compared with 33% of the placebo group ($P = .035$), with an odds ratio of 0.63. C. fungemia was documented less often in the itraconazole group compared with the control group (0.5% vs. 4%, $P = .01$). There was no difference in survival between the two groups.

Morgenstern et al. conducted a multicenter study, however, comparing the efficacy of itraconazole and fluconazole in a randomized, open-label fashion.[61] Patients (n = 445) receiving chemotherapy for hematologic malignancy, including recipients of autologous or allogeneic HSCT, were randomly (according to the treatment strata) assigned to itraconazole oral solution, 2.5 mg/kg BID (n = 218), or fluconazole suspension, 100 mg daily (n = 227), during 591 episodes of neutropenia. The patients in the chemotherapy, autologous HSCT, and allogeneic HSCT arms numbered 178, 88, and 22, respectively, in the itraconazole arm and 173, 91, and 29, respectively, in the fluconazole arm. Fewer proven systemic fungal infections occurred in the

itraconazole arm compared with the fluconazole arm (1 vs. 6, $P = .03$). The use of intravenous amphotericin B was significantly higher in the fluconazole group (58 vs. 39, $P = .043$).

These studies show that the bioavailability of the oral solution of itraconazole is reliable and that monitoring of the serum level is no longer required. The desired serum level, however, is achieved only after day 8 of itraconazole administration at 2.5 mg/kg, twice daily, although the rate of invasive pulmonary aspergillosis increases progressively after day 6 of neutropenia.[41] Achieving the desired serum level is especially relevant in patients who have experienced previous fungal infection, because there is a high chance of relapse during any subsequent neutropenic period.[62] Boogaerts et al., however, have shown that the steady state can be achieved by day 1 when itraconazole, 200 mg BID, is given intravenously as a loading dose for 2 days followed by once a day from days 3–7; thereafter, it can be switched to the oral solution.[63] The intravenous formulation of itraconazole is currently under evaluation as prophylaxis in allogeneic HSCT.

Voriconazole

Voriconazole is a new monotriazole with a wide spectrum of antifungal activity, including *Aspergillus*. In an animal model, voriconazole was highly efficacious in the prevention and treatment of *Aspergillus* infection and was superior to itraconazole in these respects.[64] To date, no voriconazole data are available on prophylaxis of fungal infection in humans, although voriconazole was shown to be effective in the treatment of *Aspergillus* infection in recipients of HSCT.

Amphotericin B
Intravenous Form

Although amphotericin B, despite its side effects, has been the gold standard in the treatment of fungal infection for more than 40 years, it is not licensed to be used as prophylaxis or empirical therapy in fungal infection. Amphotericin B has been studied as a low-dose intravenous infusion or as a drug for nasal administration in HSCT. Most studies were retrospective and give very limited information because the incidence of fungal infection varies from one year to another (Table 38–6).

Rousey et al. studied the use of low-dose prophylactic intravenous amphotericin B in 110 recipients of allogeneic

TABLE 38–5.   STUDIES ON PROPHYLACTIC ITRACONAZOLE SOLUTION IN HEMATOLOGIC MALIGNANCY

REFERENCE	STUDY	ITRACONAZOLE VS. CONTROL	DOSAGE (ORAL SOLUTION)	USE OF EMPIRIC AMPHOTERICIN	SYSTEMIC FUNGAL INFECTION	SUPERFICIAL FUNGAL INFECTION	MORTALITY
Menichetti et al.[60]	Randomized double-blind placebo-controlled	201 vs. 204	2.5 mg/kg BID	↓	↓	↔	↔
Morgenstern et al.[61]	Randomized open-label itraconazole vs. fluconazole	218 vs. 227	2.5 mg/kg BID	↓	↓	Not addressed	↓

TABLE 38–6. SUMMARY OF PROPHYLACTIC AMPHOTERICIN B STUDIES IN HEMATOPOIETIC STEM CELL TRANSPLANTATION

REFERENCE	STUDY	PATIENTS	DOSAGE	SYSTEMIC FUNGAL INFECTION	NEPHROTOXICITY	EMPIRIC AMPHOTERICIN B USE	OVERALL MORTALITY
Rousey et al.[65]	Retrospective study with historical control	186 allogeneic recipients	0.15–0.25 mg/ kg daily	↓	↑	↔	↓
Riley et al.[66]	Randomized double-blind placebo-controlled	17 vs. 18 amphotericin B vs. placebo; allogeneic recipients	0.1 mg/kg daily	↓	↔	Trend ↓	↔
Perfect et al.[67]	Randomized placebo-controlled	Autologous recipients	0.1 mg/kg daily	Not addressed *But* ↓ colonization ↔ superficial yeast infection	Not addressed *But* ↑ infusion-related toxity	↔	↓

HSCT for the prevention of invasive aspergillosis. Patients receiving amphotericin B were nursed in laminar air flow isolation and were compared with historical controls. The first control cohort of 28 patients was nursed in the general oncology ward, and the second cohort of 48 patients was nursed in laminar air flow isolation.[65] Amphotericin B was given at 0.15–0.25 mg/kg daily from the start of the conditioning regimen until the day of transplantation, when the dose was reduced to alternate-day administration and was continued until neutrophil recovery to 1000/mm³. Empirical use of amphotericin B was allowed when fungal infection was suspected in all three cohorts. There was a significant reduction in both the incidence and mortality of invasive aspergillosis in patients receiving amphotericin B prophylaxis compared with those cohorts without prophylaxis. Although this approach of low-dose amphotericin B was claimed not to be associated with increased renal or hepatic toxicity, baseline serum creatinine levels more than doubled in half of the patients in each cohort. The authors concluded that the risks of invasive aspergillosis in allogeneic marrow transplant recipients can be reduced by administration of prophylactic, low-dose, intravenous amphotericin B.

Another study, albeit small, was a double-blind, randomized, controlled trial in which patients undergoing HSCT received prophylactic, intravenous, low-dose amphotericin B (0.1 mg/kg/day) or placebo from the onset of neutropenia until the absolute neutrophil count remained above 500/ mm³.[66] Five of 18 patients (28%) randomized to placebo experienced documented systemic fungal infection within the first 30 days after transplantation, compared with none of 17 patients of the study arm (P = .045). There was no difference in the renal toxicity in either arm. Although there was a trend toward a shorter duration of empirical amphotericin B use in the study group, there was no difference in the number who required empirical use in the two arms.

Another prospective, randomized, placebo-controlled study assessed the efficacy, toxicity, and pharmacology of prophylactic low-dose amphotericin B given to 188 recipients of autologous HSCT.[67] The administration of low-dose amphotericin B significantly reduced the numbers of yeast colonizing the oropharyngeal area. Infusion-related side effects were significantly greater in the amphotericin B group. The mortality was higher in the placebo group, but

fungal infection as a cause of death was no different between the two groups.

Nasal or Nebulized Forms

Although it has been suggested that low-dose intravenous amphotericin B may have a beneficial effect on the prevention of fungal infection, its benefit is offset by the toxic effect of its use. Because the inhalation of fungal spores is the primary mode of pulmonary infection, it was postulated that nebulized or intranasal delivery of amphotericin B might prevent fungal infection in neutropenic patients while avoiding the side effects of this drug. Although nebulized amphotericin might be useful in preventing invasive pulmonary aspergillosis in neutropenic patients, especially those nursed on the open wards, when compared with historical controls,[68] this was not shown in a prospective, multicenter, randomized, placebo-controlled study.[69] Furthermore, 25% of patients stopped nebulized amphotericin B use because of side effects, and more bacterial pneumonia occurred in the studied group.

AmBisome

Formulation of amphotericin B in various lipid vehicles enables the delivery of a higher dosage of amphotericin B to target tissues with fewer systemic side effects. There are three such products available, and their efficacy and pharmacokinetics have been extensively reviewed.[70] Data, however, are lacking on these lipid-based amphotericin B preparations for primary prophylaxis of fungal infections in HSCT except for AmBisome (Nexstar, San Dimas, CA) (Table 38–7). A placebo-controlled, double-blind, randomized study of prophylactic intravenous AmBisome at 1 mg/ kg/day in 76 patients who underwent HSCT (36 in the AmBisome arm and 40 in the placebo arm) was carried out in Sweden.[71] The majority of the patients were recipients of allogeneic HSCT (30 and 33 in the AmBisome and placebo groups, respectively). The study drug was administered during the period of neutropenia (<500/mm³) until neutrophil recovery or an infection or toxicity end point was reached. Fungal colonization decreased in the study group (33%) and increased in the placebo group (62%, P = .05). Presumed fungal infection developed in five patients in the AmBisome arm and 7 patients in the placebo arm.

TABLE 38–7. SUMMARY OF PROPHYLACTIC LIPID-BASED AMPHOTERICIN B STUDIES IN HEMATOPOIETIC STEM CELL TRANSPLANTATION

REFERENCE	TYPE OF STUDY	PATIENTS	DOSAGE	FUNGAL COLONIZATION	SYSTEMIC FUNGAL INFECTION	SUPERFICIAL FUNGAL INFECTION	MORTALITY
Tollemar et al.[71]	Prophylactic double-blind, placebo-controlled, randomized study	AmBisome vs. placebo 36 vs. 40	1 mg/kg/day	↓	↔	Not addressed	Not addressed
Kelsey et al.[72]	Prophylactic double-blind, placebo-controlled, randomized study	AmBisome vs. placebo 75 vs. 88	2 mg/kg on alternate days	↓	↔	Not addressed	Not addressed

There was no statistical reduction of autopsy-proven fungal infection. Proven fungal infection developed in one patient receiving AmBisome (*C. guillermondi*) compared with three patients receiving placebo (*C. guillermondi*, 2; *C. albicans*, 1). The authors concluded that AmBisome at the dose of 1 mg/kg/day was well tolerated and reduced fungal colonization in recipients of HSCT.

Another double-blind, placebo-controlled study was carried out in the United Kingdom and Ireland when AmBisome, 2 mg/kg, was given on alternate days from day 1 of chemotherapy until neutrophil recovery to greater than 500/mm^3.[72] Of the 163 evaluable patients, 75 were randomized to receive AmBisome and 88 received placebo. Suspected fungal infection was no different between the two groups (32% vs. 41% in the AmBisome and placebo groups, respectively). Fungal isolates, however, were fewer in the AmBisome group (24%) compared with the placebo group (42%, $P < .05$).

EMPIRICAL THERAPY

The empirical treatment of presumed fungal infection in the febrile neutropenic patient is defined as introduction of an antifungal agent when the fever has failed to respond to broad-spectrum antibiotics for 4–7 days and appropriate investigations have failed to define a bacterial or viral cause.

Amphotericin B

A number of nonrandomized studies support the view of empirical use of amphotericin B in neutropenic fever unresponsive to broad-spectrum antibiotics; however, there were only two randomized studies on the use of amphotericin B as empirical therapy. Pizzo et al. addressed the role of continued antibiotics as well as empirical amphotericin B in 652 episodes of fever in 271 neutropenic patients.[73] After initial therapy with broad-spectrum antibiotics, 323 episodes (50%) were regarded as fever of unknown origin. Of those who had fever of unknown origin and remained febrile for 7 days on antibiotics, 50 patients were randomized either to stop antibiotics (n = 16), continue antibiotics until the fever settled (n = 16), or continue antibiotics with additional empirical amphotericin B therapy at 0.5 mg/kg daily (n = 18). There were six episodes of septic shock in the patients in whom antibiotics were discontinued compared with five fungal infections in patients who continued

to receive antibiotics. Two infections, including one fungal infection, developed in the group who received empirical amphotericin B. The authors concluded that because the risk of fungal infection remains high in febrile patients with prolonged granulocytopenia, empirical amphotericin B may be indicated.

Another randomized trial was performed by the European Organization for Research and Treatment of Cancer (EORTC) International Antimicrobial Therapy Cooperative Group.[74] In this study, 132 patients who remained febrile and granulocytopenic despite broad-spectrum antibiotics for 4 days were randomized to receive either additional empirical amphotericin B (n = 64) or the same antibiotics (n = 68). Amphotericin B was given at either 0.6 mg/kg daily or 1.2 mg/kg on alternate days. Although the mortality was no different between the two groups, there was only one case of fungemia in the empirical amphotericin B group as compared with six documented fungal infections in the antibiotic group ($P = .01$). These data suggest that it is beneficial to give amphotericin B to neutropenic patients who remain febrile despite broad-spectrum antibiotic use.

AmBisome

AmBisome has been used for the empirical treatment of febrile neutropenia in a number of trials and has proved to be far better tolerated and to produce fewer signs of nephrotoxicity than amphotericin B.[75] Furthermore, two large, randomized studies compared AmBisome with conventional amphotericin B (Table 38–8).

One such randomized study was conducted by Prentice et al. using AmBisome at 1 mg/kg/day and 3 mg/kg/day in comparison with amphotericin B at 1 mg/kg/day in two prospective trials involving 204 neutropenic children and 104 adults.[76] The study was primarily designed to determine the comparative safety of the formulations, and results showed clearly that there was an almost complete absence of severe adverse events with AmBisome (1% incidence vs. 12% with amphotericin B). There were also significantly fewer ($P < .01$) adverse events overall with AmBisome. Nephrotoxicity was significantly reduced in both AmBisome groups ($P < .01$), even in patients who were receiving other nephrotoxic drugs concomitantly. The overall clinical response to AmBisome at both dose levels was better than that in the amphotericin B group. Although there was no statistical difference when the 1-mg and 3-mg dosages of AmBisome combined were compared with conventional

TABLE 38–8. SUMMARY OF EMPIRIC USE OF LIPID-BASED AMPHOTERICIN B IN NEUTROPENIC FEVER

	PRENTICE ET AL.[76]			**WALSH ET AL.**[77]		**WHITE ET AL.**[78]	
Study type	Randomized empiric AmBisome vs. conventional amphotericin B			Double-blind empiric AmBisome vs. conventional amphotericin B		Double-blind empiric Amphocil vs. conventional amphotericin B	
Study drug and dosage	AmBisome 1 mg/kg	AmBisome 3 mg/kg	Amphotericin B 1 mg/kg	AmBisome 3 mg/kg	Amphotericin B 0.6 mg/kg	Amphocil 4 mg/kg	Amphotericin B 0.8 mg/kg
Number of patients	118	118	118	343	344	98	95
Response	58% ↔	64% ↑	49%	50% ↔	49%	50% ↔	43%
Survival	89.8% ↔	89.8% ↔	87.5%	93% ↔	90%	↔	
Infusion-related toxicity	1% ↓	1% ↓	12%	17–18% ↓	44–54%	80% ↑	65%
Nephrotoxicity	10% ↓	12% ↓	24%	19% ↓	34%	↓	

amphotericin B (*P* = .09), there was a significant difference between the 3-mg dose and conventional amphotericin B (*P* = .03).

Another well-designed, randomized, double-blind, multicenter study comparing the empirical use of AmBisome, 3 mg/kg/day, with amphotericin B, 0.6 mg/kg/day, in 687 neutropenic patients, approximately half of whom had received HSCT, was completed in 1997.[77] The composite rates of success were similar in the two groups studied (50% of patients who received AmBisome [n = 343] and 49% of patients who received conventional amphotericin B [n = 344]). There was no difference in the outcome of the empirical treatment with AmBisome and conventional amphotericin groups with regard to survival (93% vs. 90%) and resolution of fever (58% for both groups). Proven breakthrough fungal infection, however, was less in the AmBisome group (3%) compared with the conventional amphotericin B group (8%, *P* = .009). Infusion-related toxicity was far less in the AmBisome-treated patients, with the incidence of fever and chills or rigors after infusion being 17% and 18% compared with 44% and 54% in the amphotericin B group, respectively. Nephrotoxicity was also significantly higher after amphotericin B administration (19% vs. 34%, *P* < .001). The authors concluded that AmBisome is as effective as conventional amphotericin B for empirical antifungal therapy in febrile neutropenia and is associated with fewer breakthrough fungal infections, less nephrotoxicity, and less infusion-related toxicity. After this study, AmBisome at 3 mg/kg daily became the only antifungal agent to have a licensed indication as empirical therapy in febrile neutropenia.

Amphocil

Another lipid-based form of amphotericin is amphotericin B colloidal dispersion (ABCD; Amphocil, Sequus Pharmaceuticals, Menlo Park, CA). A prospective, randomized, double-blind clinical trial comparing Amphocil and conventional amphotericin B in the empirical treatment of neutropenic fever for more than 3 days despite broad-spectrum antibiotics was published in 1998.[78] Of the 193 evaluable patients, 98 received Amphocil, 4 mg/kg daily,

and 95 received conventional amphotericin B, 0.8 mg/kg daily. There was no difference in therapeutic response: 50% of Amphocil-treated patients and 43% of amphotericin B–treated patients responded (*P* = .31). The development of renal toxicity was more frequent in amphotericin B recipients (*P* < .001). Infusion-related adverse effects, however, were more common in patients who received Amphocil. Chills were more common in Amphocil-treated patients (80%) compared with amphotericin-treated patients (65%, *P* = .018). Hypoxia was noted more in Amphocil-treated patients (13 of 98) compared with amphotericin-treated patients (3 of 95, *P* = .013). This study showed no benefit of Amphocil over conventional amphotericin B in the outcome of empirical therapy except less nephrotoxicity. Furthermore, Amphocil caused more infusion-related adverse effects and was more costly.

Abelcet

No data are available on primary prophylaxis or empirical therapy regarding the lipid formulation Abelcet despite its therapeutic use in the treatment of fungal infection.[79–82] The result of an ongoing trial in North America on the use of low-dose Abelcet as primary prophylaxis of fungal infection in recipients of allogeneic HSCT is eagerly awaited.

Up to the end of 1998, there were no data on the head-to-head comparison of lipid-based formulations of amphotericin B in the management of fungal infection. Wingard et al., however, presented such data at the focus group of a fungal infection meeting in March 1999 from a double-blind study comparing AmBisome and Abelcet as empirical therapy in febrile neutropenic patients.[83] In this study, patients were randomized to receive AmBisome, 3 mg/kg (n = 85), AmBisome, 5 mg/kg (n = 81), or Abelcet, 5 mg/kg (n = 78), every day. Both mean and trough levels of serum amphotericin B were higher in the AmBisome arms compared with the Abelcet arm. The overall success rate was no different in the three groups (40%, 42%, and 33% in the AmBisome 3 mg/kg, AmBisome 5 mg/kg, and Abelcet 5 mg/kg arms, respectively). Side effects, however, including infusion-related toxicity and nephrotoxicity, were higher in the Abelcet group compared with the AmBisome groups. The authors concluded that AmBisome, either 3 mg/kg or 5 mg/kg daily, is associated with significantly less toxicity than Abelcet, 5 mg/kg daily.

SECONDARY PROPHYLAXIS

Recurrence of invasive fungal infection during subsequent chemotherapy or HSCT has become increasingly common. Treatment of acute leukemia often includes high-dose cytosine arabinoside during remission induction, which leads to prolonged neutropenia and which in turn increases the likelihood of invasive fungal infection. Fungal pneumonia recurred during 52% of neutropenic episodes due to subsequent chemotherapy.[62] Therefore, patients who have previously had invasive fungal infections are at high risk for recurrence of infection during subsequent chemotherapy or HSCT. Although various modalities of prevention of recurrence have been tried, including intravenous amphotericin B, intravenous lipid-based amphotericin B, itraconazole, and surgical excision of the fungal infection, the best approach to secondary prophylaxis remains to be determined.[84–86]

The landmark paper on secondary prophylaxis was published in 1988.[87] The authors used a combination of conventional amphotericin B, 1 mg/kg daily, with 5-flucytosine started 2 days before subsequent chemotherapy as secondary prophylaxis in 9 of 10 patients with acute myeloid leukemia and previous invasive fungal infection. Seven patients did not experience recurrence of invasive fungal infection despite the fact that only a partial response was achieved with primary antifungal therapy in two patients. One patient who had not received secondary prophylaxis experienced a fatal reactivation of invasive fungal infection. Two of the remaining nine patients who received secondary prophylaxis experienced a recurrence but responded to further antifungal therapy.

Despite the fact that the risk of fungal reactivation is well known, large studies on the prevention of fungal infections in HSCT recipients have not addressed the issue of previous fungal infection.[49, 50] Furthermore, this variable is not analyzed in studies aimed at risk factors involved in the development of invasive fungal infection after HSCT.[8, 48, 88]

Because the actual risk of reactivation of fungal infection during HSCT is unknown and there are no guidelines on the ethical acceptability of HSCT in recipients with previous invasive fungal infections, the European Blood and Marrow Transplant Registry (EBMT) performed a retrospective analysis in conjunction with the EORTC on this issue.[86] In this retrospective study, the authors found recurrence in 16 of 48 HSCT recipients who previously had invasive fungal infection (33%). This is lower than the expected number of recurrences. Reactivation, however, was fatal in 14 of 16 patients (88%). The authors concluded that a history of previous invasive fungal infection is not a formal contraindication to subsequent HSCT. Furthermore, they found that there was no clear role of surgical resection of residual lesions.[89, 90] The authors could not determine the best prophylactic approach, but they suggested that secondary

prophylaxis with either itraconazole or some form of intravenous amphotericin B might lead to a lower incidence of recurrence.

Hoover et al. also found no recurrence in seven of eight pediatric patients who underwent HSCT with ongoing antifungal prophylaxis after receiving aggressive antifungal therapy for invasive fungal infections with or without surgical excision of residual fungal infections.[91] In contrast, Martino et al. suggested resection of residual cavities or nodules, which invariably contain viable fungi, prior to HSCT and giving antifungal prophylaxis during the peritransplant period.[92]

Our own series of 14 patients received Abelcet, 1 mg/kg, daily (n = 6), on alternate days (n = 11), or both (n = 8) as secondary prophylaxis during 25 subsequent episodes of prolonged neutropenia (chemotherapy n = 19, autologous HSCT n = 4, sibling allogeneic HSCT n = 1, matched unrelated donor transplantation n = 1).[93] The duration of neutropenia was 4–34 days (median, 17 days). With this approach, we managed to prevent recurrence of pulmonary fungal infection during 24 episodes of neutropenia in 11 patients, including 2 patients who had undergone surgical resection for residual lesions and who had previously received Abelcet, 5 mg/kg/day, for the treatment of invasive fungal infections, although either *Aspergillus fumigatus* was cultured from the serum or the *Aspergillus* antigen test result was positive in 4 patients. The one patient who experienced recurrence had previously been treated with conventional amphotericin B for primary fungal pneumonia, and the recurrence was successfully treated with a therapeutic dose of Abelcet (5 mg/kg/day) during autologous HSCT.

In summary, patients with a previous history of invasive fungal infection can safely receive further intensive chemotherapy and even proceed to HSCT (sibling donor or matched unrelated donor allogeneic transplantation or autologous peripheral blood progenitor cell transplantation), provided they have recovered from fungal infection after antifungal therapy with radiologic and clinical resolution. The role of surgery and secondary prophylaxis need to be defined with prospective randomized studies.

GROWTH FACTORS

The administration of recombinant colony-stimulating factors (CSF) such as granulocyte CSF (G-CSF) and granulocyte-macrophage CSF (GM-CSF) has been shown to shorten the duration of neutropenia. Furthermore, GM-CSF might be useful as an adjunctive treatment of fungal infection.[31, 94–96] No data, however, are available on the prophylactic use of growth factors in invasive fungal infection.

SUMMARY OF THE REVIEWS OF PREVENTION OF FUNGAL INFECTION IN HSCT

Numerous review papers have examined the role of prophylaxis of fungal infections in HSCT recipients.[84, 97–107] Furthermore, the Working Party of the British Society for Antimicrobial Chemotherapy published guidelines on the chemoprophylaxis[108] and therapy[109] of deep fungal infection in neutropenia and transplantation. Likewise, a consensus paper on the management and prevention of severe candidal infections has been published.[110] By and large, most of the review papers agreed on the use of either high-efficiency particulate air (HEPA) ventilation or laminar air flow (LAF) ventilation in the prevention of *Aspergillus* infection, especially in the presence of construction sites in the vicinity. Fluconazole, 400 mg daily, is recommended starting from day 1 of neutropenia until neutrophil recovery for the prevention of fluconazole-sensitive *Candida* infections.[105, 110]

The most controversial publication is the meta-analysis of prophylactic or empirical antifungal treatment versus placebo or no treatment in patients with cancer complicated by neutropenia.[111] Gotzsche et al. reviewed 24 randomized trials with 2758 patients and found 434 deaths, concluding that antifungal prophylaxis had no effect on mortality (odds ratio, 0.92; 95% CI, 0.74–1.14), although amphotericin B decreased mortality in their analysis. They also found that both amphotericin B and fluconazole decreased the incidence of invasive fungal infections. They went on and questioned the current approach of prophylactic or empirical treatment with antifungal agents for fear of death if treatment is delayed. They recommended the use of antifungal agents only in patients with proved fungal infections or in patients participating in the randomized trials. Their meta-analysis combined prophylaxis, different empirical approaches, and earlier trials of oral nonabsorbable amphotericin with empirical intravenous amphotericin; hence, it is not a surprise to find prophylaxis ineffectiveness. Kibbler et al. rightly questioned the validity of the meta-analysis because it is inappropriate to combine different antifungal strategies in the same systematic review.[112] They suggest that empirical intravenous amphotericin reduces mortality and that prophylactic fluconazole reduces both superficial and invasive fungal infections but not mortality. In addition, this superficial meta-analysis was superseded by a more comprehensive analysis that confirmed the effectiveness of fluconazole in reducing the rate of systemic fungal infection and mortality compared with nonabsorbable polyenes and placebo.[113]

PNEUMOCYSTIS CARINII PNEUMONIA

Pneumocystis carinii, long believed to be a protozoan, is today classified as a lower order fungus.[114] *P. carinii* pneumonia (PCP) occurs in 85% of patients with AIDS, although in patients with hematologic disorders it is most commonly associated with HSCT, leukemia, lymphoma, primary immunodeficiency, and treatment with steroids. Mycophenylate mofetil, which has become a first-line agent for the prevention of GVHD although it has been used in solid organ transplantation for some time, may have intrinsic anti–*P. carinii* activity, in contrast with tacrolimus (FK506), which increases its growth in vitro.[115] Without effective prophylaxis, PCP occurs in 5–15% of HSCT recipients with a mortality rate of 60%.[116] In recent years, the prophylactic use of co-trimoxazole (trimethoprim-sulfamethoxazole, or TPM/SMX) has almost completely eliminated this disease in recipients of HSCT. Documented PCP predominantly occurs only when chemoprophylaxis is interrupted because of poor compliance or intolerance of TMP/SMX.

Asymptomatic infection with *Pneumocystis* occurs early in life. Circulating antibodies are detected in children by the age of 2–3 years, presumably via airborne transmission. Hence, lifelong latency is established in the pulmonary alveoli. If immunity does not develop from asymptomatic infection, when the host becomes immunocompromised reinfection occurs in the absence of adequate host defense.

In hematologic patients undergoing chemotherapy and in HSCT recipients, infection typically presents as a rapidly progressive disease, with severe hypoxia and dyspnea developing within 5–10 days of initial manifestations. Patients receiving immunosuppressive drugs frequently experience these clinical manifestations after steroids have been tapered. In contrast, in patients with AIDS, the onset is more subtle than in cancer patients, with symptoms lasting from weeks to months.

The mainstay of prevention of PCP is medical prophylaxis starting around 7 days after sustained engraftment (i.e., day +30) until day +180 in recipients of autologous bone marrow or peripheral blood progenitor cell transplants but longer in recipients of allogeneic HSCT if the patients are on immunosuppressive therapy for chronic GVHD.

TMP/SMX remains the drug of choice for prophylaxis of PCP. With a single-strength TMP/SMX tablet daily (TMP, 80 mg with SMX, 400 mg) or a double-strength tablet daily (TMP, 80 mg with SMX, 800 mg), a wide variety of opportunistic infections are prevented: those caused by *P. carinii*, *Toxoplasma gondii*, *Listeria monocytogenes*, *Isospora belli*, and many other pathogens. One double-strength TMP/SMX tablet three times a week is equally effective. TMP/SMX, however, is associated with adverse side effects, including nausea, vomiting, bone marrow suppression, renal toxicity, and skin rashes. A meta-analysis of 35 randomized trials of PCP prophylaxis have shown that the risk of discontinuation of TMP/SMX decreased by 43% if one double-strength tablet was given three times a week instead of daily.[117] Aerosolized pentamidine is well tolerated and is used frequently if patients experience side effects from TMP/SMX but is inferior to TMP/SMX as a prophylactic agent.[117] Furthermore, oral prophylaxis including regimens based on TMP/SMX and dapsone reduced the number of cases of toxoplasmosis by 30% when compared with aerosolized pentamidine.[117] The agents used for prophylaxis of PCP are summarized in Table 38–9, and the indications for their use are given in Table 38–10.

PREVENTION OF FUNGAL INFECTION IN THE MILLENNIUM: PRACTICAL GUIDELINES

Systemic fungal infection remains an increasing problem in patients with immunosuppressive chemotherapy or undergoing HSCT. Associated mortality had come down to a rate of 40–50% from more than 90% when Denning and Stevens reviewed the literature in 1990.[85] Furthermore, 25–40% of neutropenic patients with persistent or recurrent fever without prophylactic antifungal therapy have evidence of fungal invasion in the bloodstream and/or the tissues.[118] Therefore, strategies for prevention of fungal infection

TABLE 38–9. PROPHYLAXIS OF *PNEUMOCYSTIS CARINII* PNEUMONIA

Trimethoprim/sulfamethoxazole (TMP/SMX)	One double-strength tablet daily *or* One single-strength tablet daily *or* One double-strength tablet 3 times/week
Dapsone (second choice)	100 mg daily PO once a week
Atovaquone (Mepron)	750-mg suspension daily PO
Pentamidine	300 mg every 4 wk (nebulized)
Dapsone plus pyrimethamine	200 mg/wk plus 75 mg/wk (weekly dose of leukovorin)

should include removal of the potential environmental source, including careful hand washing, housing of high-risk patients in HEPA or LAF ventilation, primary medical prophylaxis involving fluconazole and/or itraconazole, empirical therapy with intravenous conventional or lipid formulations of amphotericin B, and secondary prophylaxis with prophylactic amphotericin B or oral itraconazole solution.

WHICH PATIENTS REQUIRE PROPHYLAXIS?

1. Antifungal prophylaxis is recommended for patients who are expected to have severe neutropenia (neutrophil count below 100/mm^3 for 1 week) or neutropenia (neutrophil count between 100 and 500/mm^3 for 2 weeks). These should include patients with acute leukemia or myelodysplastic syndrome undergoing intensive chemotherapy.
2. Because the incidence of invasive fungal infection depends not only on the severity of neutropenia but on the type of transplantation, antifungal prophylaxis may not be required for patients undergoing autologous peripheral blood progenitor cell transplantation, especially for solid tumors. If, however, the patient has a previous history of fungal infection during chemotherapy for acute leukemia, secondary prophylaxis is essential during autologous peripheral blood progenitor cell or BMT to prevent reactivation of invasive fungal infection.
3. For patients undergoing either allogeneic sibling donor transplantation or matched unrelated donor transplantation, antifungal prophylaxis is of vital importance, including housing patients in either HEPA or LAF ventilation and medical prophylaxis.

TABLE 38–10. INDICATIONS FOR PROPHYLAXIS OF *PNEUMOCYSTIC CARNII* PNEUMONIA

All recipients of allogeneic HSCT for 6 months; longer in patients with chronic graft-versus-host disease on immunosuppression
All recipients of autologous bone marrow or PBPC for 6 months
Acute lymphoblastic leukemia patients during induction and maintenance therapy
Trimethoprim/sulfamethoxazole must be stopped 2 weeks prior to high-dose methotrexate therapy for central nervous system prophylaxis in acute lymphoblastic leukemia
Patients on fludarabine or 2-chlorodeoxyadenosine therapy; continue prophylaxis for 1–2 yr, depending on recovery of CD4 count

PHYSICAL MEASURES

No amount of sophisticated measures are of any use in the prevention of invasive fungal infection in patients undergoing HSCT if doctors, nurses, other health care workers, and visitors do not wash their hands adequately.

The current trend is to perform autologous peripheral blood progenitor cell transplantation as an outpatient procedure, and sooner or later minitransplant (allogeneic HSCT after nonmyeloablative conditioning) will be performed as an outpatient procedure. In the meantime, patients undergoing conventional allogeneic bone marrow or peripheral blood progenitor cell transplantation from either a sibling or a matched unrelated donor should ideally be housed in a place with HEPA or LAF ventilation.

The value of surveillance cultures in the prediction of *Aspergillus* infections is controversial. The conclusion drawn from several studies, however, is that a positive culture for *Aspergillus* in a profoundly immunocompromised patient is highly suggestive of invasive disease.[102] The value of surveillance cultures in prediction of *Candida* infections has been the subject of debate. It has been shown, however, that in recipients of HSCT and patients with leukemia, there is a strong correlation between the development of systemic candidiasis and positive surveillance cultures.

FLUCONAZOLE OR ITRACONAZOLE

Autologous Bone Marrow or Peripheral Blood Progenitor Cell Transplantation

In autologous BMT, it is advisable to give fluconazole for *albicans* species or itraconazole for non-*albicans* species to patients in whom surveillance cultures are positive. Despite the results of two large randomized studies of fluconazole, 400 mg daily, in prophylaxis of fungal infection in recipients of HSCT,[49, 50] it may suffice to use half the dose in a majority of the cases.[119–122]

Fluconazole should be started with the conditioning regimen and should be continued either well after hematologic recovery is maintained (usually day 35) or when amphotericin B is given empirically or therapeutically. It must be used with caution in patients with liver impairment. Because it is predominantly excreted in the urine as unchanged drug, a dose adjustment of fluconazole is required in patients with renal impairment. There is no significant impairment of fluconazole absorption, even after total body irradiation, when it is taken with food, antacids, and cimetidine. The dosage of certain drugs, however, should be adjusted—including cyclosporine and phenytoin—after monitoring the drug level. Co-administration of terfenadine and cisapride is contraindicated in patients receiving fluconazole.

Allogeneic Bone Marrow or Peripheral Blood Progenitor Cell Transplantation (Sibling or Unrelated Donor)

Fluconazole, even at the dose of 400 mg/day, will not prevent *Aspergillus* infection in recipients of allogeneic

HSCT. Furthermore, it has been suggested that the incidence of *Aspergillus* infection may increase in patients who receive prophylactic fluconazole during HSCT. Therefore, itraconazole oral solution is preferable, despite the lack of randomized studies, in recipients of allogeneic HSCT because of its broader spectrum of activity against fungi.[61, 108, 123]

It is known that itraconazole in capsule form is associated with erratic absorption. Because the itraconazole molecule is virtually insoluble, the liquid is prepared by addition of hydroxypropyl-β-cyclodextrin, resulting in better absorption,[59–61] and therapeutic monitoring is no longer required. One caution of note is that the desired serum level is achieved only after day 8 of itraconazole, 2.5 mg/kg, and the achievement of the desired level is especially relevant in patients who have had previous fungal infection because of a high rate of reactivation. The steady state of itraconazole, however, can be achieved by day 1 after a loading dose of intravenous itraconazole, 200 mg BID for 2 days, followed by once-a-day administration from days 3–7. Thereafter, the oral solution of itraconazole is maintained at 200 mg daily.[63]

Itraconazole liquid should be taken without food. Itraconazole appears to have more gastrointestinal side effects than fluconazole. Itraconazole is predominantly metabolized in the liver, and liver enzymes should be monitored regularly. The following drugs should not be given concurrently with itraconazole: terfenadine, astemizole, cisapride, pimozide, and HMG-CoA reductase inhibitors.[123] Midazolam is contraindicated in patients receiving itraconazole.[124] When it is co-administered with enzyme-inducing drugs such as phenytoin (busulfan-cyclophosphamide conditioning regimen) and rifampicin, the itraconazole level may be subtherapeutic; therefore, it is essential to monitor the level. Cyclosporine and tacrolimus dosages need to be monitored and reduced if necessary when itraconazole is given concomitantly. Itraconazole can also lead to toxic effects of vincristine[125, 126] as well as busulfan.[127]

Although it is customary to give antifungal prophylaxis during the period of neutropenia, only the following patients may require long-term prophylaxis: patients with GVHD, patients undergoing unrelated donor transplantation, patients who have received profoundly immunosuppressive chemotherapy (e.g., a fludarabine-containing regimen such as FLAG or induction chemotherapy for acute lymphocytic leukemia), patients receiving corticosteroids, and patients with a history of previous invasive fungal infection.

Amphotericin B

Until tools for the diagnosis of invasive fungal infection are improved, empirical therapy with amphotericin will remain an important part of prevention of fungal infection in recipients of HSCT.[73, 74, 76, 77, 109] The timing of starting empirical therapy varies among the different investigators, but there is enough evidence to start after 72–96 hours of neutropenic fever of unknown origin unresponsive to broad-spectrum antibiotics.[76, 77, 109] The role of prophylactic amphotericin B in different routes, including intravenous low-dose prophylaxis, nasal, or nebulized forms, is unknown.

In patients with normal renal function, intravenous amphotericin B remains the drug of choice as empirical therapy. Amphotericin should be started at a dose of 0.6–1 mg/kg body weight given daily in 500 mL of 5% dextrose over 4 hours as an intravenous infusion after a test dose of 1 mg in 80 mL of 5% dextrose over 30–60 minutes to identify hypersensitive patients.[109] The rate of infusion may be increased after 7 days so that it can be given over 1–2 hours. Although it is possible to give a 2-hour infusion instead of a 4-hour infusion with hydrocortisone and antihistamine cover,[128] the widespread use of steroids should be discouraged because it is one of the risk factors for invasive fungal infection. Furthermore, it has been suggested that the transfusion of platelets at least 2 hours after the completion of amphotericin B administration decreases the detrimental effect of this antifungal agent on transfused platelet recovery and survival.[129]

Acute side effects such as chills and fever, albeit common, can be prevented or lessened by a slow intravenous injection of pethidine, 25–50 mg, and a slow intravenous injection of chlorpheniramine, 10–20 mg.

Renal side effects are common. Hypokalemia and hypomagnesemia may be prevented by oral administration of amiloride, 10–20 mg daily, but intravenous potassium and magnesium may be required. Thirty to forty percent of patients may experience a reversible increased serum creatinine level that requires careful monitoring, especially if concomitant nephrotoxic drugs such as cyclosporine, tacrolimus, and aminoglycoside antibiotics are used. When the serum creatinine exceeds two to three times the pretreatment baseline (less in children), a change to AmBisome or Abelcet is recommended (see later).

LIPID FORMULATIONS OF AMPHOTERICIN B

AmBisome appears to be the drug of choice for empirical therapy in recipients of HSCT.[76, 77, 83] Abelcet may have more side effects than AmBisome,[83] and Amphocil is associated with more side effects than conventional amphotericin B.[78] Furthermore, AmBisome is the only licensed drug to be used as empirical therapy at a dose of 3 mg/kg daily. AmBisome at 1 mg/kg/day, however, is as effective as 3 mg/kg/day as empirical therapy in neutropenic fever of unknown origin.[76] In addition, it is economically viable to use AmBisome, 1 mg/kg/day, as empirical therapy according to current evidence. Therefore, AmBisome, 1 mg/kg/day, is recommended as empirical therapy if renal insufficiency either exists at the outset or ensues after initial amphotericin B therapy (Fig. 38–1). A higher dose of AmBisome (3–5 mg/kg daily),[130–132] Abelcet (5 mg/kg daily),[79–82] or Amphocil (4–6 mg/kg daily)[133] is recommended for therapeutic use.

SECONDARY PROPHYLAXIS

Patients with a previous history of invasive fungal infection can safely receive further intensive chemotherapy and even proceed to HSCT provided they have recovered from fungal infection. Although the definite role of surgery and secondary prophylaxis need to be defined with prospective ran-

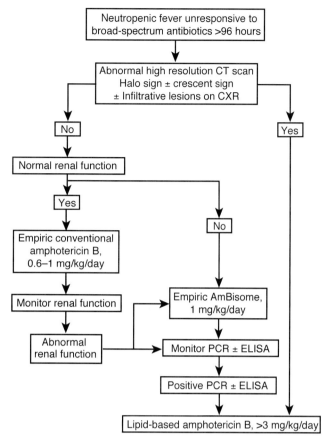

FIGURE 38–1. Flow chart for empiric antifungal therapy in hematopoietic stem cell transplant recipients.

domized studies, the residual cavitary lesions in the lungs should be removed surgically before HSCT is attempted. Intravenous amphotericin B appears to be the drug of choice in this situation,[87] but itraconazole oral solution could be an alternative.

CONCLUSION

The prevention of invasive fungal infection remains a challenge for physicians performing HSCT. No single measure is adequate to prevent invasive fungal infection. Therefore, the strategy includes a combination of physical measures, including housing patients in HEPA or LAF ventilation and careful hand washing; medical prophylaxis, including fluconazole and itraconazole; empirical therapy, including intravenous amphotericin B and AmBisome; and secondary measures, including intravenous amphotericin B use and surgical excision of residual fungal lesions. The results of ongoing clinical trials with newer antifungal agents such as voriconazole, SCH 56592, echinocandins (MK 0991, FK 463), pradimicin, and nikkomycin are eagerly awaited.

REFERENCES

1. Castagnola E, Bucci B, Montinaro E, Viscoli C: Fungal infections in patients undergoing bone marrow transplantation: an approach to a rational management protocol. Bone Marrow Transplant 18(Suppl 2): 97, 1996.
2. Morrison VA, Haake RJ, Weisdorf DJ: The spectrum of non-*Candida* fungal infections following bone marrow transplantation. Medicine (Baltimore) 72:78, 1993.
3. Odds FC: *Candida* infections: an overview. Crit Rev Microbiol 15:1, 1987.
4. Coleman DC, Sullivan DJ, Bennett DE, et al: Candidiasis: the emergence of a novel species, *Candida dubliniensis*. AIDS 11:557, 1997.
5. Meis JM, Runke M, De Pauw B, et al: *Candida dubliniensis* candidemia in patients with chemotherapy-induced neutropenia and bone marrow transplantation. Emerging Infectious Disease, CDC (Electronic citation), 1999.
6. Warnock DW: Fungal complications of transplantation: diagnosis, treatment and prevention. J Antimicrob Chemother 36(Suppl B):73, 1995.
7. Goodrich JM, Reed EC, Mori M, et al: Clinical features and analysis of risk factors for invasive candidal infection after marrow transplantation. J Infect Dis 164:731, 1991.
8. Morrison VA, Haake RJ, Weisdorf DJ: Non-*Candida* fungal infections after bone marrow transplantation: risk factors and outcome. Am J Med 96:497, 1994.
9. Kuhlman JE, Fishman EK, Siegelman SS: Invasive pulmonary aspergillosis in acute leukemia: characteristic findings on CT, the CT halo sign and the role of CT in early diagnosis. Radiology 157:611, 1985.
10. Logan PM, Miuller NL: CT manifestations of pulmonary aspergillosis. Crit Rev Diagn Imaging 37:1, 1996.
11. Worthy SA, Flint JD, Mller NL: Pulmonary complications after bone marrow transplantation: high-resolution CT and pathologic findings. Radiographics 17:1359, 1997.
12. Walsh TJ, Hier DB, Caplan LR: Aspergillosis of the central nervous system: clinicopathological analysis of 17 patients. Ann Neurol 18:574, 1985.
13. Mutton KJ, Lucas TJ, Harkness JL: Disseminated *Fusarium* infection. Med J Aust 2:624, 1980.
14. Blazar BR, Hurd DD, Snover DC, et al: Invasive *Fusarium* infections in bone marrow transplant recipients. Am J Med 77:645, 1984.
15. Boutati EI, Anaissie EJ: *Fusarium*, a significant emerging pathogen in patients with hematologic malignancy: ten years' experience at a cancer center and implications for management. Blood 90:999, 1997.
16. June CH, Beatty PG, Shulman HM, Rinaldi MG: Disseminated *Fusarium moniliforme* infection after allogeneic marrow transplantation. South Med J 79:513, 1986.
17. Nelson PE, Dignani MC, Anaissie EJ: Taxonomy, biology and clinical aspects of *Fusarium* species. Clin Microbiol Rev 7:479, 1994.
18. Minor RL, Pfaller MA, Gingrich RD, Burns LJ: Disseminated *Fusarium* infections in patients following bone marrow transplantation. Bone Marrow Transplant 4:653, 1989.
19. Anaissie EJ, Kantarjian H, Ro J, et al: The emerging role of *Fusarium* infections in patients with cancer. Medicine 67:77, 1988.
20. Parfrey NA: Improved diagnosis and prognosis of mucormycosis: a clinicopathological study of 33 cases. Medicine 65:113, 1986.
21. Greenberg MR, Lippman SM, Grinnell VS, et al: Computed tomographic findings in orbital mucor. West J Med 143:102, 1985.
22. Guyotat D, Piens MA, Bouvier R, Fiere D: A case of disseminated *Scedosporium apiospermum* infection after bone marrow transplantation. Mykosen 30:151, 1987.
23. Gumbart CH: *Pseudallescheria boydii* infection after bone marrow transplantation. Ann Intern Med 99:193, 1983.
24. Salesa R, Burgos A, Ondiviela R, et al: Fatal disseminated infection by *Scedosporium inflatum* after bone marrow transplantation. Scand J Infect Dis 25:389, 1993.
25. Bouza E, Munoz P, Vega L, et al: Clinical resolution of *Scedosporium prolificans* fungemia associated with reversal of neutropenia following administration of granulocyte colony-stimulating factor. Clin Infect Dis 23:192, 1996.
26. Winston DJ, Balsley GE, Rhodes J, Linne SR: Disseminated *Trichosporon capitatum* infection in an immunosuppressed host. Arch Intern Med 137:1192, 1977.
27. Lowenthal RM, Atkinson K, Challis DR, et al: Invasive *Trichosporon cutaneum* infection: an increasing problem in immunosuppressed patients. Bone Marrow Transplant 2:321, 1987.
28. Siegert W, Henze G, Wagner J, et al: Invasive *Trichosporon cutaneum*

(beigelii) infection in a patient with relapsed acute myeloid leukemia undergoing bone marrow transplantation. Transplantation 46:151, 1988.

29. Anaissie EJ, Bodey GP: Disseminated trichosporonosis: meeting the challenge. Eur J Clin Microbiol Infect Dis 10:711, 1991.
30. Walsh TJ: Trichosporonosis. Infect Dis Clin North Am 3:43, 1989.
31. Naum S, Petursson SR, Weinbaum D, Rosenfeld CS: Long-term survival after allogeneic bone marrow transplantation complicated by trichosporonosis. South Med J 87:286, 1994.
32. Orth B, Frei R, Itin PH, et al: Outbreak of invasive mycoses caused by *Paecilomyces lilacinus* from a contaminated skin lotion. Ann Intern Med 125:799, 1996.
33. Lundstrom TS, Fairfax MR, Dugan MC, et al: *Phialophora verrucosa* infection in a BMT patient. Bone Marrow Transplant 20:789, 1997.
34. Lonial S, Williams L, Carrum G, et al: *Neosartorya fischeri:* an invasive fungal pathogen in an allogeneic bone marrow transplant patient. Bone Marrow Transplant 19:753, 1997.
35. Goss G, Grigg A, Rathbone P, Slavin M: *Hansenula anomala* infection after bone marrow transplantation. Bone Marrow Transplant 14:995, 1994.
36. Thuler LC, Faivichenco S, Velasco E, et al: Fungaemia caused by *Hansenula anomala*—an outbreak in a cancer hospital. Mycoses 40:193, 1997.
37. Tsai TW, Hammond LA, Rinaldi M, et al: *Cokeromyces recurvatus* infection in a bone marrow transplant recipient. Bone Marrow Transplant 19:301, 1997.
38. Emmens RK, Richardson D, Thomas W, et al: Necrotizing cerebritis in an allogeneic bone marrow transplant recipient due to *Cladophialophora bantiana.* J Clin Microbiol 34:1330, 1996.
39. Phillips P, Wood WS, Phillips G, Rinaldi MG: Invasive hyalohyphomycosis caused by *Scopulariopsis brevicaulis* in a patient undergoing allogeneic bone marrow transplant. Diagn Microbiol Infect Dis 12:429, 1989.
40. Neglia JP, Hurd DD, Ferrieri P, Snover DC: Invasive *Scopulariopsis* in the immunocompromised host. Am J Med 83:1163, 1987.
41. Gerson SL, Talbot GH, Hurwitz S, et al: Prolonged granulocytopenia: the major risk factor for invasive pulmonary aspergillosis in patients with acute leukaemia. Ann Intern Med 100:345, 1984.
42. Samonis G, Rolston K, Karl C, et al: Prophylaxis of oropharyngeal candidiasis with fluconazole. Rev Infect Dis 12(Suppl 3):369, 1990.
43. Toren A, Or R, Ackerstein A, Nagler A: Invasive fungal infections in lymphoma patients receiving immunotherapy following autologous bone marrow transplantation (ABMT). Bone Marrow Transplant 20:67, 1997.
44. Strausbaugh L J, Sewell DL, Ward TT, et al: High frequency of yeast carriage on hands of hospital personnel. J Clin Microbiol 32:2299, 1994.
45. De Bock R, Gyseens I, Peetermans M, Nolard N: *Aspergillus* in pepper. Lancet 2:331, 1989.
46. Sherertz RJ, Belani A, Kramer BS, et al: Impact of air filtration on nosocomial *Aspergillus* infections. Am J Med 83:709, 1987.
47. Barnes RA, Rogers TR: Control of an outbreak of nosocomial aspergillosis by laminar air-flow isolation. J Hosp Infect 14:89, 1989.
48. Wald A, Leisenring W, van Burik JA, Bowden R: Epidemiology of *Aspergillus* infections in a large cohort of patients undergoing bone marrow transplantation. J Infect Dis 175:1459, 1997.
49. Goodman JL, Winston DJ, Greenfield RA, et al: A controlled trial of fluconazole to prevent fungal infections in patients undergoing bone marrow transplantation [see comments]. N Engl J Med 326:845, 1992.
50. Slavin MA, Osborne B, Adams R, et al: Efficacy and safety of fluconazole prophylaxis for fungal infections after marrow transplantation—a prospective, randomized, double-blind study. J Infect Dis 171:1545, 1995.
51. Winston DJ, Chandrasekar PH, Lazarus HM, et al: Fluconazole prophylaxis of fungal infections in patients with acute leukemia: results of a randomized placebo-controlled, double-blind, multicenter trial. Ann Intern Med 118:495, 1993.
52. Wingard JR, Merz WG, Rinaldi MG, et al: Increase in *Candida krusei* infection among patients with bone marrow transplantation and neutropenia treated prophylactically with fluconazole. N Engl J Med 325:1274, 1991.
53. Wingard JR, Merz WG, Rinaldi MG, et al: Association of *Torulopsis glabrata* infections with fluconazole prophylaxis in neutropenic bone

marrow transplant patients. Antimicrob Agents Chemother 37:1847, 1993.
54. Hitchcock CA, Pye GW, Troke PF, et al: Fluconazole resistance in *Candida glabrata.* Antimicrob Agents Chemother 37:1962, 1993.
55. van Burik JH, Leisenring W, Myerson D, et al: The effect of prophylactic fluconazole on the clinical spectrum of fungal diseases in bone marrow transplant recipients with special attention to hepatic candidiasis: an autopsy study of 355 patients. Medicine (Baltimore) 77:246, 1998.
56. Vreugdenhil G, Van Dijke BJ, Donnelly JP, et al: Efficacy of itraconazole in the prevention of fungal infections among neutropenic patients with hematological malignancies and intensive chemotherapy. Leuk Lymphoma 11:353, 1993.
57. Tricot G, Joosten E, Boogaerts MA, et al: Ketoconazole vs. itraconazole for antifungal prophylaxis in patients with severe granulocytopenia: preliminary results of two nonrandomised studies. Rev Infect Dis 9:S94, 1987.
58. Boogaerts MA, Verhoef GE, Zachee P, et al: Antifungal prophylaxis with itraconazole in prolonged neutropenia: correlation with plasma levels. Mycoses 32:103, 1989.
59. Prentice AG, Warnock DW, Johnson SA, et al: Multiple dose pharmacokinetics of an oral solution of itraconazole in autologous bone marrow transplant recipients. J Antimicrob Chemother 34:247, 1994.
60. Menichetti F, Del Favero A, Martino P, et al: Itraconazole oral solution prophylaxis of fungal infections in neutropenic patients with haematologic malignancies: a randomised, placebo-controlled, double blind, multicentre trial. Clin Infect Dis 28:250, 1999.
61. Morgenstern GR, Prentice AG, Prentice HG, et al: A randomised controlled trial of itraconazole versus fluconazole for the prevention of fungal infections in patients with haematological malignancies. Br J Haematol 105:901, 1999.
62. Robertson MJ, Larson RA: Recurrent fungal pneumonias in patients with acute nonlymphocytic leukemia undergoing multiple courses of intensive chemotherapy. Am J Med 84:233, 1988.
63. Boogaerts MA, Michaux J-L, Bosly A, et al: Pharmacokinetics and safety of seven days' intravenous itraconazole followed by two weeks' oral itraconazole solution in patients with haematological malignancy [Abstract 387]. *In* Proceedings of the 36th Interscience Conference on Antimicrobial Agents and Chemotherapy, New Orleans, 1996.
64. Martin MV, Yates J, Hitchcock CA: Comparison of voriconazole (UK-109,496) and itraconazole in prevention and treatment of *Aspergillus fumigatus* endocarditis in guinea pigs. Antimicrob Agents Chemother 41:13, 1997.
65. Rousey SR, Russler S, Gottlieb M, Ash RC: Low-dose amphotericin B prophylaxis against invasive *Aspergillus* infections in allogeneic marrow transplantation. Am J Med 91:484, 1991.
66. Riley DK, Pavia AT, Beatty PG, et al: The prophylactic use of low-dose amphotericin B in bone marrow transplant patients. Am J Med 97:509, 1994.
67. Perfect JR, Klotman ME, Gilbert CC, et al: Prophylactic intravenous amphotericin B in neutropenic autologous bone marrow transplant recipients. J Infect Dis 165:891, 1992.
68. Conneally E, Cafferkey MT, Daly PA, et al: Nebulized amphotericin B as prophylaxis against invasive aspergillosis in granulocytopenic patients. Bone Marrow Transplant 5:403, 1990.
69. Behre GF, Schwartz S, Lenz K: Aerosol amphotericin B inhalations for prevention of invasive pulmonary aspergillosis in neutropenic cancer patients. Ann Hematol 71:287, 1995.
70. Hiemenz J, Walsh TJ: Lipid formulations of amphotericin B: Recent progress and future directions. Clin Infect Dis 22:S133, 1996.
71. Tollemar J, Ringden O, Andersson S, et al: Randomized double-blind study of liposomal amphotericin B (AmBisome) prophylaxis of invasive fungal infections in bone marrow transplant recipients. Bone Marrow Transplant 12:577, 1993.
72. Kelsey SM, Goldman JM, McCann S, et al: Liposomal amphotericin (AmBisome) in the prophylaxis of fungal infections in neutropenic patients: a randomised, double-blind, placebo controlled study. Bone Marrow Transplant 23:163–168, 1999.
73. Pizzo PA, Robichaud KJ, Gill FA, Witebsky FG: Empiric antibiotic and antifungal therapy for cancer patients with prolonged fever and granulocytopenia. Am J Med 72:101, 1982.
74. EORTC International Antimicrobial Therapy Cooperative Group:

Empiric antifungal therapy in febrile granulocytopenic patients. Am J Med 86:668, 1989.

75. Myint H. AmBisome: an overview of current use. Hospital Med 60(2):123, 1999.

76. Prentice HG, Hann IM, Herbrecht R, et al: A randomized comparison of liposomal versus conventional amphotericin B for the treatment of pyrexia of unknown origin in neutropenic patients. Br J Haematol 98:711, 1997.

77. Walsh TJ, Finberg RW, Arndt C, et al: Liposomal amphotericin B for empirical therapy in patients with persistent fever and neutropenia. N Engl J Med 340:764, 1999.

78. White MH, Bowden RA, Sandler ES, et al: Randomized, double-blind clinical trial of amphotericin B colloidal dispersion vs. amphotericin B in the empirical treatment of fever and neutropenia. Clin Infect Dis 27:296, 1998.

79. Lister J: Amphotericin B lipid complex (Abelcet) in the treatment of invasive mycoses: the North American experience. Eur J Haematol 56(Suppl 57):18, 1996.

80. Wingard JR: Efficacy of amphotericin B lipid complex injection (ABLC) in bone marrow transplant recipients with life-threatening systemic mycoses. Bone Marrow Transplant 19:343, 1997.

81. Mehta J, Kelsey S, Chu P, et al: Amphotericin B lipid complex (ABLC) for the treatment of confirmed or presumed fungal infections in immunocompromised patients with hematologic malignancies. Bone Marrow Transplant 20:39, 1997.

82. Myint H, Kyi AA, Winn R: An open, non-comparative evaluation of the efficacy and safety of amphotericin B lipid complex as treatment of neutropenic patients with presumed or confirmed pulmonary fungal infection. J Antimicrob Chemother 41:424, 1998.

83. Wingard JR, White MH, Anaissie EJ, et al: A randomized double blind safety study of AmBisome and Abelcet in febrile neutropenic patients. In Proceedings of the 9th Focus on Fungal Infections Meeting, San Diego, March 1999.

84. Denning DW, Donnelly JP, Hellreigel KP, et al: Antifungal prophylaxis during neutropenia or allogeneic bone marrow transplantation: what is the state of the art? Ad HOC Working Group. Chemotherapy 38 (Suppl 1):43, 1992.

85. Denning DW, Stevens DA: Antifungal and surgical treatment of invasive aspergillosis: review of 2121 published cases. Rev Infect Dis 12:1147, 1990.

86. Offner F, Cordonnier C, Ljungman P, et al: Impact of previous aspergillosis on the outcome of bone marrow transplantation. Clin Infect Dis 26:1098, 1998.

87. Karp JE, Burch PA, Merz WG: An approach to intensive antileukemic therapy in patients with previous invasive aspergillosis. Am J Med 85:203, 1988.

88. Jantunen E, Ruutu P, Niskanen L, et al: Incidence and risk factors for invasive fungal infections in allogeneic BMT recipients. Bone Marrow Transplant 19:801, 1997.

89. Robinson LA, Reed EC, Galbraith TA, et al: Pulmonary resection for invasive aspergillus infection in immunocompromised patients. J Thorac Cardiovasc 109:1182, 1995.

90. McWhinney PH, Kibbler CC, Hamon MD, et al: Progress in the diagnosis and management of aspergillosis in bone marrow transplantation: 13 years' experience. Clin Infect Dis 17:397, 1993.

91. Hoover M, Morgan ER, Kletzel M: Prior fungal infection is not a contraindication to bone marrow transplant in patients with acute leukemia. Med Pediatr Oncol 28:268, 1997.

92. Martino R, Lopez R, Sureda A, et al: Risk of reactivation of a recent invasive fungal infection in patients with hematological malignancies undergoing further intensive chemo-radiotherapy: a single-center experience and review of the literature. Haematologica 82:297, 1997.

93. Myint H, Bolam S, Kyi AA, Creasy T: Prevention of recurrence of fungal pneumonia with prophylactic low dose amphotericin B in lipid complex (Abelcet) following myelosuppressive chemotherapy. Bone Marrow Transplant 19:S165a, 1997.

94. Armitage JO: Emerging applications of recombinant human granulocyte-macrophage colony-stimulating factor. Blood 92:4491, 1998.

95. Nemunaitis J: A comparative review of colony-stimulating factors. Drugs 54:709, 1997.

96. Nemunaitis J: Growth factors in allogeneic transplantation. Semin Oncol 20:96, 1993.

97. Fraser IS, Denning DW: Empiric amphotericin B therapy: the need for a reappraisal. Blood Rev 7:208, 1993.

98. Gubbins PO, Bowman JL, Penzak SR: Antifungal prophylaxis to prevent invasive mycoses among bone marrow transplantation recipients. Pharmacotherapy 18:549, 1998.

99. Hiemenz JW, Greene JN: Special considerations for the patient undergoing allogeneic or autologous bone marrow transplantation. Hematol Oncol Clin North Am 7:961, 1993.

100. Lam HH, Althaus BL: Antifungal prophylaxis in bone marrow transplant. Ann Pharmacother 29:921, 1995.

101. Milliken ST, Powles RL: Antifungal prophylaxis in bone marrow transplantation. Rev Infect Dis 12 (Suppl 3):S374, 1990.

102. Richardson MD, Kokki MH: Antifungal therapy in 'bone marrow failure.' Br J Haematol 100:619, 1998.

103. Schuler US, Haag C: Prophylaxis of fungal infections. Mycoses 40 (Suppl 2):41, 1997.

104. Serody JS, Shea TC: Prevention of infections in bone marrow transplant recipients. Infect Dis Clin North Am 11:459, 1997.

105. Uzun O, Anaissie EJ: Antifungal prophylaxis in patients with hematologic malignancies: a reappraisal. Blood 86:2063, 1995.

106. Walsh TJ, Lee JW: Prevention of invasive fungal infections in patients with neoplastic disease. Clin Infect Dis 17 (Suppl 2):S468, 1993.

107. Castagnola E, Bucci B, Montinaro E, Viscoli C: Fungal infections in patients undergoing bone marrow transplantation: an approach to a rational management protocol. Bone Marrow Transplant 18 (Suppl 2):97, 1996.

108. Working Party for the British Society for Antimicrobial Chemotherapy: Chemoprophylaxis for candidosis and aspergillosis in neutropenia and transplantation: a review and recommendation. J Antimicrob Chemother 32:5, 1993.

109. Working Party for the British Society for Antimicrobial Chemotherapy: Therapy of deep infection in haematological malignancy. J Antimicrob Chemother 40:779, 1997.

110. Edwards, JE, Bowden R, Buckner T, et al: International conference for the development of a consensus on the management and prevention of severe candidal infections. Clin Infect Dis 25:43, 1997.

111. Gotzsche PC, Johansen HK: Meta-analysis of prophylactic or empirical antifungal treatment versus placebo or no treatment in patients with cancer complicated by neutropenia. BMJ 314:1238, 1997.

112. Kibbler CC, Manuel R, Prentice HG: Prophylactic and empirical antifungal treatment in cancer complicated by neutropenia: combining different antifungal strategies in same systematic review is inappropriate. BMJ 315:488, 1997.

113. Bow EJ, Laverdiere M, Lussier N, et al: Anti-fungal prophylaxis in neutropenic cancer patients—a meta-analysis. Presented at the 37th Interscience Conference on Antimicrobial Agents and Chemotherapy, Toronto, 1997.

114. Edman JC, Kovacs JA, Masur H, et al: Ribosomal RNA sequences show *Pneumocystis carinii* to be a member of the fungi. Nature 334:519, 1988.

115. Oz HS, Hughes WT: Novel anti–*Pneumocystis carinii* effects of the immunosuppressant mycophenolate mofetil in contrast to provocative effect of tacrolimus. J Infect Dis 175:901, 1997.

116. Tuan IZ, Dennison D, Weisdorf D: *Pneumocystis carinii* pneumonia following bone marow transplantation. Bone Marrow Transplant 10:267, 1992.

117. Ioannidis J, Cappelleri JC, Skolnik PR, et al: A meta-analysis of the relative efficacy and toxicity of *Pneumocystis carinii* prophylactic regimens. Arch Intern Med 156:177, 1996.

118. Karp JE, Merz WG, Dick JD, Saral R: Strategies to prevent or control infections after bone marrow transplants. Bone Marrow Transplant 8:1, 1991.

119. Alangaden G, Chandrasekar PH, Bailey E, Khaliq Y: Antifungal prophylaxis with low-dose fluconazole during bone marrow transplantation: the Bone Marrow Transplantation Team. Bone Marrow Transplant 14:919, 1994.

120. Ellis ME, Clink H, Ernst P, et al: Controlled study of fluconazole in the prevention of fungal infections in neutropenic patients with haematological malignancies and bone marrow transplant recipients. Eur J Clin Microbiol Infect Dis 13:3, 1994.

121. Quabeck K, Mller KD, Beelen DW, et al: Prophylaxis and treatment of fungal infections with fluconazole in bone marrow transplant patients. Mycoses 35:221, 1992.

122. Quirk PC, Osborne PJ, Walsh LJ: Australian Dental Research Fund Trebitsch Scholarship: efficacy of antifungal prophylaxis in bone marrow transplantation. Aust Dent J 40:267, 1995.

123. Prentice HG, Caillot D, Dupont B, et al: Oral and intravenous itraconazole for sytemic fungal infections in neutropenic haematological patients: meeting report. Acta Haematol 101:56, 1999.

124. Olkkola KT, Backman JT, Neuvonen PJ: Midazolam should be avoided in patients receiving the systemic antimycotics ketoconazole or itraconazole. Clin Pharmacol Ther 55:481, 1994.

125. Bohme A, Ganser A, Hoelzer D: Aggravation of vincristine-induced neurotoxicity by itraconazole in the treatment of adult ALL. Ann Hematol 71:311, 1995.

126. Gillies J, Hung KA, Fitzsimons E, Soutar R: Severe vincristine toxicity in combinations with itraconazole. Clin Lab Haematol 20:123, 1998.

127. Buggia I, Zecca M, Alesandrino EP, et al: Itraconazole can increase systemic exposure to busulfan in patients given bone marrow transplantation (GITMO). Anticancer Res 16:2083, 1996.

128. Nicholl TA, Nimmo CR, Shepherd JD, et al: Amphotericin B infusion-related toxicity: comparison of two- and four-hour infusions. Ann Pharmacother 29:1081, 1995.

129. Hussein MA, Fletcher R, Long TJ, et al: Transfusing platelets 2 h after the completion of amphotericin-B decreases its detrimental effect on transfused platelet recovery and survival. Transfus Med 8:43, 1998.

130. Leenders AC, Daenen S, Jansen RLH: Liposomal amphotericin B (AmBisome) compared with amphotericin B deoxycholate in the treatment of documented and suspected neutropenia-associated invasive fungal infections. Br J Haematol 103:205, 1998.

131. Conkell AJ, Brogden RN: Liposomal amphotericin B: therapeutic use in the management of fungal infections and visceral leishmaniasis. Drugs 55:585, 1998.

132. Mills W, Chopra R, Linch DC, Goldstone AH: Liposomal amphotericin B in the treatment of fungal infections in neutropenic patients: a single centre experience of 133 episodes in 116 patients. Br J Haematol 86:754, 1994.

133. Oppenheim BA, Herbrecht R, Kusne S: The safety and efficacy of amphotericin B colloidal dispersion in the treatment of invasive mycoses. Clin Infect Dis 21:1145, 1995.

CHAPTER THIRTY-NINE

Prevention of Acute Graft-Versus-Host Disease

Donna Przepiorka, M.D., Ph.D.

When the syndrome of acute graft-versus-host disease (GVHD) was recognized early in the development of the field of clinical marrow transplantation,[1, 2] its occurrence and etiology had already been the subject of animal studies for several decades.[3] Billingham, on the basis of these animal studies, outlined the principles for development of GVHD: (1) the recipient is not immunologically competent to reject the donor cells, (2) the recipient possesses an antigenic target to which donor cells can react, and (3) the donor cells are competent to mediate an immunologic response.[3]

In animal models, the reproducible induction of GVHD by transplantation of lymphohematopoietic tissue between inbred strains that differed at the major histocompatibility complex (MHC) proved that antigens encoded by this region were major stimuli for the host-reactive immune response.[4] The identity and nature of these antigens in humans are now well-known,[5] and their role in the development of GVHD in humans is supported by the observation that the severity of GVHD increases with the degree of human leukocyte antigen (HLA) disparity[6] and by the isolation of T-cell clones with specific HLA reactivity from patients with GVHD.[7] GHVD, however, also occurred in animal models in which the donor and host were matched at the MHC,[8, 9] suggesting that other "minor" histocompatibility antigens (mHA) act as stimuli for the induction of GVHD. The importance of human mHA was inferred from the occurrence of GVHD in HLA-identical marrow transplant recipients not receiving immunosuppression[10] and the isolation of mHA-reactive T-cell clones from patients with GVHD,[11, 12] but investigators have only recently appreciated the spectrum of potential mHA in humans.[13]

PATHOGENESIS OF ACUTE GRAFT-VERSUS-HOST DISEASE

It has been well established in animal systems[14, 15] that GVHD is mediated by T lymphocytes, and the fact that a similar mechanism is active in humans was supported by results of initial clinical trials in which T-cell depletion of marrow allografts led to a decreased risk of acute GVHD.[16] The identity of the T-cell subset responsible for GVHD has been the subject of intense investigation. In the murine system, it is clear that whether CD4 or CD8 cells mediate GVHD depends on the strains and the direction of transplantation,[17] and it is likely that both CD4 and CD8 subsets are involved in GVHD in humans.

Natural killer (NK) cells have also been implicated in the pathophysiology of GVHD. In animal experiments, GVHD can be induced by transplantation of spleen cells from nude mice that are devoid of T cells but include NK cells.[18-20] In humans, NK cells have been found to predominate in skin and peripheral blood of patients with acute GVHD.[21] It is not clear that NK cells alone are sufficient to cause GVHD in humans, but upregulation of NK activity during GVHD may intensify the process, either by direct cell-mediated cytotoxicity or through release of cytokines.[23]

Allospecific suppressor cells have been detected in murine and canine as well as human radiation chimeras.[23-25] Because they usually are detected late after transplantation, these suppressor cells do not provide protection against the development of acute GVHD, but they may have an active immunoregulatory role in GVHD after delayed donor lymphocyte infusions.[26] MHC-nonrestricted suppressor cells, or natural suppressor cells, are detectable transiently during the first few weeks after transplantation.[27] This is a time during which murine recipients of T-cell–poor mHA-disparate marrow demonstrate tolerance to donor spleen cell infusion,[28] suggesting that these cells may have an active role in control of acute GVHD. In humans, such nonspecific suppressor cells have been associated with chronic GVHD when they persist, and these cells may be Th2 in nature.[29, 30]

The final phase of the graft-versus-host reaction is the tissue damage in target organs. The mechanisms by which this occurs is multifactorial. Abundant preclinical data indicate that lymphocyte-mediated cell death in target organs is brought about by (1) the perforin/granzyme pathway, (2) the Fas/FasL (Fas ligand) pathway, or (3) the tumor necrosis factor (TNF) pathway. Lymphocytes from murine strains deficient in perforin, granzyme, or FasL (*gld* -/-), inducers of apoptosis, show a reduced capacity to cause GVHD in normal hosts.[31-34] Recipients deficient in the Fas receptor (*lpr* -/-) or the TNF receptor, receptors that transduce the signal for programmed cell death, develop a moderated level of GVHD when transplanted with normal spleen cells.[35, 36] The roles of the perforin/granzyme and Fas/FasL pathways in human GVHD have not been investigated, but the importance of TNF is well established in that neutralization of TNF has been at least partially effective in the prevention and amelioration of acute GVHD in humans.[37-40]

Other cytokines may also play a role in the pathophysiology of acute GVHD.[37, 38] Patients with acute GVHD have variably been found to have elevated serum levels of interleukin-6 (IL-6) as well as TNF. In addition, patients with GVHD have a CD4 subset imbalance favoring Th1 cells, which secrete these and other inflammatory cytokines (IL-1, IL-2, and interferon-γ [IFN-γ]).[41–44] These cytokines are released by lymphocytes in response to specific alloantigen stimulation, by tissues injured by the conditioning regimen, or by monocytes stimulated by infection.[39, 45] Both the incidence and severity of acute GVHD may be modified by inflammatory cytokines through upregulation of MHC or costimulatory molecules in the target organs and by enhancement of proliferation or activation of the effector cells.[37, 38]

RISK FACTORS FOR ACUTE GVHD

Histoincompatibility is the strongest risk factor for acute GVHD (Fig. 39–1). For patients receiving standard GVHD prophylaxis with or without T-cell depletion, the rate of moderate-to-severe acute GVHD is 29–42% with HLA-identical transplants, 35–42% with HLA–phenotypically matched related donor transplants, 44–73% with one-antigen–mismatched related donor transplants, 54–88% with HLA–phenotypically matched unrelated donor transplants, 56–84% with two- or three-antigen–mismatched related donor transplants, and 63–95% with one-antigen–mismatched unrelated donor transplants.[6, 46–48]

Several studies have explored the effect of type and locus of HLA mismatch on GVHD when using alternative donors. For patients with one-antigen–mismatched related donors, whether the serologic mismatch is in class I or class II does not affect GVHD,[46] and with modern GVHD prophylaxis, there is also no difference whether the mismatch is major or minor.[49] For patients with serologically matched unrelated

donors, mismatches at HLA-DP do not alter GVHD risk.[50] Preliminary reports suggest that serologic or low-resolution mismatches in HLA-C increase the risk of GVHD, although evaluation of this observation is not yet complete.[51–53] Molecular matching for HLA-DRB1 in this group has been associated with a reduction in severe but not moderate GVHD, and this effect is lost when T-cell depletion is used.[54, 55] Molecular matching for class I is likely to also result in a reduction in GVHD after matched unrelated donor marrow transplantation and will almost certainly replace serologic methods in time.

For patients with HLA-identical donors, early analyses indicated that the risk of GVHD was increased with specific HLA-A, -B, and -DR alleles, but more recent studies have failed to confirm this.[56–58] Preliminary data, however, suggest that GVHD is increased with mismatching for certain mHA presented in an HLA-allele–restricted fashion.[9, 59] Thus, GVHD risk may be associated with specific HLA alleles for HLA-identical transplant recipients, but only in concert with mismatches for the mHA presented by that specific allele.

A number of in vitro assays for alloreactivity, including the mixed lymphocyte culture and limiting dilution assays, have been evaluated as predictors for GVHD. The relative response rate in the mixed lymphocyte culture was not found to be more useful than class II typing when assessing unrelated or class I–mismatched related patient-donor pairs.[60, 61] Also, an increased relative response rate was not always associated with a higher risk of GVHD with HLA-identical transplants.[62, 63] Similarly, in multivariate analyses of GVHD in alternative donor transplant recipients, limiting dilution assays to quantitate the frequency of precursors of host-reactive cytotoxic T lymphocytes or helper T lymphocytes (HTLp) were not consistently found to be independent prognostic factors.[64–66] Several investigators, however, have reported a strong correlation between HTLp and GVHD in HLA-identical transplant recipients, but whether HTLp is an independent prognostic factor has not been tested in a multivariate analysis.[67–69] With HLA-identical transplants, the alloreactivity detected is likely directed against mHA. A correlation between alloreactivity and GVHD was also detected using a skin explant model for mHA,[70] but its clinical application was not tested prospectively.

Of the characteristics of the graft, only T-cell dose correlated with the risk of GVHD for patients with either HLA-identical or alternative donors, but this was observed only with T-cell depletion of marrow.[71–73] Interestingly, the correlation was not observed in studies using pan–T-cell depletion, which were associated with a high rate of graft failure.[74] These results are consistent with the hypothesis that the linear portion of the T-cell dose/GVHD response curve is limited. Unmanipulated grafts have a T-cell burden that falls on the plateau above the upward linear slope, and in series with deep depletions, the T-cell burden falls below the threshold for GVHD. Concurrent immunoprophylaxis may also affect this observation. Total nucleated cell dose is not an adequate surrogate for T-cell dose. A high total nucleated cell dose was associated with a decrease in GVHD in unrelated donor marrow transplant recipients,[75] but there was no relationship between total nucleated cell dose or lymphocyte subset dose and GVHD after HLA-identical

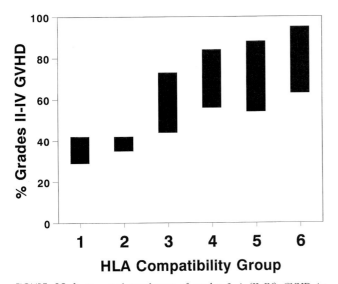

FIGURE 39–1. Reported incidences of grades 2–4 (II–IV) GVHD in recipients of marrow from (1) HLA-identical related donors, (2) HLA-phenotypically matched related donors, (3) one-antigen–mismatched related donors, (4) two- or three-antigen–mismatched related donors, (5) HLA-matched unrelated donors, or (6) one-antigen–mismatched unrelated donors. Data from large comparative studies (Szydlo et al.,[6] Beatty et al.,[46, 48] and Ash et al.[47]).

marrow or peripheral blood progenitor cell transplantation without T-cell depletion.[56, 76–78]

An increase in GVHD was noted with increasing intensity of the conditioning regimen.[79] It was suggested that this was due to a lack of compliance with immunoprophylaxis dosing as a result of regimen-related organ toxicity, but in a multivariate analysis, conditioning regimen intensity as defined by the dose of TBI was an independent risk factor for GVHD.[58] Others have postulated that cytokines, especially TNF, produced during the conditioning regimen cause subclinical organ toxicity that magnifies the effects of GVHD. This is supported by the finding of an association between early elevated TNF levels and GVHD post transplantation in both animal models and clinical studies.[43, 80] Patients with aplastic anemia receiving cyclophosphamide alone have the lowest risk of GVHD. This risk increases with increasing intensity of the conditioning regimen.[81] The increase in GVHD in these patients may be due to elimination of the protective effect of mixed chimerism as well.[82]

Numerous demographic characteristics have been cited as independent risk factors for GVHD (Table 39–1). There is a clear association between age and risk of GVHD independent of the degree of histocompatibility.[54, 56–58, 76, 83–87] The strength of this association is greatest when both adults and pediatric patients are included in an analysis. With improvements in supportive care and immunoprophylaxis, even as the upper age limit of transplant candidates increases, whether age will continue to be a risk factor for GVHD within the adult population remains to be seen. Other factors, such as donor sex, donor parity, and viral serology, were identified as risk factors for GVHD in early studies, but these seem to have inconsistent significance in the modern era of immunoprophylaxis or with T-cell depletion.[54–58, 76–78, 83–88]

TABLE 39–1. INDEPENDENT CLINICAL RISK FACTORS FOR ACUTE GRAFT-VERSUS-HOST DISEASE

HLA-IDENTICAL DONOR	HLA-MATCHED UNRELATED DONOR	HLA-MISMATCHED RELATED DONOR
Patient-donor sex-mismatch	Patient age	Patient age
Female donor for male recipient	Serologic HLA major mismatch	Increasing degree of histoincompatibility
Parous donor	Serologic HLA minor mismatch	
Alloimmunized donor	Class II micromismatch	
Patient age		
Donor seropositive for herpes simplex virus		
Donor seropositive for cytomegalovirus (CMV)		
Patient seropositive for CMV		
TBI dose >12 Gy		
Minor histoincompatibility		

HLA, human leukocyte antigen; TBI, total body irradiation.
Data from references 54–58, 76–78, and 83–88.

PHARMACOLOGIC PROPHYLAXIS FOR ACUTE GVHD

The ultimate goal of immune manipulation in allogeneic transplant recipients is to induce a state of specific tolerance. Prevention of GVHD after allogeneic transplantation requires methods to delete alloreactive effector cells and prevent activation of naive lymphocytes. Thus, common approaches to GVHD prophylaxis involve combination drug therapy, depletion of T cells plus an activation inhibitor, or an extensive T-cell depletion. Methods for removal of lymphocytes from allografts are reviewed in Chapter 30.

Activation of T cells is initiated by engagement of the T-cell receptor by antigen, usually in the context of MHC on the antigen-presenting cell, with subsequent transduction of the signal through a calcium-dependent pathway for transcription of the early activation genes. Concurrent signaling through costimulatory molecules enhances T-cell responsiveness. With upregulation of IL-2 and IL-2 receptor expression, a second signal is transduced via a calcium-independent pathway, and cell cycling begins. End-organ damage is mediated by cytokines released by the activated lymphocytes or by FasL upregulated on the activated lymphocytes. A number of immunosuppressive drugs interfere with one of these steps in T-cell activation (Fig. 39–2).

Cyclosporine is a cyclic undecapeptide.[89] In the cytoplasm, cyclosporine combines with cyclophilin and inhibits the phosphatase activity of calcineurin. As a result, the transcription factor NF-AT is trapped in the cytoplasm, and transcription of the earliest activation genes in T cells cannot proceed. No effects on activated T cells have been identified. Clearance of cyclosporine is by hepatic metabolism, and it decreases with age. For most adults, the terminal half-life is about 8 hours.[90] Disposition of cyclosporine is altered by a number of drugs that affect the hepatic P450 system. Imidazole antibiotics, macrolide antibiotics, metronidazole, protease inhibitors, calcium channel blockers, estrogens, and grapefruit juice decrease clearance of cyclosporine, and rifampin, isoniazid, phenobarbital, phenytoin, primidone, and carbamazepine increase cyclosporine clearance. Drugs excreted renally may have reduced clearance when administered to patients with cyclosporine-induced nephrotoxicity.

Renal insufficiency is the major toxicity of cyclosporine. Mild renal insufficiency is usually reversible. Other common toxic events include magnesium wasting, hirsutism, and hypertension. Hyperkalemia, glucose intolerance, and tremor occur frequently. Fewer patients have experienced allergic reactions, chest pain, headache, insomnia, hyperchloremic metabolic acidosis, hyperuricemia, hyperlipidemia, cholestasis, gynecomastia, nausea, microangiopathic hemolytic anemia, hemolytic-uremic syndrome, seizures, confusion, leukoencephalopathy, cortical blindness, and palmar-plantar dysesthesia with the use of cyclosporine. Some toxic events are idiosyncratic or precipitated by rapid infusion of the drug, but the risk of nephrotoxicity is clearly increased with elevated steady-state or trough blood concentrations of cyclosporine.[91]

The dose schedule of cyclosporine for prevention of GVHD has not been standardized.[92, 93] Most regimens begin on day −1 or −2 with 3–5 mg/kg/day IV over 20–24 hours or 1.5–2.5 mg/kg IV over 6 hours twice daily (Table

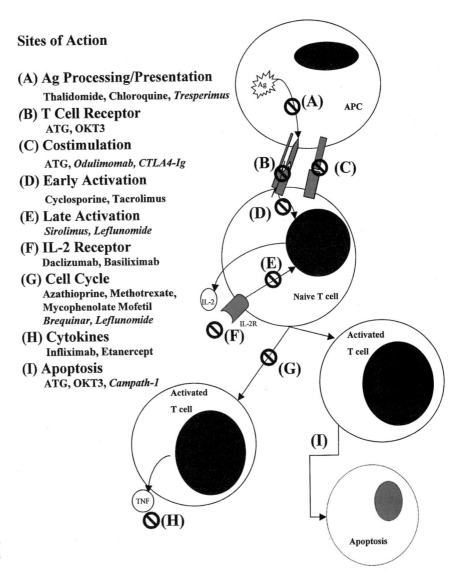

Sites of Action

(A) Ag Processing/Presentation
   Thalidomide, Chloroquine, *Tresperimus*

(B) T Cell Receptor
   ATG, OKT3

(C) Costimulation
   ATG, *Odulimomab, CTLA4-Ig*

(D) Early Activation
   Cyclosporine, Tacrolimus

(E) Late Activation
   Sirolimus, Leflunomide

(F) IL-2 Receptor
   Daclizumab, Basiliximab

(G) Cell Cycle
   Azathioprine, Methotrexate,
   Mycophenolate Mofetil
   Brequinar, Leflunomide

(H) Cytokines
   Infliximab, Etanercept

(I) Apoptosis
   ATG, OKT3, *Campath-1*

FIGURE 39–2. Immunosuppressive drugs for prevention of GVHD. Drugs listed in italics are investigational.

39–2),[94] but lower doses have been advocated in order to avoid the higher risk of relapse associated with the higher dose schedules.[95] The oral preparations of cyclosporine are not bioequivalent,[96] and the conversion ratio (1:4 IV:oral or 1:2 IV:oral) depends on which formulation is used. Commonly used cyclosporine assays measure either parent compound (RIA or HPLC) or parent plus metabolites (TDx), but the therapeutic target range for either type of assay has not been firmly established for HSCT recipients.[93, 97] Although the risk of GVHD is inversely proportional to the steady-state or trough concentration of cyclosporine,[91] because of the lack of consensus on therapeutic monitoring, some centers use a wide therapeutic target range and modify cyclosporine doses more routinely for renal insufficiency or other toxic events.

Cyclosporine is most commonly administered for at least 6 months after transplantation. Taper schedules vary from 5% per week starting on day 50 to 10% per week starting on day 180. A randomized study concluded that cyclosporine could be discontinued safely at day 60 after HLA-identical marrow transplantation,[98] but in a prospective study of tapering between day 30 and day 60, the risk of severe GVHD was high, and almost all patients experienced chronic GVHD.[99] Early discontinuation of cyclosporine is largely successful in pediatric patients, and even in that population, it has been reserved for patients at high risk for relapse with HLA-identical donors in the absence of acute GVHD.[94] The risk of chronic GVHD is clearly higher when cyclosporine is tapered before day 150.[100] Use of cyclosporine for as long as 9 months after transplantation delayed the onset of chronic GVHD but did not appear to reduce the overall risk.[101] Chronic GVHD can be especially severe in unrelated donor marrow transplant recipients and in allogeneic blood progenitor cell transplant recipients when immunoprophylaxis is discontinued early. For patients with aplastic anemia, extending the duration of cyclosporine use[102] reduces the risk of graft rejection.

Tacrolimus is a macrolide lactone.[103] The combination of tacrolimus and FKBP, its cytosolic binding protein, also inhibits calcineurin and prevents the transcription of early activation factors in T cells. Tacrolimus has no activity in activated T cells. The terminal half-life of tacrolimus in marrow transplant recipients is about 8 hours,[104] although the half-life is shorter in young children than in adults.

TABLE 39–2. COMMONLY USED DRUG REGIMENS FOR PREVENTION OF ACUTE GVHD*

REGIMEN	DOSING SCHEDULE
Long Methotrexate	
Methotrexate	IV 15 mg/m² day 1, 10 mg/m² days 3, 6, 11, and weekly through day 100
Cyclosporine-Methotrexate	
Methotrexate	IV 15 mg/m² day 1, 10 mg/m² days 3, 6, and 11
Cyclosporine†	IV 1.5 mg/kg BID from day −1, taper 5% weekly starting day 60
Cyclosporine/Very Short Methotrexate	
Methotrexate	IV 10 mg/m² days 1, 3, 6
Cyclosporine	IV 3 mg/kg/day infusion from day −1, taper 10% weekly starting day 180
Cyclosporine/Steroids	
Cyclosporine†	IV 3 mg/kg/day infusion from day −2, taper 10% weekly starting day 180
Methylprednisolone	IV 0.25 mg/kg BID days 7–14, 0.5 mg/kg BID days 15–28, 0.4 mg/kg BID days 29–42, 0.25 mg/kg BID days 43–56, 0.1 mg/kg BID days 57–119, 0.1 mg/kg daily days 120–180
Triple-Drug Prophylaxis	
Methotrexate	IV 15 mg/m² day 1, 10 mg/m² days 3 and 6
Cyclosporine	IV 5 mg/kg/day infusion from day −2, taper 20% every 2 weeks starting day 84
Methylprednisolone	IV 0.25 mg/kg BID days 7–14, 0.5 mg/kg BID days 15–28, 0.4 mg/kg BID days 29–42, 0.25 mg/kg BID days 43–56, 0.1 mg/kg BID days 57–119, 0.1 mg/kg daily days 120–180
Antithyroid Globulin (ATG)/Cyclosporine/Methotrexate	
ATG	IV 20 mg/kg days −3, −2, and −1
Methotrexate	IV 10 mg/m² days 1, 3, 6, and 11
Cyclosporine	IV 5 mg/kg/day infusion from day −1, taper 10% weekly starting day 180
Tacrolimus/Minimethotrexate	
Methotrexate	IV 5 mg/m² days 1, 3, 6, and 11
Tacrolimus†	IV 0.03 mg/kg/day infusion from day −2, taper 20% every 2 weeks from day 180

*Individuals not experienced in the administration of immunosuppressive drugs for prevention of acute GVHD should consult the primary reference 94 or the references cited in Tables 39–4 through 39–8 regarding premedications, precautions, and monitoring during use of these regimens.

†Tacrolimus and cyclosporine have been used interchangeably with this methotrexate or steroid dose schedule.

Clearance is through hepatic metabolism, and drug interactions are similar to those reported with cyclosporine. The side effect profile of tacrolimus is also similar to that of cyclosporine except that tacrolimus does not cause hirsutism, gingival hyperplasia, chondrodysplasia, or hyperlipidemia. Tacrolimus has also been associated with less hypertension after transplantation but occasionally more glucose intolerance.

Use of tacrolimus for allogeneic marrow transplantation was standardized by consensus.[105] The recommended starting dose of tacrolimus is 0.03 mg/kg/day IV by 20- to 24-hour infusion beginning on day −1 or −2, and dosing is based on ideal body weight. Tacrolimus is converted to oral drug in a 1:4 IV:oral ratio, and oral drug is administered twice daily in divided doses. The therapeutic steady state or trough whole blood concentration range is 10–20 ng/mL, although some have used a range of 5–15 ng/mL successfully. Therapeutic monitoring is required. Doses of

tacrolimus are also modified for renal toxicity, with changes made for as little as a 25% increase from baseline creatinine.[105] For prevention of GVHD, tacrolimus has been used in combination with standard methotrexate or minimethotrexate (see Table 39–2). The duration of therapy with tacrolimus and taper schedule at individual centers are generally similar to those of cyclosporine.

Sirolimus is a macrolide.[106] It is structurally related to tacrolimus, but the mechanism of action of sirolimus is quite different. The combination of sirolimus and FKBP inhibits S6 protein kinase (p70^{s6k}) and possibly other cell cycle proteins, blocking the signal transduction cascade initiated by growth factors such as IL-2. The terminal half-life of sirolimus is approximately 60 hours. The parent compound has poor absorption and stability, but a new derivative, SDZ RAD, is active orally. Clearance is by hepatic metabolism. Combined use of sirolimus and tacrolimus is neutral to antagonistic because both drugs act via the same binding protein. Sirolimus and cyclosporine are synergistic, but close therapeutic monitoring is required because sirolimus delays the clearance of cyclosporine. Reported side effects of sirolimus in solid organ transplant recipients and patients with autoimmune disorders include hyperlipidemia, thrombocytopenia, leukopenia, and capillary leak syndrome. Sirolimus has not been evaluated completely for prevention of GVHD in humans. Preliminary studies in mice indicate that sirolimus is effective GVHD prophylaxis but may abrogate the graft-versus-leukemia effect.[107]

Methotrexate is a folic acid analog. The drug inhibits dihydrofolate reductase, blocking purine synthesis and DNA replication. The disposition of methotrexate is triphasic, with a terminal half-life in excess of 8–10 hours, although the polyglutamated form can remain intracellularly for extended periods. Methotrexate is cleared renally, and clearance may be prolonged in patients with renal insufficiency or effusions. Under these circumstances, doses are modified, and methotrexate levels are drawn 24 hours after dosing to determine whether the drug level is within the safe range; patients may require leucovorin to reduce the risk of toxicity. The most common toxic events associated with methotrexate use are mucositis and myelosuppression. Routine use of leucovorin does not abrogate the immunosuppressive effect of methotrexate and may reduce toxicity.[108]

The original schedule of methotrexate given through day 100 after transplantation was derived in a dog model.[109] When used in combination with cyclosporine or tacrolimus, the standard four-dose or "short" methotrexate regimen is sufficient (see Table 39–2). Several variations of the standard regimen are used regularly.[93] In the "minimethotrexate" regimen (see Table 39–2), the doses have been reduced substantially with less toxicity and no change in the risk of GVHD.[110] In the "very short" methotrexate regimen, the day 11 dose is omitted. Reports of retrospective evaluation of the need for the day 11 dose of methotrexate have yielded conflicting conclusions.[58, 111] Prospective evaluation has not been performed.

Mycophenolate mofetil is the prodrug of mycophenolic acid, which inhibits inosine monophosphate dehydrogenase, blocking synthesis of purines in the de novo pathway.[112] The half-life of mycophenolic acid is about 18 hours. The active form of the drug is metabolized in the liver by glucuronidation, and the metabolite is excreted renally. Drugs that are eliminated by tubular secretion may compete with the metabolite for clearance, which may prolong the half-life of the metabolite; drugs that inhibit tubular secretion may reduce the clearance of the metabolite. Antacids delay absorption of mycophenolate mofetil, and cholestyramine interferes with its enterohepatic recirculation. The most common toxicities of mycophenolate mofetil are nausea, vomiting, anorexia, diarrhea, and leukopenia. For prevention of GVHD, mycophenolate mofetil has been administered at 15 mg/kg (up to 1 g) orally, twice daily, for 14–28 days after transplantation in combination with cyclosporine or tacrolimus. Absorption of mycophenolate mofetil is variable, and therapeutic monitoring may be necessary as is done for solid organ transplantation. The intravenous formulation has not been evaluated fully for GVHD prevention.

Corticosteroids combine intracellularly with the glucocorticoid receptor and alter transcription of genes having a glucocorticoid response element.[113] Actions mediated by glucocorticoids include downregulation of cytokine expression in lymphocytes and phagocytes, downregulation of adhesion molecules and alteration of cell trafficking, induction of apoptosis of activated lymphocytes, decreased antigen processing and presentation, decreased phagocytosis, inhibition of degranulation, and membrane stabilization. The 11-keto group on prednisone requires reduction by the liver for activity of the drug, so an active form, methylprednisolone, is preferred when hepatic function is impaired. The plasma half-life of methylprednisolone is about 3 hours. Clearance is by metabolism. Side effects of corticosteroids include hyperglycemia, hypertension, hyperlipidemia, hypokalemia, edema, myopathy, nausea, and gastric ulceration and/or bleeding. Corticosteroids may also cause headaches, pseudotumor cerebri, and psychiatric disturbances, and they may accelerate development of cataracts, aseptic necrosis, and osteoporosis. Methylprednisolone, 0.5 mg/kg twice daily, has been used as sole GVHD prophylaxis when patients have become intolerant of other agents, but this strategy is not successful in the long term. More frequently, methylprednisolone has been used for prevention of GVHD in conjunction with cyclosporine or tacrolimus beginning 5–7 days after transplantation for a short term in the periengraftment period (see Table 39–2).

Antilymphocyte globulin (ATG) is a polyclonal antibody preparation from horses or rabbits immunized with human lymphoid tissue. Different types of ATG and different lots from the same manufacturer may not be bioequivalent.[114, 115] ATG is thought to be lymphocytotoxic by virtue of endogenous complement fixation or opsonization, but it may also induce partial anergy.[116] Fever, chills, rash, leukopenia, thrombocytopenia, arthralgias, myalgias, and interstitial pneumonitis are potential side effects. Anaphylaxis may occur, and skin testing prior to the first dose is routine at many centers. Many of the side effects can be reduced in intensity or prevented by premedication and concurrent infusion with corticosteroids. The optimal dose schedule of ATG for prevention of GVHD has not been determined. Doses of 5–30 mg/kg/day for 2–14 days have been used. Substantial amounts of ATG can be detected in the peripheral blood for 1–2 months after administration,[117]

so ATG administered before transplantation to prevent graft rejection may still be circulating after transplantation and prevent GVHD.

The *Campath-1* series of monoclonal antibodies recognizes CD52, a glycophosphotiylinositol-anchored glycoprotein on lymphocytes.[118] Campath-1M, a rat IgM, has a high potency for cell lysis by complement fixation, and it has been used largely for in vitro T-cell depletion. Campath-1G, a rat IgG$_{2b}$, also fixes complement. Campath-1H is the humanized version. Campath-1G has been administered in vivo for GVHD prophylaxis at 20 mg/day IV for 5 days beginning before transplantation.[119] A first-dose reaction is the most common side effect.

CLINICAL ADVANCES IN GVHD PROPHYLAXIS

Prevention of GVHD has been a major focus of clinical transplantation research, but it was not until the 1994 Consensus Conference that recommendations for results reporting were standardized (Table 39–3).[120] Despite the lack of consistency in reporting prior to that time, several major advances in GVHD prophylaxis have been recognized and accepted.

MATCHED RELATED DONOR MARROW TRANSPLANTATION (HLA-IDENTICAL BMT)

It is clear in the adult population that GVHD prophylaxis is required to prevent moderate-to-severe GVHD after HLA-identical bone marrow transplantation (BMT).[121] A number of randomized trials have addressed the question of optimal

TABLE 39–3. CONSENSUS RECOMMENDATION FOR REPORTING RESULTS OF ACUTE GVHD PREVENTION TRIALS

1. Details of the grading system should be described or referenced accurately.
2. The criteria for initiation of treatment of acute GVHD and the drugs used for first-line therapy of acute GVHD should be reported.
3. The rates of grades 2–4 and grades 3–4 GVHD should be reported.
4. When calculating the actuarial estimates of acute GVHD, patients should be censored at:
   (a) the date of graft failure.
   (b) the date GVHD prophylaxis is discontinued for relapse.
   (c) the date of hematologic relapse or treatment of relapse if it occurred off prophylaxis.
5. When evaluating acute GVHD as the end-point, data should be reported separately for subgroups with acknowledged potential differences in risk of GVHD (e.g., pediatric vs. adult, T-cell–depleted vs. unmanipulated transplant, HLA-identical vs. alternative donor).
6. When evaluating survival as the end-point, data should be reported separately for subgroups with acknowledged potential differences in survival (e.g., pediatric vs. adult, early vs. intermediate or advanced leukemia).

GVHD, graft-versus-host disease; HLA, human leukocyte antigen.
Adapted from reference 120.

prophylaxis (Table 39–4). Long methotrexate was the initial standard prophylaxis, but with its introduction in the 1980s,[148] cyclosporine became the drug of choice despite the fact that only some of the studies demonstrated that cyclosporine was more effective than long methotrexate for prevention of GVHD and none demonstrated a survival advantage on long-term follow-up.[149, 150] The equivalence of cyclosporine and methotrexate for prevention of GVHD was also confirmed in a large registry analysis.[151] Some authors observed a lower relapse rate with methotrexate, and at present, long methotrexate is generally reserved for subgroups with a low potential for GVHD and a high risk of relapse, such as pediatric patients with advanced acute lymphocytic leukemia.[94]

TABLE 39–4. GVHD PROPHYLAXIS FOR HLA-IDENTICAL ALLOGENEIC MARROW TRANSPLANTATION: RANDOMIZED TRIALS

REFERENCE	NO. OF PATIENTS	REGIMEN	GRADE 2–4 GVHD	GRADE 3–4 GVHD	SURVIVAL ADVANTAGE
122	27	Long methotrexate	19%	—	No
	29	Long methotrexate/ATG	7%	—	
123	42	Long methotrexate	21%	—	No
	30	Long methotrexate/ATG	27%	—	
124	35	Long methotrexate	31%*	17%	No
	32	Long methotrexate/ATG/steroids	9%	3%	
125	44	Long methotrexate	25%*	—	No
	40	Methotrexate	59%	—	
	25	Long methotrexate + buffy coat cells	82%	—	
126	39	Long methotrexate	56%	41%*	No
	36	Cyclosporine	33%	16%	
127	23	Long methotrexate	46%	—	No
	25	Cyclosporine	42%	—	
128	29	Long methotrexate	22%	15%	No
	30	Cyclosporine	40%	20%	
129	30	Long methotrexate	71%*	—	No
	26	Cyclosporine	45%	—	
130	16	Long methotrexate	21%	—	No
	18	Cyclosporine	41%	—	
131	31	Long methotrexate	39%	6%	No
	26	Cyclosporine	46%	15%	
132	53	Long methotrexate/steroids	47%*	25%	—
	54	Cyclosporine/steroids	28%	11%	
133	40	Cyclophosphamide/steroids	68%*	—	—
	42	Cyclosporine/steroids	32%	—	Yes†
134	60	Cyclosporine	73%*	40%	No
	62	Cyclosporine/steroids	60%	34%	
135	24	Long methotrexate	53%*	38%	No
	22	Cyclosporine/methotrexate	18%	0%	
136	39	Cyclosporine	51%*	—	—
	37	Cyclosporine/methotrexate	25%	—	Yes†
137	50	Cyclosporine	54%*	26%	—
	43	Cyclosporine/methotrexate	33%	7%	Yes†
138	28	Cyclosporine	61%*	—	No
	32	Cyclosporine/methotrexate	34%	—	
139	55	Cyclosporine/methotrexate	36%*	—	No
	53	Cyclosporine/methotrexate/steroids	13%	—	
140	21	Cyclosporine/methotrexate	15%	—	No
	20	Cyclosporine/methotrexate/steroids	10%	—	
141	63	Cyclosporine/methotrexate	25%*	—	No
	24	Cyclosporine/methotrexate/late steroids	25%	9%	
	59	Cyclosporine/methotrexate/early steroids	46%	4%	
142	74	Cyclosporine/steroids	23%*	17%	No
	75	Cyclosporine/methotrexate/steroids	7%	13%	
143	164	Cyclosporine/methotrexate	44%*	22%	No‡
	165	Tacrolimus/methotrexate	32%	14%	
144	50	Cyclosporine/methotrexate	46%*	11%	Yes+
	51	Cyclosporine/methotrexate/anti-IL-2	38%	7%	—
145	20	Long methotrexate or cyclosporine	73%	—	No
	20	CD2 depletion/long methotrexate or cyclosporine	15%	—	
146	25	Cyclosporine/methotrexate	12%	4%	No
	23	CD6/CD8 depletion	23%	4%	
147	19	Cyclosporine	80%*	44%*	No
	19	CD8 depletion/cyclosporine	20%	5%	

*P < .05.
†Yes indicates which arm had a survival advantage. The advantage was not always long-lasting.[152]
‡Initially reported with a survival advantage, but not when corrected for disease and disease status at transplantation.[174]

Subsequent randomized trials and the registry analysis showed both a treatment benefit and a survival benefit for the combination of cyclosporine and methotrexate over single-agent cyclosporine (see Table 39–3). The combination of cyclosporine and methotrexate thus became the standard of care for prevention of GVHD after HLA-identical BMT. Long-term follow-up of the randomized trials, however, failed to demonstrate improvement in the prevention of chronic GVHD or in disease-free survival.[152, 153] The combination of cyclosporine and corticosteroids has been used frequently,[154] especially with busulfan-based conditioning regimens, because methotrexate was associated with a higher risk of veno-occlusive disease when administered with busulfan-based regimens.[155] Although not formally tested in a randomized trial, the risk of grade 2–4 GVHD after HLA-identical BMT with cyclosporine and corticosteroids appears to be similar to that with cyclosporine and methotrexate, but grade 3 or 4 GVHD occurs more frequently when methotrexate is not used. Mycophenolate mofetil has arisen as another alternative to methotrexate for use in combination with cyclosporine (Table 39–5). Preliminary results suggest that this combination is also active as GVHD prophylaxis,[159] but absorption of mycophenolate mofetil using the oral preparation is sometimes unpredictable.

Triple-drug prophylaxis with cyclosporine, methotrexate, and corticosteroids has been tested in randomized trials, but an advantage for the three-drug regimen has not been consistent (see Table 39–4), and no long-term benefits have been reported.[139, 172] Furthermore, concerns have been raised regarding the increase in infections when corticosteroids are used for the prevention of GVHD.[173] Adding anti–IL-2 to the standard combination delayed the onset of GVHD significantly, but it was also associated with a higher risk of relapse and lower disease-free survival.[144] Anti-TNF

also delayed the onset of GVHD, but it appeared to have an adverse effect on engraftment.[39]

Tacrolimus is the first drug demonstrated to be superior to cyclosporine for the prevention of acute GVHD after HLA-identical BMT. In a randomized trial, the risk of grade 2–4 GVHD was significantly lower with tacrolimus and methotrexate than with cyclosporine and methotrexate (see Table 39–4),[143] whereas engraftment and relapse were not affected. Although the original study showed a survival disadvantage for tacrolimus when the outcome of all patients was assessed, there was no difference in long-term disease-free survival when assessed specifically by disease and disease status at the time of transplantation.[174]

T-cell depletion has been explored extensively for prevention of GVHD after HLA-identical BMT (see Tables 39–4 and 39–5). The original randomized trial of CD8 depletion was encouraging,[147] but subsequent trials have reported a high incidence of "cytokine syndrome" mimicking GVHD and a high rate of pulmonary hemorrhage in patients receiving CD8-depleted marrow transplants.[161–163] Pan–T-cell depletion using anti-CD6 or one of the antibodies of the Campath series was effective in preventing GVHD without additional pharmacologic therapy (Table 39–5), but the risk of graft failure was substantial. Increasing the intensity of the conditioning regimen or administering additional CD34+ cells reduced the graft failure rate associated with elutriation for prevention of GVHD.[169, 170] Elutriation, lectin + E-rosette depletion, and CD34+ selection all appear to be promising approaches, but randomized trials are lacking.

T-cell depletion for HLA-identical marrow transplantation has been associated with an increase in infection, relapse, and graft failure with no survival advantage.[175] Preliminary reports using T-cell depletion with planned T-cell add-back post transplantation have not been encouraging. This strategy was still associated with substantial infec-

TABLE 39–5. GVHD PROPHYLAXIS FOR HLA-IDENTICAL ALLOGENEIC MARROW TRANSPLANTATION: NEW AND INVESTIGATIONAL APPROACHES

REFERENCE	NO. OF PATIENTS	REGIMEN	GRADE 2–4 GVHD	GRADE 3–4 GVHD	REJECTION
156	27	Tacrolimus	41%	4%	0%
157	28*	Tacrolimus/methotrexate	15%	7%	—
158	43	Tacrolimus/minimethotrexate	18%	0%	0%
159	14	Cyclosporine/mycophenolate mofetil	47%	7%	0%
39	21*	Cyclosporine/methotrexate/anti-TNF	70%	30%	10%
160	4	CD4 depletion/cyclosporine	75%	75%	0%
161	36	CD8 depletion/cyclosporine	28%	8%	3%
162	29*	CD8 depletion/cyclosporine	20%	5%	0%
163	57	CD8 depletion/cyclosporine ± other	61%	—	0%
164	112	CD6 depletion	18%	9%	3%
165	41	CD6 depletion	15%	2%	7%
118	34	Campath-1G	27%	17%	6%
	53	Campath-1G depletion	9%	2%	4%
	46	Campath-1G depletion/Campath-1G	3%	0%	22%
	290	Campath-1M depletion	20%	8%	21%
	161	Campath-1M depletion/Campath-1G	11%	9%	8%
166	31	Lectin + E-rosette depletion	8%	0%	16%
167	70	Lectin + E-rosette depletion	37%	0%	0%
168	39	Lectin + E-rosette depletion	0%	0%	0%
169	181	Elutriation/cyclosporine ± other	20%	5%	5%
170	110	Elutriation/cyclosporine	11%	—	4%
171	14	CD34 selection	29%	0%	0%

*Series includes occasional alternative donor marrow transplant recipient.

tion, and the risk of GVHD increased when lymphocyte infusions were given.[176, 177]

ALLOGENEIC PERIPHERAL BLOOD PROGENITOR CELL TRANSPLANTATION (PBPCT)

Cyclosporine-based regimens were used for the first large studies of HLA-identical allogeneic PBPCT; rates of grade 2–4 acute GVHD were 37–57% in the largest studies using cyclosporine in combination with methotrexate or methylprednisolone (Table 39–6).[78, 178–180, 191] The risk of GVHD after allogeneic PBPCT was significantly lower with tacrolimus-based prophylaxis than with cyclosporine and methylprednisolone,[78] and the combination of tacrolimus and minimethotrexate was more effective than tacrolimus alone.[181]

Cyclosporine has also been evaluated in combination with mycophenolate mofetil for the prevention of GVHD after HLA-identical allogeneic PBPCT. Animal studies have demonstrated that mycophenolate mofetil is potent in enabling engraftment of allogeneic stem cells without a myeloablative regimen.[192] In clinical studies using a regimen of cyclosporine 6.25 mg/kg PO BID days −1 to +35, and mycophenolate mofetil 15 mg/kg PO BID days 0 to +28, mixed chimerism was achieved without a substantial risk of moderate-to-severe acute GVHD.[193] In a pilot study using cyclosporine and mycophenolate mofetil with a myeloablative conditioning regimen, however, 8 of 10 patients experienced grade 2–4 GVHD, indicating that oral mycophenolate mofetil may not be sufficiently immunosuppressive in this circumstance.[194]

Ex vivo T-cell depletion has not proved to be clinically effective for HLA-identical allogeneic PBPCT. Density gradient separation of allogeneic stem cells reduced CD3+ content by approximately 1 log and did not confer a significant reduction in GVHD.[195, 196] The risk of GVHD also remained high in recipients of CD8-depleted allogeneic stem cells,[163] and with elutriation.[182] With use of Campath-1G "in the bag" as sole GVHD prophylaxis, only 17% of HLA-identical PBPCT recipients experienced grade 2–4 GVHD, but as with many T-cell–depletion procedures, engraftment was delayed and infectious complications were a problem.[184] The rate of GVHD was also low with Campath-1M "in the bag" and a short course of cyclosporine, but there was a high rate of mixed chimerism with this approach.[183]

CD34+ selection has been studied extensively for HLA-identical allogeneic PBPCT (see Table 39–7).[186–190] CD34+ selection results in about a 2-log depletion of CD3+ cells and is used in conjunction with cyclosporine- or tacrolimus-based immunosuppression. The rates of grade 2–4 GVHD with CD34+-selected allogeneic PBPCT are 0–86%. High doses of CD34+ cells are associated with a high incidence of GVHD after allogeneic PBPCT,[78] and this may account for the results in the two studies with the highest rates of GVHD in CD34+-selected allogeneic PBPCT recipients.[185, 186] Although CD34+ selection of PBPC results in a decrease in severe GVHD, there was also a trend for increased relapse,[190] as was predicted by preclinical studies.[197]

The risk of moderate-to-severe GVHD after transplantation of stem cells from partially matched donors is nearly prohibitive using standard cyclosporine-based[198] or tacrolimus-based[199] immunosuppression, with rates in excess of 70% for one-antigen–mismatched transplants. Extensive T-cell depletion in combination with CD34+ selection reduced the T-cell content of the grafts by greater than 4 logs, and when used as sole GVHD prophylaxis for haploidentical PBPCT recipients, this deep T-cell depletion essentially eliminated the risk of GVHD.[200] This approach, however, greatly delays immune reconstitution and predisposes patients to a higher risk of fatal opportunistic infections.

In contrast, the risk of GVHD after PBPCT from HLA-A, -B, and -DRB1–matched unrelated donors is similar to that with unrelated donor marrow transplantation.[201] The risk of GVHD was even lower with CD34+ selection of the matched unrelated donor PBPC, but this was also

TABLE 39–6. GVHD PROPHYLAXIS FOR HLA-IDENTICAL ALLOGENEIC BLOOD PROGENITOR CELL TRANSPLANTATION

REFERENCE	NO. OF PATIENTS	REGIMEN	GRADE 2–4 GVHD	GRADE 3–4 GVHD	REJECTION
178	37	Cyclosporine/methotrexate	37%	14%	0%
179	33	Cyclosporine/methotrexate	54%	21%	3%
180	21	Cyclosporine/minimethotrexate	57%	24%	0%
78	50	Cyclosporine/steroids	45%	22%	0%
	55	Tacrolimus/steroids	30%	13%	0%
	55	Tacrolimus/micromethotrexate	21%	7%	4%
181	48	Tacrolimus/minimethotrexate	24%	—	—
	49	Tacrolimus	39%	—	—
182	12	Elutriation/cyclosporine	42%	17%	0%
183	17	Campath-1M "in the bag"/cyclosporine	6%	0%	6%
184	25	Campath-1G "in the bag"	16%	4%	4%
185	16	CD34+/cyclosporine ± methotrexate	86%	43%	0%
186	10	CD34+/cyclosporine ± methotrexate	60%	50%	0%
187	10	CD34+/cyclosporine	30%	0%	0%
188	20	CD34+/cyclosporine/steroids	0%	0%	0%
189	62	CD34+/cyclosporine ± methotrexate/steroids	10%	2%	3%
190	25	CD34+/cyclosporine ± methotrexate/antithyroid globulin (ATG)	—	0%	—
	25	Cyclosporine ± methotrexate/ATG	—	27%	—

associated with an increase in graft failure from 5% to 22%.[201]

PARTIALLY MATCHED RELATED DONOR MARROW TRANSPLANTATION (MISMATCHED RELATED BMT)

Using long methotrexate[46] or cyclosporine/methotrexate,[49] the rates and severity of acute GVHD increase with increasing HLA disparity. For patients with one-antigen–mismatched related donors, grade 2–4 acute GVHD occurs in 47–73%, with the lowest rate reported using tacrolimus and minimethotrexate[199] (Table 39–7). With either cyclosporine-based or tacrolimus-based prophylaxis, there is only a trend for less GVHD with single HLA-A or -B incompatibility than with HLA-DR mismatches.[199, 213] In fact, the combination of cyclosporine and methotrexate is no better than long methotrexate when there is an HLA-DR mismatch.[49] Nevertheless, combination prophylaxis has become standard for one-antigen–mismatched related BMT.

The markedly high rates of grade 2–4 GVHD with mismatched related BMT, especially with two- and three-antigen mismatches (>70%), clearly warrant evaluation of new methods for T-cell depletion for these patients. Using current techniques, ex vivo depletion of marrow T-cell subsets has diminished the risk of acute GVHD only modestly. Furthermore, this decrease has been accompanied by a mild increase in graft rejection.[208, 209] By contrast, GVHD prophylaxis using T10B9 for depletion of αβ+ T cells in combination with cyclosporine and ATG after transplantation was highly effective in reducing the risk of GVHD without a marked increase in graft rejection (see Table 39–7).[207] As with chemoprophylaxis, T-cell–subset depletion is most effective with one-antigen–mismatched transplants; with greater degrees of histoincompatibility, rates of grade 2–4 GVHD may still be in excess of 60%.[47, 206, 209]

Extensive lymphocyte depletion using Campath-1M or lectin + E-rosette depletion reduced the risk of GVHD

without the need for additional immunosuppressive drugs after mismatched related BMT, but the high rates of graft rejection (32–54%) made this approach ineffectual (see Table 39–7).[118, 210] Use of "megadoses" of selected CD34+ cells from peripheral blood augmenting marrow allografts has been used to overcome the problem with graft rejection associated with extensive lymphocyte depletion. CD34+ selection was not as effective in reducing GVHD as CD34+ selection in combination with lectin + E-rosette depletion.[211, 212] Both methods, however, were associated with profound and prolonged immunodeficiency.

More recently, induction of tolerance has been attempted by ex vivo blockade of costimulation during incubation of donor marrow with recipient cells in the presence of CTLA4-Ig. Patients also received cyclosporine and methotrexate after transplantation. Preliminary results suggest that this is a feasible approach for reducing GVHD in haploidentical marrow transplant recipients without increasing graft rejection,[205] but longer follow-up is needed to assess the effect on graft-versus-leukemia activity and survival.

Haploidentical marrow transplantation for severe combined immunodeficiency is a special circumstance. These patients have no malignancy to eradicate, no risk of graft rejection, and no need for repletion of myeloid hematopoiesis. For these patients, a conditioning regimen may not be needed, and extensive lymphocyte depletion of the haploidentical marrow using Campath-1M or lectin + E-rosette depletion is generally sufficient to prevent GVHD.[214–217] Additional posttransplant immunosuppressive therapy may be needed with lesser degrees of T-cell depletion.

UNRELATED DONOR MARROW TRANSPLANTATION (MATCHED UNRELATED BMT)

Cyclosporine and methotrexate have been used most commonly for prevention of GVHD after matched unrelated

TABLE 39–7. GVHD PROPHYLAXIS FOR PARTIALLY MATCHED RELATED DONOR MARROW TRANSPLANTATION

REFERENCE	NO. OF PATIENTS	REGIMEN	GRADES 2–4 GVHD WITH MISMATCH AT			
			1 Antigen	2 Antigens	3 Antigens	Rejection
46	93	Long methotrexate	73%	76%	84%	5%
202	15	Methotrexate, antithyroid globulin (ATG), prednisone		(75%)*		25%
203	19	Cyclosporine		(89%)*		5%
	14	Cyclosporine/methotrexate		(79%)*		7%
204	19	Cyclosporine/methotrexate (children)		(58%)*		21%
199	22	Tacrolimus/methotrexate	47%	—	—	9%
205	12	CTLA4-Ig incubation/cyclosporine/methotrexate		(27%)*		9%
206	40	T10B9 depletion/immunotoxin/steroids	33%	37%	67%	7%
207	58	T10B9 depletion/cyclosporine/steroids/ATG	18%	12%	18%	12%
208	23	CD5 depletion/methotrexate		(50%)*		15%
209	27	CD6 depletion		(40%)*		11%
118	124	Campath-1M depletion or -1G "in the bag"/other		(16%)*		54%
	40	Campath-1M depletion or -1G/other		(20%)*		32%
210	20	Lectin + E-rosette depletion		(5%)*		40%
211	10	CD34+/cyclosporine†		(80%)*		0%
212	17	CD34+/lectin + E-rosette depletion†		(6%)*		6%

*Data reported for patients as a group without regard to degree of HLA disparity.
†Marrow and peripheral blood progenitor cells used.

BMT (Table 39–8). With this combination, rates of 60–85% grade 2–4 GVHD and 35–55% grade 3–4 GVHD have been reported with HLA-A, -B, and -DR matched donors. With serologic mismatches, the risk of GVHD after matched unrelated BMT rises[48, 223] even with combination prophylaxis and is nearly as high as that reported for long methotrexate alone.[238] The risk of GVHD is reduced with molecular matching of class II, but grade 3–4 GVHD rates as high as 50% have still been reported despite such matching.[54]

The combination of tacrolimus and methotrexate has been shown to be superior to cyclosporine and methotrexate in a randomized trial for matched unrelated BMT.[222] Using tacrolimus-based prophylaxis, grade 2–4 GVHD was reported in 42–51%, and grade 3–4 in 12–31% of cases (see Table 39–8). The risk of GVHD is increased with molecular mismatching using tacrolimus-based immunoprophylaxis as well.[219] In a phase II multicenter study of combination regimens, the risk of GVHD was highest using tacrolimus and steroids, whereas there was little difference in GVHD between tacrolimus and standard methotrexate or minimethotrexate.[221] The combination of tacrolimus and minimethotrexate is currently favored because it produces less mucositis.

Others have evaluated additional agents in combination with cyclosporine and methotrexate to reduce GVHD after matched unrelated BMT. The addition of steroids provided better control of GVHD with molecularly matched donors,[225] but the beneficial effects of steroids were not consistent.[224] Low rates of GVHD were also reported using ATG, especially when administration began prior to transplantation,[226, 227] but randomized studies are lacking. Use of anti–IL-2 receptor antibodies has not been effective in the prevention of GVHD when used with cyclosporine and methotrexate, likely because IL-2 receptor blockade prohibits activation-induced programmed cell death and prevents clonal deletion of alloreactive T cells.[228, 229] Campath-1G, a broadly lympholytic antibody, does reduce the risk of GVHD, but its use also resulted in substantial graft rejection.[118] Anti-CD5 immunotoxin, another broadly reactive agent, was both ineffective and toxic. When combined with cyclosporine and T-cell depletion, however, anti-CD5 immunotoxin was much more effective in preventing GVHD and less toxic, but the relapse rate was markedly increased.[231]

T-cell depletion has been tested using a number of lymphocyte subset or broadly reactive antibodies or elutriation

TABLE 39–8. GVHD PROPHYLAXIS FOR UNRELATED DONOR MARROW TRANSPLANTATION

REFERENCE	NO. OF PATIENTS	REGIMEN	GRADE 2–4 GVHD	GRADE 3–4 GVHD	REJECTION†
218	43*	Tacrolimus/methotrexate	42%	12%	—
219	68*	Tacrolimus/minimethotrexate	43%	22%	0%
	100	Tacrolimus/minimethotrexate	51%	31%	1%
220	43	Tacrolimus/minimethotrexate	40%	22%	0%
221	44	Tacrolimus/methotrexate	43%	14%	—
	37	Tacrolimus/minimethotrexate	41%	19%	—
	16	Tacrolimus/steroids	50%	19%	—
222	90	Tacrolimus/methotrexate	56%	19%	—
	90	Cyclosporine/methotrexate	74%	27%	—
54	305*	Cyclosporine/methotrexate	88%	48%	1%
223	42*	Cyclosporine/methotrexate (children)	83%	37%	0%
224	16	Cyclosporine/methotrexate	56%	—	—
	13	Cyclosporine/methotrexate/steroids	77%	—	—
225	30*	Cyclosporine/methotrexate/steroids	38%	24%	0%
226	132	Antithyroid globulin (ATG)/OKT3-cyclosporine/methotrexate	23%	8%	4%
227	48	ATG/cyclosporine/methotrexate/others	39%	11%	2%
228	64	Cyclosporine/methotrexate/anti-IL-2R	58%	40%	9%
	89	Cyclosporine/methotrexate/other	61%	43%	7%
229	65	Cyclosporine/methotrexate	66%	—	8%
	69	Cyclosporine/methotrexate/low anti-IL-2R	72%	—	9%
	76	Cyclosporine/methotrexate/high anti-IL-2R	75%	—	8%
118	60	Cyclosporine/methotrexate/Campath-1G	31%	19%	12%
230	31	Cyclosporine/methotrexate/anti-CD5-RAC	58%	19%	0%
231	16	Cyclosporine/steroids/anti-CD5-RAC	86%	86%	10%
	13	CD3 depletion/cyclosporine/steroids	86%	52%	0%
	39	CD3 depletion/cyclosporine/steroids/anti-CD5-RAC	36%	13%	8%
232	20	T10B9 depletion/cyclosporine	37%	10%	0%
233	30	ATG-CD5/8 depletion/cyclosporine/methotrexate/steroids	—	24%	—
	31	ATG-cyclosporine/methotrexate/steroids	—	67%	—
234	23*	CD6 depletion	39%	—	—
118	30	Campath-1M depletion/Campath-1G	39%	9%	27%
235	27	Campath-1M or -1G depletion/cyclosporine (children)	7%	0%	—
236	12	Elutriation/cyclosporine/steroids/ATG	25%	—	17%
237	23	CD34+/cyclosporine/steroid ± methotrexate	20%	—	9%
	37	Cyclosporine/methotrexate ± other	60%	—	0%

*Predominantly or exclusively HLA-A, -B, and -DRB1 matched. In the remainder of the studies, patient/donor pairs are predominantly serologically matched for HLA-A, -B, and -DR.
†May include patients with graft failure not due to immunologic rejection if the reason for graft failure was not provided.

(see Table 39–8). The individual studies as well as large registry analyses[85, 239] have repeatedly demonstrated that the risk of GVHD is lower after matched unrelated BMT when T-cell depletion is used. This benefit, however, was offset by an increase in infection and graft rejection in many cases, and no survival advantage was demonstrated in a randomized trial[233] or in the registry studies.[239] Less rejection and infectious complications have been reported using T-cell depletion with T10B9, currently being tested in a randomized protocol for matched unrelated BMT. T10B9 depletion has also been used for mismatched unrelated donor marrow transplantation, but the results have been inconsistent.[232, 240, 241]

A small study has been conducted using CD34+ selection of marrow with cyclosporine-based immunosuppression for matched unrelated BMT.[237] There was less GVHD with CD34+ selection than with cyclosporine/methotrexate and unmanipulated marrow, but more than 60% of patients had mixed chimerism after CD34+ selected matched unrelated BMT and 9% experienced graft rejection. Whether this portends loss of the graft-versus-leukemia effect using CD34+ selection remains to be determined.

UMBILICAL CORD BLOOD TRANSPLANTATION

The optimal regimen for prevention of GVHD after umbilical cord blood transplantation (UCBT) has not been determined. Cyclosporine, cyclosporine/steroids, cyclosporine/high-dose steroids (methylprednisolone, 10 mg/kg/day), cyclosporine/methotrexate, and tacrolimus/minimethotrexate have been used, with grade 3–4 GVHD occurring in less than 10% of cases after related UCBT[242, 243] and in 0–29% of cases after unrelated matched or mismatched UCBT.[243–246] Standard-dose methotrexate has been avoided in view of the already prolonged period of neutropenia common after UCBT. Inclusion of steroids in the GVHD prophylaxis regimen was associated with significantly lower mortality.[247] At present, however, no specific GVHD prophylaxis regimen appears superior to the others for UCBT.

DONOR LYMPHOCYTE INFUSION

Without pharmacologic prophylaxis, GVHD is reported to occur in almost 50% of patients who receive a donor lymphocyte infusion (DLI).[248, 249] CD8 depletion has been used to reduce the risk of GVHD, and the occurrence of GVHD has been shown to correlate with the number of CD4+ cells infused.[250, 251] CD8 depletion did not appear to abrogate the graft-versus-leukemia effect of DLI, but no randomized studies have been performed to confirm this. Ex vivo depletion of IL-2R+ cells after activation with recipient cells is under evaluation.[252, 253] In vivo depletion of activated alloreactive cells has been accomplished using donor lymphocytes transduced with the herpes simplex virus thymidine kinase genes,[254] but whether alloreactive T cells can be controlled reliably using gene therapy remains to be determined.

CONCLUSION

Acute GVHD is a complex reaction dependent on T-lymphocytes and other immunocompetent cells in the marrow or PBPC allograft. The incidence and severity of acute GVHD are related to the degree of mismatch in both major and minor histocompatibility antigens. Combination chemoprophylaxis is currently the standard of care for HLA-identical BMT. Ex vivo manipulations to deplete T-lymphocytes are favored when there is a substantial degree of histoincompatibility. Although T-cell depletion reduces the risk of GVHD, the associated increase in graft failure, relapse, and prolonged immunodeficiency may limit the benefit of this approach over standard combination chemoprophylaxis. Thus, GVHD remains a major cause of morbidity and mortality after BMT. A number of new immunosuppressive drugs have become available, and new methods for lymphocyte removal and adoptive immunotherapy are being evaluated to achieve specific tolerance induction with allogeneic BMT.

REFERENCES

1. Mathé G, Bernard J, de Vries MJ, et al: Nouveaux essais de greffe de moelle osseuse homologue après irradiation totale chez des enfants atteints de leucémie aige en rémission: le problème due syndrome secondaire chez l'homme. Rev Hematol 15:115–161, 1960.
2. Thomas ED, Herman EC, Greenough WB, et al: Irradiation and marrow infusion in leukemia. Arch Intern Med 107:829–845, 1961.
3. Billingham RE: The biology of graft-versus-host reactions. Harvey Lecture 62:21–78, 1966.
4. Trentin JJ: Mortality and skin transplantibility in X-irradiated mice receiving isologous, homologous or heterologous bone marrow. Proc Soc Exp Biol Med 92:688–693, 1956.
5. Bodmer JG, Marsh SGE, Albert ED, et al: Nomenclature for factors of the HLA system, 1998. Hum Immunol 60:361–395, 1999.
6. Szydlo R, Goldman JM, Klein JP, et al: Results of allogeneic bone marrow transplants for leukemia using donors other than HLA-identical siblings. J Clin Oncol 15:1767–1777, 1997.
7. Nishimura M, Uchida S, Mitsuaga S, et al: Identification of HLA class II antigens as the targets of effector clones which may cause transfusion-associated graft-versus-host disease. Transfus Med 7:89–94, 1997.
8. Storb R, Rudolph RH, Kolb HJ, et al: Marrow grafts between DL-A-matched canine littermates. Transplantation 15:92–100, 1973.
9. Bevan MJ: The major histocompatibility complex determines susceptibility to cytotoxic T cells directed against minor histocompatibility antigens. J Exp Med 142:1349–1364, 1975.
10. Sullivan KM, Deeg HJ, Sanders J, et al: Hyperacute graft-v-host disease in patients not given immunosuppression after allogeneic marrow transplantation. Blood 67:1172–1175, 1986.
11. Niederwieser D, Grassegger A, Aubock J, et al: Correlation of minor histocompatibility antigen-specific cytotoxic T lymphocytes with graft-versus-host disease status and analyses of tissue distribution of their target antigens. Blood 81:2200–2208, 1993.
12. Faber LM, van Luxemburg-Heijs SA, Veenhof WF, et al: Generation of CD4+ cytotoxic T-lymphocyte clones from a patient with severe graft-versus-host disease after allogeneic bone marrow transplantation: implications for graft-versus-leukemia reactivity. Blood 86:2821–2828, 1995.
13. Goulmy E: Human minor histocompatibility antigens: new concepts for marrow transplantation and adoptive immunotherapy. Immunol Rev 157:125–140, 1997.
14. Gallagher MT, Richie ER, Heim LR, et al: Inhibition of the graft-versus-host reaction: I. Reduction of the graft-versus-host potential of mouse spleen cells (with sparing of stem cells) by treatment with antilymphocyte globulin-derived Fab fragments. Transplantation 14:597–602, 1972.
15. Korngold B, Sprent J: Lethal graft-versus-host disease after bone marrow transplantation across minor histocompatibility barriers in mice: prevention by removing mature T cells from marrow. J Exp Med 148:1687–1698, 1978.
16. Reisner Y, Kapoor N, Kirkpatrick D, et al. Transplantation for acute leukemia with HLA-A and B non-identical parenteral marrow cells fractionated with soybean agglutinin and sheep red blood cells. Lancet 2:327–331, 1981.

17. Sykes M, Harty MW, Pearson DA: Strain dependence of interleukin-2 induced graft-versus-host disease protection: evidence that interleukin-2 inhibits selected CD4 functions. J Immunother 15:11–21, 1994.

18. O'Kunewick JP, Meredith RF, Raikow RB, et al: Possibility of three distinct and separable components to fatal graft-vs-host reaction. Exp Hematol 10:277–291, 1982.

19. Ferrara JL, Guillen FJ, van Dijken PJ, et al: Evidence that large granular lymphocytes of donor origin mediate acute graft-versus-host disease. Transplantation 47:50–54, 1989.

20. Mowat AM, Felstein MV: Experimental studies of immunologically mediated enteropathy: II. Role of natural killer cells in the intestinal phase of murine graft-versus-host reaction. Immunology 61:179–183, 1987.

21. Rhoades JL, Cibull ML, Thompson JS, et al: Role of natural killer cells in the pathogenesis of human acute graft-versus-host disease. Transplantation 56:113–120, 1993.

22. Ghayur T, Seemayer TA, Lapp WS: Kinetics of natural killer cell cytotoxicity during graft-versus-host reaction: relationship between natural killer cell activity, T and B cell activity, and development of histopathological alterations. Transplantation 44:254–260, 1987.

23. Tutschka PJ, Ki PF, Beschorner WE, et al: Suppressor cells in transplantation tolerance: II. Maturation of suppressor cells in the bone marrow chimera. Transplantation 32:321–325, 1981.

24. Deeg HJ, Severns E, Raff RF, et al: Specific tolerance and immunocompetence in haploidentical, but not completely allogeneic, canine chimeras treated with methotrexate and cyclosporine. Transplantation 44:621–632, 1987.

25. Tsoi MS, Storb R, Dobbs S, et al: Specific suppressor cells in graft-host tolerance of HLA-identical marrow transplantation. Nature 292:355–357, 1981.

26. Weiden PL, Storb R, Tsoi MS, et al: Infusion of donor lymphocytes into stable canine radiation chimeras: implications for mechanism of transplantation tolerance. J Immunol 116:1212–1219, 1976.

27. Strober S: Natural suppressor (NS) cells, neonatal tolerance, and total lymphoid irradiation: exploring obscure relationships. Ann Rev Immunol 2:219–237, 1984.

28. Johnson BD, Truitt RL: Delayed infusion of immunocompetent donor cells after bone marrow transplantation breaks graft-host tolerance allows for persistent antileukemic reactivity without severe graft-versus-host disease. Blood 85:3302–3312, 1995.

29. Tsoi MS, Storb R, Dobbs S, et al: Specific suppressor cells and immune response to host antigens in long-term human allogeneic marrow recipients: implications for the mechanisms of graft-host tolerance and chronic graft-versus-host disease. Transplant Proc 13:237–240, 1981.

30. Reinherz EL, Parkman R, Rappeport J, et al: Aberrations of suppressor T cells in human graft-versus-host disease. N Engl J Med 300:1061–1068, 1979.

31. Pham CT, Ley TJ: The role of granzyme B cluster proteases in cell-mediated cytotoxicity. Semin Immunol 9:127–133, 1997.

32. Graubert TA, DiPersio JF, Russell JH, et al: Perforin/granzyme-dependent and independent mechanisms are both important for the development of graft-versus-host disease after murine bone marrow transplantation. J Clin Invest 100:904–911, 1997.

33. Blazar BR, Taylor PA, Vallera DA: CD4+ and CD8+ T cells each can utilize a perforin-dependent pathway to mediate lethal graft-versus-host disease in major histocompatibility complex-disparate recipients. Transplantation 64:571–576, 1997.

34. Baker MB, Riley RL, Podack ER, et al: Graft-versus-host-disease-associated lymphoid hypoplasia and B cell dysfunction is dependent upon donor T cell-mediated Fas-ligand function, but not perforin function. Proc Natl Acad Sci U S A 94:1366–1371, 1997.

35. Hosaka N, Nagata N, Nakagawa T, et al: Analyses of lpr-GVHD by adoptive transfer experiments using MRL/lpr-Thy-1.1 congenic mice. Autoimmunity 17:217–224, 1994.

36. Speiser DE, Bachmann MF, Frick TW, et al: TNF receptor p55 controls early acute graft-versus-host disease. J Immunol 158:5185–5190, 1997.

37. Jadus MR, Wepsic HT: The role of cytokines in graft-versus-host reactions and disease. Bone Marrow Transplant 10:1–14, 1992.

38. Ferrara JL, Cooke KR, Pan L, et al: The immunopathophysiology of acute graft-versus-host disease. Stem Cells 14:473–489, 1996.

39. Holler E, Kolb HJ, Mittermuller J, et al: Modulation of acute graft-versus-host disease after allogeneic bone marrow transplantation by

40. Herve P, Flesch M, Tiberghien P, et al: Phase I–II trial of a monoclonal anti-tumor necrosis factor antibody for the treatment of refractory severe acute graft-versus-host disease. Blood 79:3362–3368, 1992.

41. Holler E, Kolb HJ, Hintermeier-Knabe R, et al: Role of tumor necrosis factor alpha in acute graft-versus-host disease and complications following allogeneic bone marrow transplantation. Transplant Proc 25:1234–1236, 1993.

42. Imamura M, Hashino S, Kobayashi H, et al: Serum cytokine levels in bone marrow transplantation: interaction of interleukin-6, interferon gamma, and tumor necrosis factor-alpha in graft-versus-host disease. Bone Marrow Transplant 13:745–751, 1994.

43. Abdallah AN, Boiron JM, Attia Y, et al: Plasma cytokines in graft-vs-host disease and complications following bone marrow transplantation. Hematol Cell Ther 39:27–32, 1997.

44. Tanaka J, Imamura M, Kasai M, et al: Cytokine gene expression in the mixed lymphocyte culture in allogeneic bone marrow transplants as a predictive method for transplantation-related complications. Br J Haematol 87:415–418, 1994.

45. Vossen JM, Heidt PJ, van den Berg H, et al: Prevention of infection and graft-versus-host disease by suppression of intestinal microflora in children treated with allogeneic bone marrow transplantation. Eur J Clin Microbiol Infect Dis 9:14–23, 1990.

46. Beatty PG, Clift RA, Mickelson EM, et al: Marrow transplantation from related donors other than HLA-identical siblings. N Engl J Med 313:765–771, 1985.

47. Ash RC, Horowitz MM, Gale RP, et al: Bone marrow transplantation from related donors other than HLA-identical siblings: effect of T cell depletion. Bone Marrow Transplant 7:443–452, 1991.

48. Beatty PG, Anasetti C, Hansen JA, et al: Marrow transplantation from unrelated donors for treatment of hematologic malignancies: effect of mismatching for one HLA locus. Blood 81:249–253, 1993.

49. Anasetti C, Hansen J: Bone marrow transplantation from HLA-partially matched related donors and unrelated volunteer donors. In Forman SJ, Blume KG, Thomas ED (eds): Bone Marrow Transplantation. Cambridge, MA, Blackwell Scientific, 1994, pp 665–679.

50. Petersdorf EW, Smith AG, Mickelson EM, et al: The role of HLA-DPB1 disparity in the development of acute graft-versus-host disease following unrelated donor marrow transplantation. Blood 8l:1923–1932, 1993.

51. Nagler A, Brautbar C, Slavin S, et al: Bone marrow transplantation using unrelated and family related donors: the impact of HLA-C disparity. Bone Marrow Transplant 18:891–897, 1996.

52. Sasazuki T, Juji T, Morishima Y, et al: Effect of matching of class I HLA alleles on clinical outcome after transplantation of hematopoietic stem cells from an unrelated donor. N Engl J Med 339:1177–1185, 1998.

53. Senitzer D, Schaub B, Dagis A, et al: Mismatching for HLA-C in 107 unrelated bone marrow transplants: effects on the risk of the occurrence of acute graft-versus-host disease. Blood 90:397a, 1997.

54. Petersdorf EW, Longton GM, Anasetti C, et al: The significance of HLA-DRB1 matching on clinical outcome after HLA-A, B, DR identical unrelated donor marrow transplantation. Blood 86:1606–1613, 1995.

55. Gajewski J, Gjertson D, Cecka M, et al: The impact of T-cell depletion on the effects of HLA DRB1 and DQB allele matching in HLA serologically identical unrelated donor bone marrow transplantation. Biol Blood Marrow Transplant 3:76–82, 1997.

56. Bross DS, Tutschka PJ, Farmer ER, et al: Predictive factors for acute graft-versus-host disease in patients transplanted with HLA-identical bone marrow. Blood 63:1265–1270, 1984.

57. Weisdorf D, Hakke R, Blazar B, et al: Risk factors for acute graft-versus-host disease in histocompatible donor bone marrow transplantation. Transplantation 51:1197–1203, 1991.

58. Nash RA, Pepe MS, Storb R, et al: Acute graft-versus-host disease: analysis of risk factors after allogeneic marrow transplantation and prophylaxis with cyclosporine and methotrexate. Blood 80:1838–1845, 1992.

59. Goulmy E, Schipper R, Pool J, et al: Mismatches of minor histocompatibility antigens between HLA-identical donors and recipients and the development of graft-versus-host disease after bone marrow transplantation. N Engl J Med 334:281–285, 1996.

60. Mickelson EM, Guthrie LA, Etzioni R, et al: Role of the mixed lymphocyte culture (MLC) reaction in marrow donor selection: matching for transplants from related haploidentical donors. Tissue Antigens 44:83–92, 1994.

61. Mickelson EM, Longton G, Anasetti C, et al: Evaluation of the mixed lymphocyte culture (MLC) assay as a method for selecting unrelated donors for marrow transplantation. Tissue Antigens 47:27–36, 1996.

62. Johnsen HE, Beatty PG, Michelson E, et al: Donor alloreactivity may predict acute graft-versus-host disease in HLA-matched bone marrow transplantation for leukemia in early remission. Eur J Haematol 48:249–253, 1992.

63. Johnsen HE, Bostrom L, Moller J, et al: A study of alloreactivity, which may predict acute graft-versus-host disease in HLA identical bone marrow transplantation for early leukemia. Scand J Immunol 35:353–360, 1992.

64. Spencer A, Szydlo RM, Brookes PA, et al: Bone marrow transplantation for chronic myeloid leukemia with volunteer unrelated donors using ex vivo or in vivo T-cell depletion: major prognostic impact of HLA class I identity between donor and recipient. Blood 86:3590–3597, 1995.

65. Pei J, Martin PJ, Longton G, et al: Evaluation of pretransplant donor anti-recipient cytotoxic and helper T lymphocyte responses as correlates of acute graft-versus-host disease and survival after unrelated marrow transplantation. Biol Blood Marrow Transplant 3:142–149, 1997.

66. Keever-Taylor CA, Passweg J, Kawanishi Y, et al: Association of donor-derived host-reacting cytolytic and helper T cells with outcome following alternative donor T cell-depleted bone marrow transplantation. Bone Marrow Transplant 19:1001–1009, 1997.

67. Theobald M, Nierle T, Bunjes D, et al: Host-specific interleukin-2-secreting donor T-cell precursors as predictors of acute graft-versus-host disease in bone marrow transplantation between HLA-identical siblings. N Engl J Med 327:1613–1617, 1992.

68. Schwarer A, Jiang Y, Brookes P, et al: Frequency of anti-recipient alloreactive helper T-cell precursors in donor blood and graft-versus-host disease after HLA-identical sibling bone-marrow transplantation. Lancet 341:203–205, 1993.

69. Lachance S, Gouvello SL, Roudot F, et al: Predictive value of host-specific donor helper T-cell precursor frequency for acute graft-versus-host disease and relapse in HLA-identical siblings receiving allogeneic bone marrow transplantation for hematologic malignancies. Transplantation 64:1147–1152, 1997.

70. Vogelsang GB, Hess AD, Berkman AW, et al: An in vitro test for graft-versus-host disease in patients with genotypic HLA-identical bone marrow transplants. N Engl J Med 313:645–650, 1985.

71. Kernan NA, Collins NH, Juliano L, et al: Clonable T lymphocytes in T cell-depleted bone marrow transplants correlate with development of graft-versus-host disease. Blood 68:770–773, 1986.

72. Filipovich AH, Vallera D, McGlave P, et al: T cell depletion with anti-CD5 immunotoxin in histocompatible bone marrow transplantation. Transplantation 50:410–415, 1990.

73. Przepiorka D, Huh YO, Khouri I, et al: Graft failure and graft-versus-host disease after subtotal T-cell-depleted marrow transplantation: correlations with marrow hematopoietic and lymphoid subsets. Prog Clin Biol Res 389:557–563, 1994.

74. Martin PJ, Hansen JA, Torok-Storb B, et al: Graft failure in patients receiving T cell-depleted HLA-identical allogeneic marrow transplants. Bone Marrow Transplant 3:445–456, 1988.

75. Sierra J, Storer B, Hansen JA, et al: Transplantation of marrow cells from unrelated donors for treatment of high-risk acute leukemia: the effect of leukemic burden, donor HLA-matching and marrow cell dose. Blood 89:4226–4235, 1997.

76. Atkinson K, Farrel C, Chapman G, et al: Female marrow donors increase the risk of acute graft-versus-host disease: effect of donor age and parity and analysis of cell subpopulations in the donor marrow inoculum. Br J Haematol 63:231–239, 1986.

77. Hagglund H, Bostrom L, Remberger M, et al: Risk factors for acute graft-versus-host disease in 291 consecutive HLA-identical bone marrow transplant recipients. Bone Marrow Transplant 16:747–753, 1995.

78. Przepiorka D, Smith TL, Folloder J, et al: Risk factors for acute graft-vs-host disease after allogeneic blood stem cell transplantation. Blood 94:1465–1470, 1999.

79. Deeg HJ, Spitzer TR, Cottler-Fox M, et al: Conditioning-related toxicity and acute graft-versus-host disease in patients given methotrexate/cyclosporine prophylaxis. Bone Marrow Transplant 7:193–198, 1991.

80. Hill GR, Crawford JM, Cooke KR, et al: Total body irradiation and acute graft-versus-host disease: the role of gastrointestinal damage and inflammatory cytokines. Blood 90:3204–3213, 1997.

81. Gluckman E, Horowitz MM, Champlin RE, et al: Bone marrow transplantation for severe aplastic anemia: influence of conditioning and graft-versus-host disease prophylaxis regimens on outcome. Blood 79:269–275, 1992.

82. Hill RS, Petersen FB, Storb R, et al: Mixed hematologic chimerism after allogeneic marrow transplantation for severe aplastic anemia is associated with a higher risk of graft rejection and a lessened incidence of acute graft-versus-host disease. Blood 67:811–816, 1986.

83. Gale RP, Bortin MM, van Bekkum DW, et al: Risk factors for acute graft-versus-host disease. Br J Haematol 67:397–406, 1987.

84. Anasetti C, Beatty PG, Storb R, et al: Effect of HLA incompatibility on graft-versus-host disease, relapse, and survival after marrow transplantation for patients with leukemia or lymphoma. Hum Immunol 29:79–91, 1990.

85. Kernan NA, Bartsch G, Ash RC, et al: Analysis of 462 transplantations from unrelated donors facilitated by the National Marrow Donor Program. N Engl J Med 328:593–602, 1993.

86. Davies SM, Shu XO, Blazar BR, et al: Unrelated donor bone marrow transplantation: influence of HLA A and B incompatibility on outcome. Blood 86:1636–1642, 1995.

87. Gaziev D, Polchi P, Galimberti M, et al: Graft-versus-host disease after bone marrow transplantation for thalassemia. Transplantation 63:854–860, 1997.

88. Flowers ME, Pepe MS, Longton G, et al: Previous donor pregnancy as a risk factor for acute graft-versus-host disease in patients with aplastic anaemia treated by allogeneic marrow transplantation. Br J Haematol 74:492–496, 1990.

89. Bierer B: Biology of cyclosporin A and FK506. Prog Clin Biol Res 390:203–223, 1994.

90. Schwinghammer TL, Przepiorka D, Venkataramanan R, et al: The kinetics of cyclosporine and its metabolites in bone marrow transplant patients. Br J Pharmacol 32:323–328, 1991.

91. Wingard JR, Nash RA, Przepiorka D, et al: Relationship of tacrolimus (FK506) whole blood concentrations and efficacy and safety after HLA identical sibling bone marrow transplantation. Biol Blood Marrow Transplant 4:157–163, 1998.

92. Caudell KA, Adams J: Cyclosporine administration practices on bone marrow transplant units: a national survey. Oncol Nursing Forum 17:563–568, 1990.

93. Ruutu T, Niederwieser D, Gratwohl A, et al: A survey of the prophylaxis and treatment of acute GVHD in Europe: a report of the European Group for Blood and Marrow Transplantation (EBMT). Bone Marrow Transplant 19:759–764, 1997.

94. Peters C, Minkov M, Gadner H, et al: Proposal for standard recommendatons for prophylaxis of graft-versus-host disease in children. Bone Marrow Transplant 21:S57–S60, 1998.

95. Bacigalupo A, van Lint MT, Occhini D, et al: Increased risk of leukemia relapse with high-dose cyclosporine A after allogeneic marrow transplantation for acute leukemia. Blood 77:1423–1428, 1991.

96. Kahan BD: Considerations concerning generic formulations of immunosuppressive drugs. Transplant Proc 31:1635–1641, 1999.

97. Atkinson K, Downs K, Ashby M, et al: Clinical correlations with cyclosporine blood levels after allogeneic bone marrow transplantation: an analysis of four different assays. Transplant Proc 22:1331–1334, 1990.

98. Storb R, Leisenring W, Anasetti C, et al: Methotrexate and cyclosporine for graft-vs-host disease prevention: what length of therapy with cyclosporine? Biol Blood Marrow Transplant 3:194–201, 1997.

99. Abraham R, Szer J, Bardy P, et al: Early cyclosporine taper in high-risk sibling allogeneic bone marrow transplants. Bone Marrow Transplant 20:773–777, 1997.

100. Bacigalupo A, Maiolino A, van Lint MT, et al: Cyclosporin A and chronic graft-versus-host disease. Bone Marrow Transplant 6:341–344, 1990.

101. Schwinghammer TL, Bloom EJ, Rosenfeld CS, et al: High-dose cyclosporine and corticosteroids for prophylaxis of acute and chronic graft-versus-host disease. Bone Marrow Transplant 16:147–154, 1995.

102. Hows J, Palmer S, Gordon-Smith EC: Cyclosporine and graft failure following bone marrow transplantation for severe aplastic anemia. Br J Haematol 60:611–617, 1985.

103. Jacobson P, Uberti J, Davis W, et al: Tacrolimus: a new agent for the prevention of graft-versus-host disease in hematopoietic stem cell transplantation. Bone Marrow Transplant 22:217–225, 1998.

104. Boswell GW, Bekersky I, Fay J, et al: Tacrolimus pharmacokinetics in BMT patients. Bone Marrow Transplant 21:23–28, 1998.

105. Przepiorka D, Devine SM, Fay JW, et al: Practical considerations in the use of tacrolimus for allogeneic marrow transplantation. Bone Marrow Transplant 24:1053–1056, 1999.

106. Kelly PA, Gruber SA, Behbod F, et al: Sirolimus, a new potent immunosuppressive agent. Pharmacotherapy 17:1148–1156, 1997.

107. Blazar BR, Taylor PA, Panoskaltsis-Mortari A, et al: Rapamycin inhibits the generation of graft-versus-host disease- and graft-versus-leukemia-causing T cells by interfering with the production of Th1 or Th1 cytotoxic cytokines. J Immunol 160:5355–5365, 1998.

108. Nevill TJ, Tirgan MH, Deeg HJ, et al: Influence of post-methotrexate folinic acid rescue on regimen-related toxicity and graft-versus-host disease after allogeneic bone marrow transplantation. Bone Marrow Transplant 9:349–354, 1992.

109. Storb R, Epstein RB, Graham TC, et al: Methotrexate regimens for control of graft-versus-host disease in dogs with allogeneic marrow grafts. Transplantation 9:240, 1970.

110. Yau JC, Dimopoulos MA, Huan SD, et al: An effective acute graft-vs-host disease prophylaxis with minidose methotrexate, cyclosporine, and single-dose methylprednisolone. Am J Hematol 38:288–292, 1991.

111. Atkinson K, Downs K: Omission of day 11 methotrexate does not appear to influence the incidence of moderate to severe acute graft-versus-host disease, chronic graft-versus-host disease, relapse rate or survival after HLA-identical sibling bone marrow transplantation. Bone Marrow Transplant 16: 755–758, 1995.

112. Pirsch JD, Sollinger HW: Mycophenolate mofetil—clinical and experimental experience. Ther Drug Monit 18:357–361, 1996.

113. Boumpas DT, Chrousos GP, Wilder RL, et al: Glucocorticoid therapy for immune-mediated diseases: basic and clinical correlates. Ann Intern Med 119:1198–1208, 1993.

114. Bonnefoy-Berard N, Vincent C, Revillard J-P: Antibodies against functional leukocyte surface molecules in polyclonal antilymphocyte and antithymocyte globulins. Transplantation 51:669–673, 1991.

115. Bourdage JS, Hamlin DM: Comparative polyclonal antithymocyte globulin and antilymphocyte/antilymphoblast globulin anti-CD antigen analysis by flow cytometry. Transplantation 59:1194–1200, 1995.

116. Merion RM, Howell T, Bromberg JS: Partial T-cell activation and anergy induction by polyclonal antithymocyte globulin. Transplantation 65:1481–1489, 1998.

117. Baurmann H, Revillard JP, Bonnefor-Berard N, et al: Potent effects of ATG used as part of the conditioning in matched unrelated donor (MUD) transplantation. Blood 92:290a, 1998.

118. Hale G, Waldmann H: Campath-1 monoclonal antibodies in bone marrow transplantation. J Hematother 3:15–31, 1994.

119. Hale G, Zhang M-J, Bunjes D, et al: Improving the outcome of bone marrow transplantation by using CD52 monoclonal antibodies to prevent graft-versus-host disease and graft rejection. Blood 92:4581–4590, 1998.

120. Przepiorka D, Weisdorf D, Martin P, et al: Consensus conference on acute GVHD grading. Bone Marrow Transplant 15:825–828, 1995.

121. Sullivan KM, Deeg HJ, Sanders J, et al: Hyperacute graft-v-host disease in patients not given immunosuppression after allogeneic marrow transplantation. Blood 67:1172–1175, 1986.

122. Weiden PL, Doney K, Storb R, et al: Antihuman thymocyte globulin for prophylaxis of graft-versus-host disease. Transplantation 27:227–230, 1979.

123. Doney KC, Weiden PL, Storb R, et al: Failure of early administration of antithymocyte globulin to lessen graft-versus-host disease in human allogeneic marrow transplant recipients. Transplantation 31:141–143, 1981.

124. Ramsay NKC, Kersey JH, Robison LL, et al: A randomized study of the prevention of acute graft-versus-host disease. N Engl J Med 306:392–397, 1982.

125. Sullivan KM, Storb R, Buckner CD, et al: Graft-versus-host disease as adoptive immunotherapy in patients with advanced hematologic neoplasms. N Engl J Med 320:828–834, 1989.

126. Deeg HJ, Storb R, Thomas ED, et al: Cyclosporine as prophylaxis for graft-versus-host disease: a randomized study in patients undergoing marrow transplantation for acute nonlymphoblastic leukemia. Blood 65:1325–1334, 1985.

127. Storb R, Deeg HJ, Thomas ED, et al: Marrow transplantation for chronic myelocytic leukemia: a controlled trial of cyclosporine versus methotrexate for prophylaxis of graft-versus-host disease. Blood 66:698–702, 1985.

128. Ringden O, Backman L, Lonnqvist B, et al: A randomized trial comparing use of cyclosporin and methotrexate for graft-versus-host disease prophylaxis in bone marrow transplant recipients with haematologic malignancies. Bone Marrow Transplant 1:41–51, 1986.

129. Irle C, Deeg HJ, Buckner CD, et al: Marrow transplantation for leukemia following fractionate total body irradiation: a comparative trial of methotrexate and cyclosporine. Leuk Res 9:1255–1261, 1985.

130. Atkinson K, Biggs JC, Concannon A, et al: A prospective randomised trial of cyclosporin versus methotrexate after HLA-identical sibling marrow transplantation for patients with acute leukemia in first remission: analysis 2.5 years after last patient entry. Aust N Z J Med 18:594–599, 1988.

131. Torres A, Martinez F, Gomez P, et al: Cyclosporin A versus methotrexate, followed by rescue with folinic acid as prophylaxis of acute graft-versus-host disease after bone marrow transplantation. Blut 58:63–68, 1989.

132. Forman SJ, Blume KG, Krance RA, et al: A prospective randomized study of acute graft-v-host disease in 107 patients with leukemia: methotrexate/prednisone v cyclosporine A/prednisone. Transplant Proc 19:2605–2607, 1987.

133. Santos GW, Tutschka PJ, Brookmeyer R, et al: Cyclosporine plus methylprednisolone versus cyclophosphamide plus methylprednisolone as prophylaxis for graft-versus-host disease: a randomized double-blind study in patients undergoing allogeneic marrow transplantation. Clin Transplant 1:21–28, 1987.

134. Deeg HJ, Lin D, Leisenring W, et al: Cyclosporine or cyclosporine plus methylprednisolone for prophylaxis of graft-versus-host disease: a prospective, randomized trial. Blood 89:3880–3887, 1997.

135. Storb R, Deeg HJ, Farewell V, et al: Marrow transplantation for severe aplastic anemia: methotrexate alone compared with a combination of methotrexate and cyclosporine for prevention of acute graft-versus-host disease. Blood 68:119–125, 1986.

136. Mrsic M, Labar B, Bogdanic V, et al: Combination of cyclosporin and methotrexate for prophylaxis of acute graft-versus-host disease after allogeneic bone marrow transplantation for leukemia. Bone Marrow Transplant 6:137–141, 1990.

137. Storb R, Deeg HJ, Whitehead J, et al: Methotrexate and cyclosporine compared with cyclosporine alone for prophylaxis of acute graft versus host disease after marrow transplantation for leukemia. N Engl J Med 314:729–735, 1986.

138. Zikos P, van Lint MT, Frassoni F, et al: Low transplant mortality in allogeneic bone marrow transplantation for acute myeloid leukemia: a randomized study of low-dose cyclosporin versus low-dose cyclosporin and low-dose methotrexate. Blood 91:3503–3508, 1998.

139. Ruutu T, Volin L, Parkkali T, et al: Cyclosporine and methotrexate with or without methylprednisolone in the prophylaxis of graft-versus-host disease: long-term follow-up of a randomized study. Blood 92:685a, 1998.

140. Atkinson K, Biggs J, Concannon A, et al: A prospective randomised trial of cyclosporin and methotrexate versus cyclosporin, methotrexate and prednisolone for prevention of graft-versus-host disease after HLA-identical sibling marrow transplantation for haematologic malignancy. Aust N Z J Med 21:850–856, 1991.

141. Storb R, Pepe M, Anasetti C, et al: What role for prednisone in prevention of acute graft-versus-host disease in patients undergoing marrow transplants? Blood 76:1037–1045, 1990.

142. Chao NJ, Schmidt GM, Niland JC, et al: Cyclosporine, methotrexate, and prednisone compared with cyclosporine and prednisone for prophylaxis of acute graft-versus-host disease. N Engl J Med 329:1225–1230, 1993.

143. Ratanatharathorn V, Nash RA, Przepiorka D, et al: Phase III study comparing methotrexate and tacrolimus (Prograf, FK506) with methotrexate and cyclosporine for graft-versus-host disease prophylaxis after HLA-identical sibling bone marrow transplantation. Blood 92:2303–2314, 1998.

144. Blaise D, Olive D, Michallet M, et al: Impairment of leukemia-free

survival by addition of interleukin-2-receptor antibody to standard graft-versus-host prophylaxis. Lancet 345:1144–1146, 1995.

145. Mitsuyasu RT, Champlin RE. Gale RP, et al: Treatment of donor bone marrow with monoclonal anti-T-cell antibody and complement for the prevention of graft-versus-host disease: a prospective randomized double-blind trial. Ann Intern Med 105:20–26, 1986.

146. Ringden O, Pihlstedt P, Markling L, et al: Prevention of graft-versus-host disease with T cell depletion or cyclosporin and methotrexate: a randomized trial in adult leukemic marrow recipients. Bone Marrow Transplant 7:221–226, 1991.

147. Nimer SD, Giorgi J, Gajewski JL, et al: Selective depletion of CD8+ cells for prevention of graft-versus-host disease after bone marrow transplantation: a randomized controlled trial. Transplantation 57:82–87, 1994.

148. Powles RL, Clink HM, Spence D, et al: Cyclosporin A to prevent graft-versus-host disease in man after allogeneic bone-marrow transplantation. Lancet 1:327–329, 1980.

149. Backman L, Ringden O, Tollemar J, et al: An increased risk of relapse in cyclosporin-treated compared with methotrexate-treated patients: long-term follow-up of a randomized trial. Bone Marrow Transplant 3:463–471, 1988.

150. Storb R, Deeg HJ, Fisher L, et al: Cyclosporine v methotrexate for graft-v-host disease prevention in patients given marrow grafts for leukemia: long-term follow-up of three controlled trials. Blood 71:293–298, 1988.

151. Ringden O, Horowitz MM, Sondel P, et al: Methotrexate, cyclosporine, or both to prevent graft-versus-host disease after HLA-identical sibling bone marrow transplants for early leukemia? Blood 81:1094–1101, 1993.

152. Storb R, Deeg HJ, Pepe M, et al: Methotrexate and cyclosporine versus cyclosporine alone for prophylaxis of graft-versus-host disease in patients given HLA-identical marrow grafts for leukemia: long-term follow-up of a controlled trial. Blood 73:1729–1734, 1989.

153. Storb R, Deeg HJ, Pepe M, et al: Graft-versus-host disease prevention by methotrexate combined with cyclosporin compared to methotrexate alone in patients given marrow grafts for severe aplastic anemia: long-term follow-up of a controlled trial. Br J Haematol 72:567–572, 1989.

154. Shepherd JD, Shore TB, Reece DE, et al: Cyclosporine and methylprednisolone for prophylaxis of acute graft-versus-host disease. Bone Marrow Transplant 3:553–558, 1988.

155. Essell JH, Thompson JM, Harman GS, et al: Marked increase in veno-occlusive disease of the liver associated with methotrexate use for graft-versus-host disease prophylaxis in patients receiving busulfan/cyclophosphamide. Blood 79:2784–2788, 1992.

156. Fay JW, Wingard JR, Antin JH, et al: FK506 (tacrolimus) monotherapy for prevention of graft-versus-host disease after histocompatible sibling allogeneic bone marrow transplantation. Blood 87:3514–3519, 1996.

157. Uberti JP, Silver SM, Adams PT, et al: Tacrolimus and methotrexate for the prophylaxis of acute graft-versus-host disease in allogeneic bone marrow transplantation in patients with hematologic malignancies. Bone Marrow Transplant 19:1233–1238, 1997.

158. Nasr F, Cleary K, Ippoliti C, et al: Tacrolimus and reduced dose methotrexate for prevention of GVHD after HLA-identical marrow or blood stem cell transplantation. Blood 92:450a, 1998.

159. Bornhauser M, Schuler U, Porken G, et al: Mycophenolate mofetil and cyclosporine as graft-versus-host disease prophylaxis after allogeneic blood stem cell transplantation. Transplantation 67:499–504, 1998.

160. Nagler A, Condiotti R, Nabet C, et al: Selective CD4+ depletion does not prevent graft-versus-host disease. Transplantation 66:138–131, 1998.

161. Champlin R, Ho W, Gajewski J, et al: Selective depletion of CD8+ T lymphocytes for prevention of graft-versus-host disease after allogeneic bone marrow transplantation. Blood 76:418–423, 1990.

162. Jansen J, Hanks S, Akard L, et al: Selective T cell depletion with CD8-conjugated magnetic beads in the prevention of graft-versus-host disease after allogeneic bone marrow transplantation. Bone Marrow Transplant 15:271–278, 1995.

163. Giralt S, Mirza N, Mehra R, et al: Results of CD8-depleted allogeneic peripheral blood stem cell transplantation for chronic myelogenous leukemia. Blood 90:372a, 1997.

164. Soiffer RJ, Murray C, Mauch P, et al: Prevention of graft-versus-host disease by selective depletion of CD6-positive T lymphocytes from donor bone marrow. J Clin Oncol 10:1191–1200, 1992.

165. Soiffer RJ, Fairclough D, Robertson M, et al: CD6-depleted allogeneic bone marrow transplantation for acute leukemia in first complete remission. Blood 89:3039–3047, 1997.

166. Young JW, Papadopoulos EB, Cunningham I, et al: T-cell-depleted allogeneic bone marrow transplantation in adults with acute non-lymphocytic leukemia in first remission. Blood 79:3380–3387, 1992.

167. Verdonck LF, Dekker AW, de Gast GC, et al: Allogeneic bone marrow transplantation with a fixed low number of T cells in the marrow graft. Blood 83:3090–3096, 1994.

168. Papadopoulos EB, Carabasi MH, Castro-Malaspina H, et al: T-cell-depleted allogeneic bone marrow transplantation as postremission therapy for acute myelogenous leukemia: freedom from relapse in the absence of graft-versus-host disease. Blood 91:1083–1090, 1998.

169. Schaaf N, Schattenberg A, Bar B, et al: Outcome of transplantation for standard-risk leukemia with grafts depleted of lymphocytes after conditioning with an intensified regimen. Br J Haematol 98:750–759, 1997.

170. O'Donnell PV, Jone RJ, Vogelsang GB, et al: CD34+ stem cell augmentation of elutriated allogeneic bone marrow grafts: results of a phase II clinical trial of engraftment and graft-versus-host disease prophylaxis in high-risk hematologic malignancies. Bone Marrow Transplant 22:947–955, 1998.

171. Cornetta K, Gharpure V, Mills B, et al: Rapid engraftment after allogeneic transplantation using CD34-enriched marrow cells. Bone Marrow Transplant 21:65–71, 1998.

172. Ross M, Forman SJ, Wong RM, et al: A prospective randomized trial comparing cyclosporin A and prednisone versus cyclosporin A, methotrexate and prednisone for the prevention of acute graft-versus-host disease: effect on chronic graft-versus-host disease and long-term survival. Blood 90:590a, 1997.

173. Sayer HG, Longton G, Bowden R, et al: Increased risk of infection in marrow transplant patients receiving methylprednisolone for graft-versus-host disease prevention. Blood 84:1328–1332, 1994.

174. Horowitz MM, Przepiorka D, Bartels P, et al: Tacrolimus vs. cyclosporine immunosuppression: results in advanced-stage disease compared with historical controls treated exclusively with cyclosporine. Biol Blood Marrow Transplant 5:180–186, 1999.

175. Marmont AM, Horowitz MM, Gales RP, et al: T-cell depletion of HLA-identical transplants in leukemia. Blood 78:2120–2130, 1991.

176. Barrett AJ, Mavroudis D, Tisdale J, et al: T-cell-depleted bone marrow transplantation and delayed T cell add-back to control acute GVHD and conserve a graft-versus-leukemia effect. Bone Marrow Transplant 21:543–551, 1998.

177. Lee C-K, Gingrich RD, de Magalhaes-Silverman M, et al: Prophylactic reinfusion of cells for T cell-depleted allogeneic bone marrow transplantation. Biol Blood Marrow Transplant 5:15–27, 1999.

178. Bensinger WI, Clift R, Martin P, et al: Allogeneic peripheral blood stem cell transplantation in patients with advanced hematologic malignancies: a retrospective comparison with marrow transplantation. Blood 88:2794–2800, 1996.

179. Schmitz N, Bacigalupo A, Hasenclever D, et al: Allogeneic bone marrow transplantation vs filgrastim-mobilised peripheral blood progenitor cell transplantation in patients with early leukemia: first results of a randomised multicentre trial of the European Group for Blood and Marrow Transplantation. Bone Marrow Transplant 21:995–1003, 1998.

180. Pavletic ZS, Bishop MR, Tarantolo SR, et al: Hematopoietic recovery, after allogeneic blood stem-cell transplantation compared with bone marrow transplantation in patients with hematologic malignancies. J Clin Oncol 15:1608–1616, 1997.

181. Reynolds C, Ratanatharathorn V, Adams P, et al: Comparative analysis of tacrolimus/methotrexate versus tacrolimus in allogeneic peripheral blood stem cell transplants: engraftment, GVHD, relapse, and survival outcomes. Blood 92:449a, 1998.

182. Preijers FWMB, van Hennik PB, Schattenberg A, et al: Counterflow centrifugation allows addition of appropriate numbers of T cells to allogeneic marrow and blood stem cell grafts to prevent severe GVHD without substantial loss of mature and immature progenitor cells. Bone Marrow Transplant 23:1061–1070, 1999.

183. Starobinski M, Roosnek E, Hale G, et al: T cell depletion of allogeneic peripheral blood stem cells. Bone Marrow Transplant 21:429–430, 1998.

184. Fibbe WE, Brouwer R, Hale G, et al: Accelerated marrow reconstitution and earlier CMV infections in patients receiving T cell-depleted

allogeneic blood cell grafts using "Campath-1G in the bag." J Hematother 7:270, 1998.

185. Bensinger WI, Buckner CD, Shannon-Dorcy K, et al: Transplantation of allogeneic CD34+ peripheral blood stem cells in patients with advanced hematologic malignancy. Blood 88:4132–4138, 1996.

186. Link H, Arseniev L, Bahre O, et al: Transplantation of allogeneic CD34+ blood cells. Blood 87:4903–4909, 1996.

187. Finke J, Brugger W, Bertz H, et al: Allogeneic transplantation of positively selected peripheral blood CD34+ progenitor cells from matched related donors. Bone Marrow Transplant 18:1081–1086, 1996.

188. Urbano-Ispizua A, Rozman C, Martinez C, et al: Rapid engraftment without significant graft-versus-host disease after allogeneic transplantation of CD34+ selected cells from peripheral blood. Blood 89:3967–3973, 1997.

189. Urbano-Ispizua A, Solano C, Brunet S, et al: Allogeneic transplantation of selected CD34+ cells from peripheral blood: experience of 62 cases using immunoadsorption or immunomagnetic technique. Spanish Group of Allo-PBT. Bone Marrow Transplant 22:519–525, 1998.

190. Brugger W, Scheding S, Faul C, et al: Direct comparison of CD34+ selected vs. unselected peripheral blood progenitor cells (PBPC) for matched related allogeneic transplantation. Blood 92:112a, 1998.

191. Schmitz N, Bacigalupo A, Labopin M, et al: Transplantation of peripheral blood progenitor cells from HLA-identical sibling donors. Br J Haematol 95:715, 1996.

192. Storb R, Yu C, Wagner JL, et al: Stable mixed hematopoietic chimerism in DLA-identical littermate dogs given sublethal total body irradiation before and pharmacological immunosuppression after marrow transplantation. Blood 89:3048–3054, 1997.

193. McSweeney PA, Wagner JL, Maloney DG, et al: Outpatient PBSC allografts using immunosuppression with low-dose TBI before and cyclosporine and mycophenolate mofetil after transplant. Blood 92:519a, 1998.

194. Bornhauser M, Thiede HM, Schuler U, et al: GVHD prophylaxis with mycophenolate mofetil and cyclosporin A after allogeneic blood stem cell transplantation: results of a pilot study. Blood 90:105a, 1997.

195. Vij R, Brown R, Haug JS, et al: CD34+ selection using density gradient separation does not reduce the risk of graft-vs-host disease after allogeneic peripheral blood stem cell (PBSC) transplant. Blood 92:649a, 1998.

196. Przepiorka D, Van Vlasselaer P, Lu J-G, et al: Safety and feasibility of ultralight density gradient separation of blood stem cells for allogeneic transplantation. Blood 92:651a, 1998.

197. Uharek L, Glass B, Zeis M, et al: Abrogation of graft-vs-leukemia activity after depletion of CD3+ T cells in a murine model of MHC-matched peripheral blood progenitor cell transplantation (PBPCT). Exp Hematol 26:93–99, 1998.

198. Russell JA, Desai S, Herbut B, et al: Partially mismatched blood cell transplants for high-risk hematologic malignancy. Bone Marrow Transplant 19:861–866, 1997.

199. Przepiorka D, Khouri I, Ippoliti C, et al: Tacrolimus and minidose methotrexate for prevention of acute graft-vs-host disease after HLA-mismatched marrow or blood stem cell transplantation. Bone Marrow Transplant 24:763–768, 1999.

200. Aversa F, Tabilio A, Velardi A, et al: Treatment of high-risk acute leukemia with T-cell-depleted stem cells from related donors with one fully mismatched HLA haplotype. N Engl J Med 339:1186–1193, 1998.

201. Ringden O, Remberger M, Runde V, et al: Peripheral blood stem cell transplantation from unrelated donors: a comparison with marrow transplantation. Blood 94:455–464, 1999.

202. Filipovich AH, Ramsay NKC, Arthur DC, et al: Allogeneic bone marrow transplantation with related donors other than HLA MLC-matched siblings, and the use of antithymocyte globulin, prednisone, and methotrexate for prophylaxis of graft-versus-host disease. Transplantation 39:282–285, 1985.

203. Powles RL, Morgenstern GR, Kay HEM, et al: Mismatched family donors for bone-marrow transplantation as treatment of acute leukemia. Lancet 1:612–615, 1983.

204. Polchi P, Galimberti M, Lucarelli G, et al: Mother as HLA haploidentical marrow donor for children with advanced leukemia. Bone Marrow Transplant 7:124, 1991.

205. Guinan EC, Boussiotis VA, Neuberg D, et al: Transplantation of anergic histoincompatible bone marrow allografts. N Engl J Med 340:1704–1714, 1999.

206. Henslee-Downey P J, Parrish RS, MacDonald JS, et al: Combined in vitro and in vivo T lymphocyte depletion for the control of graft-versus-host disease following haploidentical marrow transplant. Transplantation 61:738–845, 1996.

207. Henslee-Downey PJ, Abhyankar SH, Parrish RS, et al: Use of partially mismatched related donors extends access to allogeneic marrow transplant. Blood 89:3864–3872, 1997.

208. Antin JH, Bierer BE, Smith BR, et al: Selective depletion of bone marrow T lymphocytes with anti-CD5 monoclonal antibodies: effective prophylaxis for graft-versus-host disease in patients with hematologic malignancies. Blood 78:2139–2149, 1991.

209. Soiffer RJ, Mauch P, Fairclough D, et al: CD6+ T cell depleted allogeneic bone marrow transplantation from genotypically HLA non-identical related donors. Biol Blood Marrow Transplant 3:11–17, 1997.

210. O'Reilly RJ, Collins NH, Kernan N, et al: Transplantation of marrow-depleted T cells by soybean lectin agglutination and E-rosette depletion: major histocompatibility complex-related graft resistance in leukemic transplant recipients. Transplant Proc 17:455–459, 1985.

211. Bacigalupo A, Mordini N, Pitto A, et al: Transplantation of HLA-mismatched CD34+ selected cells in patients with advanced malignancies: severe immunodeficiency and related complications. Br J Haematol 98:760–766, 1997.

212. Aversa F, Tabilio A, Terenzi A, et al: Successful engraftment of T-cell-depleted haploidentical "three-loci" incompatible transplants in leukemia patients by addition of recombinant human granulocyte colony-stimulating factor-mobilized peripheral blood progenitor cells to bone marrow inoculum. Blood 84:3948–3955, 1994.

213. Servida P, Gooley T, Hansen JA, et al: Improved survival of haploidentical related donor marrow transplants mismatched for HLA-A or -B versus HLA-DR. Blood 88:484a, 1996.

214. Reisner Y, Kapoor N, Kirkpatrick D, et al: Transplantation for severe combined immunodeficiency with HLA-A,B,D,DR incompatible parental marrow cells fractionated by soybean agglutinin and sheep red blood cells. Blood 61:341–348, 1983.

215. Fischer A, Landais P, Friedrich W, et al: European experience of bone-marrow transplantation for severe combined immunodeficiency. Lancet 336:850–854, 1990.

216. Dror Y, Gallagher RM, Wara DW, et al: Immune reconstitution in severe combined immunodeficiency disease after lectin-treated, TCD haplo-identical bone marrow transplantation. Blood 81:2021–2030, 1993.

217. Buckley RH, Schiff SE, Schiff RI, et al: Hematopoietic stem-cell transplantation for the treatment of severe combined immunodeficiency. N Engl J Med 340: 508–516, 1999.

218. Nash RA, Pineiro LA, Storb R, et al: FK506 in combination with methotrexate for the prevention of graft-versus-host disease after marrow transplantation from matched unrelated donors. Blood 88:3634–3641, 1996.

219. Przepiorka D, Ippoliti C, Khouri I, et al: Double Class II micromismatches increase the risk of acute graft-vs-host disease after unrelated donor marrow transplantation with tacrolimus and minimethotrexate for prophylaxis. Biol Blood Marrow Transplant 4:1, 1998.

220. Geller RB, Devine SM, O'Toole K, et al: Allogeneic bone marrow transplantation with matched unrelated donors for patients with hematologic malignancies using a preparative regimen of high-dose cyclophosphamide and fractionated total body irradiation. Bone Marrow Transplant 20:219–225, 1997.

221. Fay JW, Nash RA, Wingard JR, et al: FK506-based immunosuppression for prevention of graft versus host disease after unrelated donor marrow transplantation. Transplant Proc 27:1374, 1995.

222. Nash RA, Antin JH, Karanes C, et al: A phase III study comparing methotrexate and tacrolimus with methotrexate and cyclosporine for prophylaxis of acute graft-versus-host disease after marrow transplantation from unrelated donors. Blood 90:561a, 1997.

223. Balduzzi A, Gooley T, Anasetti C, et al: Unrelated donor marrow transplantation in children. Blood 86:3247–3256, 1995.

224. Leelasiri A, Greer JP, Stein RS, et al: Graft-versus-host disease prophylaxis for matched unrelated donor bone marrow transplantation: comparison between cyclosporine-methotrexate and cyclosporine-methotrexate-methylprednisolone. Bone Marrow Transplant 15:401–405, 1995.

225. Nademanee A, Schmidt GM, Parker P, et al: The outcome of matched

unrelated donor bone marrow transplantation in patients with hematologic malignancies using molecular typing for donor selection and graft-versus-host disease prophylaxis regimen of cyclosporine, methotrexate, and prednisone. Blood 86:1228–1234, 1995.

226. Ringden O, Reinberger M, Carlens S, et al: Low incidence of acute graft-versus-host disease using unrelated HLA-A, HLA-B and HLA-DR-compatible donors and conditioning including anti-T-cell antibodies. Transplantation 66:620–625, 1998.

227. Zander AR, Zabelina T, Kroger N, et al: Use of a five-agent GVHD prevention regimen in recipients of unrelated donor marrow. Bone Marrow Transplant 23:889–893, 1999.

228. Belanger C, Esperou-Bourdeau H, Bordigoni P, et al: Use of an anti-interleukin-2 receptor monoclonal antibody for GVHD prophylaxis in unrelated donor BMT. Bone Marrow Transplant 11:293–297, 1993.

229. Anasetti C, Lin A, Nademanee A, et al: A phase II/III randomized, double-blind, placebo-controlled multicenter trial of humanized anti-Tac for prevention of acute graft-versus-host disease (GVHD) in recipients of marrow transplants from unrelated donors. Blood 86:621a, 1995.

230. Phillips GL, Nevill TJ, Spinelli JJ, et al: Prophylaxis for acute graft-versus-host disease following unrelated donor bone marrow transplantation. Bone Marrow Transplant 15:213–219, 1995.

231. Przepiorka D, Gajewski J, Ippoliti C, et al: The combination of partial T-cell depletion and immunotoxin is optimal GVHD prophylaxis after MUD BMT. Proc First Ann Mtg ASBMT: 114, 1995.

232. Drobyski WR, Ash RC, Casper JT, et al: Effect of T-cell depletion as graft-versus-host disease prophylaxis on engraftment, relapse, and disease-free survival in unrelated marrow transplantation for chronic myelogenous leukemia. Blood 83:1980–1987, 1994.

233. Gajewski J, Wall D, Adkins D, et al: A randomized double blind trial of T cell depletion with CD5/8 CELLector in addition to cyclosporine, methotrexate and steroids for acute graft-versus-host disease prevention in HLA mismatched or unrelated bone marrow transplant. Blood 90:396b, 1997.

234. Soiffer R, Alyea E, Weller E, et al: Impact of CD6+ T-cell depletion on GVHD, engraftment, and outcome in patients undergoing allogeneic BMT from unrelated donors. Blood 92:290a, 1998.

235. Oakhill A, Pamphilon H, Potter MN, et al: Unrelated donor bone marrow transplantation for children with relapsed acute lymphoblastic leukemia in second complete remission. Br J Haematol 94:574–578, 1996.

236. Neudorf SM, Rybka W, Ball E, et al: The use of counterflow centrifugal elutriation for the depletion of T cells from unrelated donor bone marrow. J Hematother 6:351–359, 1997.

237. Socie G, Cayuela JM, Raynal B, et al: Influence of CD34 cell selection on the incidence of mixed chimaerism and minimal residual disease after allogeneic unrelated donor transplantation. Leukemia 12:1440–1446, 1998.

238. Gingrich RD, Ginder GD, Goeken NE, et al: Allogeneic marrow grafting with partially mismatched unrelated marrow donors. Blood 71:1375–1381, 1988.

239. Wagner JE, King R, Kollman C, et al: Unrelated donor bone marrow transplantation (UBMT) in 5075 patients with malignant and non-malignant disorders: impact of marrow T cell depletion (TCD). Blood 92:686a, 1998.

240. Ash RC, Casper JT, Chitambar CR, et al: Successful allogeneic transplantation of T-cell-depleted bone marrow from closely HLA-matched unrelated donors. N Engl J Med 322:485–494, 1990.

241. Casper J, Camitta B, Truitt R, et al: Unrelated bone marrow donor transplants for children with leukemia or myelodysplasia. Blood 85:2354–2363, 1995.

242. Wagner JE, Kernan NA, Steinbuch M, et al: Allogeneic sibling umbilical-cord-blood transplantation in children with malignant and non-malignant disease Lancet 346:214–219, 1995.

243. Gluckman E, Rocha V, Boyer-Chammard A, et al: Outcome of cord-blood transplantation from related and unrelated donors. N Engl J Med 337:373–381, 1997.

244. Kurtzberg J, Laughlin M, Graham ML, et al: Placental blood as a source of hematopoietic stem cells for transplantation into unrelated recipients. N Engl J Med 335:157–166, 1996.

245. Rubinstein P, Carrier C, Scaradavou A, et al: Outcomes among 562 recipients of placental-blood transplants from unrelated donors. N Engl J Med 339:1565–1577, 1998.

246. Przepiorka D, Petropoulos D, Mullen C, et al: Tacrolimus for prevention of graft-vs-host disease after mismatched unrelated donor cord blood transplantation. Bone Marrow Transplant 23:1291, 1999.

247. Gluckman E, Rocha V, Chastang C: European results of unrelated cord blood transplants. Bone Marrow Transplant 21:S87–S91, 1998.

248. Collins RH, Shpilberg O, Drobyski WR, et al: Donor leukocyte infusions in 140 patients with relapsed malignancy after allogeneic bone marrow transplantation. J Clin Oncol 15:433–444, 1997.

249. Mackinnon S, Papadopoulos EB, Carabasi MH, et al: Adoptive immunotherapy evaluating escalating doses of donor leukocytes for relapse of chronic myeloid leukemia after bone marrow transplantation: separation of graft-versus-leukemia responses from graft-versus-host disease. Blood 86:1261–1268, 1995.

250. Giralt S, Hester J, Huh Y, et al: CD8-depleted donor lymphocyte infusion as treatment for relapsed chronic myelogenous leukemia after allogeneic bone marrow transplantation. Blood 86:4337–4343, 1995.

251. Alyea EP, Soiffer RJ, Canning C, et al: Toxicity and efficacy of defined doses of CD4+ donor lymphocytes for treatment of relapse after allogeneic bone marrow transplant. Blood 91:3671–3780, 1998.

252. Garderet L, Snell V, Przepiorka D, et al: Effective depletion of alloreactive lymphocytes from peripheral blood mononuclear cell preparations. Transplantation 67:124–130, 1999.

253. Montagna D, Yvon E, Calcaterra V, et al: Depletion of alloreactive T cells by a specific anti-interleukin-2 receptor p55 chain immunotoxin does not impair in vitro antileukemia and antiviral activity. Blood 93:3550–3557, 1999.

254. Bonini C, Ferrari G, Verzeletti S, et al: HSV-TK gene transfer into donor lymphocytes for control of allogeneic graft-versus-leukemia. Science 276:1719–1724, 1997.

CHAPTER FORTY

Use of Hematopoietic Growth Factors

John R. Wingard, M.D., and
Alison A. Bartfield, M.D.

Tremendous strides have been made in recent decades in the understanding of hematopoiesis. Hematopoietic stem cells (HSC) occupy the central role, but increasingly we recognize the important contributions of the stromal microenvironment and various cytokines in the regulation of blood cell production. It is now known that hematopoietic progenitors differentiate along different lineages. This process is regulated by a number of low-molecular-weight glycoprotein molecules collectively known as hematopoietic growth factors (HGF). Although much has been learned about proliferation and differentiation of hematopoietic progenitors, the interplay among HGF, the hematopoietic progenitors, and the stromal microenvironment remains uncertain. This is further compounded by the enormous number of cytokines that both positively and negatively regulate proliferation and differentiation by direct action or through intermediates.

Currently available for clinical use are several HGF whose biologic actions are relatively restricted to hematopoietic cells of one or another differentiation lineage (called *lineage-specific*). Erythropoietin is currently available for stimulation of erythropoiesis. Granulocyte colony-stimulating factor (G-CSF) and granulocyte-macrophage colony-stimulating factor (GM-CSF) are available for bolstering the production of myeloid progenitors. Thrombopoietin is currently under clinical investigation as an agent to stimulate thrombopoiesis. In addition, there are a variety of multilineage HGF with biologic activity on target hematopoietic progenitors of more than one lineage (e.g., interleukin-3 [IL-3], IL-6, IL-11, stem cell factor). Several engineered molecules in which portions of one molecule have been combined with another in the hope of achieving novel stimulatory properties are also being evaluated (e.g., PIXY321).

In this chapter, the biology of the three commercially available HGF is briefly reviewed, the rationale for their use in hematopoietic transplantation is presented, the data from various clinical trials conducted to evaluate their role in hematopoietic transplantation are analyzed, and issues for future study are discussed.

BIOLOGY OF HEMATOPOIETIC GROWTH FACTORS

The bone marrow is metabolically highly active, continuously producing large numbers of blood cells. Any perturbation of the homeostasis of this process, such as loss of red blood cells through hemorrhage or hemolysis, deployment of granulocytes to tissues to counter infection, consumption of platelets through hemorrhage or an autoimmune process, requires the bone marrow to respond by greater production of one or more cell lineages. The HGF serve crucial roles in rapidly stimulating the production of needed blood cells.

Our current understanding of hematopoiesis suggests that there are pluripotent HSC with the capability for multilineage differentiation and expansion as well as self-renewal.[1-4] The regulation of the initial division of these stem cells and characterization of the events that take place in the transition from a quiescent, nondividing state to one of replication, further proliferation, and then return to quiescence are poorly understood. It is believed that the HGF currently used in clinical practice do not influence the transition of the pluripotent HSC from its usual quiescent state to active division and the subsequent earliest steps of lineage determination. Although puzzling, this is fortuitous because it is self-protective, ensuring that pluripotent HSC would not be depleted through pharmacologic use of one or another HGF. The progeny of the pluripotent HSC, however, depend on HGF for survival, proliferation, and continued differentiation. Hematopoietic progenitors have large numbers of receptors for multiple HGF. The mechanisms by which binding of the ligands to these receptors leads to the intracellular signals that produce biologic response are not fully elucidated, but important insights have emerged in recent years (reviewed in Shivdasani and Orkin[5]).

Each HGF may have multiple biologic activities. For example, a given HGF may simultaneously stimulate proliferation of one cell population and differentiation of another. It may also enhance the functional capacity of a third while inducing apoptosis in a fourth cell population. Other HGF may be more limited and lineage-restricted in their effects. HGF have both direct and indirect effects whereby the cells that are targeted for their primary activity may in turn stimulate other cells (even those of another tissue) to produce other cytokines with different biologic consequences. This "amplifying" effect may increase the magnitude of the direct effects of HGF or broaden their spectrum of activities.

Some malignant cells express receptors for HGF on their cell membranes. This has posed a concern that HGF potentially stimulate neoplastic cells as well as normal HSC. To date, most studies have failed to demonstrate this to be a clinically relevant problem.[6] Most clinical trials of HGF in hematologic malignancies have failed to show greater relapse rates in patients receiving HGF (reviewed in ref. 7), but not all.[8] This concern requires additional research and continued vigilance.

G-CSF is an O-glycosylated polypeptide produced by fibroblasts, endothelial cells, and monocytes.[9, 10] This 18- to 22-kD protein is encoded by genes on the long arm of chromosome 17 (17q11.2-21). The in vitro target in tissue culture is the colony-forming unit granulocyte (CFU-G). In vivo, it appears to principally affect late myeloid progenitors. G-CSF appears to have only modest influence on the functionality of monocytes or macrophages.

GM-CSF is an N-glycosylated glycoprotein produced by fibroblasts, endothelial cells, and activated T cells.[10] The molecule is 14–32 kD in weight (depending on its glycosylation state) and is encoded by genes located on chromosome 5(5q23-31) in a region where other HGF genes, including IL-3, M-CSF, IL-4, IL-5, and the M-CSF receptor, are also located. Although both G-CSF and GM-CSF in their natural state are glycosylated, glycosylation does not appear to be required for biologic activity because nonglycosylated synthetic forms of GM-CSF are biologically active. GM-CSF has a broader stimulatory effect than G-CSF. In vitro, this molecule promotes the development of granulocyte and macrophage colonies, but it also has effects on erythroid and thrombopoietic colonies. Moreover, in contrast with G-CSF, GM-CSF has potent effects on the function of macrophages.[10] The use of GM-CSF has been wider,[11] as with ex vivo expansion and development of immunocompetent cells,[12, 13] as vaccine adjuvant,[14] and immunotherapy against acute myelogenous leukemia.[15]

Erythropoietin (Epo) is a glycoprotein produced largely by the interstitial peritubular cells of the kidneys in adults and to a much lesser degree by other organs such as the liver (reviewed in ref. 16). This 165-amino-acid molecule is encoded by genes located on chromosome 7. It serves as the principal regulator of erythrocyte production. It stimulates erythroid progenitors to differentiate into mature erythrocytes and maintains their survival. Under the stress conditions of tissue hypoxia, Epo production increases. The target cells of Epo in in vitro systems are known as burst-forming units erythroid (BFU-E) and colony-forming units erythroid (CFU-E). Other HGF, including IL-3 and GM-CSF, also influence erythropoiesis, especially in the earliest committed erythroid progenitors (BFU-E).

RATIONALE FOR THE USE OF HEMATOPOIETIC GROWTH FACTORS IN HEMATOPOIETIC STEM CELL TRANSPLANTATION

The conditioning regimen for allogeneic HSC transplantation (HSCT) is designed to eradicate the underlying malignancy, to provide adequate immunosuppression to prevent graft rejection, and to provide "space" (a term not referring to physical space but rather an effect on the microenvironment to facilitate hematopoiesis of the new graft).[17] In the setting of autologous transplantation, the conditioning regimen needs only to eradicate the underlying neoplastic disease. All conditioning regimens employ the use of cytotoxic agents to achieve these ends. A consequence of these

TABLE 40–1. COMPLICATIONS OF APLASIA AND ADJUNCTIVE TREATMENT MEASURES

PARAMETER	COMPLICATIONS	MANAGEMENT STRATEGY
Neutropenia	Bacterial infections (first week)	Antibiotics
	Fungal infections (second week)	Antifungal agents Granulocyte transfusion
Anemia	Impaired quality of life (mild to moderate)	Erythrocyte transfusion
	Congestive heart failure	
Thrombocytopenia	Hemorrhage	Platelet transfusion

cytoreductive regimens is ablation of normal hematopoiesis (Table 40–1).

In the case of some less-intensive autologous HSCT regimens, only suppression of the host hematopoiesis occurs; aplasia would reverse over time even in the absence of an infusion of HSC. In the latter case, HSC hasten the recovery of blood counts. In addition to the effects on hematopoiesis, damage to other normal tissues and organs occurs, including mucosal barrier damage and frequently hepatic, pulmonary, cardiac, renal, and other organ toxicity. The peritransplant period (during the first 2–4 weeks after transplantation) is marked by the occurrence of these toxic events and their clinical management. Treatment-related mortality from infection, hemorrhage, or toxicity to normal tissue occurs in up to 10% of patients treated with many of the commonly used conditioning regimens. Morbidity, prolonged hospitalization, intensive use of health care resources, and severe short-term compromise in quality of life are also sequelae. Severe neutropenia occurs in all cases. During the first week of neutropenia, a majority of patients experience fever. Although a source of infection is identified in only a minority of patients, broad-spectrum antibiotics are instituted empirically because experience has demonstrated that such agents confer a lower rate of bacteremia, morbidity from infection, and mortality. Further, given enough time, the ability to document an infection as the underlying reason for the fever increases; however, the severity of infection also increases.

When an infection is identified during the first week of neutropenia, bacterial pathogens predominate. As the duration of the neutropenic interval increases, the risk of infection increases[18, 19]; however, the spectrum of infectious pathogens also expands. The risk of invasive fungal infections increases during the second or third week.[20] Thus, for neutropenic intervals exceeding 1 week, clinicians must employ antifungal agents either prophylactically, empirically, or as treatment for documented fungal infections in addition to the antibacterial agents employed during the first week. In severe infections not responding to antibiotics, granulocyte transfusions are occasionally employed to bolster host defenses.

The vast majority of infections occur during severe neutropenia when the circulating neutrophil count is less than 100 cells/mm[3] (Table 40–2).[18, 21–23] Although infections occur at higher levels (between 100 and 500 cells/mm[3]), their occurrence is less frequent and the life-threatening potential is lower. Once antibiotics are initiated, customarily they

TABLE 40–2. RELATIONSHIP BETWEEN NEUTROPENIA AND INFECTION AND THE EFFECTS OF MYELOID HEMATOPOIETIC GROWTH FACTOR (HGF)

LEVEL OF CIRCULATING NEUTROPHILS (CELLS/mm³)	RELATIVE OCCURRENCE OF INFECTION	RELATIVE MAGNITUDE OF HGF RESPONSE
0–100	+ + + +	+
101–500	+	+ +
501–1500	+/−	+ + +
>1500	−	+ + + +

are continued until neutropenia resolves (or longer if the infection has not been satisfactorily controlled). This has been variously defined as between 500 and 1500 cells/mm³. In recent years, most clinicians have used 500 neutrophils/mm³ as the guide for antibiotic discontinuation. This definition is arbitrary, however, and more recently several clinical trials have used 250 neutrophils/mm³ with comparably acceptable results.

Since the late 1970s, it has been customary to manage febrile neutropenia within the hospital. With the advent of home care companies, computerized information systems, effective monotherapy antibiotic regimens, implantable central venous catheters, and programmable portable infusion pumps, it is now possible to manage many cases with neutropenic fever in the outpatient setting. Several clinical trials have identified subgroups of patients at low risk for life-threatening complications of neutropenic fever. These febrile episodes can be managed wholly in the outpatient setting; otherwise, after a short inpatient stay of 24–48 hours, discharge to the outpatient setting with continued antibiotics is a suitable alternative to inpatient stay.[24–30] Although most of these studies were of patients not undergoing HSCT, effective outpatient antibiotic regimens have been described for patients undergoing HSCT as well.[31, 32]

Thrombocytopenia is also an almost universal consequence of HSCT. With severe thrombocytopenia (less than 10,000–20,000 platelets/mm³), there is the potential for hemorrhage; in some cases hemorrhage may be life-threatening. The risk depends on both the depth of thrombocytopenia and its duration. Other factors, including the presence of coagulopathy or the use of medications that interfere with platelet function, may also contribute. Platelet transfusions are generally given when the circulating platelet count falls below 5000–20,000 platelets/mm³. Different transplant centers use different thresholds for transfusion, although 20,000/mm³ is the most commonly used one. Questions have been raised as to whether lower thresholds would be just as suitable.[33–37] To date, there have been no randomized trials to establish the optimal transfusion threshold. Reducing the units of transfused platelets is important because transfusions are associated with the potential for allergic reactions, febrile reactions, and exposure to viral pathogens (especially cytomegalovirus). They may increase the risk for alloimmunization and thereby reduce the responsiveness to later transfusions if and when hemorrhage control becomes vital. Moreover, platelet products are a costly and limited commodity in community blood banks.

Interruption of erythropoiesis, as well as repeated phlebotomy during the peritransplant period, produces profound anemia that in most cases requires multiple erythrocyte transfusions. Erythrocyte transfusions carry similar risks and problems as with platelets. Different centers use different transfusion thresholds, generally allowing hemoglobin to drop to 7–9 g/dL or awaiting the onset of symptoms. As with the platelet transfusion threshold, controversy exists over the erythrocyte transfusion threshold.[38] In patients undergoing renal dialysis who have severe anemia, quality of life is compromised at very low hemoglobin concentrations.[39] Elevation of the hemoglobin level can substantially improve quality of life.

Although HGF have been primarily intended as an adjunct to the management of aplasia, the potential for beneficial effects on other HSCT complications have been proposed. The neutrophils are an important component of the mucosal barrier. Neutrophils are present in the saliva of chemotherapy-treated patients several days prior to their appearance in the circulation.[40] These phagocytic effectors control infectious pathogens at the mucosal surface and can reduce the severity and duration of chemotherapy-induced mucositis. Furthermore, infections cause the release of a variety of proinflammatory cytokines. Several of these cytokines have been implicated in the pathogenesis of graft-versus-host disease (GVHD), hepatic veno-occlusive disease, and other treatment-related toxicities (IL-1, IL-6, IL-2, tumor necrosis factor, interferon-γ).[41–51]

Because of the morbidity and mortality from aplasia as well as the significant compromise in the quality of life and the intensive use of health care resources, there is tremendous potential for benefit from the use of HGF during HSCT. Of theoretic concern have been issues such as the potential for increasing the risk of GVHD, growth of residual myeloid leukemia, and an increased potential for relapse in autologous HSCT.

STRATEGIES FOR HEMATOPOIETIC GROWTH FACTOR USE

HGF use has been evaluated in several ways (Table 40–3). The most frequently evaluated approach is administration of HGF immediately post transplantation with the goal of

TABLE 40–3. STRATEGIES FOR HEMATOPOIETIC GROWTH FACTOR USE IN HEMATOPOIETIC STEM CELL TRANSPLANTATION

STRATEGY	INTENDED EFFECT
To speed engraftment	Decrease resource utilization, morbidity
For delayed engraftment	Decrease resource utilization, morbidity, mortality
To treat infection as an adjunct to antimicrobial agents	Decrease morbidity, mortality
To enhance the stem cell product (in vivo and ex vivo)	Decrease resource utilization
To facilitate tandem transplants using dose-intensive treatment regimens	Maintain dose-intensive chemotherapy schedule to maximize tumor cell kill; optimize control of cancer

hastening recovery of blood counts and reducing treatment-related toxicity. A second strategy is its use for delayed engraftment, the goal being to facilitate the recovery of blood counts. A third use is as an adjunct to antibiotics for treatment of infection to speed recovery, shorten the duration of antibiotic therapy, reduce morbidity, and improve survival. A fourth use is to give HGF prior to transplantation to enrich the HSC content of the marrow graft or to mobilize HSC from the bone marrow to the peripheral blood. A fifth strategy under evaluation is to facilitate tandem transplantations in which HGF are used to maintain treatment schedules. This strategy is a combination of the first and fourth, but its intent is to permit the use of repeated dose-intensive chemotherapy cycles to speed engraftment in anticipation for the next course of chemotherapy, a treatment strategem that is being evaluated in several solid tumors.

PARAMETERS USED TO EVALUATE THE BENEFITS OF HEMATOPOIETIC GROWTH FACTORS

Three categories of parameters have been used to characterize the effects and quantify the benefits of HGF: (1) laboratory values, (2) resource utilization, and (3) clinical events (Table 40–4). The most widely used and easily quantifiable is the effect on laboratory parameters: hemoglobin, reticulocyte count, neutrophil count, platelet count, or in vitro assays of the function of mature blood cells. Although readily quantifiable, these parameters are only useful as surrogate markers for the latter two categories: to identify patients that are likely to use a great deal of resources or at the risk for clinical events. It seems apparent that the achievement of a certain neutrophil count is somewhat arbitrary and is not biologically a particularly relevant endpoint. More important than a given number of circulating neutrophils is the process of recovery (Fig. 40–1). Thus, evidence of increasing numbers of neutrophils over time or the demonstration of neutrophils mobilized to tissues (such

TABLE 40–4. PARAMETERS USED TO EVALUATE THE EFFICACY OF HEMATOPOIETIC GROWTH FACTORS

Laboratory values
  Hemoglobin, hematocrit, reticulocyte count
  Leukocyte count, neutrophil count
  Platelet count
  Functional assays of neutrophils, monocytes, platelets
Resource utilization
  Erythrocyte transfusion
  Antibiotics, antifungal agents, granulocyte transfusion
  Platelet transfusion
  Length of hospitalization
  Diagnostic procedures
  Cost
Clinical events
  Exercise tolerance, level of energy/fatigue
  Documented infection, fever, sepsis syndrome, morbidity
  Hemorrhage
  Disease control
  Survival
  Quality of life
  Mucositis, other toxic events

as the demonstration of neutrophils in saliva, which typically occurs several days prior to their appearance in the circulation) may be better gauges of neutrophil recovery and more useful clinical guideposts for discontinuation of antibiotics.

In reality, the more important parameters to assess are the latter two categories. The second category, resource utilization, includes the various diagnostic procedures, transfusions, antibiotics, and stay in the hospital, which are used as supportive care in the management of aplasia. Utilization of resources can be burdensome to the patient and is costly. The imperative to control health care costs has placed a greater emphasis on resource utilization as an important end-point of any medical intervention, and resource utilization is subject to changes in supportive care. For example, as noted earlier, the number of transfusions given is very dependent on the threshold for transfusion. Similarly, the number of days of antibiotic use depends on the milestone determination of neutropenia recovery. The number of days in the hospital is irrelevant in some autologous HSCT centers because care traditionally provided in the hospital has now been moved to the outpatient setting.

The third category, clinical events, is truly important. These events include exercise tolerance, level of energy, infection, fever, sepsis syndrome, morbidity, hemorrhage, disease control, survival, quality of life, and the occurrence of mucositis or other toxic events.

Such considerations of the impact of HGF on different end-points and the clinical significance of these end-points are important in the application of clinical trial recommendations to each institutional practice guideline. Moreover, results must be periodically reinterpreted to reflect changing health care practices.

DOSING, ADMINISTRATION, AND TOXICITY OF HEMATOPOIETIC GROWTH FACTORS

Both G-CSF and yeast-derived GM-CSF are approved by the Food and Drug Administration (FDA) in the United States for application in the HSCT setting. Their use has been the subject of several reviews.[52–59] The approved dose schedule for GM-CSF is 250 $\mu g/m^2$/day for 21 days given as a 2-hour IV infusion beginning 2–4 hours after autologous HSC infusion but not less than 24 hours after the last dose of chemotherapy or 12 hours after the last dose of radiotherapy. Should the circulating neutrophil count exceed 20,000/mm³, GM-CSF should be discontinued or dose reduced. The approved dose schedule for G-CSF is 10 μg/kg/day intravenously over 4–24 hours or as a continuous 24-hour subcutaneous infusion starting at least 24 hours after the last dose of chemotherapy or HSC infusion. The G-CSF dose should be reduced to 5 μg/kg/day if the circulating neutrophil count exceeds 1000/mm³ for 3 consecutive days and stopped when the neutrophil count continues to exceed 1000/mm³. If the neutrophil count falls below 1000/mm³, G-CSF can be resumed at 5 μg/kg/day.

If the doses for GM-CSF and G-CSF were converted to a uniform expression as either dose per body weight or dose per body surface area, the manufacturers' recommended dose for G-CSF would be greater than that for

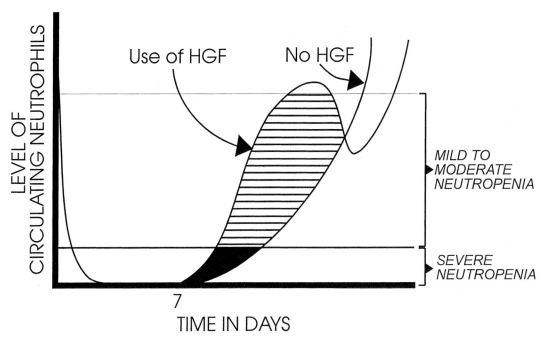

FIGURE 40–1. Schematic representation of neutrophil recovery after HSCT with and without myeloid HGF use. The rapidity of recovery (depicted as the steepness of the slope of the curve after 7 days) is hastened by HGF. The duration of mild to moderate neutropenia (*striped area*) is most affected by HGF, but the duration of severe neutropenia is only marginally affected (*black area*).

GM-CSF. In the absence of comparative trials, the rationale in terms of efficacy is uncertain. Indeed, many centers have adopted an alternative-dose strategy. Lower-than-recommended doses may be adequate to speed neutrophil engraftment at a lower cost. Unfortunately, no randomized trials have been performed to determine which dose schedule is most efficacious. Moreover, to reduce waste (and to optimize cost), many centers round the dose to the nearest vial size. For example, a patient whose weight is 75 kg or less may receive 300 μg/day of G-CSF and heavier patients may be given 480 μg/day.[57] Alternatively, patients weighing 60 kg or less may be given 250 μg/day of GM-CSF and heavier patients would receive 500 μg/day.

There is no biologic rationale for the different intervals between the HSC infusion and the start of G-CSF or GM-CSF. Moreover, as discussed later, delayed infusion of HGF may offer as much efficacy at a lower cost because the clinically relevant benefits appear to be optimized when more differentiated progenitor cells are present in sufficient numbers. Larger numbers of progenitor cells are usually present approximately 1 week after the HSC infusion.

Although a number of routes of administration have been evaluated, continuous intravenous infusion may be associated with more toxicity. Once- or twice-daily subcutaneous injections have been found to be efficacious and well tolerated. Moreover, such injections are easier to administer either in the outpatient setting or by the patient or a caregiver and may be more cost effective.

The duration of therapy has not been sufficiently studied to optimize HGF exposure. Most clinical trials have given the HGF over a defined interval such as 2 or 3 weeks. Several studies have tapered the dose in an effort to minimize the fall in neutrophil count after discontinuing the HGF altogether. Individualized termination in which the patient's own neutrophil count is used as a gauge for stopping (typically when the circulating neutrophil count exceeds 1000 or 1500/mm³ for 1 or more days) has also been evaluated and is used in many centers. Even when a tapering schedule is used, 10–20% of patients still experience a fall in the circulating neutrophil count to a level below 500/mm³. Generally, this second fall is short-lived and often does not pose a danger of infection because a second, more-gradual rebound follows within several days without any additional intervention. If the fall is excessive or the interval prolonged, the HGF can be restarted. At the FDA-approved doses, toxicity from either G-CSF or GM-CSF is minor and generally not serious. Most controlled clinical trials have found little or no difference in toxicity profiles between GM-CSF or G-CSF treatment and the control groups. At higher doses, the incidence of toxicity is greater for both G-GSF and GM-CSF and is dose related.

The most common toxicity for both G-CSF and GM-CSF is bone pain, which is generally mild to moderate but at times can be severe. Some clinicians have noted an association of pain and the recovery of neutrophils, suggesting that the pain may be a manifestation of marrow "crowding" that has irritated pain receptors in the marrow cavity. Pain can also be problematic at the start of HGF therapy. This can be ameliorated by analgesics.

Fever is another side effect of HGF, and care must be taken to distinguish a fever produced by infection versus the side effect. In controlled studies, febrile episodes are generally comparable between the HGF-treated group and the control group. The fever associated with HGF, however, may be more common near the time of neutrophil recovery rather than in the midst of deep neutropenia.

Other side effects are much less common but can include weight gain, headache, injection site reaction, fatigue, rash, and serositis. With *Escherichia coli*–derived GM-CSF (in contrast with the yeast-derived GM-CSF product, which is

TABLE 40–5. EFFECT OF G-CSF AND GM-CSF ON ENGRAFTMENT AFTER HSCT AS EVALUATED IN RANDOMIZED TRIALS

AUTHOR	REF. NO.	EVIDENCE LEVEL	NO. PTS	HSCT TYPE	HSC SOURCE	GROWTH FACTOR	Neutropenia 100/MM³	500/MM³	1000/MM³	Hosp. Stay	Platelet Transfusion	Erythrocyte Transfusion	Antibiotic Duration	Ampho B Duration
Khwaja	23	I	61	Auto	BM	GM-CSF	−	+ +	NA	−	−	−	−	−
Gorin	61	I	91	Auto	BM	GM-CSF	NA	+ +	NA	+	−†	−†	−	NA
Gulati	62	II	24	Auto	BM	GM-CSF	NA	NA	+	+ +	−	−	NA	NA
Link	63	I	81	Auto	BM	GM-CSF	NA	+ +	+ +	−	−†	−†	−	NA
Nemunaitis	64	I	128	Auto	BM	GM-CSF	−	+ +	+ +	+	−†	+	+ +	−
Schmitz	65	I	54	Auto	BM	G-CSF	NA	+ +	+ +	−	−	−	−	NA
Stahel	66	II	43	Auto	BM	G-CSF	NA	+ +	NA	−	−	−	−	NA
Advani	67	I	69	Auto	PB, BM	GM-CSF	NA	+	+ +	−	−†	NA	NA	NA
Legros	68	I	50	Auto	PB	GM-CSF	NA	−	NA	−	−†	NA	−	NA
Spitzer	69	II	37	Auto	PB	G & GM-CSF	+ +	+ +	+ +	+	−	−	NA	NA
Klumpp	70	II	41	Auto	PB	G-CSF	NA	+ +	NA	+ +	−†	−	+	NA
Linch	71	I	63	Auto	PB	G-CSF	NA	+ +	NA	+ +	−	NA	NA	NA
Gisselbrech	72	I	315	Allo & auto	PB, BM	G-CSF	NA	+ +	+ +	+	−	NA	+ +	NA
de Witte	73	I	57	Allo	BM	GM-CSF	+ +	−	NA	−	−	−	−	NA
Nemunaitis	74	I	109	Allo	BM	GM-CSF	+ +	+ +	+ +	+	−†	−	−	−
Powles	75	II	40	Allo	BM	GM-CSF	NA	−	NA	−	−	<	<	NA
Linch	22	I	121	Allo & auto	BM	G-CSF	NA	+ +	+ +	+	−	−	+	−

+, $P < 0.05$; + +, $P < 0.01$; −, not significantly different; NA, not assessed; <, HGF group inferior to control.

*Laboratory parameters abnormal but no adverse clinical events.

†Days to reach platelet or RBC recovery reported; numbers of platelet or RBC transfused not assessed.

Allo, allogeneic; auto, autologous; BM, bone marrow; G-CSF, granulocyte colony-stimulating factor; GM-CSF, granulocyte macrophage colony-stimulating factor; GVHD; graft-versus-host disease; PB, peripheral blood progenitor cells.

commercially available in the United States), there was also a "first-pass" phenomenon manifested by fever, serositis, and capillary leak syndrome, especially at higher doses. The phenomenon does not appear to be associated with yeast-derived GM-CSF. Other toxic events occasionally described include reduction in platelet count (not associated with hemorrhage), elevation of lactic dehydrogenase, uric acid, alkaline phosphatase, capillary leak syndrome, and dyspnea (with the first dose of GM-CSF). Anti–G-CSF antibodies have not been reported, whereas neutralizing antibodies to GM-CSF have been detected in fewer than 5% of treated patients. The clinical significance of these antibodies is uncertain.

Epo is typically given in a dose of 150–300 U/kg subcutaneously for 3 days weekly or daily, but a wide variety of doses and schedules have been used. Treatment is generally started during the first week after transplantation and continued until transfusion independence and achievement of an acceptable hemoglobin level established by each center. Toxicity can include hypertension, headache, arthralgia, nausea, vomiting, diarrhea, and the potential for thrombosis. Fever and peripheral edema are symptoms more frequently reported in patients with cancer receiving Epo than in patients with chronic renal failure. When sluggish erythrocyte recovery is expected, an endogenous Epo level can be measured to ascertain the utility of starting exogenous Epo. In general, patients with lower baseline serum Epo levels respond more than those with higher levels. After 8 weeks of therapy, if the desired response is not achieved, the dose can be increased to 300 U/kg three times weekly or daily. If no response occurs at this higher level, a response is unlikely.

USE OF HEMATOPOIETIC GROWTH FACTORS TO HASTEN ENGRAFTMENT

A number of clinical reports have evaluated the use of G-CSF, GM-CSF, and Epo in the post-transplant setting to hasten engraftment. The evidence in each report was graded as to its relative strength in providing evidence for or against a particular benefit.[60] Level I evidence was obtained from data from a randomized controlled trial. Level II evidence was obtained from randomized controlled trials with low power. Level III evidence was from a well-designed concurrent cohort or case-controlled analysis. Level IV evidence was data collected from multiple intervals with or without the growth factor. Level V evidence was case reports without controls.

G-CSF/GM-CSF

Seventeen level I or II reports evaluated G-CSF or GM-CSF in the post-transplant setting to hasten engraftment (Table 40–5).[22, 23, 61–75] Twelve of the clinical trials were conducted in the autologous setting (seven used marrow, four employed peripheral blood progenitor cell (PBPC), and one

EFFECT ON CLINICAL EVENTS

Fever Duration	Infection	Bacteremia	Fungal Infection	GVHD	Toxicity	Mucositis	Relapse	Survival
−	−	−	−	NA	NA	NA	−	−
−	−	−	−	NA	−	NA	−	−
NA	−	−	−	NA	−	NA	−	−
−	+	−	−	NA	<	NA	−	−
−	−	−	−	NA	−	−	−	−
−	−	−	−	NA	−	NA	−	−
+	−	−	−	NA	−	NA	−	−
NA	+	−	−	NA	−	NA	−	−
+	−	NA	NA	NA	−	−	NA	NA
−	−	−	NA	NA	NA	NA	NA	NA
−	NA	NA	NA	NA	NA	NA	−	−
NA	NA	NA	NA	NA	NA	NA	NA	NA
+	+	−	NA	−	−	−	NA	−
−	−	−	−	−	<	NA	−	−
−	+ +	+	−	−	−	+	−	−
<	−	−	NA	−	<*	NA	−	−
−	−	−	NA	NA	−	−	−	−

used the combination of PBPC and marrow). Two trials studied both allogeneic and autologous bone marrow transplantation (BMT). Three studies evaluated the use of HGF in allogeneic BMT.

In these clinical trials, the primary outcome studied was most often the median number of days to reach an absolute neutrophil count greater than 500 cells/mm^3. In all but one of the studies of autologous HSCT, there was a statistically significant shortening of time to neutrophil recovery (the number of circulating neutrophils exceeding 500/mm^3). In two of the five studies of allogeneic BMT, however, there was no significantly shortened neutrophil engraftment interval. In the nine studies in which recovery to a circulating neutrophil count exceeding 1000/mm^3 was also assessed, all showed this milestone to be reached significantly sooner. The utility of these milestones (as well as resources utilization) is uncertain as we shift more of the HSCT care to the outpatient arena, as discussed earlier. A more important end-point relating to the risk of infection is the median days to reach an absolute neutrophil count greater than 100/mm^3, the period during which the patient is at the greatest risk for infection. Unfortunately, this end-point was reported in only five of the studies and did not consistently reach statistical significance.

Resource utilization was not as substantially affected as the achievement of neutrophil recovery. The number of days of intravenous antibiotics was not shortened in most studies, the use of amphotericin B was not reduced in the four studies in which it was assessed, and the length of hospital stay was shortened in only 9 of the 17 studies. The number of units of platelet transfusions and erythrocyte transfusions was not shortened in most studies in which these parameters were enumerated. Many of these second-

ary end-points are subject to differences in standards of care, making it more difficult to elucidate a clear advantage in the treated cohort (see Table 40–5). For instance, the second most common milestone shown to be statistically shorter in the treated cohort was the median length of hospitalization after transplantation. This end-point is arbitrary, depending on the discharge criteria at the various transplant centers. Not only were the discharge criteria incongruent among the different studies, they often were different among the various centers participating in the same study.

The impact of G-CSF or GM-CSF on clinical events was similarly marginal in most studies. In three studies there was a reduction in the number of days with fever, in four studies the number of infections was reduced, and in only one study was the number of episodes of bacteremia reduced. No study reported a reduction in the number of fungal infections. There was no significant impact on relapse or survival in any of the studies. There were no documented reductions in toxicity to other tissues except for reduced severe mucositis in one trial,[74] despite anecdotal evidence[76–79] and one level I trial in patients not undergoing HSCT[80] suggesting a potential to reduce mucositis and other toxic events. On the other hand, there was no evidence for greater incidence or severity of GVHD. An increase in adverse events in matched unrelated donor BMT was suggested in two reports,[81, 82] one level II, the other level IV.

Opinion is divided as to whether G-CSF or GM-CSF is needed after transplantation if the HGF was used for mobilization in PBPC collection.[68–70, 83–85] Some data suggest that if the HSC content is optimal, the benefit of post-transplantation HGF is marginal.[84]

An alternative to "priming" the peripheral blood to enhance HSC content is to administer HGF to patients prior to bone marrow harvest. In a trial that evaluated G-CSF, GM-CSF, or IL-3 administered prior to bone marrow harvest, there was an increase in the myeloid progenitors, although the time to myeloid engraftment was not shortened compared with historical controls.[86] In a randomized trial comparing primed bone marrow to mobilize PBPC as the source of HSC, times to recovery of neutrophil and platelet counts were equivalent.[87] These data suggest that, at least in terms of engraftment, the source of HSC may be less important than the numbers of progenitors. Certainly, other issues such as extent of tumor contamination and characteristics of lymphoid cell populations may be quite different between the HSC sources, which may be important considerations in the overall choice on the source of cells.

In one study, the effect of delayed initiation of HGF was compared with early HGF.[88] No difference was found, suggesting that substantial cost savings might be realized by delaying administration until more progenitors are present. Other noncontrolled historical comparisons support this concept.[89–93]

It is common for transplant recipients to receive G-CSF or GM-CSF routinely after HSCT to speed engraftment; however, review of the controlled trials indicates that this practice offers fewer benefits than was hoped for. Although there certainly is a role for HGF in the early post-transplantation setting to hasten the patient's recovery from neutropenia, more emphasis is placed on the patient's clinical status and less on arbitrary parameters such as the neutrophil count; thus, the use of HGF will need to be continually reassessed.

ERYTHROPOIETIN

A number of studies have measured endogenous Epo levels in the post-transplantation interval to evaluate the basis for its use (Table 40–6).[94–101] In several studies, inappropriately low Epo levels were detected for the level of anemia (as compared with that expected in a patient with iron-deficiency anemia at a similar hematocrit level), but in others there did not appear to be a correlation between the Epo and the hematocrit. In general, endogenous Epo levels were low in most patients undergoing allogeneic HSCT but appropriate for the degree of anemia in most patients undergoing autologous HSCT.

Epo was studied in seven level I or II clinical trials (see Table 40–6).[102–108] Four of the studies were conducted in the allogeneic setting, two in the autologous setting, and one trial studied both allogeneic and autologous BMT. In two of these studies (one of allogeneic BMT and one of autologous and allogeneic BMT), Epo produced a significantly shorter time to erythrocyte transfusion independence. In three studies, fewer units of erythrocyte transfusions were required in allogeneic BMT. After autologous HSCT (using marrow and/or PBPC), Epo yielded no clinical benefits.[106–108] Not surprisingly, the time to neutrophil and platelet recovery was not affected. Similarly, there was no shortening of the time to discharge.

Quality-of-life considerations with Epo have been evalu-

ated to a much greater extent than with myeloid HGF. Patients who respond to Epo have been shown to have an improved level of energy, an improved level of daily activity, and a greater quality of life by self-report. These changes have been noted in different patient groups. Remarkably, improvement in quality of life exceeds the expectation based on hematocrit change. Although Epo has been shown to improve quality-of-life parameters in other settings, this was not assessed in any of the seven BMT trials (see Table 40–6).

USE OF HEMATOPOIETIC GROWTH FACTORS TO TREAT DELAYED ENGRAFTMENT

Patients in whom recovery of blood count is poor after transplantation are ideal candidates for HGF administration. There are no randomized controlled trials (either level I or level II studies) to demonstrate the efficacy of HGF in this setting. Several studies, however, have reported responses to GM-CSF in a proportion of patients with poor graft function after either autologous or allogeneic transplantation.[109–114] GM-CSF was generally given at a dose of 250 μg/m²/day for 2 or more weeks. There was no advantage to giving GM-CSF followed by G-CSF compared with GM-CSF alone.[109] Generally, response occurs within 2 weeks after start of the HGF. Several studies suggested an improvement in survival and reduction in infection. In one study,[113] doses were escalated weekly until a response was seen. Issues related to delayed engraftment are discussed in Chapter 44.

USE OF HEMATOPOIETIC GROWTH FACTORS AS TREATMENT OF INFECTION

It has long been recognized that the effectiveness of antimicrobial therapy is highly dependent on the host immunologic response. For example, treatment for bacteremia has a substantially higher mortality rate in patients with persistent neutropenia than in patients whose neutrophil count recovers.[18, 19, 115] Similar observations for invasive *Candida*[116] and *Aspergillus*[117] infections have been noted. Moreover, a number of antibiotics and antifungal agents have only marginal killing activity in severe neutropenia, thus compromising their efficacy. Based on these observations, a number of early trials evaluated the use of granulocyte transfusions given to patients with life-threatening infection not responding to antimicrobial therapy or given "prophylactically" to patients with prolonged neutropenia in whom the risk of life-threatening infection was estimated to be very high. This latter approach has been largely abandoned because of the marginal effect on the number of circulating neutrophils, difficulty in demonstrating that patients had better outcomes, and, in patients undergoing HSCT, the risk of transmitting cytomegalovirus (CMV) via the transfusions (which were often obtained from CMV-seropositive persons, which a majority of adults are), which increased the transplant risk for CMV morbidity and mortality.

With the introduction of myeloid HGF, the potential for restoring host defenses by improving neutrophil recovery

TABLE 40–6. EFFECTS OF ERYTHROPOIETIN ON ENGRAFTMENT AFTER BMT AS EVALUATED IN RANDOMIZED CONTROLLED TRIALS

AUTHOR	REF. NO.	EVIDENCE LEVEL	NO. PTS.	BMT TYPE	STEM CELL SOURCE	EFFECT ON LABORATORY PARAMETERS					EFFECT ON RESOURCE UTILIZATION			EFFECT ON CLINICAL EVENTS				
						Reticulocyte Recovery	Hgb Recovery	Neutrophil Recovery	Platelet Recovery	Erythrocyte Recovery	Hospital Stay	Platelet Transfusion	Erythrocyte Transfusion	Hemorrhage	GVHD	Toxicity	Survival	Quality of Life
Biggs	102	I	91	Allo	BM	++	++	–	–	NA	–	–	–	NA	–	–	–	NA
Fleming	103	I	50	Allo	BM	NA	NA	–	NA	–	–	–	–	NA	–	–	NA	NA
Klaesson	104	I	50	Allo	BM	–	+	–	–	+	–	+	+	–	NA	+	+	NA
Steegmann	105	II	28	Allo	BM	+	–	–	+	NA	NA	+	+	NA	NA	–	–	NA
Link	106	I	329	Allo/Auto	BM	+	NA	–	–	++	NA	–	++	NA	NA	–	–	NA
Chao	107	II	35	Auto	BM, PB	NA	NA	–	–	NA	NA	–	–	NA	NA	–	NA	NA
Miller	108	I	50	Auto	BM	–	–	NA	–	–	NA	–	–	NA	NA	–	NA	NA

+, $P < .05$; ++, $P < .01$; –, not significant; NA, not assessed; <, HGF group inferior to control.
*Time to neutrophil recovery refers to achieving circulating neutrophil count of 500 per microliter; time to platelet and erythroid recovery refers to transfusion independence.
Allo, allogeneic; Auto, autologous; BM, bone marrow; BMT, blood and marrow transplantation; GVHD, graft-versus-host disease; PB, peripheral blood.

as well as enhancing the functionality of neutrophils and macrophages can be re-explored. Several reports have evaluated the role of G-CSF, GM-CSF, or monocyte-colony stimulating factor (M-CSF) as an adjunct to antimicrobial therapy for treatment of infection during neutropenia.[118–120] M-CSF appears to be particularly appealing with respect to its effects on monocytes and macrophages where, in in vitro assays, macrophage migration, expression of Fc receptors, cytotoxicity, respiratory burst activity, and bacterial and fungal killing were enhanced. Moreover, in a murine model, animals were protected by M-CSF against a lethal challenge of *Candida*.[121] Initial trials of M-CSF appeared promising,[119, 120] but this molecule is no longer under clinical development. Thrombocytopenia was noted in many patients.[119]

GM-CSF and G-CSF potentiate the function and survival of neutrophils by enhanced killing of microorganisms via increased phagocytosis and superoxide production. There has been considerable interest in evaluating the commercially available HGF as adjuncts to antimicrobial therapy for documented infection. Although randomized controlled trials have not been conducted in the HSCT setting, there are a number of randomized trials in cancer patients who are receiving less-intensive chemotherapy treatment.[122–127] In general, these studies have found, in most cases, a shortening of time to neutrophil recovery (with the exception of ref. 124). In two studies the duration of antibiotic therapy was shortened,[123, 126] but no reduction occurred in other trials. None of the studies found a reduction in the duration of fever. Most importantly, there was no reduction in infectious mortality. In one study, quality-of-life scores and hospital charges were greater in the group receiving GM-CSF than in the placebo group.[127] Thus, data have not been supportive of this practice. It should be noted that there was considerable heterogeneity among the patients and, thus, for the risk of severe and life-threatening infections. Whether the benefit would be more substantial in higher-risk patients, such as those undergoing HSCT with prolonged neutropenia (especially those receiving ex vivo purged marrows, those given PBPC with low progenitor cell content, or those with poor graft function), or in patients with life-threatening, invasive fungi or antibiotic-resistant bacteria infections, remains to be addressed.

The use of neutrophil transfusions from normal donors after HGF stimulation is also being considered as an adjunct to life-threatening infection. To date, no clinical trial has proven its efficacy, but preliminary reports have indicated the ability to generate substantially larger numbers of phagocytes with this technique.[128, 129]

USE OF HEMATOPOIETIC GROWTH FACTORS TO ENHANCE THE STEM CELL PRODUCT

Efforts to enhance the progenitor content of the HSC product have emphasized "priming" the peripheral blood or bone marrow in vivo prior to collection. In recent years, investigations have also focused on enriching the progenitor cell content after collection ex vivo.

Numerous observations have noted enhanced numbers of hematopoietic progenitors in the peripheral blood during the recovery phase after chemotherapy and in normal persons given HGF. The use of HGF after chemotherapy produces even greater numbers of hematopoietic progenitors in the blood during recovery. Through improvements in cell separation techniques and advances in apheresis technology, it is now possible to collect large numbers of hematopoietic progenitors from peripheral blood as an alternative to bone marrow. Before autologous PBPC collection, chemotherapy, HGF, or the combination of chemotherapy plus HGF is given. In general, the combination of chemotherapy plus HGF has been shown to produce a larger number of hematopoietic progenitors collected by each apheresis, but this combination is associated with a greater utilization of health care resources (the costs of chemotherapy and management of aplasia, which frequently requires hospitalization or parenteral antibiotics) than mobilization by HGF alone; the optimal day of PBPC collection is also less predictable, making utilization of apheresis staff more problematic.[130] These concerns may offset the advantages of higher yields of progenitor cells. Data from several reports suggest that G-CSF may be more effective than GM-CSF in providing a higher PBPC content.[131–133] Randomized trials in allogeneic PBPC transplantation show that G-CSF is more efficacious than GM-CSF in mobilizing sufficient qualities of HSC.[134]

This technique of "in vivo" enrichment of HSC involves not only proliferation of hematopoietic progenitors within the bone marrow but also movement of the progenitors from one compartment (the bone marrow) to another (the blood). It is clear that these two facets are quite different and that some HGF are proficient at increasing proliferation but less proficient at mobilizing them from the marrow compartment to the peripheral blood. Indeed, adhesion molecule antibodies have been used to enhance the number of hematopoietic progenitors in the peripheral blood even though there is no effect on their proliferation; this is accomplished presumably by shifting progenitors between compartments.[135]

Mobilization by HGF also permits the collection of hematopoietic progenitors for allogeneic HSCT. The procedure may be more acceptable to donors than marrow harvesting because general anesthesia is avoided.[136] A number of studies have demonstrated the feasibility of successful long-term engraftment.[137–140] Although there are concerns about higher numbers of T lymphocytes than with marrow grafts, leading to more severe GVHD, early reports suggest that rates of acute GVHD are not higher. Several preliminary reports, however, suggest that there may be a higher rate of chronic GVHD. Randomized trials comparing PBPC with bone marrow as HSC source in allogeneic transplantation are underway. Mobilization and collection of autologous and allogeneic PBPC are discussed in detail in Chapter 25.

EX VIVO EXPANSION OF HEMATOPOIETIC PROGENITORS

Expansion of hematopoietic progenitors ex vivo is attractive for several reasons. Adequate numbers of hematopoietic progenitors cannot be harvested in some patients. Also, it is desirable to reduce the volume of blood processed or bone marrow removed to enhance the safety and the tolerability of the stem cell collection. Smaller volumes of blood or marrow might translate into a lower risk of contamination by tumor cells. These considerations have led to a search for ways to expand the number of hematopoietic precursors ex vivo. Current strategies of hematopoietic stem and progenitor cell expansion are discussed in detail in Chapter 32.

HEMATOPOIETIC GROWTH FACTORS BEING EVALUATED IN CLINICAL TRIALS

THROMBOPOIETIN

Since the isolation and cloning of thrombopoietin, reported in 1994,[141-145] a large number of studies have evaluated the biologic effects of several forms of this molecule. Phase I clinical trials have been conducted and reported in abstract form.[146-148] This molecule appears to be highly capable of increasing platelet counts in chemotherapy-treated patients. Increased "stickiness" does not appear to be problematic in the early reports, although some clots have been noted. Clinical trials in PBPC and BMT settings are underway to evaluate capacity of thrombopoietin to speed platelet engraftment as well as to treat delayed engraftment. Anti-thrombopoietin antibodies have been reported in the serum of treated patients, thus limiting the potential use of this molecule.[149]

MULTILINEAGE HEMATOPOIETIC GROWTH FACTORS

Several multilineage HGF are in various stages of evaluation. IL-3, IL-6, IL-11, and stem cell factor (SCF) have been most studied. Each of these has shown promise in preclinical studies to speed not only myeloid recovery but platelet recovery. Randomized studies for use after HSCT have not yet been published. An area of ongoing interest is their use in combination with G-CSF, GM-CSF, or other HGF. In particular, their use in mobilization of PBPC appears attractive. A variety of dose schedules is being evaluated. One potential concern is the toxicity profile. Several, such as IL-6, cause release of acute phase proteins, and one randomized trial was terminated because of excessive toxicity.[150] If one or more of these molecules ultimately are found to have unacceptable toxicity, they still might find important uses in ex vivo expansion of HSC.

SCF is a ligand for c-kit receptor. SCF acts in concert with other HGF to augment the proliferative response of primitive hematopoietic progenitors.[151] In preclinical models, the combination of SCF and G-CSF have added to the effects of mobilization of bone marrow progenitors into the circulation. SCF by itself appears to have poor mobilizing properties,[152] but several studies[152-161] have shown that the combination of SCF plus G-CSF increases the number of progenitors in the peripheral circulation. In a murine model of sublethal irradiation (a scenario to mimic an accidental exposure), HGF were used to test whether blood counts could be increased and life-threatening infection reduced

by the use of HGF. With G-CSF and the combination of G-CSF plus SCF, a higher survival rate was noted.[162]

The flt3 ligand acts on very early hematopoietic progenitors and is synergistic with multiple other HGF in its effects.[163-165] Recent trials have shown that administration of the flt3 ligand is safe in healthy persons. Although its effect on HSC mobilization was minimal, it could cause a substantial increase in circulating dendritic cells.

IL-3 is produced by T lymphocytes. The gene, producing a glycoprotein with a molecular weight of 14–30 kD, is encoded by DNA on the long arm of chromosome 5, a region close to the GM-CSF gene. IL-3 stimulates multilineage progenitors, including CFU-granulocyte, erythrocyte, macrophage, and megakaryocyte (GEMM), CFU-GM, CFU-G, CFU-M, CFU-eosinophil, CFU-basophil, CFU-megakaryocyte, and burst-forming units—erythrocyte (BFU-E).[166] IL-3 supports proliferation and differentiation of undifferentiated as well as early committed progenitor cells. IL-3 has stimulatory effects on early progenitors of several lineages, both by itself and synergistically with other HGF,[167] as well as enhanced thrombopoiesis.[166, 168, 169] In some clinical trials, stimulatory effects on neutrophil and platelet recovery have been observed,[170] other studies have seen no similar benefits.[170-175] Toxic events were substantial in a randomized trial.[176] Several studies have evaluated the combination of IL-3 plus G-CSF or GM-CSF.[170-173, 175, 177-180] In normal volunteers, IL-3 plus G-CSF was found to increase the number of circulating CD34+ cells, suggesting that the combination might enhance engraftment after transplantation.[181] In one pilot study of lymphoma patients with low progenitor numbers due to heavy prior chemotherapy, sequential IL-3 followed by G-CSF produced higher CD34+ cell yields than did G-CSF alone.[182] In two studies, the combination of IL-3 plus G-CSF[183, 184] made no difference in the number of harvested PBPC compared with G-CSF alone. In both cases, however, there was a faster rate of platelet engraftment (neutrophil engraftment was comparable). Thus, qualitative differences in the PBPC product were produced by this combination.

Another genetically engineered IL-3 molecule is being studied in which the moieties that confer hematopoietic stimulatory properties have been retained and those conferring pro-inflammatory properties have been altered.[185, 186] This molecule has shown potent hematopoietic stimulatory effects in preclinical models, and clinical trials are now underway.[187]

IL-6 is a cytokine that has regulatory effects both early and late in hematopoietic differentiation.[188] It appears to prime HSC to become more receptive to other HGF. It also stimulates the terminal differentiation of megakaryocytes and plays a role in the production of platelets. Its effect on thrombopoiesis is enhanced in combination with other HGF, such as IL-3 and GM-CSF. IL-6 also has other effects on the differentiation of T and B cells. In primates, IL-6 accelerates platelet recovery after irradiation.[189] In early clinical trials, IL-6 has been shown to have an effect on platelet production.[190-192] Side effects include fatigue, malaise, and hepatocellular dysfunction. IL-6 also may have a role in mobilization of progenitors into the circulation.[193] One randomized clinical trial in the autologous BMT setting was terminated prematurely because of a high rate of hepatotoxicity.[150] Whether the beneficial effects of IL-6 will outweigh its toxicity remains the subject of future clinical trials.

IL-11 has pleiotropic effects, stimulating HSC proliferation and affecting multiple cell lineages. In preclinical models, beneficial effects on thrombopoiesis and amelioration of gastrointestinal mucositis have been noted.[194, 195] More-rapid return of neutrophil and platelet counts has been demonstrated.[196] Expansion of plasma volume with a concomitant fall in hemoglobin concentration has been noted. Randomized clinical trials concluded that both the proportion of cancer patients receiving platelet transfusions and the number of platelet transfusions were reduced compared with the placebo group.[197, 198] Results from a randomized trial in breast cancer patients following HSCT showed that IL-11 administration did not improve platelet recovery or platelet transfusion requirements.[200] Fatigue and cardiovascular symptoms were noted. Most reported adverse events were mild to moderate and were reversible. Some beneficial effects on mucosal healing have been noted in preliminary studies.[199] A report from an animal study showed that IL-11 may be used to separate graft-versus-leukemia effects from GVHD after BMT.[201] IL-11 has been approved by the FDA for treatment of chemotherapy-induced thrombocytopenia.

COST CONSIDERATIONS

HGF are expensive and thus without substantial clinical benefit their use would not be cost-effective. Several studies have attempted to evaluate the cost and health care resource utilization in comparable groups of patients with or without the use of HGF.[202–209] Benefits are implicated in several settings, but it is important to note that many of the advantages depended on standards of care that are continually changing. Moreover, these analyses depend on the type of health care system, making cost analysis variable from one country to another. For example, the use of a particular neutrophil count to determine whether or not a patient remains in the hospital or is discharged may not be justified in many cases. As noted earlier, a number of studies have identified a variety of criteria that permit continued care in an outpatient setting. Thus, much of the cost savings associated with HGF use may disappear when newer, more-liberal discharge criteria are employed. This is particularly true in light of the fact that HGF have no proven impact on overall survival or disease control. For this reason, the decision as to whether HGF use is justified in one setting or another may change over time as advances in supportive care continue.

CONCLUSION

G-CSF and GM-CSF have assumed important roles in HSCT, especially in the autologous setting. Both G-CSF and GM-CSF shorten the neutropenia associated with autologous transplantation, as demonstrated in controlled randomized trials. Their effects on resource utilization and clinical events are much less certain. After autologous PBPC transplantation, the benefit of G-CSF and GM-CSF may depend on the HSC content, and are more substantial when the HSC content is low but only marginal when optimal numbers of HSC are collected. G-CSF and GM-CSF are safe in allogeneic siblings BMT and do not appear to exacerbate the risk of GVHD, but the magnitude of benefit is smaller than after autologous transplantation. Their benefits are less clear in BMT using matched unrelated donors. Opinion is divided as to whether the benefit justifies the high cost of HGF. Questions have been raised as to the safety of GM-CSF in unrelated donor marrow transplantation, further study is needed. Although of theoretical concern, evidence for an increased rate of relapse is lacking, although it would be useful to have more long-term follow-up data in patients receiving transplants for myeloid malignancy.

Epo levels are low in many patients after allogeneic transplant according to some (but not all) studies, suggesting that benefit may accrue with its use. In contrast, Epo levels after autologous transplantation are appropriate for the level of anemia, and benefits from exogenous Epo administration have not been consistant.

G-CSF and GM-CSF have been shown to be beneficial for a substantial proportion of patients with delayed engraftment. A 2-week trial of either molecule appears justified in such patients. Those who do not respond should be considered for investigational cytokine trials.

Although attractive conceptually, the use of HGF as adjunctive therapy to antimicrobial agents for treatment of infection has not been proven. Further studies should be conducted to address this role for HGF.

G-CSF and GM-CSF both have been found to be effective mobilizing agents for the collection of large numbers of PBPC. Early studies suggest that combinations of newer investigational multilineage HGF that act earlier in the differentiation hierarchy along with G-CSF or GM-CSF may enhance mobilization of PBPC, which may hasten platelet recovery.

REFERENCES

1. Till JE, McCulloch EA: A direct measurement of the radiation sensitivity of normal mouse bone marrow cells. Radiat Res 14:213–222, 1961.
2. Leary AG, Strauss LC, Civin KC, Ogawa M: Disparate differentiation in hemopoietic colonies derived from human paired progenitors. Blood 66:327–332, 1985.
3. Lemishka IR, Raulet DH, Mulligan RC: Developmental potential and dynamic behavior of hematopoietic stem cells. Cell 45:917–924, 1986.
4. Metcalf D: Clonal Culture of Hemopoietic Cells. Amsterdam, Elsevier/North American Biomedical Press, 1984.
5. Shivdasani RA, Orkin SH: The transcriptional control of hematopoiesis. Blood 87:4025–4039, 1996.
6. Foulke RS, Marshall MH, Trotta PP, Von Hoff DD: In vitro assessment of the effects of granulocyte-macrophage colony-stimulating factor on primary human tumors and derived lines. Cancer Res 50:6264–6267, 1990.
7. Geller JC: Use of cytokines in the treatment of acute myelocytic leukemia: a critical review. J Clin Oncol 14:1371–1382, 1996.
8. Zittoun R, Suciu S, Mandelli F, et al: Granulocyte-macrophage colony-stimulating factor associated with induction treatment of acute myelogenous leukemia: a randomized trial by the European Organization for Research and Treatment of Cancer Leukemia Cooperative Group. J Clin Oncol 14:2150–2159, 1996.
9. Metcalf D: The molecular biology of the granulocyte/macrophage colony-stimulating factors. Blood 67:257–267, 1986.
10. Cannistra SA, Griffin JD: Regulation of the production and function of granulocytes and monocytes. Semin Hematol 25:173–188, 1988.

11. Armitage JO: Emerging applications of recombinant human granulo-cyte-macrophage colony-stimulating factor. Blood 92:4491–4508, 1998.

12. Baxevanis CN, Dedoussis GVZ, Papdopoulos NG, et al: Enhanced human lymphokine activated killer cell function after brief exposure to GM-CSF. Cancer 76:1253, 1995.

13. Epling-Burnette PK, Wei S, Blanchard DK, et al: Coinduction of granulocyte-macrophage colony-stimulating factor release and lymphokine-activated killer cell susceptibility in monocytes by interleukin-2 via interleukin-2 receptor beta. Blood 81:3130–3137, 1993.

14. Disis ML, Bernhard H, Shiota FM, et al: Granulocyte-macrophage colony-stimulating factor: an effective adjuvant for protein and peptide-based vaccines. Blood 88:202–210, 1996.

15. Richard C, Baro J, Bello-Fernandez C, et al: Recombinant human granulocyte-macrophage colony-stimulating factor (rhGM-CSF) administration after autologous bone marrow transplantation for acute myeloblastic leukemia enhances activated killer cell function and may diminish leukemic relapse. Bone Marrow Transplant 15:721–726, 1996.

16. Spivak JL: Recombinant human erythropoietin and the anemia of cancer. Blood 84:997–1004, 1994.

17. Santos GW: Immunosuppression for clinical marrow transplantation. Semin Hematol 11:341–351, 1974.

18. Bodey GP, Buckley M, Sathe YS, et al: Quantitative relationship between circulating leukocytes and infection in patients with acute leukaemia. Ann Intern Med 64:328–340, 1966.

19. Gurney H: The problem of neutropenia resulting from cancer therapy. Clinician 7:2–10, 1989.

20. Winston DJ, Gale RP, Meyer DV, et al: Infectious complications of human bone marrow transplantation. Medicine 58:1–31, 1979.

21. Tsakona CP, Khwaja A, Goldstone AH: Does treatment with haemopoietic growth factors affect the incidence of bacteraemia in adult lymphoma transplant recipients? Bone Marrow Transplant 11:433–436, 1993.

22. Linch DC, Scarffe H, Proctor S, et al: Randomized vehicle-controlled dose-finding study of glycosylated rhG-CSF after bone marrow transplantation. Bone Marrow Transplant 11:307, 1993.

23. Khwaja A, Linch DC, Goldstone AH, et al: rhG-CSF after bone marrow transplantation for malignant lymphoma: a BNLI double-blind placebo-controlled trial. Br J Haematol 82:317, 1992.

24. Talcott JA, Finberg R, Mayer RJ, Goldman L: The medical course of cancer patients with fever and neutropenia: clinical identification of a low-risk subgroup at presentation. Arch Intern Med 148:2561–2568, 1988.

25. Mullen CA, Buchanan GR: Early hospital discharge of children with cancer treated for fever and neutropenia: identification and management of the low-risk patient. J Clin Oncol 8:1998–2004, 1990.

26. Talcott JA, Siegel RD, Finberg R, Goldman L: Risk assessment in cancer patients with fever and neutropenia: a prospective, two-center validation of a prediction rule. J Clin Oncol 10:316–322, 1992.

27. Rubenstein EB, Rolston K, Benjamin RS, et al: Outpatient treatment of febrile episodes in low-risk neutropenic patients with cancer. Cancer 71:3640–3646, 1993.

28. Buchanan GR: Approach to treatment of the febrile cancer patient with low-risk neutropenia. Hematol Oncol Clin North Am 7:919–935, 1993.

29. Weiser MA, Frisbee-Hume S, Manzullo E, et al: Identification and outpatient management of the low-risk febrile neutropenic patient with cancer. Home Health Care Consult 3:35–49, 1996.

30. Rubenstein EB, Rolston KV: Outpatient treatment of febrile neutropenic patients with cancer. European J Cancer 31A:2–4, 1995.

31. Gilbert C, Meisenberg B, Vrendenburgh J, et al: Sequential prophylactic oral and empiric once-daily parenteral antibiotics for neutropenia and fever after high-dose chemotherapy and autologous bone marrow support. J Clin Oncol 12:1005–1011, 1994.

32. Meisenberg B, Gollard R, Brehm T, et al: Prophylactic antibiotics eliminate bacteremia and allow safe outpatient management following high-dose chemotherapy and autologous stem cell rescue. Support Care Cancer 4:364–369, 1996.

33. Gmur J, Burger J, Schanz U, et al: Safety of stringent prophylactic platelet transfusion policy for patients with acute leukaemia. Lancet 338:1223–1226, 1991.

34. Schiffer CA: Prophylactic platelet transfusion. Transfusion 32:295–297, 1992.

35. Baer MR, Bloomfield CD: Controversies in transfusion medicine: prophylactic platelet transfusion therapy: pro. Transfusion 32:377–380, 1992.

36. Patten E: Controversies in transfusion medicine: prophylactic platelet transfusion revisited after 25 years: con. Transfusion 32:381–385, 1992.

37. Beutler E: Platelet transfusions: the 20,000/μL trigger. Blood 81:1411–1413, 1993.

38. Kitchens CS: Are transfusions overrated? Surgical outcome of Jehovah's Witnesses. Am J Med 94:117–119, 1993.

39. Evans RW, Rader B, Manninen DL: Cooperative multicenter EPO clinical trial group: the quality of hemodialysis recipients treated with recombinant human erythropoietin. JAMA 263:825, 1990.

40. Lieschke GJ, Ramenghi U, O'Connor MP, et al: Studies of oral neutrophil levels in patients receiving G-CSF after autologous marrow transplantation. Br J Haematol 82:589–595, 1992.

41. Jadus MR, Wepsic HT: The role of cytokines in graft-versus-host reaction and disease. Bone Marrow Transplant 10:1–14, 1992.

42. Mowat AM: Antibodies to IFN-γ prevent immunologically mediated intestinal damage in murine graft-versus-host reaction. Immunology 68:18–23, 1989.

43. McCarthy PL, Abhyankar S, Neben S, et al: Inhibition of interleukin-1 by an interleukin-1 receptor antagonist prevents graft-versus-host disease. Blood 78:1915–1918, 1991.

44. Ferrara JLM: Cytokine dysregulation as a mechanism of graft versus host disease. Immunology 5:794–799, 1993.

45. Via CS, Finkelman FD: Critical role of interleukin-2 in the development of acute graft-versus-host disease. Int Immunol 5:565–572, 1993.

46. Holler E, Thierfelder S, Behrends U, et al: Anti-TNF-alpha and pentoxifylline for prophylaxis of aGvHD in murine allogeneic bone marrow transplantation. Onkologie 15:31–35, 1992.

47. Beelen DW, Haralambie E, Brandt H, et al: Evidence that sustained growth suppression of intestinal anaerobic bacteria reduces the risk of acute graft-versus-host disease after sibling marrow transplantation. Blood 80:2668–2676, 1992.

48. Blaise D, Olive D, Hirn P, et al: Prevention of acute GVHD by in vivo use of anti-interleukin-2 receptor monoclonal antibody (33B3.1): a feasibility trial in 15 patients. Bone Marrow Transplant 8:105–111, 1991.

49. van Bekkum DW, Roodenburg J, Heidt PJ, van der Waaij D: Mitigation of secondary disease of allogeneic mouse radiation chimeras by modification of the intestinal microflora. J Natl Cancer Inst 52:401–404, 1974.

50. Holler E, Kolb HJ, Hintermeier-Knaabe J, et al: Role of tumor necrosis factor alpha in acute graft-versus-host disease and complications following allogeneic bone marrow transplantation. Transplant Proc 25:1234–1236, 1993.

51. Symington FW, Symington BE, Liu PY, et al: The relationship of serum IL-6 levels to acute graft-versus-host disease and hepatorenal disease after human bone marrow transplantation. Transplantation 54:457–462, 1992.

52. ASCO Ad Hoc Colony-Stimulating Factor Guideline Expert Panel: American Society of Clinical Oncology Recommendations for the use of hematopoietic colony-stimulating factors: evidence-based, clinical practice guidelines. J Clin Oncol 12:2471–2508, 1994.

53. Anderson JR, Anderson PN, Armitage JO, et al: Update of recommendations for the use of hematopoietic colony-stimulating factors: evidence-based clinical practice guidelines. J Clin Oncol 14:1957–1960, 1996.

54. Nemunaitis J: Growth factors in allogeneic transplantation. Semin Oncol 20:96–101, 1993.

55. Lazarus HM, Rowe JM: Clinical use of hematopoietic growth factors in allogeneic bone marrow transplantation. Blood Rev 8:169–178, 1994.

56. Vose JM, Armitage JO: Clinical applications of hematopoietic growth factors. J Clin Oncol 13:1023–1035, 1995.

57. Dix SP, Gilmore CE: Cytokine therapy after bone marrow transplantation: review of GM-CSF and G-CSF. Pharmacotherapy 16:593–608, 1996.

58. Wingard JR, Elfenbein GJ: Host immunologic augmentation for the control of infection. Infect Dis Clin North Am 10:345–364, 1996.

59. Bociek RG, Armitage JO: Hematopoietic growth factors. Cancer J Clin 46:165–184, 1996.

60. Cook DJ, Guyatt GH, Laupacis A, et al: Rules of evidence and

clinical recommendations on the use of antithrombotic agents. Chest 102(Suppl 4):305S–311S, 1992.

61. Gorin NC, Coiffier B, Hayat M, et al: rhGM-CSF after high dose chemotherapy and ABMT with unpurged and purged marrow in non-Hodgkin's lymphoma: a double-blind placebo-controlled trial. Blood 80:1149, 1992.

62. Gulati SC, Bennett CL: GM-CSF as adjunct therapy in relapsed Hodgkin disease. Ann Intern Med 116:177, 1992.

63. Link H, Boogaerts MA, Carella AM, et al: A controlled trial of rhGM-CSF after TBI, high-dose chemotherapy, and ABMT for ALL or malignant lymphoma. Blood 80:2188, 1992.

64. Nemunaitis J, Rabinowe SN, Singer JW, et al: rhGM-CSF after ABMT for lymphoid cancer. N Engl J Med 324:1773, 1991.

65. Schmitz N, Dreger P, Zander AR, et al: Results of a randomized controlled multicenter study of rhG-CSF in patients with Hodgkin's disease and non-Hodgkin's lymphoma undergoing ABMT. Bone Marrow Transplant 15:261, 1995.

66. Stahel RA, Jost LM, Cerny T, et al: Randomized study of rhG-CSF after high-dose chemotherapy and ABMT for high-risk lymphoid malignancies. J Clin Oncol 12:1931, 1994.

67. Advani R, Chao NJ, Horning SJ, et al: GM-CSF as an adjunct to autologous hemopoietic stem cell transplantation for lymphoma. Ann Intern Med 116:183, 1992.

68. Legros M, Fleury J, Bay J, et al: rhGM-CSF vs placebo following rhGM-CSF-mobilized PBPC transplantation: a phase III double-blind randomized trial. Bone Marrow Transplant 19:209–213, 1997.

69. Spitzer G, Adkins DR, Spencer V, et al: Randomized study of growth factors post PBPC transplant: neutrophil recovery is improved with modest clinical benefit. J Clin Oncol 12:661, 1994.

70. Klumpp TR, Mangan KF, Goldberg SL, et al: G-CSF accelerates neutrophil engraftment following PBSC transplantation: a prospective, randomized trial. J Clin Oncol 13:1323, 1995.

71. Linch DC, Milligan DW, Winfield DA, et al: G-CSF after peripheral blood stem cell transplantation in lymphoma patients significantly accelerated neutrophil recovery and shortened time in hospital: results of a randomized BNLI trial. Br J Haematol 99:933–938, 1997.

72. Gisselbrecht C, Prentice HG, Bacigalupo A, et al: Placebo-controlled phase III trial of lenograstim in bone marrow transplantation. Lancet 343:696, 1994.

73. DeWitte T, Gratwohl A, Van Der Lely N, et al: rhGM-CSF accelerates neutrophil and monocyte recovery after allogeneic T-cell-depleted bone marrow transplantation. Blood 79:1359, 1992.

74. Nemunaitis J, Rosenfeld CS, Ash R, et al: Phase III randomized, double-blind placebo-controlled trial of rhGM-CSF following allogeneic bone marrow transplantation. Bone Marrow Transplant 15:949, 1995.

75. Powles R, Smith C, Milan S, et al: rhGM-CSF in allogeneic bone-marrow transplantation for leukaemia: double-blind, placebo-controlled trial. Lancet 336:1417, 1990.

76. Wardley AM, Scarffe JH: Role of granulocyte-macrophage colony-stimulating factor in chemoradiotherapy-induced oral mucositis. J Clin Oncol 14:1741–1744, 1996.

77. Gordon B, Spadinger A, Hodges E, et al: Effect of granulocyte-macrophage colony-stimulating factor on oral mucositis after hematopoietic stem-cell transplantation. J Clin Oncol 12:1917–1922, 1994.

78. Peters WP: The effect of recombinant human colony-stimulating factors on hematopoietic reconstitution following autologous bone marrow transplantation. Semin Hematol 26:18–23, 1989.

79. Singer JW: Role of colony-stimulating factors in bone marrow transplantation. Semin Oncol 19:27–31, 1992.

80. Pettengell R, Gurner H, Radford JA, et al: Granulocyte colony-stimulating factor to prevent dose-limiting neutropenia in non-Hodgkin's lymphoma: a randomized controlled trial. Blood 80:1430–1436, 1992.

81. Schriber JR, Chao NJ, Long GD, et al: Granulocyte colony-stimulating factor after allogeneic bone marrow transplantation. Blood 84:1047–1050, 1989.

82. Anasetti C, Anderson G, Appelbaum FR, et al: Phase III study of rhGM-CSF in allogeneic marrow transplantation from unrelated donors. Blood 82:154a, 1993.

83. Cortelazzo S, Viero P, Bellavita P, et al: G-CSF following PBPC transplant in non-Hodgkin's lymphoma. J Clin Oncol 13:935, 1995.

84. Szilvassy SF, Hoffman R: Hematopoietic growth factors do not accelerate neutrophil recovery after transplantation of optimally mobi-

85. Brandwein JM, Callum J, Sutcliffe SB, et al: Analysis of factors affecting hematopoietic recovery after ABMT. Bone Marrow Transplant 6:291, 1990.

86. Hansen PB, Knudsen H, Gaarsdal E, et al: Short-term in vivo priming of bone marrow haematopoiesis with rhG-CSF, rhGM-CSF or rhIL-3 before marrow harvest expands myelopoiesis but does not improve engraftment capability. Bone Marrow Transplant 16:373–379, 1995.

87. Janssen WE, Smilee RC, Elfenbein GJ: A prospective randomized trial comparing blood vs. marrow derived stem cells for hematopoietic replacement following high dose chemotherapy. J Hematother 4:139–140, 1995.

88. Faucher C, Le Corroller AG, Chabannon C, et al: Administration of G-CSF can be delayed after transplantation of autologous G-CSF-primed blood stem cells: a randomized study. Bone Marrow Transplant 17:533–536, 1996.

89. Sobrevilla-Calvo P, Cortes P, Solano P, et al: Starting G-CSF on day + 7 or on day 0 is equally effective in accelerating neutrophil recovery after autologous peripheral blood stem cell transplantation [Abstract 724]. J Clin Oncol 15:272, 1996.

90. Vey N, Molnar S, Faucher C, et al: Delayed administration of granulocyte colony-stimulating factor after autologous bone marrow transplantation: effect of granulocyte recovery. Bone Marrow Transplant 14(5):779, 1994.

91. Khwaja A, Mills W, Leveridge K, et al: Efficacy of a delayed granulocyte colony-stimulating factor after autologous bone marrow transplantation. Bone Marrow Transplant 11:479–482, 1993.

92. Viret F, Molina L, Plantaz D, et al: Impact of delayed start (day + 5) G-CSF after allogeneic bone marrow transplantation: a pilot study [Abstract 369]. Blood 84 (Suppl 1):63, 1994.

93. Masaoka T, Takaku F, Kato S, et al: rhG-CSF in allogeneic bone marrow transplantation. Exp Hematol 17:1047, 1989.

94. Schapira L, Antin JH, Ransil BJ, et al: Serum erythropoietin levels in patients receiving intensive chemotherapy and radiotherapy. Blood 76:2354–2359, 1990.

95. Miller CV, Jones RJ, Zahurak ML, et al: Impaired erythropoietin response to anemia after bone marrow transplantation. Blood 80:2677–2682, 1992.

96. Ireland RM, Atkinson K, Concannon A, et al: Serum erythropoietin changes in autologous and allogeneic bone marrow transplant patients. Br J Haematol 76:128–134, 1990.

97. Beguin Y, Clemons GK, Oris R, et al: Circulating erythropoietin levels after bone marrow transplantation: inappropriate response to anemia in allogeneic transplants. Blood 77:868–873, 1991.

98. Bosi A, Vannucchi AM, Gross A, et al: Serum erythropoietin levels in patients undergoing autologous bone marrow transplantation. Bone Marrow Transplant 7:421–425, 1991.

99. Lazarus HM, Goodnough LT, Goodwasser E, et al: Serum erythropoietin levels and blood component therapy after autologous bone marrow transplantation: implications for erythropoietin in this setting. Bone Marrow Transplant 10:71–75, 1992.

100. Bosi A, Vannucchi Am, Grossi A, et al: Serum erythropoietin levels in allogeneic, non T-depleted bone marrow transplantation, and the effects of rhEPO administration. Bone Marrow Transplant 7(Suppl 2):87, 1991.

101. Vannucchi AM, Bosi A, Grossi A, et al: Stimulation of erythroid engraftment by recombinant human erythropoietin in ABO-compatible, HLA-identical, allogeneic bone marrow transplant patients. Leukemia 6:215–219, 1992.

102. Biggs JC, Atkinson KA, Booker V, et al: Prospective randomized double-blind trial of the in vivo use of rhEPO in bone marrow transplantation from HLA-identical sibling donors: the Australian Bone Marrow Transplant Study Group. Bone Marrow Transplant 15(1):129, 1995.

103. Fleming WH, Alvernas J, Fleming NC, et al: A randomized study of EPO in patients undergoing HLA-matched allogeneic bone marrow transplantation. Blood (Abstract Suppl):212a, 1995.

104. Klaesson S, Ringden O, Ljungman P, et al: Reduced blood transfusions requirements after allogeneic bone marrow transplantation: results of a randomized, double-blind study with high-dose EPO. Bone Marrow Transplant 13(4):397, 1994.

105. Steegmann JL, Lopez J, Otero MJ, et al: Erythropoietin treatment in allogeneic bone marrow transplant accelerated erythroid reconstitu-

tion: results of a prospective controlled randomized trial. Bone Marrow Transplant 10:541, 1992.

106. Link H, Boogaerts MA, Fauser AA, et al: A controlled trial of rhEPO after bone marrow transplantation. Blood 84:3327, 1994.

107. Chao NH, Schriber JR, Long GD, et al: A randomized study of erythropoietin and granulocyte colony-stimulating factor (G-CSF) versus placebo and G-CSF for patients with Hodgkin's and non-Hodgkin's lymphoma undergoing autologous bone marrow transplantation. Blood 83:2823–2828, 1994.

108. Miller CB, Mills SR, Barnett AG, et al: A randomized trial of recombinant human erythropoietin (rhuEPO) after purged autologous bone marrow transplant (BMT) [Abstract 1126]. Blood 82:285a, 1993.

109. Weisdorf DJ, Verfaillie CM, Davies SM, et al: Hematopoietic growth factors for graft failure after bone marrow graft failure: a randomized trial of granulocyte macrophage colony stimulating factor (GM-CSF) plus granulocyte CSF. Blood 85:3452–3456, 1995.

110. Nemunaitis J, Singer JW, Buckner CD, et al: Use of rhGM-CSF in graft failure after BMT. Blood 76:245, 1990.

111. Vose JM, Bierman PJ, Kessinger A, et al: The use of rhGM-CSF for the treatment of delayed engraftment following high dose therapy and autologous hematopoietic stem cell transplantation for lymphoid malignancies. Bone Marrow Transplant 7:139, 1991.

112. Brandwein JM, Nayar R, Baker MA, et al: GM-CSF therapy for delayed engraftment after ABMT. Exp Hematol 19:191, 1991.

113. Ippoliti C, Przepiorka D, Giralt S, et al: Low-dose non-glycosylated rhGM-CSF is effective for the treatment of delayed hematopoietic recovery after ABMT or PBSC transplantation. Bone Marrow Transplant 11:55, 1993.

114. Klingemann HG, Eaves AC, Barnett MJ, et al: rGM-CSF in patients with poor graft function after bone marrow transplantation. Clin Invest Med 13:77, 1990.

115. Dejongh CA, Joshi JH, Newman KI, et al: Antibiotic synergism and response in gram-negative bacteraemia in granulocytopenic cancer patients. Am J Med 80:96–100, 1986.

116. Maksymiuk AW, Thongprasert S, Hopfer R, et al: Systemic candidiasis in cancer patients. Am J Med 77 (Suppl 40):22–27, 1984.

117. Bodey GP, Vartivarian S: Aspergillosis. Eur J Clin Microbiol Infect Dis 8:413–437, 1989

118. Bodey GP, Anaissie E, Gutterman J, et al: Role of GM-CSF as adjuvant therapy for fungal infection in patients with cancer. Clin Infect Dis 17:705–707, 1993.

119. Nemunaitis J, Meyers JD, Buckner CD, et al: Phase I trial of recombinant human macrophage colony-stimulating factor in patients with invasive fungal infections. Blood 78:907–913, 1991.

120. Nemunaitis J, Shannon-Dorcy K, Appelbaum FR, et al: Long-term follow-up of patients with invasive fungal disease who received adjunctive therapy with recombinant human macrophage colony-stimulating factor. Blood 82:1422–1427, 1993.

121. Cenci E, Bartocci A, Puccetti P, et al: Macrophage colony-stimulating factor in murine candidasis: serum and tissue levels during infection and protective effect of exogenous administration. Infect Immun 59:868, 1991.

122. Maher DW, Lieschke GJ, Green M, et al: Filgrastim in patients with chemotherapy-induced febrile neutropenia. A double-blind, placebo-controlled trial [see comments]. Ann Intern Med 121:492–501, 1994.

123. Mayordomo JI, Rivera F, Díaz-Puente MT, et al: Improving treatment of chemotherapy-induced neutropenic fever by administration of colony-stimulating factors [see comments]. J Natl Cancer Inst 87:803–808, 1995.

124. Anaissie E, Vartivarian S, Bodey GP, et al: Randomized comparison between antibiotics alone and antibiotics plus granulocyte-macrophage colony stimulating factor (E. coli–derived) in cancer patients with fever and neutropenia. Am J Med 100:17–23, 1996.

125. Biesma B, de Vries ER, Willemse PH, et al: Efficacy and tolerability of recombinant human granulocyte-macrophage colony-stimulating factor in patients with chemotherapy-related leukopenia and fever. Eur J Cancer 26:932–936, 1990.

126. Riikonen P, Saarinen UM, Makipernaa A, et al: rhGM-CSF in the treatment of fever and neutropenia: a double-blind, placebo-controlled study in children with malignancy. Proc Am Soc Clin Oncol 12:442, 1993.

127. Valenga E, Uyl-de Groat CA, de Wit R, et al: Randomized placebo controlled trial of granulocyte-macrophage colony-stimulating factor in patients with chemotherapy-related febrile neutropenia. J Clin Oncol 14:619–627, 1996.

128. Bensinger WI, Price TH, Dale DC, et al: The effects of daily recombinant human granulocyte colony-stimulating factor administration on normal granulocyte donors undergoing leukapheresis. Blood 81:1883–1889, 1993.

129. Caspar CB, Seger RA, Burger J, Gmor J: Effective stimulation of donors for granulocyte transfusions with recombinant methionyl granulocyte colony-stimulating factor. Blood 81:2866–2871, 1993.

130. Masauzi N, Kobayashi N, Suzuki G, et al: Comparison of the collection efficiency and characteristics of peripheral blood progenitor cells mobilized by G-CSF administration in the steady state versus postmyelosuppressive chemotherapy. Transplant Proc 28:1741–1745, 1996.

131. Bolwell BJ, Goormastic M, Yanssens T, et al: Comparison of G-CSF with GM-CSF for mobilizing peripheral blood progenitor cells and for enhancing marrow recovery after autologous bone marrow transplant. Bone Marrow Transplant 14:913–918, 1994.

132. Lane TA, Law P, Maruyama M, et al: Harvesting and enrichment of hematopoietic progenitor cells mobilized into the peripheral blood of normal donors by GM-CSF or G-CSF: potential role in allogeneic marrow transplantation. Blood 85:275, 1995.

133. Peters WP, Rosner G, Ross M, et al: Comparative effects of GM-CSF and G-CSF on priming PBPC for use with ABMT after high-dose chemotherapy. Blood 81:1709, 1993.

134. Bachier C, Gokmen E, Teale J, et al: Randomized trial of granulocyte colony stimulating factor (G-CSF) versus granulocyte-macrophage colony stimulating factor (GM-CSF) for mobilization of peripheral blood stem cells (PBSC) for allogeneic transplantation in patients with hematological disorders [abstract]. Blood 92:683, 1998.

135. Papayannopoulou T, Nakamoto B: Peripheralization of hematopoietic progenitors in primates treated with anti-VLA4 integrin. Proc Natl Acad Sci U S A 90:9374–9378, 1993.

136. Aquier P, Macquart-Moulin G, Moatti JP, et al: Comparison of anxiety, pain and discomfort in two procedures of hematopoietic stem cell collection: leukocytapheresis and bone marrow harvest. Bone Marrow Transplant 16:541–547, 1995.

137. Baumann I, Test HG, Lange C, et al: Haematopoietic cells mobilized by lenograstim as an alternative to bone marrow for allogeneic transplants. Lancet 341:369, 1993.

138. Korbling M, Przepiorka D, Huh YO: Allogeneic blood stem cell transplantation for refractory leukemia and lymphoma: potential advantage of blood over marrow allografts. Blood 85:1659–1665, 1995.

139. Russell NH, Hunter A, Rogers S, et al: Peripheral blood stem cells as an alternative to marrow for allogeneic transplantation. Lancet 341:1482, 1993.

140. Bensinger WI, Weaver CH, Appelbaum FR, et al: Transplantation of allogeneic peripheral blood stem cells mobilized by recombinant human granulocyte colony-stimulating factor. Blood 85:1655–1658, 1995.

141. Lok S, Kaushansky K, Holly RD, et al: Cloning and expression of murine thrombopoietin cDNA and stimulation of platelet production in vivo. Nature 369:565–568, 1994.

142. Kaushansky K, Lok S, Holly RD, et al: Promotion of megakaryocyte progenitor expansion and differentiation by the c-Mpl ligand thrombopoietin. Nature 369:568–571, 1994.

143. De Sauvage FJ, Hass PE, Spencer SD, et al: Stimulation of megakaryocytopoiesis and thrombopoiesis by the c-Mpl ligand. Nature 369:533–538, 1994.

144. Metcalf D: Thrombopoietin—at last. Nature 369:519–520, 1994.

145. Wendling F, Maraskovsky E, Bebill N, et al: C-Mpl ligand is a humoral regulator of megakaryocytopoiesis. Nature 369:571–574, 1994.

146. Basser RL, Rasko JE, Clarke K, et al: Randomized, blinded, placebo-controlled phase I trial of pegylated recombinant human megakaryocyte growth and development factor with filgrastim after dose-intensive chemotherapy in patients with advanced cancer [published erratum appears in Blood 90:2513, 1997]. Blood 89:3118–3128, 1997.

147. Fanucchi M, Glaspy J, Crawford J, et al: Effects of polyethylene glycol-conjugated recombinant human megakaryocyte growth and development factor on platelet counts after chemotherapy for lung cancer [see comments]. N Engl J Med 336:404–409, 1997.

148. Vadhan-Raj S, Murray LJ, Bueso-Ramos C, et al: Stimulation of megakaryocyte and platelet production by a single dose of recombinant human thrombopoietin in patients with cancer [see comments]. Ann Internal Med 126:673–681, 1997.

149. Shiojaki H, Kuwaki T, Hagiwara T, et al: Presence of antibodies that can neutralize the biological activity of thrombopoietin in a patient with amegakaryocytic thrombocytopenic purpura [abstract]. Blood 92:472, 1998.

150. Devine SM, Winton EF, Holland HK, et al: Simulatneous administration of IL-6 and rhG-CSF following ABMT for breast cancer. Blood 84:89a, 1994.

151. Toksoz D, Zsebo KM, Smith KA, et al: Support of human hematopoiesis in long-term bone marrow cultures by murine stromal cell selectively expressing the membrane-bound and secreted forms of the human homolog of the steel gene product, stem cell factor. Proc Natl Acad Sci U S A 89:7350, 1992.

152. Shpall EJ, Wheeler CA, Turner SA, et al: A randomized phase 3 study of peripheral blood progenitor cell mobilization with stem cell factor and filgrastim in high-risk breast cancer patients. Blood 93:2491–2501, 1999.

153. DeRevel T, Appelbaum FR, Storb R, et al: Effects of granulocyte colony-stimulating factor and stem cell factor, alone and in combination, on the mobilization of peripheral blood cells that engraft lethally irradiated dogs. Blood 83:3795–3799, 1994.

154. Andrews RG, Briddell RA, Knitter GH, et al: Rapid engraftment by peripheral blood progenitor cells mobilized by recombinant human stem cell factor and recombinant human granulocyte colony-stimulating factor in nonhuman primates. Blood 85:15–20, 1995.

155. Morstyn G, Glaspy J, Shpall E, et al: Clinical application of filgrastim and stem cell factor in vivo and in vitro. J Hematother 3:353–355, 1994.

156. Glaspy JA, Shpall EJ, LeMaistre CF, et al: Peripheral blood progenitor cell mobilization using stem cell factor in combination with filgrastim in breast cancer patients. Blood 90:2939–2951, 1997.

157. Briddell R, Glaspy J, Shpall EJ, et al: Recombinant human stem cell factor (rhSCF) and filgrastim (rhG-CSF) synergize to mobilize myeloid, erythroid, and megakaryocyte progenitors in patients with breast cancer [Abstract 361]. Br J Haematol 87:92, 1994.

158. Weaver A, Testa NG: Stem cell factor leads to reduced blood processing during apheresis or the use of whole blood aliquots to support dose-intensive chemotherapy. Bone Marrow Transplant 22:33, 1998.

159. Weaver A, Chang J, Wrigley E, et al: Randomized comparison of progenitor-cell mobilization using chemotherapy, stem-cell factor, and filgrastim or chemotherapy plus filgrastim alone in patients with ovarian cancer. J Clin Oncol 16:2601, 1998.

160. Geissler K, Kabrna E, Stengg S, et al: Recombinant human megakaryocyte growth and development factor increases levels of circulating haemopoietic progenitor cells post chemotherapy in patients with acute myeloid leukaemia. Br J Haematol 102:535, 1998.

161. Basser RL, To LB, Begley CG, et al: Rapid hematopoietic recovery after multicycle high-dose chemotherapy: enhancement of filgrastim-induced progenitor-cell mobilization by recombinant human stem-cell factor. J Clin Oncol 16:1899, 1998.

162. Storb R, Raff RF, Appelbaum FR, et al: DLA-identical bone marrow grafts after low-dose total body irradiation: the effect of canine recombinant hematopoietic growth factors. Blood 84:3558–3566, 1994.

163. Jacobsen SEW, Veiby OP, Myklebust J, et al: Ability of flt3 ligand to stimulate the in vitro growth of primitive murine hematopoietic progenitors is potently and directly inhibited by transforming growth factor-β and tumor necrosis factor. Blood 87:5016–5026, 1996.

164. Rusten LS, Lyman SD, Veiby OP, Jacobsen SEW: The FLT3 ligand is a direct and potent stimulator of the growth of primitive and committed human CD34⁺ bone marrow progenitor cells in vitro. Blood 87:1317–1325, 1996.

165. Shah AJ, Smogorzewska EM, Hannum C, Crooks GM: Flt3 ligand induces proliferation of quiescent human bone marrow CD34⁺ CD38⁻ cells and maintains progenitor cells in vitro. Blood 87:3563–3570, 1996.

166. Yang YC, Clark SC: Interleukin-3: molecular biology and biologic activities. Hematol Oncol Clin North Am 3:441–452, 1989.

167. Donahue RE, Seehra J, Metzger M, et al: Human IL-3 and GM-CSF act synergistically in stimulating hematopoiesis in primates. Science 241:1820, 1988.

168. Donajue RE, Seehra J, Metzger M, et al: Human IL-3 and GM-CSF act synergistically in stimulating hematopoiesis in primates. Science 241:1820–1823, 1988.

169. Lindemann A, Ganser A, Hermann F, et al: Biologic effects of recombinant interleukin-3 in vivo. J Clin Oncol 9:2120–2127, 1991.

170. Fibbe WE, Raemaekers J, Verdonck LF, et al: Recombinant human interleukin-3 after autologous bone marrow transplantation for malignant lymphoma: a phase I/II multicenter study [Abstract]. Blood 78:163a, 1991.

171. Lindemann A, Ganser A, Herrmann F, et al: Biologic effects of recombinant human interleukin-3 in vivo. J Clin Oncol 9:2120–2127, 1991.

172. Kurzrock R, Talpaz M, Estrov Z, et al: Phase I study of recombinant human interleukin-3 in patients with bone marrow failure. J Clin Oncol 9:1241–1250, 1991.

173. Fay JW, et al: Sequential administration of recombinant human interleukin-3 and granulocyte-macrophage colony-stimulating factor after autologous bone marrow transplantation for malignant lymphoma: a phase I/II multicenter study. Blood 84:2151–2157, 1994.

174. Sosman JA, Stiff PJ, Bayer RA, et al: A phase I trial of interleukin 3 (IL-3) pre-bone marrow harvest with granulocyte-macrohage colony stimulating factor (GM-CSF) post-stem cell infusion in patients with solid tumors receiving high-dose combination chemotherapy. Bone Marrow Transplant 16:655–661, 1995.

175. Brugger W, Rumbeger B, Bertz H, et al: Randomized phase II trial of hematopoietic growth factor support (IL-3 + GM-CSF) after peripheral blood progenitor cell transplantation in patients with solid tumors and lymphomas [Abstract 349]. Blood 84:90a, 1994.

176. Fibbe WE, Velenga E, Bezwoda WR, et al: Thrombopoietic effect of interleukin-3 (IL-3) after autologous bone marrow transplantation (ABMT) in patients with non-Hodgkin lymphoma (NHL) or Hodgkin's disease (HD): results from a phase III placebo-controlled study [Abstract 355]. Blood 84:92a, 1994.

177. Rosenfeld CS, Bolwell B, LeFever A, et al: Comparison of four cytokine regimens for mobilization of peripheral blood stem cells: IL-3 alone and combined with GM-CSF or G-CSF. Bone Marrow Transplant 17:179–183, 1996.

178. Hogge DE, Eaves CJ, Sutherland HJ, et al: Administration of IL-3 with GM-CSF after high dose cyclophosphamide mobilizes blood progenitors which enhance platelet recovery following ABMT. Blood 84:106a, 1994.

179. Nemunaitis J, Rosenfeld C, Bolwell B, et al: Phase II randomized trial comparing SDZ ILE 965 (rhIL-3) to sequential and combination administration of rhIL-3 and leukine or neupogen in the mobilization of peripheral blood progenitor cells for autologous transplant (PBSCT) in patient with lymphoid malignancy or breast cancer [Abstract 1446]. Blood 82:365a, 1993.

180. Rosenfeld CS, Bolwell B, LeFever A, et al: Comparison of four cytokine regimens for mobilization of peripheral blood stem cells: IL-3 alone and combined with GM-CSF or G-CSF. Bone Marrow Transplant 17:179–183, 1995.

181. Huhn RD, Yurkow EJ, Tushinski R, et al: Recombinant human interleukin-3 (rhIL-3) enhances the mobilization of peripheral blood progenitor cells by recombinant human granulocyte colony-stimulating factor (rhG-CSF) in normal volunteers. Exp Hematol 24:839–847, 1996.

182. Geissler K, Peschel C, Niederwieser D, et al: Potentiation of granulocyte colony-stimulating factor-induced mobilization of circulating progenitor cells by seven-day pretreatment with interleukin-3. Blood 87:2732–2739, 1996.

183. Bolwell B, Rosenfeld C, LeFever A, et al: A phase II trial of G-CSF with or without SDZ ILE 964 (IL-3) for the mobilization of peripheral blood progenitor cells (PBPC) for autologous progenitor cell transplantation [Abstract 411]. Blood 84:106a, 1994.

184. Engel H, Korbling M, Palmer J, et al: Randomized trial of G-CSF alone vs sequential interleukin-3 (IL-3) and G-CSF treatment to peripheralize progenitor cells for apheresis and blood stem cell autotransplantation in patients with advanced stage breast cancer [Abstract 420]. Blood 84:108a, 1994.

185. MacVittie TJ, Farese AM, Herodin F, et al: Combination therapy for radiation-induced bone marrow aplasia in nonhuman primates using synthokine SC-55494 and recombinant human granulocyte colony-stimulating factor. Blood 87:4129–4135, 1996.

186. Farese AM, Herodin F, McKearn JP, et al: Acceleration of hematopoietic reconstitution with a synthetic cytokine (SC-55494) after radiation-induced bone marrow aplasia. Blood 87:581–591, 1996.

187. Thomas JW, Baum CM, Hood WE, et al: Potent interleukin 3 receptor agonist with selectively enhanced hematopoietic activity relative to recombinant human interleukin 3. Proc Natl Acad Sci U S A 92:3779, 1995.

188. Weber J: Interleukin-6: multifunctional cytokine. Biol Ther Cancer Updates 3(2):1–9, 1993.
189. MacVittie TJ, Farese AM, Patchen ML, et al: Therapeutic efficacy of recombinant interleukin-6 (IL-6) alone and combined with recombinant human IL-3 in a nonhuman primate model of high-dose, sublethal radiation-induced marrow aplasia. Blood 84:2515–2522, 1994.
190. Demetri GD, Samuels B, Gordon M, et al: Recombinant human interleukin-6 (IL-6) increases circulating platelet counts and C-reactive protein levels in vivo: initial results of a phase I trial in sarcoma patients with normal hemopoiesis [Abstract 344]. Blood 80:88a, 1992.
191. Gameren MM, Velenga E, Willemse PHB, et al: The effects of recombinant human interleukin-6 (RhIL-6) on in vivo hematopoiesis in cancer patients [Abstract 985]. Blood 80:249a, 1992.
192. Van Doren B, Saez RA, Burstein SA, et al: Clinical and laboratory evaluation of rIL-6 in ABMT. Blood 84:96a, 1994.
193. Pettengell R, Luft T, de Wynter E, et al: Effects of interleukin-6 on mobilization of primitive haemopoietic cells into the circulation. Br J Haematol 89:237–242, 1995.
194. Neben TY, Loebelenz J, Hayes L, et al: Recombinant human interleukin-11 stimulates megakaryocytopoiesis and increases peripheral platelets in normal and splenectomized mice. Blood 81:901–908, 1993.
195. Ritch PS, Schiller J, Ribkin S, et al: Phase I evaluation of recombinant human interleukin-6 [Abstract 1453]. Blood 82:367a, 1993.
196. Du XX, Neben T, Goldman S, Williams DA: Effects of recombinant human interleukin-11 on hematopoietic reconstitution in transplant mice: acceleration of recovery of peripheral blood neutrophils and platelets. Blood 81:27–34, 1993.
197. Tepler I, Elias L, Smith JW, et al: A randomized placebo-controlled trial of recombinant human interleukin-11 in cancer patients with severe thrombocytopenia due to chemotherapy. Blood 87:3607–3614, 1996.
198. Isaacs C, Robert NJ, Bailey FA, et al: Randomized placebo-controlled study of recombinant human interleukin-11 to prevent chemotherapy-induced thrombocytopenia in patients with breast cancer receiving dose-intensive cyclophosphamide and doxorubicin. J Clin Oncol 15:3368, 1997.
199. Du XX, Doerschuk CM, Orazi A, Williams DA: A bone marrow stromal-derived growth factor, interleukin-11, stimulates recovery of small intestinal mucosal cells after cytoablative therapy. Blood 83:33–37, 1994.
200. Vredenburg JJ, Hussein A, Fisher D, et al: A randomized trial of recombinant human interleukin-11 following autologous bone marrow transplantation using peripheral blood progenitor cell support in patients with breast cancer. Biol Blood Marrow Transplant 4:134–141, 1998.
201. Teshima T, Hill GR, Pan L, et al: IL-11 separates graft-versus-leukemia effects from graft-versus-host disease after bone marrow transplantation. J Clin Invest 104:317–325, 1999.
202. Wells PS, Crump M: GM-CSF following ABMT: a meta-analysis and cost effectiveness evaluation [Abstract 1565]. Blood 84:146, 1994.
203. Gulati SC, Bennett CL: GM-CSF as adjunct therapy in relapsed Hodgkin disease. Ann Intern Med 116:177, 1992.
204. Finley RS: Measuring the cost-effectiveness of hematopoietic growth factor therapy. Cancer 67:2727, 1991.
205. Brice P, Godin S, Libert O, et al: Effect of lenograstim on the cost of ABMT. Pharmaco Econ 7:238, 1995.
206. Luce BR, Singer JW, Wescheler JM, et al: rhGM-CSF after ABMT for lymphoid cancer. Pharmaco Econ 6:42, 1994.
207. Peters WP, Rosner G: A bottom-line analysis of the financial impact of hematopoietic colony stimulating factors and CSF-primed peripheral blood progenitor cells. Blood 78:6a, 1991.
208. Degroot CAU, Velenga E, Rutter FFH: An economical model to assess the savings from a clinical application of hematopoietic growth factors. Eur J Cancer 32A:57–62, 1996.
209. Petros WP, Peters WP: Cost implications of hematopoietic growth factors in BMT setting. Bone Marrow Transplant 11:36, 1993.

Coagulation Issues

CHAPTER FORTY-ONE

Coagulopathy During Transplantation
William D. Haire, M.D., and
Stefano R. Tarantolo, M.D.

BACKGROUND

Since the mid-19th century, physicians have recognized that patients with cancer are unusually predisposed to thrombosis. For generations it was presumed that the tumor or its products were the major, if not the sole, cause of these thrombi. In 1980, evidence began to appear suggesting that some of our treatments for cancer, particularly chemotherapy, might add an independent risk of thrombosis in patients with cancer.[1-18] Later in the 1980s, evidence began to mount that some supportive care measures, particularly the use of colony-stimulating factors to hasten recovery from chemotherapy-induced granulocytopenia, posed an additional risk of thrombosis.[19-24]

Administration of a variety of chemotherapeutic agents was found to result in acute and more long-term changes in the coagulation system. Infusion of chemotherapy was found to cause an abrupt increase in the level of fibrinopeptide A, the activation peptide cleaved by thrombin from fibrinogen as it is converted to fibrin.[25-27] Because this rise in fibrinopeptide A level was abolished by heparin it was thought that chemotherapy, through unknown mechanisms, activated the coagulation system, thereby putting the patient at risk for acute thrombotic events.[27] Long-term impairment of the fibrinolytic system and a decrease in the levels of the natural anticoagulants antithrombin III and proteins C and S with the protracted administration of hormonal and cytostatic chemotherapy were noted, putting patients at risk for thrombosis long after the acute administration of the chemotherapy had ceased.[28-31]

Though less well studied, there is evidence that colony-stimulating factors (CSF) activate the coagulation system and perturb vascular endothelial cells. In normal persons, granulocyte-CSF (G-CSF) use is associated with generation of thrombin and increases in vascular endothelial cell proteins, possibly in a dose-related manner.[32, 33] When given to patients after peripheral blood stem cell transplantation, granulocyte macrophage CSF (GM-CSF) predisposes to deficiency in both antithrombin III and protein C.[34]

At the same time that conventional doses of chemotherapy were found to activate coagulation and predispose to thrombosis, investigators were beginning to appreciate that high-dose therapy with hematopoietic stem cell rescue was also associated with a variety of complications that could be related to the activation of coagulation. Nonbacterial thrombotic endocarditis, focal ischemia of the ocular fundus, stroke, catheter-induced subclavian vein thrombosis (occasionally with superior vena cava thrombosis), purpura fulminans, small bowel infarction, and hepatic veno-occlusive disease (associated with fibrin and factor VIII in the walls of the hepatic central venules) became recognized complications of high-dose therapy.[35-42]

Taken in aggregate, these observations strongly suggested that cytotoxic and cytokine therapy both acutely activate coagulation and cause long-term prothrombotic changes in the hemostatic system. Both of these events could predispose cancer patients, particularly those undergoing hematopoietic stem cell transplantation (HSCT), to all of the adverse consequences of a "procoagulant state." As will be shown later, these consequences potentially included not only macrovascular thrombus formation but a variety of other problems not classically associated with overt vascular occlusive thrombi. The mechanism and the precise outcome of this procoagulant state, however, were not clear and are the subject of active investigation.

HEMOSTATIC CHANGES DURING TRANSPLANTATION

In an attempt to understand the mechanism of the procoagulant state, many investigators measured levels of procoagulant and anticoagulant proteins during marrow transplantation. The best documented of these changes are shown in Figure 41–1. In general, global screening studies, such as prothrombin time and partial thromboplastin time, do not change during transplantation. Factor II, total and free protein S, and plasminogen activator inhibitor levels show no predictable changes during transplantation.[43] Fibrinogen, factor V, and factor VIII levels increase moderately after beginning the preparative regimen.[43, 44] Levels of protein C, antithrombin III, and factors VII, IX, X, and XII all drop during transplantation.[43-48] Albumin levels also drop during transplantation, and the fall in albumin correlates strongly with the fall in factor VII, protein C, and antithrombin III levels.[43, 44, 48] Generally, the levels of the proteins reach a nadir approximately 2 weeks after the preparative regimen is begun, at which time they gradually begin to return toward normal. Some of the changes, however, may last for a protracted period of time, particularly the changes in protein C.[49]

The mechanism of the drop in these various coagulation-related parameters is not precisely known. The association of the drop in albumin with the drop in factor VII, protein

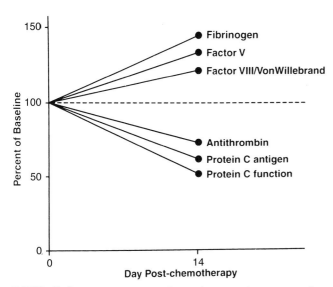

FIGURE 41–1. Changes in procoagulant and anticoagulant proteins after beginning the preparative regimen during hematopoietic stem cell transplantation.

C, and antithrombin III levels suggests a component of impaired hepatic synthesis and/or extravascular redistribution due to an increase in vascular permeability. Another possibility is the "consumption" of these proteins, either by their conversion to active enzymes with subsequent removal from the intravascular space (in the cases of the hemostatically active proenzymes, such as factors XII, X, IX, and VII and protein C) or by their complexing with activated enzymes and subsequent removal from the plasma (such as antithrombin III).

Some of the proenzymes whose levels drop during transplantation require vitamin K for production of a fully functional protein, such as protein C and factors VII, IX, and X. In the absence of vitamin K, dysfunctional molecules are produced. This is precisely what occurs in the case of protein C, a proenzyme whose functional anticoagulant activity drops further than its antigenic level during transplantation.[43] This observation, plus the observation that vitamin K levels drop precipitously during transplantation, lent credence to the hypothesis that evolving vitamin K deficiency during transplantation (caused by impaired oral intake and impaired intestinal absorption due to mucositis and broad-spectrum antibiotic use impairing production of vitamin K by the intestinal flora) might play a role in the deficiency of these proteins.[50] This hypothesis was tested by giving patients daily vitamin K (5 mg) or weekly vitamin K (10 mg) in their parenteral nutrition formula and monitoring the protein C antigen and anticoagulant activities.[51] Patients receiving daily vitamin K had almost the same degree of drop in protein C as the patients who received weekly vitamin K, but the specific activity of their protein C was significantly higher. Thus, it is felt that vitamin K deficiency plays a small but definite role in the changes in some of the hemostatic parameters during transplantation. Consequently, daily supplementation of vitamin K (in doses of approximately 5 mg of vitamin K1) after the preparative regimen is begun and continuing until the patient is able to consume an adequate oral diet has been recommended.

Vitamin K deficiency is not the entire explanation for the

hemostatic changes in HSCT. Daily vitamin K supplementation does not entirely prevent the fall of protein C, and aggressive vitamin K replacement does not substantially improve its activity once deficiency has been established.[50] Vitamin K is also not required for the production of antithrombin III, another protein whose levels drop during transplantation. Obviously, other explanations are required. Unfortunately, studies meant to determine the rate of synthesis of the various hemostatic proteins have not been done, making this part of the equation an unknown. Studies looking at the rate of loss of at least antithrombin III from the intravascular space during transplantation have been done, however. Increasing requirements for supplemental antithrombin III concentrate to keep the plasma level above 90% activity along with high levels of thrombin/antithrombin III complexes have been reported in transplant recipients given GM-CSF.[52] A more formal analysis of the pharmacokinetics of antithrombin III concentrate in hematopoietic stem cell transplantation has shown that although the immediate recovery of infused antithrombin is normal and remains constant during transplantation, the half-life drops progressively after beginning the preparative regimen, reaching a nadir roughly 2 weeks later (Table 41–1).[53]

These reports confirm that the rate of removal of antithrombin from the intravascular space is increased during transplantation, but the mechanism for this remains unclear. The increased levels of thrombin/antithrombin III complexes suggest that the inactivation of thrombin (and possibly other serine proteases) is at least part of the cause of the rapid loss of antithrombin from the circulation. The possibility of extravascular redistribution also remains a viable explanation, however. Antithrombin III has a molecular weight of approximately 45 daltons (similar to that of albumin), making "leakage" from the vascular space possible if there was an increase in vascular permeability—a common occurrence during transplantation.

Changes in vascular permeability during transplantation may also indirectly involve the coagulation system. Factor XII, when activated, can activate the complement system via the classic pathway by activating the first component of the complement system, C1.[54] Both activated factor XII

TABLE 41–1. RECOVERY AND HALF-DISAPPEARANCE TIMES OF ANTITHROMBIN III CONCENTRATE (37.5 U/KG) INFUSED PRIOR TO AND WEEKLY AFTER BEGINNING THE PREPARATIVE REGIMEN IN 11 PATIENTS WITH NON-HODGKIN LYMPHOMA UNDERGOING HEMATOPOIETIC STEM CELL TRANSPLANTATION

	RECOVERY (%/UNIT-KG)	50% DISAPPEARANCE TIME (hr)
0	2.2 + 0.1	19.0 + 1.8
7	1.9 + 0.1	21.8 + 2.7
14	1.8 + 0.1	12.2 + 1.8*†
21	2.1 + 0.3	15.5 + 2.5*

*$P < .05$ compared with day 0.
†$P < .05$ compared with day 7.
From Haire WD, Stevens LC, Kotulak GD, et al: Pharmacokinetics of antithrombin concentrate during autologous hematopoietic stem cell transplantation. Bone Marrow Transplant 15:505, 1995.

and activated C1 interact with and are inhibited by C1-esterase inhibitor. Interestingly, during bone marrow transplantation, the complement system is activated and C1-esterase inhibitor levels fall.[55] These changes in the complement system are associated with an increase in vascular permeability, resulting in the "vascular leak syndrome" (generalized edema, pleural/pericardial effusions, weight gain, tachycardia, prerenal azotemia). The mechanism of activation of the complement system is unknown, but may be partly the result of the activation of factor XII (with resultant fall in factor XII levels, as previously mentioned). Activated factor XII can also activate prekallikrein, which subsequently can cleave high-molecular-weight kininogen to yield bradykinin.[56] Bradykinin has diverse biologic effects, one of which is increasing vascular permeability.[57]

Thus, the activation of coagulation can set into motion a series of events that promotes an increase in vascular permeability, which in turn can lower the levels of antithrombin III, allowing continued activation of coagulation to proceed relatively unopposed, ultimately creating a vicious circle that may be difficult for the organism to control. Just how difficult this whole process is to control is illustrated by the fact that the vascular leak syndrome is a component of the syndrome of hepatic veno-occlusive disease—a disorder associated with a high incidence of multiple organ dysfunction and death.[58–60]

Activation of the coagulation cascade potentially has biologic consequences far beyond formation of a fibrin-based thrombus. The serine protease thrombin has a variety of direct and indirect effects on vascular endothelial cells throughout the body, effects generally detrimental to their function. Thrombin stimulates these cells to release plasminogen activator inhibitor, an inhibitor of fibrinolysis found in high concentrations in patients with liver dysfunction, during transplantation.[61, 62] Thrombin also induces expression of P-selectin, an adhesion molecule that facilitates polymorphonuclear leukocyte adhesion to endothelial cells and their subsequent degranulation.[63, 64] Neutrophil degranulation releases elastase and proteinase 3, serine proteases that can mediate endothelial cell death by apoptosis.[65] Apoptotic endothelial cells become procoagulant, causing further activation of coagulation in a potentially self-propagating manner.[66] As mentioned earlier, activation of factor XII can indirectly generate bradykinin and activate the complement cascade, systems that not only affect the vascular endothelial cell but are involved in the generation of many of the observed cellular and physiologic effects of inflammation.[57] The importance of these aspects of the coagulation system will become evident later in the chapter.

In addition to the changes in hemostatic proenzymes and their inhibitors, platelet counts routinely drop after administration of the preparative regimen. In most patients, this is thought to be due to simple impairment of platelet production due to marrow damage from the preparative regimen. In some patients, however, this is not necessarily the sole problem. A minority of patients experience thrombocytopenia that is not corrected with platelet transfusion—"platelet refractoriness." Although alloimmune mechanisms for this phenomenon are occasionally found, more often they are absent and the patient does not respond to standard therapy empirically directed at an allo-

immune process. In these patients, platelet "consumption" in an ongoing activation of the coagulation system—in the vascular space or at the level of the vascular endothelial cell—may explain the limited response to platelet transfusion. This is currently a hypothetical explanation, but there is circumstantial evidence to support it. As will be discussed, patients receiving large numbers of platelet transfusions are more likely to experience a variety of organ dysfunction and have lower levels of protein C and antithrombin III, levels that may be low due to consumption.

Significance of the Hemostatic Changes During Transplantation

Although the changes in the hemostatic system can be readily used to explain the thrombotic complications of transplantation, such as subclavian vein thrombosis or nonbacterial thrombotic endocarditis, these changes have more far-reaching implications in the pathogenesis of other transplant-related complications—complications not thought to be due to vascular occlusive thrombi. To understand the actual and potential significance of these hemostatic changes during hematopoietic stem cell transplantation, one has to become familiar with the current concepts of systemic inflammation and its contribution to various complications of severe illness. This understanding is important because the inflammatory system interacts significantly with the hemostatic system and is probably involved in the pathogenesis of many transplant-related complications. This chapter is not intended to be an exhaustive review of these concepts, but a short synopsis of them will be helpful.

The human body's response to a variety of noxious stimuli is to generate what has been known generically as "inflammation." The noxious stimuli that can induce this response are as diverse as infection (e.g., bacterial, fungal, viral), trauma, burns, and pancreatitis.[67] The "inflammatory reaction" induced by these stimuli is mediated by a complex, and poorly understood, interplay of cytokines, hemostatic factors, the complement cascade, lymphocytes, phagocytes, vascular endothelial cells, and probably other elements not currently recognized.[68] This inflammatory reaction has been formally dubbed the systemic inflammatory response syndrome (SIRS) and is defined as the presence of two or more of the following:

Temperature $> 38°$ or $< 36°C$
Heart rate > 90
Respiratory rate > 20
Granulocytosis ($> 12.0 \times 10^9/L$) or granulocytopenia ($< 4.0 \times 10^9/L$) or the presence of $> 10\%$ band forms[67]

If SIRS is due to the presence of an infection (not necessarily bacteremic infection), the process is called sepsis. It is assumed that SIRS begins as a beneficial reaction whose goal is to eliminate the noxious stimulus that generated it. In the majority of patients, this is probably true. In a minority of patients, however, the mediators of SIRS get "out of control" and begin to mediate reactions throughout the body that are harmful to the function of many organs. Again, the precise mechanism for the generation of these harmful reactions is poorly understood but often involves changes in vascular endothelial cells of organs throughout the body. When the mediators of SIRS begin to impair the function of various organs to the point that the impairment can be detected clinically, the patient has entered the multiple organ dysfunction syndrome (MODS). Adult respiratory distress syndrome, acute tubular necrosis, "shock liver," and other conditions are thought to be manifestations of MODS in a variety of settings. MODS affects up to 40% of critically ill patients and is the leading cause of mortality in intensive care units. The salient points to remember as we begin to discuss hematopoietic stem cell transplantation are as follows:

The noxious stimuli that can induce SIRS are diverse and are not limited to infection (they may well include components of the preparative regimen).

SIRS is a systemic process whose effects are not limited to one organ but affect all organs (probably via damage to the vascular endothelium).

MODS evolving from SIRS can involve virtually any organ, and when it does so the cause is not an abnormality limited to that specific organ but a generalized problem involving other organs to some extent. The corollary is that diagnostic evaluation of and treatment directed only at that specific organ are doomed to failure because the basic problem is systemic.

SIRS and resultant MODS involve changes in the hemostatic system. As mentioned earlier, one of the inciting causes of SIRS and MODS is infection. Consequently, an understanding of the hemostatic changes occurring in these syndromes can be gained by evaluating animal models and human examples of sepsis.

Changes in the hemostatic system in SIRS and MODS have been the subject of several reviews.[69–74] This complex and incompletely understood interplay between coagulation and inflammation is summarized in Figure 41–2. Human sepsis involves activation of coagulation with subsequent generation of soluble fibrin.[75] Additionally, low levels of antithrombin III and protein C are found.[75–85] Similar changes occur after surgical or accidental trauma uncomplicated by infection.[76, 79, 81, 86–88] The degree of abnormality of the hemostatic parameters, particularly of antithrombin III and protein C, correlate well with outcome—lower levels correlating with worse prognosis in patients with infection or trauma-related SIRS.[76, 79, 81, 82, 84, 86–88] Animal and human studies also show activation of the complement system with low levels of total hemolytic complement and C1-esterase inhibitor.[77, 89] Additionally, platelet sequestration in the microvasculature occurs in patients with sepsis and predicts a poor outcome.[90] Thus, in the nontransplantation setting, SIRS is associated with hemostatic changes similar to those occurring during hematopoietic stem cell trans-

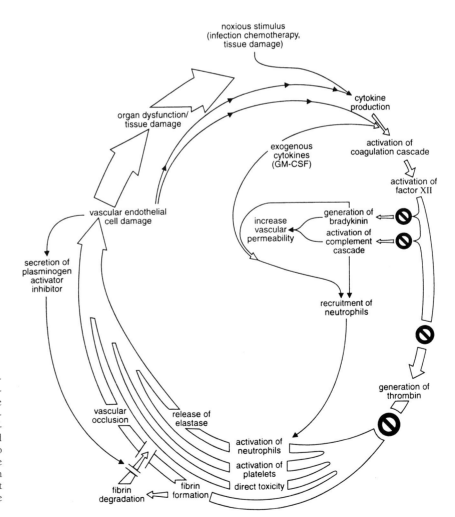

FIGURE 41–2. Diagram of the inter-relationships of the coagulation and inflammatory systems. The noxious stimuli that initially activate the systems can set up a positive feedback system, or "vicious circle," which can lead to self-propagating tissue injury that does not need continued exposure to the original stimulus to maintain itself. The "stop" signs illustrate the areas where antithrombin III concentrate in pharmacologic doses could potentially interrupt this cycle. GM-CSF, granulocyte macrophage colony-stimulating factor.

plantation. In patients not undergoing transplantation, changes in the hemostatic parameters correlate with outcome, suggesting at least a predictive value for these studies and possibly suggesting a role for the hemostatic system in the pathogenesis of SIRS and MODS.

The reason for discussing the concept of SIRS and MODS in non–transplant recipients is that the conceptual framework of SIRS and MODS is valid in hematopoietic stem cell transplant recipients as well. Importantly, when these concepts are applied clinically to transplant recipients, the hemostatic changes of SIRS have therapeutic implications. SIRS is a universal occurrence during transplantation. It is generally detectable within the first few days of the preparative regimen.[60, 91] Organ dysfunction (CNS, pulmonary, or hepatic) develops approximately 2 weeks later, followed by bacteremia a week or so after that. Patients who ultimately experience dysfunction of one or more organs have had more manifestations of SIRS for longer periods of time than those who do not experience organ dysfunction. Thus, in transplant recipients, the preparative regimen is a universal stimulus of SIRS, organ dysfunction from all causes is preceded by stronger manifestations of SIRS (raising the possibility of an etiologic relationship), and bacteremia is not required for the development of either SIRS or organ dysfunction.

Organ dysfunction in HSCT has been given names, such as hepatic veno-occlusive disease or interstitial pneumonitis, that imply that their etiology is understood or that they are unique to transplant recipients. That this is not correct is being increasingly recognized by the coining of new names for these entities such as "the syndrome of hepatic veno-occlusive disease after marrow transplantation" and "idiopathic pneumonia syndrome."[59, 92] Although it is tempting to go with the latter name, there is a dearth of data comparing the complications of transplantation to those encountered in other groups of critically ill patients, making it an unproved hypothesis open to testing.

Investigators have been impressed with the similarity between what happens to marrow transplant recipients after being given their preparative regimens and what happens to patients after major trauma, serious infection, or obstetric catastrophes. They all tend to get progressively ill a few days after they are medically stabilized from their acute injury. Despite aggressive efforts, an etiology to account for their deterioration is generally not found and they too often get progressively worse, dying with hypoten-

sion, on vasopressive agents, obtunded, on a ventilator, and after a period of anuria and dialysis. Postmortem examination is generally dissatisfying, with the pathologist being unable to identify a cause for these patients' progressive organ failure and death—often with evidence that the original pathology (e.g., cancer, infection) was improving.

As an outgrowth of these clinical observations, a hypothesis was developed that the complications of marrow transplantation were similar in pathogenesis to those in other populations of critically ill patients. With a growing body of information suggesting a potential role for the hemostatic system in the genesis of complications in these other populations, studies were organized to correlate changes in hemostasis with complications of transplantation and to define the relationship between the various complications.[60] The clinical course of 199 patients admitted for hematopoietic stem cell transplantation was closely followed. Protein C and antithrombin III levels were performed prior to beginning the preparative regimen and weekly thereafter until hospital dismissal. Patients were monitored for the development of serious complications of transplantation. Because of the limited accuracy of premortem diagnostic procedures in determining an etiology of most complications, however, we defined the complications in generic, organ-specific terms rather than classic diagnostic entities. *Pulmonary dysfunction* was the term used for patients needing supplemental oxygen (generally because of documented hypoxia) independent of the clinical diagnosis. *Central nervous system (CNS) dysfunction* was the term given lethargic or disoriented patients, again independent of any clinical diagnosis. Hepatic dysfunction was defined using the standard criteria for the syndrome of hepatic veno-occlusive disease (VOD). Renal dysfunction was defined as changes from baseline creatinine and urea levels.

Of the 199 patients entering the study, 14 died. Two died of progressive malignancy during transplantation, one died of CNS aspergillosis, and one died of idiopathic sudden death on day 3 of the preparative regimen. The other 10 died of unexplained progressive multiple organ dysfunction. Of these 10, 6 underwent postmortem examination. In none of these 6 could a cause for the progressive multiple organ dysfunction be found. This observation supported the hypothesis that most deaths, and by inference, many of the nonfatal complications during transplantation do not have an etiology definable by current techniques and may be part of MODS.

TABLE 41–2. COX PROPORTIONAL HAZARDS MODEL EVALUATING THE LIKELIHOOD OF SUBSEQUENT COMPLICATIONS IN PATIENTS PRESENTING WITH PULMONARY OR CENTRAL NERVOUS SYSTEM (CNS) DYSFUNCTION RELATIVE TO THOSE WITHOUT PULMONARY OR CNS DYSFUNCTION*

| | PRESENTING DYSFUNCTION | | | |
| | Pulmonary | | CNS | |
COMPLICATION	P	RR (95% CI)	P	RR (95% CI)
Any subsequent organ dysfunction	.02	2.2 (1.1–4.39)	.03	2.2 (1.06–4.53)
Subsequent hepatic VOD	.02	3.7 (1.29–10.55)	.002	5.0 (1.79–14.19)
Subsequent CNS dysfunction	<.001	4.9 (2.83–8.33)	. . .	. . .
Subsequent pulmonary dysfunction	. . .	. . .	<.001	3.7 (2.22–6.30)
Death	.006	18.4 (2.30–147.41)	.03	4.9 (1.22–19.53)

*RR indicates relative risk, which is the hazard ratio determined by the Cox analysis; CI, confidence interval; VOD, veno-occlusive disease; ellipses, no data available.
From Haire WD et al: Multiple organ dysfunction syndrome in bone marrow transplantation. JAMA 274:1289, 1995.

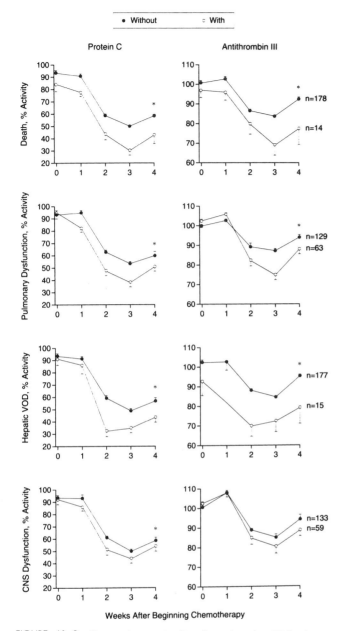

FIGURE 41-3. Changes in protein C and antithrombin III levels in patients with and without organ dysfunction and death during hematopoietic stem cell transplantation. Differences are measured with repeated measures analysis of variance. The asterisk indicates significance at P = .05. (From Haire WD et al: Multiple organ dysfunction syndrome in bone marrow transplantation. JAMA 274:1289, 1995.)

Of the 199 patients, 93 experienced organ dysfunction during transplantation. Ultimately, pulmonary dysfunction occurred in 63 patients, CNS dysfunction in 59, hepatic dysfunction in 15, and renal dysfunction in 39. The significance of organ dysfunction is summarized in Table 41-2. Patients presenting with either pulmonary or CNS dysfunction were up to five times more likely to subsequently experience other organ dysfunction and as much as 18 times more likely to die than patients without pulmonary or CNS dysfunction. This mirrors the experience in patients with the syndrome of VOD—patients with single organ dysfunction (be it pulmonary, CNS, or hepatic) have

a high likelihood of subsequent organ dysfunction and death.[58, 59] Changes in several hemostatic parameters correlated with single-organ dysfunction and death. Protein C and antithrombin III levels were lower or dropped further in patients with pulmonary, CNS, and hepatic dysfunction and those who died compared with those without organ dysfunction (Fig. 41-3). Patients with organ dysfunction also had a significantly greater number of platelet transfusions than those without (Fig. 41-4; Table 41-3), possibly related to "consumption" in a generalized or localized activation of coagulation.[93] Levels of protein C and antithrombin III early in the transplant course were associated with a greater likelihood of pulmonary or CNS dysfunction later in the transplant period (Table 41-4). Indeed, patients whose antithrombin III level was less than 84% of normal at the time of development of any type of organ dysfunction had a 71% likelihood of going on to multiple-organ dysfunction compared with a 31% likelihood in patients whose antithrombin III level was greater than that.

Although protein C levels did not have quite this strong a predictive value, other investigators have found that protein C levels of less than 88% of normal prior to beginning the preparative regimen are associated with a 91% likelihood of hepatic dysfunction during the transplant period.[94] There were differences in organ dysfunction rates that depended on the preparative regimen, the type of transplantation (allogeneic, autologous bone marrow, and autologous peripheral stem cell), and whether or not there was a positive blood culture, but levels of protein C and/or antithrombin III were the only consistent independent predictors of pulmonary and CNS dysfunction (Table 41-5). Despite many efforts to do so, we were unable to find any

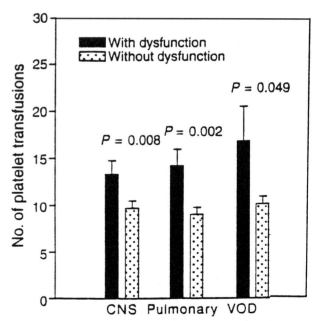

FIGURE 41-4. Mean number of platelet weekly transfusions after beginning the preparative regimen in 199 patients undergoing hematopoietic stem cell transplantation who did or did not experience central nervous system (CNS), pulmonary, or hepatic (veno-occlusive disease [VOD]) dysfunction. (From Gordon B et al: Increased platelet transfusion requirement is associated with multiple organ dysfunctions in patients undergoing hematopoietic stem cell transplantation. Bone Marrow Transplant 22:999, 1998.)

consistent association between antithrombin III or protein C levels and renal dysfunction, though these patients showed significantly greater utilization of platelets than patients without renal dysfunction (see Fig. 41–3).

These data, along with those from other institutions, show that single-organ dysfunction during hematopoietic stem cell transplantation—whether it is first recognized as hepatic, pulmonary, or CNS dysfunction—has similar correlates (low levels of antithrombin III and protein C with a higher rate of platelet transfusion) and similar outcomes (a high likelihood of progression to multiple-organ dysfunction and death).[59, 95] This suggests, with the possible exception of renal dysfunction, that the organ dysfunction during transplantation does not represent a process confined to a specific organ but does have a common systemic etiology. The correlation of organ dysfunction with the clinical manifestations of SIRS, the changes in protein C and antithrombin III, and the consumption of transfused platelets and the sequential failure of other vital organs leading to death are all sufficiently reminiscent of MODS in the nontransplant setting to warrant consideration of the hypothesis that they are similar, if not identical, syndromes. Changes in hemostatic parameters are at least strong markers of this systemic syndrome and may be involved in its pathogenesis. The conspicuous lack of correlation of renal dysfunction to other systemic abnormalities suggests that there may be other, possibly additive, mechanisms of renal damage in this setting. A similar concept has been proposed by other investigators, noting a lack of correlation between urinary markers of renal tubular damage and renal dysfunction in patients with the syndrome of hepatic VOD and, by inference, other organ dysfunction.[96]

Another observation made in the transplant population deserves elaboration. As has been previously mentioned, use of CSF has been associated with thrombotic complications in nontransplant settings.[19–24] This suggests that these

TABLE 41–3. MEAN AND ZENITH NUMBER OF WEEKLY PLATELET TRANSFUSIONS DURING PREPARATIVE REGIMEN IN 199 PATIENTS UNDERGOING HSCT WHO DID OR DID NOT EXPERIENCE ORGAN DYSFUNCTION OR DIE DURING TRANSPLANT-RELATED HOSPITALIZATION

		WEEKLY PLATELET TRANSFUSIONS	
		Mean	**Zenith**
CNS dysfunction	Yes	13.3 ± 1.5	21.6 ± 2.6
	No	9.6 ± 0.9	14.6 ± 1.6
	P	.008	.004
Pulmonary dysfunction	Yes	14.2 ± 1.8	24.0 ± 3.4
	No	9.0 ± 0.7	13.2 ± 1.1
	P	.002	.002
Hepatic dysfunction	Yes	17.8 ± 4.4	28.5 ± 7.6
	No	10.5 ± 0.8	16.4 ± 1.4
	P	.049	.042
Death	Yes	14.2 ± 2.9	23.6 ± 5.4
	No	10.4 ± 0.8	16.2 ± 1.4
	P	.056	.038

From Gordon B, et al: Increased platelet transfusion requirement is associated with multiple organ dysfunctions in patients undergoing hematopoietic stem cell transplantation. Bone Marrow Transplant 22:999, 1998.

TABLE 41–4. RISK OF ORGAN DYSFUNCTION DURING TRANSPLANT DAYS 15–28 OF PATIENTS WITH ANTITHROMBIN III (ATIII) LEVELS <80% OR PROTEIN C (PC) LEVELS <60% DURING TRANSPLANTATION RELATIVE TO DAYS 0–14 IN PATIENTS WHOSE LEVELS WERE HIGHER DURING THAT TIME

ANTICOAGULANT LEVELS DURING TRANSPLANTATION DAYS 0–14		ORGAN DYSFUNCTION DURING TRANSPLANTATION DAYS 15–28	
		Pulmonary	**CNS**
ATIII <80%	RR	3.4	1.8
	(95% CI)	(1.38–8.50)	(0.70–4.53)
	P	.005	.22
PC <60%	RR	3.8	2.7
	(95% CI)	(1.72–8.28)	(1.24–6.00)
	P	<.001	.01

CNS, central nervous system; RR, relative risk; CI, confidence interval.
From Haire WD, et al: Multiple organ dysfunction syndrome in bone marrow transplantation. JAMA 274:1289, 1995.

molecules, either alone or in combination with chemotherapy (or other events that occur during cancer therapy, such as infection), either predispose to activation of the hemostatic system or prevent the physiologic limitation of the consequences of activation of the hemostatic system by other stimuli (or both). As mentioned previously, there is evidence that GM-CSF activates coagulation in a dose-related manner.[32, 33] With G-CSF pretreatment, the clinical and biochemical response to endotoxemia is grossly exaggerated in humans and experimental animals, suggesting that these molecules can, in fact, potentiate the inflammatory reaction to certain stimuli.[97, 98] When GM-CSF is given after transplantation, it predisposes to the capillary leak syndrome with weight gain (one of the clinical manifestations of the syndrome of hepatic VOD) and hypoalbuminemia (a correlate of protein C and antithrombin III deficiency).[99] When given after peripheral blood stem cell transplantation, it predisposes to protein C and antithrombin III deficiency.[34]

The significance of these diverse observations is not completely clear, but together they suggest that some of the CSF may contribute to the development of clinically significant organ dysfunction by potentiating the clinical effects of the mediators of SIRS when given to transplant recipients. This contention is supported by the observation that when given to allogeneic transplant recipients (known to be predisposed to frequent inflammatory stimuli) in a double-blind trial, GM-CSF was associated with a disturbing trend to higher mortality despite earlier phagocyte recovery.[100]

Having developed the concept that hemostatic changes, not classically thought to be related to coagulation or thrombosis, are part of the inflammatory process that contributes to the complications of hematopoietic stem cell therapy (HSCT), let us consider the syndrome of thrombotic microangiopathy (TM). This syndrome is postulated to have thrombosis as a fundamental part of its pathogenesis. As with many of the complications of HSCT, transplant-related TM has many parallels with non–transplant-related

TABLE 41-5. LOGISTIC REGRESSION MODELING OF INDEPENDENT ASSOCIATIONS BETWEEN PULMONARY AND CENTRAL NERVOUS SYSTEM (CNS) DYSFUNCTION DURING TRANSPLANTATION

| | TRANSPLANT DAYS | | | | | |
| | 7–13 | | 14–20 | | 21–28 | |
DYSFUNCTION	RR	*P*	RR	*P*	RR	*P*
Pulmonary						
ATIII < 70%	. . .	.10	2.9	.01	3.2	.04
PC < 50%	5.7	.003	4.6	<.001	3.5	.006
CNS						
ATIII < 70%	3.1	.055	2.4	.053	6.0	.007
Treatment 4	0.1	.058	. . .	.26	. . .	.40
Treatment 6	.04	.01	. . .	.59	. . .	.19
Positive blood culture	8.4	.001	. . .	.82	. . .	.90
Autologous transplant	. . .	.87	0.21	.01	. . .	.66

RR, relative risk; ellipses, not computed.
From Haire WD, et al: Multiple organ dysfunction syndrome in bone marrow transplantation. JAMA 274:1289, 1995.

syndromes. In the non-transplant population, TM represents a spectrum encompassing thrombotic thrombocytopenic purpura (TTP) to the hemolytic-uremic syndrome (HUS). Clinically, these are overlapping syndromes with similar pathogenesis, differing mainly in the degree of systemic involvement. Both syndromes are thought to be due to consequences of vascular endothelial cell damage, either due to or as the result of intravascular hyaline thrombi.

The process is clinically confined to the renal vasculature in HUS, whereas the process is systemic in TTP, involving potentially all organ systems. The diagnostic hallmark of non-transplant TM is the presence of microangiopathic hemolysis (caused by the physical breakage of red blood cells as they are sheared across the intravascular thrombi) and thrombocytopenia (caused by the consumption of platelets in the generation of the thrombi) accompanied by organ dysfunction. In these patients, enteric infections with a variety of organisms, most notably *Escherichia coli* serotype O157:H7, is increasingly recognized as an inciting factor. The pathogenesis of non–transplant-related TM is thought to be the presence of intravascular platelet-aggregating factor that causes intravascular platelet activation with subsequent formation of hyaline thrombi and vascular endothelial cell damage, ultimately progressing to organ dysfunction. Von Willebrand factor of unusually large multimeric structure is one of the most promising candidates for this intravascular platelet-aggregating factor.

As mentioned previously, HSCT is often complicated by multiple-organ dysfunction. This occasionally coexists with a greater or lesser amount of evidence for microangiopathic hemolysis (generally, varying degrees of schistocytosis) and increased platelet transfusion. In a small number of biopsies, these changes have also been found to coexist with glomerular capillary thrombi.[101] Because of these similarities with non–transplant-related TM syndromes, transplant recipients with organ dysfunction, schistocytosis, and increasing platelet transfusion utilization are thought to have a thrombotic microangiopathy syndrome similar to non–transplant-related TTP or HUS. This inference has allowed practitioners to postulate that the two syndromes have a similar pathogenesis and would respond well to the same types of treatment. Transplant-related TM, however, has characteristics not shared with non–transplant-related TM.

Transplant-related TM was originally described in patients undergoing allogeneic transplantation using cyclosporin as graft-vs.-host disease (GVHD) prophylaxis.[101, 102] The importance of cyclosporin was highlighted in a report of allogeneic marrow transplant recipients treated with cyclosporin or methotrexate as GVHD prophylaxis.[103] Though the diagnostic criteria were liberally defined, 49 of 66 cyclosporin-treated patients had TM, compared with none of the 11 methotrexate-treated patients. In these patients, von Willebrand factor antigen levels rose in relation to the evolution and severity of the TM. Although cyclosporin is generally accepted as a contributor to transplant-related TM, it is not a requirement for the development of this syndrome. There are many reports of TM complicating autologous transplantation or allogeneic transplantation without cyclosporin use.[35, 104, 105] Increasingly, the use of tacrolimus (FK-506) as an immunomodulatory agent to prevent or treat GVHD has been associated with transplant-related TM.

The relative roles of the components of the preparative regimen, the use of immunomodulating agents, and other unknown factors (e.g., infection, SIRS) in the genesis of transplant-related TM are unknown. Chemotherapy and radiation are directly toxic to vascular endothelial cells, as is cyclosporin.[106–108] Cyclosporin enhances thromboxane A2 release from platelets and inhibits prostacyclin production by vascular endothelial cells—both stimuli being potentially prothrombotic.[109] In experimental situations, cyclosporin increases vascular endothelial cell permeability.[110] The milieu of allogeneic HSCT, with its use of immunomodulating agents such as cyclosporin and FK506, is almost universally associated with a mild degree of microangiopathic hemolysis (<5% of red blood cells).[111] At autopsy, 54% of allogeneic transplant recipients are found to have vascular thromboses.[112] The clinical significance of this is unknown, but it suggests that vascular endothelial cell damage with resultant red blood cell trauma is a common occurrence that can progress to vascular occlusion in severely ill patients.

The chemotherapy and radiation of the preparative regimens and the use of potentially toxic immunomodulating agents are not part of the pathogenesis of non–transplant-related TM, suggesting that the similarities between the transplant- and non–transplant-related TM syndromes may be more apparent than real. Zeigler et al. reported a study of plasma von Willebrand antigen and thrombomodulin levels comparing TTP/HUS patients and patients with TM associated with transplant.[113] Results were divergent in the two groups and suggested a stronger role for endothelial damage in TM associated with transplant. As will be discussed later, the hypothesis that TTP/HUS and TM differ in pathogenesis is supported by the observation that transplant-related TM does not respond to treatment like its spontaneously appearing counterpart. Indeed, the notion that they are different syndromes is so strong that at least one cooperative group study of TTP therapy specifically excluded transplant-related TM from enrollment.

The vascular endothelial cell damage that appears to be part of transplant-related TM may be one part of the spectrum of MODS induced by the preparative regimen, immunomodulating agents (or the GVHD they are meant to control), and intercurrent infections. More research on the pathogenesis of transplant-related TM, concentrating on transplant-specific variables and their relationship to MODS and other coexistent causes of vascular endothelial cell damage, is warranted.

THERAPEUTIC IMPLICATIONS

If the hypothesis that MODS in transplant and nontransplant settings is the same disorder incited by different stimuli, it would be expected that they respond in the same way to therapeutic intervention. Because MODS is routinely associated with alterations in the hemostatic system, one could postulate that changes in the hemostatic system would result in alteration of the clinical manifestations of MODS. This approach has been taken in a variety of animal models of MODS using sepsis or trauma as the inciting stimuli. Changing the hemostatic system to enhance activation of hemostasis worsens the response to infection.[114] Limiting the activity of the coagulation system with naturally occurring inhibitors such as antithrombin III, protein C, and thrombomodulin improves the clinical and biochemical response to infection.[115–119] Similar outcomes can be obtained with pharmacologic limitation of the activity of the coagulation system by heparin or by enhancing the activity of the fibrinolytic system with tissue plasminogen activator.[120–122] The beneficial effects of these interventions may not be due entirely to their ability to inhibit the activity of thrombin. In models in which these interventions are helpful, use of specific thrombin inhibitors does not have

significant activity.[123] This suggests that alterations at other levels of the coagulation system, perhaps at levels at which the coagulation enzymes act on the complement cascade, the kinin-generating proteins and other effector arms of the inflammatory system may be important.

Similar interventions have been used in the treatment of human MODS in the nontransplant setting. Antithrombin III concentrate has been shown to result in a trend to lower mortality in patients with sepsis.[124] In multisystem trauma patients, the use of antithrombin III concentrates results in lower levels of proinflammatory cytokines and fewer days on the ventilator and in the intensive care unit.[125] In patients undergoing marrow transplantation, limiting hemostatic activity with heparin (either unfractionated or low-molecular-weight) has been found to be potentially effective in preventing hepatic dysfunction manifesting as the syndrome of VOD.[126–128] Enhancing the activity of the fibrinolytic system with tissue plasminogen activator has been successfully used to treat established hepatic VOD.[129, 130] Combining tissue plasminogen activator with antithrombin III concentrate has also been anecdotally successful in treating hepatic VOD, as has use of antithrombin III concentrate alone.[131, 132]

If the syndrome of hepatic VOD is, as suggested previously, one manifestation of the spectrum of MODS, it is possible that these therapeutic alterations in the hemostatic system can favorably modify the clinical course of other manifestations of SIRS and MODS in hematopoietic stem cell transplantation. The problem with all of these interventions is that they have not been rigorously tested in double-blind studies, they have not been tested for outcomes other than hepatic VOD, and they have potential bleeding complications or (generally) all three. An ideal therapy would address these issues.

A prospective, randomized, double-blind trial of antithrombin III concentrate in the treatment of MODS in hematopoietic stem cell transplantation was reported in 1998.[133] In this trial, 186 patients entering the hospital for transplantation were followed daily for organ dysfunction (CNS, pulmonary, or hepatic) associated with antithrombin deficiency (Table 41–6). If a patient was found to have one of these dysfunctions, the likelihood of early MODS was estimated via an antithrombin III assay. If the concomitant antithrombin III activity was less than 84% of normal, the patient was considered to have a high likelihood of being in early MODS. At that point the patient was randomly assigned to aggressive antithrombin III replacement or albumin placebo (Table 41–7).

After randomization, the patients' clinical outcomes were

TABLE 41–6. DEFINITIONS OF ORGAN DYSFUNCTION USED FOR INITIATION OF ANTITHROMBIN III REPLACEMENT THERAPY

Central nervous system dysfunction	A drop of 4 or more points from baseline in the score of the standardized Mini-Mental Status Examination.[147] This represents slightly more than 2 SD from the mean of the differences in test/retest scores with this tool. This definition has been shown to have a specificity of 100% for diagnosing delirium in subjects with an education level of at least 8th grade.[148]
Pulmonary dysfunction	A finger oximetry reading of S_AO_2 <90% on two occasions on the same day at least 2 hours apart.
Hepatic dysfunction	A combination of bilirubin >2.0 mg/dL, a weight gain of >5% over pre-chemotherapy weight, and abdominal pain of possible hepatic origin.

From Haire WD, et al: A prospective randomized double-blind trial of antithrombin III concentrate in the treatment of multiple-organ dysfunction syndrome during hematopoietic stem cell transplantation. Biol Blood Marrow Transplant 4:142, 1998.

TABLE 41–7. ANTITHROMBIN III TREATMENT PROTOCOL USED IN THERAPY OF EARLY MULTIPLE ORGAN DEFICIENCY SYNDROME

ANTITHROMBIN III CONCENTRATE
70 units/kg within 24 hours of recognition of organ dysfunction
50 units/kg 8, 16, 48, and 72 hours after the initial dose
Total dose: 270 units/kg over 72 hours

From Haire WD, et al: A prospective randomized double-blind trial of antithrombin III concentrate in the treatment of multiple-organ dysfunction syndrome during hematopoietic stem cell transplantation. Biol Blood Marrow Transplant 4:142, 1998.

followed, including an overall severity-of-illness score. This score simply summed the number of organs involved on each day of hospitalization, with the final score being the total for each patient's hospitalization. A total of 54 patients with organ dysfunction were found. Of this group, 24 died compared with no deaths in the group of patients who never were found to fill these definitions of organ dysfunction. This demonstrated the clinical significance of organ dysfunction being treated in this study. As shown in Table 41–8, 49 patients had single-organ dysfunction with a low antithrombin III level and were randomized. The patients who received antithrombin III had a significantly lower severity-of-illness score, spent fewer days in the hospital, and had a strong trend to lower hospital charges ($P = .06$ between control and antithrombin III groups). This was accomplished with a trend to lower mortality ($P = .19$) in the antithrombin III group. No bleeding or other complications were observed.

Although this is the only study of this type of intervention in transplant-related MODS, it was a rigorously performed, high-quality study that could be replicated in any transplant unit. It did not require technology or medication that is not readily available, the therapy employed has never been associated with any significant toxicity (in either animal or human studies), it addressed all clinically significant organ dysfunction syndromes, and it did so in a prospective, double-blind manner. Consequently, it seems reasonable to suggest that the methodology of this study be considered for clinical use. At the very least, transplant recipients should be monitored daily for organ dysfunction using the definitions outlined in Table 41–6.

When organ dysfunction is found, serious consideration

should be given to estimating the patient's likelihood of proceeding to multiple-organ dysfunction and death by quantifying the plasma antithrombin III activity. If the level is much below the 80% range, the patient has a sufficiently high likelihood of adverse outcome that antithrombin III therapy should be strongly considered. Indeed, the question, "Why should the patient not be given antithrombin III supplementation?" might be asked. Such therapy is now standard practice at the University of Nebraska Medical Center using the protocol outlined in Table 41–7. Although it is not known, the likelihood of a response may well decrease with increasing duration and severity of MODS. If this type of therapy is to be used, it seems logical that it be given early in the course of MODS rather than as a "last ditch" attempt to improve the outcome of a patient with several severely dysfunctional organs in whom protracted attempts at standard supportive care have failed.

The therapeutic implications of other alterations of hemostasis are much less clear. The issue of "platelet refractoriness" that coexists with MODS and the hemostatic changes associated with the use of CSF deserve comment. Platelet transfusion recovery in transplant recipients is lower than in other groups of patients with marrow damage.[134, 135] It is even worse in transplant recipients with fever or on antibiotics (including amphotericin)—precisely the subgroup of patients with the greatest likelihood of having or later experiencing MODS.[134, 136] The mechanism for this refractoriness and for the increased use of platelets in transplant recipients with MODS is not known, but it is postulated to be due to widespread vascular endothelial cell damage with resultant consumption of platelets on the endothelial cell surface.[134, 135]

The clinical consequences of this potential interaction are not well understood but may be adverse.[137–140] Intravascular platelet aggregation releases factors that can mediate vascular endothelial cell injury.[137] Vascular endothelial cells acted upon by tumor necrosis factor and/or other cytokines express platelet-binding ligands; when bound to these molecules, platelets mediate changes resulting in endothelial cell death, which can lead to hemorrhagic necrosis of the skin and possibly other organ injury.[138–140] Induction of thrombocytopenia can prevent some of these complications in experimental settings.[140] Consequently, the hypothesis that transfused platelets may mediate some of the manifestations of MODS in transplant recipients is not far-fetched. When

TABLE 41–8. OUTCOMES OF PATIENTS WITH MULTIPLE ORGAN DYSFUNCTION SYNDROME DURING TRANSPLANTATION TREATED WITH ANTITHROMBIN III CONCENTRATE OR ALBUMIN PLACEBO*

	ATIII (n = 24)	PLACEBO (n = 25)	P VALUE
Death	9	14	.19
Duration (days)			
1st Organ dysfunction	3.5 (1.0–63.0)	8 (0–66.0)	.37
2nd Organ dysfunction	5.0 (1.0–56.0)	18.5 (1.0–50.0)	.15
3rd Organ dysfunction	16.0 (1.0–34.0)	28.5 (8.0–51.0)	.24
Severity of illness score	5.5 (1.0–77.0)	21 (3.0–66.0)	.03
Hospital length of stay (days post randomization)	7.5 (1.0–62.0)	2.01 (3.0–66.0)	.03
Hospital charges (thousands of dollars)	96.1 (35.0–46.5)	118.0 (51.0–630.3)	.06

*Results are reported as medians with minimum and maximum values in parentheses.
From Haire WD et al: A prospective randomized double-blind trial of antithrombin III concentrate in the treatment of multiple-organ dysfunction syndrome during hematopoietic stem cell transplantation. Biol Blood Marrow Transplant 4:142, 1998.

patients are experiencing organ dysfunction and an increasingly poor response to transfused platelets, consideration should be given to minimizing (or even withholding) prophylactic platelet transfusions. In these cases, transfusion of one "dose" (8 whole-blood units or 1 apheresis unit) of platelets daily seems a reasonable recommendation. This is more than enough platelets required for maintenance of vascular integrity under physiologic circumstances.[141] Any more than that may not be effective in raising the platelet count above the "standard" 20,000/mm³, may not be more effective at preventing bleeding complications, and may be more toxic. Much more clinical research should be directed at this issue. This group of patients would be a good target for a trial of infusible platelet membranes rather than intact platelets to prevent or treat the hemorrhagic complications of transplantation.[142, 143]

In the generic category of platelet refractoriness, the syndrome of transplant-related thrombotic microangiopathy (TM) should be considered. This syndrome should be considered in patients experiencing an increase in platelet transfusion utilization, especially those allogeneic transplant recipients taking immunomodulating agents known to predispose to vascular endothelial cell damage (e.g., cyclosporin) because they may respond to alteration in the dose or type of therapy. Universally accepted diagnostic criteria for this syndrome do not exist. Grading systems, however, have been devised that can be used for both diagnosis and, more importantly, predicting response to therapy.

The grading system that appears to have the greatest degree of clinical utility has been devised by Zeigler and colleagues.[144] This simple grading system incorporates the percentage of fragmented red blood cells (FC) on peripheral smear and the lactate dehydrogenase (LDH) level. In their report of 33 patients with transplant-related TM, 17 were found to have grade 0–1 disease (<1.3% FC or ≥1.3% FC, a normal LDH level, and no organ dysfunction), 10 had grade 2 disease (1.3–4.8% FC, increased LDH), 6 had grade 3 disease (4.9–9.6% FC, increased LDH), and 6 had grade 4 disease (>9.6% FC, increased LDH). All patients were on cyclosporin. Cyclosporin levels did not correlate with the grade of disease. Seventy percent of patients with grade 2 disease experienced resolution spontaneously or upon withdrawal of cyclosporin; none of the patients with grades 3 or 4 disease responded to only cyclosporin withdrawal, suggesting that elimination of cyclosporin or another potentially contributory immunomodulating agent should be considered early in the evolution of this syndrome.

Therapy for patients not responding to withdrawal of an immunomodulating agent or with grade 3/4 disease is not standardized. Treatment is based on successful modalities used in non–transplant-related TM and generally consists of a variety of plasma exchange procedures, which result in remission in more than 70% of these spontaneous cases. Partial response was obtained in patients with grades 3 and 4 disease with fresh-frozen plasma exchange, exchange with cryoprecipitate supernatant (to remove von Willebrand factor), exchange with staphylococcal protein A extracorporeal immunoadsorption, or exchange with sequential combinations of exchange types.[145] Splenectomy, intravenous immunoglobulin, vincristine, and various combinations of these measures have been anecdotally reported to be associated with clinical improvement. Unfortunately, there have been no formal comparisons of these various treatment regimens in transplant-related TM from which one could rationally determine a "treatment of choice." Treatment of this syndrome as a variant of MODS by withdrawal of an inciting agent such as cyclosporin and infusion of antithrombin III supplementation in it earliest stages, progressing to therapeutic plasma exchange with cryoprecipitate supernatant in refractory cases, is reasonable. Plasma exchange procedures often have to be performed daily over protracted periods of time before improvement occurs. Therapy for patients whose condition deteriorates while undergoing plasma exchange must be individualized to the patient and institution.

The contribution of hemostatic changes associated with the use of CSF, particularly GM-CSF, to complications in HSCT is even less clear from a clinical point of view than the contributions associated with platelet transfusion. The association of CSF with thrombosis and changes in levels of antithrombin and protein C after transplantation has been outlined. Although this does not constitute hard evidence that they are clinically detrimental in all transplant recipients, they do raise suspicions about their safety profile in patients who already have marked abnormalities in their inflammatory pathways, such as patients undergoing unrelated allogeneic transplantation or other patient populations who have experienced MODS. In these transplant settings, CSF may fuel the "cytokine storm" that may be causing critical illness.

The effects of CSF in these situations have not been widely studied, but in the one study their use in unrelated allogeneic transplants was associated with a sufficiently high mortality that the authors concluded, "Use of cytokines for accelerating hematopoietic recovery after allogeneic transplants remains to be proven safe and effective and it should not be considered outside controlled clinical trials."[100] A similar statement could be made about their routine use in autologous transplant recipients who experience MODS or other inflammation-related complications. The potential risks of CSF precipitating organ dysfunction in these populations should be weighed against their potential benefit, which to date does not include a reduction in short- or long-term mortality.[146] As with platelet transfusion, the use of CSF in ill (or potentially ill) transplant recipients deserves much more clinical research.

CONCLUSION

Perturbation of the coagulation system by HSCT and its complications may have dire consequences. SIRS, MODS, TM, VOD, and IPS may be the end result of an unregulated interaction between the coagulation and complement systems, with attendant endothelial cell damage. These often-fatal complications might be reversible with early identification and therapy. Further clinical and laboratory work is needed to accurately define the useful parameters for diagnosis and how they should be monitored. Therapeutically the use of antithrombin III for the direct treatment of organ dysfunction has demonstrated clinical utility. Judicious avoidance of CSF treatment in patients with organ dysfunction might also be justified on the available evidence. Further investigation in this area has the potential to reduce transplant-related morbidity and mortality.

REFERENCES

1. Weiss RB, Tormey DC, Holland JF, Weinberg VE: Venous thrombosis during multimodal treatment of primary breast carcinoma. Cancer Treat Rep 65:677, 1981.
2. Goodnough LT, Saito H, Manni A, et al: Increased incidence of thromboembolism in stage IV breast cancer patients treated with a five-drug chemotherapy regimen: a study of 159 patients. Cancer 54:1264, 1984.
3. Seifter EJ, Young RC, Longo DL: Deep venous thrombosis during therapy for Hodgkin's disease. Cancer Treat Rep 69:1011, 1985.
4. Schreiber DP, Kapp DS: Axillary-subclavian vein thrombosis following combination chemotherapy and radiation therapy in lymphoma. Int J Radiat Oncol Biol Phys 12:391, 1986.
5. Samuels BL, Vogelzang NJ, Kennedy BJ: Severe vascular toxicity associated with vinblastine, bleomycin, and cisplatin chemotherapy. Cancer Chemother Pharmacol 19:253, 1987.
6. Doll DC, List AF, Greco FA, et al: Acute vascular ischemic events after cisplatin-based combination chemotherapy for germ-cell tumors of the testis. Ann Intern Med 105:48, 1986.
7. Wall JG, Weiss RB, Norton L, et al: Arterial thrombosis associated with adjuvant chemotherapy for breast carcinoma: a Cancer and Leukemia Group B Study. Am J Med 87:501, 1989.
8. Cantwell BM, Mannix KA, Roberts JT, et al: Thromboembolic events during combination chemotherapy for germ-cell-malignancy [Letter]. Lancet 2:1086, 1988.
9. Cantwell BM, Carmichael J, Ghani SE, Harris AL: Thromboses and thromboemboli in patients with lymphoma during cytotoxic chemotherapy. BMJ 297:179, 1988.
10. Levine MN, Gent M, Hirsh J, et al: The thrombogenic effect of anticancer drug therapy in women with stage II breast cancer. N Engl J Med 318:404, 1988.
11. Tannock I, Gospodarowicz M, Connolly J, Jewett M: M-VAC (methotrexate, vinblastine, doxorubicin and cisplatin) chemotherapy for transitional cell carcinoma: the Princess Margaret Hospital experience. J Urol 142:289, 1989.
12. Berliner S, Rahima M, Sidi Y, et al: Acute coronary events following cisplatin-based chemotherapy. Cancer Invest 8:583, 1990.
13. Zurborn KH, Gram J, Glander K, et al: Influence of cytostatic treatment on the coagulation system and fibrinolysis in patients with non-Hodgkin's lymphomas and acute leukemias. Eur J Haematol 47:55, 1991.
14. Dreicer R, Messing EM, Loehrer PJ, Trump DL: Perioperative methotrexate, vinblastine, doxorubicin and cisplatin (M-VAC) for poor risk transitional cell carcinoma of the bladder: an Eastern Cooperative Oncology Group pilot study. J Urol 144:1123, 1990.
15. Saphner T, Tormey DC, Gray R: Venous and arterial thrombosis in patients who received adjuvant therapy for breast cancer. J Clin Oncol 9:286, 1991.
16. Clahsen PC, van de Velde CJ, Julien JP, et al: Thromboembolic complications after perioperative chemotherapy in women with early breast cancer: a European Organization for Research and Treatment of Cancer Breast Cancer Cooperative Group study. J Clin Oncol 12:1266, 1994.
17. Blomback M, Hedlund PO, Sawe U: Changes in blood coagulation and fibrinolysis in patients on different treatment regimens for prostatic cancer: predictors for cardiovascular complications? Thromb Res 49:111, 1988.
18. Pritchard KI, Paterson AH, Paul NA, et al: Increased thromboembolic complications with concurrent tamoxifen and chemotherapy in a randomized trial of adjuvant therapy for women with breast cancer: National Cancer Institute of Canada Clinical Trials Group Breast Cancer Site Group. J Clin Oncol 14:2731, 1996.
19. Nissen C, Tichelli A, Gratwohl A, et al: Failure of recombinant human granulocyte-macrophage colony-stimulating factor therapy in aplastic anemia patients with very severe neutropenia. Blood 72:2045, 1988.
20. Antman KS, Griffin JD, Elias A, et al: Effect of recombinant human granulocyte-macrophage colony-stimulating factor on chemotherapy-induced myelosuppression [see comments]. N Engl J Med 319:593, 1988.
21. Hoekman K, Wagstaff J, van Groeningen CJ, et al: Effects of recombinant human granulocyte-macrophage colony-stimulating factor on myelosuppression induced by multiple cycles of high-dose chemotherapy in patients with advanced breast cancer. J Natl Cancer Inst 83:1546, 1991.
22. Conti JA, Scher HI: Acute arterial thrombosis after escalated-dose methotrexate, vinblastine, doxorubicin, and cisplatin chemotherapy with recombinant granulocyte colony-stimulating factor: a possible new recombinant granulocyte colony-stimulating factor toxicity. Cancer 70:2699, 1992.
23. Tolcher AW, Giusti RM, O'Shaughnessy JA, Cowan KH: Arterial thrombosis associated with granulocyte-macrophage colony-stimulating factor (GM-CSF) administration in breast cancer patients treated with dose-intensive chemotherapy: a report of two cases. Cancer Invest 13:188, 1995.
24. Stephens LC, Haire WD, Schmit-Pokorny K, et al: Granulocyte macrophage colony stimulating factor: high incidence of apheresis catheter thrombosis during peripheral stem cell collection. Bone Marrow Transplant 11:51, 1993.
25. Zurborn KH, Bruhn HD: Hypercoagulability in cytostatic tumor therapy: Blut 53:179, 1986.
26. Kuzel T, Esparaz B, Green D, Kies M: Thrombogenicity of intravenous 5-fluorouracil alone or in combination with cisplatin. Cancer 65:885, 1990.
27. Edwards RL, Klaus M, Matthews E, et al: Heparin abolishes the chemotherapy-induced increase in plasma fibrinopeptide A levels. Am J Med 89:25, 1990.
28. Ruiz MA, Marugan I, Estelles A, et al: The influence of chemotherapy on plasma coagulation and fibrinolytic systems in lung cancer patients. Cancer 63:643, 1989.
29. Enck RE, Rios CN: Tamoxifen treatment of metastatic breast cancer and antithrombin III levels. Cancer 53:2607, 1984.
30. Love RR, Surawicz TS, Williams EC: Antithrombin III level, fibrinogen level, and platelet count changes with adjuvant tamoxifen therapy. Arch Intern Med 152:317, 1992.
31. Rogers JSd, Murgo AJ, Fontana JA, Raich PC: Chemotherapy for breast cancer decreases plasma protein C and protein S. J Clin Oncol 6:276, 1988.
32. Kadar JG, Arseniev L, Schnitger K, et al: Technical and safety aspects of blood and marrow transplantation using G-CSF mobilized family donors. Transfus Sci 17:611, 1996.
33. Falanga A, Marchetti M, Evangelista V, et al: Neutrophil activation and hemostatic changes in healthy donors receiving granulocyte colony-stimulating factor. Blood 93:2506, 1999.
34. Gordon B, Haire W, Ruby E, et al: Factors predicting morbidity following hematopoietic stem cell transplantation. Bone Marrow Transplant 19:497, 1997.
35. Guinan EC, Tarbell NJ, Niemeyer CM, et al: Intravascular hemolysis and renal insufficiency after bone marrow transplantation. Blood 72:451, 1988.
36. Patchell RA, White CLD, Clark AW, et al: Nonbacterial thrombotic endocarditis in bone marrow transplant patients. Cancer 55:631, 1985.
37. Jerman MR, Fick RB Jr: Nonbacterial thrombotic endocarditis associated with bone marrow transplantation. Chest 90:919, 1986.
38. Bernauer W, Gratwohl A, Keller A, Daicker B: Microvasculopathy in the ocular fundus after bone marrow transplantation [see comments]. Ann Intern Med 115:925, 1991.
39. Gordon BG, Haire WD, Patton DF, et al: Thrombotic complications of BMT: association with protein C deficiency. Bone Marrow Transplant 11:61, 1993.
40. Haire WD, Lieberman RP, Edney J, et al: Hickman catheter-induced thoracic vein thrombosis: frequency and long-term sequelae in patients receiving high-dose chemotherapy and marrow transplantation. Cancer 66:900, 1990.
41. Haire WD, Lieberman RP, Lund GB, et al: Thrombotic complications of silicone rubber catheters during autologous marrow and peripheral stem cell transplantation: prospective comparison of Hickman and Groshong catheters. Bone Marrow Transplant 7:57, 1991.
42. Shulman HM, Gown AM, Nugent DJ: Hepatic veno-occlusive disease

after bone marrow transplantation: immunohistochemical identification of the material within occluded central venules. Am J Pathol 127:549, 1987.

43. Gordon B, Haire W, Kessinger A, et al: High frequency of antithrombin 3 and protein C deficiency following autologous bone marrow transplantation for lymphoma. Bone Marrow Transplant 8:497, 1991.

44. Haire W, Gordon B, Stephens L, et al: Protein C (PC) deficiency during marrow transplantation: a frequent occurrence associated with a decrease in PC antigen and production of a dysfunctional PC molecule. Blood 78:288a, 1996.

45. Harper PL, Jarvis J, Jennings I, et al: Changes in the natural anticoagulants following bone marrow transplantation. Bone Marrow Transplant 5:39, 1990.

46. Kaufman PA, Jones RB, Greenberg CS, Peters WP: Autologous bone marrow transplantation and factor XII, factor VII, and protein C deficiencies: report of a new association and its possible relationship to endothelial cell injury. Cancer 66:515, 1990.

47. Leblond V, Salehian BD, Borel C, et al: Alterations in natural anticoagulant levels during allogeneic bone marrow transplantation: a prospective study in 27 patients. Bone Marrow Transplant 11:299, 1993.

48. Collins P, Roderick A, O'Brien D, et al: Factor VIIa and other haemostatic variables following bone marrow transplantation. Thromb Haemostat 72:28, 1994.

49. Gordon B, Haire W, Ruby E, et al: Prolonged deficiency of protein C following hematopoietic stem cell transplantation. Bone Marrow Transplant 17:415, 1996.

50. Elston TN, Dudley JM, Shearer MJ, Schey SA: Vitamin K prophylaxis in high-dose chemotherapy [Letter]. Lancet 345:1245, 1995.

51. Gordon BG, Haire WD, Stephens LC, et al: Protein C deficiency following hematopoietic stem cell transplantation: optimization of intravenous vitamin K dose. Bone Marrow Transplant 12:73, 1993.

52. Nurnberger W, Michelmann I, Gehentges S, et al: Increased consumption of antithrombin III in patients receiving granulocyte-macrophage colony-stimulating factor after bone marrow transplantation [Letter]. Blood 84:3986, 1994.

53. Haire WD, Stephens LC, Kotulak GD, et al: Pharmacokinetics of antithrombin concentrate during autologous hematopoietic stem cell transplantation. Bone Marrow Transplant 15:505, 1995.

54. Ghebrehiwet B, Silverberg M, Kaplan AP: Activation of the classical pathway of complement by Hageman factor fragment. J Exp Med 153:665, 1981.

55. Nurnberger W, Michelmann I, Petrik K, et al: Activity of C1 esterase inhibitor in patients with vascular leak syndrome after bone marrow transplantation. Ann Hematol 67:17, 1993.

56. DeLa Cadena RA, Wachtfogel YT, Colman RW: Contact activation pathway: inflammation and coagulation. In Colman RW, Hirsh J, Marder VJ, Salzman EW (eds): Hemostasis and Thrombosis: Basic Principles and Clinical Practice, 3rd ed. Philadelphia, JB Lippincott, 1994, p 219.

57. Fein AM, Bernard GR, Criner GJ, et al: Treatment of severe systemic inflammatory response syndrome and sepsis with a novel bradykinin antagonist, deltibant (CP-0127): results of a randomized, double-blind, placebo-controlled trial. CP-0127 SIRS and Sepsis Study Group. JAMA 277:482, 1997.

58. McDonald GB, Hinds MS, Fisher LD, et al: Veno-occlusive disease of the liver and multiorgan failure after bone marrow transplantation: a cohort study of 355 patients. Ann Intern Med 118:255, 1993.

59. Bearman SI: The syndrome of hepatic veno-occlusive disease after marrow transplantation. Blood 85:3005, 1995.

60. Haire WD, Ruby EI, Gordon BG, et al: Multiple organ dysfunction syndrome in bone marrow transplantation. JAMA 274:1289, 1995.

61. Gelehrter TD, Sznycer-Laszuk R: Thrombin induction of plasminogen activator-inhibitor in cultured human endothelial cells. J Clin Invest 77:165, 1986.

62. Salat C, Holler E, Kolb HJ, et al: Plasminogen activator inhibitor-1 confirms the diagnosis of hepatic veno-occlusive disease in patients with hyperbilirubinemia after bone marrow transplantation. Blood 89:2184, 1997.

63. Lorant DE, Patel KD, McIntyre TM, et al: Coexpression of GMP-140 and PAF by endothelium stimulated by histamine or thrombin: a juxtacrine system for adhesion and activation of neutrophils. J Cell Biol 115:223, 1991.

64. Wright DG, Gallin JI: Secretory responses of human neutrophils: exocytosis of specific (secondary) granules by human neutrophils during adherence in vitro and during exudation in vivo. J Immunol 123:285, 1979.

65. Yang JJ, Kettritz R, Falk RJ, et al: Apoptosis of endothelial cells induced by the neutrophil serine proteases proteinase 3 and elastase. Am J Pathol 149:1617, 1996.

66. Bombeli T, Karsan A, Tait JF, Harlan JM: Apoptotic vascular endothelial cells become procoagulant. Blood 89:2429, 1997.

67. Bone RC, Balk RA, Cerra FB, et al: Definitions for sepsis and organ failure and guidelines for the use of innovative therapies in sepsis: the ACCP/SCCM Consensus Conference Committee. American College of Chest Physicians/Society of Critical Care Medicine [see comments]. Chest 101:1644, 1992.

68. Bone RC: Immunologic dissonance: a continuing evolution in our understanding of the systemic inflammatory response syndrome (SIRS) and the multiple organ dysfunction syndrome (MODS) [see comments]. Ann Intern Med 125:680, 1996.

69. Esmon CT, Taylor FB Jr, Snow TR: Inflammation and coagulation: linked processes potentially regulated through a common pathway mediated by protein C. Thromb Haemost 66:160, 1991.

70. Bone RC: Modulators of coagulation: a critical appraisal of their role in sepsis. Arch Intern Med 152:1381, 1992.

71. Hasegawa N, Husari AW, Hart WT, et al: Role of the coagulation system in ARDS. Chest 105:268, 1994.

72. Bone RC: Sepsis and coagulation: an important link [Editorial; Comment]. Chest 101:594, 1992.

73. Levi M, ten Cate H, van der Poll T, van Deventer SJ: Pathogenesis of disseminated intravascular coagulation in sepsis [see comments]. JAMA 270:975, 1993.

74. Carvalho AC, Freeman NJ: How coagulation defects alter outcome in sepsis. J Crit Ill 9:51, 1994.

75. Bredbacka S, Blomback M, Wiman B: Soluble fibrin: a predictor for the development and outcome of multiple organ failure. Am J Hematol 46:289, 1994.

76. Brandtzaeg P, Sandset PM, Joo GB, et al: The quantitative association of plasma endotoxin, antithrombin, protein C, extrinsic pathway inhibitor and fibrinopeptide A in systemic meningococcal disease. Thromb Res 55:459, 1989.

77. Carvalho AC, DeMarinis S, Scott CF, et al: Activation of the contact system of plasma proteolysis in the adult respiratory distress syndrome. J Lab Clin Med 112:270, 1988.

78. Schipper HG, Roos J, van der Meulen F, ten Cate JW: Antithrombin III deficiency in surgical intensive care patients. Thromb Res 21:73, 1981.

79. Hesselvik JF, Blomback M, Brodin B, Maller R: Coagulation, fibrinolysis, and kallikrein systems in sepsis: relation to outcome. Crit Care Med 17:724, 1989.

80. Hesselvik JF, Malm J, Dahlback B, Blomback M: Protein C, protein S and C4b-binding protein in severe infection and septic shock. Thromb Haemost 65:126, 1991.

81. Lorente JA, Garcia-Frade LJ, Landin L, et al: Time course of hemostatic abnormalities in sepsis and its relation to outcome. Chest 103:1536, 1993.

82. Fijnvandraat K, Derkx B, Peters M, et al: Coagulation activation and tissue necrosis in meningococcal septic shock: severely reduced protein C levels predict a high mortality. Thromb Haemost 73:15, 1995.

83. Fourrier F, Lestavel P, Chopin C, et al: Meningococcemia and purpura fulminans in adults: acute deficiencies of proteins C and S and early treatment with antithrombin III concentrates. Intensive Care Med 16:121, 1990.

84. Fourrier F, Chopin C, Goudemand J, et al: Septic shock, multiple organ failure, and disseminated intravascular coagulation: compared patterns of antithrombin III, protein C, and protein S deficiencies [see comments]. Chest 101:816, 1992.

85. Wilson RF, Farag A, Mammen EF, Fujii Y: Sepsis and antithrombin III, prekallikrein, and fibronectin levels in surgical patients. Am Surg 55:450, 1989.

86. Nedorn E, Wosegien F, Kemmler G: Antithrombin III and early prognosis in polytraumatized patients: a pilot study. Klin Wochenschr 69:817, 1991.

87. Miller RS, Weatherford DA, Stein D, et al: Antithrombin III and trauma patients: factors that determine low levels. J Trauma 37:442, 1994.

88. Owings JT, Bagley M, Gosselin R, et al: Effect of critical injury on plasma antithrombin activity: low antithrombin levels are associated with thromboembolic complications. J Trauma 41:396, 1996.

89. Zimmermann T, Laszik Z, Nagy S, et al: The role of the complement system in the pathogenesis of multiple organ failure in shock. Prog Clin Biol Res 308:291, 1989.

90. Sigurdsson GH, Christenson JT, el-Rakshy MB, Sadek S: Intestinal platelet trapping after traumatic and septic shock: an early sign of sepsis and multiorgan failure in critically ill patients? Crit Care Med 20:458, 1992.

91. Haire WD: The multiple organ dysfunction syndrome in cancer patients undergoing hematopoietic stem cell transplantation [in process citation]. Semin Thromb Hemost 25:223, 1999.

92. Clark JG, Hansen JA, Hertz MI, et al: NHLBI workshop summary. Idiopathic pneumonia syndrome after bone marrow transplantation. Am Rev Respir Dis 147:1601, 1993.

93. Gordon B, Tarantolo S, Ruby E, et al: Increased platelet transfusion requirement is associated with multiple organ dysfunctions in patients undergoing hematopoietic stem cell transplantation. Bone Marrow Transplant 22:999, 1998.

94. Faioni EM, Krachmalnicoff A, Bearman SI, et al: Naturally occurring anticoagulants and bone marrow transplantation: plasma protein C predicts the development of veno-occlusive disease of the liver. Blood 81:3458, 1993.

95. Wingard JR, Mellits ED, Jones RJ, et al: Association of hepatic veno-occlusive disease with interstitial pneumonitis in bone marrow transplant recipients. Bone Marrow Transplant 4:685, 1989.

96. Fink JC, Cooper MA, Burkhart KM, et al: Marked enzymuria after bone marrow transplantation: a correlate of veno-occlusive disease-induced "hepatorenal syndrome." J Am Soc Nephrol 6:1655, 1995.

97. Pollmacher T, Korth C, Mullington J, et al: Effects of granulocyte colony-stimulating factor on plasma cytokine and cytokine receptor levels and on the in vivo host response to endotoxin in healthy men. Blood 87:900, 1996.

98. King J, Deboisblanc BP, Mason CM, et al: Effect of granulocyte colony-stimulating factor on acute lung injury in the rat. Am J Respir Crit Care Med 151:302, 1995.

99. Link H, Boogaerts MA, Carella AM, et al: A controlled trial of recombinant human granulocyte-macrophage colony-stimulating factor after total body irradiation, high-dose chemotherapy, and autologous bone marrow transplantation for acute lymphoblastic leukemia or malignant lymphoma. Blood 80:2188, 1992.

100. Anasetti C, Anderson G, Appelbaum FR, et al: Phase III study of rhGM-CSF in allogeneic marrow transplantation from unrelated donors: Blood 82:454a, 1993.

101. Shulman H, Striker G, Deeg HJ, et al: Nephrotoxicity of cyclosporin A after allogeneic marrow transplantation: glomerular thromboses and tubular injury. N Engl J Med 305:1392, 1981.

102. Powles RL, Clink HM, Spence D, et al: Cyclosporin A to prevent graft-versus-host disease in man after allogeneic bone-marrow transplantation. Lancet 1:327, 1980.

103. Holler E, Kolb HJ, Hiller E, et al: Microangiopathy in patients on cyclosporine prophylaxis who developed acute graft-versus-host disease after HLA-identical bone marrow transplantation. Blood 73:2018, 1989.

104. Juckett M, Perry EH, Daniels BS, Weisdorf DJ: Hemolytic uremic syndrome following bone marrow transplantation. Bone Marrow Transplant 7:405, 1991.

105. Rabinowe SN, Soiffer RJ, Tarbell NJ, et al: Hemolytic-uremic syndrome following bone marrow transplantation in adults for hematologic malignancies. Blood 77:1837, 1991.

106. Grace AA, Barradas MA, Mikhailidis DP, et al: Cyclosporine A enhances platelet aggregation. Kidney Int 32:889, 1987.

107. Allen JB, Sagerman RH, Stuart MJ: Irradiation decreases vascular prostacyclin formation with no concomitant effect on platelet thromboxane production. Lancet 2:1193, 1981.

108. Rosenthal RA, Chukwuogo NA, Ocasio VH, Kahng KU: Cyclosporine inhibits endothelial cell prostacyclin production. J Surg Res 46:593, 1989.

109. Voss BL, Hamilton KK, Samara EN, McKee PA: Cyclosporine suppression of endothelial prostacyclin generation: a possible mechanism for nephrotoxicity. Transplantation 45:793, 1988.

110. Moore LC, Mason J, Feld L, et al: Effect of cyclosporine on endothelial albumin leakage in rats. J Am Soc Nephrol 3:51, 1992.

111. Schriber JR, Herzig GP: Transplantation-associated thrombotic thrombocytopenic purpura and hemolytic uremic syndrome. Semin Hematol 34:126, 1997.

112. Nizze H, Mihatsch MJ, Zollinger HU, et al: Cyclosporine-associated nephropathy in patients with heart and bone marrow transplants. Clin Nephrol 30:248, 1988.

113. Zeigler ZR, Rosenfeld CS, Andrews DF III, et al: Plasma von Willebrand factor antigen (vWF:AG) and thrombomodulin (TM) levels in adult thrombotic thrombocytopenic purpura/hemolytic uremic syndromes (TTP/HUS) and bone marrow transplant-associated thrombotic microangiopathy (BMT-TM). Am J Hematol 53:213, 1996.

114. Taylor F, Chang A, Ferrell G, et al: C4b-binding protein exacerbates the host response to Escherichia coli. Blood 78:357, 1991.

115. Kessler CM, Tang Z, Jacobs HM, Szymanski LM: The suprapharmacologic dosing of antithrombin concentrate for Staphylococcus aureus–induced disseminated intravascular coagulation in guinea pigs: substantial reduction in mortality and morbidity. Blood 89:4393, 1997.

116. Redens TB, Emerson TE Jr: Antithrombin-III treatment limits disseminated intravascular coagulation in endotoxemia. Circ Shock 28:49, 1989.

117. Murakami K, Okajima K, Uchiba M, et al: Activated protein C attenuates endotoxin-induced pulmonary vascular injury by inhibiting activated leukocytes in rats. Blood 87:642, 1996.

118. Taylor FB Jr, Chang A, Esmon CT, et al: Protein C prevents the coagulopathic and lethal effects of Escherichia coli infusion in the baboon. J Clin Invest 79:918, 1987.

119. Uchiba M, Okajima K, Murakami K, et al: Recombinant human soluble thrombomodulin reduces endotoxin-induced pulmonary vascular injury via protein C activation in rats. Thromb Haemost 74:1265, 1995.

120. Meyer J, Cox CS, Herndon DN, et al: Heparin in experimental hyperdynamic sepsis. Crit Care Med 21:84, 1993.

121. Hardaway RM, Williams CH, Marvasti M, et al: Prevention of adult respiratory distress syndrome with plasminogen activator in pigs. Crit Care Med 18:1413, 1990.

122. Paloma MJ, Paramo JA, Rocha E: Endotoxin-induced intravascular coagulation in rabbits: effect of tissue plasminogen activator vs urokinase of PAI generation, fibrin deposits and mortality. Thromb Haemost 74:1578, 1995.

123. Taylor FB Jr, Chang AC, Peer GT, et al: DEGR-factor Xa blocks disseminated intravascular coagulation initiated by Escherichia coli without preventing shock or organ damage. Blood 78:364, 1991.

124. Fourrier F, Chopin C, Huart JJ, et al: Double-blind, placebo-controlled trial of antithrombin III concentrates in septic shock with disseminated intravascular coagulation. Chest 104:882, 1993.

125. Jochum M: Influence of high-dose antithrombin concentrate therapy on the release of cellular proteinases, cytokines, and soluble adhesion molecules in acute inflammation. Semin Hematol 32:19, 1995.

126. Attal M, Huguet F, Rubie H, et al: Prevention of hepatic veno-occlusive disease after bone marrow transplantation by continuous infusion of low-dose heparin: a prospective, randomized trial [see comments]. Blood 79:2834, 1992.

127. Demuynck H, Vandenderghe P, Verhoef GEG, et al: Prevention of veno-occlusive disease (VOD) of the liver after marrow and blood progenitor cell transplantation: a prospective, randomized study of different prophylactic regimens. Blood 86:620a, 1995.

128. Or R, Nagler A, Shpilberg O, et al: Low molecular weight heparin for the prevention of veno-occlusive disease of the liver in bone marrow transplantation patients. Transplantation 61:1067, 1996.

129. Bearman SI, Shuhart MC, Hinds MS, McDonald GB: Recombinant human tissue plasminogen activator for the treatment of established severe veno-occlusive disease of the liver after bone marrow transplantation. Blood 80:2458, 1992.

130. Yu LC, Malkani I, Regueira O, et al: Recombinant tissue plasminogen activator (rt-PA) for veno-occlusive liver disease in pediatric autologous bone marrow transplant patients. Am J Hematol 46:194, 1994.

131. Patton DF, Harper JL, Wooldridge TN, et al: Treatment of veno-occlusive disease of the liver with bolus tissue plasminogen activator and continuous infusion antithrombin III concentrate. Bone Marrow Transplant 17:443, 1996.

132. Morris J, Hashmi R, Sambrano J, et al: Treatment of regimen related toxicity following bone marrow transplant (BMT) with antithrombin III (ATIII). Blood 86:219a, 1995.

133. Haire WD, Ruby EI, Stephens LC, et al: A prospective randomized double-blind trial of antithrombin III concentrate in the treatment of multiple-organ dysfunction syndrome during hematopoietic stem cell transplantation. Biol Blood Marrow Transplant 4:142, 1998.

134. Bishop JF, McGrath K, Wolf MM, et al: Clinical factors influencing the efficacy of pooled platelet transfusions. Blood 71:383, 1988.

135. Hussein MA, Long T, Zuccaro K: Platelet transfusion recovery and survival in stable bone marrow transplant patients: a prospective study: Blood 86:103a, 1995.

136. Benson K, Fields K, Hiemenz J, et al: The platelet-refractory bone marrow transplant patient: prophylaxis and treatment of bleeding. Semin Oncol 20:102, 1993.

137. Fujimoto T, Suzuki H, Tanoue K, et al: Cerebrovascular injuries induced by activation of platelets in vivo. Stroke 16:245, 1985.

138. Heffner JE, Sahn SA, Repine JE: The role of platelets in the adult respiratory distress syndrome: culprits or bystanders? Am Rev Respir Dis 135:482, 1987.

139. Grau GE, Lou J: TNF in vascular pathology: the importance of platelet-endothelium interactions. Res Immunol 144:355, 1993.

140. Piguet PF, Vesin C, Ryser JE, et al: An effector role for platelets in systemic and local lipopolysaccharide-induced toxicity in mice, mediated by a CD11a- and CD54-dependent interaction with endothelium. Infect Immun 61:4182, 1993.

141. Hanson SR, Slichter SJ: Platelet kinetics in patients with bone marrow hypoplasia: evidence for a fixed platelet requirement. Blood 66:1105, 1985.

142. Goodnough LT, Kolodziej M, Ehlenbeck C, et al: A phase I study of safety and efficacy for infusible platelet membrane in patients. Blood 86:610a, 1995.

143. Scigliano E, Fruchtman S, Tsola L, et al: Infusible platelet membrane (IPM) for control of bleeding in thrombocytopenic patients. Blood 86:446a, 1995.

144. Zeigler ZR, Shadduck RK, Nemunaitis J, et al: Bone marrow transplant–associated thrombotic microangiopathy: a case series. Bone Marrow Transplant 15:247, 1995.

145. Zeigler ZR, Shadduck RK, Nath R, Andrews DF: Pilot study of combined cryosupernatant and protein A immunoadsorption exchange in the treatment of grade 3–4 bone marrow transplant–associated thrombotic microangiopathy. Bone Marrow Transplant 17:81, 1996.

146. Demetri GD: Beyond supportive care: what are the next questions in the use of hematopoietic cytokines with cytotoxic chemotherapy? [Editorial; Comment]. Blood 82:2278, 1993.

147. Folstein MF, Folstein SE, McHugh PR: "Mini-mental state": a practical method for grading the cognitive state of patients for the clinician. J Psychiatry Res 12:189, 1975.

148. Anthony JC, LeResche L, Niaz U, et al: Limits of the "Mini-Mental State" as a screening test for dementia and delirium among hospital patients. Psychol Med 12:397, 1982.

Nutritional Support

CHAPTER FORTY-TWO

Nutritional Issues and Management in Hematopoietic Stem Cell Transplantation

Cheryl L. Rock, Ph.D., R.D.

Nutrition is an important part of the management of patients who undergo hematopoietic stem cell transplantation (HSCT). As a component of medical care, nutritional assessment, management, and monitoring can affect many patient outcomes and may influence the risk of complications and the overall costs of the procedure. Because of the gastrointestinal symptoms that result from high-dose chemotherapy and radiation therapy and other aspects of HSCT, patients who do not receive nutrition support or specialized nutritional care typically eat poorly for a prolonged period and exhibit indicators of poor nutritional status.[1-3] A positive effect on overall survival has been associated with nutrition support, even in patients not considered to be at nutritional risk prior to transplantation.[2] Prevention of malnutrition and correction of energy and nutrient inadequacies has been incorporated into the standardized post-transplantation treatment at most (if not all) transplant centers, although many of the details of nutritional management are more empirical than evidence-based.

This chapter reviews the basic principles, major issues, and current general guidelines that are applicable to the nutritional management of patients undergoing HSCT. Rather than attempt to comprehensively review all of the evidence on the topic, this chapter instead focuses on the basic concepts and most salient issues for the HSCT clinician with limited training and expertise in clinical nutrition.

NUTRITIONAL PROBLEMS

Some of the nutritional problems that occur in patients undergoing HSCT may be a consequence of a pre-existing disease or condition, particularly in patients who present for treatment after a period of chronic illness. Some patients with malignant or nonmalignant disease who undergo HSCT have been ill for some time prior to the procedure, with a history of frequent hospitalizations and symptoms that may have interfered with the ability to eat an adequate diet and maintain a healthy body weight. Nutritional problems also result from adverse effects of various drug therapies, such as oral immunosuppressive agents and antibiotics, that may be necessary for post-transplant management.[4] Both immunosuppressive regimens and antibiotics are associated with metabolic and gastrointestinal side effects that can alter nutri-

tional requirements or status or that may interfere with the ability to obtain adequate nutrients from foods.

Most notably, however, the conditioning regimen of intensive chemotherapy, often in conjunction with total body irradiation, is associated with several specific side effects that have significant adverse nutritional consequences, such as nausea, vomiting, diarrhea, oropharyngeal mucositis, and esophagitis. Total body irradiation damages the gastrointestinal mucosa, resulting in malabsorption and diarrhea, because these epithelial cells are highly susceptible to the effects of radiation. Finally, the common complication of graft-versus-host disease (GVHD) in patients who undergo allogeneic transplantation results in abdominal pain, nausea, severe diarrhea, malabsorption, and substantial nitrogen losses due to gastrointestinal damage.[1, 5, 6]

Using isotopic dilution technology to assess body composition, Cheney et al.[7] documented decreased body cell mass and negative nitrogen balance in patients undergoing HSCT for acute lymphocytic leukemia. Thiamin deficiency, a significant reduction in the plasma pool of vitamin E, and electrolyte and trace-element deficiencies have also been observed in clinical studies of patients undergoing HSCT.[6, 8, 9]

NUTRITIONAL REQUIREMENTS

Energy is required for normal metabolism, for growth, and for any additional anabolic processes, such as tissue healing; however, the catabolic state induced by the conditioning regimen and the presence of infection further increases the energy expenditure of the patient undergoing HSCT. To illustrate the effect of infection, the basal metabolic rate increases approximately 7% for each 1°F increase in body temperature. If portable gas exchange equipment is available, indirect calorimetry may be used to actually measure the energy requirement of the patient. An alternative and common approach used to estimate the energy requirement is based on an estimate of the basal energy requirement (BEE), using the Harris-Benedict equations[10]:

For women, BEE = 655.10 + 9.56W + 1.85H − 4.68A
For men, BEE = 66.47 + 13.75W + 5.00H − 6.76A

where W = weight (kg), H = height (cm), and A = age

503

(years). Total daily energy requirement can then be estimated as BEE $\times$ 1.2–1.5 to allow for energy necessary for physical activity and other needs. In adult HSCT patients, 30–50 kcal/kg body weight per day has been found to be required to maintain energy balance,[11] which is higher than the level usually required for energy balance in healthy individuals or hospitalized patients (usually $\leq$35 kcal/kg per day). One can obtain a comparable estimate using the figure derived with a factor of 1.5 in the Harrison-Benedict equations. Energy requirements of pediatric transplant patients are higher, ranging from 80–100 kcal/kg per day. Typically, 70–90% of energy provided in a parenteral solution used in nutrition support is derived from dextrose and 10–30% is derived from a lipid emulsion when a parenteral solution is being used to meet the energy and nutrient needs of these patients.

Protein requirements also appear to be increased in the transplant recipient, partly because of intestinal losses associated with protein-losing enteropathy.[1, 6] Protein requirements are usually estimated at 1.5 g/kg body weight for adults (range, 1.2–1.5 g/kg) and 1.5–2.5 g/kg for pediatric patients. Providing adequate amino acids via nutritional support may help to improve nitrogen balance, although some degree of negative nitrogen balance may be unavoidable because of the metabolically catabolic state promoted by the conditioning regimen, immunosuppressive therapy, and other aspects of HSCT. Improved nitrogen balance and protein status is also inextricably linked with the provision of adequate energy, because if energy intake is inadequate, dietary protein and amino acids are simply metabolized as energy substrates and not spared for tissue repair and healing. Thus, the potential energy contribution of amino acids that are added to parenteral nutrition solutions to meet protein needs is not included in the calculation of total energy provided to the patient, as is usually done when evaluating the diets of persons obtaining energy and nutrients from oral diets.

In addition to energy and protein, requirements may also be increased for the micronutrients involved in metabolism and the minerals that may be lost at increased rates because of diarrhea-related intestinal losses. Levels of micronutrients in formulations added to parenteral solutions or used in enteral formula diets are set to meet or exceed requirements for hospitalized patients under typical circumstances, but indicators of nutritional status should also be monitored to ensure adequacy.

APPROACHES TO NUTRITION SUPPORT

Because many patients undergoing HSCT are unable to eat enough food to achieve the estimated energy requirement (or maintain the level of intake reported at admission), alternative routes to nutrition support are often considered. In addition to strategies and assistance to optimize oral intake, enteral (primarily via nasogastric tube) and parenteral (via central venous catheter because peripheral venous access constrains the ability to provide sufficient energy) are the two major approaches to nutrition support. Both of these approaches have distinct advantages and disadvantages.

Historically, parenteral nutrition has been considered the

method of choice for ensuring nutritional adequacy in HSCT, mainly because of the likelihood of severe gastrointestinal symptoms. Because of the high risk of nutritional problems in these patients, parenteral nutrition support may even be initiated and used as prophylaxis and is usually not discontinued until the patient demonstrates the ability to consume a sufficient amount of the oral diet to achieve a predetermined goal level of nutritional requirements (ranging from 50% to 70%).

The usefulness of tube feeding is often limited by the presence of mucosal and esophageal ulceration, nausea and vomiting, and local infection of the mouth and esophagus, even when gut function appears normal. In clinical trials, total parenteral nutrition has been shown to result in significantly higher energy and protein intake when compared with allowing patients to consume an oral diet ad libitum.[2]

Parenteral nutrition, however, has not been consistently associated with favorable effects on duration of hospitalization, episodes of bacteremia, or total number of complications, and it has been suggested that intestinal mucosal integrity is better maintained by using enteral rather than parenteral nutrition support.[6, 12] The theory, described as bacterial translocation, is that bowel rest (which results from reliance on parenteral nutrition) may enable the intestinal tract to serve as a portal of entry for bacteria into the bloodstream and visceral organs, particularly in patients who are physiologically stressed or immunocompromised. In practice, aggressive parenteral nutrition is also more likely to result in fluid overload, hyperglycemia, and catheter-related complications.[13]

The goal is always to promote the progression toward achieving regular oral intake as a component of normal functioning and recovery, which may be impeded or delayed when patients are discharged on parenteral nutrition. In a controlled trial in which outpatient parenteral nutrition was compared with intravenous hydration, parenteral nutrition was associated with delayed resumption of oral intake after transplantation while failing to substantially improve patient outcome.[14]

In another prospective randomized study,[15] total parenteral nutrition was compared with an individualized enteral feeding program that involved close monitoring, snacks, and/or tube feeding. Approximately 25% of the patients assigned to the enteral nutrition group ultimately had to receive parenteral nutrition because of intolerance of the tube feeding, but parenteral nutrition did not shorten the duration of marrow aplasia and was associated with more complications related to feeding route (i.e., fluid overload requiring diuretics). Also, the cost of the enteral nutrition intervention (which included individualized attention and snacks) for the 28-day feeding period was less than half that of the parenteral nutrition approach. Results from other studies of enteral nutrition support suggest that, when tolerated, this approach is effective, is probably underused, and may even impart some special protective effects.[6, 12]

Modifications is the parenteral nutrition solutions used in the nutrition support of patients undergoing HSCT, such as the addition of certain amino acids (i.e., glutamine, arginine) or omega-3 fatty acids, are also currently under study. The addition of glutamine, which is not considered an essential amino acid, is based on the rationale that it

TABLE 42–1. DIETARY STRATEGIES TO MANAGE COMMON PROBLEMS

	NOT WELL TOLERATED	BETTER TOLERATED
Nausea	Very sweet; greasy; strong odors; meats	Cold, clear liquids: flat soda, Koolaid; watermelon; cold folds; salty foods
Mucositis	Fruit juice; acidic foods/beverages; hot spices; highly salted foods; crunchy snacks/grainy cereals and breads; too hot/too cold; fresh, raw fruits and vegetables	Canned fruit; cold, clear liquids; melon
Dry mouth	Meats; grainy cereals and breads; crackers; potatoes	Lemonade; gravies, broths; sauces added to foods; eggs/omelettes; cured meat/lunch meat; grapes, melon; canned fruit
Taste changes	Meats; potatoes	Salty foods; highly flavored foods (e.g., lasagna, BBQ)
Thick saliva	Gelatin; oily foods; thick cream soup; nectars; hot cereals; breads	Club soda; hot tea with lemon; lemon drops; increase fluids

Modified from American Dietetic Association: Nutrition management following bone marrow transplantation. *In* Manual of Clinical Dietetics, 5th ed. Chicago, American Dietetic Association, 1996.

may improve intestinal mucosal integrity, reduce the incidence of bacterial translocation, and improve nitrogen balance. In one small clinical trial, Ziegler et al.[16] demonstrated that glutamine-supplemented parenteral nutrition after HSCT was associated with improved nitrogen balance, reduced incidence of clinical infection, lower rates of microbial colonization, and reduced hospital stay compared with standard parenteral nutrition support. No differences in the incidence of fever or time of recovery from myelosuppression were observed, however.

The importance of providing individualized guidance with food choices may often be unrecognized, but several strategies can be helpful when reduced appetite and taste changes, in addition to mild or moderate mucositis, xerosoma, and dysgeusia, appear to be interfering with adequate oral intake.[17] Examples of these dietary strategies are listed in Table 42–1. Diet counseling from knowledgeable and skilled dietitians, particularly when their involvement is initiated early in the HSCT process, may help to prevent severe debilitation and enhance nutritional complications of the procedure.[5, 18]

NUTRITIONAL MANAGEMENT OF GRAFT-VERSUS-HOST DISEASE

One complication specifically associated with allogeneic HSCT, graft-versus-host disease (GVHD), can have a significant adverse effect on nutritional status because of the involvement of the gastrointestinal tract in the clinical presentation. Damage to the enterocytes and epithelium results in voluminous diarrhea related to deficiency of epithelial cell enzymes required for absorption of sugars, abnormal transport mechanisms, and protein and water exudation through the epithelium. The presence of acute or chronic GVHD usually precludes the ability to obtain adequate nutrients via the enteral route or from a regular oral diet.

In clinical practice, a phased dietary approach has been shown to be useful in the nutritional management of this complication,[18] as summarized in Table 42–2. The first phase consists of bowel rest with complete reliance on total parenteral nutrition to meet the needs for energy, protein, and micronutrients. When abdominal cramping is minimal and diarrhea is less than 500 mL/day, an oral diet of

isotonic clear liquids is initiated in the second phase of the regimen. If this second phase of nutrition management is tolerated for 4 or more days, progression can continue, although any resumption of cramping or increased gastrointestinal symptoms suggests the need to return to bowel rest. Solid foods are initiated in the third phase when minimal or no abdominal cramping is present and formed stool is observed, although the composition of the foods provided should be low in lactose, fiber, and fat (<20 g/day). Dairy foods (with the exception of aged cheese) are the primary source of dietary lactose, and fiber is found in whole-grain breads and cereals, bran, nuts, legumes, and vegetables and fruit. Foods that are high in total acidity or contain gastric irritants should also be avoided, particularly if patients complain that these foods irritate the mouth, so in practice the diet usually consists of bland and soft foods.

Throughout this progression, intravenous nutrition support should continue at a rate that ensures the provision of adequate energy and protein to enable tissue healing. When

TABLE 42–2. PHASED DIETARY MANAGEMENT OF GRAFT-VERSUS-HOST DISEASE

PHASE	DIET
I	Bowel rest (nothing by mouth), parenteral nutrition support
II	Oral, isosmotic, clear liquid diet (residue-free liquid nutritional supplements and dilute beverages, broth, and clear juice), continue parenteral nutrition support
III	Introduction of solid foods but low in lactose, fiber, and fat (<20 g/day), total acidity, and gastric irritants; continue parenteral nutrition support
IV	Continue expansion of diet but maintain low-lactose and low-fiber emphasis, limit foods high in total acidity and gastric irritants; continue parenteral nutrition support to meet energy and nutrient requirements
V	Expand diet to achieve a regular diet, introducing formerly restricted foods at a rate of one per day; discontinue parenteral nutrition when energy and nutrient requirements are met by the liberalized oral diet

Data from American Dietetic Association: Nutrition management following bone marrow transplantation. *In* Manual of Clinical Dietetics, 5th ed. Chicago, American Dietetic Association, 1996; Aker SN: Bone marrow transplantation: nutrition support and monitoring. *In* Bloch AS (ed): Nutrition Management of the Cancer Patient. Rockville, MD, Aspen Publishers, 1990.

the third phase is tolerated for 3–4 days, the diet may be expanded to the fourth phase but should continue to consist of foods that are low in lactose and fiber. In the fifth and final phase of this dietary approach, which is appropriate when no cramping is present and the stool and transit time are normal, a regular diet may be instituted, but the formerly restricted foods should be introduced at a rate of one per day so that tolerance can be monitored. Any evidence of steatorrhea indicates that regular dietary fat should be restricted, and more easily digested lipids such as medium-chain triglyceride oil may be used to supplement the diet. The intravenous (parenteral) nutrition support should continue until it has been demonstrated that adequate energy, protein, and other nutrients are being provided from the oral diet.

Patients with acute GVHD typically progress to a regular diet by 3–4 months after transplantation, although the rate of progression varies from patient to patient. In the management of chronic GVHD, the nutritional approach is basically what would be used in malabsorption syndrome, involving careful and consistent attention to nutritional monitoring with the goal of meeting the energy and nutritional requirements to promote recovery and prevent secondary problems due to nutrient inadequacies. Corticosteroids, typically used in the management of chronic GVHD, can cause glucose intolerance and hypertriglyceridemia, which should be managed with the dietary approaches used in the management of type II diabetes mellitus.

ROLE OF LOW-MICROBIAL DIETS

As an infection prevention strategy, low-microbial or sterile diets may be helpful in the management of immuncompromised transplant recipients. In the HSCT setting, neutropenia results from underlying disease, chemotherapy, or radiation therapy. By definition, a sterile diet consists of food and water that have no bacterial or fungal growth on culture[19] and is based on foods that have been steam-autoclaved or oven-baked for a prolonged period. In the provision of a sterile diet, food preparation and assembly of the meal must also be done aseptically in a laminar airflow hood, which imposes a substantial burden on a food service operation. In practice, the low-microbial or low-bacteria diet, which is less rigorous and is based primarily on empiric knowledge of the distribution of microorganisms in the food supply, is the nutritional approach usually used to reduce risk of infection that could be caused by foods. These diets are primarily cooked-food diets because the major limitation imposed is on fresh or uncooked food items.

In a few previous studies, the microbiologic content of several food items has been evaluated. In a study examining the foods appropriate for patients undergoing gastrointestinal decontamination who were maintained in protective isolation, Pizzo et al.[20] evaluated the microbial content of 236 foods and applied a criterion of less than 500 *Bacillus* organisms per mL as defining acceptability. Almost all beverages and breads, 70% or less of canned foods, cereals, frozen foods, and snack items, and less than 30% of processed meats and fresh fruits and vegetables were deemed acceptable. Foods given to patients undergoing HSCT have

also been evaluated for acceptability using a criterion of less than 10^3 colony-forming units of *Bacillus* organisms, diptheroids, or micrococci per milliliter and less than 10^3 colony-forming units of coagulase-negative staphylococci or *Streptococcus viridans* per milliliter.[21] Using these criteria more than 80% of beverages, starches, breads and cereals, cooked fresh meats, and mixed cooked entrees and frozen vegetables were found acceptable. In comparison, only 36% of pasteurized diary products and 42% of dessert and snack items met the criteria.

For most hospital food service operations, the low-microbial diet is basically the regular diet but served first off the tray assembly line and without fresh, raw vegetables and fresh fruits. Eliminating dairy foods, spices, nuts, and food items prepared with condiments from multiserving containers can further reduce risk for exposure to pathogen-containing foods. In addition to modification of the food choices, tray service items such as utensils and condiments are sterile and wrapped individually to reduce the risk of contamination.

Only a few previous studies have evaluated the acceptability and efficacy of low-microbial diets in the HSCT setting. The large variability in how these diets are actually defined across different medical facilities contributes to the difficulty of examining the clinical impact. One review of studies on immunosuppressed cancer patients treated with sterile, low-microbial, or regular diets concluded that current evidence cannot address the question of whether infection, morbidity, mortality, and response to therapy are affected.[22] Because many food restrictions are imposed with this strategy, the nutrient adequacy of actual food intake of patients who are prescribed the low-microbial diet should be monitored.

NUTRITIONAL ASSESSMENT AND MONITORING

No routine laboratory test is specific for nutrition, so the key to accurate nutritional assessment is to use information collectively. Data from anthropometric measurements, circulating hepatic secretory protein concentrations, nutrient intake assessment, and clinical features should all contribute to the assessment and monitoring of nutritional status. Although body weight is universally available, fluid balance can be markedly altered because of pathophysiologic condition and medications; thus, changes in body weight must be interpreted as a reflection of overall nutritional status in the context of the total clinical situation. Measurements of skinfold thickness and midarm muscle circumference are better indicators of the body compartments of greatest interest (i.e., adipose tissue, muscle mass). The use of electrical conductance, popularized as bioelectrical impedance, is based on the nature of the conduction of an applied electrical current, and estimates from these measures can be useful under controlled conditions. Alterations in body fluids and electrolytes (which are usually abnormal in the clinically ill patient and are modified by activity, meals, and other factors) can adversely influence the validity of the figures derived from bioelectrical impedence measurements, however.

Circulating concentrations of the hepatic secretory proteins can theoretically reflect energy balance, and the measurement usually available is the serum albumin concentration. This protein fraction accounts for 50–60% of the total serum protein concentration but has a relatively long half-life and is substantially affected by sepsis, edema, blood loss, and numerous other factors. In one study,[23] serum prealbumin and retinol-binding protein concentrations (two hepatic secretory proteins present in smaller concentrations and with shorter half-lives) were shown to be useful in the evaluation of nutrition repletion among children undergoing HSCT.

Biochemical vitamin and mineral assays are occasionally useful in the identification of nutrient deficiencies. Micronutrients are partitioned or compartmentalized in the body in various pools, such as an exchangeable pool or a storage pool. Whether or not circulating concentrations of these micronutrients reflect body storage pools or overall status is the key factor in determining the usefulness of clinically available laboratory measurements. Accurate interpretation of the nutrient concentration in tissues depends on knowledge of both dietary and nondietary influencing factors. In many circumstances, a more-sophisticated functional indicator may be a better approach to biochemical assessment.

Energy and nutrient intake can be monitored fairly easily with the hospitalized patient because enteral and parenteral nutrition support formulations and infusion rates are available and "calorie counts" can be ordered to obtain estimates of the intake of oral foods and beverages. For outpatient monitoring, patients or their caregivers can be taught and encouraged to keep food records,[5] which can be evaluated by a clinical dietitian as a key approach to monitoring intake over a longer period.

CONCLUSION

Inclusion of a dietitian in the multidisciplinary management team ensures that someone with specialized training and expertise in clinical nutrition will be involved in the nutritional care, assessment, and monitoring of patients undergoing HSCT. Timely and appropriate nutritional management can contribute enormously to a good course and quality of life for these patients.

REFERENCES

1. Papadopoulous A, Lloyd DR, Williams MD, et al: Gastrointestinal and nutritional sequelae of bone marrow transplantation. Arch Dis Child 75:208, 1996.
2. Weisdorf SA, Lysne J, Wind D, et al: Positive effect of prophylactic total parenteral nutrition on long-term outcome of bone mineral transplantation. Transplantation 43:833, 1987.
3. Lenssen P, Sherry ME, Cheney CL, et al: Prevalence of nutrition-related problems among long-term survivors of allogenic marrow transplantation. J Am Diet Assoc 90:835, 1990.
4. Rowe JM, Ciobanu N, Ascensao J, et al: Recommended guidelines for the management of autologous and allogeneic bone marrow transplantation: a report from the Eastern Cooperative Oncology Group (ECOG). Ann Intern Med 120:143, 1994.
5. Dickson TC: Clinical pathway nutrition management for outpatient bone marrow transplantation. J Am Diet Assoc 97:61, 1997.
6. Herrmann VM, Petruska PJ: Nutrition support in bone marrow transplant recipients. Nutr Clin Pract 8:19, 1993.
7. Cheney CL, Abson KG, Aker SN, et al: Body composition changes in marrow transplant receipients receiving total parenteral nutrition. Cancer 59:1515, 1987.
8. Rovelli A, Bonomi M, Murano A, et al: Severe lactic acidosis due to thiamine deficiency after bone marrow transplantation in a child with acute monocytic leukemia. Haematologica 75:579, 1990.
9. Clemens MR, Ladner C, Ehninger G, et al: Plasma vitamin E and β-carotene concentrations during radiochemotherapy preceding bone marrow transplantation. Am J Clin Nutr 51:216, 1990.
10. Harris JA, Benedict FG: A Biometric Study of Basal Metabolism in Man. Washington, DC, Carnegie Institute, 1919.
11. Szeluga DJ, Stuart RK, Brookmeyer R, et al: Energy requirements of parenterally fed bone marrow transplant patients. J Parenter Enteral Nutr 9:139, 1985.
12. Papadopoulou A, MacDonald A, Williams MD, et al: Enteral nutrition after bone marrow transplantation. Arch Dis Child 77:131, 1997.
13. Taveroff A, McArdle AH, Rybka WB: Reducing parenteral energy and protein intake improves metabolic homeostasis after bone marrow transplantation. Am J Clin Nutr 54:1087, 1991.
14. Charuhus PM, Fosberg KL, Bruemmer B, et al: A double-blind randomized trial comparing outpatient parenteral nutrition with intravenous hydration: effect on resumption of oral intake after marrow transplantation. J Parent Enteral Nutr 21:157, 1997.
15. Szeluga PJ, Stuart RK, Brookmayer R, et al: Nutritional support of bone marrow transplant recipients: a prospective, randomized clinical trial comparing total parenteral nutrition to an enteral feeding program. Cancer Res 47:3309, 1987.
16. Ziegler TR, Young LS, Benfell K, et al: Clinical and metabolic efficacy of glutamine-supplemented parenteral nutrition after bone marrow transplantation. Ann Intern Med 116:821, 1992.
17. American Dietetic Association: Nutrition management following bone marrow transplantation. In Manual of Clinical Dietetics, 5th ed. Chicago, American Dietetic Association, 1996, p 605.
18. Aker SN: Bone marrow transplantation: nutrition support and monitoring. In Bloch AS (ed): Nutrition Management of the Cancer Patient. Rockville, MD, Aspen Publishers, 1990, p 199.
19. Moe G: Enteral feeding and infection in the immunocompromised patient. Nutr Clin Pract 6:55, 1991.
20. Pizzo PA, Purvis DS, Waters C: Microbiological evaluation of food items. J Am Diet Assoc 81:272, 1982.
21. Moe GL: Low-microbial diets for patients with granulocytopenia. In Bloch AS (ed): Nutrition Management of the Cancer Patient. Rockville, MD, Aspen Publishers, 1990, p 125.
22. Aker SN, Cheney CL: The use of sterile and low microbial diets in ultraisolation environments. J Parent Enteral Nutr 7:390, 1983.
23. Uderzo C, Rovelli A, Bonomi M, et al: Total parenteral nutrition and nutritional assessment in leukaemic children undergoing bone marrow transplantation. Eur J Cancer 27:758, 1991.

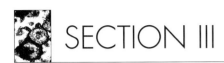

SECTION III

Complications

The Immediate Post-transplant Period

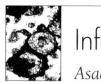

CHAPTER FORTY-THREE

Infection
Asad Bashey, M.D., Ph.D.

Increased susceptibility to infections has been a challenge to the clinical practice of hematopoietic stem cell (HSC) transplantation (HSCT) since its inception. Infections are a major cause of post-transplantation mortality in patients after allogeneic and autologous HSCT. Advances in infection therapy and prophylaxis have helped improve the results of HSCT. They have also led to shifts in the relative frequency of infections caused by different organisms and the time periods of susceptibility to the infections. This chapter focuses on the management of infective complications of HSCT in the first 3 months after transplantation. Prevention of infections and management of late infections are discussed in Chapters 36, 38, and 53.

FACTORS LEADING TO INCREASED SUSCEPTIBILITY TO INFECTIONS

Several sequelae of HSCT are responsible for the increased susceptibility to infections characteristic of the post-transplantation period. Recognition of these factors is essential to the management of infections in the patient undergoing HSCT because eradication of specific infections (e.g., invasive aspergillosis) often depends on abrogation of the causes of increased susceptibility (e.g., neutropenia). Often the infection can only be controlled until endogenous host defenses recover. The intensity and duration of these breaches in host defense are related to the nature of the conditioning regimen, the type of grafts (e.g., autologous vs. allogeneic, bone marrow vs. peripheral blood progenitor cells [PBPC]), and the occurrence of other transplant complications and their management.

NEUTROPENIA

Neutropenia is an expected complication of both autologous and allogeneic HSCT. The depth and the duration of neutropenia are independent risk factors for bacterial and fungal infections. Risk increases significantly when the absolute neutrophil count (ANC) is less than 500/mm^3, and most life-threatening bacterial infections occur when the ANC is less than 100/mm^3.[1, 2] The duration of neutropenia is related to the infused HSC dose, the occurrence of infections in the post-transplantation setting, and the use of post-HSCT hematopoietic growth factors.[3] For autologous HSCT, the use of ex vivo purging of tumor cells with cytotoxic agents or antibodies can further slow engraftment.[4] For allogeneic HSCT, the use of cytotoxic agents (e.g., methotrexate) after HSCT for immunosuppression

and factors increasing the possibility of immunologic rejection (e.g., increased human leukocyte antigen [HLA] disparity between donor and recipient, inadequate immunosuppressive conditioning of the recipient, or T-cell depletion of the graft) can also prolong the period of neutropenia.[5, 6] The median duration of neutropenia (ANC < 500/mm^3) is shorter after HSCT derived from PBPC than after bone marrow transplant.[7, 8]

BREAKDOWN OF PHYSICAL BARRIERS

Mucositis produced by chemotherapy and radiation aids the entry of endogenous bacteria from the gastrointestinal tract into the blood stream. Although mucositis is most evident in the buccal and pharyngeal mucosa, it is indicative of loss of mucosal integrity throughout the gastrointestinal tract. The degree of mucositis differs with different conditioning regimens—regimens including etoposide, melphalan, thiotepa, busulfan, cytarabine, anthracyclines, and taxanes as well as total body irradiation—are particularly likely to produce clinically significant mucosal toxicity. The use of methotrexate after allogeneic HSCT can further exacerbate mucositis.[9] Reactivation of herpes simplex virus type 1 in the immediate post-transplantation period can produce severe oropharyngeal and esophageal ulceration. Prophylactic acyclovir can effectively prevent this complication.[10] Neutrophils are an important component of mucosal integrity, and full recovery from mucositis is often associated with recovery from neutropenia. Mucosal integrity can be breached by active gastrointestinal graft-versus-host disease (GVHD) after recovery from the conditioning regimen.[11] Sepsis from enteric organisms is often the cause of death in patients with severe acute GVHD of the gastrointestinal tract.

The use of indwelling venous catheters for HSCT is routine. Venous catheter–associated sepsis from gram-positive organisms is among the most common infections acquired in neutropenic patients.[12] The use of fluoroquinolone prophylaxis against gram-negative organisms during the neutropenic period has also contributed to this complication.

DEFECTS IN CELLULAR AND HUMORAL IMMUNITY

Defects in T- and B-cell reconstitution are present for months to years after allogeneic HSCT and are exacerbated by the presence of GVHD.[13, 14] CD4+ cell numbers and the CD4/CD8 ratio are depressed for 6–9 months after uncomplicated allogeneic HSCT and may not recover adequately in the presence of chronic GVHD. This is accompanied by functional defects in T-cell responses to mitogen and susceptibility to viral infections, especially herpes simplex, varicella zoster, cytomegalovirus, and Epstein-Barr virus.[14, 15] Although B-cell numbers return to pretransplantation levels by 1–2 months after HSCT, functional abnormalities are detectable for much longer. This is partly related to the deficiency in T-helper cell function during this period.[16, 17] Immunoglobulin IgG levels are diminished for 6–9 months unless replaced using intravenous immunoglobulin; IgM and IgA levels are diminished for longer periods of time. This produces a predisposition to infections with encapsulated bacteria, which can be prolonged by chronic GVHD.[18]

Immune reconstitution after autologous HSCT has been less well studied. Although diminished CD4+ numbers and ratios may be present for 4–9 months and perturbations in immunoglobulin production can also be detected for 2–3 months, these patients are much less susceptible to the associated infections than patients undergoing allogeneic HSCT.[19]

BACTERIAL INFECTIONS

The type of bacterial infections varies with time after HSCT. During the neutropenic phase, more than 90% of infections are bacterial. Enteric gram-negative pathogens (e.g., *Escherichia coli*, *Klebsiella*, *Enterobacter*, and *Pseudomonas aeruginosa*) are among the most life-threatening infections during this period. Their propensity to induce rapidly progressive hemodynamic collapse necessitates empirical antibiotic therapy in all patients with neutropenic fever.[20] The use of prophylactic antibiotics that target gram-negative organisms and the almost universal use of indwelling venous catheters has led to the emergence of gram-positive organisms, especially *Staphylococcus epidermidis* and α-hemolytic *Streptococcus*, as the most common causes of bacteremia in the neutropenic period.[12, 21] *Staphylococcus aureus* remains among the most potentially life-threatening of these organisms but is encountered less frequently. Recurrent fevers occurring after treatment of the first febrile episode are more likely to involve antibiotic-resistant organisms. Resistant gram-negative organisms and vancomycin-resistant *Enterococcus* organisms can be rapidly life-threatening unless recognized early and appropriately treated.

Bacterial infections in the mid- to late post-transplantation period (or days after HSCT) are usually catheter-acquired (*Staphylococcus* species or gram-negative species) or enteric organisms acquired in the presence of ongoing gastrointestinal GVHD. In the presence of chronic GVHD, pneumonias and septicemia caused by encapsulated organisms are frequent in the absence of adequate prophylaxis.

MANAGEMENT OF FEBRILE NEUTROPENIA IMMEDIATELY AFTER HSCT

The majority of initial febrile episodes exceeding 101°F (38.3°C) in neutropenic patients (ANC < 500/mm³ or

500–1000/mm³ and expected to fall below 500/mm³) result from bacterial infections. Furthermore, these infections have a potential to be rapidly life-threatening in the context of neutropenia. Recognition of these factors has led to the widespread acceptance of the need for rapid institution of empirical broad-spectrum antibiotic coverage for neutropenic patients experiencing their first febrile episode.

Blood cultures obtained from both the central venous catheter and a peripheral vein are mandatory prior to institution of therapy. Evaluation for a potential site of origin of the sepsis includes physical examination of the oropharynx, skin, intravenous catheter sites, perianal area, and chest with directed cultures if abnormalities are detected at these sites. A chest radiograph is routinely performed to evaluate the possibility of pneumonia.

Many factors are considered in determining the appropriate regimen for the individual patient. They include the type, frequency, and antibiotic sensitivities of bacteria isolated in similar patients at the same hospital, organ dysfunction (e.g., renal, ocular, or hepatic), and known drug allergies. The nature of the initial antibiotic regimen has been an area of debate for some time. The guidelines developed by the Infectious Diseases Society of America for the management of neutropenic patients with unexplained fever, however, are helpful.[22] A schema based on the Society's recommendations is shown in Figure 43–1. Three main approaches are feasible.

Monotherapy with broad-spectrum agents (i.e., ceftazidime or imipenem) has been demonstrated to be statistically equivalent to multidrug combinations in several randomized comparisons.[23–25] Advantages of this approach include simplicity, lack of major toxicity, and cost. These agents, however, show little activity against *Staphylococcus epidermidis* or methicillin-resistant *S. aureus*, penicillin-resistant streptococci, or enterococci. They often neccesitate the addition of further antibiotics once positive cultures have been obtained. Few data support the use of quinolone monotherapy in this context, and it cannot be regarded as the standard of care. The "fourth-generation" cephalosporin, cefepime, has enhanced coverage of both gram-positive and gram-negative organisms and is undergoing trials for this indication, as is the new carbapenem, meropenem.

Duotherapy with the combination of an aminoglycoside with an antipseudomonal β-lactam antibiotic is another potential approach. Advantages include potential synergy against some gram-negative bacteria and decreased likelihood of the emergence of resistant organisms during therapy. The major disadvantages are the need for serum level monitoring, nephrotoxicity, ototoxicity, electrolyte disturbances, and failure to cover some gram-positive species, especially methicillin-resistant staphylococci and enterococci.

The third commonly used strategy is to combine vancomycin with one of the other two approaches as a means of providing more comprehensive gram-positive coverage from the start of therapy. The rationale for this approach is based on the increased frequency of gram-positive infections that are susceptible only to vancomycin. Vancomycin, however, is expensive, may cause cytopenia and nephrotoxicity as well as the infusion-associated "red man syndrome," and may lead to the development of nosocomial vancomy-

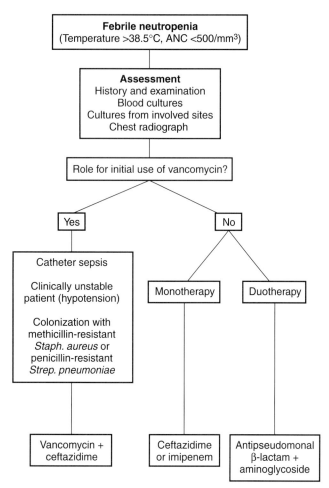

FIGURE 43–1. Schema for the initial management of the patient with febrile neutropenia undergoing hematopoietic stem cell therapy. Note that aminoglycosides should be avoided in patients with renal dysfunction or who are receiving concurrent nephrotoxic or ototoxic medication. Empiric therapy should be reassessed after 72 hours in the light of culture results and clinical response. ANC, absolute neutrophil count. (Adapted from Hughes WT et al: 1997 Guidelines for the use of antimicrobial agents in neutropenic patients with unexplained fever: Infectious Diseases Society of America. Clin Infect Dis 25[3]:551–573, 1997.)

cin-resistant or -dependent organisms, especially enterococci. Although vancomycin appears to increase the response rates when used to treat febrile neutropenias as part of the initial empirical regimen, toxicity is also increased. Overall survival of patients treated in this way appears no better than those treated with a more conventional empirical regimen.[26] A major factor in these findings is that the majority of gram-positive infections encountered by neutropenic patients are not immediately life-threatening and respond readily to the addition of vancomycin once they are identified. Given the seriousness of the emergence of vancomycin resistance,[27] the empirical use of vancomycin in all patients with neutropenia-associated fever cannot be routinely recommended. Instead, the judicious empirical use of vancomycin when clinically indicated (e.g., obvious catheter-related infections, seriously ill patients with hypotension or other signs of hemodynamic compromise in which a gram-positive infection is suspected or in institutions where virulent gram-positive organisms are prevalent) is a more prudent approach.

SUBSEQUENT MANAGEMENT OF THE EMPIRICAL ANTIBIOTIC REGIMEN

Because 2–7 days (median, 5 days) are normally required to effect defervescence in patients with febrile neutropenia secondary to chemotherapy, it is important that the initial empirical regimen be allowed at least 3 days to prove efficacy. Culture results are usually available at this stage to allow informed reassessment. An exception to this practice is the patient who deteriorates rapidly within 3 days, necessitating earlier reassessment. If an organism has been identified, a guided change in antibiotics to provide optimal coverage with minimal cost should be made, if necessary. Broad-spectrum coverage is usually maintained until neutrophil recovery, however. If defervescence is observed but no organism is identified, it is recommended that the empirical regimen be continued for at least 7 days or until the ANC is greater than 500/mm³.

If the patient has persistent fever after 3 days and no organism has been identified, other causes should be considered. These include drug-resistant bacterial infection, bacterial infection at a "privileged" site (e.g., poorly perfused abcess, intravenous catheter site) nonbacterial infection, and fever caused by medications. Assessment at this stage usually includes a repeat of the initial evaluation, chest and sinus radiographs, and serum drug levels. Abdominal computed tomography or sonography may help to identify loculated infections. Changes in therapy can be made between 4 and 7 days after starting the initial regimen, depending on the patient's condition and the results of reassessment. Replacement of ceftazidime with imipenem provides a broader spectrum of coverage. Addition of an aminoglycoside to a β-lactam–based regimen may provide synergy against resistant gram-negative organisms. Addition of vancomycin is appropriate if a gram-positive organism is suspected or the patient is clinically unstable.

Patients who remain febrile and profoundly neutropenic after 5–7 days of broad-spectrum antibiotics should be considered for the introduction of empirical antifungal therapy with systemic amphotericin B. Such therapy is directed at occult *Candida* infections. It must be noted, however, that less than one third of febrile neutropenia patients who do not respond to a week of broad-spectrum antibiotic therapy have a systemic fungal infection.[28]

Interest in outpatient management of febrile neutropenia has increased in recent years. The shortened duration of neutropenia associated with peripheral blood progenitor cell (PBPC) transplantation, the widespread availability of home infusion services and ambulatory infusion pumps, and considerations of cost and patient comfort have led to autologous HSCT in an outpatient setting. A number of studies in both transplant recipients and non–transplant-related febrile neutropenia have demonstrated the safety and efficacy of this approach when used for selected patients.[29–32] This approach is suitable for patients defined as having low risk (i.e., no clinical evidence of immediately life-threatening septicemia [e.g., hypotension], no serious focal infection [e.g., pneumonia], stable underlying malignancy, no major comorbidity). Regimens using once-daily intravenous antibiotics (e.g., ceftriaxone, vancomycin) and oral antibiotics (e.g., ofloxacin) have been evaluated in this context and found to be effective in some studies.[30–32] More detailed studies are necessary before such regimens can be generally recommended, however.

OTHER SUPPORTIVE MEASURES DURING FEBRILE NEUTROPENIA

Hematopoietic growth factors are widely used after autologous and allogeneic HSCT. Although several randomized studies have demonstrated a statistically significant acceleration of neutrophil recovery, benefits in reduction of morbidity or antibiotic use have been more difficult to demonstrate.[33–35] Further, it is unclear whether these benefits also occur when growth factors are added to patients in established febrile neutopenia after HSCT. No study has demonstrated a reduction in infection-related mortality. Thus, the routine addition of hematopoietic growth factors in patients with fever and neutropenia cannot be recommended, especially when PBPC are used as the source of HSCT. Instead, their use must be based on judicious assessment of the importance of the relatively small acceleration of neutrophil engraftment that is achievable by this approach.

The use of granulocyte transfusions in febrile neutropenic patients after HSCT is also of uncertain benefit. Whereas such transfusion was once relatively common, it has been used less frequently since the mid-1980s because of the risk of cytomegalovirus (CMV) transmission and lack of clearly demonstrable efficacy. The use of CMV-screened donors and the potential of using large numbers of granulocytes derived from donors treated with granulocyte colony-stimulating factor (G-CSF) or granulocyte macrophage colony-stimulating factor (GM-CSF) has rekindled interest in this therapy. Comprehensive studies assessing the efficacy of this approach after HSCT are lacking.

FUNGAL INFECTIONS

The frequency of post-HSCT fungal infections has been increasing since the 1980s. This is particularly apparent after allogeneic HSCT, with which the incidence of fungal infection is approximately 10 times greater than that after autologous HSCT.[36, 37] Among the factors associated with this epidemiologic shift is the successful prophylaxis and treatment of bacterial and viral infections, especially CMV, after HSCT. Aspergillosis is now the most common cause of death from infection after allogeneic HSCT.

The four main categories of fungal pathogens are listed in Table 43–1. Infections caused by *Candida* and infections of the respiratory tract caused by *Aspergillus* are the most common fungal infections encountered after HSCT. They are discussed in more detail later. The other listed pathogens are much less common as causes of disease in the post-HSCT setting. They may be more frequently encountered in institutions that use prophylactic regimens targeting *Candida* and *Aspergillus*, however.

Cryptococcus causes subacute or acute infections typically involving the meninges and brain. Patients with severe deficiency of cellular immunity (e.g., HIV-infected patients) are more susceptible than patients with neutropenia. Occasional infections occur in allogeneic HSCT recipients on immunosuppressive therapy for acute or chronic GVHD.

TABLE 43–1. CLASSIFICATION OF FUNGAL PATHOGENS IN PATIENTS UNDERGOING HEMATOPOIETIC CELL TRANSPLANTATION

Yeast pathogens	Moulds (dematiaceous)
Candida spp.	*Pseudoallescheria boydii*
Cryptococcus neoformans	*Bipolaris* spp.
Trichosporon beigelii	*Scedosporium* spp.
Moulds (hyaline)	Dimorphic fungi
Aspergillus spp.	*Coccidioides immitis*
Fusarium spp.	*Histoplasma capsulatum*
Mucormycosis	*Blastomyces dermatitidis*
organisms	

Although the organism is usually sensitive to fluconazole, amphotericin B with 5-fluorocytosine remains the choice for active disease in the post-transplantation setting.

Trichosporon organisms are responsible for superficial infections of the hair shaft in immunocompetent patients. Rarely does disseminated and rapidly fatal infection (trichosporonosis) occur in neutropenic patients on corticosteroids. Renal infection with urinary involvement is characteristic. The organism has only limited sensitivity to amphotericin.[38] Fluconazole has been found to be active, but detailed studies of its use in this context are not available.

Mucormycosis refers to severe angiocentric necrotizing infections originating in the respiratory tract caused by hyaline molds of *Rhizopus, Rhizomucor,* and *Cunninghamella*.[39] Patients with uncontrolled diabetes are most at risk, but sporadic infections occur in neutropenic or steroid-treated HSC recipients. Prior long-term therapy with desferrioxamine is an added risk factor. Amphotericin B in maximally tolerated doses is the treatment of choice. Surgical excision of sinus and facial lesions may aid the therapy. Survival is rare in pulmonary mucormycosis.

Pseudoallescheria boydii and *Fusarium* organisms cause respiratory tract infections with clinical patterns similar to those seen with *Aspergillus*. They are substantially less sensitive to amphotericin B, requiring greatly increased dosing or the use of investigational agents. *Pseudoallescheria* may respond to high-dose combinations of amphotericin with a triazole drug.

Infections caused by *Malassezia* in patients undergoing HSCT are usually associated with hyperalimentation using intravenous lipids. Clinical manifestations can include fever, thrombocytopenia, and pulmonary infiltrates.[40] Discontinuation of the lipid preparation and removal of the catheter are important components of therapy.

Endemic mycoses caused by the dimorphic fungi (e.g., *Histoplasma capsulatum* and *Coccidioides immitis*) are relatively uncommon after HSCT.[41] Occasional cases occur in persons from the southwestern United States or the Ohio and Mississipi river valleys. Amphotericin B is the treatment of choice.

CANDIDIASIS

Candida organisms are normal commensals of mucous membranes of the gastrointestinal tract in more than half of normal persons.[42] The organism can behave as an opportunistic pathogen when factors that maintain the normal host-commensal relationship are disturbed. *C. albicans* is the most common cause of candidiasis, but *C. tropicalis, C. krusei, C. glabrata, C. parapsilosis,* and *C. lusitaniae* infections are well recognized.[37, 43, 44] Risk factors for candidiasis are prolonged neutropenia (especially for *C. albicans, C. tropicalis,* and *C. krusei*), impaired cellular immunity after allogeneic HSCT (especially in patients on therapy for GVHD), diabetes mellitus, mucositis, indwelling intravenous catheters (especially for *C. parapsilosis*), and broad-spectrum antibiotic use. Only *C. albicans* and *C. tropicalis* are sensitive to fluconazole—these species were responsible for more than 70% of all candidal infections in earlier series.[37] Infections with the other *Candida* species are assuming greater importance following the widespread use of fluconazole prophylaxis in patients undergoing HSCT.[43, 44]

Candida infections are mostly encountered in the neutropenic phase after HSCT. Prior to the use of fluconazole prophylaxis, median time of onset of *Candida* infections was day 15 after HSCT.[37] Patients undergoing allogeneic HSCT on immunosuppressive therapy after engraftment face a second, prolonged risk period. Clinical syndromes vary with severity of predisposing illness and species, and they range from superficial mucosal infection to deeply invasive infection that may be limited to a single organ or be widely disseminated.[37] *Oropharyngeal candidiasis (thrush)* presents as discrete and confluent adherent white mucosal plaques. Although the clinical appearance is often characteristic, definitive diagnosis can be made using microscopic examination of a wet-mount or Gram stain for fungal forms. Thrush has become relatively rare in the post-HSCT setting because of the frequent use of prophylactic fluconazole or clotrimazole troches. Both agents are highly effective in treating candidiasis limited to this site. *Esophageal candidiasis* presents as dysphagia and retrosternal pain. It is difficult to distinguish clinically from severe esophageal mucositis caused by the conditioning regimen, herpes simplex virus, or CMV esophagitis or bacterial infections. Thus, endoscopy may be necessary to establish the diagnosis. Treatment of esophageal candidiasis is with fluconazole or amphotericin B until symptoms and neutropenia resolve.

Blood-stream infection with *Candida* may present with fever and systemic symptoms but few localizing symptoms. Up to 45% of candidemia may occur without documented tissue involvement.[37] The mortality rate of such patients is lower than when candidemia is a component of multiorgan involvement. Specialized blood culture techniques (e.g., the lysis centrifugation system) have increased the sensitivity of blood culture for *Candida*. False-positive results are rare, and therefore an initial course of amphotericin B is the treatment of choice in all neutropenic patients with documented candidemia.[45] A starting dose of 0.5–1 mg/kg/day is usually recommended.

A prospective observational study of candidemia not limited to patients undergoing HSCT found no difference in mortality between lower (<500 mg total dose) and higher (> 500 mg) doses.[46] However, patients at risk for infection with non-*albicans* species of *Candida* (e.g., patients experiencing candidemia while on fluconazole prophylaxis) may require higher doses (up to 1.5 mg/kg/day). No convincing evidence favors a gradual escalation of amphotericin dosage in patients with candidemia—such an approach may allow for the persistence of candidemia after the commencement of therapy and lead to more advanced infections.

Although removal of the central venous catheter was associated with an improved outcome in the analysis by Nguyen et al.,[46] most practitioners remove the catheter only if the blood cultures remain positive for more than 48 hours during therapy. Patients with persistent candidemia and those with *Candida tropicalis* infections may benefit from the addition of 5-flucytosine to their regimen.[45] Flucytosine, however, can suppress hematopoiesis and engraftment. Thus, its use must be carefully balanced against the risk of prolonging neutropenia.

Some existing data indicate that fluconazole may be an effective substitute for amphotericin B in the treatment of candidiasis for patients who are clinically stable and not expected to have prolonged neutropenia.[46] Multiorgan involvement by *Candida* in neutropenic patients may include central nervous system, ophthalmic, and cardiac disease.[37] Such patients have a universally poor prognosis, with mortality rates close to 100% in most series. *Hepatosplenic candidiasis* is a relatively chronic infection syndrome that is typically subclinical during the neutropenic phase, when it is presumably seeded. After the patient recovers from neutropenia, the condition may present as fever, abdominal discomfort, nausea, vomiting, and a rising white blood cell count.[37, 47] These patients are usually less unwell than neutropenic patients with systemic candidiasis. Although radiologic appearances obtained through magnetic resonance imaging (MRI) or computed tomography (CT) can be suggestive, definitive diagnosis requires a liver biopsy. The lesions are often difficult to treat. It is thought that the organism enters a vegetative state that is relatively resistant to agents that target the cell wall. Amphotericin B (1.0–1.5 mg/kg/day) plus flucytosine has been the standard of care. There are some reports of the activity of fluconazole in this disease in cases resistant to amphotericin and flucytosine.[48]

INVASIVE ASPERGILLOSIS

Aspergillus pathogens normally grow in septate hyphal forms on dead and decaying vegetation. The conidiospores of these fungi are 3- to 5-μm ubiquitous airborne particles. Inhalation of spores by any individual is common. Invasive infection, however, usually only occurs in immunosuppressed hosts who possess a combination of the following risk factors: neutropenia (typically, ANC < 500/mm^3 for longer than 7–10 days), supraphysiologic doses of glucocorticoid drugs, and a history of cytotoxic drug therapy.[36, 49]

Patients undergoing HSCT have two major risk periods: the neutropenic phase and GVHD with immunosuppressive medication. Although most *Aspergillus* infections in HSCT are sporadic events, outbreaks of infection may be associated with construction work or contamination of ventilation systems. *A. fumigatus* and *A. flavus* are the most commonly involved species. *A. niger* is encountered only rarely as a pathogen.[36] The lungs are the most commonly involved site. Fever and cough productive of clear or blood-tinged sputum is common. Dyspnea and frank hemoptysis are typically late features associated with fatal progression of the disease.[36]

Radiologic features include nodular infiltrates and bronchopneumonia. Although cavitation of nodules is characteristic, it may be associated with neutrophil recovery and healing of the lesions.[50] Sputum culture and microscopy may be helpful but they are insensitive. Bronchoalveolar lavage (BAL) is the investigation of choice—any positive isolate of *Aspergillus* from BAL has a high degree of correlation with invasive infection,[51] and differences in outcome are insignificant whether BAL or tissue biopsy is used for diagnosis.[36] BAL results may be negative in up to 50% of patients with invasive aspergillosis. Thus, open-lung biopsy is usually indicated in patients with radiologic features of aspergillosis but negative BAL results.

The respiratory sinuses are less commonly the portal of infection with *Aspergillus*. Because *Aspergillus* organisms are inherently less sensitive to amphotericin than *Candida*, high-dose therapy—1.0–1.5 mg/kg/day for a total dose of 3–5 g—is standard. Some clinicians add flucytosine or rifampin to the therapy, but the efficacy of such measures has not been proven in clinical trials. Resection of isolated pulmonary lesions may be beneficial,[52] and surgery is an important component of the treatment of sinus infections. Amelioration of the predisposing factors, especially neutropenia and high-dose corticosteroids, is important to recovery from invasive aspergillosis.

NEWER ANTIFUNGAL DRUGS

Three preparations of amphotericin B in association with lipid vehicles are now available in the United States. AmBisome is the only liposomal formulation, whereas Abelcet and Amphotec are complexed with lipid in ribbon- and disk-like structures, respectively. Randomized studies show that these preparations appear to have at least equivalent efficacy but reduced nephrotoxicity compared with standard amphotericin B deoxycholate.[53, 54] AmBisome appears to have a significantly reduced incidence of infusion-related toxicities. Although these agents have not been shown to produce superior outcomes when used from the start in proven fungal infections, some data indicate a reduced incidence of emergent fungal infections when these agents are used in the empirical setting.[54] Furthermore, some studies have demonstrated a response to the lipid formulations in patients whose condition progresses during standard amphotericin therapy.[55] The significantly increased drug costs of the lipid formulations, however, have limited their use in most centers to patients intolerant of, or worsening on, standard amphotericin therapy.

Itraconazole is a newer triazole antifungal that demonstrates activity against *Candida* and *Aspergillus*. Although the clinical activity of this drug against *Aspergillus* has been documented,[56] no randomized prospective studies of its use in active fungal infection have been reported. In practice, its use has been limited by the lack of a parenteral preparation, the erratic absorption of the drug (improved by the newer cyclodextrin formulation), and the potential for drug interactions through modulations of the cytochrome P450 system. Its widest use in HSCT has been in the prevention of fungal infections in at-risk but clinically stable patients.

Voriconazole is a new triazole drug that demonstrates very broad antifungal activity in vitro, including *Aspergillus* species and *Candida krusei*,[57] which are highly resistant to fluconazole. Although only case reports have documented the efficacy of this drug against *Aspergillus*, larger studies are underway.

VIRAL INFECTIONS

Although viral infections have now been supplanted by *Aspergillus* as the most common cause of infection-related death after allogeneic HSCT, they remain an important cause of post-HSCT morbidity and mortality. The Herpesviridae are the most prominent viral pathogens in the post-HSCT setting. The risk periods for the three main herpes virus infections are sequential. Herpes simplex infections predominate in the first 30 days following both allogeneic and autologous HSCT in the absence of adequate prophylaxis. After allogeneic HSCT in which either the donor or the recipient is seropositive for CMV, infections with this virus were common between 1 and 3 months in patients not receiving prophylactic or pre-emptive therapy.[58] Infections caused by Varicella zoster typically occur after day 100 but occur occasionally in the early post-HSCT period.

CYTOMEGALOVIRUS INFECTIONS

CMV is the largest of the herpesviruses known to infect humans. It has a 240-kb genome that encodes nearly 200 proteins.[59] After clinical infection, the virus can exist in a latent phase or a phase of active replication with the production of infectious virus. CMV infection is not known to cause any recognized illness in immunocompetent persons. A number of clinical disease states have been described in immunocompromised persons, however. The nature of the immunocompromise dictates the type of disease. In the HSCT setting, interstitial pneumonitis, enteritis, and bone marrow suppression are the major clinical phenomena attributed to CMV infection. The neurotropic syndromes in patients with HIV disease are rare in HSCT patients.

Approximately 30–45% of the adult population is seropositive for CMV.[60] In previously exposed persons, the virus exists in a latent state in several cell types, including endothelial cells and monocytes.[61, 62] CMV infection can follow HSCT as a primary infection in seronegative patients, reactivation of latent virus in seropositive patients, or reinfection/superinfection with a new strain in seropositive patients.[63] CMV infection is defined as the isolation or identification of CMV from any site or seroconversion in the absence of passive transfer of antibodies. CMV disease refers to clinical manifestations that can be attributed to CMV that occur in conjunction with evidence of infection.

Current practice in blood banking has decreased the risk of transfusion-related CMV infection of seropositive persons undergoing HSCT to negligible levels. Strategies include use of blood products from CMV-screened donors and depletion of leukocytes by filtration.[64] Furthermore, the use of pharmacologic prophylaxis of CMV infection or early-detection strategies with pre-emptive therapy in transplant recipients wherein either the recipient or the donor is seropositive has led to a decline in CMV disease and associated mortality in the first 100 days following HSCT.[65, 66] These approaches, however, may have resulted in an increase in late (beyond day 100) infections with CMV. In patients undergoing autologous or syngeneic HSCT, evidence of reactivation of CMV can readily be found in seropositive persons; however, the incidence of CMV disease is much lower than it is after allogeneic HSCT.[67] Other risk factors associated with development of CMV disease include increasing age of recipient and the occurrence of GVHD requiring increased doses of immunosuppressive drugs.[68]

CMV Interstitial Pneumonitis

CMV interstitial pneumonitis (CMV-IP) is potentially the most life-threatening of the disease states associated with CMV reactivation in the setting of HSCT. Prior to the use of preventive strategies, CMV-IP occurred in 15–25% of patients.[69] Time of onset was typically between days 30 and 100 following allogeneic HSCT. The disease presents with hypoxia, often with fevers and cytopenia. Chest radiology typically demonstrates infiltrates in an interstitial pattern with a basilar predominance. The radiologic appearance can be quite variable, however. The diagnosis is confirmed using BAL with demonstration of cytologic or antigenic evidence of CMV.[70] If left untreated, the disease has an anticipated mortality rate of greater than 80%.[71] Although several antiviral agents show good inhibitory activity against CMV in vitro, the use of antiviral drugs alone has been unable to significantly improve outcomes in established CMV-IP (reviewed in reference 72). These results implied that the mortality of CMV-IP was aided by factors other than the direct cytopathic effect of the virus.

The combination of ganciclovir and high doses of intravenous immunoglobulin (IVIG) (normal or CMV-hyperimmune) has reduced the mortality rate in patients with established CMV-IP to 30–50%.[73, 74] Combination therapy with ganciclovir and IVIG has now become the recommended standard in patients with established CMV-IP. The recommended schedule is ganciclovir, 10 mg/kg daily, with IVIG, 500 mg/kg every other day, for 21 days followed by ganciclovir, 5 mg/kd/day for 5 days per week and IVIG, 500 mg/kg weekly, until day 180 following HSCT. Using this schedule, 80% survival was achieved at 6 weeks after the start of therapy.[75]

Therapy usually causes rapid resolution of fever and hypoxia, although radiologic lesions can persist for several weeks. Clinical deterioration on therapy may be a sign of ganciclovir resistance and should be investigated with repeat BAL. Persistence of CMV on BAL specimens after 14–21 days of adequate ganciclovir-based therapy is usually an indication of resistant disease. In such patients, foscarnet may be used at a dose of 60 mg/kg, three times daily for 7 days, followed by 90 mg/kg/day until day 180 following HSCT.[76, 77] Primary toxicities of ganciclovir are neutropenia and renal impairment.[65] It is customary to add G-CSF or GM-CSF if the ANC falls to less than 1000/mm³ and to hold the drug if the ANC is less than 500 mm³. Dose reductions are also necessary for patients with a creatinine clearance of less than 60 mL/min. Renal toxicity is the main adverse event associated with the use of foscarnet.[76, 77]

This necessitates careful monitoring of renal function and dose adjustments based on creatinine clearance.

CMV Enteropathy

Infection by CMV in the patient undergoing HSCT can affect both the lower and the upper gastrointestinal tract.[78] Dysphagia, abdominal pain, nausea/vomiting, diarrhea, and gastrointestinal bleeding can all be presenting symptoms and have a wide differential diagnosis in the setting of HSCT.[78] Mucosal ulceration with characteristic inclusion bodies in epithelial and endothelial cells are the pathognomonic histologic findings. Treatment of CMV enteropathy has been based on regimens found to be effective against CMV-IP. Most clinicians use a combination of ganciclovir and immunoglobulin in symptomatic infection. Systematic studies of therapy in CMV enteropathy have been infrequent, and the outcome with therapy is uncertain.

Pre-emptive Therapy

The mortality of symptomatic CMV disease in the HSCT setting remains high even with the use of combination therapy.[73–75] Although universal prophylaxis with ganciclovir can effectively prevent reactivation of CMV during the period of its use, it is associated with significant neutropenia and its cost can be prohibitive. The use of monitoring for CMV infection post HSCT (using culture, polymerase chain reaction, or antigenemia methods) followed by pre-emptive therapy upon virus detection has been shown to effectively prevent CMV disease in patients undergoing HSCT. Ganciclovir is used at a dose of 5 mg/kg twice daily for 7–14 days, followed by 5 mg/kg/day until day 100 or 120 following transplantation.[79, 80] In patients who are intolerant of ganciclovir, foscarnet at a dose of 60 mg/kg twice daily for 14 days followed by maintenance therapy can be used instead. Prophylaxis against viral infection is discussed in Chapter 36.

HERPES SIMPLEX

More than 80% of adults are seropositive for herpes simplex virus (HSV).[81] Prior to the use of acyclovir prophylaxis in the peri-HSCT period, more than 70% of these patients would demonstrate virologic evidence of reactivation of latent virus (median, 17 days after commencement of preparative regimen).[82] A substantial proportion of these patients had symptomatic HSV infection. Infections of the lips, buccal cavity, pharynx, and esophagus occurred in 85%, with 15% of patients experiencing genital disease. Ulceration at these sites provides a portal for potentially serious bacterial infections during the neutropenic period. HSV-induced encephalitis, pneumonia, and hepatitis were more rarely witnessed.

Acyclovir, when used prophylactically, is highly effective in suppressing reactivation-induced disease in the post-HSCT setting.[83] Most centers use acyclovir (oral, 800 mg twice daily or 200 mg four times daily; intravenous, 5 mg/kg two or three times daily) from a few days prior to HSCT until hematopoietic recovery or patient discharge. HSV resistant to acyclovir is more likely to emerge if the drug is used to treat symptomatic disease than if used prophylactically.[84] In patients who experience symptomatic disease when not on prophylaxis, acyclovir (400 mg five times daily po; 5–10 mg/kg three times daily IV for 7–10 days) may shorten the duration of symptomatic disease and viral shedding.[85] Newer prodrugs (e.g., valacyclovir, famciclovir) have greater bioavailability and more convenient schedules than acyclovir when administered orally, and they may increase the effectiveness of oral antiviral therapy.[86] Ganciclovir is also effective against HSV infections, yet is not usually used specifically in this context. These drugs are ineffective in treating acyclovir-resistant strains because of their common mode of action.

Acyclovir-resistant strains are infrequently encountered in the post-HSCT setting. Resistance usually arises through a mutation in the viral thymidine kinase gene, although mutations in viral DNA polymerase conferring reduced sensitivity to acyclovir can also occur. Foscarnet (40 mg/kg three times daily) is the drug of choice for infections with acyclovir-resistant strains of HSV, especially in life-threatening infections.[87] In less severe disease, increased doses of acyclovir (500 mg/m^2 three times daily) are sometimes effective.

VARICELLA ZOSTER VIRUS

Approximately 85% of persons undergoing HSCT are seropositive for varicella zoster virus (VZV), indicating past infection and the presence of latent virus. Twenty-five to 50% of patients undergoing HSCT experience a clinical reactivation of VZV at a median of 4–5 months after transplantation.[88, 89] A significant risk of reactivation is present between 2 and 10 months after HSCT. The risk stands for both allogeneic and autologous transplantation.[90] Patients undergoing allogeneic HSCT wherein donor and recipient are HLA-mismatched and patients with chronic GVHD are at increased risk. Localized herpes zoster is the most common clinical manifestation in the HSCT setting. Cutaneous dissemination (defined as more than five vesicular lesions beyond the primary dermatome) and visceral dissemination following localized reactivation, however, are more common in patients undergoing HSCT than in immunocompetent persons. Visceral dissemination occurred in up to 20% of HSCT patients with herpes zoster prior to the availability of acyclovir and can occasionally precede dermatomal involvement or occur in its absence.[88]

Primary infection with herpes zoster can occur in seronegative persons during the post-HSCT period. Because of the significant immunosuppression of HSCT patients, the risk of proceeding to visceral dissemination is particularly high.[88] Intravenous acyclovir (10 mg/kg or 500 mg/m^2), three times daily for 7 days, is the treatment of choice for both herpes zoster and varicella in the first 12 months post HSCT. Such therapy has been shown to prevent cutaneous and systemic progression with reduced fatality.[91] The newer analogues of acyclovir (valacyclovir, famciclovir—see earlier discussion of herpes simplex) can potentially be used orally to achieve sufficient concentrations of drug to inhibit VZV replication.[92] They have not been tested in controlled trials against acyclovir in the HSCT setting, however, and their use is limited to relatively stable patients with no gastrointestinal dysfunction.

COMMUNITY-ACQUIRED RESPIRATORY VIRUS INFECTION

Enhanced techniques for viral culture and detection have led to the increasing appreciation of the significance of post-HSCT community-acquired respiratory viral infections.[93–95] Respiratory syncytial virus is the most common respiratory viral pathogen in the HSCT setting, affecting approximately 5% of patients. A peak of infection is encountered in the winter months. At the Fred Hutchinson Cancer Research Center, approximately 58% of patients with respiratory syncytial virus infection experienced viral pneumonia, with a mortality rate of 78%.[93] The most serious infections occurred in the pre-engraftment phase. Intravenous ribavirin was not effective in treating established pneumonia. Aerosolized ribavirin in combination with IVIG appeared to reduce mortality in a noncontrolled study at the M.D. Anderson Cancer Center.[94] Parainfluenza, influenza, and rhinovirus infections can also proceed to serious pneumonia in the post-HSCT period. Experience with antiviral therapy is limited—although ribavirin is effective in vitro, efficacy in patients with established pneumonia is not well documented.

Adenovirus infections occur in 5–20% of patients undergoing HSCT, depending on the center.[96] Infections often occur between 30 and 100 days after HSCT and may be more common in children. Pneumonitis is common, with a mortality rate exceeding 70%. Fulminant hepatitis, encephalitis, and hemorrhagic cystitis have also been described. The primary disease site varies with viral serotype. IgG and ribavirin have been used, but their efficacy has not been proven. Because of the poor outcomes of therapy in established pneumonia and other systemic diseases caused by these emerging viral complications of HSCT, the best current practice is directed at prevention of exposure and infection.

CONCLUSION

Myeloablative conditioning regimens cause severe neutropenia, breakdown of physical barriers, and defects in immunity, leading to an increased susceptibility to infections immediately after HSCT. The immunosuppressive nature of treatments for GVHD also increases the incidences and severity of infection. Prophylaxis and empiric therapy of bacterial infections is now established practice during the neutropenic phase following HSCT. Antibiotics with broad-spectrum gram-negative coverage are the mainstay of empiric therapy of febrile neutropenia. Because of the cost and the patient's potential for developing resistance, vancomycin usage can generally be limited to suspected or proven gram-positive infections or persistence of fever after the use of first-line empiric therapy. Although the impact of candidiasis has been successfully limited by adequate prophylaxis, *Aspergillus* remains an important cause of mortality and morbidity in HSCT. Amphotericin B preparations remain the mainstay of therapy against *Aspergillus* infection, but newer agents, such as voriconazole, may provide an effective alternative in the future. Viral infections, such as CMV, HSV, and VZV, are common in the immediate post-HSCT period. Prevention of CMV infection by screening and/or leukocyte depletion of transfused blood components in seronegative donor-recipient pairs or pre-emptive therapy with ganciclovir is the most effective strategy, but active CMV infections can also be treated with ganciclovir and IVIG. Treatment with foscarnet is an alternative to ganciclovir in ganciclovir-intolerant individuals with CMV infection. Prophylactic ancyclovir is effective against HSV. VZV infection can also be treated with newer agents, such as valacyclovir or famciclovir, which have improved bioavailability in oral formulation. Despite significant recent progress, further clinical studies are necessary to assess the efficacy and cost-effectiveness of therapeutic strategies against infections in the post-HSCT period.

REFERENCES

1. Bodey GP, Buckley M, Sathe YS, Freireich EJ: Quantitative relationships between circulating leukocytes and infection in patients with acute leukemia. Ann Intern Med 64(2):328–340, 1966.
2. Winston DJ, Gale RP, Meyer DV, Young LS: Infectious complications of human bone marrow transplantation. Medicine (Baltimore) 58(1):1–31, 1979.
3. Linch DC, Milligan DW, Winfield DA, et al: G-CSF after peripheral blood stem cell transplantation in lymphoma patients significantly accelerated neutrophil recovery and shortened time in hospital: results of a randomized BNLI trial [see comments]. Br J Haematol 99(4):933–938, 1997.
4. Rowley SD, Jones RJ, Piantadosi S, et al: Efficacy of ex vivo purging for autologous bone marrow transplantation in the treatment of acute nonlymphoblastic leukemia. Blood 74(1):501–506, 1989.
5. Anasetti C, Amos D, Beatty PG, et al: Effect of HLA compatibility on engraftment of bone marrow transplants in patients with leukemia or lymphoma. N Engl J Med 320(4):197–204, 1989.
6. Ash RC, Horowitz MM, Gale RP, et al: Bone marrow transplantation from related donors other than HLA-identical siblings: effect of T cell depletion. Bone Marrow Transplant 7(6):443–452, 1991.
7. Beyer J, Schwella N, Zingsem J, et al: Hematopoietic rescue after high-dose chemotherapy using autologous peripheral-blood progenitor cells or bone marrow: a randomized comparison. J Clin Oncol 13(6):1328–1335, 1995.
8. Hartmann O, Le Corroller AG, Blaise D, et al: Peripheral blood stem cell and bone marrow transplantation for solid tumors and lymphomas: hematologic recovery and costs. A randomized, controlled trial. Ann Intern Med 126(8):600–607, 1997.
9. Storb R, Deeg HJ, Whitehead J, et al: Methotrexate and cyclosporine compared with cyclosporine alone for prophylaxis of acute graft versus host disease after marrow transplantation for leukemia. N Engl J Med 314(12):729–735, 1986.
10. Hann IM, Prentice HG, Blacklock HA, et al: Acyclovir prophylaxis against herpes virus infections in severely immunocompromised patients: randomised double blind trial. Br Med J (Clin Res Ed) 287(6389):384–388, 1983.
11. Snover DC, Weisdorf SA, Vercellotti GM, et al: A histopathologic study of gastric and small intestinal graft-versus-host disease following allogeneic bone marrow transplantation. Hum Pathol 16(4):387–392, 1985.
12. Lowder JN, Lazarus HM, Herzig RH: Bacteremias and fungemias in oncologic patients with central venous catheters: changing spectrum of infection. Arch Intern Med 142(8):1456–1459, 1982.
13. Ault KA, Antin JH, Ginsburg D, et al: Phenotype of recovering lymphoid cell populations after marrow transplantation. J Exp Med 161(6):1483–1502, 1985.
14. Reusser P, Riddell SR, Meyers JD, Greenberg PD: Cytotoxic T-lymphocyte response to cytomegalovirus after human allogeneic bone marrow transplantation: pattern of recovery and correlation with cytomegalovirus infection and disease. Blood 78(5):1373–1380, 1991.
15. Atkinson K, Farewell V, Storb R, et al: Analysis of late infections after human bone marrow transplantation: role of genotypic nonidentity between marrow donor and recipient and of nonspecific suppressor cells in patients with chronic graft-versus-host disease. Blood 60(3):714–720, 1982.
16. Friedrich W, O'Reilly RJ, Koziner B, et al: T-lymphocyte reconstitution in recipients of bone marrow transplants with and without GVHD: imbalances of T-cell subpopulations having unique regulatory and cognitive functions. Blood 59(4):696–701, 1982.
17. Witherspoon RP, Goehle S, Kretschmer M, Storb R: Regulation of immunoglobulin production after human marrow grafting: the role of helper and suppressor T cells in acute graft-versus-host disease. Transplantation 41(3):328–335, 1986.
18. Lum LG, Seigneuret MC, Storb RF, et al: In vitro regulation of immunoglobulin synthesis after marrow transplantation: I. T-cell and B-cell deficiencies in patients with and without chronic graft-versus-host disease. Blood 58(3):431–439, 1981.
19. Guillaume T, Rubinstein DB, Symann M: Immune reconstitution and immunotherapy after autologous hematopoietic stem cell transplantation. Blood 92(5):1471–1490, 1998.
20. Sickles EA, Greene WH, Wiernik PH: Clinical presentation of infection in granulocytopenic patients. Arch Intern Med 135(5):715–719, 1975.
21. Rubin M, Hathorn JW, Marshall D, et al: Gram-positive infections and the use of vancomycin in 550 episodes of fever and neutropenia. Ann Intern Med 108(1):30–35, 1988.
22. Hughes WT, Armstrong D, Bodey GP, et al: 1997 guidelines for the use of antimicrobial agents in neutropenic patients with unexplained fever. Infectious Diseases Society of America. Clin Infec Dis 25(3):551–573, 1997.
23. Pizzo PA, Hathorn JW, Hiemenz J, et al: A randomized trial comparing ceftazidime alone with combination antibiotic therapy in cancer patients with fever and neutropenia. N Engl J Med 315(9):552–558, 1986.
24. De Pauw BE, Deresinski SC, Feld R, et al: Ceftazidime compared with piperacillin and tobramycin for the empiric treatment of fever in neutropenic patients with cancer: a multicenter randomized trial. The Intercontinental Antimicrobial Study Group [see comments]. Ann Intern Med 120(10):834–844, 1994.
25. Winston DJ, Ho WG, Bruckner DA, Champlin RE: Beta-lactam antibiotic therapy in febrile granulocytopenic patients: a randomized trial comparing cefoperazone plus piperacillin, ceftazidime plus piperacillin, and imipenem alone [see comments]. Ann Intern Med 115(11):849–859, 1991.
26. Vancomycin added to empirical combination antibiotic therapy for fever in granulocytopenic cancer patients: European Organization for Research and Treatment of Cancer (EORTC) International Antimicrobial Therapy Cooperative Group and the National Cancer Institute of Canada—Clinical Trials Group [published erratum appears in J Infect Dis 164(4):832; 1991] [see comments]. J Infect Dis 163(5):951–958, 1991.
27. Mayhall CG: Prevention and control of vancomycin resistance in gram-positive coccal microorganisms: fire prevention and fire fighting [editorial; comment]. Infect Control Hosp Epidemiol 17(6):353–355, 1996.
28. Pizzo PA, Robichaud KJ, Gill FA, Witebsky FG: Empiric antibiotic and antifungal therapy for cancer patients with prolonged fever and granulocytopenia. Am J Med 72(1):101–111, 1982.
29. Mullen CA, Buchanan GR: Early hospital discharge of children with cancer treated for fever and neutropenia: identification and management of the low-risk patient. J Clin Oncol 8(12):1998–2004, 1990.
30. Gilbert C, Meisenberg B, Vredenburgh J, et al: Sequential prophylactic oral and empiric once-daily parenteral antibiotics for neutropenia and fever after high-dose chemotherapy and autologous bone marrow support [see comments]. J Clin Oncol 12(5):1005–1011, 1994.
31. Hidalgo M, Hornedo J, Lumbreras C, et al: Outpatient therapy with oral ofloxacin for patients with low risk neutropenia and fever: a prospective, randomized clinical trial. Cancer 85(1):213–219, 1999.
32. Karthaus M, Egerer G, Kullmann KH, et al: Ceftriaxone in the outpatient treatment of cancer patients with fever and neutropenia. Eur J Clin Microbiol Infect Dis 17(7):501–504, 1998.
33. Kawano Y, Takaue Y, Mimaya J, et al: Marginal benefit/disadvantage of granulocyte colony-stimulating factor therapy after autologous blood stem cell transplantation in children: results of a prospective randomized trial. The Japanese Cooperative Study Group of PBSCT. Blood 92(11):4040–4046, 1998.
34. Klumpp TR, Mangan KF, Goldberg SL, et al: Granulocyte colony-stimulating factor accelerates neutrophil engraftment following peripheral-blood stem-cell transplantation: a prospective, randomized trial. J Clin Oncol 13(6):1323–1327, 1995.
35. Nemunaitis J, Rosenfeld CS, Ash R, et al: Phase III randomized,

double-blind placebo-controlled trial of rhGM-CSF following allogeneic bone marrow transplantation. Bone Marrow Transplant 15(6):949–954, 1995.

36. Wald A, Leisenring W, van Burik JA, Bowden RA: Epidemiology of *Aspergillus* infections in a large cohort of patients undergoing bone marrow transplantation [see comments]. J Infect Dis 175(6):1459–1466, 1997.

37. Goodrich JM, Reed EC, Mori M, et al: Clinical features and analysis of risk factors for invasive candidal infection after marrow transplantation. J Infect Dis 164(4):731–740, 1991.

38. Walsh TJ, Melcher GP, Rinaldi MG, et al: *Trichosporon beigelii*, an emerging pathogen resistant to amphotericin B. J Clin Microbiol 28(7):1616–1622, 1990.

39. Gaziev D, Baronciani D, Galimberti M, et al: Mucormycosis after bone marrow transplantation: report of four cases in thalassemia and review of the literature. Bone Marrow Transplant 17(3):409–414, 1996.

40. Guého E, Boekhout T, Ashbee HR, et al: The role of *Malassezia* species in the ecology of human skin and as pathogens. Med Mycol 36(Suppl 1):220–229, 1998.

41. Peterson MW, Pratt AD, Nugent KM: Pneumonia due to *Histoplasma capsulatum* in a bone marrow transplant recipient. Thorax 42(9):698–699, 1987.

42. Slavin MA, Osborne B, Adams R, et al: Efficacy and safety of fluconazole prophylaxis for fungal infections after marrow transplantation—a prospective, randomized, double-blind study. J Infect Dis 171(6):1545–1552, 1995.

43. Abi-Said D, Anaissie E, Uzun O, et al: The epidemiology of hematogenous candidiasis caused by different *Candida* species [see comments] [published erratum appears in Clin Infect Dis 1997 Aug;25(2):352]. Clin Infect Dis 24(6):1122–1128, 1997.

44. Wingard JR: Importance of *Candida* species other than *C. albicans* as pathogens in oncology patients. Clin Infect Dis 20(1):115–125, 1995.

45. Edwards JE Jr, Bodey GP, Bowden RA, et al: International Conference for the Development of a Consensus on the Management and Prevention of Severe *Candidal* Infections [see comments]. Clin Infect Dis 25(1):43–59, 1997.

46. Nguyen MH, Peacock JE Jr, Tanner DC, et al: Therapeutic approaches in patients with candidemia: evaluation in a multicenter, prospective, observational study. Arch Intern Med 155(22):2429–2435, 1995.

47. Rossetti F, Brawner DL, Bowden R, et al: Fungal liver infection in marrow transplant recipients: prevalence at autopsy, predisposing factors, and clinical features. Clin Infect Dis 20(4):801–811, 1995.

48. Kauffman CA, Bradley SF, Ross SC, Weber DR: Hepatosplenic candidiasis: successful treatment with fluconazole. Am J Med 91(2):137–141, 1991.

49. Morrison VA, Haake RJ, Weisdorf DJ: Non-*Candida* fungal infections after bone marrow transplantation: risk factors and outcome. Am J Med 96(6):497–503, 1994.

50. Albelda SM, Talbot GH, Gerson SL, et al: Pulmonary cavitation and massive hemoptysis in invasive pulmonary aspergillosis: influence of bone marrow recovery in patients with acute leukemia. Am Rev Respir Dis 131(1):115–120, 1985.

51. Yu VL, Muder RR, Poorsattar A: Significance of isolation of *Aspergillus* from the respiratory tract in diagnosis of invasive pulmonary aspergillosis: results from a three-year prospective study. Am J Med 81(2):249–254, 1986.

52. Csekeo A, Agocs L, Egervary M, Heiler Z: Surgery for pulmonary aspergillosis. Eur J Cardiothorac Surg 12(6):876–879, 1997.

53. Prentice HG, Hann IM, Herbrecht R, et al: A randomized comparison of liposomal versus conventional amphotericin B for the treatment of pyrexia of unknown origin in neutropenic patients. Br J Haematol 98(3):711–718, 1997.

54. Walsh TJ, Finberg RW, Arndt C, et al: Liposomal amphotericin B for empirical therapy in patients with persistent fever and neutropenia: National Institute of Allergy and Infectious Diseases Mycoses Study Group. N Engl J Med 340(10):764–771, 1999.

55. Walsh TJ, Hiemenz JW, Seibel NL, et al: Amphotericin B lipid complex for invasive fungal infections: analysis of safety and efficacy in 556 cases. Clin Infect Dis 26(6):1383–1396, 1998.

56. Stevens DA, Lee JY: Analysis of compassionate use itraconazole therapy for invasive aspergillosis by the NIAID Mycoses Study Group criteria. Arch Intern Med 157(16):1857–1862, 1997.

57. Sanati H, Belanger P, Fratti R, Ghannoum M: A new triazole, voriconazole (UK-109,496), blocks sterol biosynthesis in *Candida albicans* and *Candida krusei*. Antimicrob Agents Chemother 41(11):2492–2496, 1997.

58. Neiman PE, Reeves W, Ray G, et al: A prospective analysis interstitial pneumonia and opportunistic viral infection among recipients of allogeneic bone marrow grafts. J Infect Dis 136(6):754–767, 1977.

59. Chee MS, Bankier AT, Beck S, et al: Analysis of the protein-coding content of the sequence of human cytomegalovirus strain AD169. Curr Top Microbiol Immunol 154:125–169, 1990.

60. Zhang LJ, Hanff P, Rutherford C, et al: Detection of human cytomegalovirus DNA, RNA, and antibody in normal donor blood. J Infect Dis 171(4):1002–1006, 1995.

61. Soderberg-Naucler C, Fish KN, Nelson JA: Reactivation of latent human cytomegalovirus by allogeneic stimulation of blood cells from healthy donors. Cell 91(1):119–126, 1997.

62. Fish KN, Soderberg-Naucler C, Mills LK, et al: Human cytomegalovirus persistently infects aortic endothelial cells. J Virol 72(7):5661–5668, 1998.

63. Drew WL, Sweet ES, Miner RC, Mocarski ES: Multiple infections by cytomegalovirus in patients with acquired immunodeficiency syndrome: documentation by Southern blot hybridization. J Infect Dis 150(6):952–953, 1984.

64. Gilbert GL, Hayes K, Hudson IL, James J: Prevention of transfusion-acquired cytomegalovirus infection in infants by blood filtration to remove leucocytes. Neonatal Cytomegalovirus Infection Study Group [see comments]. Lancet 1(8649):1228–1231, 1989.

65. Goodrich JM, Bowden RA, Fisher L, et al: Ganciclovir prophylaxis to prevent cytomegalovirus disease after allogeneic marrow transplant. Ann Intern Med 118(3):173–178, 1993.

66. Boeckh M, Gooley TA, Myerson D, et al: Cytomegalovirus pp65 antigenemia-guided early treatment with ganciclovir versus ganciclovir at engraftment after allogeneic marrow transplantation: a randomized double-blind study. Blood 88(10):4063–4071, 1996.

67. Wingard JR, Chen DY, Burns WH, et al: Cytomegalovirus infection after autologous bone marrow transplantation with comparison to infection after allogeneic bone marrow transplantation. Blood 71(5):1432–1437, 1988.

68. Miller W, Flynn P, McCullough J, et al: Cytomegalovirus infection after bone marrow transplantation: an association with acute graft-v-host disease. Blood 67(4):1162–1167, 1986.

69. Reusser P: Cytomegalovirus infection and disease after bone marrow transplantation: epidemiology, prevention, and treatment. Bone Marrow Transplant 7(Suppl 3):52–56, 1991.

70. Stover DE, Zaman MB, Hajdu SI, et al: Bronchoalveolar lavage in the diagnosis of diffuse pulmonary infiltrates in the immunosuppressed host. Ann Intern Med 101(1):1–7, 1984.

71. Meyers JD, Flournoy N, Thomas ED: Risk factors for cytomegalovirus infection after human marrow transplantation. J Infect Dis 153(3):478–488, 1986.

72. Zaia JA, Forman SJ: Cytomegalovirus infection in the bone marrow transplant recipient. Infect Dis Clin North Am 9(4):879–900, 1995.

73. Emanuel D, Cunningham I, Jules-Elysee K, et al: Cytomegalovirus pneumonia after bone marrow transplantation successfully treated with the combination of ganciclovir and high-dose intravenous immune globulin. Ann Intern Med 109(10):777–782, 1988.

74. Reed EC, Bowden RA, Dandliker PS, et al: Treatment of cytomegalovirus pneumonia with ganciclovir and intravenous cytomegalovirus immunoglobulin in patients with bone marrow transplants. Ann Intern Med 109(10):783–788, 1988.

75. Schmidt GM, Kovacs A, Zaia JA, et al: Ganciclovir/immunoglobulin combination therapy for the treatment of human cytomegalovirus-associated interstitial pneumonia in bone marrow allograft recipients. Transplantation 46(6):905–907, 1988.

76. Aschan J, Ringden O, Ljungman P, et al: Foscarnet for treatment of cytomegalovirus infections in bone marrow transplant recipients. Scand J Infect Dis 24(2):143–150, 1992.

77. Bacigalupo A, van Lint MT, Tedone E, et al: Early treatment of CMV infections in allogeneic bone marrow transplant recipients with foscarnet or ganciclovir. Bone Marrow Transplant 13(6):753–758, 1994.

78. Page MJ, Dreese JC, Poritz LS, Koltun WA: Cytomegalovirus enteritis: a highly lethal condition requiring early detection and intervention. Dis Colon Rectum 41(5):619–623, 1998.

79. Goodrich JM, Mori M, Gleaves CA, et al: Early treatment with ganciclovir to prevent cytomegalovirus disease after allogeneic bone marrow transplantation. N Engl J Med 325(23):1601–1607, 1991.

80. Schmidt GM, Horak DA, Niland JC, et al: A randomized, controlled trial of prophylactic ganciclovir for cytomegalovirus pulmonary infec-

tion in recipients of allogeneic bone marrow transplants: the City of Hope–Stanford–Syntex CMV Study Group [see comments]. N Engl J Med 324(15):1005–1011, 1991.

81. Terzin AL, Masic MG: Age-specific incidence of neutralization antibodies of herpes simplex virus. J Hyg (Lond) 77(2):155–160, 1976.

82. Meyers JD, Flournoy N, Thomas ED: Infection with herpes simplex virus and cell-mediated immunity after marrow transplant. J Infect Dis 142(3):338–346, 1980.

83. Saral R, Burns WH, Laskin OL, et al: Acyclovir prophylaxis of herpes-simplex-virus infections. N Engl J Med 305(2):63–67, 1981.

84. Ambinder RF, Burns WH, Lietman PS, Saral R: Prophylaxis: a strategy to minimise antiviral resistance. Lancet 1(8387):1154–1155, 1984.

85. Wade JC, Newton B, McLaren C, et al: Intravenous acyclovir to treat mucocutaneous herpes simplex virus infection after marrow transplantation: a double-blind trial. Ann Intern Med 96(3):265–269, 1982.

86. Schacker T, Hu HL, Koelle DM, et al: Famciclovir for the suppression of symptomatic and asymptomatic herpes simplex virus reactivation in HIV-infected persons: a double-blind, placebo-controlled trial. Ann Intern Med 128(1):21–28, 1998.

87. Safrin S, Crumpacker C, Chatis P, et al: A controlled trial comparing foscarnet with vidarabine for acyclovir-resistant mucocutaneous herpes simplex in the acquired immunodeficiency syndrome: the AIDS Clinical Trials Group. N Engl J Med 325(8):551–555, 1991.

88. Locksley RM, Flournoy N, Sullivan KM, Meyers JD: Infection with varicella-zoster virus after marrow transplantation. J Infect Dis 152(6):1172–1181, 1985.

89. Han CS, Miller W, Haake R, Weisdorf D: Varicella zoster infection after bone marrow transplantation: incidence, risk factors and complications. Bone Marrow Transplant 13(3):277–283, 1994.

90. Schuchter LM, Wingard JR, Piantadosi S, et al: Herpes zoster infection after autologous bone marrow transplantation. Blood 74(4):1424–1427, 1989.

91. Meyers JD, Wade JC, Shepp DH, Newton B: Acyclovir treatment of varicella-zoster virus infection in the compromised host. Transplantation 37(6):571–574, 1984.

92. Tyring S, Barbarash RA, Nahlik JE, et al: Famciclovir for the treatment of acute herpes zoster: effects on acute disease and postherpetic neuralgia. A randomized, double-blind, placebo-controlled trial. Collaborative Famciclovir Herpes Zoster Study Group [see comments]. Ann Intern Med 123(2):89–96, 1995.

93. Bowden R: Respiratory virus infections after marrow transplant: the Fred Hutchison Cancer Center experience. Am J Med 102(Suppl 3A):27–30, 1997.

94. Garcia R, Raad I, Abi-Said D, et al: Nosocomial respiratory syncytial virus infections: prevention and control in bone marrow transplant patients. Infect Control Hosp Epidemiol 18(6):412–416, 1997.

95. Ljungman P: Respiratory virus infections in bone marrow transplant recipients: the European experience. Am J Med 102(Suppl 3A):44–47, 1997.

96. Carrigan D: Adenovirus infections in immunocompromised patients. Am J Med 107(Suppl 3A):71–74, 1997.

CHAPTER FORTY-FOUR

Failure of Engraftment

Jian Chen, M.D., Ping Law, Ph.D., and Edward D. Ball, M.D.

Hematopoietic stem cell (HSC) transplantation (HSCT) is an effective treatment for a variety of malignant and nonmalignant hematologic diseases and solid tumors. A successful transplant requires an adequate number of HSC in the graft, an optimal conditioning or immunosuppressive regimen for the recipient, a complex interaction between the graft and the marrow microenvironment, and hematopoietic growth factors either administered ex vivo or produced at different time intervals in vivo. A compromise in any of these conditions can lead to graft failure (early or late), which is an uncommon but serious complication of HSCT.

Graft failure is defined as the lack of functional hematopoiesis after transplantation and is classified as either primary or secondary graft failure. Primary graft failure, also called *early graft failure* or *failure of initial engraftment,* is diagnosed when donor hematopoiesis is not established in the recipient by an arbitrary date ranging from 14 to 42 days post transplantation. Primary graft failure also occurs in autologous HSCT.

The diagnostic criteria for primary graft failure vary among institutions. It is, however, almost exclusively based on post-transplantation absolute neutrophil counts (ANC). Severe acute graft-versus-host disease (GVHD) and overwhelming infections in the early post-transplantation days should be excluded as the cause of delayed engraftment. In some institutions, primary graft failure is diagnosed only after the patient fails to respond to a course of hematopoietic growth factor. The mechanism of graft failure is different for autologous and allogeneic transplantation. In autologous HSCT, damage to HSC and the marrow microenvironment by chemotherapy or irradiation prior to transplantation is the most important cause of graft failure. In allogeneic HSCT, the HSC are usually normal. The human leukocyte antigen (HLA) disparity between donor and recipient leading to rejection of the graft by residual host immune effect cells is one of the most important mechanisms of graft failure. The common causes of graft failure are listed in Table 44–1. The incidence of primary graft failure from several large series is listed in Table 44–2.

A number of risk factors have been identified, including human histocompatibility antigen (HLA) incompatibility, inadequate numbers of infused HSC, T-cell depletion, severity of GVHD, suboptimal conditioning regimens, alloimmunization in the recipient, damaged HSC or marrow stroma prior to transplantation, and infections. In the early experience with HSCT for severe aplastic anemia, the incidence of graft failure was as high as 50% with patients who received no conditioning regimen. The incidence has declined significantly since the 1970s because of better patient selection and HLA matching, more-defined conditioning regimens, increased use of hematopoietic growth factors, and infusion of an adequate dose of HSC.

Early graft failure can also be caused by a deficiency in the homing of infused HSC into the marrow microenvironment. Although the understanding of HSCT biology has improved considerably, little is known about how infused HSC home into the marrow and the role of stroma in the support of hematopoiesis. The adhesion receptor expression on the HSC surface has been shown to play an important role for homing after transplantation. A number of cytokines (interleukin-3 [IL-3], IL-6, IL-11, and stem cell factor) can increase or decrease the expression of selective adhesion receptors, including alpha-L, alpha-1, alpha-2, alpha-3, alpha-4, alpha-5, alpha-6, beta-1, L-selectin, CD44, and platelet endothelial cell adhesion molecule (PECAM). These changes in adhesion receptor expression and function with cytokines and during cell cycle are involved in the process of rolling, attachment to endothelium, endothelial transmigration, and cell migration within the marrow space.[1]

ALLOGENEIC HSCT

HLA INCOMPATIBILITY

The correlation between the degree of HLA incompatibility and success of HSCT has been extensively studied.[2–12] Anasetti et al. at the Fred Hutchinson Cancer Research Center (FHCRC) summarized results from 269 patients with hematologic malignancies who received HLA-haploidentical marrow from family members and compared them with 930 patients who received HLA-identical marrow from siblings.[13] Overall graft failure occurred in 12.3% of patients who received HLA-haploidentical marrow compared with 2.0% of patients who received HLA-identical marrow. The incidence of graft failure was directly correlated to the degree of HLA disparity. Primary graft failure occurred in

TABLE 44–1. COMMON CAUSES OF GRAFT FAILURE

HLA incompatibility between donor and recipient
Poor quality or quantity of stem cells
T-cell depletion
Inadequate conditioning regimen
Alloimmunization
Stromal cell dysfunction
Infections
Medications

HLA, human leukocyte antigen.

521

TABLE 44–2. INCIDENCE OF PRIMARY GRAFT FAILURE FOR ALLOGENEIC HSCT

INSTITUTION	NO.	CRITERIA	INCIDENCE	YEAR (REFERENCE)
HLA-Identical, Related Donor				
FHCRC	50	Donor markers	10%	1986 (2)
FHCRC	930	ANC<100/mm³ by day 14	1.6%	1989 (13)
IBMTR	625	Not specified	11%	1989 (14)
UK, multicenter	51	ANC<500/mm³	10%	1990 (3)
Hammersmith	57	ANC<500/mm³	1.8%	1993 (4)
U. Minnesota	211	ANC<500/mm³ by day 42	5%	1994 (5)
EBMTR	618	Not specified	16%	1994 (16)
FHCRC	39	ANC <100/mm³ by day 14	5%	1994 (15)
HLA-Identical, Unrelated Donor				
Hammersmith	46	ANC<500/mm³	11%	1993 (4)
NMDP	462	ANC<500/mm³	6%	1993 (6)
U. Minnesota	32	ANC<500/mm³ by day 42	6%	1994 (5)
FHCRC	192	ANC<500/mm³ by day 28	3%	1998 (7)
HLA Nonidentical Donor				
FHCRC	269	ANc<100/mm³ by day 14	8.5%	1989 (13)
UK, multi-center	51	ANC<500/mm³	25%	1990 (3)
U. Wisconsin	55	ANC<1000/mm³	5.6%	1990 (8)
U. Minnesota	54	ANC<500/mm³ by day 42	15%	1994 (5)
FHCRC	40	Not specified	22.5%	1996 (9)
U. Perugia, Italy	43	ANC<100/mm³ by day 21	4.6%	1998 (10)

ANC, absolute neutrophil count; EBMTR, European Bone Marrow Transplant Registry; FHCRC, Fred Hutchinson Cancer Research Center; NMDP, National Marrow Donor Program.

9% of patients who had one incompatible locus and in 21% of patients who had two incompatible loci. In multivariate analysis, parameters such as age and sex of the donor and recipient; disease diagnosis and staging, ABO blood type compatibility, conditioning regimen, GVHD prophylaxis, and the number of infused marrow cells were not significantly correlated to graft failure. The mean marrow cell dose was 2.75 × 10⁸ cells/kg, with 84% of patients receiving more than 1.5 × 10⁸ cells/kg. The history of blood transfusion was not associated with increased incidence of graft failure. Nevertheless, the alloimmunization detected by positive donor cross-match and persistent host lymphocytes in the circulation after transplantation was correlated with increased incidence of graft failure. The results showed that HLA incompatibility was the most important risk factor and that immunologic rejection of the graft was the primary cause of engraftment failure.

Bone marrow transplantation (BMT) from unrelated donors is being performed more frequently to overcome the limited availability of HLA-identical bone marrow from siblings. It is expected that graft failure will occur with increased frequency because of the degree of HLA incompatibility. The hypothesis is confirmed from a retrospective analysis concerning recipients of matched sibling HSC compared with recipients of HSC from unrelated donors by Davies et al. from the University of Minnesota.[15] One hundred and eight patients who underwent allogeneic HSCT from a fully HLA-matched or a partially HLA-matched unrelated donor were compared with 236 patients who received HLA-identical marrow from their siblings. Primary graft failure occurred in 5% of patients with HLA-identical sibling donors, 6% of patients with fully matched unrelated donors, and 15% of patients with partially matched unrelated donors. All 108 patients underwent transplantation for hematologic malignancies, and 97 of them received

total body irradiation (TBI) as part of the conditioning regimens. In univariate and multivariate analysis, parameters such as disease type, disease staging, patient age, donor age and sex, GVHD prophylaxis, marrow cell dose, and ABO compatibility were not significantly associated with graft failure. The higher marrow cell dose (median, 3.0 × 10⁸/kg), however, was associated with faster engraftment compared with lower cell dose (median, 2 × 10⁸/kg). The report concluded that the primary graft failure was a significantly more frequent event in recipients of bone marrow from partially HLA-matched unrelated donors and hence extended the observation in the report from the FHCRC to unrelated donors.

A retrospective review by Howard et al. summarizing data from four centers in the United Kingdom also reported a higher incidence of graft failure associated with HLA incompatibility.[13] Fifty-one patients who underwent allogeneic BMT from unrelated donors were compared with 51 transplants using HLA-identical sibling donors. The incidence of graft failure was 25% for unrelated graft and 5% for HLA-identical graft. Similar results were reported from the FHCRC and the International Blood and Marrow Transplantation Registry (IBMTR).[2, 14, 15]

In 1998, Hansen et al. from the FHCRC reported results for 196 patients with Philadelphia chromosome–positive chronic myelogenous leukemia who received marrow from unrelated donors between 1985 and 1994.[7] One hundred and fifty-two patients received fully matched unrelated donor marrow. Patients under 36 years of age who had no HLA-matched unrelated donor received marrow with a single minor mismatch. Results from a pretransplantation cross match between the patient's serum and donor's cells were negative in all cases, however. The median marrow cell dose was 3.0 × 10⁸/kg. All patients received TBI and cyclophosphamide. Primary graft failure occurred in only six patients. A logistic-regression analysis suggested that patients who received the lower cell dose were more likely to experience graft failure, with a relative risk of 4.9 for each decrement of 1.0×10^8 cells/kg. Nevertheless, the cell doses for individual patients who experienced graft failure were not reported. Survival was adversely affected by the interval from diagnosis to transplantation of 1 year or more, mismatch of HLA-DRβ1, and patient age of 50 years or older. Hansen et al. concluded that transplantation using HLA-matched unrelated donors was a safe and effective treatment for selective patients with chronic myelogenous leukemia. A graft failure rate of 5% was an acceptable risk for patients who had no HLA-identical sibling donors.

The outcome of graft failure in patients with aplastic anemia was analyzed from IBMTR data by Champlin et al.[14] A total of 625 patients who underwent transplantation from HLA-identical sibling donors at 98 centers worldwide from 1978 to 1986 were included. The number of pretransplantation transfusions ranged from zero to 158, with a median of 22. Graft failure occurred in 11% of patients. All 19 patients who experienced primary graft failure died, including 10 patients who received a second transplant. The risk factors included conditioning regimens without TBI, GVHD prophylaxis without cyclosporin A, and T-cell depletion (4 failures in 10 patients). The inclusion of TBI in the conditioning regimens reduced the incidence of graft failure but did not improve overall survival.

An analysis of European Blood and Marrow Transplantation Registry (EBMTR) data included 618 patients with aplastic anemia who underwent BMT from HLA-identical siblings between 1976 and 1990 in eight European centers.[16] Overall incidence of graft failure was 16%. A significant decline of graft failure was noted, from 32% prior to 1980, to 8.8% between 1980 and 1984, to 7.6% after 1984. The factors contributing to graft failure included pretransplantation blood transfusion, lower marrow cell dose, GVHD prophylaxis without cyclosporin A, T-cell depletion, prior alloimmunization, and conditioning regimens without TBI. It was of interest that the incidence of graft failure for patients with post-hepatitis aplastic anemia was significantly lower than that for patients with idiopathic aplastic anemia—4% versus 16%, respectively. Among 85 patients experiencing graft failure, 17 patients underwent a second BMT within 60 days. The prognosis was significantly poor, with an overall survival rate of 17% at 8 years, when compared with 24 patients who received a second BMT after 60 days. The findings from these analyses of two large registries are remarkably similar.

HEMATOPOIETIC STEM CELL DOSE

The dose of infused HSC is critical for engraftment in both animal models and clinical studies.[17–23] In a murine model, Uharek et al. observed 88% graft failure when 1×10^5 cells were infused into each mouse, and 0% graft failure when the cell dose was increased to 4×10^8 cells per mouse.[23] The biologic mechanism behind the difference is unknown. It is generally accepted that a few pluripotent HSC are required to establish hematopoiesis and that the number of true pluripotent HSC may be lower than 0.1% in infused marrow cells. It is unclear why more marrow

cells enhance engraftment. The alternative explanation is that, although the pluripotent HSC have the capacity of self-renewal, a minimal number of self-renewing HSC are required to sustain hematopoiesis. Currently, there is no established or accepted in vitro assay for human pluripotent HSC.

In clinical studies, a dose of $2–3 \times 10^8$ marrow cells/kg of recipient body weight provided rapid engraftment and stable long-term hematopoiesis.[17, 24, 25] The risk of graft failure was significantly increased if the cell dose was less than 1×10^8/kg.[7, 17, 20, 22]

Counting nucleated marrow cells is the easiest method, but it is unreliable because of the wide variations in the proportion of progenitor cells among individuals. The number of colony-forming units—granulocyte and macrophage (CFU-GM) has also been used as a determinant. Theoretically, CFU-GM determines the functional status of hematopoietic progenitor cells committed to myeloid differentiation.[26–28] It is impractical to use CFU-GM as a guide for marrow harvest or peripheral blood progenitor cell (PBPC) collections, especially in allogeneic HSCT, because of the time required to complete the assay (14 days), screening of reagents, standards for scoring colonies, and considerable variations among different laboratories. As the CD34 surface marker was discovered in 1984 and the use of flow cytometry in clinical laboratories has been more common since the late 1980s, the number of CD34+ cells per kilogram of body weight has been used routinely as a guide for PBPC collection.[29, 30] Currently, most transplantation centers aim at harvesting 5×10^6 CD34+ cells/kg for rapid and sustained engraftment.

Additional discussion on colony culture can be found in Chapter 28. Chapter 27 is devoted to the measurement of CD34+ cells.

T-CELL DEPLETION

T-cell depletion is associated with significantly increased risk of graft failure. With HLA-identical T-cell depleted BMT, the incidence of graft failure ranges from 5% to 75%.[31–37] A review of earlier experience with T cell–depleted BMT before 1990 is summarized in Table 44–3. These data led to the hypothesis that T cells, by producing a number of cytokines, were required for HSC to proliferate.[38] Successful engraftment of T cell–depleted marrow in clinical trials and animal models, however, indicated that T cells are not absolutely required. There is a complex interaction between donor and recipient cells after HSCT, which eventually leads to the elimination of residual host

TABLE 44–3. INCIDENCE OF GRAFT FAILURE BEFORE 1990 USING POOLED DATA

T-cell depletion using monoclonal antibodies	
HLA-identical BMT	55/460 (12%)
HLA-mismatched BMT	30/111 (27%)
T-cell depletion using physical techniques	
HLA-identical BMT	15/160 (9%)
HLA-mismatched BMT	21/59 (36%)

BMT, bone marrow transplantation; HLA, human leukocyte antigen.

HSC and immune-competent cells. With a less than 2-log depletion of T cells, engraftment occurs in most cases, concomitant with an increase in GVHD.[36] In recent studies, when large numbers of CD34+ cells (>10[7]/kg recipient body weight) were infused, prompt and sustained engraftment was achieved without GVHD, even when the T-cell dose was less than 1×10^5/kg.[10, 39]

Successful engraftment can be achieved by infusing a large dose of HSC in T cell–depleted transplants and/or a more intensive immunosuppressive regimen.[10, 33, 40, 41] Forty-three patients with high-risk acute leukemia received HLA-haploidentical marrow from their relatives.[10] Fifteen patients received allogeneic PBPC only, and 28 patients received both PBPC and marrow. All patients underwent an intensive conditioning regimen including TBI, thiotepa, fludarabine, and antithymocyte globulin. No prophylaxis for GVHD was given. The mean dose of CD34+ cells was 1.4×10^7/kg for patients who received PBPC only and 1.06×10^7/kg for patients who received both PBPC and marrow. Only two patients suffered primary graft failure, and no secondary graft failure was reported. The same group also reported 54 patients with acute leukemia who received T cell–depleted marrow from HLA-identical sibling donors. All patients received TBI, thiotepa, antithymocyte globulin, and cyclophosphamide as conditioning regimen. Again, no prophylaxis against GVHD was given. All patients achieved sustained engraftment with full donor-type chimerism.[39]

T cell–depleted marrow has been successfully transplanted to infants with severe combined immunodeficiency. Buckley et al. reported their results of 89 infants who underwent transplantation at Duke University between 1982 and 1998.[42] Seventy-two infants received T cell–depleted marrow from HLA-haploidentical parents with a mean cell dose of 3.13×10^8/kg after processing. None of these patients received chemotherapy prior to transplantation and prophylaxis for GVHD. The incidence of primary graft failure was not reported, but a number of patients received booster marrow infusion. Only one patient failed to engraft after four T cell–depleted marrow transplantations. Four patients received two booster transplants, and 14 received one booster transplant. Sixty patients achieved long-term survival. The result is encouraging in that none of the patients died from graft failure. The report concluded that T cell–depleted, HLA-haploidentical marrow could be successfully transplanted to patients with severe combined immunodeficiency disorders.

Several other approaches have been developed to overcome the higher incidence of graft failure in T cell–depleted allografts. Controlled depletion is used to adjust the T-cell dose to limit GVHD but not promote graft failure.[36] Total lymphoid irradiation has been added to conditioning regimens for prevention of rejection.[43] Depletion of T-cell subsets (CD6+ or CD8+ cells) has been shown to be effective in preventing GVHD without compromising engraftment.[44, 45] It is also feasible to give donor lymphocyte infusion with carefully controlled T-cell doses and scheduling after T cell–depleted transplants.[46] Some of the common procedures for T-cell depletion are discussed in detail in Chapter 30.

In summary, T cell–depleted HSCT has improved significantly in the 1990s. The graft failure rate has steadily declined to less that 5% since 1990 with less-severe acute GVHD. It will remain an active field of clinical trials.

CONDITIONING REGIMENS

The pretransplantation conditioning regimen is important in reducing the incidence of graft failure, especially in HLA-mismatched allografts. An analysis of 40 patients undergoing allogeneic BMT for severe aplastic anemia at the FHCRC demonstrated the importance of including TBI as part of the conditioning regimen for HLA-mismatched transplantation.[9] Nine patients received HLA-identical marrow using cyclophosphamide, 200 mg/kg, and TBI as the conditioning regimen. Eight of them were alive and disease-free 3–18 years post transplantation. Fifteen patients received HLA-mismatched marrow from their relatives and were prepared with the same dose of cyclophosphamide without TBI. None became a long-term survivor. Nine patients in the latter group experienced graft failure. Since 1984, TBI has been added to the conditioning regimen for HLA-mismatched allografts for aplastic anemia. Sixteen patients received the combined conditioning regimen, and eight of them remained disease free 1.5–11.3 years after their transplantation. The report concluded that TBI should be included in conditioning regimen for marrow transplants using mismatched related donors, especially for aplastic anemia.[9]

The addition of TBI is associated with higher toxicity. Other conditioning regimens without TBI have been extensively studied in other disease settings. A randomized trial comparing TBI/cyclophosphamide with busulfan/cyclophosphamide was reported from the FHCRC in patients receiving marrow from HLA-matched siblings for treatment of chronic myelogenous leukemia. Although the disease-free survival in the two groups was similar, the busulfan/cyclophosphamide combination was superior in all other aspects with significantly less toxicity. Patients who received TBI/cyclophosphamide experienced more renal failure, more acute GVHD, and more infectious complications, and they spent longer times in the hospital.[47] The same regimen of busulfan/cyclophosphamide was used in 25 patients who received HLA-identical marrow from unrelated donors for treatment of a variety of hematologic malignancies.[48] Nineteen of them received transplants for chronic myelogenous leukemia. All patients had cyclosporine and methotrexate for GVHD prophylaxis as well as granulocyte-macrophage colony-stimulating factor (GM-CSF) from the day of infusion. All patients achieved initial engraftment, and there was no secondary graft failure. The projected disease-free survival and overall survival at 1 year were comparable to such values in other reports.[48] The results demonstrated that conditioning regimens without TBI can be effective for diseases other than aplastic anemia.

STROMAL DAMAGE

Stromal cells in the marrow provide an important matrix for cellular communication through direct cell-cell contact and through elaboration of hematopoietic growth factors. They have to survive intensive conditioning regimens and remain functional for the incoming HSC. Experimental evidence showed that stromal cells have retained host origin after an intensive conditioning regimen. Infused marrow contains stromal cell elements but does not replace the microenvironment of the patient.[49]

Stroma damage in allogeneic HSCT is primarily the result of donor cells reacting to the existing marrow microenvironment. The HLA disparity between donor and recipient is a cause of compromise in the marrow microenvironment. In one retrospective analysis of 171 recipients of HLA-matched transplants, grade II–IV acute GVHD was identified as a major risk factor for graft failure.[50] Lysis of host stromal cells by donor's reactive lymphocytes may represent one extreme graft-versus-host effect. Some in vitro studies did demonstrate the presence of alloreactive cytotoxic T lymphocytes that were able to lyse stromal cells.[51]

The morphologic change of the marrow in patients who experience graft failure after transplantation has not been studied in detail. Laboratory studies have shown that the alteration of microenvironment can lead to decreased production of stimulatory growth factors such as granulocyte colony stimulating factor (G-CSF) and increased production of inhibitory cytokines such as transforming growth factor β.[52] There is a report that G-CSF production is reduced in long-term marrow culture from patients experiencing graft failure.[53] Adhesion receptor expression plays a critical role for HSC homing and migration after transplantation. A number of cytokines can selectively regulate their expression.[1] The exact mechanisms as to how the marrow microenvironment interacts with HSC are not clear and require further study.

ALLOIMMUNIZATION PRIOR TO HSCT

Alloimmunization is an important contributing factor to primary graft failure, especially in patients with aplastic anemia. Anasetti et al. reported on 50 patients with severe aplastic anemia who received no blood transfusion until just before their allogeneic BMT. All patients underwent transplantation with HLA-identical marrow from siblings and were conditioned with cyclophosphamide alone. The median interval between diagnosis and transplantation was 2 weeks. The median marrow cell dose was 3.49×10^8/kg. Cyclosporine and methotrexate were given for GVHD prophylaxis. There was no primary graft failure in this cohort of patients. The 10-year probability of survival rate was 82% after a median follow-up of 7 years. This was significantly better compared with historical data of 50% long-term survival for patients who had undergone blood transfusions prior to transplantation in the same institution.[2]

Graft failure usually is the result of immunologic rejection of the donor's marrow by host-derived cytotoxic T cells or natural killer cells. The presence of antidonor antibodies has been documented as the cause of primary graft failure. There are two classes of antidonor antibodies, one with specificity for HLA and the other against the ABO blood group. The presence of ABO blood type antibodies usually results in prolonged erythroid hypoplasia, leaving the recipient transfusion-dependent. A few cases of primary graft failure have been reported in the presence of anti-

HLA antibody.[54, 55] In some cases, patients failed to achieve engraftment despite aggressive plasmapheresis before and after BMT. One patient died after aggressive plasmapheresis to decrease the antibody titer from 1:16 to 1:1, an additional conditioning regimen, and three separate marrow grafts.[55]

AUTOLOGOUS HSCT

In autologous HSCT, the number of infused cells, the accumulation of cytotoxic treatment prior to transplantations, and ex vivo purging to remove contaminating cancer cells are critical factors for successful engraftment.[20, 22, 56–60]

HEMATOPOIETIC STEM CELL DOSE

Just as in the allografts, HSC dose is an important factor in primary graft failure. Early studies of cell dose were mainly conducted using the CFU-GM assay. Juttner et al. reported that a CFU-GM dose of more than 5×10^5/kg was associated with rapid and sustained engraftment in 10 of 10 patients receiving autologous PBPC.[61] In contrast, three patients receiving less than 5×10^5 CFU-GM/kg did not achieve sustained engraftment. Although the correlation between CFU-GM and CD34+ cells is not always well established, the number of CD34+ cells/kg correlates well with the clinical outcome of transplantation.[22, 56–60]

In one study, 30 women with breast cancer were treated with high-dose chemotherapy followed by autologous HSCT using PBPC. There was a significant delay in neutrophil recovery in those patients who received less than 0.75×10^6 CD34+ cells/kg (median, 22 days), compared with those who received more than 0.75×10^6 CD34+ cells/kg (median, 12 days). A significant delay in platelet recovery occurred between those who received less than 2×10^6 CD34+ cells/kg (median, 75 days) and those who received more than 2×10^6 CD34+ cells/kg (median, 15 days).

In a retrospective analysis by Kiss et al., 17 patients received autologous PBPC for solid tumors.[56] Ten patients who received more than 5×10^6 CD34+ cells/kg experienced significantly earlier recovery of neutrophils and platelets compared with seven patients who received less than 5×10^6 CD34+ cells/kg. At 180 days post transplantation, the median hemoglobin level was 12.4 g/dL versus 8.8 g/dL, platelet count was 202,000/mm³ versus 25,000/mm³, and neutrophil count was 3100/mm³ versus 1400/mm³ in those two cohorts of patients. The report concluded that the number of CD34+ cells/kg is a reliable indicator for early as well as late hematopoietic function.[56] The minimal and optimal doses of CD34+ cells are still under study. Engraftment can be achieved with a lower CD34+ cell content. In one report, 48 patients were infused with less than 2.5×10^6 CD34+ cells/kg after high-dose chemotherapy for various malignancies. Although all patients achieved neutrophil levels of greater than 500/mm³ at a median of 11 days, 9 patients experienced delayed platelet recovery.[57] Currently, CD34+ cell content has gained worldwide acceptance and most transplantation centers aim at harvesting 5×10^6 CD34+ cells/kg from PBPC for rapid and sustained engraftment.

A recent report demonstrated that the CD33− subset of CD34+ cells influenced the success of engraftment in autologous transplantation.[62] Mobilization and engraftment was analyzed in 410 patients. A majority mobilized CD34+CD33− cells, which were usually collected in the greatest quantity on the first day of apheresis. Patients who were mobilized with growth factor alone had the highest percentage of CD34+CD33− cells, whereas extensive prior chemotherapy limited the collection of CD34+CD33− cells. The diagnosis of underlying malignancy, CD34+ cell dose, CD34+CD33− cell dose, and percentage of CD34+CD33− cells were identified as independent factors significantly predictive of engraftment kinetics. A CD34+ cell dose of more than 5×10^6/kg and a CD34+CD33− cell dose of more than 1.0×10^6/kg were associated with significantly earlier neutrophil engraftment and sustained platelet engraftment.[62] Detailed discussion of mobilization and collection of HSC can be found in Chapter 25.

Although the CD34+ cell population has been consistently shown to have the capacity to reconstitute hematopoiesis, the debate about the phenotype of the most primitive HSC continues. Different investigators have demonstrated in a murine model that the true primitive HSC were CD34−.[63–65] Primitive CD34− HSC have been demonstrated in xenografts of human cells into SCID mice[66] or in utero into sheep fetuses.[62] A 1999 report suggested that there was an interconvertible change in CD34 expression. The marker was expressed upon activation of the HSC and then became negative when HSC returned to a resting self-renewing phase.[68] The implication and the significance of such an observation remain to be explored.

Ex vivo purging of autologous marrow using pharmacologic agents has led to delayed neutrophil and platelet engraftment.[69–71] Chemicals such as 4-hydroperoxycyclophosphamide (4-HC) and mafosfamide damage tumor cells as well as CFU-GM, which is the main cause of delayed engraftment. Detailed discussion of various purging procedures and clinical results can be found in Chapter 29.

THERAPIES PRIOR TO HSCT

Most autologous HSCT candidates usually received several cycles of chemotherapy with multiple agents and sometimes localized radiation as well. Their HSC compartment and bone marrow microenvironment may be extensively damaged. An unfavorable marrow microenvironment has long been suspected to be a contributing factor to graft failure, especially in autologous transplantation. One study of four patients who experienced graft failure showed marked hypocellular marrow containing histiocytes with foamy eosinophilic cytoplasm distributed diffusely throughout the marrow biopsy specimen. Marrow fibrosis was not evident. Three of the four patients had undergone autologous BMT and received GM-CSF after marrow infusion. Similar profuse histiocytic proliferation is observed among patients with severe immunodeficiency and other storage diseases such as Gaucher disease, suggesting extensive stro-

mal cell damage.[72] The quality of HSC can be affected by prior chemotherapy. Although the minimum PBPC dose can be collected by multiple sessions of leukapheresis, some data suggest that long-term platelet engraftment is delayed in patients receiving grafts with a low percentage (<0.3%) of CD34+ cells.[73]

MISCELLANEOUS CAUSES

Delayed engraftment should be considered in differential diagnosis during the early post-transplantation period. A number of routinely used medications can cause marrow suppression, including trimethoprim/sulfamethoxazole (TMP/SMZ), acyclovir, ganciclovir, and methotrexate. Acute GVHD should be excluded by appropriate laboratory studies, including skin biopsy at the site of rash and gastrointestinal mucosal biopsy in case of diarrhea. Hematopoietic growth factors, such as G-CSF and GM-CSF, are used routinely in the immediate post-transplantation period to promote engraftment, although the evidence to support their effectiveness is not well documented. Acute viral infections (e.g., cytomegalovirus [CMV]), are less common in the early post-transplantation period. They should be actively investigated before primary graft failure is diagnosed. A weekly polymerase chain reaction (PCR) test for CMV antigenemia is a reliable screening test for early diagnosis of CMV infection. Bone marrow aspirate and biopsy should be performed to evaluate marrow cellularity in case of persistent cytopenia and to rule out gross malignancy in the marrow. Finally, molecular studies (such as fluorescence-labeled X and Y chromosome probe, PCR amplification of individual-specific short-tandem-repeat or variable-number tandem-repeat [VNTR] assay) can be performed to evaluate cell origin in peripheral blood and bone marrow.

STUDIES IDENTIFYING PREDICTIVE FACTORS

Primary graft failure is a devastating complication of HSCT and is almost always fatal if left untreated. Several groups have attempted to identify the risk factors and early predictive signs of graft failure. A retrospective review of 712 patients who underwent allogeneic BMT between 1980 and 1994 in a single institute was reported.[74] Fifty-two patients died primarily because of hemorrhage, infection, or graft failure within 3 months of BMT but prior to relapse. Another 47 patients required second infusion of allogeneic or autologous marrow as rescue for primary graft failure or delayed engraftment within 2 months of the first transplantation. Serial blood counts from days 2–22 after the first BMT were analyzed. In univariate and multivariate analysis, the persistent low leukocyte count of less than 200/mm³ from day 12 onward was significantly associated with increased risk of death and the requirement of second marrow infusion. The authors noted that the absolute neutrophil count of under 100/mm³ might be a better index than total leukocyte count. Unfortunately, reliable data on neutrophils were missing for a large number of patients in their analysis. The authors concluded that a low white blood cell count of less than 200/mm³ between days 12 and 22 was strongly predictive of subsequent graft failure or death.

A quantitative assessment of chimerism in circulation leukocytes is reported to be predictive of graft failure as early as day +5 after allogeneic BMT.[75] Using fluorescence in situ hybridization with mixed X and Y chromosome probes, Gyger et al.[75] monitored chimerism of neutrophils and lymphoid cells from day 1 to day 100 in 28 consecutive patients. All patients received sex-mismatched, unmanipulated marrow. Twenty-one patients experienced engraftment by day 21, and their circulating neutrophils were entirely from donor origin after day +5. Five patients who experienced delayed engraftment at day 20 responded well to G-CSF treatment. Their neutrophils, although below 100/mm³, were entirely of donor origin at day +20. Two patients experienced persistent graft failure and did not respond to G-CSF treatment. Their neutrophils were undetectable at day +20. The proportion of donor-type CD3+, CD56− cells was 0% and 14%, respectively, at day +20. The authors concluded that quantitative molecular monitoring of blood cell chimerism could predict irreversible graft failure.

In a prospective study, 23 patients who received umbilical cord blood or marrow transplants from unrelated donors were monitored by PCR amplification of individual-specific VNTR loci. Sustained engraftment with full donor chimerism occurred in 9 of 9 patients who received bone marrow and 10 of 14 patients who received cord blood. Four patients experienced graft failure characterized by persistent autologous hematopoiesis. In three patients, autologous neutrophils were less than 500/mm³ at days 27, 33, and 37 after transplantation.[76] The authors suggested that molecular analysis of chimerism could predict graft failure in allogeneic transplantation. The clinical application of molecular monitoring needs to be studied in the future.

MANAGEMENT OF PRIMARY GRAFT FAILURE

Management of primary graft failure is difficult. Most patients die from complications of progressive pancytopenia. All patients should be treated initially with hematopoietic growth factors. Autologous back-up cells can be infused first to achieve rapid recovery of hematopoiesis. Prolonged remission from autologous marrow rescue for two patients with chronic myelogenous leukemia after graft failure of allogeneic transplantation has been reported.[77] Second allogeneic marrow transplantation is an option if a donor is available. The second marrow graft or G-CSF mobilized PBPC can come from the same or a different donor.[78, 79] It appears that the source of second marrow grafts may not be critical for engraftment,[14, 16, 77–86] although data are limited. The long-term survival of second marrow transplants for primary graft failure is not promising. Several important issues remain unresolved, including the type and intensity of reconditioning regimen, the choice of marrow (from the same donor or from a different donor), and the timing for second marrow infusion.

Individual case reports of second transplants for graft failure can be found throughout the literature.[83–85] A review of second transplants for relapsed leukemia and graft failure using a different donor has been published.[78] All eight patients who underwent second transplantation for graft failure received additional conditioning regimen prior to the second graft. One patient died from interstitial pneumonia. Seven patients experienced successful engraftment. Although these encouraging results could merely reflect the reporting bias for positive outcome and patient selection in individual case reports, these reports do support the feasibility of second transplants using different donors.

Ten patients experiencing primary graft failure after receiving allografts were treated with autologous marrow (8 of 10) or PBPC (2 of 10) as rescue. These autologous cells were harvested 1–8 weeks prior to transplantation. No reconditioning regimen was given prior to second infusion. Cyclosporine was rapidly tapered in all patients and discontinued 2 weeks after the second infusion. The time from first allograft to second infusion ranged from 21 to 40 days with a median of 22 days. All patients experienced engraftment after second infusion. Four patients died from their recurrent leukemia. Six patients experienced complete remission and survived at 228–3382 days after second transplantation. The authors concluded the autologous rescue was safe and effective treatment for patients with primary graft failure and that the collection of autologous cells should be considered for all patients who were to receive mismatched or unrelated donor marrow.[79] Some practical considerations for collection of autologous marrow or PBPC for possible use as a back-up are listed in Table 44–4.

The outcome of patients in whom first HSCT for aplastic anemia failed was analyzed from EBMTR data.[16] Among 85 patients who experienced graft failure, 41 underwent second HSCT and 44 patients did not. Eighteen patients died from rejection of the second marrow grafts. The long-term survival rate for those who underwent second HSCT was 33%, and for those who did not get second HSCT it was 8%. The timing of second HSCT was an important prognostic factor in the analysis. Patients undergoing second HSCT within 60 days of their initial transplantation experienced an actuarial survival rate of 17% at 8 years, whereas those undergoing second HSCT more than 60 days after the first graft experienced a significantly better outcome with a 43% actuarial survival rate at 12 years. The authors did not specify how many patients received conditioning regimen prior to second HSCT or the agents used in conditioning regimens.

TABLE 44–4. CONSIDERATIONS FOR COLLECTION OF AUTOLOGOUS BACK-UP MARROW AND/OR PERIPHERAL BLOOD PROGENITOR CELLS (PBPC)

Histologic remission in hematologic malignancies
Absence of marrow involvement in nonhematologic malignancies
Conditions that put patients at risk for graft failure:
HLA-mismatched unrelated donor
Haplo-mismatched related donors
Necessity of T-cell depletion
Difficulty anticipated in re-collection of marrow and/or PBPC from same donor due to geographic location, health status, age, or psychosocial issues
Cord blood transplantation in adult setting
Purging of autologous marrow grafts

HLA, human leukocyte antigen.

A similar analysis was performed from IBMTR data.[14] All patients received marrow from HLA-identical sibling donors for treatment of severe aplastic anemia. Graft failure occurred in 68 patients. Nineteen experienced primary and 47 experienced secondary graft failure. A total of 37 patients received an additional transplant, 23 from the same donor and 14 from a different HLA-identical sibling donor. The outcome differed significantly between patients with primary and secondary graft failure. All 19 patients with primary graft failure did not survive for the long term, including 10 patients who had undergone second transplantation. In contrast, 16 of 27 patients with secondary graft failure who received a subsequent allograft achieved engraftment and long-term survival. A majority of patients who received a second transplant were treated with a conditioning regimen. The median interval between the first and second graft was 2.6 months. The type of conditioning regimen for the second HSCT and the type of donor did not significantly influence survival.

Recombinant hematopoietic growth factors have been used routinely in the immediate post-transplantation period. They can be administered in combination to improve graft survival. In one report, six patients who experienced graft failure were treated with a variety of growth factor combinations. All patients were receiving G-CSF before the diagnosis of graft failure. One patient with primary graft failure was successfully treated with daily G-CSF plus IL-1α and was switched to IL-1α/G-CSF in a regimen of 4 days off, 3 days on until engraftment. Five patients with secondary graft failure were treated with a variable combination of IL-1α, G-CSF, M-CSF, GM-CSF, erythropoietin, pulse glucocorticoids, and donor lymphocyte infusion. All six patients experienced engraftment and five of them survived 11–36 months post-transplantation.[78]

CONCLUSION

Primary graft failure is a serious complication of HSCT with very high mortality. Using HLA-identical sibling donors, the overall incidence is about 1–2% of patients receiving transplants for hematologic malignancies and 5–10% of patients given transplants for aplastic anemia and congenital immunodeficiency. The incidence is increased to 10–20% when an unrelated donor is the source of HSC. The mechanism of primary allograft failure is immunologic rejection of infused HSC.

Several measures can be taken to decrease the risk of graft failure, including better patient selection, optimal HLA matching, avoidance of blood transfusion for patients with aplastic anemia prior to transplantation, harvesting an adequate number of HSC, a more effective immunosuppressive regimen, judicious use of hematopoietic growth factors, and careful monitoring after transplantation. Second transplantation is an effective treatment of primary graft failure, although the mortality remains high for such patients. The source of HSC for the second transplant can come from the same donor, another donor, or the patient's own back-up cells.

REFERENCES

1. Becker PS, Nilsson SK, Quesenberry PJ, et al: Adhesion receptor expression by hematopoietic cell lines and murine progenitors: modulation by cytokines and cell cycle status. Exp Hematol 27:533, 1999.
2. Anasetti C, Doney KC, Storb R, et al: Marrow transplantation for severe aplastic anemia: long-term outcome in fifty untransfused patients. Ann Intern Med 104:461, 1986.
3. Howard MR, Hows JM, Gore SM, et al: Unrelated donor marrow transplantation between 1977 and 1987 at four centers in the United Kingdom. Transplantation 49:547, 1990.
4. Marks DI, Cullis JO, Ward KN, et al: Allogeneic bone marrow transplantation for chronic myeloid leukemia using sibling and volunteer unrelated donors. Ann Intern Med 119:207, 1993.
5. Davies SM, Ramsay NRC, Haake RJ, et al: Comparison of engraftment in recipients of matched sibling or unrelated donor marrow allografts. Bone Marrow Transplant 13:51, 1994.
6. Kernan NA, Bausch G, Ash RC, et al: Analysis of 462 transplantations from unrelated donors facilitated by the National Marrow Donor Program. N Engl J Med 328:593, 1993.
7. Hansen JA, Gooley TA, Martin PJ, et al: Bone marrow transplants from unrelated donors for patients with chronic myeloid leukemia. N Engl J Med 338:962, 1998.
8. Ash RC, Casper JT, Chitambar CR, et al: Successful allogeneic transplantation of T-cell-depleted bone marrow from closely HLA-matched unrelated donors. N Engl J Med 322:485, 1990.
9. Wagner JL, Deeg HJ, Seidel K, et al: Bone marrow transplantation for severe aplastic anemia from genotypically ULA-nonidentical relatives: an update of the FRCRC experience. Transplantation 15:54, 1996.
10. Aversa F, Tabilio A, Velardi A, et al: Treatment of high-risk acute leukemia with T-cell-depleted stem cells from related donors with one fully mismatched HLA haplotype. N Engl J Med 339:1186, 1998.
11. Beatty PG, Clift RAT, Mickelson EM, et al: Marrow Transplantation from related donors other than HLA-identical siblings. N Engl J Med 313:765, 1985.
12. Bacigalupo A, Hows J, Gordon-Smith BC, et al: Bone marrow transplantation for severe aplastic anemia from donors other than HLA identical siblings: a report of the BMT Working Party. Bone Marrow Transplant 3:531, 1988.
13. Anasetti C, Amos D, Beatty PG, et al: Effect of HLA compatibility on engraftment of bone marrow transplants in patients with leukemia and lymphoma. N Engl J Med 320:197, 1989.
14. Champlin RE, Horowitz MM, van Bekkum DW, et al: Graft failure following bone marrow transplantation for severe aplastic anemia: risk factors and treatment results. Blood 73:606, 1989.
15. Storb R, Etzioni R, Anasetti C, et al: Cyclophosphamide combined with antithymocyte globulin in preparation for allogeneic marrow transplants in patients with aplastic anemia. Blood 84:941, 1994.
16. McCann SR, Bacigalupo A, Gluckman E, et al: Graft rejection and second bone marrow transplants for acquired aplastic anemia: a report from the Aplastic Anemia Working Party of the European Bone Marrow Transplant Group. Bone Marrow Transplant 13:233, 1994.
17. Thomas ED, Storb R, Clift RA, et al: Bone marrow transplantation. N Engl J Med 292:832, 1975.
18. Storb R: Graft rejection and GVHD in marrow transplantation. Transplant Proc 21:2915, 1989.
19. Bolger GB, Sullivan KM, Storb R, et al: Second marrow infusion for poor graft function after allogeneic marrow transplantation. Bone Marrow Transplant 1:21, 1986.
20. To LB, Dyson PG, Juttner CA: Cell-dose effect in circulating stem cell autografting. Lancet 2:404, 1986.
21. Juttner CA, To LB, Ho JQK, et al: Early lymphohematopoietic recovery after autografting using peripheral blood stem cell in acute non-lymphoid leukemia. Transplant Proc 20:40, 1988.
22. Bender J, To JB, Williams S, et al: Defining a therapeutic dose of peripheral blood stem cells. J Hematother 1:329, 1992.
23. Uharek L, Glass B, Gaska, et al: Influence of donor lymphocytes on the incidence of primary graft failure after allogeneic bone marrow transplantation in a murine model. Br J Haematol 88:79, 1994.
24. O'Reilly RJ: Allogeneic bone marrow transplantation: current and future directions. Blood 62:941, 1983.
25. Santos GW: Bone marrow transplantation in hematologic malignancies. Cancer 65:786, 1990.
26. Pike BL, Robinson WA: Human bone marrow colony growth in agar gel. J Cell Physiol 76:77, 1976.
27. Fauser AA, Messner HA: Granuloerythropoietic colonies in human bone marrow, peripheral blood, and cord blood. Blood 52:1243, 1978.
28. Messner HA, Curtis JE, Minden MD, et al: Clonogenic hemopoietic precursors in bone marrow transplantation. Blood 70:1425, 1987.

29. Civin CI, Strauss LC, Brovall C, et al: Antigenic analysis of hematopoiesis III: a hematopoietic progenitor cell surface antigen defined by a monoclonal antibody raised against KG-1a cells. J Immunol 133:157, 1984.

30. Siena S, Bregni M, Brando B, et al: Flow cytometry for clinical estimation of circulating hematopoietic progenitors for autologous transplantation in cancer patients. Blood 77:400, 1991.

31. Patterson J, Prentice HG, Brenner MK, et al: Graft rejection following HLA-matched T lymphocyte depleted bone marrow transplantation. Br J Haematol 63:221, 1986.

32. Martin PJ, Hansen JA, Buckner CD, et al: Effects of in vitro depletion of T cells in HLA-identical allogeneic marrow grafts. Blood 66:664, 1985.

33. Filipovich AH, Ramsay NKC, Arthor DC, et al: allogeneic bone marrow transplantation with related donors other than HLA MLC-matched siblings, and the use of antithymocyte globulin, prednisone, and methotrexate for prophylaxis of GVHD. Transplantation 39:282, 1985.

34. Kernan NA, Flomenberg N, Dupont B, et al: Graft rejection in recipients of T-cell-depleted HLA-nonidentical marrow transplants for leukemia. Transplantation 43:842, 1987.

35. Champlin R: T-cell depletion to prevent GVHD after bone marrow transplantation. Bone Marrow Transplant 4:687, 1990.

36. Drobyski WR, Ash RC, Casper JT, et al: Effect of T-cell depletion as GVHD prophylaxis on engraftment, relapse, and disease-free survival in unrelated marrow transplantation for CML. Blood 83:1980, 1994.

37. Hamplin RE: T-cell depletion to prevent GVHD after bone marrow transplantation. Hematol Oncol Clin North Am 4:687, 1990.

38. Moore MAS: The clinical use of colony stimulating factors. Ann Rev Immunol 9:159, 1991.

39. Aversa F, Terenzi A, Carotti A, et al: Improved outcome with T-cell-depleted bone marrow transplantation for acute leukemia. J Clin Oncol 17:1545, 1999.

40. Patterson J, Prentice HG, Brenner MK, et al: Graft rejection following HLA-matched T lymphocyte depleted bone marrow transplantation. Br J Haematol 63:221, 1986.

41. Niederwieser D, Pepe M, Storb R, et al: Improvement in rejection, engraftment rate and survival without increase in GVHD by high marrow cell dose in patients transplanted for aplastic anemia. Br J Haematol 69:23, 1988.

42. Buckley RH, Schiff SE, Schiff RI, et al: Hematopoietic stem-cell transplantation for the treatment of severe combined immunodeficiency. N Engl J Med 340:508, 1999.

43. Slavin S, Naparstek E, Aker M, et al: The use of total lymphoid irradiation for prevention of rejection of T-lymphocyte deleted bone marrow allografts in non-malignant hematological disorders. Transplant Proc 21:3053, 1989.

44. Soiffer RJ, Fairclough D, Roberton M, et al: CD6+-depleted allogeneic bone marrow transplantation for acute leukemia in first complete remission. Blood 89:3039, 1997.

45. Garderet L, Snell V, Champlin RE, et al: Effective depletion of alloreactive lymphocytes from peripheral blood mononuclear cell preparations. Transplantation 67:124, 1999.

46. Drobyski WR, Hessner MJ, Klein JP, et al: T-cell depletion plus salvage immunotherapy with donor leukocyte infusions as a strategy to treat chronic-phase chronic myelogenous leukemia patients undergoing HLA-identical sibling marrow transplantation. Blood 94:434, 1999.

47. Clift RA, Buckner CD, Thomas ED, et al: Marrow transplantation for chronic myeloid leukemia: a randomized study comparing cyclophosphamide and total body irradiation with bulsulfan and cyclophosphamide. Blood 84:2036, 1994.

48. Topolsky D, Crilley P, Styler MJ, et al: Unrelated donor bone marrow transplantation without T cell depletion using a chemotherapy only conditioning regimen: low incidence of failed engraftment and severe acute GVHD. Bone Marrow transplant 17:549, 1996.

49. Simmons PJ, Przepiorka D, Thomas ED, et al: Host origin of marrow stromal cells following allogeneic bone marrow transplantation. Nature 328:429, 1987.

50. Peralvo J, Bacigolupo A, Pittaluga PA, et al: Poor graft function associated with GVHD after allogeneic marrow transplantation. Bone Marrow Transplant 2:279, 1987.

51. Torok-Storb B, Simmons PJ, Przepiorka D: Impairment of hemopoiesis in human allografts. Transplant Proc 19(Suppl 7):33, 1987.

52. Greenberger JS: Toxic effects on the hematopoietic microenvironment. Exp Hematol 19:1101, 1991.

53. Storb R: Graft rejection and graft-versus-host disease in marrow transplantation. Transplant Proc 21:2915, 1989.

54. Barge AJ, Johnson G, Witherspoon R, et al: Antibody-mediated marrow failure after allogeneic bone marrow transplantation. Blood 74:1477, 1989.

55. Scornik JC, Elfenbein G, Graham-Pole J, et al: Role of anti-donor antibodies in bone marrow transplant rejection: evaluation by flow cytometry and effect of plasma exchanges. Transplant Proc 21:2974, 1989.

56. Kiss JE, Rybka WB, Winkelstein A, et al: Relationship of CD34+ cell dose to early and late hematopoiesis following autologous peripheral blood stem cell transplantation. Bone Marrow Transplant 19:303, 1997.

57. Weaver CH, Potz J, Redmond J, et al: Engraftment and outcomes of patients receiving myeloablative therapy followed by autologous peripheral blood stem cells with a low CD34+ cell content. Bone Marrow Transplant 19:1103, 1997.

58. Zimmerman TM, Lee WJ, Bender JG, et al: Quantitative CD34 analysis may be used to guide peripheral blood stem cell harvest. Bone Marrow Transplant 9:439, 1995.

59. Bensinger W, Singer J, Applebaum F, et al: Autologous transplantation with peripheral blood mononuclear cells collected after administration of recombinant granulocyte stimulating factor. Blood 81:3158, 1993.

60. Dercksen MW, Rodenhuis S, Dirkson MKA, et al: Subsets of CD34+ cells and rapid hematopoietic recovery after peripheral blood stem cell transplantation. J Clin Oncol 13:1922, 1995.

61. Juttner CA, To LB, Haylock DN, et al: Autologous blood stem cell transplantation. Transplant Proc 21:2929, 1989.

62. Pecora AL, Preti RA, Gleim GW, et al: CD34+ CD33− cells influence days to engraftment and transfusion requirements in autologous blood stem-cell recipients. J Clin Oncol 16:2093, 1998.

63. Osawa M, Hanada K, Hamada H, et al: Long-term lymphohematopoietic reconstitution by single CD34-low/negative hematopoietic stem cell. Science 273:242–245, 1996.

64. Goddel M, Brose K, Paradis G, et al: Isolation and functional properties of murine hematopoietic stem cells that are replicating in vitro. J Exp Med 183:1797, 1996.

65. Goodell M, Rosenzweig M, Kim H, et al: Dye efflux studies suggest that hematopoietic stem cells expressing low or undetectable levels of CD34 antigen exist in multiple species. Nature Med 3:1337, 1997.

66. Dick JE: Absence of CD34 on some human SCID-repopulating cells. Ann N Y Acad Sci 872(9):211–217, 1999.

67. Zanjani ED, Almeida-Porada G, Livingston AG, et al: Human bone marrow CD34− cells engraft in vivo and undergo multilineage expression that includes giving rise to CD34+ cells. Exp Hematol 26(4):353–360, 1998.

68. Sato T, Laver JH, Ogawa M: Reversible expression of CD34 by murine hematopoietic stem cells. Blood 94:2548, 1999.

69. Miller CB, Rowlings PA, Jones RJ, et al: Autotransplants for acute myelogenous leukemia (AML) effects of purging with 4-hydroperoxy-cyclophosphamide (4-HC). Proc Am Soc Clin Oncol 15:338, 1996.

70. Gorin NC, Aegerter P, Auvert B, et al: Autologous bone marrow transplantation for acute myelocytic leukemia in first remission: a European survey of the role of marrow purging. Blood 75:1606–1614, 1990.

71. Chao NJ, Stein AS, Long GD, et al: Busulfan/etoposide initial experience with a new preparatory regimen for autologous bone marrow transplantation in patients with acute nonlymphocytic leukemia. Blood 81:319–323, 1993.

72. Rosenthal NS, Farhi DC: Failure to engraft after bone marrow transplantation: bone marrow morphologic findings. Am J Clin Pathol 102:821, 1994.

73. Bashey A, Lane TA, Mullen M, et al: Value of percentage of CD34 positive cells in leukapheresis product as a predictor of platelet engraftment in autologous transplants. Blood 90(Suppl 1):370a, 1997.

74. Mehta J, Powles R, Singhal S, et al: Early identification of patients at risk of death due to infections, hemorrhage, or graft failure after allogeneic bone marrow transplantation on the basis of the leukocyte counts. Bone Marrow Transplant 19:349, 1997.

75. Gyger M, Baron C, Forest L, et al: Quantitative assessment of hematopoietic chimerism after allogeneic bone marrow transplantation has predictive value for the occurrence of irreversible graft failure and graft-vs.-host disease. Exp Hematol 26:426, 1998.

76. Cimino G, Rapanotti MC, Elia L, et al: A prospective molecular study of chimerism in patients with hematological malignancies receiving

unrelated cord blood or bone marrow transplants: detection of mixed chimerism predicts graft failure with or without early autologous reconstitution in cord blood recipients. Br J Haematol 104:770, 1999.

77. Redei I, Waller BK, Holland, et al: Successful engraftment after primary graft failure in aplastic anemia using G-CSF mobilized peripheral stem cell transfusions. Bone Marrow Transplant 19:175, 1997.

78. Yokota T, Tsuboi A, Okjima Y, et al: Treatment of graft failure after bone marrow transplantation. Leuk Res 18:875, 1994.

79. Mehta J, Powles R, Singhal S, et al: Outcome of autologous rescue after failed engraftment of allogeneic marrow. Bone Marrow Transplant 17:213, 1996.

80. Fouillard L, Deconinck E, Tiberghien P, et al: Prolonged remission and autologous recovery in two patients with CML after graft failure of allogeneic bone marrow transplantation. Bone Marrow Transplant 21:943, 1998.

81. Lipton JH, Messner H: The role of second bone marrow transplant using a different donor for relapsed leukemia or graft failure. Eur J Haematol 58:133, 1997.

82. Zecca M, Perotti C, Marradi P, et al: Recombinant human G-CSF mobilized peripheral blood stem cells for second allogeneic transplant after bone marrow graft rejection in children. Br J Haematol 92:432, 1996.

83. Miflin G, Russel NH, Haynes A, et al: Second allogeneic transplant for severe aplastic anemia following late graft rejection. Br J Haematol 105:570, 1999.

84. Bentley SA, Brecher ME, Powell E, et al: Long-term engraftment failure after marrow ablation and autologous hematopoietic reconstitution: differences between peripheral blood stem cell and bone marrow recipients. Bone Marrow Transplant 19:557, 1997.

85. Remberger M, Ringden O, Ljungman P, et al: Booster marrow or blood cells for graft failure after allogeneic bone marrow transplantation. Bone Marrow Transplant 27:73, 1998.

86. Grandage VL, Cornish JM, Pamphilon DH, et al: Second allogeneic bone marrow transplants from unrelated donors for graft failure following initial unrelated donor bone marrow transplantation. Bone Marrow Transplant 21:687, 1998.

CHAPTER FORTY-FIVE

Therapy of Acute Graft-vs.-Host Disease

*Donna Przepiorka, M.D., Ph.D., and
Karen Cleary, M.D.*

CLINICAL ASPECTS OF ACUTE GVHD

The most common clinical manifestations of acute graft-vs.-host disease (GVHD) are fever, rash, nausea, diarrhea, and abnormal liver function test results.[1] A proportion of patients may experience mucositis, conjunctivitis, or serositis. Endothelialitis may present as microangiopathic hemolytic anemia.[2] Because microangiopathic hemolytic anemia has many causes in the transplant recipient, however, other causes of hemolysis should be excluded in patients with active GVHD. Thrombocytopenia, largely due to consumption, is frequent,[3] and marrow aplasia may occur even in the absence of evidence of host-mediated graft rejection.[4] Elevations of serum and/or peripheral blood leukocyte type 1 cytokines have been reported, but these findings in isolation have a low predictive value.[5–7]

Onset of acute GVHD generally occurs between 14 and 60 days post transplantation. When methotrexate is not used for GVHD prophylaxis, onset may be as early as the first week post transplantation. Neutrophil recovery is not required for GVHD to occur; GVHD may develop prior to hematopoietic engraftment. By convention, the usual clinical manifestations are considered acute GVHD only through post-transplantation day 100; however, a similar clinical syndrome, called early generalized chronic GVHD, may develop well after day 100 and should be managed as acute GVHD.

CUTANEOUS GVHD

Classically, the rash begins as erythema or a maculopapular eruption on the shoulders and back that then extends around the trunk and to the head and extremities (Fig. 45–1).[1] A purpuric eruption similar to small-vessel vasculitis has also been seen. The rash may coalesce to or present as generalized erythroderma, with formation of bullae and desquamation of the epidermis. Pain and erythema of the

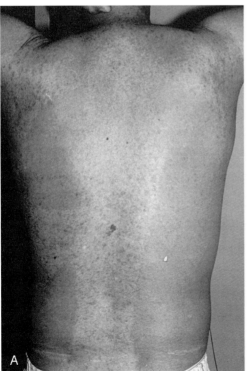

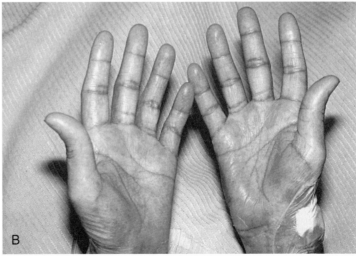

FIGURE 45–1. Acute GVHD of the skin. There may be a maculopapular rash that coalesces to diffuse erythroderma. Note that there is sparing of the total lymphoid irradiation (TLI) field (A). Painful palmar erythema is also seen (B).

palms and soles may be due to GVHD, but when these occur in isolation, acral erythema induced by the preparative regimen must be excluded as the cause.[8] Histologic abnormalities are visible in skin biopsies in the absence of a rash early after transplantation, and biopsy findings may be normal even in the presence of an overt rash.[9, 10] Thus, clinical acumen remains the mainstay for diagnosis of cutaneous GVHD. The major use of the biopsy is to exclude other causes of rash, such as drug allergy, infection, and damage due to chemoradiotherapy.

HEPATIC GVHD

Liver involvement by GVHD is manifested by elevated serum bilirubin and alkaline phosphatase with lesser abnormalities of the serum transaminases,[1, 11] although with hyperacute onset, the laboratory abnormalities may be similar to those of acute hepatitis. Patients with long-standing unresponsive hepatic GVHD may experience liver failure. Liver function abnormalities that wax and wane with biopsy-proven GVHD in other organs are likely due to hepatic involvement, but isolated acute GVHD of the liver can occur, though infrequently. Biopsy of the liver is most helpful in patients with persistent liver function abnormalities when GVHD is absent in other organs, when GVHD in other organs is responding to immunosuppressive therapy, and when liver function abnormalities occur late after the onset of GVHD in other organs.

Other potential causes of post-transplantation liver function abnormalities that may mimic or confound the diagnosis of acute GVHD include infection, drug effects, veno-occlusive disease, hemosiderosis, steatosis, and relapse.[11–16] It is prudent to attempt noninvasive diagnostic procedures, but if a treatable problem cannot be excluded by these means in a patient in stable condition, biopsy should not be delayed beyond the window of opportunity for successful therapy. In one series, results of liver biopsy altered treatment in 31% of patients studied.[16] The morbidity of liver biopsy in transplant recipients has been reduced by the use of laparoscopic and transjugular approaches, but the procedure is not without hazard in a thrombocytopenic patient.

GASTROINTESTINAL GVHD

The distal small bowel and colon are the most common sites of GVHD in the gastrointestinal tract, and some patients may have intestinal involvement without GVHD elsewhere. Patients present with crampy lower abdominal pain and mucoid-to-watery, frequently greenish diarrhea.[1, 11] The diarrhea is secretory, and several liters may be produced daily even in a patient who is not undergoing oral alimentation, resulting in severe fluid and electrolyte imbalances. Protein-losing enteropathy may also occur, with marked hypoalbuminemia and third-spacing of fluids. Life-threatening hemorrhage can accompany extensive denudation and ulceration of the bowel.

The presentation of viral infection and Epstein-Barr virus lymphoma of the gastrointestinal tract can be very similar to that of acute GVHD, and biopsy of the lower tract is necessary for diagnosis,[11, 17] although adenovirus infection

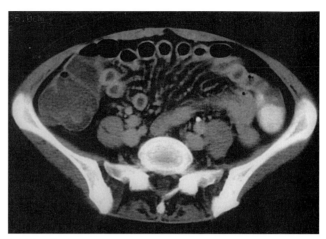

FIGURE 45–2. Acute GVHD of the small bowel. Thickened bowel wall that enhances with contrast is visible on computed tomographic scan of the abdomen. Involvement may be segmental.

and *Clostridium difficile* toxin can be detected by culture of the stool. If diarrhea persists or recurs rapidly after treatment with immunosuppressives, rebiopsy to exclude secondary infection is warranted. When the small bowel alone is involved, biopsy is not possible. In this circumstance, if the patient has recovered from the acute effects of the preparative regimen, characteristic changes on radiographic imaging may aid diagnosis (Fig. 45–2).[18–20]

Patients with upper gastrointestinal GVHD have anorexia, persistent nausea, vomiting, and abdominal pain.[21, 22] These symptoms may also be caused by infection, pancreatitis, peptic ulcer, drugs, acalculous cholecystitis, and subdural hematoma. Biopsies of the stomach and duodenum generally provide diagnostic material. A negative biopsy of the lower gastrointestinal tract is not reliable for excluding upper gastrointestinal GVHD.[23]

OTHER SETTINGS FOR ACUTE GVHD

Acute GVHD may occur after infusion of donor leukocytes for treatment of relapse after transplantation.[24, 25] The clinical manifestations are the same as when GVHD develops post transplantation, except that a proportion of patients also become aplastic, as occurs in patients with transfusion-associated GVHD. Median time to onset of GVHD is approximately 1 month after infusion of donor leukocytes. In large retrospective reviews, 41–46% of patients experienced grade II–IV GVHD. The incidence was highest for recipients with unrelated or human leukocyte antigen (HLA)-nonidentical donors.[24, 25] For patients treated for post-transplantation relapse of chronic myelogenous leukemia, the incidence of GVHD increased with T-cell dose,[26] but reports of other risk factors for GVHD after donor leukocyte infusion have been inconsistent.[24, 25]

A syndrome similar to the acute GVHD that occurs after allogeneic transplantation has also been observed in recipients of autologous or syngeneic marrow.[27] Onset of the syndrome in these patients occurs at the time of engraftment and is heralded by fever. In syngeneic transplant recipients, the syndrome has generally been mild, involving usually the skin,[28] but patients may also experience nausea, diarrhea, jaundice, alveolar hemorrhage, and multiorgan failure.[27–30] In one series, 0.5% of all autologous transplant recipients experienced a severe or fatal course.[27] Unlike classic GVHD, which is thought to be mediated by donor lymphocytes, the syndrome in syngeneic and autologous transplant recipients is thought to be mediated by cytokines released during rapid expansion of the hematopoietic compartment at the time of engraftment[31] and is sometimes called the *cytokine syndrome*.

HISTOLOGY OF ACUTE GVHD

CUTANEOUS HISTOPATHOLOGY

The histologic changes of GVHD reflect the single-cell injury induced by the immune system and are manifested by apoptosis and necrosis.[32, 33] In the skin, basal vacuolization is the earliest change detected by biopsy, but this abnormality is nonspecific because it can also occur early after transplantation in the absence of GVHD and may be an effect of the preparative regimen. Necrotic keratinocytes or "eosinophilic bodies" are visible in the epidermis and hair follicle (Fig. 45–3), occasionally surrounded by one or more lymphocytes (satellitosis). With increasing necrosis along the epidermis, there is focal acantholysis, which may progress to complete loss of the epidermis. The latter is histologically indistinguishable from toxic epidermal necrolysis induced by drugs or bacterial exotoxin. A histologic grading system has been published, but it does not correlate with prognosis.[32, 33]

HEPATIC HISTOPATHOLOGY

With GVHD of the liver, damage to the interlobular bile ducts, the most typical feature, is manifested as cytoplasmic

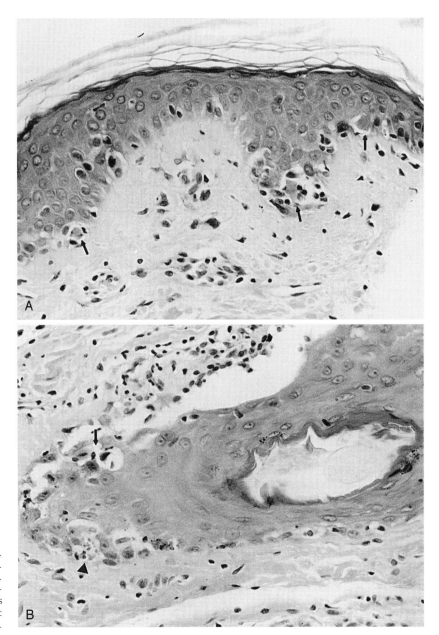

FIGURE 45–3. Acute GVHD of the skin (× 20). *A,* Scattered lymphocytes infiltrate the epidermis. Three necrotic keratinocytes (*arrows*) are present. Two of them have associated lymphocytes (satellitosis). *B,* A hair follicle underlying the epidermis has subepidermal clefting in addition to necrotic keratinocytes with residual pyknotic nuclei (*arrow*).

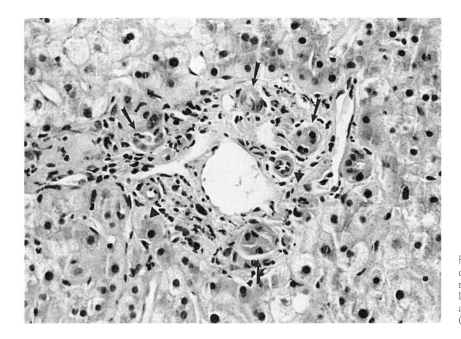

FIGURE 45–4. Acute GVHD of the liver. Bile ducts are damaged. All have abnormal nuclei, nuclear dropout, cytoplasmic eosinophilia, and lymphocytic infiltration. Arterioles (*arrowheads*) are prominent, but there is little inflammation. (× 20.)

vacuolization and eosinophilia in addition to nuclear atypia, pseudostratification, or drop-out with or without a mild lymphocytic infiltrate in the portal region and within the ductal epithelium itself (Fig. 45–4).[32, 33] There is generally a lesser degree of lobular damage, with mild ballooning degeneration of hepatocytes and rare acidophilic bodies. Cholestasis is variable. Isolated cholestatic changes in the liver may occur with severe GVHD of the gut. They are thought to be due to the effect of cytokines transported from the area of inflammation in the gut through the portal system to the liver. The major differential diagnoses are viral hepatitis and drug effects. With endothelialitis, lymphocytes are attached to portal or central vein endothelial cells. The presence of endothelialitis or moderate-to-severe damage to more than 50% of the bile ducts with little hepatocellular change is most predictive of GVHD.[12, 33] In

long-standing or advanced disease, there is ductopenia and cholestasis with a variable degree of portal inflammation and fibrosis.

GASTROINTESTINAL HISTOPATHOLOGY

Single-cell necrosis or apoptotic bodies at the base of large bowel crypts and gastric or small bowel glands are most characteristic of acute GVHD of the gastrointestinal tract (Fig. 45–5).[32, 34] This early lesion may also occur with cytomegalovirus infection, however, and in the absence of intranuclear inclusions, specific immunohistochemical staining may be required to detect the viral infection.[35] If cytomegalovirus is found in biopsies with apoptosis, GVHD cannot be excluded because the two may occur simultane-

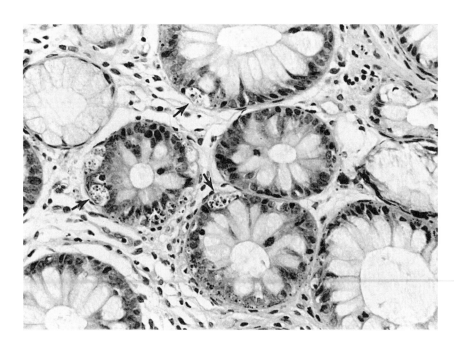

FIGURE 45–5. Acute GVHD of the gut. Several large bowel crypts contain single-cell necrosis (apoptotic bodies) (*arrows*). A normal crypt is in the upper left corner. (× 20.)

TABLE 45–1. CONSENSUS CRITERIA FOR CLINICAL STAGING AND GRADING OF ACUTE GRAFT-VERSUS-HOST DISEASE

	Skin	Liver	Gut
Stage			
1	Rash <25%*	Bilirubin 2–3 mg/dL†	Diarrhea >500 mL/day‡ or persistent nausea§
2	Rash 25–50%	Bilirubin 3–6 mg/dL	Diarrhea >1000 mL/day
3	Rash >50%	Bilirubin 6–15 mg/dL	Diarrhea >1500 mL/day
4	Generalized erythroderma with bullae	Bilirubin >15 mg/dL	Severe abdominal pain with or without ileus
Grade¶			
I	Stage 1–2	None	None
II	Stage 3 *or*	Stage 1 *or*	Stage 1
III	—	Stage 2–3 *or*	Stage 2–4
IV	Stage 4 *or*	Stage 4 *or*	Stage 4‖

*Use "rule of nines" or burn chart to determine extent of rash.
†Range given as total bilirubin. Downgrade one stage if an additional cause of elevated bilirubin has been documented.
‡Volume of diarrhea applies to adults. For pediatric patients, the volume of diarrhea should be based on body surface area. Downgrade one stage if an additional cause of diarrhea has been documented.
§Persistent nausea with histologic evidence of GVHD in the stomach or duodenum.
¶Criteria for grading given as degree of organ involvement required to confer that grade.
‖Grade IV may also include lesser organ involvement with Karnofsky performance status <50%, so patients with stage 4 gut GVHD are usually grade IV.
From Przepiorka D, Weisdorf D, Martin P, et al: Consensus conference on acute GVHD grading. Bone Marrow Transplant 15:825–828, 1995.

ously. Necrosis of an entire crypt ("crypt abscess") and glands with intraluminal debris also occurs in early GVHD. This progresses to complete loss of crypts and glands with denudation of the mucosa. The diagnosis of GVHD is difficult to make at the end-stage of the process because mucosal denudation also occurs with other inflammatory or infectious disorders such as adenoviral enteritis. Cytoreductive treatment may produce similar epithelial destruction, so interpretation of biopsies within the first 21 days after transplantation must be undertaken with caution.

CLINICAL GRADING CRITERIA FOR ACUTE GVHD

Although it is currently well appreciated that the short-term outcome for patients with acute GVHD varies with the severity of disease, the original GVHD grading system proposed by Glucksberg et al.[36] in 1974 and subsequently modified by Thomas et al.[1] was largely a descriptive classification based on degree of organ involvement. There was no significant difference in outcomes for patients with grade II, III, or IV GVHD. The system allowed for comparisons among studies and became widely accepted, however.

After an additional 20 years of experience, both the European Group for Blood and Marrow Transplantation and the International Bone Marrow Transplant Registry reported that the grading system does, in fact, distinguish groups of patients with increasing risks of treatment-related mortality. For patients with chronic myelogenous leukemia in chronic phase receiving transplants from HLA-identical donors, the relative risks of treatment-related mortality were 1.2, 2.1, 4.0, and 8.5, respectively, for patients with grades I–IV GVHD.[37] For patients with acute leukemia or chronic myelogenous leukemia receiving transplants from HLA-identical donors using cyclosporine and methotrexate as prophylaxis, the relative risks of treatment-related mortality were 1.1, 2.2, and 5.3 for patients with grades I, II, and III/IV GVHD, respectively.[38]

On review of the grading system in 1994, it was con-

cluded that the experience available did not support modification of the grading system for pediatric patients, patients with HLA-nonidentical donors, or patients receiving T cell–depleted transplants.[39] Treatment-related mortality in each of these populations appeared to correlate with grade of GVHD. Data also suggested that the outcome for patients with isolated upper gastrointestinal GVHD was similar to that of patients with grade II GVHD,[22] and persistent nausea was incorporated into the staging system at this level (Table 45–1). Consensus could not be reached regarding objective criteria for distinguishing grades III and IV GVHD, and performance status remains a major criterion for assignment of grade IV. For reporting purposes, the incidences or actuarial estimates of grades III and IV GVHD are combined.

Further evaluation of the GVHD grading system showed substantial heterogeneity in outcomes within a grade for patients with different combinations of organ stages.[38] Patterns of organ involvement in patients with similar outcomes were combined to devise a Severity Index System based solely on objective criteria and having greater homogeneity within an index (Table 45–2). This was accomplished by a retrospective analysis of HLA-identical marrow transplant recipients using cyclosporine and methotrexate

TABLE 45–2. CRITERIA FOR INTERNATIONAL BONE MARROW TRANSPLANT REGISTRY SEVERITY INDEX FOR ACUTE GRAFT-VS.-HOST DISEASE

Index*	Extent of Rash		Total Bilirubin		Volume of Diarrhea
A	<25%	*or*	<2.0 mg/dL	*or*	<500 mL/day
B	25–50	*or*	2.0–6.0 mg/dL	*or*	500–1500 mL/day
C	>50%	*or*	6.1–15.0 mg/d	*or*	>1500 mL/day
D	Bullae	*or*	>15 mg/dL	*or*	Severe pain or ileus

*Index assigned based on maximum organ involvement.
From Rowlings PA, Przepiorka D, Klein JP, et al: IBMTR Severity Index for grading acute graft-versus-host disease: retrospective comparison with Glucksberg grade. Br J Haematol 97:855–864, 1997.

for GVHD prophylaxis, and the system was validated retrospectively for a cohort of HLA-identical T cell–depleted marrow transplant recipients. The relative risks of treatment-related mortality were 0.8, 1.9, 4.3, and 11.9, respectively, for patients in indices A–D. Isolated upper gastrointestinal GVHD is not included in the system but would fall into index B.

PRIMARY TREATMENT OF ACUTE GVHD

TREATMENT OF MILD ACUTE GVHD

Patients with stage I cutaneous GVHD are often observed; minimal erythema can be confused with acute radiation changes of the skin. Alternatively, stage I and stage II cutaneous GVHD may be treated with topical steroids. Selected patients, such as those with HLA-mismatched or unrelated donors, have been treated with systemic therapy even when only grade 1 GVHD is present because of the perceived high risk of rapid development of life-threatening GVHD.

CORTICOSTEROIDS

High-dose corticosteroids are well established as first-line treatment of acute GVHD.[40–49] Complete response rates reported varied from 20% to 76% for doses of methylprednisolone of 2 mg/kg/day to as high as 2 g/m^2/day. Treatment with more than 2 mg/kg/day did not improve response rates, but infectious complications were increased.[40, 49] Although most patients with moderate-to-severe GVHD are treated with intravenous corticosteroids, oral treatment can be successful for those with mild-to-moderate involvement using methylprednisolone or a bioequivalent corticosteroid. Once a response is achieved, steroids are tapered 20–50% every 3–7 days; tapering more slowly has not resulted in a significant decrease in GVHD flares, incidence of chronic GVHD, or early mortality.[50]

OTHER AGENTS

A number of agents have been compared with corticosteroids as first-line treatment of acute GVHD. When long methotrexate was used for prophylaxis, the response rate with cyclosporine was not different from that with methylprednisolone.[51] In the current era, however, cyclosporine or tacrolimus is usually used as prophylaxis. For such patients, two randomized studies of anti–T cell reagents have been performed. In the first study, it was found that in comparison to corticosteroids alone, the response to therapy was no better when monoclonal anti-CD25 was added.[52] In the second randomized study, although short-term response was improved with monoclonal anti-CD5 immunotoxin and corticosteroids, this combination did not show any intermediate or long-term advantage over corticosteroids alone.[53]

Few studies have evaluated monoclonal[54, 55] or polyclonal[40, 44, 48, 56, 57] anti–T cell antibodies as single agents for first-line treatment of acute GVHD. Antithymocyte globulin

(ATG) was used most frequently. The limited experience with ATG provided highly variable results, but even if it were equivalent to corticosteroids in efficacy, the cost and toxicities of ATG have precluded its routine use as first-line therapy for uncomplicated GVHD.[40, 57]

TREATMENT OF REFRACTORY ACUTE GVHD

For patients with GVHD refractory to corticosteroids, a number of treatment options have emerged. Anecdotally, escalating the dose of corticosteroid from 2 to 10 mg/kg/day has been reported to alleviate GVHD, but controlled trials testing this strategy are lacking, and toxicities of prolonged use of very high-dose corticosteroids can be prohibitive.

Newer therapies are aimed at abrogating the ongoing inflammatory response and inhibiting T-cell reactivity. These include inhibitors of antigen processing and presentation, inhibitors of early T-cell activation, antimetabolites, broad antilymphocyte antibodies, cytokine antagonists, and monoclonal antibodies directed against the T-cell receptor, co-stimulatory molecules, and activation molecules (Table 45–3).

CYTOKINE ANTAGONISTS

The cytokine antagonists are especially attractive for treatment of GVHD because they may reduce inflammation directly and generally have fewer side effects than corticosteroids. The initial clinical trials targeting individual cytokines, however, yielded unenthusiastic results, probably because the remainder of the multiple cytokines active in GVHD were left unaffected.[93–95] If GVHD were mediated by a cytokine cascade rather than a cytokine storm, tar-

TABLE 45–3. AGENTS TESTED FOR TREATMENT OF STEROID-REFRACTORY ACUTE GRAFT-VS.-HOST DISEASE

Class	Drug	References
Inhibitors of antigen processing and presentation	Thalidomide	58, 59
	Hydroxychloroquine	60
	Deoxyspergualin	61
Inhibitors of early T-cell activation	Tacrolimus	62–65
Antimetabolites	Mycophenolate mofetil	66–68
Antilymphocyte antibodies	Antithymocyte globulin	69–71
	Campath-1	72
Anti–T-cell receptor antibody	Muromonab (OKT3)	54, 73, 74
	Anti-CD3	55, 75, 76
Antibodies against T-cell activation antigens	Murine anti-CD25	77–82
	Dacliximab	83–85
	CBL-1	86
Antibodies against T-cell co-stimulatory and adhesion molecules	Anti-CD4	87
	Anti-LFA-1	88
	Anti-CD5 immunotoxin	89
	Anti-CD2	90–92
Cytokine antagonists	Anti-TNFα	93
	rhuIL-1 receptor antagonist	94
	Soluble rhuIL-1 receptor	95

geting the individual cytokine at the beginning of the cascade might be effective. It remains to be determined whether etanercept or infliximab, currently available drugs that neutralize tumor necrosis factor-α, will be useful for steroid-sparing as an adjunct with an anti–T cell reagent.

T-CELL ACTIVATION INHIBITORS

Tacrolimus is the only T-cell activation inhibitor evaluated for treatment of GVHD in the modern era of transplantation.[62–65] Preclinical studies in a major histocompatibility complex–mismatched rat model demonstrated that tacrolimus was more effective than cyclosporine for treatment of GVHD.[96] Tacrolimus, however, is known to have no activity against activated T cells, and in clinical trials of steroid-refractory GVHD, response rates were only 12–38%.[63–65]

ANTIMETABOLITES

Mycophenolate mofetil given orally has been evaluated in few patients with acute GVHD. Response rates have been only 18–30%,[66–68] although a steroid-sparing effect was demonstrated in one report.[67] Neutropenia and nausea were cited as the most common complications.

LYMPHOCYTE IMMUNE GLOBULIN

Although no controlled studies have been performed, horse ATG is widely accepted as first-line treatment of steroid-refractory acute GVHD. A number of dose-schedules have been used (Table 45–4), with overall response rates of 20–54%.[50, 69, 70] Complete responses occur in only about a third of patients. Side effects of ATG included fever, chills, myalgias, thrombocytopenia, leukopenia, fluid overload, dyspnea, pulmonary infiltrates, and rash. Thymoglobulin, a rabbit preparation of ATG, is also active for treatment of GVHD, but the dose schedules evaluated led to a high rate of adverse events, including post-transplantation lymphoproliferative disorders.[71]

TABLE 45–4. COMMERCIALLY AVAILABLE DRUGS FOR TREATMENT OF ACUTE GRAFT-VS.-HOST DISEASE*

Drug	Regimen
Primary treatment	
Methylprednisolone	0.5 mg/kg IV or PO every 6 hr
Salvage therapy	
Antithymocyte globulin	15 mg/kg IV every other day × 6
	10 mg/kg IV daily × 14
	30–40 mg/kg IV daily × 4
Muromonab	5 mg IV daily × 10–14 days
Dacliximab	1 mg/kg IV on days 1, 4, 8, 15, and 22
Mycophenolate mofetil	1 g PO twice daily × 21–35 days

*Individuals not experienced in the administration of immunosuppressive drugs for treatment of acute GVHD should consult the primary references regarding premedications, precautions, and monitoring during use of these agents.

ANTI-CD3 ANTIBODY

The complete response rate reported for muromonab (OKT3) has been 12–50%.[54, 73, 74] Toxicity has been common, however. Almost all patients experience a "first-dose reaction" that is thought to be mediated by tumor necrosis factor, and this may exacerbate the underlying clinical symptoms.[97] The dose schedule used is the one approved for organ allograft rejection; different dose schedules have not been evaluated specifically for treatment of acute GVHD.

INTERLEUKIN-2 RECEPTOR BLOCKADE

The strategy of targeting CD25, the chain of the interleukin-2 receptor, was based on the fact that CD25 was up-regulated on activated T cells, so blockade of activated T cells in a patient with acute GVHD would affect only the alloreactive cells. Complete response rates with the murine anti-CD25 antibodies were 10–88%.[77–82] For daclizumab, the humanized form of anti-CD25, complete responses occurred in 28–47% of patients. Few side effects were noted with use of dacliximab.

PHOTOTHERAPY

For treatment of acute GVHD, extracorporeal photopheresis is performed on 2 consecutive days every 2 weeks. Using oral 8-methoxypsoralen as the photosensitizer proved ineffective for treatment of liver GVHD,[98] but five of six patients responded when photopheresis was conducted with ex vivo 8-methoxypsoralen.[99] The procedure has been well tolerated, although it requires a substantial time commitment on the part of the patient.

SUPPORTIVE CARE

Symptomatic support can greatly improve the quality of life for patients with acute GVHD. Skin care should address the inflammation and potential for cellulitis that occur with denudation of the epidermis, and cutaneous pain may require local anesthetics such as pramoxine. The abdominal pain of intestinal GVHD may require systemic narcotics, and octreotide has been found to be helpful with the secretory diarrhea.[100]

Infection is the most common cause of death in patients with acute GVHD,[43, 48] and acute GVHD is an independent risk factor for post-transplantation bacterial, fungal, and cytomegalovirus infections.[101–103] Fungal prophylaxis is clearly warranted for all patients on intensive immunosuppressive therapy, and many centers initiate ganciclovir prophylaxis for patients who experience acute GVHD rather than rely only on high-sensitivity monitoring for cytomegalovirus. Bacterial prophylaxis is frequently used for patients with intestinal GVHD, but use of intravenous immunoglobulin for prevention of bacterial infections in the absence of hypogammaglobulinemia remains controversial.[104]

CAVEATS IN THE TREATMENT OF ACUTE GVHD

When managing moderate-to-severe acute GVHD, the transplant physician frequently looks to the literature to assess prognosis and identify the best available treatment option. In several large retrospective studies of the treatment of acute GVHD, factors consistently predictive of response to therapy were low initial organ severity score, lack of liver involvement, and minimal degree of histoincompatibility.[44, 46, 48, 50, 69] Initial overall grade, a heterogeneous categorization at best, was not an independent prognostic factor. It is therefore difficult to compare results among treatment studies without knowing how the patient populations compare in terms of these predictive factors. This situation is confounded further by the lack of consensus on the definition of response to therapy for acute GVHD.

Once a treatment option has been identified, the transplant physician must also decide whether to use the new agent in addition to or instead of a current drug. Although it is commonly assumed that adding therapy would be most beneficial, there is evidence that oversuppression of immune function may have a negative impact on survival.[105] Optimal management of acute GVHD, although a challenge, is clearly a worthy goal, since response to therapy is associated with a significant reduction in treatment-related mortality.[43, 44, 48, 50, 69]

REFERENCES

1. Thomas ED, Storb R, Clift RA, et al: Bone-marrow transplantation. N Engl J Med 292:895–902, 1975.
2. Holler E, Kolb HJ, Hiller E, et al: Microangiopathy in patients on cyclosporine prophylaxis who developed acute graft-versus-host disease after HLA-identical bone marrow transplantation. Blood 73:2018–2024, 1989.
3. Anasetti C, Rybka W, Sullivan KM, et al: Graft-v-host disease is associated with autoimmune-like thrombocytopenia. Blood 73:1054–1058, 1989.
4. Torok-Storb B, Simmons P, Przepiorka D: Impairment of hemopoiesis in human allografts. Transplant Proc 19(Suppl 7):33–37, 1987.
5. Holler E, Kolb HJ, Möller A, et al: Increased serum levels of tumor necrosis factor precede major complications of bone marrow transplantation. Blood 75:1011–1016, 1990.
6. Jadus MR, Wepsic HT: The role of cytokines in graft-versus-host reactions and disease. Bone Marrow Transplant 10:1–14, 1992.
7. Imamura M, Hashino S, Kobayashi H, et al: Serum cytokine levels in bone marrow transplantation: synergistic interaction of interleukin-6, interferon-γ, and tumor necrosis factor-α in graft-versus-host disease. Bone Marrow Transplant 13:745–751, 1994.
8. Reynaert H, DeConinck A, Neven AM, et al: Chemotherapy-induced acral erythema and acute graft-versus-host disease after allogeneic bone marrow transplantation. Bone Marrow Transplant 10:185–187, 1992.
9. Elliott CJ, Sloane JP, Sanderson KV, et al: The histological diagnosis of cutaneous graft-versus-host disease: relationship of skin changes to marrow purging and other clinical variables. Histopathology 11:145–155, 1987.
10. Kohler S, Hendrickson MR, Chao NJ, et al: Value of skin biopsies in assessing prognosis and progression of acute graft-versus-host disease. Am J Surg Pathol 21:988–996, 1997.
11. McDonald GB, Shulman HM, Sullivan KM, et al: Intestinal and hepatic complications of human bone marrow transplantation. part I. Gastroenterology 90:460–477, 1986.
12. Snover DC, Weisdorf SA, Ramsay NK, et al: Hepatic graft-versus-host disease: a study of the predictive value of liver biopsy in diagnosis. Hepatology 4:123–130, 1984.
13. Shulman HM, Sharma P, Amos D, et al: A coded histologic study of hepatic graft-versus-host disease after human bone marrow transplantation. Hepatology 8:463–470, 1988.
14. Einsele H, Waller HD, Weber P, et al: Cytomegalovirus in liver biopsies of marrow transplant recipients: detection methods, clinical, histological and immunohistological features. Med Microbiol Immunol 183:205–216, 1994.
15. Forbes GM, Davies JM, Herrmann RP, et al: Liver disease complicating bone marrow transplantation: a clinical audit. J Gastroenterol Hepatol 10:1–7, 1995.
16. Iqbal M, Creger RJ, Fox RM, et al: Laparoscopic liver biopsy to evaluate hepatic dysfunction in patients with hematologic malignancies: a useful tool to effect changes in management. Bone Marrow Transplant 17:655–662, 1996.
17. Terdiman JP, Linker CA, Ries CA, et al: The role of endoscopic evaluation in patients with suspected intestinal graft-versus-host disease after allogeneic bone-marrow transplantation. Endoscopy 28:680–685, 1996.
18. Fisk JD, Shulman HM, Greening RR, et al: Gastrointestinal radiographic features of human graft-versus-host disease. Am J Radiol 136:329–336, 1981.
19. Worawattanakul S, Semelka RC, Kelekis NL, et al: MR findings of intestinal graft-versus-host disease. Magnetic Res Imag 14:1221–1223, 1996.
20. Donnelly LF, Morris CL: Acute graft-versus-host disease in children: abdominal CT findings. Radiology 199:265–268, 1996.
21. Spencer GD, Hackman RC, McDonald GB, et al: A prospective study of unexplained nausea and vomiting after marrow transplantation. Transplantation 42:602–607, 1986.
22. Weisdorf DJ, Snover DC, Haake R, et al: Acute gastrointestinal graft-versus-host disease: clinical significance and response to immunosuppressive therapy. Blood 76:624–629, 1990.
23. Roy J, Snover D, Weisdorf S, et al: Simultaneous upper and lower endoscopic biopsy of intestinal graft-versus-host disease. Transplantation 51:642–626, 1991.
24. Kolb HJ, Schattenberg A, Goldman JM, et al: Graft-versus-leukemia effect of donor lymphocyte transfusions in marrow grafted patients. Blood 86:2041–2050, 1995.
25. Collins RH, Shpilberg O, Drobyski WR, et al: Donor leukocyte infusions in 140 patients with relapsed malignancy after allogeneic bone marrow transplantation. J Clin Oncol 15:433–444, 1997.
26. Mackinnon S, Papadopoulos EB, Carabasi MH, et al: Adoptive immunotherapy evaluating escalating doses of donor leukocytes for relapse of chronic myeloid leukemia after bone marrow transplantation: separation of graft-versus-leukemia responses from graft-versus-host disease. Blood 86:1261–1268, 1995.
27. Miller CB, Hayashi RJ, Vogelsang GB, et al: Aseptic shock syndrome after bone marrow transplantation. Blood 80(Suppl 1):140a, 1992.
28. Einsele H, Ehninger G, Schneider EM, et al: High frequency of graft-versus-host-like syndromes following syngeneic bone marrow transplantation. Transplantation 45:579–585, 1988.
29. Cahill RA, Spitzer TR, Mazumder A: Marrow engraftment and clinical manifestations of capillary leak syndrome. Bone Marrow Transplant 18:177–184, 1996.
30. Moreb JS, Kubilis PS, Mullins DL, et al: Increased frequency of autoaggression syndrome associated with autologous stem cell transplantation in breast cancer patients. Bone Marrow Transplant 19:101–106, 1997.
31. Pechumer H, Leinisch E, Bender-Gotze C, et al: Recovery of monocytes after bone marrow transplantation—rapid reappearance of tumor necrosis factor alpha and interleukin 6 production. Transplantation 52:698–704, 1991.
32. Sale GE, Shulman HM: The Pathology of Bone Marrow Transplantation. New York, Masson, 1984.
33. Snover DC: Biopsy interpretation in bone marrow transplantation. In Rosen PP, Fechner RE (eds): Pathology Annual, Part 2. Hartford, CT, Appleton & Lange, 1989, pp 63–101.
34. Snover DC: Graft-vs-host disease of the gastrointestinal tract. Am J Surg Pathol 14:101–108, 1990.
35. Einsele H, Ehninger G, Hebart H, et al: Incidence of local CMV infection and acute intestinal graft-versus-host disease in marrow transplant recipients with severe diarrhoea. Bone Marrow Transplant 14:955–963, 1994.
36. Glucksberg H, Storb R, Fefer A, et al: Clinical manifestations of graft-versus-host disease in human recipients of marrow from HLA-matched sibling donors. Transplantation 18:295–304, 1974.

37. Gratwohl A, Hermans J, Apperley J, et al: Acute graft-versus-host disease: grade and outcome in patients with chronic myelogenous leukemia. Blood 86:813–818, 1995.

38. Rowlings PA, Przepiorka D, Klein JP, et al: IBMTR Severity Index for grading acute graft-versus-host disease: retrospective comparison with Glucksberg grade. Br J Haematol 97:855–864, 1997.

39. Przepiorka D, Weisdorf D, Martin P, et al: Consensus conference on acute GVHD grading. Bone Marrow Transplant 15:825–828, 1995.

40. Tutschka PJ, Farmer E, Beschorner WE, et al: Therapy of acute graft-versus-host diease (GVHD)—Baltimore experience. Exp Hematol 9:126, 1981.

41. Kendra J, Barrett AJ, Lucas C, et al: Response of graft versus host disease to high doses of methylprednisolone. Clin Lab Haematol 3:19–26, 1981.

42. Kanojia MD, Anagnostou AA, Zander AR, et al: High-dose methyl-prednisolone treatment for acute graft-verus-host disease after bone marrow transplantation in adults. Transplantation 37:246–251, 1984.

43. Weisdorf D, Haake R, Blazar B, et al: Treatment of moderate/severe acute graft-versus-host disease after allogeneic bone marrow transplantation: an analysis of clinical risk features and outcome. Blood 75:1024–1030, 1990.

44. Martin PJ, Schoch G, Fisher L, et al: A retrospective analysis of therapy for acute graft-versus-host disease: initial treatment. Blood 76:1464–1472, 1990.

45. Oblon DJ, Felker D, Coyle K, et al: High-dose methylprednisolone therapy for acute graft-versus-host disease associated with matched unrelated donor bone marrow transplantation. Bone Marrow Transplant 10:355–357, 1992.

46. Roy J, McGlave PB, Filipovich AH, et al: Acute graft-versus-host disease following unrelated donor marrow transplantation: failure of conventional therapy. Bone Marrow Transplant 10:77–82, 1992.

47. Hings IM, Filipovich AH, Miller WJ, et al: Prednisone therapy for acute graft-versus-host disease: short- versus long-term treatment. Transplantation 56:577–580, 1993.

48. Aschan J: Treatment of moderate to severe acute graft-versus-host disease: a retrospective analysis. Bone Marrow Transplant 14:601–607, 1994.

49. Van Lint MT, Uderzo C, Locasciulli A, et al: Early treatment of acute graft-versus-host disease with high- or low-dose 6-methylprednisolone: a multicenter randomized trial from the Italian Group for Bone Marrow Transplantation. Blood 92:2288–2293, 1998.

50. Hings IM, Severson R, Filipovich AH, et al: Treatment of moderate and severe acute GVHD after allogeneic bone marrow transplantation. Transplantation 58:437–442, 1994.

51. Kennedy MS, Deeg HJ, Storb R, et al: Treatment of acute graft-versus-host disease after allogeneic marrow transplantation. Am J Med 78:978–983, 1985.

52. Cahn JY, Bordigoni P, Tiberghien P, et al: Treatment of acute graft-versus-host disease with methylprednisolone and cyclosporine with or without an anti-interleukin-2 receptor monoclonal antibody. Transplantation 60:939–942, 1995.

53. Martin PJ, Nelson BJ, Appelbaum FR, et al: Evaluation of a CD5-specific immunotoxin for treatment of acute graft-versus-host disease after allogeneic marrow transplantation. Blood 88:824–830, 1996.

54. Gratama JW, Jansen J, Lipovich RA, et al: Treatment of acute graft-versus-host disease with monoclonal antibody OKT3. Transplantation 38:469–473, 1983.

55. Beelen DW, Grosse-Wilde H, Ryschka U, et al: Initial treatment of acute graft-versus-host disease with a murine monoclonal antibody directed to the human / T cell receptor. Cancer Immunol Immunother 34:97–102, 1991.

56. Storb R, Gluckman E, Thomas ED, et al: Treatment of established human graft-versus-host disease by antithymocyte globulin. Blood 44:57, 1974.

57. Doney KC, Weiden PL, Storb R, et al: Treatment of graft-versus-host disease in human allogeneic marrow graft recipients: a randomized trial comparing antithymocyte globulin and corticosteroids. Am J Hematol 11:1–8, 1981.

58. Lim SH, McWhannell A, Vora AJ, et al: Successful treatment with thalidomide of acute graft-versus-host disease after bone-marrow transplantation. Lancet 1:117, 1988.

59. Ringden O, Aschan J, Westerberg L: Thalidomide for severe acute graft-versus-host disease. Lancet 2:568, 1988.

60. Schultz KR, Gilman AL: The lysomotropic amines, chloroquine and hydroxychloroquine: a potentially novel therapy for graft-versus-host disease. Leuk Lymphoma 24:201–210, 1997.

61. Kasia M, Higa T, Naohara T, et al: 15-Deoxyspergualin controls cyclosporin- and steroid-resistant intestinal acute graft-versus-host disease after allogeneic bone marrow transplantation. Bone Marrow Transplant 14:315–317, 1994.

62. Masaoka T, Shibata H, Kakishita E, et al: Phase II study of FK 506 for allogeneic bone marrow transplantation. Transplant Proc 23:3228–3231, 1991.

63. Kanamaru A, Takemoto Y, Kakishita E, et al: FK506 treatment of graft-versus-host disease developing or exacerbating during prophylaxis and therapy with cyclosporin and/or other immunosuppressants. Bone Marrow Transplant 15:885–889, 1995.

64. Koehler MT, Howrie D, Mirro J, et al: FK506 (tacrolimus) in the treatment of steroid-resistant acute graft-versus-host disease in children undergoing bone marrow transplantation. Bone Marrow Transplant 15:895–899, 1995.

65. Furlong T, Storb R, Anasetti C, et al: Conversion to FK506 for cyclosporine (CSP)-resistant acute GVHD or CSP-associated toxicity. Blood 90:104a, 1997.

66. Nash RA, Furlong T, Storb R, et al: Mycophenolate mofetil as salvage treatment for graft-versus-host disease after allogeneic hematopoietic stem cell transplantation: safety analysis. Blood 90:105a, 1997.

67. Basara N, Blau WI, Romer E, et al: Mycophenolate mofetil for the treatment of acute and chronic GVHD in bone marrow transplant patients. Bone Marrow Transplant 22:61–65, 1998.

68. Abhyankar S, Godder K, Christiansen N, et al: Treatment of resistant acute and chornic graft-versus-host disease with mycophenolate mofetil. Blood 92:454a, 1998.

69. Martin PJ, Schoch G, Fisher L, et al: A retrospective analysis of therapy for acute graft-versus-host disease: secondary treatment. Blood 77:1821–1828, 1991.

70. Kienast J, Ippoliti C, Mehra R, et al: Dose-intensified antithymocyte globulin in steroid-resistant graft-versus-host disease after allogeneic marrow or blood stem cell transplantation. Blood 90:104a, 1997.

71. McCaul K, Nevill TJ, Klingermann HG, et al: Treatment of steroid-resistant graft-versus-host disease (GVHD) following allogeneic bone marrow transplantation (BMT) with rabbit anti-thymocyte globulin (ATG). Blood 92:335b, 1998.

72. Varadi G, Or R, Slavin S, et al: In vivo CAMPATH-1 monoclonal antibodies: a novel mode of therapy for acute graft-versus-host disease. Am J Hematol 52:236–237, 1996.

73. Gluckman E, Devergie A, Varin F, et al: Treatment of steroid resistant severe acute graft-versus host disease with a monoclonal pan T OKT3 antibody. Exp Hematol 12(S):66–67, 1984.

74. Hebart H, Gscheidle H, Holler E, et al: OKT3 for steroid-resistant acute GVHD: a three-center experience. Blood 92:451a, 1998.

75. Martin PJ, Hansen JA, Anasetti C, et al: Treatment of acute graft-versus-host disease with anti-CD3 monoclonal antibodies. Am J Kidney Dis 11:149–152, 1988.

76. Anasetti C, Martin PJ, Storb R, et al: Treatment of acute graft-versus-host disease with a nonmitogenic anti-CD3 monoclonal antibody. Transplantation 54:844–851, 1992.

77. Hervè P, Wijdenes J, Bergerat JP, et al: Treatment of corticosteroid resistant acute graft-versus-host disease by in vivo administration of anti-interleukin-2 receptor monoclonal antibody (B-B10). Blood 75:1017, 1990.

78. Anasetti C, Martin PJ, Hansen JA, et al: A phase I–II study evaluating the murine anti-IL-2 receptor antibody 2A3 for treatment of acute graft-versus-host disease. Transplantation 50:49, 1990.

79. Tiley C, Powles R, Teo CP, et al: Treatment of acute graft-versus-host disease with a murine monoclonal antibody to the IL-2 receptor. Bone Marrow Transplant 7:151, 1991.

80. Cuthbert RJG, Phillips GL, Barnett MJ, et al: Anti-interleukin-2 receptor monoclonal antibody (BT563) in the treatment of severe acute GVHD refractory to systemic corticosteroid therapy. Bone Marrow Transplant 10:451, 1991.

81. Herbelin C, Stephan J-L, Donadieu J, et al: Treatment of steroid resistant acute graft-versus-host disease with an anti-IL-2-receptor monoclonal antibody (BT563) in children who received T cell–depleted, partially matched, related bone marrow transplants. Bone Marrow Transplant 13:563, 1994.

82. Hertenstein B, Stefanic M, Sandherr M, et al: Treatment of steroid-resistant acute graft-vs-host disease after allogeneic marrow transplantation with anti-interleukin-2 receptor antibody (BT563). Transplant Proc 26:3114, 1994.

83. Anasetti C, Hansen JA, Waldmann TA, et al: Treatment of acute graft-versus-host disease with humanized anti-Tac: an antibody that binds to the interleukin-2 receptor. Blood 84:1320, 1994.

84. Pinto RM, Arcese W, Fattore P, et al: A phase I study of humanized anti-TAC (HAT) in patients with acute GVHD refractory to cyclosporine and corticosteroid. Bone Marrow Transplant 15:S142, 1998.

85. Przepiorka D, Kernan N, Ippoliti C, et al: Phase II study of daclizumab for treatment of acute graft-versus-host disease. Exp Hematol 26:691, 1998.

86. Heslop HE, Benaim E, Brenner MK, et al: Response of steroid-resistant graft-versus-host disease to lymphoblast antibody CBL1. Lancet 346:805–806, 1995.

87. Bacigalupo A, Corte G, Ramarli D, et al: Intravenous monoclonal antibody (BT5/9) for the treatment of acute graft-versus-host disease. Acta Haematol 73:185–186, 1985.

88. Stoppa AM, Maraninchi D, Blaise B, et al: Anti-LFA 1 monoclonal antibody (25.3) for treatment of steroid-resistant grade III–IV acute graft-versus-host disease. Transplant Int 4:3–7, 1991.

89. Byers VS, Henslee PJ, Kernan NA, et al: Use of an anti-pan T-lymphocyte ricin A chain immunotoxin in steroid-resistant acute graft-versus-host disease. Blood 75:1426–1432, 1990.

90. Remlinger K, Martin PJ, Hansen JA, et al: Murine monoclonal anti–T cell antibodies for treatment of steroid-resistant acute graft-versus-host disease. Hum Immunol 9:21–35, 1984.

91. Racadot E, Milpied N, Bordigoni, et al: Sequential use of three monoclonal antibodies in corticosteroid-resistant acute GVHD: a multicentric pilot study including 15 patients. Bone Marrow Transplant 15:669–677, 1995.

92. Przepiorka D, Phillips GL, Ratanatharathorn V, et al: A phase II study of BTI-322, a monoclonal anti-CD2 antibody, for treatment of steroid-resistant acute graft-versus-host disease. Blood 92:4066–4071, 1998.

93. Herve P, Flesch M, Tiberghien P, et al: Phase I–II trial of a monoclonal anti-tumor necrosis factor antibody for the treatment of refractory severe acute graft-versus-host disease. Blood 79:3362–3368, 1992.

94. Antin JH, Weinstein HJ, Guinan EC, et al: Recombinant human interleukin-1 receptor antagonist in the treatment of steroid-resistant graft-versus-host disease. Blood 84:1342–1348, 1994.

95. McCarthy PL, Williams L, Harris-Bacile M, et al: A clinical phase I/II study of recombinant human interleukin-1 receptor in glucocorticoid-resistant graft-versus-host disease. Transplantation 62:626–631, 1996.

96. Markus PM, Cai XC, Ming W, et al: FK 506 reverses acute graft-versus-host disease after allogeneic bone marrow transplantation in rats. Surgery 110:357–364, 1991.

97. Gleixner B, Kolb HJ, Holler E, et al: Treatment of aGVHD with OKT3: clinical outcome and side-effects associated with release of TNF alpha. Bone Marrow Transplant 8:93–98, 1991.

98. Smith EP, Sniecinski I, Dagis AC, et al: Extracorporeal photochemotherapy for treatment of drug-resistant graft-vs-host disease. Biol Blood Marrow Transplant 4:27–37, 1998.

99. Greinix HT, Volc-Platzer B, Rabitsch W, et al: Successful use of extracorporeal photochemotherapy in the treatment of severe acute and chronic graft-versus-host disease. Blood 92:3098–3104, 1998.

100. Ely P, Dunitz J, Rogosheske J, et al: Use of a somatostatin analogue, octreotideacetate, in the management of acute gastrointestinal graft-versus-host disease. Am J Med 90:707–10, 1991.

101. Yuen KY, Woo PC, Hui CH, et al: Unique risk factors for bacteraemia in allogeneic bone marrow transplant recipients before and after engraftment. Bone Marrow Transplant 21:1137–1143, 1998.

102. O'Donnell MR, Schmidt GM, Tegtmeier BR, et al: Prediction of systemic fungal infection in allogeneic marrow recipients: impact of amphotericin prophylaxis in high-risk patients. J Clin Oncol 12:827–834, 1994.

103. Manteiga R, Martino R, Sureda A, et al: Cytomegalovirus pp65 antigenemia-guided pre-emptive treatment with ganciclovir after allogeneic stem cell transplantation: a single-center experience. Bone Marrow Transplant 22:899–904, 1998.

104. Sullivan KM: Immunomodulation in allogeneic marrow trasnplantation: use of intravenous immune globulin to suppress acute graft-versus-host disease. Clin Exp Immunol 104(S):43–48, 1996.

105. Deeg HJ, Loughran TP, Storb R, et al: Treatment of human acute graft-versus-host disease with antithymocyte globulin and cyclosporine with or without methylprednisolone. Transplantation 40:162–166, 1985.

CHAPTER FORTY-SIX

Liver Disease in Hematopoietic Stem Cell Transplant Recipients

Rakesh Vinayek, M.D., Jake Demetris, M.D., and Jorge Rakela, M.D.

Liver disease is a major cause of morbidity and mortality after hematopoietic stem cell transplantation (HSCT) because more than 80% of patients experience liver dysfunction with variable etiology.[1, 2] After HSCT, the most frequent liver diseases are veno-occlusive disease (VOD), drug toxicity, and complications of sepsis. In patients surviving more than 3 months, liver pathology is dominated by graft-versus-host disease (GVHD) and viral hepatitis, even though drug-related hepatitis and chronic VOD may occur.

VENO-OCCLUSIVE DISEASE OF THE LIVER

VOD is the nonthrombotic obliteration of small intrahepatic veins affecting zone 3 of the liver acinus (also called the centrilobular region). It is characterized by painful hepatomegaly, hyperbilirubinemia, and fluid retention. VOD can be fatal. Although this syndrome was initially described as an epidemic form after ingestion of bush tea containing pyrrolizidine alkaloids,[3–7] it has since been described in multiple clinical settings, including hepatic irradiation,[8–10] and the administration of various chemotherapeutic agents.[11–14]

In 1979, VOD following allogenic HSCT was first reported.[15] It is now recognized as a common complication of high-dose cytoreductive therapy and a major cause of morbidity and mortality during the first 80–100 days after HSCT.[16–24] Various conditioning regimens containing single or combination of chemotherapeutic agents with or without radiation have been implicated. The frequency of VOD varies from 1% to 2% among allogeneic recipients who received grafts after T-cell depletion as well as GVHD prophylaxis[25] to 64% among patients who received a second HSCT for recurrent malignancy.[26] The expected mortality rate is 20–40%.[16–26] Several explanations for this broad range in frequency include differences in the intensity of conditioning regimens, individual pharmacokinetic metabolism of antineoplastic agents, type of donor, and presence or absence of certain risk factors such as pretransplantation hepatitis and fever.[20–22, 26]

HISTOPATHOLOGY

Shulman et al first described the histopathologic features of VOD in the setting of HSCT.[18] They found concentric narrowing or fibrous obliteration of terminal hepatic venules and sublobular veins; dilatation and ultimately fibrosis of centrilobular sinusoids; and necrosis of Rappaport zone 3 hepatocytes (Fig. 46–1). The earliest observed changes from autopsy series included massive hemorrhage in zone 3 of the acinus and narrowing of small venule lumens secondary to an edematous subendothelial zone containing red blood cell fragments and hemosiderin-laden macrophages. Immunohistochemical and ultrastructural studies have further characterized the injury.[27] There was intense immunostaining of the adventitia portion of the central venules for factor VIII and fibrinogen at the interface of hepatic sinusoids and terminal hepatic venules. Some cases of early VOD have also demonstrated deposition of type I and III collagens in zone 3 sinusoids. Positive immunostaining with antibodies against albumin, immunoglobulin G(IgG), IgA, or C3 have not been observed. The early clinical stages of VOD also demonstrated marked loss of zone 3 hepatocyte cytokeratin. Late clinical stage VOD cases, defined as autopsy findings in patients who died after day 50 following HSCT, have demonstrated increased type III collagen within the occluded venules and type II and IV in zone 3 sinusoids. Platelet deposition is usually not evident in early VOD cases, and these observations have been confirmed by electron microscopy.[15]

The clinical syndrome of VOD results from extensive damage to structures in zone 3 of the liver acinus. No single histologic gold standard for the diagnosis of VOD exists, but two autopsy series by McDonald et al.[22] and Shulman et al.[23] showed that clinically severe VOD was significantly correlated with a constellation of histologic lesions involving structures in zone 3 of the hepatic acinus and the hepatic venules into which sinusoidal blood flows. These lesions included occluded hepatic venules with variable degrees of occlusion, eccentric luminal narrowing with phlebosclerosis, zone 3 sinusoidal fibrosis, and zone 3 hepatocyte necrosis.

There was a significant relationship between the number of these histologic abnormalities and the severity of VOD. The presence of ascites significantly correlated with zone 3 sinusoidal fibrosis and zone 3 hepatocyte necrosis, and maximum serum bilirubin in the first 20 days after HSCT significantly correlated with sinusoidal fibrosis, hepatocyte necrosis, and eccentric luminal sclerosis/phlebosclerosis but not with venular occlusion. The severity of clinical VOD

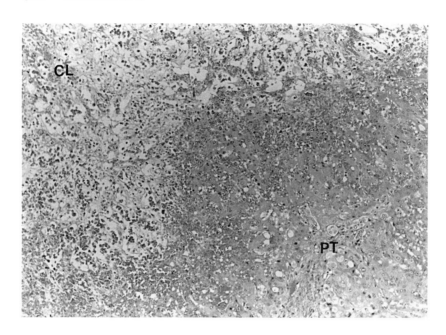

FIGURE 46–1. Veno-occlusive disease after allogeneic bone marrow transplantation is characterized by centrilobular (CL) hepatocellular necrosis and dropout, sinusoidal congestion, and sinusoidal deposition of fibrin in affected areas. Note the absence of portal tract (PT) inflammation and intact bile ducts (H&E; × 20).

appeared to be proportional to number of such histologic changes and not solely to occlusion of small hepatic venules.

PATHOPHYSIOLOGY

Although historically, the syndrome was first described after ingestion of pyrrolizidine alkaloids in contaminated cereals or herbal teas,[3–7] nowadays VOD is usually related to pre-transplantation conditioning regimen.[16–24] Cellular events that lead to the clinical presentation of VOD are presently unknown, but there is evidence that (1) hepatic and endothelial cell glutathione depletion predisposes to injury, (2) cytokines such as tumor necrosis factor-α (TNF-α) and markers of inflammation are involved, (3) transforming growth factor-β (TGF-β) is associated with hepatic fibrosis in these patients, (4) the degree of impairment of zone 3 cytochrome P-450 function is important, (5) in situ thrombosis contributes to altered sinusoidal blood flow, and (6) altered pharmacokinetics of antineoplastic agents also correlate with liver injury.[22–24, 28]

Injury to hepatic venular and sinusoidal endothelium is believed to be one of the earliest events in the pathogenesis of VOD. Indirect evidence suggests that endothelial injury and activation of clotting mechanisms may result in the eventual obstruction of the hepatic venule. Endothelial cells are more susceptible to damage from radiation or chemotherapy than are hepatocytes. Administration of monocrotaline, a pyrrolizidine alkaloid, to monkeys results in denudation of hepatic venular endothelium within 6–12 hours.[29] Hepatic sinusoidal endothelial cells are also damaged by dacarbazine, a known cause of VOD in humans,[30] whereas hepatocytes are not.[31]

MORPHOLOGIC CHANGES

The first morphologic changes are endothelial damage and extravasation of erythrocytes into the space of Disse[29, 32, 33]

and deposition of fibrinogen and factor VIII.[34] When endothelial cells are perturbed, a number of events may contribute to pathogenesis of VOD. First, a hypercoagulable state is formed locally. Tissue factor, which promotes factor VIIa–mediated activation of factor X, is synthesized and expressed by endothelial cells in response to injury and to selected cytokines.[35, 36] Tissue factor synthesis is accompanied by down-regulation of thromomodulin, which is necessary for the efficient anticoagulant function of protein C–protein S complex[37] and release of von Willebrand factor, which facilitates platelet aggregation.[38] Elevated levels of thrombomodulin,[39] von Willebrand factor, and serum angiotensin converting enzyme[38, 40, 41] have been demonstrated in patients prepared for HSCT.

The significance of these findings or whether these alterations either contribute to or are markers for patients who will experience VOD is uncertain. Furthermore, the role of endothelins, vasoactive peptides produced in response to endothelial injury in the pathogenesis of VOD, is not clear. The sites at which this process occurs are the sinusoids and pores that connect sinusoids to terminal hepatic venules. This has been demonstrated by immunohistochemical localization of fibrin and factor VIII in subendothelial zones of affected venules and electron microscopic studies showing irregularity and reduction in the number of these pores.[27, 42]

Zone 3 hepatocyte necrosis is visible in liver biopsy specimens obtained shortly after the clinical onset of VOD even without venular occlusion in the corresponding acinus.[23] The hepatocyte necrosis has been found to be more extensive and pronounced than venular occlusion in patients who died with VOD before day 50 after HSCT than in control patients without VOD lesions.[27]

The basis for predilection of zone 3 to endothelial injury is presumably linked to two major biochemical pathways that may promote endothelial cell damage.[23] First, zone 3 of the hepatic acinus is the primary site of the glutathione S transferase family of enzymes, which catalyze the reaction of glutathione with electrophilic compounds and constitute the major pathway for the detoxification of oxygen free radicals. Various conditioning agents (busulfan, carmustine [BCNU], total body irradiation) as well as pyrrolizidine alkaloids deplete glutathione in experimental models, resulting in accumulation of oxygen free radicals with subsequent zone 3 necrosis. Second, cytochrome P-450 enzymes that metabolize many of the drugs used in conditioning regimens are present, predominantly in zone 3, giving higher concentrations of reactive metabolites of drugs in this region.[43] Therefore, reactive metabolites of cyclophosphamide in combination with commonly used drugs such as busulfan cause depletion of glutathione, leading to sinusoidal and hepatocyte injury in zone 3.[44, 45]

ROLE OF CYTOKINES

The role of cytokines in the development of VOD remains to be defined. TNF-α, interleukin-1 (IL-1), and other cytokines are produced by macrophages, Kupffer cells, and other reticuloendothelial cells in response to cytoreductive therapy and infection,[46] ionizing radiation, and hypoxia.[47, 48] Studies have shown an association between serum levels of inflammatory cytokines (especially TNF-α) and the toxic effects of cytoreductive therapy.[49–51]

In a study reported by Holler et al., increased serum levels of TNF-α preceded major complications of HSCT, including GVHD, interstitial pneumonia, endothelial leak syndrome, and VOD.[49] A role for TNF-α in the pathogenesis of VOD is consistent with several known effects of the factor, notably the down-regulation of thrombomodulin, prostaglandin E_1 and E_2, and protein S, and up-regulation of cellular adhesion molecules and platelet-derived growth factors.[52–54]

Because several studies have clearly demonstrated that an intrahepatic prothrombotic state contributes to the obstruction of sinusoidal blood flow in VOD,[27, 40, 55, 56] the procoagulant effects of TNF-α are of particular interest. These include effects on protein C (through decreases in thrombomodulin), increased local synthesis of tissue factors, and initiation of the coagulation cascade.[52–54, 57] TNF-α also causes increased capillary permeability, a prominent feature of multiorgan failure in patients with severe VOD, and hemorrhagic necrosis, and TNF-α is directly toxic to endothelial cells.[58, 59] Fever, an independent risk factor for VOD, is produced by TNF-α and IL-1, both of which induce endothelial procoagulant activity.[35, 36] Although, in initial studies,[51–61] inhibition of TNF-α release with pentoxifylline has been reported to alleviate toxicity in marrow recipients, subsequent studies showed no benefit with this agent.[62, 63]

TGF-β, a cytokine that stimulates migration of fibroblasts into sites of injury and promotes production of collagen, has also been implicated as a causal agent for VOD or pulmonary fibrosis in patients who underwent autologous HSCT for advanced breast cancer.[64] In addition, IL-6 administration to patients who underwent autologous HSCT for breast cancer resulted in a greater than 50% incidence of VOD, compared with a historical incidence of only 5%.[65] These data suggest that cytokines play a causative role in VOD.

COAGULATION SYSTEM

Several groups have examined the causal relationship between coagulation and VOD, and apart from the immunohistochemical evaluation of hepatic tissue by Shulman et al. demonstrating fibrinogen and factor VIII within the subendothelial zones,[27] the evidence for this relationship is indirect. Scrobohaci et al. found that preconditioning levels of protein C and factor VII were lower in patients who experienced VOD than in patients who did not.[40] Values of protein C and factor VII continued to fall after conditioning therapy.

Faioni et al. measured naturally occurring anticoagulants protein C, protein S, and antithrombin III as well as factor VII levels in 45 patients undergoing HSCT.[56] Levels of protein C, antithrombin III, and factor VII decreased and protein S increased over time more in patients who experienced VOD than in patients without VOD. Decrease in protein C level was demonstrated to be an independent risk factor for VOD.

Collins et al. reported that protein C, protein S, factor VII, and factor X fell after high-dose cytoreductive therapy but that there were differences depending on the conditioning regimen used and type of transplantation performed.[41] These parameters were not of any predictive value in VOD. On the other hand, Catani et al. serially assessed prothrombin time, partial prothrombin time, fibrinogen, levels of natural anticoagulants, markers of hypercoagulabilty, and fibrinolytic parameters before the start of cytoreductive therapy, on day zero, and weekly for 5 weeks and found no parameters associated with development of VOD.[66] It is currently unclear whether changes in coagulation parameters are involved in the pathogenesis of VOD or are epiphenomena of this disease process.

von Willebrand factor, endothelin, and cytokines implicated in the pathogenesis of VOD can result in platelet aggregation and adhesion. Several groups have shown an increased platelet requirement in patients who subsequently experienced VOD.[22] Elevated serum procollagen type III has been shown to precede the clinical manifestations of VOD.[67, 68] In one study, serum levels were found to be consistently elevated beginning at day 0 through 49 days after HSCT and were highly predictive of the development of VOD.[68] Elevated serum procollagen type III levels have been associated with fibrotic liver disease, suggesting that serum procollagen type III is a surrogate marker for intrahepatic accumulation of type III collagen.[69]

RISK FACTORS

Pretransplantation

Various pretransplantation risk factors have been associated with the development of VOD after HSCT. Most groups have shown that elevated serum aminotransferases before the conditioning regimen predispose patients to VOD.[20–22] Two independent studies from Johns Hopkins Oncology Center (JHOC)[21] and Fred Hutchinson Cancer Research Center (FHCRC)[22] have found that the risk of VOD is proportional to the degree of aspartate aminotransferase elevation. Other investigators, however, have found no association between pretransplantation aminotransferase elevations and VOD.[25, 70–72]

Patients undergoing HSCT are also at high risk for acquiring viral infections from blood transfusion or other parenteral exposure. The role of hepatitis C virus (HCV) or hepatitis B virus (HBV) infection in causing severe liver disease or VOD after HSCT is uncertain. A study by Frickhofen et al. linked HCV infection prior to transplantation with subsequent development of VOD.[73] Five of the six patients infected with HCV died from VOD, compared with 9 of 52 patients not infected with HCV. Other risk factors for VOD were balanced between the two groups. Furthermore, primary infection by HCV after transplantation resulted in an increased risk of VOD. The mechanism responsible for the increased risk by HCV is not known. In another study, however, despite the 47% prevalence of HCV infection, HCV-RNA positivity was neither a predictor of VOD nor a marker for life-threatening liver disease.[74] On the other hand, it has been long known that reactivation of HBV can occur in chronic carriers who receive immunosuppressive therapy[75] or cancer chemotherapy.[76] Fulminant hepatitis, however, or the recently described fibrosing cholestatic hepatitis is rare in patients undergoing HSCT.[77, 78] Overall, HBV is not clearly associated with increased risk of VOD after HSCT.

Patients who receive conditioning regimen while they are being treated for bacterial or viral infections appear to be at increased risk for fatal VOD. Although earlier studies demonstrated that older age,[20] female gender,[79, 80] a diagnosis other than acute lymphocytic leukemia,[23] and leukemia in relapse[21] were associated with a higher incidence of VOD, a more-recent prospective analysis failed to confirm these earlier results.[22] Other risk factors identified included prior radiation therapy for liver metastases[22] and second HSCT.[26]

Antimicrobial Therapy

Several antimicrobial agents, including acyclovir, amphotericin B, and vancomycin, have been incriminated in the development of VOD. VOD has been reported with prolonged use of broad-spectrum antibiotics and the use of amphotericin B given for either documented fungal infection or empirical treatment for febrile neutropenia during and after conditioning regimen, irrespective of the duration of amphotericin treatment.[80] Amphotericin B use strongly correlated with the development of VOD in one study, although it was not an independent risk factor after multivariate analysis.[22] In this study, pretransplantation acyclovir and vancomycin use during cytoreductive therapy proved to be independent risk factors.

Preparative Regimens

Certain conditioning regimens have been associated with a higher incidence of severe VOD. Regimens reported to have a higher incidence of VOD than standard therapy with cyclophosphamide (120 mg/kg) and total body irradiation (12 Gy) (8%) include those incorporating higher doses of total body radiation (23%) or cyclophosphamide (23%), busulfan plus cyclophosphamide (24–32%), and carmustine, cyclophosphamide, and etoposide (33%).[21–22]

Altered pharmacokinetics of cytoreductive agents have been implicated in the pathogenesis of VOD. Patients who experienced VOD after receiving busulfan and cyclophosphamide had a higher busulfan area under the concentration curve versus time (AUC) than patients who did not.[81] The subsequent clinical trial by the same group demonstrated that busulfan AUC greater than 1500 μmol/min/L was associated with a higher incidence of VOD and increased mortality.[82] A 1996 study confirmed these results with subsequent recommendations that routine determination of busulfan pharmacokinetics should guide busulfan dosing.[83] Adjusting busulfan dose on this basis would prevent elevated AUC exposure to busulfan and, as a consequence, VOD.

GVHD Prophylaxis

The choice of GVHD prophylaxis may adversely influence development of VOD. The use of methotrexate for prophylaxis of GVHD might be associated with an increased risk of VOD.[84] In 87 patients treated with cyclophosphamide and total body radiation who received methotrexate as part of their GVHD prophylaxis, the incidence of VOD increased from 18% in the control group to 70% in the methotrexate group, and the rate of severe VOD went from 4.5% to 25%, respectively.[84] Overall long-term survival, however, was comparable in both groups. Several large multivariate analyses have failed to show an influence of GVHD prophylaxis on the incidence of VOD.[20–22]

Source of Marrow

Although two reports from FHCRC suggested that comparably treated autologous marrow recipients experience VOD less frequently than allogeneic transplant recipients,[85, 86] these results have been refuted by three large multivariate analyses.[20–22] VOD has been reported to be more likely in patients receiving marrow from a mismatched family donor or from an unrelated donor than from fully matched, related donors.

Miscellaneous Factors

The development of VOD has been strongly associated with oral mucositis and interstitial pneumonitis. In a prospective study in 47 patients undergoing HSCT, patients with oral mucositis were 6.5 times more likely to experience VOD than patients who did not experience ulcerative mucositis.[87] The authors concluded that VOD was unusual without a concomitant history of mucositis and that other causes of hepatic dysfunction should be evaluated in patients lacking oral lesions. The same group also reported an association between interstitial pneumonitis and VOD in patients undergoing HSCT.[88] One hundred fifty-four patients were retrospectively evaluated, 68 of whom experienced interstitial pneumonitis and 39 of whom experienced VOD. The actuarial incidence of interstitial pneumonitis was 71% in patients with VOD and 45% in those without VOD.

CLINICAL FEATURES

VOD is an illness characterized by hyperbilirubinemia, painful hepatomegaly, and fluid retention. The incidence of

TABLE 46–1. CLINICAL CRITERIA FOR DIAGNOSING VENO-OCCLUSIVE DISEASE

JHOC CRITERIA (JONES ET AL.[21])	FHCRC CRITERIA (MCDONALD ET AL.[20])
Hyperbilirubinemia ≥ 2 mg/dL with at least 2 of 3 other findings occurring within 21 days of transplantation: 1. Hepatomegaly and right upper quadrant pain 2. Ascites 3. Weight gain greater than 5% of baseline bodyweight	Occurrence of at least 2 of the following events within 20 days of transplantation: 1. Hyperbilirubinemia ≥ 2 mg/dL 2. Hepatomegaly with right upper quadrant pain of liver origin 3. Weight gain greater than 2% of baseline bodyweight

VOD in patients undergoing HSCT has been reported to be as high as 50–55% with an associated mortality rate of up to 40%.

Two sets of criteria are widely used (Table 46–1). The first set was developed from review of autopsy data on 255 consecutive patients undergoing HSCT for malignancy from 1978 through 1980.[20] The predictive criteria for the clinical diagnosis were based on the results of liver histology from a cohort of 64 patients. The incidence of VOD was 21%, with death from VOD in 45%. The predictive value of a clinical diagnosis of VOD in the cohort was 89%, and the predictive value of non-VOD or uncertain classification was 92%. According to these criteria, two of the three clinical manifestations (jaundice, painful hepatomegaly, ascites, and/or unexplained weight gain) must be present by day 20. This requirement, however, may be inappropriate because VOD can develop later than day 20 with some regimens.

The second set was developed from a review of 235 consecutive patients undergoing HSCT in order to define the clinical syndrome of VOD.[21] Of the 158 patients who died, autopsy was performed in 57. Analysis of all patients with histologic proof of VOD revealed a consistent syndrome of liver dysfunction occurring within the first 3 weeks after HSCT. This was characterized by hyperbilirubinemia greater than or equal to 2 mg/dL with at least two of three other findings: hepatomegaly, ascites, and 5% or greater weight gain. VOD developed in 22% of patients, with an associated mortality rate of 47%.

The clinical criteria for VOD were modified by the group at FHCRC according to their 9-year experience in 355 consecutive patients who underwent HSCT.[22] The modified clinical criteria included the occurrence of two of the following within 20 days of transplantation: hyperbilirubinemia with total serum bilirubin over 2 mg/dL (34.2 μmol/L), hepatomegaly or right upper quadrant pain of hepatic origin, and sudden weight gain greater than 2% of body weight. Patients who experienced both mild hyperbilirubinemia (total serum bilirubin <2 mg/dL or <34.2 μmol/L) and weight gain below the threshold criteria of 2% were placed in the "uncertain cause" category.

The severity of the disease was defined retrospectively according to the outcome. Patients who met the criteria of VOD but had no apparent clinical adverse effects from liver disease and experienced complete resolution of signs and symptoms and of laboratory abnormalities had mild VOD. Those whose VOD resolved but had symptoms of fluid retention and required salt restriction and diuretics to control their edema and ascites, or who required analgesics for hepatic pain, had moderate VOD. Patients who died of VOD or whose symptoms did not resolve by day 100 post

transplantation were considered to have severe VOD. In this series, the overall incidence of VOD was 54%, with 54 patients (15%) experiencing severe VOD and 136 (38%) experiencing mild or moderate disease.

The clinical manifestations of VOD vary with the severity of the disease and in some cases occur before transplantation.[1, 2, 20–22, 89] In the majority of patients, however, laboratory evidence of liver dysfunction begins between day 6 and 7 post transplantation, peaks approximately 10 days after the onset of the initial rise and, in those whose VOD resolves, tends to return to baseline values approximately 10 days later.[21] Bilirubin values for patients with severe VOD usually peak on the day of their demise.[89] There is considerable overlap in the range of hyperbilirubinemia, weight gain, and other features of VOD among patients with mild, moderate, and severe disease. No data suggest that any therapy prevents the progression of VOD.

The incidence of VOD varies from 4% to 54%, with the mortality rate ranging from 3% to 67% in all the reported series with more than 100 patients.[20–22, 68, 77, 90–93] The marked variability in both the reported incidence and mortality of VOD is most probably attributable to the use of different conditioning regimens, patient selection, and definitions of VOD. Multiorgan failure has been reported to be more common among patients with VOD than among patients without it.[20, 22, 89]

In a series by McDonald et al., over half of the patients with severe VOD experienced cardiopulmonary and renal failure.[22] The onset of jaundice and weight gain preceded the failure of these organs by several days, and both hyperbilirubinemia and fluid retention were significant predictors of late onset of pleural effusion, heart failure, pulmonary infiltrates, confusion, renal failure, and bleeding. A retrospective review showed that both hyperbilirubinemia and amphotericin use were independent risk factors for renal failure after HSCT.

Other series have also shown a high incidence of multiorgan failure in marrow transplant recipients as well as evidence that pulmonary dysfunction and pleural effusions are related to VOD.[24, 85, 88] Hepatorenal syndrome is a manifestation of the multiorgan failure that may develop in patients with VOD.[22, 94, 95] Sodium retention is an early event, followed by edema, congestion, heart failure, pulmonary infiltrates, and hypoxia requiring supplemental oxygen. Fluid retention and jaundice precede the development of azotemia, and approximately half of these patients require hemodialysis for azotemia or fluid overload.[94, 95] The high mortality rate of patients with severe VOD is, therefore, not surprising given the high prevalence of cardiopulmonary and renal failure in these patients.

In the series at JHOC, VOD resolved in 48% of patients,

47% of the patients died, and VOD blended into GVHD in 5% of patients.[21] In the earlier series at FHCRC, 45% of patients with VOD died of or with liver dysfunction.[20] In a more-recent series by the same group, the results were more favorable, with a mortality rate of 9% in patients with mild VOD, 23% in patients with moderate VOD, and 98% in patients with severe VOD by day 100 post transplantation.[22] Fifty-six percent of patients with liver dysfunction of uncertain etiology died by day 100 post transplantation, and only 19% of patients who did not experience VOD died by day 100. In both series, early mortality was correlated with maximum bilirubin.

In the JHOC series, all patients with VOD who experienced encephalopathy died. Survival was also correlated with the requirement for hemodialysis. Only 14% of patients who required hemodialysis survived. In a retrospective analysis of 101 patients who underwent HSCT that compared survival according to whether patients met either the FHCRC or the JHOC clinical criteria for VOD,[96] the incidence of VOD by the JHOC criteria was 8% but was 32% by the FHCRC criteria. Early mortality (prior to 50 days post transplantation) was 75% (6 of 8) in patients who fulfilled the JHOC criteria but only 28% (9 of 32) in the FHCRC criteria (P = 0.005), although the overall mortality rate was 75% and 66%, respectively. The authors concluded that the JHOC criteria of VOD, which require three clinical signs, identified a group of patients who experienced clinical liver dysfunction earlier and were likely to have an unfavorable outcome.

DIAGNOSTIC STUDIES

Ultrasonographic Studies

A variety of ultrasonographic findings have been reported in patients with VOD, including thickening of the gallbladder wall, ascites, hepatomegaly, reversal of portal venous blood flow, changes in velocity of the portal venous flow, and resistive index in the hepatic artery, none of which is sensitive or specific for VOD.[97, 98] A prospective study from FHCRC failed to identify any sonographic findings that were strongly associated with VOD in the early phase of the illness.[99]

^{99}Tcm-Sulphur Colloid Liver Spleen Scan

Increased lung uptake on liver/spleen scintography in the early post-transplantation period may be useful for identifying patients likely to experience significant VOD and for assessing their prognosis. A study by Jacobson et al. prospectively evaluated marrow transplant recipients with serial ^{99}Tc-sulphur colloid liver/spleen scintigraphy to determine whether quantification of lung uptake would aid in early identification of patients with VOD.[100] Anterior lung/liver (L/L) and geometric mean spleen/liver ratios were determined prior to conditioning chemotherapy/total body radiation and at 104 days (n = 17), 11–14 days (n = 18), and 27–33 days (n = 15) post transplantation, and these findings correlated with the presence of VOD post transplantation employing standard clinical criteria. Of 17 patients studied 1–4 days post transplantation, at which time

no patient had objective evidence of VOD, an L/L ratio of 0.075 or greater predicted subsequent development of moderate or severe VOD with a sensitivity of 100% (4 of 4) and a specificity of 85% (11 of 13). An increase in lung uptake at 4 weeks post transplantation was associated with a poor prognosis because the four patients with L/L ratios of 0.085–0.115 died during the first year and two patients with L/L ratios of 0.032 and 0.078 survived. Larger prospective trials are required to further evaluate the sensitivity and specificity of this diagnostic modality.

Liver Biopsy and Hepatic Venous Pressure Gradient

Thrombocytopenia and coagulopathy are contraindications to percutaneous liver biopsy. Even so, recent results from two groups on the use of transjugular liver biopsy and hepatic venous pressure gradient (HPVG) measurement have shown that adequate specimens can be obtained for histology and culture without life-threatening complications. Liver biopsy and pressure measurements provide useful diagnostic information in marrow transplant recipients with liver dysfunction.[101, 102] Liver biopsy may confirm the clinical suspicion of VOD, justifying potentially dangerous treatment with recombinant tissue plasminogen activator (r-tPA), but may also help to determine other causes of hepatic dysfunction in these patients. Two studies,[101, 102] however, failed to identify a large proportion of patients with biopsy-proven VOD who did not meet clinical criteria. Furthermore, tissue confirmation might delay therapy or, in cases of hemorrhagic complications, preclude potentially beneficial therapy.

On the other hand, the measurement of HVPG alone can be performed safely as long as balloon-tipped catheters are used. Both studies showed that an HVPG greater than 10 mm Hg is highly specific for the diagnosis of VOD. HVPG was significantly higher in patients with VOD than in patients without VOD but with GVHD. Furthermore, the mean HVPG was statistically much higher in patients who died of VOD compared with those who survived.

PROPHYLAXIS AND TREATMENT

At present, no therapy for moderate to severe VOD has been evaluated in a prospective randomized clinical trial. Investigators have evaluated models in an attempt to predict the severity and risk of VOD. These models might then be used to guide therapy.

Using the FHCRC database of 355 consecutive patients, Bearman et al. developed a mathematical model to predict the clinical outcome early in the transplant course.[103] Logistic regression models were developed to estimate probabilities of severe VOD based on total serum bilirubin and weight gain at each of six time intervals from day −7 through day +16 post transplantation. Regression models were used to generate coefficients (β_0, β_1, β_2) for the equation $P = 1/(1 + e^{-z})$, where P is the probability of severe VOD and $z = \beta_0 + \beta_1$ (ln total serum bilirubin [mg/dL] + β_2 (percent weight gain). β_0, β_1, β_2 are fixed constants whose values are specific to a given time interval from day −1 through day +16. Subsequent application of this mathematical model in 392 consecutive patients demonstrated a high specificity, but the overall sensitivity was less than 50% for predicting severe VOD. The authors suggested that such probability estimates may be useful when considering potentially risky interventions such as r-tPA. The model could also be used to evaluate the effectiveness of treatment algorithms by selecting only those patients who are at high risk for VOD.

Prophylaxis

Prophylactic measures include recognizing patients who are at high risk for VOD, such as patients with hepatitis, and delaying transplantation in them until the hepatitis has resolved; treating patients with medications that reduce the incidence of VOD; and finally, early and aggressive treatment of patients who experience VOD in the hope that the early intervention might alter the natural history of VOD. Because endothelial injury leading to deposition of coagulation factors is believed to be the key event in the pathogenesis of VOD, various investigators have advocated prophylactic measures aimed at reducing the hypercoagulable state. A number of clinical trials have been conducted with this intent, and several agents have been evaluated.

Heparin

A number of studies have investigated the use of heparin by continuous infusion with contradictory results. In a retrospective study, Chen et al. reviewed 63 patients who received continuous infusion of heparin, none of whom experienced VOD.[104] In another study, 28 patients were treated with heparin at four different dose levels.[105] Heparin was given from the onset of the preparative regimen until day 14 post transplantation. VOD developed in 20 patients (71%) and was severe or fatal in four patients (14%). This trial was hampered by the inability to complete treatment in 21 of 28 patients because of bleeding in 14 patients and thrombocytopenia in 7 patients.

In a study by Marsa-Vila et al, patients randomized to receive heparin experienced an overall incidence of VOD of 7%, compared with 2% for those randomized not to receive heparin.[106] They concluded that heparin was ineffective as prophylaxis of VOD.

Attal et al. conducted a prospective randomized controlled trial using low-dose heparin at a dose of 100 U/kg/day by continuous infusion in 161 patients.[107] The patients were randomized to either a control group or to receive heparin starting on day −8 until day +30 post transplantation. VOD developed in 13% of patients in the control group and in 3% of patients in the heparin group (P < .01). There was no increased risk of bleeding in the patients treated with heparin; however, there was no significant difference in the incidence of severe VOD, 100-day survival, or mortality from VOD in both groups. Furthermore, none of the patients who was at high risk for VOD (based on elevated serum aminotransferases at the time of transplantation) experienced VOD irrespective of whether heparin was administered. Therefore, the role of heparin in VOD prophylaxis is uncertain, and larger randomized trials are required to determine whether heparin confers a significant survival benefit.

Prostaglandins

Prostaglandin E_1 (PGE$_1$) has both vasodilator and antithrombotic activity. Antithrombotic activity includes inhibition of platelet aggregation, activation of fibrinolysis, and inhibition of superoxide anion generation. Gluckman et al. prophylactically treated 50 leukemic patients undergoing allogeneic BMT using PGE$_1$ at a dose of 0.03 μg/kg/hour from day −8 through day +30.[108] Mild VOD occurred in 12% of patients in the treated group and in 26% of patients in the nonrandomized control group (P = .05). This treatment was more beneficial in patients with a prior history of hepatitis, with an incidence of 16% in the treated group compared with 63% in the nontreated group (P = .05). No side effects of PGE$_1$ were observed in this study.

In another study by Bearman et al., PGE$_1$ was administered to patients with one or more risk factors for VOD.[109] The dose of PGE$_1$ ranged from 1.25 to 10 ng/kg/min. Unlike with the previous report, severe toxicity in the form of painful erythematous, bullous skin lesions, peripheral edema, and hypotension was observed at all dose levels. Furthermore, severe VOD developed in 67% of patients. Other studies of PGE$_1$ reported a high incidence of bilateral systemic arthritis, painful angioedema of the extremities, and painful periostitis. These side effects forced the conclusion that PGE$_1$ could not be safely administered in this setting. Further trials need to be conducted to determine the safety and efficacy of PGE$_1$ in reducing the severity of VOD.

Bile Salts

The prophylactic use of ursodeoxycholic acid (UDCA), a hydrophilic nonhepatotoxic bile salt, has been explored in a pilot trial of 22 consecutive patients undergoing BMT.[110] It has been postulated that the administration of UDCA alters the accumulation of hydrophilic bile salts known to be cytotoxic to hepatocytes and decreases the observed hepatotoxicity associated with VOD. UDCA, 600–900 mg/day PO, was begun on the day 1 of the conditioning regimen consisting of busulfan and cyclophosphamide. The incidence of VOD was 2 of 22 (9%) in the UDCA group and 18 of 28 (64%) in controls (P = .0001). More recently, a prospective, randomized, placebo-controlled trial from the same group reported that patients randomized to UDCA had significantly less VOD than patients randomized to placebo.[111]

Pentoxifylline

Pentoxifylline is a methylxanthine analogue that has been shown to inhibit the transcription of TNF-α. Pentoxifylline was studied in HSCT recipients because some studies implicated inflammatory mediators such as TNF-α in the pathogenesis of VOD.[49–51] Although initial studies showed pentoxifylline to be beneficial,[51, 60, 61] prospective randomized trials showed no benefit of pentoxifylline alone in the prevention of VOD,[62, 63] and therefore its use has been abandoned in most centers.

Treatment

A number of agents are being used in the treatment of VOD, but none of them has been evaluated in a prospective randomized clinical trial.

Thrombolytic Therapy

Thrombolytic therapy may reduce the severity of VOD. r-tPA was first used by Baglin et al., who successfully treated a patient with VOD using 50 mg of r-tPA/day for 4 consecutive days.[112] Because of concern that such a high dose of r-tPA in a patient population already affected by profound thrombocytopenia would be likely to cause bleeding, Bearman et al. treated seven patients who were thought to be at high risk for dying from multiorgan failure secondary to VOD with 10 mg r-tPA/day for 2 consecutive days and an infusion of heparin (1000-U bolus followed by continuous infusion of 150 U/kg/day for 10 days).[113] Five patients responded with a significant and persistent reduction in bilirubin within 96 hours of beginning the infusion, and three patients were alive without VOD 178–379 days post transplantation at the time the study was published. No significant bleeding complications were observed; however, the platelet count had to be maintained at greater than 15,000/μL to be eligible for the study. Since this original report, an additional 25 patients have been treated, 45% of whom responded to r-tPA, including the patients reported initially.[24]

Yu et al. reported reversal of VOD in two of three pediatric HSCT recipients treated with r-tPA at a low dose of 0.25–0.5 mg/kg for 4 days.[114] There have been several reports of patients treated with r-tPA who experienced catastrophic bleeding complications. Therefore, caution should be used in patient selection and monitoring, and only patients who are at high risk for VOD should be enrolled in clinical trials of r-tPA. Even though hemodialysis has been considered a contraindication to this therapy in view of the potential hemostatic complication, a 1994 case report of successful treatment with r-tPA at a dose of 10 mg/day while on peritoneal dialysis[115] suggests that the requirement for dialysis may not preclude the use of r-tPA in established VOD, and therefore this therapy warrants further study.

In an attempt to treat established VOD, Ibrahim et al. treated nine patients with PGE$_1$ at a dose of 500 μg/day with improvement in 4–7 days and with resolution of right upper quadrant pain, fluid retention, and reduction in serum bilirubin.[116] The time of onset of VOD in these patients ranged from 8 to 33 days post transplantation. In the FHCRC experience, most patients within that time period experience reversible disease. Therefore, it is difficult to state whether these patients responded to PGE$_1$ or their VOD resolved spontaneously.

None of the patients treated by Gluckman et al. responded to PGE$_1$.[108] Therefore, the role of PGE$_1$ in the treatment of VOD is uncertain. Other thrombolytic agents such as urokinase may be of some therapeutic value. In a 1993 case report, a patient with non-Hodgkin lymphoma who experienced VOD after HSCT was successfully treated with urokinase.[117]

Surgical Treatment

Several surgical approaches have been attempted to treat VOD. Surgical intervention with either splenorenal or portacaval shunts or the LeVeen shunt have been used to alleviate massive ascites. In some cases, side-to-side portacaval or splenorenal shunt led to reversal of massive ascites

and hyperbilirubinemia.[118, 119] Transjugular intrahepatic portosystemic shunt should be considered in patients who are not considered to be good surgical candidates.[120] Orthotopic liver transplantation for severe VOD has been performed.[121] Even though the operations were technically successful, there were no long-term survivors.

Supportive Treatment

Patients with VOD are fluid overloaded but may be intravascularly volume depleted. The goal of the treatment is to minimize accumulation of extracellular fluid without compromising renal function, particularly when patients are receiving nephrotoxic medications such as amphotericin B, aminoglycosides, and cyclosporine or FK506. Central hemodynamic monitoring usually shows a high cardiac output and high systemic vascular resistance. After the initial vigorous hydration required for high-dose chemotherapy, these patients should be treated with diuretics in an attempt to keep their weight at or near their admission weight. Paracentesis may be required for the treatment of refractory ascites. Some patients may experience respiratory failure from pulmonary edema or infection or renal failure and require mechanical ventilation, broad-spectrum antibiotics, and hemodialysis. In patients who experience renal failure and require hemodialysis, the mortality rate is high.[94, 95] In a study from FHCRC, 85% of patients requiring dialysis for renal failure after HSCT died.[95]

HEPATIC GRAFT-VERSUS-HOST DISEASE

Among the complications of BMT, GVHD is unique, both as a disease entity and as a possible iatrogenic model of autoimmune disease. It is the end-result of a complex immunologic reaction mediated by T cells from the grafted allogeneic marrow or blood.[122–125] Patients who receive an allograft from a matched unrelated donor, older donors, and female donor/male recipient pairs are at high risk for GVHD. It can occur in up to 70% of successful allogeneic grafts and is a major cause of mortality. Human leukocyte antigen disparity between marrow donor and recipient is the most important factor in determining the incidence and severity of the acute GVHD.[122–125] Acute and chronic GVHD are discussed in Chapters 45 and 54, respectively.

Hepatic involvement with GVHD usually occurs when there is already skin and intestinal involvement. The diagnosis of hepatic GVHD in individual patients, however, is often uncertain, and unlike hepatic VOD, well-described clinical and laboratory manifestations do not easily distinguish hepatic GVHD from other causes of hepatic dysfunction, including VOD, viral hepatitis, infection, and drug-induced or TPN-associated cholestasis.[123–125] Biopsy is usually required to confirm the clinical diagnosis, although the histologic changes early in the course of GVHD may not be as specific as in later stages.[126–128]

CLINICAL MANIFESTATIONS

Early liver involvement with GVHD usually manifests as cholestatic jaundice, characterized by increased serum alkaline phosphatase followed by hyperbilirubinemia and mild hepatomegaly.[123–125] The hepatic manifestations are usually preceded by or concurrent with skin and/or intestinal GVHD. Hepatic GVHD can develop without apparent skin and gut GVHD, but this is unusual.

The average day of onset of acute GVHD is day 19—earlier if the patient has not received GVHD prophylaxis or has received mismatched marrow or peripheral blood progenitor cells (PBPC) and later if prophylaxis has been effective. The alkaline phosphatase values may rise steadily to 10- to 20-fold above normal with parallel rises in serum bilirubin. When GVHD develops in the presence of VOD, the slope of the bilirubin rise is steep. When hemolysis, renal failure, or sepsis develops in patients with GVHD, the level of serum bilirubin may exceed 50 mg/dL. The serum levels of asparate aminotransferase and alanine aminotransferase frequently elevated, but they seldom exceed 10–times above normal.

Features of severe hepatocellular dysfunction such as ascites, coagulopathy, and encephalopathy are unusual except when acute GVHD has progressed to multiorgan end-stage disease. Hypoalbuminemia is not usually due to severe liver disease but rather secondary to protein-losing enteropathy and a negative nitrogen balance. The development of hepatic dysfunction without skin or intestinal disease should make the diagnosis suspect and requires histologic confirmation.

The clinical onset for hepatic GVHD may be as early as the second week following allogeneic HSCT. Although it is unusual to observe its development later than 6 months after transplantation, hepatic GVHD must always be considered in the differential diagnosis of hepatic dysfunction. Chronic liver disease may occur in 90% of patients with chronic GVHD, either as a part of an extensive chronic GVHD process involving several organs such as skin, mouth, eyes, esophagus, liver, and lung or as more-favorable limited disease involving just skin or liver. Because several hepatic disorders, including hepatic VOD, viral hepatitides, drug-induced liver disease, or cholestatic jaundice, infection, and shock may occur concurrently, liver biopsy is generally required to distinguish among these possibilities.[123–125, 129] Because of the relatively common occurrence of hepatic VOD and hepatic GVHD, the two can occur simultaneously.

The severity of hepatic GVHD varies considerably from isolated elevation of the serum alkaline phosphatase level without jaundice, to slowly progressive liver disease culminating in death from liver failure. Patients with less-severe GVHD may respond to steroids, antithymocyte globulin, CSA, or FK506, but normalization of liver tests may take weeks to months.[130–134] Patients who experience refractory acute GVHD with liver, skin, and/or intestinal involvement generally die of multiorgan system failure or from infection associated with the immunosuppressive therapy before progression of severe liver involvement leads to liver failure. More than 50% of patients with severe acute GVHD become long-term survivors, with frequent liver involvement.[123–125]

HISTOPATHOLOGY AND PATHOGENESIS

The histologic diagnosis of hepatic GVHD is potentially confounded by the large number of agents that can affect liver function in HSCT recipients. Portal inflammation is a hallmark feature of acute GVHD, although portal inflammation can be mild because of the conditioning regimen and subsequent marrow suppression.

Within a week of the onset of biochemical abnormalities in the serum, biopsy demonstrates a mild nonspecific lobular hepatitis with mild anisonucleosis and anisocytosis throughout the lobule and infiltration of mononuclear cells and eosinophils into portal triads. Small numbers of acidophil bodies and areas of hepatocyte dropout can be found. Bile duct injury is usually not observed in this early stage.[126–128]

Histologic changes are more obvious in liver biopsy specimens obtained 1–2 weeks after the onset of the disease. At this stage, cholestasis, infiltration of lymphocytes in the portal triads, and degenerative changes in small septal or interlobular bile ducts are visible. Abnormal interlobular bile ducts constitute the most characteristic feature of liver GVHD, but as the disease progresses, there is highly variable destruction of small bile ducts and proliferation of ductules. Abnormal ducts are characterized by irregular shapes, cytoplasmic eosinophilia, segmental nuclear loss, nuclear pleomorphism, and rarely necrotic duct epithelial cells (Fig. 46–2).[126–128] Although these findings are reminiscent of primary biliary cirrhosis, the two disorders are rarely mistaken for each other by experienced pathologists.

Bile duct lesions have also been reported in a number of other conditions, including pericholangitis associated with ulcerative colitis, acute viral hepatitis, chronic active hepatitis, cirrhosis, drug reaction, and extrahepatic biliary obstruction; the latter five of these are potential problems in the differential diagnosis of liver disease in the setting of HSCT. Endotheliitis of either central or portal veins occurs in about 30–40% of patients with acute GVHD. If present, it is a strong positive predictor of GVHD, particularly in the acute phase. Taken in conjunction with bile duct damage, whose absence is a strong negative predictor, this may be the most specific feature of GVHD.[126–128]

After weeks to months of acute GVHD, liver histology is dominated by changes of profound cholestasis with hepatocellular injury in zone 1 and loss of bile ducts. Hepatocytes in zone 1 show extensive ballooning degeneration and heavy pigmentation with lipofuscins, iron, and bile. There is also extensive hepatocyte dropout, sinusoidal fibrosis, and Kupffer cell hyperplasia. There may be bridging necrosis (portal-to-portal and portal-to-central bands), piecemeal necrosis with erosion of limiting plates, and dilated periportal cholangioles filled with dense pigments. Fibrosis develops and may progress with bridging between portal areas or from portal to central areas. Fibrosis and mononuclear cellular infiltration expand the portal triads and may be associated with bile duct proliferation and loss of interlobular bile ducts at the periphery.

The histologic findings of periportal bile thrombi, triaditis, and extensive lobular cholestasis are strongly associated with severe multisystem GVHD in HSCT recipients. If immunosuppressive therapy is ineffective in controlling the disease process, hepatocyte dropout, collapse, and fibrosis lead to cirrhosis with portal hypertension and hepatic failure.[135] Cirrhosis is rare in GVHD.

Bile duct loss, with relative paucity of portal tract inflammation and minimal interface activity, is a characteristic

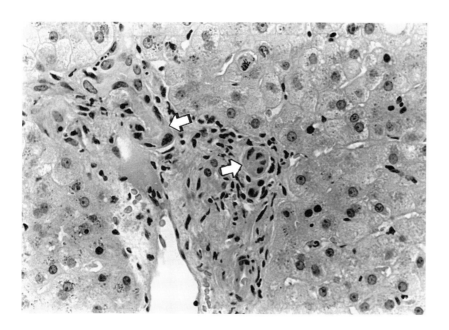

FIGURE 46–2. Atypia and degenerative changes of the small bile ductules is the pathognomonic feature of acute graft-versus-host disease. In this photomicrograph, the relative paucity of portal inflammation is likely related to the myeloablative conditioning regimen. There are, however, marked bile ductular abnormalities, including cytoplasmic eosinophilia, uneven nuclear spacing, and ducts only partially lined by epithelial cells (*arrows*) and nuclear pyknosis (H&E; × 400). Despite the extensive duct damage, periductal granulomas, like those seen with primary biliary cirrhosis, are not visible.

feature of chronic GVHD (Fig. 46–3). Interestingly, despite the duct loss, a marginal doctoral reaction is uncommon in chronic GVHD. Bile duct loss also occurs with chronic liver allograft rejection, but the characteristic obliterative arteriopathy does not occur with chronic GVHD.

MECHANISMS OF DAMAGE

Pathologically, the sine qua non of acute GVHD is selective epithelial damage of target organs. It is hypothesized that in the liver, the bile duct epithelium is the target of donor T-cell lymphocytes.[128] Death of liver cells in GVHD occurs by apoptosis as a result of cell-cell interaction between lymphoid cells and target liver cells. The molecular events leading to apoptosis in GVHD are not well understood.

The immunopathophysiologic process of GVHD involves two consecutive phases. Donor T lymphocytes are presum-

ably activated by alloantigens from host tissues (afferent phase): The activated T cells release cytokines, which recruit additional cells to areas of T cell infiltration. Subsequently, the expression of major histocompatibility antigens and adhesion molecules is increased on target tissues, which focuses the attack of donor effector cells on recipient targets (efferent phase). Experimental data challenge the hypothesis that the cytolytic function of the cytotoxic T cells directly causes tissue damage and necrosis and emphasizes the role of cytokines, particularly TNF-α, as central mediators of GVHD.[122]

Although normal bile epithelium does not express class II antigens, it is postulated that the intensive conditioning regimen causes a "cytokine storm" that up-regulates tissue HLA-DR, adhesion, and costimulatory molecule expression, which contributes to the sensitization phase of the reaction. Once initiated, the alloresponse can be amplified by recruited "nonspecific" effector cells such as eosinophils,

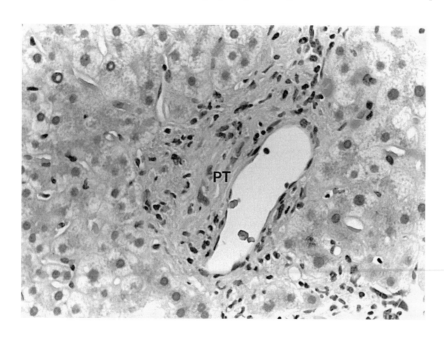

FIGURE 46–3. Bile duct loss, as shown in this photomicrograph, is a characteristic feature of chronic graft-versus-host disease (GVHD). Note the relative paucity of portal tract (PT) inflammation and minimal interface activity. Bile duct loss is also visible with chronic liver allograft rejection. In fact, the histopathologic appearance of chronic GVHD is indistinguishable from that of chronic liver allograft rejection, except for the presence of obliterative arteriopathy, which is not visible with chronic GVHD. Interestingly, despite the duct loss, a marginal ductular reaction is uncommon in chronic GVHD (H&E; × 400).

macrophages, and neutrophils. The bile ducts appear to be selectively injured. In general, the smaller the duct, the more severe the injury, with ducts smaller than 150 μm in diameter the most severely damaged. Donor cytotoxic T cells are adjacent to damaged bile duct epithelium. Cytokines, particularly IL-2, interferon-γ, TNF-α released locally by donor T cells, and recruited nonspecific effector cells are postulated to cause injury to bile duct epithelium and hepatocytes.

PROGNOSIS AND TREATMENT

Liver involvement, which occurs in 73–86% of patients with GVHD, responds more slowly than abnormalities in other organs and in many patients becomes the primary manifestation of chronic GVHD. Studies show that three features of chronic GVHD at presentation appear to be predictive of death: progressive disease (chronic GVHD evolving from acute GVHD), lichenoid skin or mucous membrane changes, and hepatic dysfunction.[138, 139] Patients with no such risk factors experienced an actuarial survival rate of 70% at 6 years, whereas patients with two or more risk factors ("high-risk" chronic GVHD) experienced a projected survival rate of 20%.

A series of reports on the natural history and treatment of chronic GVHD have emphasized the need for immunosuppressive therapy.[136–139] Less than 20% of untreated patients recover completely. In a study published in 1992, therapy with UDCA was found to be safe, well tolerated, and efficacious in the short-term treatment of refractory chronic GVHD of the liver.[140]

The mechanisms by which UDCA exerts its protective effect on the liver are not well understood. It has been postulated that UDCA protects hepatocytes from cholestatic injury by inducing hypercholeresis.[140] This process, in turn, may prevent the retention of more-hepatotoxic bile acids such as chenodeoxycholic acids and lithocholic acids. In addition, when UDCA is given orally to humans, it replaces the native, more-hydrophobic (hepatotoxic) bile acids and becomes the predominant bile acid. UDCA therapy may also have an immune-mediated mechanism, as indicated by the fact that UDCA therapy is associated with reduction of class I HLA expression on hepatocytes. Reduction in hepatocyte HLA class I expression could, by suppressing the cytotoxic T-cell target, block immune-mediated hepatocellular necrosis and, in turn, slow the progression of liver disease. Moreover, UDCA may directly modulate lymphocyte function. Further investigation is needed to evaluate the long-term effects of UDCA therapy in chronic GVHD.

OTHER LIVER DISEASES IN HSCT RECIPIENTS

Hepatic dysfunction after HSCT is a diagnostic challenge for both the clinician and pathologist (Table 46–2). Other hepatic diseases may mimic VOD or GVHD or, more commonly, coexist with them.[123–125, 129] Viral hepatitis is a relatively common event after HSCT.[71, 72, 129, 141] Most cases of viral hepatitis are caused by HCV and cytomegalovirus (CMV), with sporadic cases due to HBV, adenovirus, herpes

TABLE 46–2. OTHER LIVER DISEASES IN HSCT

Viral hepatitis (e.g., hepatitis C, V, and D virus; cytomegalovirus; Epstein-Barr virus; herpes simplex virus; varicella-zoster virus; adenovirus; papovavirus; parvovirus)
Fungal diseases (e.g., *Candida, Aspergillus, Trichosporon, Fusarium, Histoplasma*)
Bacterial infection (liver abcess, microabcesses, cholangitis)
Micobacterial infection (e.g., *M. tuberculosis, M. avium*)
Cholecystitis
Cholangitis lenta (hyperbilirubinemia associated with sepsis syndrome)
Nodular regenerative hyperplasia
Drug-induced liver diseases (e.g., cyclosporine, trimethoprim-sulfamethoxazole, mezlocillin, fluconazole, itraconazole, methotrexate)

simplex virus, varicella-zoster virus, parvovirus, and papovavirus.

VIRAL INFECTIONS

Distinguishing chronic viral hepatitis due to HCV infection from GVHD can be difficult histopathologically. A diagnosis of chronic GVHD is more likely if extensive bile duct damage is found with minimal inflammatory changes. Severe bile duct damage is unusual with chronic HCV infection. On the other hand, extensive portal inflammation favors chronic HCV infection. Although the distinction between GVHD and chronic viral hepatitis can be difficult, atypical and destructive bile duct changes favor GVHD.

Acute infection with HBV may occur in some patients in the absence of detectable hepatitis B surface antigen in the serum, and spontaneous exacerbation of chronic HBV infection may be due to superinfection with delta virus agent[142] or intense immunosuppression that may lead to reactivation of HBV infection.[76] Although there are case reports of reactivation of HBV leading to death from liver failure,[75] surveys of three large studies indicate that this severe complication is infrequent.[143–145] Fibrosing cholestatic hepatitis is a recently described lesion that develops in some patients undergoing orthotopic liver transplantation. It is characterized by periportal fibrosis, cholangiolar proliferation, ballooning degeneration of hepatocytes, prominent cholestasis, and paucity of inflammation, and it is rare in marrow transplant recipients.[77, 78]

CMV infection should be considered in the differential diagnosis in either a seropositive recipient or a patient who received marrow or PBPC from a seropositive donor.[146] Histologic features of CMV hepatitis include multiple foci of spotty acidophilic hepatocyte necrosis, mononuclear cells in the sinusoids, portal infiltration with lymphocyte and plasma cells, granuloma, and massive necrosis. In immunosuppressed patients, additional features include polymorphonuclear leukocyte aggregates, microabscesses, and cholestasis. CMV inclusions may be found in hepatocytes, Kupffer cells, endothelium, bile duct cells, gallbladder, and extrahepatic biliary endothelium.

Hepatitis with herpes simplex virus, varicella-zoster virus, and adenovirus may cause widespread necrosis and hepatic failure.[147, 148] Transient elevation of liver enzymes was also been linked to excretion of papoviruses in one series.[149] Parvovirus can be an important infective complication of HSCT, and in any susceptible patient with unexplained anemia, investigation should include a search for parvovirus B 19 DNA because treatment is easily instituted.[150] Epstein-Barr virus (EBV) may produce clinical hepatitis or a spectrum of B-cell lymphoproliferative disorders ranging from an infectious mononucleosis type of picture to immunoblastic B-cell lymphoma infiltrating the liver and other viscera.[151, 152] Rarely, the gallbladder and nodes in the porta hepatis are involved, causing biliary obstruction.

The diagnosis of viral infection is usually based on other manifestations of the infection and identification of the virus in the serum or tissue samples. Culture of liver biopsy specimens, staining or in situ hybridization for viral antigens or nucleic acids, and serum tests confirm most of the diagnoses. Herpes simplex and varicella zoster viruses can be treated with acyclovir, and CMV can be treated with ganciclovir or foscarnet.[148, 149] There is no proven effective therapy for adenovirus infection, although ribavirin and ganciclovir have activity against this virus.[149] EBV may respond to infusion of EBV-immune donor lymphocytes.[152] There is no effective treatment for HBV or HCV in the immediate post-transplantation setting.

BACTERIAL AND FUNGAL INFECTION

Fungal infection of the liver usually occurs as part of widely disseminated infection. Since the advent of fungal prophylaxis with fluconazole, fungal infection is less common and confined to patients with persistent granulocytopenia and fungal colonization. Although *Candida* species accounts for most cases of liver infection in marrow transplant recipients, a variety of other fungi, including *Aspergillus, Trichosporon, Fusarium, Histoplasma capsulatum, Pseudallescheria boydii*, and *Scedosporium prolificans* have caused severe infections in these patients.[141]

Over half the patients with disseminated fungal infection have liver involvement. Fungal lesions include granuloma, small abscesses, large cysts, massive fungi in the biliary ducts, and infarcts from vascular occlusion. Fungal obstruction of hepatic veins may mimic VOD. The reported manifestations of fungal liver infection (liver tenderness, elevated serum alkaline phosphatase) are insensitive markers in transplant recipients because of the high prevalence of other hepatic disorders. Imaging of the liver with ultrasonography or computed tomography can be useful, but a negative result should not delay liver biopsy. Ultrasound-guided fine-needle aspiration can confirm a diagnosis without the risk of biopsy. Empirical amphotericin is usually given if there is a high likelihood of visceral fungal infection rather than pursuing a tissue diagnosis.

Bacterial liver abscess, microabscesses, and cholangitis are less frequent in HSCT recipients, perhaps because of infection prophylaxis and prompt empirical antibiotic use for fever.[162] Both calculous and acalculous cholecystitis can occur in HSCT recipients.[128, 153] The combination of cytoreductive therapy, prolonged gallbladder stasis from lack of oral intake, and increased biliary excretion of precipitatable material (calcium bilirubinate, CSA, antibiotics) leads to a 60–70% prevalence of gallbladder sludge by 2 weeks.[128, 154, 155]

The exfoliation of mucus-containing cells from the gallbladder caused by cytoreductive therapy may provide nucleation material. The biliary stasis may be related to prolonged parenteral nutrition[156] and perhaps to intrahepatic cholestasis of GVHD.[154] Symptoms may result when gallbladder sludge becomes lodged in the cystic duct, common bile duct, or ampulla of Vater (biliary sludge syndrome).

Mycobacterial liver infection may occur in HSCT recipients and should be included in the differential diagnosis.[157] Nodular regenerative hyperplasia of the liver, characterized by the development of regenerative nodules alternating with areas of parenchymal atrophy, has been found in these patients, although infrequently.[158] It causes portal hypertension and can simulate moderately severe VOD, but it usually appears later after transplantation.

Extrahepatic biliary obstruction is rare in HSCT recipients and is usually related to biliary sludge, CMV/cryptosporidia-associated papillitis or stricture, or EBV lymphoproliferative disease involving portahepatis nodes or biliary tract.[141, 146]

CHOLESTASIS

Cholangitis lenta, a cholestatic liver disease that follows sepsis and other causes of cytokine release, is a common cause of jaundice in febrile transplant recipients who are neutropenic, particularly before day 30 but also when the patient is receiving high-dose immunosuppressive therapy for acute GVHD.[156] The classic presentation is usually that of hyperbilirubinemia that follows persistent fever or sepsis syndrome by days or weeks. The total serum bilirubin level may rise to 50 mg/dL if the patient already has hepatic dysfunction. Liver synthetic function is preserved and portal hypertension, hepatorenal syndrome, and ascites are unusual. Liver biopsy shows either pericentral canalicular cholestasis or cholangiolar cholestasis, but the portal inflammation often accompanying this condition in "septic" patients may be absent because of pancytopenia or immunosuppressive drugs for acute GVHD. In most cases, the diagnosis of cholangitis lenta is made in retrospect.

DRUG TOXICITIES

Drug-induced liver injury can occur any time after transplantation and can account for significant hepatic dysfunction in these patients.[129] CSA causes a defect in bilirubin excretion at the level of the bile canaliculus through its effect on transport protein, even at therapeutic blood levels.[159, 160] Toxicity has been reported to be dose dependent. At high levels, cholestasis is more prominent, and serum levels above 400 ng/mL are more commonly associated with hepatocellular damage.[160–162] The incidence of CSA toxicity has been between 15% and 50%.[159, 160] Liver injury from other medications used in the transplant setting (e.g., trimethoprim-sulfamethoxazole, mezlocillin, fluconazole, itraconazole, and methotrexate) and from parenteral nutrition can also cause liver dysfunction (both cholestasis and hepatocellular injury).[129]

Histologically, the diagnosis of drug-induced hepatitis is

suggested when the amount of hepatocellular necrosis is significant compared with the presence of inflammatory infiltrates or when some other feature, such as an eosinophilic infiltrate or granulomas, is present; however, these changes are not common and, when present, are not specific.[129]

CONCLUSION

Liver complications are a major cause of morbidity and mortality after HSCT. VOD and liver GVHD are two major problems. Currently, there are no reports of prospective clinical trials evaluating prophylaxis and therapy for both complications. For VOD, risk factors have been identified, and clinical criteria have been established by JHOC and FHCRC. Prophylaxis measures include the use of heparin, PGE_1, UDCA, and pentoxifylline. Therapeutic options include drugs such as r-tPA and PGE_1 and surgical procedures to remove ascites. For hepatic GVHD, diagnosis is less certain than for VOD, and it usually requires biopsy for confirmation. Therapy using UDCA, in addition to immunosuppressive treatment of GVHD, appears to be effective. Hepatic complications can also be caused by viral, bacterial, and/or fungal infections. Infections are less frequent and the clinical outcome is not as serious as in VOD and liver GVHD. The problem of hepatitis should be minimized by careful screening and selection of donors. Future advances in prophylaxis and therapy of both VOD and GVHD are expected and will be welcome.

REFERENCES

1. Shuhart MC, McDonald GB: Gastrointestinal and hepatic complications. *In* Forman SJ, Blume KG, Thomas ED (eds): Bone Marrow Transplantation. Cambridge, MA, Blackwell Scientific, 1994, p 454.
2. Singh C, McDonald GB: Intestinal and liver complications of marrow transplantation. *In* Taylor MB, Gollan JL, Steer ML, et al (eds): Gastrointestinal Emergencies, 2nd ed. Baltimore, Williams & Wilkins, 1997, p 859.
3. Seltzer G, Peter RGF: Senecio poisoning exhibiting as Chiari's syndrome. Am J Pathol 27: 885, 1951.
4. Valla D, Benhamou JP: Disorders of the hepatic veins and venules. *In* Mcintyre N, Benhamou JP, Bircher J, et al (eds). Oxford Textbook of Clinical Hepatology, vol 2. Oxford, England, Oxford University Press, 1991, p 1004.
5. Tandon BN, Tandon RK, Tandon HD, et al: An epidemic of veno-occlusive disease of liver in central India. Lancet 2:271, 1976.
6. Ridker PM, McDermott WV: Comfrey tea and hepatic veno-occlusive disease. Lancet 1:657, 1989.
7. Bras G, Jelliffe, DB, Stuart KL: Veno-occlusive disease of liver with nonportal type of cirrhosis, occuring in Jamaica. Arch Pathol 57:285, 1954.
8. Lewin K, Mills R: Human radiation hepatitis: a morphologic study with emphasis on late changes. Arch Pathol 96:21, 1973.
9. Reed GB, Cox AJ: The human liver after radiation injury: a form of veno-occlusive disease. Am J Pathol 48:597, 1996.
10. Fajardo LF, Colby TV: Pathogenesis of veno-occlusive disease after radiation. Arch Pathol Lab Med 104:584, 1980.
11. Satti MB, Weinbren K, Gordon-Smith EC: 6-thioquanine as a cause of toxic veno-occlusive disease of the liver. J Clin Pathol 35:1086, 1982.
12. Weitz H, Gokel JM, Loeschke K, et al: Veno-occlusive disease of the liver in patients receiving immunosuppressive therapy. Virchows Arch (A) 395:245, 1982.
13. Erichsen C, Jonsson PE: Veno-occlusive liver disease after dacarbazine therapy (DTIC) for melanoma. J Surg Oncol 27:268, 1984.
14. Reed AE, Weisner RH, LeBrecque R, et al: Hepatic veno-occlusive

disease associated with renal transplantation and azathioprine therapy. Ann Intern Med 104:651, 1986.
15. Jacobs P, Miller JL, Uys CJ, et al: Fatal veno-occlusive disease of the liver after chemotherapy, whole body radiation and bone marrow transplantation in refractory acute leukemia. S Afr Med J 55:5, 1979.
16. Berk PD, Popper H, Krueger GRF, et al: Veno-occlusive diseases of the liver after allogeneic bone marrow transplantation: possible association with graft-versus host disease. Ann Intern Med 90:158, 1979.
17. Wood WG, Dehner LP, Nesbit ME, et al: Fatal veno-occlusive disease of the liver following high dose chemotherapy, irradiation and bone marrow transplantation. Am J Med 68:285, 1980.
18. Shulman HM, McDonald GB, Matthews D, et al: An analysis of hepatic veno-occlusive disease and centrilobular degeneration following bone marrow transplantation. Gastroenterology 79:1178, 1980.
19. Lazarus HM, Gotfried MR, Herzig RH, et al: Veno-occlusive disease of the liver after high-dose mitomycin C therapy and autologous bone marrow transplantation. Cancer 49:1789, 1982.
20. McDonald GB, Sharma P, Matthews DE, et al: Veno-occlusive disease of the liver after bone marrow transplantation: diagnosis, incidence and predisposing factors. Hepatology 4:116, 1984.
21. Jones RJ, Lee KSK, Beschorner WE, et al: Veno-occusive disease of the liver following bone marrow transplantation. Transplantation 44:778, 1987.
22. McDonald GB, Hinds MS, Fisher LD, et al: Veno-occlusive disease of the liver and multiorgan failure after bone marrow transplantation: a cohort study of 355 patients. Ann Intern Med 118:255, 1993.
23. Sculman HM, Fisher LB, Schoch HG, et al: Veno-occlusive disease of the liver after marrow transplantation: histological correlates of clinical signs and symptoms. Hepatology 19:1171, 1994.
24. Bearman SI: The syndrome of hepatic veno-occlusive disease after marrow transplantation. Blood 85:3005, 1995.
25. Soiffer RJ, Dear K, Rabinowe SN, et al: Hepatic dysfunction following T cell depleted allogeneic bone marrow transplantation. Transplantation 52:1014, 1991.
26. Radich J, Sanders J, Buckner CD, et al: Second allogeneic marrow transplantation for patients with recurrent leukemia after initial transplant with total-body irradiation–containing regimens. J Clin Oncol 11:304, 1993.
27. Shulman HM, Gown AM, Nugent DJ: Hepatic veno-occlusive disease after bone marrow transplantation: immunohistochemical identification of the material with occluded central venules. Am J Pathol 127(3):549, 1987.
28. Anscher MS, Peters WP, Reisenbichler H, et al: Transforming growth factor B as a predictor of liver and lung fibrosis after autologous bone marrow transplantation for advanced breast cancer. N Engl J Med 328:1592, 1993.
29. Allen JR, Carstens LA, Katagiri GJ: Hepatic veins of monkeys with veno-occlusive disease: sequential ultrastructural changes. Arch Pathol 87:279, 1969.
30. Asbury RF, Rosenthal SN, Descalzi ME, et al: Hepatic veno-occlusive disease due to DTIC. Cancer 45:2670, 1980.
31. DeLeve LD: Dacarbazine toxicity in murine liver cells: a model of hepatic endothelial injury and glutathione and defense. J Pharm Exp Ther 286:1261, 1994.
32. Hess AF: Fatal obliterating endophelibitis of the hepatic veins. Am J Med Sci 130:986, 1905.
33. Allen JR, Garstens LA, Olson BE: Veno-occlusive disease in Macaca speciosa monkeys. Am J Pathol 50:653, 1967.
34. Carreras E, Granena A, Nasa M, et al: Transjugular liver biopsy in BMT. Bone Marrow Transplant 11:21, 1993.
35. Gertler JP, Abbott WM: Prothrombotic and fibrinolytic function of normal and preturbed endothelium. J Surg Res 52:89, 1992.
36. Nawroth PP, Stern DM: Endothelial cell procoagulant properties and the host response. Semin Thromb Hemost 13:391, 1987.
37. Dittman WA, Majerus PW: Structure and function of thrombomodulin: a natural anticoagulant. Blood 75:329, 1990.
38. Collins PW, Gutteridge CN, O'Driscoll A, et al: Von Willebrand factor as a marker of endothelial cell activation following BMT. Bone Marrow Transplant 10:499, 1992.
39. Bearman SI, Lefkowitz JB, Mones RB, et al: Thrombomodulin increases in patients receiving high-dose chemotherapy with autologous progenitor cell support. Blood (Suppl) 82:614a, 1993.
40. Scrobohaci ML, Drouet L, Monem-Mansi A, et al: Liver veno-occlu-

sive disease after bone marrow transplantation changes in coagulation parameters and endothelial markers. Thromb Res 63:509, 1991.

41. Collins P, Jones B, Uthayakumar S, et al: Hemostatic changes in uncomplicated bone marrow transplants. Bone Marrow Transplant 7 (Suppl):54, 1991.

42. Shirai M, Nagashima K, Iwasaki S, et al: A light and scanning electron microscopic study of hepatic venoocclusive disease. Acta Pathol Jpn 37:1961, 1987.

43. Traber PG, Chianale J, Gumucio JJ: Physiologic significance and regulation of hepatocellular heterogeneity. Gastroenterology 95:1130, 1988.

44. Ishawa T, Akerboom TPM, Sies H: Role of key defense systems in target organ toxicity. In Cohen GM (ed): Target Organ Toxicity. Boca Raton, FL, CRC Press, 1986, p 1.

45. Mitchell JR, Smith CV, Hughes H, et al: Overview of alkylation and peroxidation mechanism in acute lethal hepatocellular injury by chemically reactive metabolites. Semin Liver Dis 1:143, 1981.

46. Antin JH, Ferrara JLM: Cytokine dysregulation and acute graft-versus-host disease. Blood 80:2964, 1992.

47. Scannell G, Waxman K, Kaml GJ, et al: Hypoxia induces a human macrophage cell line to release tumor necrosis factor-alpha and its soluble receptors in vitro. J Surg Res 54:281, 1993.

48. Hallahan DE, Spriggs DR, Beckett MA, et al: Increased tumor necrosis factor-alpha mRNA after cellular exposure to ionizing radiation. Proc Natl Acad Sci U S A 86:10104, 1989.

49. Holler E, Kolb HJ, Moller A, et al: Increased serum levels of tumor necrosis factor-alpha precede major complications of bone marrow transplantation. Blood 75:1011, 1990.

50. Tanaka J, Imamura M, Kasai M, et al: Rapid analysis of tumor necrosis factor-alpha mRNA expression during veno-occlusive disease of the liver after allogeneic bone marrow transplantation. Transplantation 55:430, 1993.

51. Tanaka J, Imamura M, Kasai M, et al: Cytokine gene expression in peripheral blood mononuclear cells during graft-versus-host disease after allogeneic bone marrow transplantation. Br J Haematol 85:558, 1993.

52. Gerlach H, Esposito C, Stern DM: Modulation of endothelial hemostatic properties: an active role in the host response. Ann Rev Med 41:15, 1990.

53. Jattela M: Biologic activities and mechanism of action of tumor necrosis factor/cachexin. Lab Invest 64:724, 1991.

54. Bevilacqua MP, Pober JS, Majeau GR, et al: Recombinant tumor necrosis factor induces procoagulant activity in cultured human vascular endothelium: characterization and comparison with the actions of interleukin 1. Proc Natl Acad Sci U S A 83:4533, 1986.

55. Gordon B, Haire W, Kessinger A, et al: High frequency of antithrombin 3 and protein C deficiency following autologous bone marrow transplantation for lymphoma. Bone Marrow Transplant 8:497, 1991.

56. Faioni EM, Bearman SI, Krachmainicoff A, et al: Procoagulant imbalance due to low levels of protein C in patients with veno-occlusive (VOD) of the liver after marrow transplantation. Blood 78: 193a, 1991.

57. van der Poll T, Buller HR, ten Cate H, et al: Activation of coagulation after administration of tumor necrosis factor to normal subjects. N Engl J Med 322:1622, 1990.

58. Bret J, Gerlach H, Nawroth p, et al: Tumor necrosis factor/cachectin increases permeability of endothelial cell monolayers by a mechanism involving regulatory G proteins. J Exp Med 169:1977, 1989.

59. Mutto Y, Nouri-Aria KT, Meager A, et al: Enhanced tumor necrosis factor and interleukin-1 in fulminant hepatic failure. Lancet 2:72, 1988.

60. Bianco JA, Appelbaum FR, Nemunitis J, et al: Phase I–II trial of pentoxifylline for the prevention of transplant-related toxicities following bone marrow transplantation. Blood 78:1205, 1991.

61. Copelan EA, Avalos BR, Klein JL, et al: Reduction in the incidence of transplant related death using methotrexate, cyclosporin and pentoxifylline compared to cyclosporine and methylprednisolone for prevention of graft-versus-host disease following conditioning with BuCy. Blood Suppl 80:236a, 1992.

62. Attal M, Huguet F, Rubie H, et al: Prevention of regimen related toxicities after bone marrow transplantation by pentoxifylline: a prospective, randomized trial. Blood 82:732, 1993.

63. Clift RA, Bianco JA, Appelbaum FR, et al: A randomized controlled trial of pentoxifylline for the prevention of regimen-related toxicities

in patients undergoing allogeneic bone marrow transplantation. Blood 82:2025, 1993.

64. Anscher MS, Peters WP, Reisenbichler H, et al: Transforming growth factor B as a predictor of liver and lung fibrosis after autologous bone marrow transplantation for advanced breast cancer. N Engl J Med 328:1592, 1993.

65. Devine SM, Winton EF, Holland HK, et al: Simultaneous adminstration of interleukin-6 (rh IL-6) and neupogen (rhG-CSF) following autologous bone marrow transplantation (ABMT) for breast cancer (BCA). Blood 84:343a, 1994.

66. Catani L, Gugliotta L, Mattioli Belmonte M, et al: Hypercoagulabilty in patients undergoing autologous or allogeneic BMT for hematologic malignancies. Bone Marrow Transplant 12:253, 1993.

67. Eltumi M, Trivedi P, Hobbs JR, et al: Monitoring of veno-occlusive disease after bone marrow transplantation by serum aminopropeptide of type III procollagen. Lancet 342:518, 1993.

68. Rio B, Bauducer F, Arrago JP, et al: A marker for the development of hepatic veno-occlusive disease after BMT and a basis of determining the timing of prophylactic heparin. Bone Marrow Transplant 11:471, 1993.

69. Frei AU, Zimmerman A, Weigand K, et al: The N-terminal propeptide of collagen type III in serum reflects activity and degree of fibrosis in patients with chronic liver disease. Hepatology 4:830, 1984.

70. Locasciulli A, Bacigalupo A, Alberti A, et al: Predictability before transplant of hepatic complications following allogeneic bone marrow transplantation. Transplantation 48:68, 1989.

71. Locarelli G, Galimberti M, Polchi P, et al: Marrow transplantation in patients with advanced thalasemia. N Engl J Med 316:1050, 1987.

72. Witherspoon RP, Storb R, Shulman HM, et al: Marrow transplantation in hepatitis-associated aplastic anemia. Am J Hematol 17:269, 1984.

73. Frickhofen N, Wiesneth M, Jinta C, et al: Hepatitis C virus infectionis a risk factor for liver failure from veno-occlusive disease after bone marrow transplant recipients. Blood 83(7):1998, 1994.

74. Locasciulli A, Bacigalupo A, VanLint MT, et al: Hepatitic C virus infection and liver failure in patients undergoing allogeneic bone marrow transplantation. Bone Marrow Transplant 166(3):407, 1995.

75. Birds GLA, Smith H, Portman B, et al: Acute liver decompensation on withdrawal of cytotoxic chemotherapy in lymphoma patients. Q J Med 73:895, 1989.

76. Lok ASF, Liang RHS, Chiu EKW, et al: Reactivation of hepatitis B virus replication in patients receiving cytotoxic therapy: report of prospective study. Gastroenterology 100:182, 1991.

77. Cooskley WGE, McIvor CA: Fibrosing cholestatic hepatitis and HBV after bone marrow transplantation. Biomed Pharmacother 49:117, 1995.

78. McIvor C, Morton J, Bryant A, et al: Fatal reactivation of precore mutant hepatitis B virus associated with fibrosing cholestatic hepatitis after bone marrow transplantation. Ann Intern Med 121:274, 1994.

79. Ganem G, Saint-Marc Giardin M-F, Kuentz M, et al: Veno-occlusive disease of the liver after allogeneic bone marrow transplantation in man. Int J Radiat Oncol Biol Phys 14:879, 1988.

80. Nevill TJ, Barnett MJ, Klingemann H-G, et al: Regimen-related toxicity of busulfan-cyclophosphamide conditioning regimen in 70 patients undergoing allogeneic bone marrow transplantation. J Clin Oncol 9:1224, 1991.

81. Grochow LB, Jones RJ, Brundrett RB, et al: Pharmacokinetics of busulfan: correlation with veno-occlusive disease in patients undergoing bone marrow transplantation. Cancer Chemother Pharmacol 25:55, 1989.

82. Grochow LB, Piantadosi S, Santos G, et al: Busulfan dose adjustment decreases the risk of hepatic veno-occlusive disease in patients undergoing bone marrow transplantation. Proc AACR 33:1197, 1992.

83. Dix SP, Wingard JR, Mullins RE, et al: Association of busulfan area under the curve with veno-occlusive disease following BMT. Bone Marrow Transplant 17(2):225, 1996.

84. Essel JH, Thompson JM, Harman GS, et al: Marked increase in veno-occlusive disease of the liver associated with methotrexate use for graft-versus-host disease prophylaxis in patients receiving busulfan/cyclophosphamide. Blood 79:2784, 1992.

85. Bearman SI, Applebaum FR, Buckner CD, et al: Regimen related toxicity in patients undergoing bone marrow transplantation. J Clin Oncol 6:1562, 1988.

86. Dulley FL, Kanfer EJ, Applebaum FR, et al: Veno-occlusive disease of the liver after chemotherapy and bone marrow transplantation. Transplantation 43:870, 1987.
87. Wingard JR, Niehaus CS, Peterson DE, et al: Oral mucositis after bone marrow transplantation: a marker of treatment toxicity and predictor of hepatic veno-occlusive disease. Oral Surg Oral Med Oral Pathol 72:419, 1991.
88. Wingard JR, Mellitis ED, Jones RJ, et al: Association of hepatic veno-occlusive disease with interestitial pneumonitis in bone marrow transplant recipients. Bone Marrow Transplant 4:685, 1989.
89. Mcdonald GB, Sharma P, Matthews DE, et al: The clinical course of 53 patients with veno-occlusive disease of the liver after bone marrow transplantation. Transplantation 39:603, 1985.
90. Brugieres L, Hartmann D, Benhomou E, et al: Veno-occlusive disease of the liver following high dose chemotherapy and autologous bone marrow transplantation in children with solid tumors: incidence, clinical course and outcome. Bone Marrow Transplant 3:53, 1988.
91. Ayash LJ, Hunt M, Antman K, et al: Hepatic veno-occlusive disease in autologous bone marrow transplantation of solid tumors and lymphomas. J Clin Oncol 8:1699, 1990.
92. Meresse V, Hartmann O, Vassal G, et al: Risk factors for hepatic veno-occlusive disease after high-dose busulfan-containing regimens followed by autologous bone marrow transplantation: a study in 136 children. Bone Marrow Transplant 10:135, 1992.
93. Morgan M, Dodds A, Atkinson K, et al: The toxicity of busulfan and cyclophosphamide as the preparative regimen for bone marrow transplantation. Br J Haematol 77:529, 1991.
94. Zager RA: Acute renal failure in the setting of bone marrow transplantation. Kidney Int 46:1443, 1994.
95. Zager RA, O'Quigley J, Zager BK, et al: Acute renal failure following bone marrow transplantation: a retrospective study of 272 patients. Am J Kidney Dis 13:210, 1989.
96. Blostein MD, Paltiel OB, Thibault A, et al: A comparison of clinical criteria for the diagnosis of veno-occlusive disease of the liver after bone marrow transplantation. Bone Marrow Transplant 10:439, 1992.
97. Brown BP, Abu-Yousef M, Farner R, et al: Doppler sonography: a noninvasive method for evaluation of hepatic venocclusive disease. AJR 154:721, 1990.
98. Herberko J, Grigg AP, Buckley AR, et al: Venoocclusive liver disease after bone marrow transplantation: findings at duplex sonography. AJR 158:1001, 1992.
99. Hommeyer SC, Teefey SA, Jacobson AF, et al: Venooclusive disease of the liver: prospective study of US evaluation. Radiology 184:683, 1992.
100. Jacobson AF, Teefey SA, Higano CA, et al: Increased lung uptake of ⁹⁹Tcm-sulphur colloid as an early indicator of the development of hepatic veno-occlusive disease in bone marrow transplant patients. Nucl Med Commun 14(8):706–711, 1993.
101. Carreras E, Granena A, Navasa M, et al: Transjugular liver biopsy in BMT. Bone Marrow Transplant 11:21, 1993.
102. Shulman HM, Mcdonald GB: Transvenous liver biopsies and pressure measurements in bone marrow transplant recipients. Hepatology 16:148, 1992.
103. Bearman SI, Anderson GL, Mori M, et al: Venocclusive disease of the liver: development of a model for predicting fatal outcome after marrow transplantation. J Clin Oncol 9:1729, 1993.
104. Chen JY, Flesch M, Plouvier E, et al: Veno-occlusive disease of the liver and autologous bone marrow transplantation: preventive role for heparin? Nouv Rev Fr Hematol 27:27, 1985.
105. Bearman SI, Hinds MS, Wolford JL: A pilot study of continuous infusion heparin for the prevention of hepatic veno-occlusive disease after bone marrow transplantation. Bone Marrow Transplant 5:407, 1990.
106. Marsa-Vila L, Gorin NC, Laporte JP, et al: Prophylactic heparin does not prevent liver veno-occlusive disease following autologous bone marrow transplantation. Eur J Haematol 47:346, 1991.
107. Attal M, Huguet F, Rubie H, et al: Prevention of hepatic veno-occlusive disease of the liver by continuous infusion of low-dose heparin: a prospective, randomized trial. Blood 80:2149, 1992.
108. Gluckman E, Jolivet I, Scrobohaci ML: Use of prostaglandin E1 for prevention of liver veno-occlusive disease in leukemic patients treated by allogeneic bone marrow transplantation. Br J Haematol 74:277, 1990.
109. Bearman SI, Shen DD, Hinds MS, et al: A phase I/II study of prostaglandin E1 for the prevention of hepatic veno-occlusive disease after bone marrow transplantation. Br J Haematol 84:724, 1993.
110. Essell JH, Thompson JM, Harman GS, et al: Pilot trial of prophylactic ursodiol to decrease the incidence of veno-occlusive disease of the liver in allogeneic bone marrow transplant patients. Bone Marrow Transplant 10:367, 1992.
111. Essell J, Schroeder M, Thompson J, et al: A randomized double-blind trial of prophylactic ursodeoxycholic acid vs. placebo to prevent venocclusive disease of liver in patients undergoing allogeneic bone marrow transplantation. Blood Suppl 84:250a, 1994.
112. Baglin TP, Harper P, Marcus RE: Veno-occlusive disease of the liver complicating ABMT successfully treated with recombinant tissue plasminogen activator. Bone Marrow Transplant 5:439, 1990.
113. Bearman SI, Shuhart MC, Hinds MS, et al: Recombinant human tissue plasminogen activator for the treatment of established severe venocclusive disease of the liver after bone marrow transplantation. Blood 80:2458, 1992.
114. Yu LC, Malkani I, Regueira O, et al: Recombinant tissue plaminogen activator (rt-PA) for veno-occlusive liver disease in pediatric autologous bone marrow transplant patients. Am J Hematol 46:194, 1994.
115. Simpson DR, Browett PJ, Doak PB, et al: Successful treatment of veno-occlusive disease with recombinant tissue plasminogen activator in a patient requiring peritoneal dialysis. Bone Marrow Transplant 14(4):635, 1994.
116. Ibrahim A, Pico JL, Maraninchi D, et al: Hepatic veno-occlusive disease following bone marrow transplantation treated by prostaglandin E1. Bone Marrow Transplant 7(Suppl 2):53, 1991.
117. Fogteloo AJ, Smid WM, Kok T, et al: Successful treatment of veno-occlusive disease of the liver with urokinase in a patient with non-Hodgkin's lymphoma. Leukemia 7:760, 1993.
118. Murray JA, Labrecque DR, Gingrich RD, et al: Successful treatment of hepatic veno-occlusive disease in a bone marrow transplant patient with side-to-side portacaval shunt. Gastroenterology 92:1073, 1987.
119. Jacobson BK, Kalayoglu M: Effective early treatment of hepatic veno-occlusive disease with a central splenorenal shunt in a infant. J Pediatr Surg 27:531, 1992.
120. Fried MW, Connaghan G, Sharma S, et al: Transjugular intrahepatic portosystemic shunt for the management of severe venoocclusive disease following bone marrow transplantation. Hepatology 24(3):588, 1996.
121. Rapoport AP, Doyle HR, Starzl T, et al: Orthotopic liver transplantation for life-threatening veno-occlusive disease of the liver after allogeneic bone marrow transplant. Bone Marrow Transplant 8:421, 1991.
122. Ferrara, JL, Joachim Deeg H: Graft-versus-host disease. N Engl J Med 324(10):667, 1991.
123. McDonald GB, Shulman HM, Sullivan KM, et al: Intestinal and hepatic complicatons of human bone marrow transplantation: part I. Gastroenterology 90:460, 1986.
124. McDonald GB, Shulman HM, Sullivan KM, et al: Intestinal and hepatic complications of human bone marrow transplantation: part II. Gastroenterology 90:770, 1986.
125. Sullivan KM: Graft-versus-host disease. In Forman SJ, Blume KG, Thomas ED, (eds): Bone Marrow Transplantation. Boston, Blackwell Scientific, 1994, p 339.
126. Snover DC, Weisdorf SA, Ramsey NK, et al: Hepatic graft versus host disease: a study of the predictive value of liver biopsy in diagnosis. Hepatology 4:123, 1984.
127. Beschorner WD, Pino J, Boitnott JK, et al: Pathology of the liver with bone marrow transplantation: effects of busulfan, carmustine, acute graft-vs-host disease and cytomegalovirus. Am J Pathol 99:369, 1980.
128. Shulman HM, Mcdonald GB: Liver disease after marrow transplantation. In Sale GE, Schulman HM (eds): The Pathology of Bone Marrow Transplantation. New York, Masson, 1984, p 104.
129. Bertheau P, Hadengue A, Cazals-Hatem D, et al: Chronic cholestasis in patients after allogeneic bone marrow transplantation: several diseases are often associated. Bone Marrow Transplant 16:261, 1995.
130. Weisdorf D, Haake R, Blazar B, et al: Treatment of moderate/severe acute graft-versus host disease after allogeneic bone marrow transplantation: an analysis of clinical risk features and outcome. Blood 75:1024, 1990.
131. Deeg HJ, Loughran TP, Storb R, et al: Treatment of acute graft-versus-host disease with antithymocyte globulin and cyclosporin with or without metnylprednisolone. Transplantation 40:162, 1985.

132. Kennedy MS, Deeg HJ, Storb R, et al: Treatment of acute graft-versus-host disease after allogeneic marrow transplantation: a randomized study comparing corticosteroids and cyclosporine. Am J Med 78:978, 1985.

133. Koehler MT, Howrie D, Mirro J, et al: FK506 (tacrolimus) in the treatment of steroid-resistant acute graft-versus-host disease in children undergoing bone marrow transplantation. Bone Marrow Transplant 15:895, 1995.

134. Kanamaru A, Takemoto Y, Kakishita E, et al: FK506 treatment of graft-versus-host disease developing or exacerbating during prophylaxis and therapy with cyclosporin and/or other immunosuppressants. Bone Marrow Transplant 15:885, 1995.

135. Schulman HM, Sullivan KM, Weiden PL, et al: Chronic graft-versus-host syndrome in man: a long-term clinicopathologic study of 20 Seattle patients. Am J Med 69:204, 1980.

136. Storb R, Deeg HJ, Whitehead J, et al: Methotrexate and cyclosporine versus cyclosporine alone for prophylaxis of acute graft-versus-host disease after marrow transplantation for leukemia. N Engl J Med 314:729, 1986.

137. Sullivan KM, Shulman HM, Storb R, et al: Chronic graft-versus-host disease in 52 patients: adverse natural course and successful treatment with combination immunosuppression. Blood 57:267, 1981.

138. Wingard JR, Piantadosi S, Vogelsang GB, et al: Predictors of death from chronic graft-versus-host disease after bone marrow transplantation. Blood 74:1428, 1989.

139. Storb R, Prentice RL, Sullivan KM, et al: Predictive factors in chronic graft-versus-host disease in patients with aplastic anaemia by marrow transplantation from HLA-identical siblings. Ann Intern Med 98:461, 1983.

140. Fried RH, Murukami CS, Fisher LD, et al: Ursodeoxycholic acid treatment of refractory chronic graft-versus-host disease of the liver. Ann Intern Med 116:624, 1992.

141. Walter EA, Bowden RA: Infection in the bone marrow transplant recipient. Infect Dis Clin North Am 9(4):823, 1995.

142. Smendile A, Dentico P, Zanetti, et al: Infection with the delta agent in chronic HBs carriers. Gastroenterology 81:992, 1981.

143. Locasasciulli A, Bacigalupo A, Van Lint MT, et al: Hepatitis B virus (HBV) infection and liver disease after allogeneic bone marrow transplantation: a report of 30 cases. Bone Marrow Transplant 6:25, 1990.

144. Reed EC, Myerson D, Corey L, et al: Allogeneic marrow transplantation in patients positive for hepatitis B surface antigen. Blood 77:195, 1991.

145. Chen PM, Fan S, Liu CJ, et al: Changing of hepatitis markers in patients with bone marrow transplantation. Transplantation 49:708, 1990.

146. Zaia JA, Forman SJ: Cytomegalovirus infection in the bone marrow transplant recipient. Infect Dis Clin North Am 9(4):879, 1995.

147. Johnson Jr, Egaas S, Gleaves CA, et al: Hepatitis due to herpes simplex virus in marrow transplant patient. Clin Infect Dis 14:38, 1992.

148. Flomenberg P, Babbitt J, Drobyski WR, et al: Increasing incidence of adenovirus disease in bone marrow transplant recipients. J Infect Dis 169:775, 1994.

149. O'Reilly RJ, Lee FK, Grossbard E, et al: Papovavirus excretion following marrow transplantation: incidence and association with hepatic dysfunction. Transplant Proc 13:262, 1981.

150. Nour B, Green M, Michaels M, et al: Parvovirus B19 infection in pediatric transplant patients. Transplantation 56(40):836, 1993.

151. Zutter MM, Martin PJ, Sale GE, et al: Epstein-barr virus lymphoproliferation after BMT. Blood 72:520, 1988.

152. Papadopoulos EB, Ladanyi M, Emanuel D, et al: Infusion of donor leukocytes to treat Epstein-Barr virus–associated lymphoproliferative disorders after allogeneic bone marrow transplantation. N Engl J Med 330:1185, 1994.

153. Jardines LA, O'Donnell MR, Johnson DL, et al: Acalculous cholecystitis in bone marrow transplant patients. Cancer 71:354, 1993.

154. Frick MP, Snover DC, Feinberg SB, et al: Sonography of the gallbladder in bone marrow transplant patients. Am J Gastroenterol 79:122, 1984.

155. Roslyn JJ, Pitt HA, Mann LL, et al: Gallbladder disease in patients on long-term parentral nutrition. Gastroenterology 84:148, 1983.

156. Zimmerman HJ, Fang M, Utili R, et al: Jaundice due to bacterial infection. Gastroenterology 77:362, 1979.

157. Navari RM, Sullivan KM, Springmeyer SC, et al: Mycobacterial infections in marrow transplant patients. Transplantation 36:509, 1983.

158. Snover DC, Weisdorf S, Bloomer J, et al: Nodular regenerative hyperplasia of the liver following bone marrow transplantation. Hepatology 9:443, 1989.

159. Tuschka PJ, Beschorner LE, Hess AD, et al: Cyclosporin-A to prevent graft-versus-host disease in 22 patients receiving allogeneic marrow transplant. Blood 61:318, 1983.

160. Atkinson K, Biggs J, Dodds A, et al: Cyclosporine associated hepatotoxicity after allogeneic marrow transplantation in man: differentiation from other causes of post-transplant liver disease. Transplant Proc 15:2761, 1983.

161. The Canadian Multicenter Transplant Study Group: A randomized clinical trial of cyclosporine in cadaveric renal transplantation. N Engl J Med 309:809, 1983.

162. Keown PA, Stiller CR, Laupacis AL, et al: The effects and side effects of cyclosporine relationship to drug pharmacokinetics. Transplant Proc 14:659, 1982.

Mucositis and Other Gastrointestinal Complications

Hugo E. Vargas, M.D., and William B. Silverman, M.D.

The alimentary tract is particularly susceptible to damage in the process of hematopoietic stem cell transplantation (HSCT). Its high cellular turnover makes it very susceptible to the intense regimens of pretransplantation conditioning; graft-versus-host disease (GVHD) affects the mucosal surfaces and the liver, making gastrointestinal (GI) injury a hallmark for staging the severity of the process; and finally, its extensive mucosal surface is highly susceptible to infectious complications associated with transplantation process. In order to correctly diagnose GI complications of HSCT, it is crucial to understand the pathophysiology and the time course of the events leading to injury. The likely complications in each step of HSCT will be described with corresponding pathophysiology, clinical picture, characteristic diagnostic tests, and management.

CONDITIONING

Two GI complications that arise in the early stage of the transplantation process and are directly related to the conditioning regimen deserve special attention. They are direct mucosal damage (mucositis) and veno-occlusive disease (VOD) of the liver (see Chapter 46).[1–4]

DIRECT MUCOSAL TOXICITY

Most chemotherapy regimens tend to cause mild mucosal damage to the GI tract. Synergistic effects of chemotherapy and radiation have been described in the literature, however.[4–7] Patients may experience crampy abdominal pain, diarrhea, and oropharyngeal mucosal lesions that decrease their oral intake. Epstein et al. described the mucosal changes that occur within 10 days of bone marrow transplant (BMT) induction.[5] Their description included crypt cells that had atypical nuclei followed by cellular degeneration and abnormal surface epithelium. These characteristic changes disappeared 20 days after induction, except in those patients with acute GVHD. Drugs that have been implicated in creating mucosal damage in the oropharynx and esophagus when combined with radiation include doxorubicin, dactinomycin, bleomycin, cytarabine, 5-fluorouracil (5-FU), methotrexate, cyclophosphamide, etoposide, and cisplatin. Many of these agents are used alone or in combination in the ablation of bone marrow prior to HSCT.[1, 2, 8]

Clinical Presentation

Oropharyngeal ulceration and pain is a common symptom combination in patients undergoing HSCT.[3, 9–11] These mucosal changes are called ulcerative mucositis, and studies have shown a wide range of incidence. Two prospective studies evaluated the appropriate monitoring and care of oral mucositis and demonstrated that 69–75% of patients undergoing either allogeneic or syngeneic BMT with regimens that include cyclophosphamide, with or without total body irradiation, experience some degree of mucositis. The lesions described ranged from oral edema to frank ulceration in the nonkeratinized mucosa of the mouth.[10, 11] Woo et al. demonstrated a clear association between trauma and the severity of the ulcers.[12] The duration of absolute granulocytopenia paralleled the duration of the mucositis. All patients were receiving antiviral prophylaxis. Most were receiving antifungal prophylaxis. Prophylaxis breakthroughs throughout the study periods were excluded. The average duration of oral lesions in these patients was 15–16 days. Longer duration suggested early acute GVHD involving the mucosa or severe mucositis.[10]

Diagnosis

Usually, skin and oral findings are detected concomitantly.[3, 10, 11] The differential diagnosis should include viral and fungal infection, particularly in the esophagus and pharynx. Herpes simplex virus causes oral ulcers that may be difficult to differentiate visually from mucositis. In the period near the 20th day after transplantation, early acute GVHD disease needs to be considered. If dysphagia or diarrhea is present, esophagogastroduodenoscopy or flexible sigmoidoscopy is effective in differentiating the possible causal entities.[3, 13] Care should be taken to perform biopsies of the lesions for culture and polymerase chain reaction analysis that exclude treatable viral lesions early on.

Management

Nutritional support becomes an important management issue if the symptoms of early conditioning therapy are severe.[3, 14] Transplant centers place central venous access catheters early on to manage the nutritional impairment that may follow the appearance of mucositis. As described earlier, the changes apparent in this early injury should resolve with supportive measures alone, unless superinfection occurs. Some studies suggest that prostaglandins may play a significant role in the damage occurring with conditioning, particularly in the small intestine. This has led to trials using cyclo-oxygenase inhibition with salicylates to prevent some of the effects of chemoradiation in clinical and laboratory models.[9, 15]

GRAFT-VERSUS-HOST DISEASE

ACUTE GVHD

The diagnosis of acute GVHD is not generally difficult in that most patients present with a maculopapular rash (~ 75%), elevated bilirubin and alkaline phosphatase (60%), and hollow organ GI dysfunction (50%). These changes must occur before day 100 and generally do not occur before the third week after the bone marrow infusion.[3] Detailed discussion of GVHD can be found in Chapters 39, 45, and 54.

Clinical Presentation

Patients generally present with a maculopapular rash that initially presents in the palms of the hands and feet but extends to the trunk and rest of the lower extremities in more severe cases. Bullous skin disease with generalized erythrodermia can be the gravest grade of skin disease. Cholestatic liver tests generally show elevation of bilirubin and alkaline phosphatase. Gut manifestations include crampy abdominal pain with profuse diarrhea of significant volume implying small bowel hypersecretion, in many cases requiring aggressive rehydration to meet losses. GI bleeding arising from the extensive denudation of the gut mucosa may significantly increase the transfusion needs after BMT. Nutritionally, the secretory diarrhea induces a protein-losing enteropathy with marked decreases in total protein and albumin. Total parenteral nutrition is frequently used to maintain adequate nutritional status in these patients. Acute intestinal obstruction, either primary or secondary to narcotics and/or anticholinergics administered to manage the diarrheal symptoms, may be the presenting manifestation. Approximately 13–20% of patients undergoing BMT present with symptoms of heartburn, nausea, crampy abdominal pain, and food intolerance before diarrhea becomes evident, suggesting upper GI tract involvement that precedes the distal small bowel and colonic involvement that was classically described by McDonald et al.[3]

Pathogenesis

At the histologic level, the classic finding in acute GVHD is crypt cell apoptosis. Two caveats need to be mentioned: (1) the biopsy needs to be performed beyond the initial 20 days after conditioning so the effects of chemoradiation do not decrease the specificity of this test, and (2) if the biopsy is obtained late in the course of acute GVHD, the mucosal damage will have resulted in complete denudation of the cell layers, leading to nonspecific findings. Organ involvement in acute GVHD is frequently greatest in terminal ileum and ascending colon, with sigmoid and rectum being relatively spared. Biopsies from the rectum not only minimize the discomfort to the patient, they may be also be

accessible and occur early enough even to be of high diagnostic yield. Likewise, esophageal and gastric biopsies may show epithelial cell death that characterizes acute GVHD.[3, 16]

Stool studies and mucosal biopsies are essential in the patient who presents with the syndrome just described because acute GI infections, in particular, cytomegalovirus (CMV) or fungal disease, can present in identical fashion. Acute GVHD can coexist or predispose to GI tract infections, so early suspicion and appropriate aggressive antimicrobial treatment should accompany the management of these cases.

The liver disease in acute GVHD is usually limited to cholestasis, although bilirubin levels greater than 20 mg/dL can occur in severe cases. Increases in prothrombin time and ammonia, along with other findings of acute hepatic failure, should prompt suspicion of late VOD (especially if presenting early in the post-transplantation course) or acute viral or fungal liver infection. Liver biopsies are seldom necessary because the syndrome rarely presents without other organ involvement. If necessary, biopsy may be performed transjugularly when the patient is thrombocytopenic. This procedure should be reserved for a time when infection is suspected or when VOD may be in the differential diagnosis.[3, 17, 18]

The histologic findings of acute GVHD of the liver are nonspecific at first: a bland lobular hepatitis similar to viral hepatitis. The infiltrate consists mainly of eosinophils and monocytes. Later on, the periportal inflammation becomes less prominent and characteristic biliary tree damage occurs: segmental duct destruction, epithelial cell nuclear enlargement, and cytoplasmic swelling. If the course of acute GVHD is prolonged, bridging necrosis can occur.[17, 18]

Management

The medical management of acute GVHD is frustrating. The greatest benefit has been realized from prophylactic efforts. (See Chapter 39 for a full review of acute GVHD.) Management of crampy pain and diarrhea is supportive, and medical agents such as narcotics and anticholinergics can be of benefit. Caution must be used to avoid functional ileus. If the presenting symptoms are predominantly upper GI in nature, including nausea, vomiting, and abdominal pain, the patient should undergo upper endoscopic evaluation. This approach allows visualization of ulcers that may be due to mucosal infection (CMV, herpesvirus, fungus). Furthermore, biopsies in the esophagus and stomach may be highly useful when the diagnosis of acute GVHD is in question.[3, 13]

Gastrointestinal bleeding is a troubling problem in patients with acute GVHD. It can be the result of mucosal sloughing that characterizes moderate to severe acute GVHD. Ulceration from a coexisting infection, such as CMV or herpesvirus, can also cause acute hemorrhage. Further troubling the management is the frequent thrombocytopenia that can complicate GI bleeding.[3]

Liver disease complicating GVHD is generally different from VOD in that ascites and encephalopathy are not typical.[19] Generally, pruritus resulting from the cholestatic jaundice is a major issue that requires supportive management with cholestyramine. As with GVHD affecting the rest of the GI tract, there is no specific therapy. Glucocorticoids, cyclosporine, FK506, and antithymocyte globulin have been used as both prophylaxis and treatment.[18]

CHRONIC GVHD

As implied by the name, chronic GVHD does not become apparent until 80–100 days after HSCT. The syndrome is characterized by fibrosis and mucosal changes similar to autoimmune connective tissue disorders. Classic signs are sclerosis and discoloration of the skin as well as joint inflammation leading to arthritis. Esophageal strictures and dysmotility are the most significant abnormalities in the hollow GI organs. Chronic elevation in liver injury test results and cholestasis characterized by elevations in alkaline phosphatase and bilirubin are common in patients with chronic GVHD (see Chapter 54).[20–22]

Esophageal

Clinical Presentation

Patients with esophageal disease present with two kinds of symptoms: (1) chronic, severe retrosternal pain, and (2) dysphagia, odynophagia, or even total obstruction. The first symptom group is thought to be related to poor defenses against acid reflux, probably because of poor lower esophageal sphincter tone and poor acid clearing from the mucosa. The second set of symptoms generally represent mucosal webs and strictures generally restricted to the proximal half of the esophagus. They restrict the patient's ability to eat; thus, weight loss is another presenting sign of chronic GVHD.[4, 13, 20]

Diagnosis

Upper GI studies help to guide the diagnosis of strictures and ulcerations in the esophagus. Endoscopy not only defines the lesions but allows for several dilation techniques. Biopsies are not needed for diagnosis, but McDonald et al. reported that samples from affected patients showed infiltration of the submucosa with neutrophils, lymphocytes, and eosinophils as well as mucosal desquamation resulting from basal cell necrosis.[4, 13]

Management

Several studies have investigated the effectiveness of preventing chronic GVHD with immunosuppression. Tapering of cyclosporin A regimens that end at 6 months after HSCT have been widely used. The common outcome is appearance of chronic GVHD (to a greater degree in nonrelated, non–human leukocyte antigen [HLA]-identical donor patients and in those in whom chronic GVHD was an extension of acute GVHD).[20]

Primary treatment of chronic GVHD has included steroids, steroids and azathioprine, and weekly infusion of intravenous immunoglobulins. Strictures of the esophagus can be managed endoscopically, although perforation appears to be more common than with peptic strictures. Scarring and stricturing in the small bowel has been a problem in some patients, and in this setting surgical intervention may be the only available option.[4]

Hepatic

Hepatic dysfunction in chronic GVHD is, as with the rest of the GI tract, present in approximately 30% of patients who experience GVHD after day 100. The hallmark of liver involvement is an increase of cholestatic markers with hyperbilirubinemia. Ascites, portal hypertension, and encephalopathy are rare in chronic GVHD. The most important issue for the clinician when these findings arise is to rule out other causes of chronic liver disease and hepatotoxic reactions due to cyclosporin or methotrexate. The possibility of gallstones or bile sludge should not be overlooked. As with chronic GVHD of the hollow organs, medical management with cyclosporin, azathioprine, and steroids has met with some success. Because azathioprine and cyclosporin or FK506 can be hepatotoxic, care should be taken to withdraw these agents when systemic disease has improved and cholestasis continues to be problematic.[4, 18]

INFECTION IN THE GASTROINTESTINAL TRACT

Infection appears in the differential diagnosis of all the GI complications of HSCT. It is imperative to consider the wide spectrum of viral, bacterial, fungal, and protozoal infection that can jeopardize survival of the transplant recipient as a result of the injury incurred during HSCT.

Although the full spectrum of infection, prevention, and treatment after HSCT is discussed elsewhere (Chapters 36 through 38 and 43), it is important to focus on the time course of infection and the organs affected by the infection.

INFECTION OF THE ESOPHAGUS

Early in the course, generally after conditioning but not exclusively then, the esophagus is susceptible to fungal infection, generally with *Candida* species. The clinical presentation is one of dysphagia and odynophagia. Thrush is not a consistent finding in these patients. Endoscopic evaluation is warranted and, if necessary, biopsies and brushings should be obtained, particularly if the patient is neutropenic.[16] Fungal infections in the severely immunocompromised patient may progress to fungemia and severe systemic disease. The endoscopic picture, as shown in Figure 47–1, is that of white plaques on erythematous ulcerated mucosa. Biopsies show tissue invasion by the *Candida* hyphae. Deep ulceration and perforation have been reported.[4]

Treatment depends on the clinical scenario. In the patient with mild symptoms and superficial disease on esophagogastroduodenoscopy, oral fluconazole or itroconazole may suffice. If oral intake is compromised by fungal esophagitis, initial management with intravenous fluconazole may be warranted. Frankly septic patients with fevers and positive blood cultures should be treated with amphotericin B. In the susceptible period, prophylaxis with oral nystatin "swish and swallow" or oral ketoconazole troches is effective and used extensively.[4]

Viral infections of the esophagus are primarily due to herpes simplex virus and CMV. These can both present

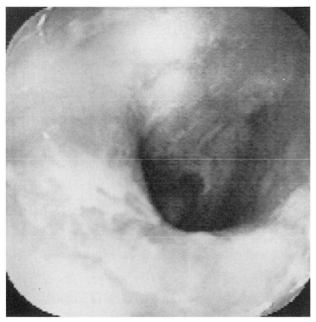

FIGURE 47–1. Endoscopic photograph of esophagus infected with *Candida* hyphae.

early in the course, but with the use of prophylaxis and effective treatment for both processes, viral infection generally presents after engraftment, approximately on day 80, when cell-mediated immunity may be deficient. Correct endoscopic diagnosis is essential because there is effective treatment. Lesions may be vesicular or ulcerative with raised, erythematous borders. Once the diagnosis is made, patients should be treated with high-dose intravenous acyclovir. CMV ulcers may vary in appearance but in general do not tend to form vesicles. Again, biopsy for histopathology and culture is essential for management. Ganciclovir is effective in the management of CMV disease.[24]

INFECTION OF THE STOMACH, DUODENUM, AND SMALL INTESTINE

Fungal infections in the gastric cavity are described, and although occasionally implicated in bleeding ulcers, this finding may not be too significant. Duodenal mucosal involvement with fungal forms generally reflects systemic disease and should prompt systemic antifungal treatment.[4]

Viral infections of the stomach and small intestine are common after engraftment, either alone or coexistent with GVHD. Gastric herpes simplex virus or CMV infection may present nonspecifically with nausea, vomiting, and hematemesis and may be difficult to diagnose, particularly in the setting of acute GVHD. Endoscopy should be performed along with biopsies, cultures, or polymerase chain reaction for rapid diagnosis. Unchecked CMV may lead to obstruction, perforation, or life-threatening GI bleeding.[4]

COLONIC INFECTIONS

The nature of colonic bacterial infections circles around the use of broad-spectrum antibiotics in these patients. The colonic flora balance is tilted toward aerobic organisms which, perhaps because of decreased host defenses, then predispose the host to sepsis. Trials of nonabsorbable antibiotics to combat this problem have not yielded any significant results in terms of patient survival.[4]

Clostridium difficile colitis is a common problem in this patient group for the same reasons. This condition should always be ruled out in the neutropenic patient. Intravenous or oral metronidazole and oral vancomycin are the agents of choice.[4]

Severely neutropenic patients may experience necrotizing colitis or "typhlitis," which is heralded by nausea, vomiting, abdominal pain, and fevers, and may progress to acute peritoneal inflammation with surgical abdomen signs.[4, 25] The etiology is believed to be primary invasion of mucosa and submucosa by aerobic organisms, although some authors think it is related to multiple factors, including CMV, ischemia, and *C. difficile* toxins. The diagnosis requires strong clinical suspicion. Plain films of the abdomen or computed tomography may reveal pneumatosis intestinalis. Figure 47–2 illustrates a typical appearance. If perforation or poorly controlled GI bleeding is found, colonic resection is indicated. Aggressive medical management with antibiotics and supportive measures until the immune function of the recipient is recovered may lead to resolution of typhlitis.

CMV colitis is common and should prompt endoscopic evaluation in patients with unexplained diarrhea, lower GI bleeding, and/or crampy abdominal pain. Typical CMV ulcers can be found endoscopically in the colon; inclusion bodies are visible in histopathology samples. Polymerase chain reaction technology allows recognition of CMV disease even in normal-appearing mucosa and should be used whenever CMV is suspected.[4, 26]

CONCLUSION

Gastrointestinal complications are very common after HSCT. The main causes are conditioning regimen–mediated

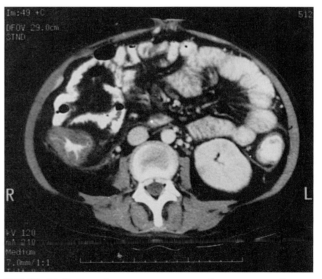

FIGURE 47–2. Typical pneumatosis intestinalis on computed tomographic scan.

damage to rapidly dividing cells of the mucosal membranes, the GI tract's being a primary target of GVHD, and infection as a result of conditioning regimen–induced neutropenia or immunosuppression in the treatment of GVHD. Nutritional support is used to alleviate GI tract injury by conditioning. Once the site of infection and the organisms are identified, individualized treatment with antibiotics and agents against fungi or viruses can be designed. The use of peripheral blood progenitor cells in autologous and allogeneic HSCT has shortened neutrophil engraftment times and decreased the risk of bacterial and fungal infections. Damage to the GI tract by acute GVHD can be prevented by prophylaxis, whereas continued immunosuppression is useful for chronic GVHD. Careful monitoring of individual patients should be maintained to balance the strength of immunosuppression against the risk of infections.

REFERENCES

1. Deeg HJ, Klingemann HG, Phillips GL: A Guide to Bone Marrow Transplantation, 2nd ed. New York, Springer-Verlag, 1992.
2. Trelaven J, Barrett J: Bone Marrow Transplantation in Practice. New York, Churchill Livingstone, 1992.
3. McDonald GB, Shulman HM, Sullivan KM, Spencer GD: Intestinal and hepatic complications of human bone marrow transplantation: part I. Gastroenterology 90:460–477, 1986.
4. McDonald GB, Shulman HM, Sullivan KM, Spencer GD: Intestinal and hepatic complications of human bone marrow transplantation: part II. Gastroenterology 90:770–784, 1986.
5. Epstein RJ, McDonald GB, Sale GE, et al: The diagnostic accuracy of the rectal biopsy in acute graft-versus-host disease: a prospective study of thirteen patients. Gastroenterology 78:764–771, 1980.
6. Shaw MT, Spector MH, Ladman AJ: Effects of cancer, radiotherapy and cytotoxic drugs on intestinal structure and function. Cancer Treat Rev 6:141–151, 1979.
7. Berthrong M, Fajardo LF: Radiation injury in surgical pathology. Part II: alimentary tract. Am J Surg Pathol 5:153–178, 1981.
8. McDonald GB, Rees GM: Approach to gastrointestinal problems in the immunocompromised patient. *In* Yamada T (ed): Textbook of Gastroenterology, 2nd ed. Philadelphia, JB Lippincott, 1995, pp 988–1022.
9. Mennie AT, Dalley VM, Dinneen LC, Collier HO: Treatment of radiation-induced gastrointestinal distress with acetylsalicylate. Lancet 2:942–943, 1975.
10. Donnelly JP, Muus P, Schattenberg A, et al: A scheme for daily monitoring of oral mucositis in allogeneic BMT recipients. Bone Marrow Transplant 9:409–413, 1992.
11. Carl W: Oral complications of local and systemic cancer treatment. Curr Opin Oncol 7:320–324, 1995.
12. Woo SB, Sonis ST, Monopoli MM, Sonis AL: A longitudinal study of oral ulcerative mucositis in bone marrow transplant recipients. Cancer 72:1612–1617, 1993.
13. Vishny ML, Blades EW, Creger RJ, Lazarus HM: Role of upper endoscopy in evaluation of upper gastrointestinal symptoms in patients undergoing bone marrow transplantation. Cancer Invest 12:384–389, 1994.
14. Herrmann VM, Petruska PJ: Nutrition support in bone marrow transplant recipients. Nutr Clin Pract 8:19–27, 1993.
15. Northway MG, Libshitz HI, Osborne BM, et al: Radiation esophagitis in the opossum: radioprotection with indomethacin. Gastroenterology 78:883–892, 1980.
16. Weisdorf DJ, Snover DC, Haake R, et al: Acute upper gastrointestinal graft-versus-host disease: clinical significance and response to immunosuppressive therapy. Blood 76:624–629, 1990.
17. Bertheau P, Hadengue A, Cazals-Hatem D, et al: Chronic cholestasis in patients after allogeneic bone marrow transplantation: several diseases are often associated. Bone Marrow Transplant 16:261–265, 1995.
18. McDonald GB, Shulman HM, Wolford JL, Spencer GD: Liver disease after human marrow transplantation. Semin Liver Dis 7:210–229, 1987.
19. Przepiorka D, Weisdorf D, Martin P, et al: 1994 Consensus Conference on Acute GVHD Grading. Bone Marrow Transplant 15:825–828, 1995.
20. Siadak M, Sullivan KM: The management of chronic graft-versus-host disease. Blood Rev 8:154–160, 1994.
21. Sullivan KM, Mori M, Sanders J, et al: Late complications of allogeneic and autologous marrow transplantation. Bone Marrow Transplant 10(Suppl 1):127–134, 1992.
22. Chao NJ, Schlegel PG: Prevention and treatment of graft-versus-host disease. Ann N Y Acad Sci 770:130–140, 1995.
23. Goodrich JM, Boeckh M, Bowden R: Strategies for the prevention of cytomegalovirus disease after marrow transplantation. Clin Infect Dis 19:287–298, 1994.
24. Reed EC, Wolford JL, Kopecky KJ, et al: Ganciclovir for the treatment of cytomegalovirus gastroenteritis in bone marrow transplant patients: a randomized, placebo-controlled trial. Ann Intern Med 112:505–510, 1990.
25. Halpert RD, Goodman P, Caroline DF: Abdominal complications in organ transplant recipients. Radiol Clin North Am 31:1345–1357, 1993.
26. Schuler U, Ehninger G: New approaches to the prophylaxis and treatment of bacterial and fungal infections in allogeneic marrow transplant recipients. Bone Marrow Transplant 14 (Suppl 4):S61–S65, 1994.

CHAPTER FORTY-EIGHT

Respiratory Complications

J.W. Kreit, M.D.

Disorders of the respiratory system are common after hematopoietic stem cell transplantation (HSCT). Respiratory complications develop in approximately 50% of patients and account for over 40% of all deaths.[1, 2] Patients requiring mechanical ventilation for respiratory failure have a particularly dismal prognosis, with a mortality rate that approaches 95%.[3, 4] Caring for patients with respiratory complications after HSCT requires a coordinated effort between the transplant physician and the pulmonologist/intensivist. This chapter discusses the respiratory disorders that occur in the immediate post-transplantation period, traditionally defined as the first 100 days after transplantation. Late respiratory complications are discussed elsewhere. The information in this chapter is based primarily on studies of bone marrow transplant (BMT) recipients.

Although peripheral blood stem cell transplantation has become increasingly common in recent years, there is relatively little information about associated respiratory complications.[5–11] The duration of neutropenia after peripheral blood stem cell transplantation is, in general, shorter than after bone marrow transplantation, and several nonrandomized studies have reported a much lower incidence of bacterial and fungal infection in the pre-engraftment period.[12–14] Information comparing the frequency of other respiratory disorders after bone marrow transplantation and peripheral blood stem cell transplantation is not available.

The respiratory complications of HSCT are listed in Table 48–1 and may be divided into two broad categories based on the presence or absence of infection.

NONINFECTIOUS COMPLICATIONS

AIRWAY DISEASE

Chemotherapy and radiation-induced injury to the mucosa of the mouth, nose, and pharynx are common after HSCT and occur very early in the post-transplantation period. Mucositis causes dysphagia and odynophagia and, when severe, may lead to recurrent aspiration of blood and saliva. In addition, involvement of laryngeal structures may cause upper airway obstruction, which may require translaryngeal intubation or tracheostomy to maintain airway patency. Mucositis typically resolves with the reappearance of neutrophils in the peripheral blood but may be prolonged because of superinfection with herpes simplex virus.

PARENCHYMAL DISEASE

Idiopathic Pneumonia Syndrome

Acute lung injury for which no infectious etiology can be found is common after HSCT, and this disorder has typically been called *idiopathic interstitial pneumonia*. A workshop sponsored by the National Institutes of Health suggested the term *idiopathic pneumonia syndrome* (IPS) to more accurately reflect the variability of its etiology and radiographic and histologic appearance.[15]

Idiopathic pneumonia syndrome occurs in approximately 15% of all patients who undergo bone marrow transplantation and is much more common in patients with an underlying hematologic malignancy than in those with nonmalignant disease.[15–20] The incidence of IPS is also much higher after allogeneic bone marrow transplantation, especially when the donor is unrelated.[21, 22] The median time to onset of IPS is approximately 50 days after transplantation.[16–18] Most cases occur within 100 days,[15, 16–20, 23] and the incidence throughout this time period is fairly constant.[17, 18] IPS is characterized clinically by the presence of nonproductive cough, fever, dyspnea, and hypoxemia. Progression to respiratory failure is common.[23] Chest radiography and computed tomography (CT) typically demonstrate diffuse or multilobar interstitial or alveolar infiltrates.[15] The diagnosis of IPS is based on the presence of compatible clinical and

TABLE 48–1. RESPIRATORY COMPLICATIONS IN THE IMMEDIATE POST-TRANSPLANTATION PERIOD

Noninfectious
  Airway disease
    Mucositis
  Parenchymal disease
    Idiopathic pneumonia syndrome
    Diffuse alveolar hemorrhage
    Pulmonary edema
    Pulmonary alveolar proteinosis
  Pulmonary vascular disease
    Pulmonary veno-occlusive disease
    Pulmonary embolism
Infectious
  Tracheobronchitis
    Aspergillus spp.
    Herpes simplex virus
  Pneumonia
    Bacterial
    Viral
      Cytomegalovirus
      Herpes simplex virus
      Respiratory syncytial virus
      Others
    Fungal
      Aspergillus spp.
      Candida spp.
      Others
    Pneumocystis carinii
    Mycobacterial

563

radiographic features and the exclusion of lower respiratory tract infection by bronchoscopy or open lung biopsy. Histologic examination reveals a wide variety of nonspecific findings ranging from interstitial inflammation and fibrosis to diffuse alveolar damage.[15]

As suggested by this variable histologic appearance, IPS is believed to be caused by multiple, and perhaps interacting, factors. There is, for example, strong evidence that IPS is associated with exposure to both radiation and chemotherapeutic agents. The incidence of IPS has been reported to increase with the total dose[15, 17, 19, 24, 25] and dose rate[16, 26] of radiation delivered to the lungs prior to transplantation, and the lower risk of IPS in patients with nonmalignant diseases may be related to the less frequent use of total body irradiation.[15, 17–20] Several drugs commonly used in pretransplantation conditioning regimens, particularly cyclophosphamide and carmustine (BCNU), are well known to cause pulmonary toxicity.[15, 27–29] Additive toxicity may occur when cytotoxic drugs are used in conjunction with total body irradiation.[28, 29] Several retrospective studies have also found an association between IPS and the use of methotrexate to prevent acute graft-versus-host disease (GVHD) after transplantation.[16, 19, 26] The results of three prospective randomized trials, however, have failed to support this association.[30–33]

Immune mechanisms also play an important role in the pathogenesis of this disease. Several studies have shown a strong association between IPS and both the presence and the severity of acute GVHD.[15–17, 19, 20, 25] This may account for the high incidence of IPS in patients receiving allogeneic transplants, especially from unrelated donors, and its relative rarity in patients undergoing autologous transplantation.[15, 17, 21]

Because the lung is typically not a target organ in acute GVHD, another inciting factor is believed to be important for the development of lung injury. There is increasing evidence that this factor may be latent viral infection.[15, 34] Using the polymerase chain reaction, several studies have demonstrated the presence of cytomegalovirus or human herpesvirus-6 DNA in lung tissue specimens that have no other microbiologic or histologic evidence of viral infection.[34–36] It has been proposed that this latent infection, in the setting of systemic GVHD, results in the activation of donor T cells. Acute lung injury may then result from cell-mediated cytotoxicity and from the effects of a "cytokine cascade" initiated by the release of tumor necrosis factor, interferon, and interleukin (IL)-2 from activated T cells.[15, 34, 36, 37] Because the diagnosis of IPS requires the exclusion of all infectious causes, additional studies are clearly required to determine the exact role of viral infection in the pathogenesis of "idiopathic" pneumonia.

Several large series have reported mortality rates of 60–82% in patients with biopsy-proven IPS.[16–18, 23] At present, therapy is primarily supportive. Although there are anecdotal reports of improvement after corticosteroid therapy,[28, 29] there is insufficient evidence to determine the effectiveness of this treatment. No studies have examined the use of antiviral therapy. A study reported in 1993 specifically investigated the natural history of this disorder and found that pulmonary or disseminated superinfection was the major or contributing cause of death in over half of patients and that only 32% died of progressive respira-

tory failure from IPS.[23] This suggests that aggressive diagnosis and treatment of infection may be the most important means of improving patient survival.

Diffuse Alveolar Hemorrhage

Although technically included within the broad definition of IPS (i.e., acute lung injury in the absence of infection), diffuse alveolar hemorrhage (DAH) has been typically described as a distinct clinical entity in patients undergoing HSCT.[5, 38–45] The reported incidence of DAH ranges between 7% and 41%, and this disorder appears to occur with equal frequency after allogeneic and autologous transplantation.[5, 38–42, 45] DAH occurs very early in the post-transplant period. The median time to onset is approximately 12 days,[5] and no cases have been reported beyond 90 days.[5, 38–40, 42–45] The clinical manifestations of DAH are dyspnea, cough, fever, and hypoxemia, and progression to respiratory failure is common.[5, 38, 45] Hemoptysis may occur but is absent in most patients.[5, 38] The appearance of the chest radiograph is nonspecific. Typically, bilateral interstitial infiltrates, most commonly involving the central and lower lung zones, appear initially and progress rapidly to a diffuse, bilateral alveolar pattern.[45] Histologic examination shows intra-alveolar hemorrhage, usually associated with features of diffuse alveolar damage.[5, 41]

The pathogenesis of DAH is unknown. Reported risk factors include radiation prior to transplantation,[5, 38, 40] age greater than 40 years,[5] solid tumors,[5] severe mucositis,[5] granulocyte recovery,[5] renal insufficiency,[5] and acute GVHD.[40] Although patients typically have marked thrombocytopenia, no difference between the platelet counts of patients with and without DAH has been demonstrated.[5, 39, 41] An association between DAH and thrombotic thrombocytopenic purpura has also been described in several BMT recipients.[46]

The clinical diagnosis of DAH is based on three criteria: (1) the presence of compatible clinical manifestations, (2) the exclusion of infectious causes by bronchoscopy, and (3) the presence of characteristic findings in bronchoalveolar lavage (BAL) fluid.[5, 38, 45, 47–49] The accuracy with which a clinical diagnosis can be made, however, is unclear.

As noted earlier, the clinical and radiographic features of this disorder are nonspecific. In addition, many pulmonary infections cannot be reliably excluded by bronchoscopy. Finally, "characteristic" findings in BAL fluid are actually of uncertain significance. For example, several studies have shown a good correlation between the presence of large quantities of hemosiderin in alveolar macrophages obtained by BAL and histologic evidence of alveolar hemorrhage.[5, 47, 48, 50] However, because small amounts of hemosiderin are nonspecific and no single, validated scoring system for quantifying hemosiderin exists, the usefulness of this finding is limited.[47, 50, 51] Based on the assumption that later aliquots reflect alveolar contents, the return of progressively bloodier fluid during BAL has also been used to diagnose DAH in several studies of BMT recipients.[5, 38, 49] Although a strong correlation between bloody lavage fluid and histologic evidence of alveolar hemorrhage has been reported,[5] this finding has been shown to lack both sensitivity and specificity by other investigators.[41] The presence of hemorrhagic lavage fluid has also been shown to have no diagnostic utility in other immunocompromised patients.[47, 51]

Making the clinical diagnosis of DAH even more difficult is the fact that alveolar hemorrhage can be caused by or coexist with bacterial, viral, and fungal pneumonia,[40, 41, 51] infections that may not be detected by BAL. This is especially of concern because high-dose corticosteroids have been advocated for the treatment of DAH (see later). Additional studies are clearly required to determine the role of bronchoscopy in the clinical diagnosis of DAH. At present, it seems prudent to obtain lung tissue for histologic and microbiologic evaluation, especially if corticosteroid therapy is planned.

In reported series, DAH has been associated with a very high mortality rate (75–100%).[5, 38, 39, 45] Supportive therapy, including aggressive platelet transfusion, has not been shown to alter this extremely poor prognosis. Two retrospective studies have reported that high-dose corticosteroid therapy (0.5–1.0 g/day of methylprednisolone) may significantly reduce both the need for mechanical ventilation and mortality in patients with DAH.[38, 49]

Pulmonary Edema

Although pulmonary edema is almost always discussed in reviews of complications after HSCT and is said to be common, there is little information regarding its incidence, pathogenesis, diagnosis, and therapy. In fact, only one study has specifically investigated pulmonary edema in the post-transplantation period. Dickout and colleagues[52] based the diagnosis of pulmonary edema on the presence of dyspnea, bibasilar rales, hypoxemia, and the radiographic findings of vascular redistribution, increased interstitial markings, and Kerley B lines. These investigators found that pulmonary edema developed in 19 (63%) of 30 patients and that almost all episodes occurred within the first 2 weeks after transplantation. Patients who experienced pulmonary edema gained a significant amount of weight after transplantation, and echocardiography, performed in a subset of these patients, revealed an increase in left ventricular end-diastolic volume. In most cases, clinical and radiographic evidence of pulmonary edema resolved over 24–48 hours with vigorous diuresis. Another group of 30 transplant recipients received prophylactic diuretic therapy, and none experienced pulmonary edema.

This study indicates that pulmonary edema in the immediate post-transplantation period is associated with volume overload, at least in some cases. This, in turn, might result from the hydration required prior to pretransplantation chemotherapy, the transfusion of multiple blood products, intravenous alimentation, and antibiotic therapy. There are, however, several other potential etiologic factors for pulmonary edema in patients undergoing HSCT. For example, systolic or diastolic heart failure may be precipitated by myocardial ischemia or dysrhythmias in the post-transplantation period, and severe myopericarditis has been described after high-dose cyclophosphamide therapy.[53, 54] In addition, serum oncotic pressure may be markedly reduced in the post-transplantation period because of malnutrition and protein losses accompanying gastrointestinal involvement by GVHD. Finally, pulmonary edema due to increased

capillary permeability may be produced by radiation and chemotherapeutic agents[27] or by extrathoracic sepsis.

A disorder consisting of noncardiogenic pulmonary edema, fever, and multiorgan dysfunction manifested primarily by azotemia and impaired hepatic function following HSCT has been described and is believed to result from diffuse capillary endothelial injury.[6, 55–57] Because this syndrome often develops within several days of engraftment, cytokine release by donor leukocytes may be important in its pathogenesis. Unlike the more benign and self-limited forms of pulmonary edema described previously, progression to respiratory failure is common and mortality is high.

Pulmonary Alveolar Proteinosis

Pulmonary alveolar proteinosis has been previously associated with hematologic malignancy, and a 1994 report described three patients who experienced this disease several weeks after bone marrow transplantation.[58] Clinical manifestations included dyspnea, hypoxemia, and diffuse alveolar infiltrates on the chest radiograph. The diagnosis of pulmonary alveolar proteinosis is based on the identification of abundant periodic acid-Schiff–positive proteinaceous material in BAL fluid or tissue specimens.

PULMONARY VASCULAR DISEASE

Pulmonary Veno-occlusive Disease

Pulmonary veno-occlusive disease (PVOD) is a rare disorder characterized histologically by partial or complete occlusion of pulmonary venules and veins by intimal fibrosis and has been reported to follow HSCT in a small number of patients.[59–62] The pathogenesis of PVOD is unknown, although reported associations include chemotherapy and viral infection. In patients undergoing HSCT, PVOD appears to be more common in the presence of IPS and hepatic veno-occlusive disease.[59] Reported cases have occurred between 40 and 60 days after transplantation. Clinical manifestations include dyspnea, hypoxemia, and signs of pulmonary hypertension and right ventricular failure.[60–62] The diagnosis of PVOD must be based on histologic examination of lung tissue obtained at open lung biopsy. Anecdotal evidence suggests that therapy with high-dose corticosteroids may be beneficial in some patients.[61, 62]

Pulmonary Embolism

Although small pulmonary emboli are commonly found at autopsy,[63] patients undergoing HSCT do not appear to be at disproportionate risk for clinically significant thromboembolic disease. Intravascular fat droplets[64] and bone fragments,[65] presumably from transfused marrow, have rarely been found in lung tissue. The clinical consequences of these forms of pulmonary embolism, if any, are unknown.

INFECTIOUS COMPLICATIONS

IMMUNOLOGIC RECOVERY AFTER TRANSPLANTATION

Patients undergoing HSCT initially have marked pancytopenia and severe combined immune deficiency. With time, the infused stem cells give rise to completely new hematopoietic and immune systems in the transplant recipient. Knowledge of both the sequence and time course of immunologic recovery and its impact on lung defense mechanisms are essential for understanding the respiratory infections that frequently complicate HSCT.[66–68]

Normal Lung Defense Mechanisms

A variety of defenses are used to protect the lung from infection.[69, 70] Microorganisms that enter the airways between the larynx and the respiratory bronchioles are coated with secretory immunoglobulin A (IgA), which inhibits adherence to the respiratory epithelium. These microorganisms are then removed by mucociliary transport. Alveolar macrophages provide the first line of defense against microbes that reach the alveoli. Alveolar macrophages both ingest the organism and release several cytokines, principally tumor necrosis factor, IL-1, and IL-8, which in turn stimulate the release of additional cytokines by epithelial cells, endothelial cells, and fibroblasts. Together, these mediators recruit circulating polymorphonuclear leukocytes into the alveolar spaces both by enhancing adhesion to endothelial cells and by providing a chemotactic gradient. This neutrophil influx is essential for the eradication of most bacteria and some fungi, particularly *Candida* and *Aspergillus.* Cell-mediated immune responses in the lung are initiated by the interaction of T cells with a microbial antigen and an "antigen-presenting cell," believed to be the dendritic cells that reside in the pulmonary interstitium. Effective cell mediated immunity is required for the control of viral, fungal, parasitic, and mycobacterial infections.

Immunologic Recovery

Repopulation of the lung by donor-derived alveolar macrophages does not occur for several weeks after transplantation, and macrophage function, as assessed by chemotaxis and phagocytosis, remains impaired for at least 4 months.[71] Typically, neutrophil recovery occurs within 2–3 weeks[67] but may be delayed by the presence of acute GVHD and the administration of myelosuppressive medications such as methotrexate, trimethoprim-sulfamethoxazole, and ganciclovir.[72–74] Although the total lymphocyte count usually approaches the normal range by 12 weeks after transplantation,[67] T-cell response to mitogens and alloantigens does not return to normal for at least 6 months after transplantation.[72, 75–77] The number of circulating B cells usually returns to normal within 1 month, although immunoglobulin production may be completely absent for up to 3 months after transplantation, and IgA levels may remain decreased for years.[72, 78, 79]

Immunologic Recovery and the Risk of Infection

The sequence of immunologic recovery largely determines the respiratory infections to which the patient is predisposed at each point in time. Based on the major type of immune deficiency, the immediate post-transplantation period can be divided into two phases by the occurrence of marrow engraftment and the resolution of neutropenia. During the pre-engraftment period, bacterial infections predominate. After neutrophil recovery, cell-mediated immunity remains abnormal, predisposing the patient to infection with viruses, fungi, mycobacteria, and parasites. In addition, impaired synthesis of immunoglobulins, including secretory IgA, results in persistent susceptibility to bacterial pneumonia.

BACTERIAL INFECTIONS

Bacterial pneumonia occurs in as many as 10% of patients during the pre-engraftment period and is associated with high mortality.[1, 68, 80–84] Pneumonia is most commonly caused by the direct spread of organisms from the oropharynx but may also be produced by septic emboli originating from an infected central venous catheter or heart valve. In the pre-engraftment period, bacterial pneumonia is most commonly caused by gram-negative bacilli, primarily *Pseudomonas aeruginosa, Klebsiella pneumoniae,* and *Enterobacter cloacae,* as well as by *Staphylococcus aureus.*[84] Anaerobic pneumonia may also occur, especially in patients with severe mucositis and recurrent aspiration. In addition, several transplant centers have reported outbreaks of pneumonia due to *Legionella pneumophila.*[82, 85] During the post-engraftment period, patients remain at risk for bacterial infections because of persistent impairment of humoral immunity. During this time, pneumonia is caused primarily by encapsulated organisms, particularly *Streptococcus pneumoniae* and *Haemophilus influenzae.*

Clinical manifestations of bacterial pneumonia include cough, fever, dyspnea, and hypoxemia. The chest radiograph usually demonstrates one or more foci of alveolar consolidation, which may progress to more diffuse involvement.[84] Septic emboli typically appear as poorly defined nodules with a peripheral distribution. Cavitation, parapneumonic effusion, and empyema may occur. Making the diagnosis of bacterial pneumonia is difficult because of the large number of alternative diagnoses in this patient population, the frequent use of empirical broad-spectrum antibiotics, and the inaccuracy of commonly used diagnostic tests. Blood cultures are usually negative in patients with bacterial pneumonia, and bacteremia, when present, often originates from sites other than the lung.[86, 87]

In hospitalized patients, cultures of sputum and endotracheal tube aspirates have been shown to have a low specificity.[88, 89] That is, cultures are often positive in patients without pneumonia and nonsignificant organisms are frequently cultured in patients with bacterial infection. In order to improve diagnostic sensitivity and specificity, several techniques have been developed to allow cultures to be obtained from the distal airways and alveoli. The most commonly used are protected specimen brushing and BAL, performed via the fiberoptic bronchoscope.[90] Therapy for bacterial pneumonia is often empirical and must provide coverage against gram-negative bacilli, including *Pseudomonas aeruginosa,* as well as gram-positive organisms. Combination therapy with an aminoglycoside and an antipseudomonal penicillin with or without vancomycin is typically used.

VIRAL INFECTIONS

Cytomegalovirus

Pulmonary infection with cytomegalovirus (CMV) accounts for approximately 40% of all pneumonias occurring after bone marrow transplantation.[16–18] Several large series have reported incidences ranging from 11–19% in allogeneic[16–18, 91–93] and 0.8–3.3% in autologous transplant recipients.[92–94] CMV pneumonia is rare in patients receiving syngeneic transplants.[18] Like IPS, CMV pneumonia is more common in patients with underlying malignancy.[17] Most cases of CMV pneumonia occur within the first 100 days after transplantation, and almost all occur within 180 days.[16–18, 92] Unlike IPS, which occurs throughout the immediate post-transplantation period, CMV pneumonia is uncommon prior to marrow engraftment and has a peak incidence at 21–80 days.[17, 18]

Risk factors for the development of CMV pneumonia have been identified, and several, including total dose[17, 18, 24, 25] and dose rate[16, 26] of total body irradiation and the presence and severity of acute GVHD,[16–20, 25, 91] are identical to those for IPS. The use of T-cell depletion and antithymocyte globulin for the prophylaxis or treatment of acute GVHD has also been shown to increase patient risk.[17, 91, 92]

The most important factor influencing the development of CMV pneumonia, however, is exposure to the virus. CMV pneumonia is much more likely to develop in patients who are seropositive prior to transplantation.[18, 91, 92] In addition, the risk of pneumonia increases dramatically when seronegative patients receive stem cells from seropositive donors or unscreened (potentially CMV-infected) blood products.[91, 95, 96] Finally, CMV pneumonia occurs much more frequently in patients with extrapulmonary infection as documented by seroconversion or recovery of CMV from the throat, urine, or blood.[91, 92] It is important to note that although the incidence is very low, CMV pneumonia does occasionally occur in seronegative patients with no history of viral exposure and no evidence of extrapulmonary infection.[17, 18, 91, 92]

Clinical manifestations of CMV pneumonia are nonspecific and include nonproductive cough, fever, and progressive dyspnea and hypoxemia. The chest radiograph typically demonstrates diffuse interstitial or alveolar infiltrates, and numerous small nodules may be evident by CT.[97]

CMV pneumonia can be diagnosed by bronchoscopy or open lung biopsy, and several techniques are used to detect the virus in BAL fluid or tissue samples. Conventional "tube" culture is performed by incubating BAL fluid or lung tissue with cells that show typical cytopathic changes when infected. Although this technique is a sensitive method for detecting CMV, cultures may not become positive for 2–6 weeks. Much more rapid detection can be achieved using centrifugation or "shell vial" cultures in which viral replication is confirmed using fluorescent monoclonal antibodies within 48 hours of innoculation.[98] Monoclonal antibodies can also be used to rapidly detect the presence of CMV antigens within infected cells obtained by BAL or lung biopsy,[99] and typical CMV inclusions may be evident by cytologic examination. Finally, DNA amplification using the polymerase chain reaction (PCR) has been shown to be a very sensitive method for detecting CMV in BAL fluid and lung tissue.[100, 101]

Because CMV may be isolated from the lower respiratory tract of both immunocompetent and immunocompromised patients in the absence of pneumonia, detection of virus in respiratory specimens does not necessarily establish the diagnosis of CMV pneumonia. Nevertheless, several lines of evidence indicate that CMV is almost always a pathogen in patients undergoing HSCT and that CMV pneumonia should be diagnosed when the virus is detected in a patient with compatible clinical findings.[16–18, 102, 103]

The mortality rate from untreated CMV pneumonia is approximately 85%,[16–18] and single-drug therapy with interferon, acyclovir, ganciclovir, corticosteroids, or immune globulin does not result in improved survival.[104–109] Combination therapy with intravenous ganciclovir and immune globulin, however, has been shown to significantly decrease patient mortality and is currently the treatment of choice.[110, 111] Unfortunately, response rates as low as 35% have been reported,[92, 110–113] relapse is common,[92, 111] and the mortality rate in patients requiring mechanical ventilation continues to approach 100%.[92] Methods designed to prevent CMV pneumonia are therefore essential in the management of patients undergoing HSCT.

In seronegative patients, the best approach is to transplant stem cells and transfuse blood products from seronegative donors.[95] This procedure has been shown to result in a very low rate of CMV infection and pneumonia.[96, 114, 115] In seropositive patients and seronegative patients who have received a transplant from a seropositive donor, administration of immune globulin significantly reduces the incidence of CMV pneumonia[115] and is recommended as prophylactic therapy.[95] Treatment with ganciclovir alone has been shown to significantly reduce the incidence of CMV pneumonia in patients with evidence of viral infection but no clinical or radiographic signs of pneumonia.[103, 116] In most centers, weekly throat, urine, and blood cultures are obtained from all seropositive patients, and those with positive cultures receive ganciclovir until at least day 100 after transplantation.[95]

Prophylactic ganciclovir therapy has also been shown to be extremely effective in asymptomatic patients with positive BAL fluid cultures, and routine bronchoscopy has been advocated for all seropositive patients.[102, 117] Because bronchoscopy is invasive and serial studies are not practical, however, this screening technique has not been widely adopted. Several studies have shown that detection of CMV DNA in blood using PCR provides an earlier and more sensitive method for detecting infection when compared with routine viral cultures.[118, 119] At the University of Pittsburgh, the need for prophylactic ganciclovir is determined solely by the results of weekly blood PCR assays.

The pathogenesis of CMV pneumonia remains unclear, although several facts have been well demonstrated. First, CMV infection in the lung is not sufficient to produce clinical pneumonia.[120] Second, eradication of CMV in the lung using ganciclovir is not accompanied by resolution of pneumonia.[107] Third, CMV pneumonia is uncommon in the absence of acute GVHD.[16–18] These findings suggest that CMV pneumonia requires both the presence of virus and an immunologic response by the host.[15, 37, 121] Infection with CMV is known to be accompanied by the expression of viral antigens and the enhanced expression of histocompatibility antigens on the surface of host cells. Donor T cells may interact with these antigens and release several cytokines, including tumor necrosis factor, interferon, and IL-2. In turn, these factors trigger the production of additional cytokines by host and donor-derived cells. Acute lung injury may then result from both direct T cell–mediated cytotoxicity and the direct and indirect effects of cytokines.[37, 121] The enhanced effectiveness of immune globulin plus ganciclovir compared with either agent alone may result from masking of viral or host antigens by the former and eradication of virus by the latter.[110, 111, 121]

Herpes Simplex Virus

Infection with herpes simplex virus (HSV), usually in the form of gingivostomatitis or esophagitis, typically occurs during the pre-engraftment period. In almost all cases, the infection is due to reactivation of latent virus. Infection has been reported to occur in as many as 80% of seropositive patients, but this incidence has been markedly reduced by the routine use of prophylactic acyclovir.[73] Although its incidence is unknown, HSV pneumonia appears to be rare.[17, 122] In almost all cases, pneumonia is preceded by mucocutaneous infection and results either from contiguous or, less commonly, hematogenous spread of infection.[122] With direct spread, herpetic tracheobronchitis is common and the chest radiograph usually demonstrates multifocal alveolar infiltrates. Hematogenous dissemination is typically associated with a diffuse interstitial pattern on the chest radiograph. In most patients, HSV pneumonia is associated with progressive respiratory failure and a very high mortality rate.[122]

The diagnosis of HSV pneumonia is based on the results of bronchoscopy or open lung biopsy. HSV may be cultured from BAL fluid or lung biopsy specimens using conventional techniques. In addition, typical intranuclear inclusions may be evident on histologic or cytologic examination of lower respiratory tract specimens. Finally, fluorescent monoclonal antibodies may be used to rapidly detect the presence of HSV antigens in infected cells obtained by BAL or biopsy.[17, 122] Although HSV may be present in the lower respiratory tract in the absence of pneumonia in patients undergoing HSCT who have compatible clinical findings, the presence of HSV should be considered diagnostic of pneumonia. Acyclovir is the treatment of choice for HSV infection.[123]

Respiratory Syncytial Virus

Respiratory syncytial virus (RSV) is a common cause of upper and lower respiratory tract infections in infants and children and may cause mild rhinitis and pharyngitis in adults. RSV infection may also cause pneumonia in immunocompromised adults. The incidence of RSV pneumonia in HSCT recipients is unknown but may be as high as 11%.[124] Like HSV infection, RSV pneumonia is most common very early after transplantation, during the pre-engraftment period. In almost all cases, pneumonia occurs in the spring and winter and is preceded by symptoms and signs of rhinitis, pharyngitis, otitis, or sinusitis.[124, 125] The chest radiograph initially shows diffuse interstitial infiltrates, and progression to diffuse air space disease is common. Despite antiviral therapy, a mortality rate approaching

50% has been reported.[124, 125] The diagnosis of RSV pneumonia can be made by bronchoscopy or open lung biopsy and is based on positive BAL fluid or tissue culture or detection of RSV antigens within infected cells using fluorescent monoclonal antibodies. Aerosolized ribavirin is effective in infants and children with severe RSV infection[126] and appears to be of benefit in some immunocompromised adults with pneumonia.[124, 127]

Other Viruses

Adenovirus,[128–130] parainfluenza virus,[129, 131, 132] influenza virus,[133] and human herpesvirus-6[35, 134] have also been reported to cause pneumonia in patients undergoing HSCT, typically during the postengraftment period. Pneumonia caused by adenovirus, parainfluenza virus, and influenza virus is often preceded by symptoms of upper respiratory tract infection. The chest radiograph most commonly shows diffuse interstitial infiltrates. Progression to respiratory failure is common, and reported mortality rates approach 100%. Diagnosis can be made by bronchoscopy or open lung biopsy and is based on isolation of these viruses in culture or detection of viral antigens using fluorescent monoclonal antibodies. Reactivation of varicella-zoster virus is common in transplant recipients and may be associated with pneumonia and other forms of visceral involvement.[68] The median time to onset, however, is 5 months, and almost all varicella-zoster virus infections occur more than 100 days after transplantation.

FUNGAL INFECTIONS

Aspergillus

Aspergillus spores are ubiquitous and, because of their small size, are commonly inhaled and reach the alveoli. Under normal circumstances, the spores are eradicated by alveolar macrophages. If germination occurs, neutrophils enter the lungs and destroy the fungal hyphae. In patients with impairment of these defenses, however, *Aspergillus* hyphae proliferate and invade the pulmonary parenchyma. Invasion of blood vessels is also common and results in thrombosis and hemorrhagic infarction of lung tissue. The major risk factors for invasive pulmonary aspergillosis are corticosteroid therapy (which impairs alveolar macrophage function) and prolonged neutropenia,[135] and patients undergoing HSCT are therefore vulnerable to infection with this organism.

Invasive pulmonary aspergillosis occurs in approximately 4% of patients after bone marrow transplantation and is most commonly caused by *A. fumigatus* and *A. flavus*.[136, 137] Infection usually becomes evident in the postengraftment period and is almost always associated with the use of corticosteroids to treat acute or chronic GVHD.[136, 137] Invasive aspergillosis may develop prior to marrow engraftment but is typically associated with prolonged neutropenia and rarely occurs less than 2 weeks after transplantation.[136, 137] Clinical manifestations are usually nonspecific, but pleuritic pain, hemoptysis, and a pleural friction rub may occur and should suggest the diagnosis. Disseminated infection is common, and symptoms and signs of meningitis, sinusitis, and space-occupying cerebral lesions may precede or accompany pulmonary infection.

The chest radiograph typically shows solitary or multiple pulmonary nodules or mass-like infiltrates, and cavitation is common.[138, 139] Peripheral, wedge-shaped densities due to large vessel thrombosis and parenchymal infarction have also been described.[138, 139] The presence of a crescent-shaped area of cavitation at the periphery of a lung nodule or infiltrate (air-crescent sign) has been reported to be a specific radiographic sign of invasive aspergillosis but appears to occur late in the course of the infection.[138, 139] CT often reveals parenchymal disease that is not evident on the chest radiograph and may demonstrate the presence of a rim of ground-glass attenuation surrounding a parenchymal nodule or mass (halo sign). This has been reported to be an early sign of invasive aspergillosis but may also occur with other fungal infections.[138, 139]

Although invasive pulmonary aspergillosis can only be diagnosed definitively when histologic specimens show characteristic hyphae in viable lung tissue, a presumptive diagnosis is often based on less-invasive tests. Sputum culture has a sensitivity of approximately 50%,[140, 141] and culture and staining of BAL fluid have a significantly higher diagnostic yield.[141, 142] Although *Aspergillus* may be present in sputum or BAL fluid in the absence of infection, this finding should be considered as strong evidence for invasive infection in patients undergoing HSCT.[143]

Invasive *Aspergillus* infection, solely or predominantly within the airways, has been reported in patients undergoing BMT and other immunocompromised patients but appears to be rare.[144–147] *Aspergillus* tracheobronchitis can range in severity from localized mucosal plaques or ulcers to diffuse erythema, edema, and ulceration. In the diffuse form of the disease, pseudomembranes consisting of fungal hyphae, inflammatory cells, and necrotic debris circumferentially line the airways and may partially or completely occlude segmental or lobar bronchi. Histologic examination reveals fungal invasion with ulceration and necrosis of the mucosa that may extend through the entire bronchial wall. Invasive tracheobronchitis may be accompanied by invasive pulmonary aspergillosis but more commonly occurs in the absence of parenchymal disease. Clinical manifestations include fever, cough, dyspnea, and hemoptysis, and wheezes and rhonchi may be evident on physical examination. The chest radiograph often appears normal but may show evidence of atelectasis from bronchial obstruction. The diagnosis of *Aspergillus* tracheobronchitis infection is based on the characteristic bronchoscopic appearance and histologic evidence of bronchial wall invasion.

The standard treatment for invasive aspergillosis is amphotericin B in a dose of 1.0–1.5 mg/kg/day. Despite this therapy, the mortality rate in patients undergoing HSCT approaches 90%.[136, 137] Amphotericin B has been coupled with various lipid vehicles, and amphotericin B lipid complex was the first lipid vehicle approved for the treatment of invasive fungal infections. Although increased efficacy has not been proven, the enhanced tissue uptake of these drugs allows much-higher doses of amphotericin to be administered with a lower risk of nephrotoxicity.[148–150] Itraconazole may be as effective or more effective than amphotericin B for the treatment of invasive aspergillosis,[151] but

randomized studies have not been performed. Prophylactic therapy with intranasal,[152] nebulized,[153] or low-dose intravenous[154] amphotericin B has been advocated, but no firm recommendations can be made because of the lack of randomized trials.[95]

Candida

Candida is a common pathogen in the immediate post-transplantation period, and invasive infection, either fungemia or visceral organ involvement, occurs in 11–16% of patients.[155, 156] Infection is most commonly caused by *C. albicans* and *C. tropicalis*, but other isolates include *C. lusitaniae*, *C. krusei*, and *C. parapsilosis*.[155, 156] *Candida* infections are most common in the pre-engraftment period, with a median time to onset of approximately 15 days, but may occur throughout the first 100 days after transplantation.[155, 156] The risk of infection increases with the duration of neutropenia and the severity of acute GVHD and is higher in allogeneic than in autologous transplant recipients.[155] Although extrathoracic infection with *Candida* is relatively common, pneumonia occurs in only 1% of patients.[155, 156] *Candida* pneumonia may result from hematogenous dissemination or from aspiration of a large inoculum from the oropharynx.[157]

Clinical manifestations are nonspecific, and chest radiography and CT typically reveal bilateral, patchy alveolar infiltrates or poorly defined nodules or masses. Cavitation and halos of ground-glass attenuation may occur but are less common than with *Aspergillus* infection.[140] The presence of *Candida* organisms is a common, nonspecific finding in sputum and BAL fluid; therefore, diagnosis of pneumonia must be based on histologic examination and culture of lung tissue. Amphotericin B is the treatment of choice for invasive *Candida* infections. Despite therapy, pneumonia and other organ infections are associated with a mortality rate of 90%.[155] Because of this high mortality rate, prophylactic fluconazole is administered throughout the pre-engraftment period,[156] and empirical amphotericin B is routinely added when neutropenic, febrile patients fail to respond to broad-spectrum antibiotics.

Other Fungi

Pneumonia due to *Trichosporon, Fusarium,* and the *Zygomycetes* organisms has been only occasionally reported in patients undergoing HSCT, but the incidence of these infections may be increasing.[158, 159] As with other fungal infections, prolonged neutropenia and corticosteroid therapy appear to be major risk factors. Infections with these organisms are most common in the postengraftment period.

Pneumocystis carinii INFECTION

Because of the routine use of prophylactic therapy, *Pneumocystis carinii* pneumonia (PCP) is uncommon in patients undergoing HSCT, and several series have reported an incidence of approximately 1%.[1, 16–18, 22, 160] PCP occurs predominantly in the postengraftment period and has a median time to onset of 2 months.[17] Clinical manifestations include nonproductive cough and rapidly progressive dyspnea and hypoxemia that often result in respiratory failure.[160, 161] Chest radiography and CT typically show diffuse interstitial or alveolar infiltrates. CT may also demonstrate areas of ground-glass attenuation and multiple small nodules.[97, 162]

The diagnosis of PCP is made by visualizing the organisms in BAL fluid or lung tissue, usually with methenamine silver stain. Although examination of sputum is often diagnostic in patients with acquired immunodeficiency syndrome (AIDS), the much lower burden of organisms in other immunocompromised patients makes this test insensitive. Bronchoalveolar lavage has been reported to have a sensitivity exceeding 90% in patients with AIDS[163] and appears to have a similar yield in other immunocompromised patients.[82, 160]

Allogeneic transplant recipients routinely receive chemoprophylaxis with trimethoprim-sulfamethoxazole starting at the time of engraftment and continuing for at least 3–6 months.[95] Based on data from patients with AIDS, patients undergoing HSCT who are allergic or intolerant to this therapy may receive dapsone or monthly aerosolized pentamidine.[95, 164, 165] The treatment of choice for PCP is high-dose trimethoprim-sulfamethoxazole. In patients with AIDS and moderate to severe PCP, the addition of corticosteroids has been shown to reduce the risk of respiratory failure and death.[166] No data are available concerning adjunctive corticosteroid therapy in other immunocompromised patients.

MYCOBACTERIAL INFECTIONS

Although pneumonia caused by *Mycobacterium tuberculosis*,[167] *M. avium* complex,[167] *M. kansasii*,[168] and *M. haemophilum*[169] has been reported in patients undergoing HSCT, these infections are uncommon. Mycobacterial infections have been most often reported in patients receiving immunosuppressive therapy for chronic GVHD and usually occur more than 6 months after transplantation.

DIAGNOSTIC EVALUATION AND MANAGEMENT OF RESPIRATORY DISEASE

A thorough, orderly, and rapid diagnostic process is required for the effective management of respiratory complications in the immediate post-transplantation period. An *initial evaluation* is essential for identifying likely disorders and allows the selection of appropriate empirical therapy. In most patients, *invasive testing* is required to establish a definitive diagnosis and institute specific therapy.

INITIAL EVALUATION

The diagnostic process must begin with a detailed history and physical examination and a careful review of the chest radiograph. In selected patients, CT of the chest may pro-

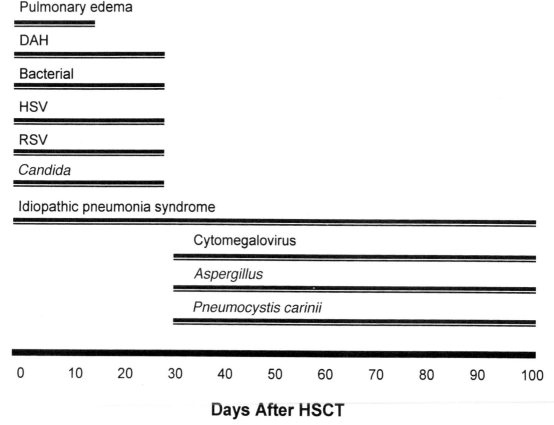

FIGURE 48–1. Approximate time of onset of respiratory disorders in the immediate post-transplantation period. DAH, diffuse alveolar hemorrhage; HSCT, hematopoietic stem cell transplantation; HSV, herpes simplex virus; RSV, respiratory syncytial virus.

TABLE 48–2. IMPORTANT HISTORICAL INFORMATION IN PATIENTS WITH RESPIRATORY DISEASE

CHARACTERISTIC	DISORDER(S)	RISK
Total body irradiation	Idiopathic pneumonia syndrome	High
	CMV pneumonia	High
CMV-positive donor	CMV pneumonia	High
Positive CMV serology, cultures, or PCR	CMV pneumonia	High
Nonmalignant disease	Idiopathic pneumonia syndrome	Low
	CMV pneumonia	Low
Negative CMV serology, cultures, and PCR	CMV pneumonia	Low
Prophylactic:		
Fluconazole	*Candida* pneumonia	Low
Acyclovir	HSV pneumonia	Low
Ganciclovir	CMV pneumonia	Low
Trimethoprim-sulfamethoxazole	*Pneumocystis carinii* pneumonia	Low

CMV, cytomegalovirus; HSV, herpes simplex virus; PCR, polymerase chain reaction.

vide additional diagnostic information.[97, 162, 170, 171] For example, CT may demonstrate unsuspected interstitial or alveolar infiltrates, nodules, cavitation, peripheral wedge-shaped infiltrates, air crescents, halos, and adenopathy. CT appears to be of greatest benefit in patients whose chest radiographs are either normal in appearance or show focal infiltrates. CT is unlikely to provide useful information in patients with diffuse interstitial or alveolar infiltrates.[170, 171]

The epidemiology, clinical manifestations, and radiographic appearance of each transplant-related respiratory disorder have previously been described in detail. Although many characteristics are nonspecific, certain details may provide important diagnostic clues and allow the selection of appropriate empirical therapy. For example, as shown in Figure 48–1, respiratory complications after HSCT tend to

TABLE 48–3. IMPORTANT CLINICAL MANIFESTATIONS IN PATIENTS WITH RESPIRATORY DISEASE

SYMPTOM/SIGN	ASSOCIATED DISORDERS
Hemoptysis	*Aspergillus* pneumonia
	Aspergillus tracheobronchitis
	Pulmonary embolism
	Diffuse alveolar hemorrhage
Rhinitis, sinusitis, otitis	Respiratory virus infection
	Aspergillus infection
Acute GVHD (grade 3 or 4)	Idiopathic pneumonia syndrome
	CMV pneumonia
Severe mucositis	Anaerobic pneumonia
	Candida pneumonia
Pleural friction rub	*Aspergillus* pneumonia
	Pulmonary embolism
Herpetic dermatitis, stomatitis, esophagitis	HSV pneumonia
	HSV tracheobronchitis
Basilar rales, S3 gallop	Pulmonary edema

CMV, cytomegalovirus; GVHD, graft-versus-host disease; HSV, herpes simplex virus.

occur in a rather well-defined temporal sequence. Knowledge of the transplantation date is therefore essential in generating a list of likely diagnoses. It is, however, important to recognize that changes in the rate of immune reconstitution may significantly alter the "usual" time at which each disorder occurs. A thorough history must also elicit characteristics of both the patient and the transplantation procedure that increase or decrease the likelihood of certain respiratory disorders. These important historical details and their potential significance are listed in Table 48–2. As shown in Tables 48–3 and 48–4, certain symptoms, physical examination findings, and radiographic signs may also aid in differential diagnosis.

INVASIVE TESTS

Bronchoscopy

Fiberoptic bronchoscopy is an extremely useful procedure in the evaluation of respiratory disease in patients undergoing HSCT. Endoscopic examination and endobronchial biopsy may be diagnostic of *Aspergillus* or HSV tracheobronchitis. In addition, samples may be obtained from the lower respiratory tract using several diagnostic techniques. *Bronchoalveolar lavage* is performed by wedging the fiberoptic bronchoscope in a subsegmental bronchus leading to an area of radiographic abnormality. Aliquots of sterile saline are instilled through the bronchoscope and then aspirated into a sterile container. The volume of saline infused is not standardized, but 3–4 aliquots of 50 mL are commonly used.

The aspirated fluid is cultured for fungi, bacteria, mycobacteria, *Legionella*, and viruses and is examined for *Legionella* spp. using the direct fluorescent antibody technique. Cytopreparation smears are made by centrifuging the lavage fluid, decanting the supernatant, and fixing the cellular material. Wright-Giemsa, Papanicolaou, methena-

TABLE 48–4. IMPORTANT RADIOGRAPHIC SIGNS IN PATIENTS WITH RESPIRATORY DISEASE

RADIOGRAPHIC SIGN	ASSOCIATED DISORDERS
Diffuse alveolar or interstitial infiltrates	Idiopathic pneumonia syndrome
	Diffuse alveolar hemorrhage
	Pulmonary edema
	Viral pneumonia
	Pneumocystis carinii pneumonia
Focal alveolar or interstitial infiltrates	Bacterial pneumonia
	Fungal pneumonia
Nodules or masses	Fungal pneumonia
	Recurrent malignancy
	Septic emboli
Cavitation	Fungal pneumonia
	Bacterial pneumonia
	Mycobacterial infection
"Air-crescent" sign	*Aspergillus* pneumonia
"Halo" sign	Fungal pneumonia
Vascular redistribution, Kerley lines	Pulmonary edema
Pleural-based density	*Aspergillus* pneumonia
	Pulmonary embolism
Hilar or mediastinal adenopathy	Fungal infection
	Mycobacterial infection
	Recurrent malignancy

mine silver, Ziehl-Neelsen, and Prussian blue stains are used to evaluate for viral inclusions, fungi, *P. carinii*, mycobacteria, and hemosiderin. In addition, fluorescein-labeled monoclonal antibodies are used to detect the presence of CMV, RSV, adenovirus, influenza virus, and parainfluenza virus within infected cells.

BAL has been extensively evaluated in immunocompromised patients who are not infected with human immunodeficiency virus (HIV),[48, 82, 83, 172–176, 177–179] and four studies have specifically examined its usefulness in patients undergoing BMT.[173, 176, 178, 179] Although all of these studies were limited by either small patient numbers, retrospective design, or, most importantly, lack of a diagnostic gold standard, several conclusions can be made from the available data. First, BAL can be safely performed even in thrombocytopenic patients with respiratory failure. Second, the overall sensitivity of BAL is somewhere between 30% and 60%.[48, 82, 83, 172–176, 178] This low diagnostic yield reflects the low incidence of PCP (for which BAL is highly sensitive) and the common occurrence of noninfectious lung disease. Finally, despite its low overall sensitivity, BAL can be an effective tool for diagnosing PCP (sensitivity, 94–100%[82, 174, 175]); CMV and other viral pneumonias (sensitivity, 69–100%[48, 82, 175]); mycobacterial infection (sensitivity, 80%[48, 175]); and *Aspergillus* pneumonia (sensitivity, 50–83%[48, 137, 141, 142, 175]).

Small samples of lung parenchyma (typically 2–3 mm) are obtained by performing *transbronchial lung biopsy* (TBBx) through the fiberoptic bronchoscope. These tissue samples may be analyzed using the same microbiologic and immunologic techniques described for BAL fluid. In addition, the biopsies may be examined histologically for viral inclusions and for noninfectious processes. Several studies have evaluated the usefulness of TBBx in immunocompromised, non–HIV-infected patients with pulmonary infiltrates.[48, 141, 142, 178, 180–182] Most researchers have concluded that TBBx has a lower sensitivity but higher specificity than BAL for the diagnosis of most respiratory infections. The sensitivity of TBBx for the diagnosis of noninfectious respiratory disorders is also low because of the small size of the tissue samples obtained. Transbronchial biopsy can be safely performed in thrombocytopenic and mechanically ventilated patients but does carry a small risk of potentially life-threatening hemorrhage and pneumothorax.[183, 184]

Protected specimen brushing is a technique used to obtain uncontaminated lower respiratory tract secretions for bacterial culture. A plugged catheter consisting of an outer cannula and an inner cannula housing a brush is inserted through the bronchoscope into an area of radiographic abnormality. The inner cannula is advanced, thereby dislodging the plug, and the brush is then advanced beyond the inner cannula. This procedure is reversed before the catheter is removed from the bronchoscope. The brush is cut aseptically and placed in 1 mL of saline or transport medium. Serial dilutions are performed, and culture results are reported as colony-forming units (cfu) per milliliter. Several studies have indicated that a quantitative culture with greater than 10³ cfu/mL effectively distinguishes pathogenic from colonizing organisms.[185, 186] Protected specimen brushing has been evaluated primarily in patients with ventilator-associated bacterial pneumonia, and the re-

ported sensitivity and specificity ranges are 58–100% and 60–100%, respectively.[90, 186–188]

Surgical Biopsy

Open-lung biopsy, usually performed through a limited thoracotomy incision, has long been considered the gold standard for diagnosing pulmonary disease in the immunocompromised host. Numerous studies have reported that a specific diagnosis is made in approximately 70% of cases, with the remaining diagnoses consisting primarily of interstitial inflammation and fibrosis and diffuse alveolar damage.[178, 189–192] In patients undergoing HSCT, the frequent occurrence of IPS increases the percentage of nonspecific biopsies, especially in the first 30 days.[178, 192] False-negative results are uncommon but have been reported in patients with fungal pneumonia.[190, 192] Open-lung biopsy is a relatively safe procedure, even in patients with thrombocytopenia and in those requiring mechanical ventilation. The most commonly reported complications are persistent air leak and delayed pneumothorax.[189–191] Hemothorax has been reported, but life-threatening hemorrhage is rare.[189–191] Although a specific diagnosis is usually made and therapy is changed in over 50% of patients,[83, 191] it is unknown whether open-lung biopsy (or any other diagnostic procedure) improves patient survival.

Video-assisted thoracoscopic surgery (VATS) has been used as an alternative to thoracotomy in patients with pulmonary infiltrates and nondiagnostic bronchoscopy.[193, 194] A double-lumen endotracheal tube is used to allow single-lung ventilation, and the lung to be biopsied is allowed to completely collapse. Three small incisions are made in the lateral chest wall to create viewing ports and access for biopsy instruments. Studies have suggested that the diagnostic yield of VATS is similar to that of thoracotomy.[193, 194] Potential advantages include decreased postoperative pain, shorter duration of chest tube drainage, and decreased postoperative morbidity. Disadvantages include increased operative time and impaired ability to manage significant hemorrhage.[193, 194] In addition, because of the requirement for single-lung ventilation, VATS cannot be performed in patients with severely impaired gas exchange. VATS has not been compared with thoracotomy in a prospective, randomized fashion, and no study has specifically examined its use in immunocompromised patients.

APPROACH TO DIAGNOSIS AND MANAGEMENT

An algorithm used at the University of Pittsburgh for the diagnosis and management of respiratory disease in the immediate post-transplantation period is outlined in Figure 48–2. Based on the history, physical examination, chest radiograph, and chest CT, likely diagnoses are identified and appropriate empirical therapy is begun. Unless pulmonary edema is strongly suspected, patients undergo immediate bronchoscopy, and specific therapy is based on the results of this procedure. If no diagnosis is made, empirical therapy is continued as long as there is evidence of clinical improvement. Surgical biopsy, either through a limited tho-

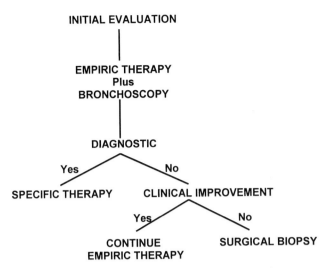

INITIAL EVALUATION

EMPIRIC THERAPY
Plus
BRONCHOSCOPY

DIAGNOSTIC

Yes — No

SPECIFIC THERAPY — CLINICAL IMPROVEMENT

Yes — No

CONTINUE
EMPIRIC THERAPY — SURGICAL BIOPSY

FIGURE 48–2. Approach to the diagnosis and management of respiratory disorders in the immediate post-transplantation period.

racotomy incision or using VATS, is performed if there is no improvement.

PROGNOSIS OF PATIENTS REQUIRING ADMISSION TO THE INTENSIVE CARE UNIT

Patients undergoing HSCT are likely to require transfer to an intensive care unit (ICU) during their hospitalization, and published series report admission rates ranging from 15–40%.[3, 4, 195, 196] In the majority of cases, ICU transfer is indicated for progressive respiratory insufficiency. The outcome of patients requiring ICU admission is generally poor, with only approximately 20% surviving to hospital discharge.[3, 4, 196] Although several factors, including multiorgan dysfunction and the need for vasoactive medications, have been shown to adversely affect survival, the most important is the need for mechanical ventilation. Patients requiring ventilatory support experience a hospital mortality rate of approximately 95%.[3, 4, 195] Recent studies suggest that this dismal prognosis is gradually improving,[195, 196] and it is hoped that aggressive approaches to the diagnosis and management of patients with respiratory disease, like the one described earlier, will favorably affect patient survival.

REFERENCES

1. Cordonnier C, Bernaudin J, Bierling P, et al: Pulmonary complications occurring after allogeneic bone marrow transplantation. Cancer 58:1047, 1986.
2. Quabeck K: The lung as a critical organ in marrow transplantation. Bone Marrow Transplant 14(Suppl 4):S19, 1994.
3. Afessa B, Tefferi A, Hoagland HC, et al: Outcome of recipients of bone marrow transplants who require intensive care unit support. Mayo Clin Proc 67:117, 1992.
4. Paz HL, Crilley P, Weinar M, Brodsky I: Outcome of patients requiring medical ICU admission following bone marrow transplantation. Chest 104:527, 1993.
5. Robbins RA, Linder J, Stahl MG, et al: Diffuse alveolar hemorrhage in autologous bone marrow transplant recipients. Am J Med 87:511, 1989.
6. Lee C-K, Gingrich RD, Hohl RJ, Ajram KA: Engraftment syndrome in autologous bone marrow and peripheral stem cell transplantation. Bone Marrow Transplant 16:175, 1995.
7. Klumpp TR: Complications of peripheral blood stem cell transplantation. Semin Oncol 22:263, 1995.
8. Kessinger A, Armitage JO, Landmark JD, et al: Autologous peripheral hematopoietic stem cell transplantation restores hematopoietic function following marrow ablative therapy. Blood 71:723, 1988.
9. Elias AD, Ayash L, Anderson KC, et al: Mobilization of peripheral blood progenitor cells by chemotherapy and granulocyte-macrophage colony-stimulating factor for hematologic support after high-dose intensification for breast cancer. Blood 79:3036, 1992.
10. Pettengell R, Morgenstern GR, Woll PJ, et al: Peripheral blood progenitor cell transplantation in lymphoma and leukemia using a single apheresis. Blood 82:3770, 1993.
11. Reiffers J, Trouette R, Marit G, et al: Autologous blood stem cell transplantation for chronic granulocytic leukaemia in transformation. Br J Haematol 77:339, 1991.
12. Nosanchuk JD, Sepkowitz KA, Pearse RN, et al: Infectious complications of autologous bone marrow and peripheral stem cell transplantation for refractory leukemia and lymphoma. Bone Marrow Transplant 18:355, 1996.
13. Bensinger WI, Clift R, Martin P, et al: Allogeneic peripheral blood stem cell transplantation in patients with advanced hematologic malignancies: a retrospective comparison with marrow transplantation. Blood 88:2794, 1996.
14. Bacigalupo A, Zikos P, Van Lint MT, et al: Allogeneic bone marrow or peripheral blood cell transplants in adults with hematologic malignancies: a single-center experience. Exp Hematol 26:409, 1998.
15. Clark JG, Hansen JA, Hertz MI, et al: Idiopathic pneumonia syndrome after bone marrow transplantation. Am Rev Respir Dis 147:1601, 1993.
16. Weiner RS, Bortin MM, Gale RP, et al: Interstitial pneumonitis after bone marrow transplantation. Ann Intern Med 104:168, 1986.
17. Meyers JD, Flournoy N, Thomas ED: Nonbacterial pneumonia after allogeneic marrow transplantation: a review of ten years' experience. Rev Infect Dis 4:1119, 1982.
18. Wingard JR, Mellits ED, Sostrin MB, et al: Interstitial pneumonitis after allogeneic bone marrow transplantation. Medicine 67:175, 1988.
19. Weiner RS, Horowitz MM, Gale RP, et al: Risk factors for interstitial pneumonia following bone marrow transplantation for severe aplastic anaemia. Br J Haematol 71:535, 1989.
20. Crawford SW, Longton G, Storb R: Acute graft-versus-host disease and the risks for idiopathic pneumonia after marrow transplantation for severe aplastic anemia. Bone Marrow Transplant 12:225, 1993.
21. Kernan NA, Bartsch G, Ash RC, et al: Analysis of 462 transplantations from unrelated donors facilitated by the national marrow donor program. N Engl J Med 328:593, 1993.
22. Wingard JR, Sostrin MB, Vriesendorp HM, et al: Interstitial pneumonitis following autologous bone marrow transplantation. Transplantation 46:61, 1988.
23. Crawford SW, Hackman RC: Clinical course of idiopathic pneumonia after bone marrow transplantation. Am Rev Respir Dis 147:1393, 1993.
24. Keane TJ, Van Dyk J, Rider WD: Idiopathic interstitial pneumonia following bone marrow transplantation: the relationship with total body irradiation. Int J Radiat Oncol Biol Phys 7:1365, 1981.
25. Pino Y Torres JL, Bross DS, Lam W-C, et al: Risk factors in interstitial pneumonitis following allogeneic bone marrow transplantation. Int J Radiat Oncol Biol Phys 8:1301, 1982.
26. Bortin MM, Kay HEM, Gale RP, Rimm AA: Factors associated with interstitial pneumonitis after bone marrow transplantation for acute leukaemia. Lancet 1:437, 1982.
27. Cooper JA, White DA, Matthay RA: Drug-induced pulmonary disease. Am Rev Respir Dis 133:321, 1986.
28. Seiden MV, Elias A, Ayash L, et al: Pulmonary toxicity associated with high dose chemotherapy in the treatment of solid tumors with autologous marrow transplant: an analysis of four chemotherapy regimens. Bone Marrow Transplant 10:57, 1992.
29. Todd NW, Peters WP, Ost AH, et al: Pulmonary drug toxicity in patients with primary breast cancer treated with high-dose combination chemotherapy and autologous bone marrow transplantation. Am Rev Respir Dis 147:1264, 1993.
30. Deeg HJ, Storb R, Thomas Ed, et al: Cyclosporine as prophylaxis for graft-versus-host disease: a randomized study in patients undergoing marrow transplantation for acute nonlymphoblastic leukemia. Blood 65:1325, 1985.

31. Storb R, Deeg HJ, Thomas ED, et al: Marrow transplantation for chronic myelocytic leukemia: a controlled trial of cyclosporine versus methotrexate for prophylaxis of graft-versus-host disease. Blood 66:698, 1985.

32. Irle C, Deeg HJ, Buckner CD, et al: Marrow transplantation for leukemia following fractionated total body irradiation: a comparative trial of methotrexate and cyclosporine. Leuk Res 9:1255, 1985.

33. Storb R, Deeg HJ, Fisher L, et al: Cyclosporin v methotrexate for graft-v-host disease prevention in patients given marrow grafts for leukemia: long-term follow-up of three controlled trials. Blood 71:293, 1988.

34. Muller CA, Hebart H, Roos A, et al: Correlation of interstitial pneumonia with human cytomegalovirus-induced lung infection and graft-versus-host disease after bone marrow transplantation. Med Microbiol Immunol 184:115, 1995.

35. Cone RW, Hackman RC, Huang M-LW: Human herpesvirus 6 in lung tissue from patients with pneumonitis after bone marrow transplantation. N Engl J Med 329:156, 1993.

36. Barbera JA, Martin-Campos JM, Ribalta T, et al: Undetected viral infection in diffuse alveolar damage associated with bone marrow transplantation. Eur Resp J 9:1195, 1996.

37. Jadus MR, Wepsic HT: The role of cytokines in graft-versus-host reactions and disease. Bone Marrow Transplant 10:1, 1992.

38. Metcalf JP, Rennard SI, Reed EC, et al: Corticosteroids as adjunctive therapy for diffuse alveolar hemorrhage associated with bone marrow transplantation. Am J Med 96:327, 1994.

39. Jules-Elysee K, Stover DE, Yahalom J, et al: Pulmonary complications in lymphoma patients treated with high-dose therapy and autologous bone marrow transplantation. Am Rev Respir Dis 146:485, 1992.

40. Wojno KJ, Vogelsang GB, Beschorner WE, Santos GW: Pulmonary hemorrhage as a cause of death in allogeneic bone marrow recipients with severe acute graft-versus-host disease. Transplantation 57:88, 1994.

41. Agusti C, Ramirez J, Picado C, et al: Diffuse alveolar hemorrhage in allogeneic bone marrow transplantation. Am J Respir Crit Care Med 151:1006, 1995.

42. Sisson JH, Thompson AB, Anderson JR, et al: Airway inflammation predicts diffuse alveolar hemorrhage during bone marrow transplantation in patients with Hodgkin disease. Am Rev Respir Dis 146:439, 1992.

43. Corso S, Vukelja SJ, Wiener D, Baker WJ: Diffuse alveolar hemorrhage following autologous bone marrow infusion. Bone Marrow Transplant 12:301, 1993.

44. Schmidt-Wolf I, Schwerdtfeger R, Schwella N, et al: Diffuse alveolar hemorrhage after allogeneic bone marrow transplantation. Ann Hematol 67:139, 1993.

45. Witte RJ, Gurney JW, Robbins RA, et al: Diffuse pulmonary alveolar hemorrhage after bone marrow transplantation: radiographic findings in 39 patients. AJR Am J Roentgenol 157:461, 1991.

46. Srivastava A, Gottlieb D, Bradstock KF: Diffuse alveolar hemorrhage associated with microangiopathy after allogeneic bone marrow transplantation. Bone Marrow Transplant 15: 863, 1995.

47. Kahn FW, Jones JM, England DM: Diagnosis of pulmonary hemorrhage in the immunocompromised host. Am Rev Respir Dis 136:155, 1987.

48. Stover DE, Zaman MB, Hajdu SI: Bronchoalveolar lavage in the diagnosis of diffuse pulmonary infiltrates in the immunosuppressed host. Ann Intern Med 101:1, 1984.

49. Chao NJ, Duncan SR, Long GD, et al: Corticosteroid therapy for diffuse alveolar hemorrhage in autologous bone marrow transplant recipients. Ann Intern Med 114:145, 1991.

50. Drew WL, Finley TN, Golde DW: Diagnostic lavage and occult pulmonary hemorrhage in thrombocytopenic immunocompromised patients. Am Rev Respir Dis 116:215, 1977.

51. de Lassence A, Fleury-Feith J, Escudier E, et al: Alveolar hemorrhage: diagnostic criteria and results in 194 immunocompromised hosts. Am J Respir Crit Care Med 151:157, 1995.

52. Dickout WJ, Chan CK, Hyland RH, et al: Prevention of acute pulmonary edema after bone marrow transplantation. Chest 92:303, 1987.

53. Gottdiener JS, Appelbaum FR, Ferrans VJ, et al: Cardiotoxicity associated with high-dose cyclophosphamide therapy. Arch Intern Med 141:758, 1981.

54. Buja LM, Ferrans VJ, Graw RG: Cardiac pathologic findings in patients treated with bone marrow transplantation. Hum Pathol 7:17, 1976.

55. McDonald GB, Hinds MS, Fisher LD, et al: Veno-occlusive disease of the liver and multiorgan failure after bone marrow transplantation: a cohort study of 355 patients. Ann Intern Med 188:255, 1993.

56. Haire WD, Ruby EI, Gordon BG, et al: Multiple organ dysfunction syndrome in bone marrow transplantation. JAMA 274:1289, 1995.

57. Cahill RA, Spitzer TR, Mazumder A: Marrow engraftment and clinical manifestations of capillary leak syndrome. Bone Marrow Transplant 18:177. 1996.

58. Cordonnier C, Fleury-Feith J, Escudier E, et al: Secondary alveolar proteinosis is a reversible cause of respiratory failure in leukemic patients. Am J Respir Crit Care Med 149:788, 1994.

59. Wingard JR, Mellits ED, Jones RJ, et al: Association of hepatic veno-occlusive disease with interstitial pneumonitis in bone marrow transplant recipients. Bone Marrow Transplant 4:685, 1989.

60. Troussard X, Bernaudin JF, Cordonnier C, et al: Pulmonary veno-occlusive disease after bone marrow transplantation. Thorax 39:956, 1984.

61. Hackman RC, Madtes DK, Petersen FB, Clark JG: Pulmonary venoocclusive disease following bone marrow transplantation. Transplantation 47:989, 1989.

62. Williams LM, Fussell S, Veith RW, et al: Pulmonary veno-occlusive disease in an adult following bone marrow transplantation. Chest 109:1388, 1996.

63. Sloane JP, Depledge MH, Powles RL, et al: Histopathology of the lung after bone marrow transplantation. J Clin Pathol 36:546, 1983.

64. Paradinas FJ, Sloane JP, Depledge MH, et al: Pulmonary fat embolism after bone marrow transplantation. Lancet 1:715, 1983.

65. Abrahams C, Catchatourian R: Bone fragment emboli in the lungs of patients undergoing bone marrow transplantation. Am J Clin Pathol 79:360, 1983.

66. Lum LG: The kinetics of immune reconstitution after human marrow transplantation. Blood 69:369, 1987.

67. Atkinson K: Reconstruction of the haematopoietic and immune systems after marrow transplantation. Bone Marrow Transplant 5:209, 1990.

68. Hiemenz JW, Greene JN: Special considerations for the patient undergoing allogeneic or autologous bone marrow transplantation. Hematol Oncol Clin North Am 7:961, 1993.

69. Shelhamer JH, Towes GB, Masur H, et al: Respiratory disease in the immunosuppressed patient. Ann Intern Med 117:415, 1992.

70. Towes GB: Pulmonary defense mechanisms. Semin Respir Infect 8:160, 1993.

71. Winston DJ, Territo MC, Ho WG: Alveolar macrophage dysfunction in human bone marrow transplant recipients. Am J Med 73:859, 1982.

72. Noel DR, Witherspoon RP, Storb R, et al: Does graft-versus-host disease influence the tempo of immunologic recovery after allogeneic bone marrow transplantation? An observation on long-term survivors. Blood 51:1087, 1978.

73. Atkinson K, Biggs JC, Ting A, et al: Cyclosporine A is associated with faster engraftment and less mucositis than methotrexate after allogeneic bone marrow transplantation. Br J Haematol 53:265, 1983.

74. Martin PJ, Hansen JA, Buckner CD, et al: Effects of in vitro depletion of T cells in HLA-identical allogeneic marrow grafts. Blood 66:664, 1985.

75. Atkinson K: T cell sub-populations defined by monoclonal antibodies after HLA-identical sibling marrow transplantation. Bone Marrow Transplant 1:121, 1986.

76. Ault KE, Antin JH, Ginsburg D, et al: Phenotype of recovering lymphoid cell populations after marrow transplantation. J Exp Med 161:1483, 1985.

77. Warren H, Atkinson K, Pembrey, et al: T lymphocyte function in human bone marrow allograft recipients: production of, and responsiveness to, interleukin 2. J Immunol 131:1771, 1983.

78. Witherspoon RP, Matthews D, Storb R, et al: Recovery of in vivo cellular immunity after human marrow grafting: influence of time post grafting and acute graft-versus-host disease. Transplantation 37:145, 1984.

79. Witherspoon RP, Storb R, Ochs HD, et al: Recovery of antibody production in human allogeneic marrow graft recipients: influence of time post transplantation, presence or absence of chronic graft-versus-host disease, and antithymocyte globulin treatment. Blood 58:360, 1981.

80. Sable CA, Donowitz GR: Infections in bone marrow transplant recipients. Clin Infect Dis 18:273, 1994.
81. Pannuti CS, Gingrich RD, Pfaller MA, Wenzel RP: Nosocomial pneumonia in adult patients undergoing bone marrow transplantation: a 9-year study. J Clin Oncol 9:77, 1991.
82. von Eiff M, Zuhlsdorf M, Roos N, et al: Pulmonary infiltrates in patients with haematologic malignancies: clinical usefulness of non-invasive bronchoscopic procedures. Eur J Haematol 54:157, 1995.
83. Ellis ME, Spence D, Bouchama A, et al: Open lung biopsy provides a higher and more specific diagnostic yield compared to broncho-alveolar lavage in immunocompromised patients. Scand J Infect Dis 27:157, 1995.
84. Lossos IS, Breuer R, Or R, et al: Bacterial pneumonia in recipients of bone marrow transplantation. Transplantation 60:672, 1995.
85. Kugler JW, Armitage JW, Helms CM, et al: Nosocomial legionnaires' disease: occurrence in recipients of bone marrow transplants. Am J Med 74:281, 1983.
86. Fagon JY, Chastre J, Hance AJ, et al: Detection of nosocomial lung infection in ventilated patients: use of a protected specimen brush and quantitative culture techniques in 147 patients. Am Rev Respir Dis 138:110, 1988.
87. Meduri GU, Mauldin GL, Wunderink RG, et al: Causes of fever and pulmonary densities in patients with clinical manifestations of ventilator-associated pneumonia. Chest 106:221, 1994.
88. Torres A, de la Bellacasa JP, Xaubet A, et al: Diagnostic value of quantitative cultures of bronchoalveolar lavage and telescoping plugged catheters in mechanically ventilated patients with bacterial pneumonia. Am Rev Respir Dis 140:306, 1989.
89. Villers D, Derriennic M, Raffi F, et al: Reliability of the bronchoscopic protected catheter brush in intubated and ventilated patients. Chest 88:527, 1985.
90. Meduri GU: Diagnosis and differential diagnosis of ventilator-associated pneumonia. Clin Chest Med 16:61, 1995.
91. Meyers JD, Flournoy N, Thomas ED: Risk factors for cytomegalovirus infection after human marrow transplantation. J Infect Dis 153:478, 1986.
92. Enright H, Haake R, Weisdorf D, et al: Cytomegalovirus pneumonia after bone marrow transplantation. Transplantation 55:1339, 1993.
93. Wingard JR, Chen DYH, Burns WH, et al: Cytomegalovirus infection after autologous bone marrow transplantation with comparison to infection after allogeneic bone marrow transplantation. Blood 71:1432, 1988.
94. Ljungman P, Biron P, Bosi A, et al: Cytomegalovirus interstitial pneumonia in autologous bone marrow transplant recipients. Bone Marrow Transplant 13:209, 1994.
95. Rowe JM, Ciobanu N, Ascensao J, et al: Recommended guidelines for the management of autologous and allogeneic bone marrow transplantation. Ann Intern Med 120:143, 1994.
96. Bowden RA, Sayers M, Flournoy N, et al: Cytomegalovirus immune globulin and seronegative blood products to prevent primary cytomegalovirus infection after marrow transplantation. N Engl J Med 314:1006, 1986.
97. Janzen DL, Padley SPG, Adler BD, Muller NL: Acute pulmonary complications in immunocompromised non-AIDS patients: comparison of diagnostic accuracy of CT and chest radiography. Clin Radiol 47:159, 1993.
98. Crawford SW, Bowden RA, Hackman RC, et al: Rapid detection of cytomegalovirus pulmonary infection by bronchoalveolar lavage and centrifugation culture. Ann Intern Med 108:180, 1988.
99. Emanuel D, Peppard J, Stover D, et al: Rapid immunodiagnosis of cytomegalovirus pneumonia by bronchoalveolar lavage using human and murine monoclonal antibodies. Ann Intern Med 104:476, 1986.
100. Cathomas G, Morris P, Pekle K, et al: Rapid diagnosis of cytomegalovirus pneumonia in marrow transplant recipients by bronchoalveolar lavage using the polymerase chain reaction, virus culture, and the direct immunostaining of alveolar cells. Blood 81:1909, 1993.
101. Goto H, Yuasa K, Sakamaki H, et al: Rapid detection of cytomegalovirus pneumonia in recipients of bone marrow transplant: evaluation and comparison of five survey methods for bronchoalveolar lavage fluid. Bone Marrow Transplant 17:855, 1996.
102. Schmidt GM, Horak DA, Niland JC, et al: A randomized, controlled trial of prophylactic ganciclovir for cytomegalovirus pulmonary infection in recipients of allogeneic bone marrow transplants. N Engl J Med 324:1005, 1991.
103. Goodrich JM, Mori M, Gleaves CA: Early treatment with ganciclovir

104. Meyers JD, McGuffin RW, Neiman PE, et al: Toxicity and efficacy of leukocyte interferon for treatment of cytomegalovirus pneumonia after marrow transplantation. J Infect Dis 141:555, 1980.
105. Wade JD, Hintz M, McGuffin R, et al: Treatment of cytomegalovirus pneumonia with high dose acyclovir. Am J Med 73:249, 1982.
106. Wade JC, McGuffin RW, Springmeyer SC, et al: Treatment of cytomegaloviral pneumonia with high-dose acyclovir and human leukocyte interferon. J Infect Dis 148:557, 1983.
107. Shepp DH, Dandliker PS, de Miranda P, et al: Activity of 9-[2-hydroxy-1-(hydroxymethyl) ethoxymethyl] guanine in the treatment of cytomegalovirus pneumonia. Ann Intern Med 103:368, 1985.
108. Reed EC, Dandliker PS, Meyers JD: Treatment of cytomegalovirus pneumonia with 9-[2-hydroxy-1-(hydroxymethyl) ethoxymethyl] guanine and high-dose corticosteroids. Ann Intern Med 105:214, 1986.
109. Reed EC, Bowden RA, Dandliker PS, et al: Efficacy of cytomegalovirus immunoglobulin in marrow transplant recipients with cytomegalovirus pneumonia. J Infect Dis 156:641, 1987.
110. Emanuel D, Cunningham I, Jules-Elysee K, et al: Cytomegalovirus pneumonia after bone marrow transplantation successfully treated with the combination of ganciclovir and high-dose intravenous immune globulin. Ann Intern Med 109:777, 1988.
111. Reed EC, Bowden RA, Dandliker PS, et al: Treatment of cytomegalovirus pneumonia with ganciclovir and intravenous cytomegalovirus immunoglobulin in patients with bone marrow transplants. Ann Intern Med 109:783, 1988.
112. Schmidt GM, Kovacs A, Zaia JA, et al: Ganciclovir/immunoglobulin combination therapy for the treatment of human cytomegalovirus-associated interstitial pneumonia in bone marrow allograft recipients. Transplantation 46:905, 1988.
113. Ljungman P, Engelhard D, Link H, et al: Treatment of interstitial pneumonitis due to cytomegalovirus with ganciclovir and intravenous immune globulin: experience of European bone marrow transplant group. Clin Infect Dis 14:831, 1992.
114. Miller WJ, McCullough J, Balfour HH, et al: Prevention of cytomegalovirus infection following bone marrow transplantation: a randomized trial of blood product screening. Bone Marrow Transplant 7:227, 1991.
115. Sullivan KM, Kopecky KJ, Jocum J, et al: Immunomodulatory and antimicrobial efficacy of intravenous immunoglobulin in bone marrow transplantation. N Engl J Med 323:705, 1990.
116. Mandanas RA, Saez RA, Selby GB, et al: Cytomegalovirus surveillance and prevention in allogeneic bone marrow transplantation: examination of a preemptive plan of ganciclovir therapy. Am J Hematol 51:104, 1996.
117. Ibrahim A, Gautier E, Roittmann S, et al: Should cytomegalovirus be tested for in both blood and bronchoalveolar lavage fluid of patients at a high risk of CMV pneumonia after bone marrow transplantation? Br J Haematol 98:222, 1997.
118. Nolte FS, Emmens RK, Thurmond C st al: Early detection of human cytomegalovirus viremia in bone marrow transplant recipients by DNA amplification. J Clin Microbiol 33:1263, 1996.
119. Hebart H, Muller C, Loffler J, et al: Monitoring of CMV infection: a comparison of PCR from whole blood, plasma-PCR, pp65-antigenemia and virus culture in patients after bone marrow transplantation. Bone Marrow Transplant 17:861, 1996.
120. Murray JF, Mills J: Pulmonary infectious complications of human immunodeficiency virus infection. Am Rev Respir Dis 141:1356, 1990.
121. Grundy JE, Shanley JD, Griffiths PD: Is cytomegalovirus interstitial pneumonitis in transplant recipients an immunopathological condition? Lancet 2:996, 1987.
122. Ramsey PG, Fife KH, Hackman RC, et al: Herpes simplex virus pneumonia. Ann Intern Med 97:813, 1982.
123. Saral R, Burns WH, Laskin OL, et al: Acyclovir prophylaxis of herpes simplex virus infections: a randomized, double-blinded, controlled trial in bone marrow transplant recipients. N Engl J Med 305:63, 1981.
124. Hertz MI, Englund JA, Snover D, et al: Respiratory syncytial virus-induced acute lung injury in adult patients with bone marrow transplants: a clinical approach and review of the literature. Medicine 68:269, 1989.
125. Englund JA, Sullivan CJ, Jordan MC, et al: Respiratory syncytial

virus infection in immunocompromised adults. Ann Intern Med 109:203, 1988.

126. Hall CB, McBride JT, Gala CL, et al: Ribavirin treatment of respiratory syncytial viral infection in infants with underlying cardiopulmonary disease. JAMA 254:3047, 1985.

127. Win M, Mitchell D, Pugh S, et al: Successful therapy with ribavirin of late onset respiratory syncytial virus pneumonitis complicating allogeneic bone marrow transplantation. Clin Lab Haematol 14:29, 1992.

128. Shields AF, Hackman RC, Fife KH, et al: Adenovirus infections in patients undergoing bone marrow transplantation. N Engl J Med 312:529, 1985.

129. Ljungman P, Gleaves CA, Meyers JD: Respiratory virus infection in immunocompromised patients. Bone Marrow Transplant 4:35, 1989.

130. Blanke C, Clark C, Broun R, et al: Evolving pathogens in allogeneic bone marrow transplantation: increased fatal adenoviral infections. Am J Med 99:326, 1995.

131. Wendt CH, Weisdorf DJ, Jordan MC, et al: Parainfluenza virus respiratory infection after bone marrow transplantation. N Engl J Med 326:921, 1992.

132. Lewis VA, Champlin R, Englund J, et al: Respiratory disease due to parainfluenza virus in adult bone marrow transplant recipients. Clin Infect Dis 23:1033, 1996.

133. Hirschhorn LR, McIntosh K, Anderson KG, Dermody TS: Influenzal pneumonia as a complication of autologous bone marrow transplantation. Clin Infect Dis 14:786, 1992.

134. Carrigan DR, Drobyski WR, Russler SK, et al: Interstitial pneumonitis associated with human herpesvirus-6 infection after marrow transplantation. Lancet 338:147, 1991.

135. Gerson SL, Talbot GH, Hurwitz S, et al: Prolonged granulocytopenia: the major risk factor for invasive pulmonary aspergillosis in patients with acute leukemia. Ann Intern Med 100:345, 1984.

136. Wingard JR, Beals SU, Santos GW, et al: *Aspergillus* infections in bone marrow transplant recipients. Bone Marrow Transplant 2:175, 1987.

137. McWhinney PHM, Kibbler CC, Hamon MD, et al: Progress in the diagnosis and management of aspergillosis in bone marrow transplantation: 13 years' experience. Clin Infect Dis 17:397, 1993.

138. Kuhlman JE, Fishman EK, Siegelman SS: Invasive pulmonary aspergillosis in acute leukemia: characteristic findings on CT, the CT halo sign, and the role of CT in early diagnosis. Radiology 157:611, 1985.

139. Mori M, Galvin JR, Barloon TJ: Fungal pulmonary infections after bone marrow transplantation: evaluation with radiography and CT. Radiology 178:721, 1991.

140. Albelda SM, Talbot GH, Gerson SL: Role of fiberoptic bronchoscopy in the diagnosis of invasive aspergillosis in patients with acute leukemia. Am J Med 76:1027, 1984.

141. Kahn FW, Jones JM, England DM: The role of bronchoalveolar lavage in the diagnosis of invasive pulmonary aspergillosis. Am J Clin Pathol 86:518, 1986.

142. Levy H, Horak DA, Tegtmeier BR, et al: The value of bronchoalveolar lavage and bronchial washings in the diagnosis of invasive pulmonary aspergillosis. Respir Med 86:243, 1992.

143. Yu VL, Muder RR, Poorsattar A: Significance of isolation of *Aspergillus* from the respiratory tract in diagnosis of invasive pulmonary aspergillosis. Am J Med 81:249, 1986.

144. Clarke A, Skelton J, Fraser RS: Fungal tracheobronchitis. Medicine 70:1, 1991.

145. Putnam JB, Dignani C, Mehra RC, et al: Acute airway obstruction and necrotizing tracheobronchitis from invasive mycosis. Chest 106:1265, 1994.

146. Hines DW, Haber MH, Yaremko L, et al: Pseudomembranous tracheobronchitis caused by *Aspergillus*. Am Rev Respir Dis 143:1408, 1991.

147. Kramer MR, Denning DW, Marshall SE, et al: Ulcerative tracheobronchitis after lung transplantation. Am Rev Respir Dis 144:552, 1991.

148. Ringden O, Meunier F, Tollemar J, et al: Efficacy of amphotericin B encapsulated in liposomes (AmBisome) in the treatment of invasive fungal infections in immunocompromised patients. J Antimicrob Chemoth 28:73, 1991.

149. Lister J: Amphotericin B lipid complex (Abelcet) in the treatment of invasive mycoses: the North American experience. Eur J Haematol 56(Suppl 57):18, 1996.

150. Bowden RA, Cays M, Gooley T, et al: Phase I study of amphotericin B colloidal dispersion for the treatment of invasive fungal infections after marrow transplant. J Infect Dis 173:1208, 1996.

151. Denning DW, Lee JY, Hostetler JS, et al: NIAID mycoses study group multicenter trial of oral itraconazole therapy for invasive aspergillosis. Am J Med 97:135, 1994.

152. Jeffery GM, Beard ME, Ikram RB, et al: Intranasal amphotericin B reduces the frequency of invasive aspergillosis in neutropenic patients. Am J Med 90:685, 1991.

153. Conneally E, Cafferkey MT, Daly PA, et al: Nebulized amphotericin B as prophylaxis against invasive aspergillosis in granulocytopenic patients. Bone Marrow Transplant 5:403, 1990.

154. Rousey SR, Russler S, Gottlieb M, Ash RC: Low dose amphotericin B prophylaxis against invasive *Aspergillus* infections in allogeneic marrow transplantation. Am J Med 91:484, 1991.

155. Goodrich JM, Reed EC, Mori M, et al: Clinical features and analysis of risk factors for invasive candidal infection after marrow transplantation. J Infect Dis 164:731, 1991.

156. Goodman JL, Winston DJ, Greenfield RA, et al: A controlled trial of fluconazole to prevent fungal infections in patients undergoing bone marrow transplantation. N Engl J Med 326:845, 1992.

157. Haron E, Vartivarian S, Anaissie, et al: Primary *Candida* pneumonia. Medicine 72:137, 1993.

158. Morrison VA, McGlave PB: Mucormycosis in the BMT population. Bone Marrow Transplant 11:383, 1993.

159. Piliero PJ, Deresiewicz RL: Pulmonary zygomycosis after allogeneic bone marrow transplantation. South Med J 88:1149, 1995.

160. Tuan I-Z, Dennison D, Weisdorf DJ: *Pneumocystis carinii* pneumonitis following bone marrow transplantation. Bone Marrow Transplant 10:267, 1992.

161. Kovacs JA, Hiemenz JW, Macher AM, et al: *Pneumocystis carinii* pneumonia: a comparison of patients with the acquired immunodeficiency syndrome and patients with other immunodeficiencies. Ann Intern Med 100:663, 1984.

162. Brown MJ, Miller RR, Muller NL: Acute lung disease in the immunocompromised host: CT and pathologic examination findings. Radiology 190:247, 1994.

163. Stover DE, White DA, Romano PA, Gellene RA: Diagnosis of pulmonary disease in acquired immune deficiency syndrome (AIDS): role of bronchoscopy and bronchoalveolar lavage. Am Rev Respir Dis 130:659, 1984.

164. Schneider MME, Hoepelman AIM, et al: A controlled trial of aerosolized pentamidine or trimethoprim-sulfamethoxazole as primary prophylaxis against *Pneumocystis carinii* pneumonia in patients with human immunodeficiency virus infection. N Engl J Med 327:1836, 1992.

165. Bozzette SA, Finkelstein DM, Spector SA, et al: A randomized trial of three antipneumocystis agents in patients with advanced human immunodeficiency virus infection. N Engl J Med 332:693, 1995.

166. Bozzette SA, Sattler FR, Chiu J, et al: A controlled trial of early adjunctive treatment with corticosteroids for *Pneumocystis carinii* pneumonia in the acquired immunodeficiency syndrome. N Engl J Med 323:1451, 1990.

167. Kurzrock R, Zander A, Vellekoop L, et al: Mycobacterial pulmonary infections after allogeneic bone marrow transplantation. Am J Med 77:35, 1984.

168. Cryer PE, Kissane JM: Pulmonary and hepatic disease after chemotherapy and bone marrow transplantation for acute leukemia. Am J Med 66:484, 1979.

169. White MH, Papadopoulos EB, Small TN, et al: *Mycobacterium haemophilum* infections in bone marrow transplant recipients. Transplantation 60:957, 1995.

170. Barloon TJ, Galvin JR, Mori M, et al: High-resolution ultrafast chest CT in the clinical management of febrile bone marrow transplant patients with normal or nonspecific chest roentgenograms. Chest 99:928, 1991.

171. Graham NJ, Muller NL, Miller RR, Shepherd JD: Intrathoracic complications following allogeneic bone marrow transplantation: CT findings. Radiology 181:153, 1991.

172. Pisani RJ, Wright AJ: Clinical utility of bronchoalveolar lavage in immunocompromised hosts. Mayo Clin Proc 67:221, 1992.

173. Cordonnier C, Bernaudin J-F, Fleury J, et al: Diagnostic yield of bronchoalveolar lavage in pneumonitis occurring after bone marrow transplantation. Am Rev Respir Dis 132:1118, 1985.

174. Martin WJ, Smith TF, Sanderson DR, et al: Role of bronchoalveolar lavage in the assessment of opportunistic pulmonary infections: utility and complications. Mayo Clin Proc 62:549, 1987.

175. Xaubet A, Torres A, Marco F, et al: Pulmonary infiltrates in immuno-

compromised patients: diagnostic value of telescoping plugged catheter and bronchoalveolar lavage. Chest 95:130, 1989.

176. Milburn HJ, Prentice HG, DuBois RM: Role of bronchoalveolar lavage in the evaluation of interstitial pneumonitis in recipients of bone marrow transplants. Thorax 42:766, 1987.

177. Weiss SM, Hert RC, Gianola FJ: Complications of fiberoptic bronchoscopy in thrombocytopenic patients. Chest 104:1025, 1993.

178. Springmeyer SC, Hackman RC, Holle R, et al: Use of bronchoalveolar lavage to diagnose acute diffuse pneumonia in the immunocompromised host. J Infect Dis 154:604, 1986.

179. Campbell JH, Blessing N, Burnett AK, Stevenson RD: Investigation and management of pulmonary infiltrates following bone marrow transplantation: an eight year review. Thorax 48:1248, 1993.

180. Springmeyer SC, Silvestri RC, Sale GE: The role of transbronchial biopsy for the diagnosis of diffuse pneumonias in immunocompromised marrow transplant recipients. Am Rev Respir Dis 126:763, 1982.

181. Puksa S, Hutcheon MA, Hyland RH: Usefulness of transbronchial biopsy in immunosuppressed patients with pulmonary infiltrates. Thorax 38:146, 1983.

182. Cazzadori A, Di Perri G, Todeschini G, et al: Transbronchial biopsy in the diagnosis of pulmonary infiltrates in immunocompromised patients. Chest 107:101, 1995.

183. Papin TA, Lynch JP, Weg JG: Transbronchial biopsy in the thrombocytopenic patient. Chest 88:549, 1985.

184. Cordasco EM, Mehta AC, Ahmad M: Bronchoscopically induced bleeding: a summary of nine years' Cleveland Clinic experience and review of the literature. Chest 100:1141, 1991.

185. Chastre J, Fagon JY, Soler P, et al: Diagnosis of nosocomial bacterial pneumonia in intubated patients undergoing ventilation: comparison of the usefulness of bronchoalveolar lavage and the protected specimen brush. Am J Med 85:499, 1988.

186. Chastre J, Viau F, Brun P, et al: Prospective evaluation of the protected specimen brush for the diagnosis of pulmonary infections in ventilated patients. Am Rev Respir Dis 130:924, 1984.

187. Chastre J, Fagon J-Y, Bornet-Lecso M: Evaluation of bronchoscopic techniques for the diagnosis of nosocomial pneumonia. Am J Resp Crit Care Med 152:231, 1995.

188. Marquette CH, Copin M-C, Wallet F, et al: Diagnostic tests for pneumonia in ventilated patients: prospective evaluation of diagnostic accuracy using histology as a diagnostic gold standard. Am J Respir Crit Care Med 151:1878, 1995.

189. Cheson BD, Samlowski WE, Tang TT, Spruance SL: Value of open-lung biopsy in 87 immunocompromised patients with pulmonary infiltrates. Cancer 55:453, 1985.

190. Haverkos HW, Dowling JN, Pasculle AW, et al: Diagnosis of pneumonitis in immunocompromised patients by open lung biopsy. Cancer 52:1093, 1983.

191. Warner DO, Warner MA, Divertie MB: Open lung biopsy in patients with diffuse pulmonary infiltrates and acute respiratory failure. Am Rev Respir Dis 137:90, 1988.

192. Crawford SW, Hackman RC, Clark JG: Open lung biopsy diagnosis of diffuse pulmonary infiltrates after marrow transplantation. Chest 94:949, 1988.

193. Harris RJ, Kavuru MS, Rice TW, Kirby TJ: The diagnostic and therapeutic utility of thoracoscopy. Chest 108:828, 1995.

194. Ferson PF, Landreneau RJ, Dowling RD, et al: Comparison of open versus thoracoscopic lung biopsy for diffuse infiltrative pulmonary disease. J Thorac Cardiovasc Surg 106:194, 1993.

195. Rubenfeld GD, Crawford SW: Withdrawing life support from mechanically ventilated recipients of bone marrow transplants: a case for evidence-based guidelines. Ann Intern Med 125:625, 1996.

196. Jackson SR, Tweeddale MG, Barnett MJ, et al: Admission of bone marrow transplant recipients to the intensive care unit: outcome, survival, and prognostic factors. Bone Marrow Transplant 21:697, 1998.

CHAPTER FORTY-NINE

Neurologic Complications

Margarida de Magalhães-Silverman, M.D., and Lisa Hammert, M.D.

Hematopoietic stem cell transplantation (HSCT) is used in the treatment of a number of genetic and acquired, neoplastic and non-neoplastic disorders. Neurologic complications are not usually considered one of the important causes of morbidity and mortality. The patient who undergoes HSCT, however, is highly susceptible to a variety of central nervous system (CNS) insults that result either from the underlying illness or untoward effects of therapy.

Research in the area of neurologic complications is limited in this patient population. The majority of studies have been retrospective or have relied on autopsy records.[1–8] The incidence of neurologic complications has varied from 37% to 70%, and such complications have been the cause of death in 6–26% of patients.[1, 5] Patients undergoing autologous transplantation generally have a lower frequency of neurologic complications than patients undergoing allogeneic transplantation.[2, 8] Neurologic complications in patients undergoing allogeneic HSCT are related to pharmacologic intervention of graft-versus-host disease (GVHD), the effects of GVHD, treatment of GVHD, and immunosuppression. Many of these complications are potentially reversible if promptly recognized and treated. A systematic approach to the differential diagnosis is key in the management of these cases. This chapter reviews the major neurologic complications, besides disease recurrence, encountered in these patients (Table 49–1).

METABOLIC ENCEPHALOPATHY

The single most common neurologic complication in patients undergoing HSCT is probably metabolic encephalopathy. The incidence of this complication has been estimated to be as high as 37%.[1] Hypoxia and/or ischemia, hepatic failure, electrolyte imbalance, and renal failure can cause metabolic encephalopathy. The clinical presentation of metabolic encephalopathy is delirium or depression of the CNS, usually without lateralizing neurologic findings.

TABLE 49–1. CAUSES OF NEUROLOGIC COMPLICATIONS

Metabolic encephalopathy
Drug toxicity
Infections
Neuromuscular immune-mediated diseases
Vascular complications
Leukoencephalopathy

An uncommon complication with severe, often fatal neurologic sequelae is hyperammonemia. The syndrome of idiopathic hyperammonemia[9, 10] occurs in patients who receive high-dose chemotherapy. This syndrome is characterized by the abrupt onset of altered mental status and respiratory alkalosis associated with markedly elevated plasma ammonium. It frequently results in intractable coma and death. This entity should be included in the differential diagnosis of any transplant recipient presenting with abnormal mental status. Because neurologic function can deteriorate rapidly, early recognition of this disorder and close monitoring of the patient are critical. It is likely multifactorial, and potential causes include ornithine transcarbamylase deficiency, glutamine synthetase deficiency, excess gastrointestinal production of ammonia, systemic catabolism, and high nitrogenous load because many patients receive intravenous alimentation.

The goal of the treatment it is to reduce the exogenous nitrogen load by holding intravenous nutrition, purging the gastrointestinal tract, and enhancing nitrogen excretion via continuous arteriovenous hemofiltration and the use of agents such as sodium benzoate or phenylbutirate.[11] It is important to diagnose and initiate therapy as soon as possible because hyperammonemia causes cerebral edema for which there is likely an early reversible phase followed by an irreversible phase. Hypoxic encephalopathy is sometimes easy to overlook if the patient is not tachypneic. Hepatic encephalopathy may occur as a consequence of severe hepatic GVHD or veno-occlusive disease. Renal failure usually results from nephrotoxic drugs used during the transplantation period (cisplatin in the conditioning regimen, cyclosporin or tacrolimus used as GVHD prophylaxis, or treatment with antibiotics such as aminoglycosides) or, more rarely, in the context of hemolytic uremic syndrome or radiation nephritis.

Simple doubling of the serum creatinine level occurs in 53% of patients, and as many as 24% may require dialysis. Initial investigation these patients should include biochemical tests designed to detect renal or hepatic impairment and arterial blood gas measurement.

Iatrogenic Wernicke encephalopathy has been described in several patients who underwent allogeneic HSCT.[12–14] It is characterized by the triad of altered mental status, ataxia, and ophthalmoplegia. Its etiology is attributed to post-transplantation failure to substitute thiamine in patients on long-term total parenteral nutrition. These patients require large amounts of thiamine to metabolize their carbohydrate intake, which can rapidly lead to depletion in thiamine stores and neurologic consequences.

DRUG TOXICITY

DRUGS USED IN THE CONDITIONING REGIMEN

Several drugs administered during and after the conditioning regimen may cause or contribute to CNS dysfunction. Among the drugs used to perform ablation, cytarabine, busulphan, ifosfamide, and carmustine can cause neurotoxicity.

Cytarabine is an analogue of deoxycytidine that is phosphorylated to its active metabolite, ara-CTP.[15] Ara-CTP inhibits DNA polymerase and is incorporated into DNA, resulting in strand breaks. It has been used mainly in the therapy of acute myeloid leukemia, either in standard dose (100–200 mg/m^2/day) or high dose (4–6 g/m^2/day). It is rarely included as part of conditioning regimens used to treat patients with myeloid leukemias and lymphomas. Somnolence, confusion, and seizures can occur with rapid infusion at high doses. Cerebellar toxicity, the principal side effect of high-dose cytosine arabinoside, can occur in 10% of patients and be irreversible in 3% of patients. A severe demyelinating neuropathy has also been associated with the use of high doses of this drug. Neurotoxicity seems to be correlated with renal function and age.

High-dose carmustine (BCNU) at doses ranging from 300 mg/m^2 to 600 mg/m^2 is currently used in conditioning regimens for patients with Hodgkin and non-Hodgkin disease.[16] It belongs to a group of compounds of nitrosoureas that are distinguished by their high lipid solubility and chemical instability. BCNU does cross the blood-brain barrier to a greater degree than similar compounds. For that reason, the drug has been used for the treatment of brain tumors. It can cause seizures, as was reported by Jagannath et al.[17] in 2 of 61 patients with relapsed Hodgkin disease treated with CBV (BCNU, cyclophosphamide, and etoposide).

Busulfan induces seizures, and two thirds of patients show epileptiform activity on electroencephalography despite prophylaxis.[17–21] Prophylaxis with phenytoin is recommended in patients receiving this drug. The incidence of busulfan-induced seizures is higher in children than adults. This drug crosses the blood-brain barrier, and it is thought to cause seizures as a direct toxic effect.

Ifosfamide can produce CNS toxicity when given at high doses.[23–25] Symptoms are usually, but not always, reversible and include mental status changes, seizures, ataxia, stupor, and even coma. There is not a clear-cut dose-toxicity relationship. Risk factors for this complication include the oral administration of the drug, renal dysfunction, hepatic disease, low serum albumin, and the presence of pelvic disease.[26] The etiology of the neurotoxicity is unclear, but it has been suggested that chloracetaldehyde, a metabolite of ifosfamide, may be involved in the pathogenesis because it is present in higher levels in patients experiencing neurotoxicity.[27] Ifosfamide should be discontinued in patients experiencing neurotoxicity, and all efforts should be made to avoid drugs that can affect the CNS such as sedatives and certain antiemetics.

IMMUNOSUPRESSANTS

Cyclosporine is a cyclic undecapeptide derived from the mycelia of two strains of *Fungi imperfecti*.[28] It is used for GVHD prophylaxis in allogeneic HSCT. Cyclosporine impairs interleukin-2 production from T-helper cells by inhibiting cytotoxic T-cell differentiation/proliferation and allowing expansion of the suppressor T-cell population. Nephrotoxicity and hypertension are common side effects of the drug.[29] Cyclosporine-related CNS toxicity is a less well-known toxic side effect of this drug. The neurologic complications are diverse (Table 49–2), ranging from tremor to coma, but are usually reversible with the discontinuation of the drug. Cyclosporine is highly lipophilic and, after either oral or intravenous administration, is rapidly distributed into both tissue and plasma stores. The majority is metabolized in the liver. Drugs that induce cytochrome P-450 (phenobarbital, phenytoin, carbamazepine, and rifampin) enhance the excretion of cyclosporine.[30]

The exact mechanism involved in cyclosporine neurotoxicity remains controversial. A direct neurotoxicity effect has been demonstrated in animals.[31] A retrospective analysis of 54 patients undergoing liver transplantation and receiving cyclosporine for antirejection purposes demonstrated an inverse relationship between cyclosporine-induced neurotoxicity and total serum cholesterol levels.[32] In 13 patients, CNS toxicity was observed during cyclosporine therapy, with a corresponding reduction in the total serum cholesterol in the first week after transplantation. It was suggested that low cholesterol levels might enable higher amounts of cyclosporine to remain unbound and pass through the blood-brain barrier, resulting in toxicity. This finding supports a direct toxic effect of cyclosporine.

There is also evidence that cyclosporine may cause endothelial damage with the release of vasoactive peptides, which may cause cerebral vasospasm.[33] Cyclosporine-induced neurotoxicity has been associated with a microangiopathic process, which may itself be triggered by endothelial injury.[34–36] Neurotoxicity has been associated most commonly with cyclosporine levels above the therapeutic range; however, a strict correlation between serum level and toxicity has not been found for individual patients over time. As previously mentioned, cyclosporine is metabolized in the liver and converted by isoenzymes of cytochrome P-450 into three major metabolites, M1, M17, and M21.[37] Monitoring M17 has been proposed as a strategy to reduce the risk of severe neurotoxicity.[38, 39] Impaired hepatic function may affect cyclosporine metabolism, allowing a slower rate of drug clearance, which compromises clearance of its metabolites and leads to increased risk of CNS toxicity. This may be observed in patients undergoing allogeneic transplantation for diseases such as thalassemia. In these patients, the liver is affected by iron overload and by blood-borne viral infections.

One of the most common CNS side effects of cyclosporine is tremor. It appears within a few days of initiation of the drug and is dose dependent. Its incidence varies from 21% to 55%. Cyclosporine has been associated

TABLE 49–2. NEUROTOXICITY OF CYCLOSPORINE

Tremor	Cortical blindness
Seizures	Neuropathy
Headaches	Mental status changes

with seizures in 5.5% of HSCT recipients.[40–42] In many cases, cyclosporine levels were elevated, but seizures have also been reported with low cyclosporine levels. They usually resolve spontaneously with reduction of the dose. Patients undergoing HSCT have a unique predisposition to seizures. Some of them may have received total body irradiation, cranial irradiation, or drugs such as high-dose cytarabine as part of or immediately before the conditioning regimen. These treatment modalities may lower the threshold for seizures. There are reports documenting seizures in patients on cyclosporine who have low levels of magnesium.[43–45] Low levels of magnesium are due to renal wasting induced by cyclosporine. Seizures have also been reported in patients who are hypertensive or receiving steroids.[29, 46]

Hypertension can occur as a direct result from cyclosporine nephrotoxicity and/or through an indirect vasoconstrictor effect of the drug.[47, 48] The treatment of seizures in patients receiving cyclosporine is problematic. Patients may be treated with phenytoin, phenobarbital, or carbamazepine. Because these drugs interfere with cytochrome P-450, however, it may be difficult to achieve a therapeutic cyclosporine level if they are used as therapy for cyclosporine-induced seizures.[49] For that reason, some investigators have recommended the use of valproic acid because this drug does not interfere with the metabolism of cyclosporine.[50, 51] Precipitating factors such as low magnesium or hypertension should be corrected.

A number of studies have reported a severe form of encephalopathy that may occur in patients taking cyclosporine. Patients may experience cortical blindness associated with confusion and sometimes even coma.[52, 53] In these cases, computed tomography (CT) and magnetic resonance imaging (MRI) results tend to be abnormal.[54] The abnormalities are mainly in the white matter and most commonly visible in the posterior temporal, parietal, and occipital lobes. These changes are thought to be focal areas of edema or ischemia, and they are radiolucent without contrast enhancement on CT. These lesions tend to resolve over a period of several weeks as clinical improvement occurs. Other clinical features in this patient population are ataxia and tremor. Other findings, although rare, include the development of paraparesis or quadraparesis.[55] In these patients, the decrease or discontinuation of cyclosporine causes clearing of all symptoms, and all patients return to their baseline neurologic status. In a few patients, reinstitution of the drug caused recurrence of their original symptoms. Other less-common reported neurologic manifestations of cyclosporine include the development of visual hallucinations, and in a few cases neuropathy has been linked to the use of cyclosporine.[56, 57]

In summary, cyclosporine is a valuable drug in patients undergoing allogeneic HSCT for the treatment of GVHD. Because of its widespread use, it is important to be familiar with the neurologic complications associated with this drug.

Tacrolimus is another drug used for prophylaxis and treatment of GVHD. Like cyclosporine, it has been associated with neurologic complications. Tacrolimus is a macrolide antibiotic produced by the soil fungus *Streptomyces tsukubaensis*. It is chemically distinct from cyclosporine, but both elicit similar immunosuppressant effects. In vitro

tacrolimus prevents activation of T-cell lymphocytes in response to mitogenic or antigenic stimulation.[58] The most common neurologic complications in patients on tacrolimus include headache, tremors, insomnia, paresthesias, and dizziness.[59, 60] Tremors and headache usually respond to a dose reduction. Other less-common neurologic complications include hallucinations, myoclonus, psychosis, incoordination, and even seizures. A reversible leukoencephalopathy very similar radiographically and pathologically to that seen with cyclosporine has been reported.[61]

Glucocorticoids are also frequently used in patients undergoing HSCT. They are used as part of antiemetic regimens and for prophylaxis and treatment of GVHD. The most common neurologic side effects from steroids include mental status changes and myopathy. As with cyclosporine, there are indirect effects of steroids on the nervous system, such as infections, complications as a consequence of steroid-induced immunosuppression, and cerebrovascular events caused by the steroid-induced hypertension. The mental status changes have been recognized for decades.[62] Mood alterations are common, and patients often experience a sense of euphoria and well-being. Less often, patients complain of dysphoria and mild agitation. Psychiatric symptoms are also frequent. Less common is mania or frank psychosis. This toxicity is often dose dependent. The most efficacious treatment for steroid-induced mental status changes is withdrawal of the drug, when possible. If not, patients usually respond well to neuroleptic and antianxiety medications.

Steroid-induced myopathy often occurs in patients undergoing allogeneic transplantation who experienced GVHD and are on long-term steroids for its treatment. Steroid myopathy is characterized by a symmetrical involvement of the proximal muscles.[63, 64] Patients usually have difficulties with tasks such as rising from a chair or climbing stairs. In these patients, reflexes are generally preserved. Serum enzyme levels are normal, and electromyography shows typical myopathic changes. Biopsy specimens usually show type IIB fiber atrophy. The treatment is to withdraw steroids, if possible, or to change to a nonfluorinated compound and physical therapy. This complication is more common with fluorinated steroids (dexamethasone) than with nonfluorinated ones (prednisone or methylprednisone).

Less frequent complications of steroid use are the development of pseudotumor cerebri and epidural lipomatosis.[65] The former can cause a syndrome of increased intracranial pressure and papilledema. The latter may cause spinal cord compression due to the abnormal fat deposition observed in patients on long-term steroids.

Thalidomide is been used to treat patients experiencing chronic GVHD.[66, 67] Drowsiness is observed frequently during the treatment with thalidomide, especially at higher doses (i.e., 200–400 mg/day) and is related to its sedative action. It can be minimized by administration at bedtime. Peripheral neuropathy has been recognized as a neurologic complication of thalidomide for some decades.[68, 69] The problem usually begins in the lower extremities with paresthesias and numbness and is often associated with hyperesthesias of the feet. In severe cases, upper motor muscle weakness may occur. Predisposing factors include high cumulative dose, older age of patients, and possibly total duration of therapy. The probable mechanism of thalido-mide-induced neuropathy is axonal degeneration without demyelination. The drug should be discontinued if pares-thesias or electrophysiologic evidence of neuropathy occurs. Withdrawal of the drug at the earliest possible stage of neuropathy increases the changes of full recovery of sensation. In some patients with severe chronic GVHD, thalido-mide has been reinstituted without recurrence of neurologic toxicity. Baseline and serial neurologic evaluations are indicated in these patients.

OTHER DRUGS

Chemotherapy and immunosuppressants are not the only drugs used during transplantation that may cause CNS toxicity. Some antibiotics have been associated with neuro-toxicity.[70, 71] Penicillins and imipenem may cause seizures.[72] Aminoglycosides and vancomycin may cause hearing loss. Neuromuscular blockade can be caused by aminoglyco-sides, causing a myasthenia-like syndrome. Of the antiviral agents used in HSCT, acyclovir has been reported to cause neurologic symptoms ranging from tremor to agitation, lethargy, disorientation, and even transient hemiparesis.[73, 74] In the setting of renal failure, seizures and reversible coma have been observed. Ganciclovir has been associated with delirium in one patient undergoing bone marrow trans-plantation, but the delirium was reversible with a dose decrease.[75] Seizures, although reported in patients with AIDS receiving the drug, have not been reported in this patient population. Foscarnet, another antiviral agent used for prophylaxis and treatment of cytomegalovirus, causes renal wasting of magnesium and calcium and has been associated with the development of muscle cramps, pares-thesias, and sometimes seizures.[76]

H_2 blockers such as cimetidine are frequently used in patients undergoing HSCT. Cimetidine has been associated with reversible confusion, delirium, depression, and even hallucinations. These complications seem to occur more often in very sick patients with impairment of renal and/ or hepatic functions. Treatment consists of withdrawing the drug.

INFECTIONS

CNS infections in HSCT recipients are related to neutro-penia and immunosuppression. For these reasons, the inci-dence of CNS infections is higher in the allogeneic setting. The incidence ranges from 2% in clinical studies to almost 14% in neuropathologic studies.[77–80] The infectious agents include a variety of bacterial, fungal, viral, and parasitic organisms. Infections in HSCT recipients may occur early in the post-transplantation period while the patient is wait-ing for neutrophil recovery. In this period, organisms in-volved include bacteria, fungi, and viruses. A second period is observed after engraftment in allogeneic transplant recipi-ents.[81] Infections are caused by the immunosuppression effects of drugs used to prevent or treat GVHD and by GVHD itself.

Clinical presentation is usually an alteration in the men-tal status. The clinical presentation is often more occult

than in immunocompetent patients. This is due to the decreased inflammatory response that is partly due to asso-ciated neutropenia and/or immunosuppression. Meningeal signs are often lacking, as are lateralizing signs. Work-up may include CT or MRI and spinal fluid examination, as in a nonimmunocompromised host. Brain biopsies are rarely performed.

BACTERIAL INFECTIONS

The incidence of bacterial infections involving the CNS ranges between 1.3% and 5.3%.[5, 6, 80] The low frequency may in part be due to the antimicrobial prophylaxis that is routinely used in the early transplantation period. No single bacterial organism has been predominantly responsible for the CNS infections in any series. Meningitis due to penicil-lin-resistant *Streptococcus pneumoniae* has been reported in two patients receiving long-term prophylaxis with trimeth-oprim-sulfamethoxazole.[81] Detailed discussions of bacterial infection can be found in Chapters 37 (Prevention) and 43 (Treatment).

FUNGAL INFECTIONS

Fungal infections mostly occur in allogeneic transplant re-cipients. Patients with acute or chronic GVHD have an increased risk of infectious episodes due the immunosup-pressive treatment and to delayed immunologic reconstitu-tion. Of the fungal organisms, *Aspergillus* (Fig. 49–1) is the most common and accounts for 30–50% of the CNS infections in this patient population.[1, 6] Antifungal prophy-

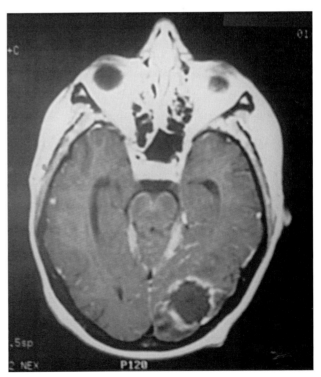

FIGURE 49–1. Computed tomograph of aspergillosis of the central ner-vous system.

laxis has been disappointing. *Aspergillus* has a tendency to invade blood vessels and frequently causes luminal thrombosis and parenchymal infarction. Invasive aspergillosis, whether involving the CNS or not, has a fatality rate approaching 100%. The literature decribes a few cases of resolution of CNS aspergillosis using an aggressive neurosurgical approach combined with antifungal therapy.[84, 85] The other major fungal pathogens include *Candida* and *Torulopsis*.[86–89] These organisms have been known to cause meningoencephalitis and multiple brain abscesses in these patients. Their frequency, however, is much lower than with *Aspergillus*. Interestingly, no abscesses or meningeal infections with *Histoplasma*, *Coccidioides*, or *Nocardia* have been reported. Other aspects of fungal infection are in Chapters 38 (Prevention) and 43 (Treatment).

PARASITIC INFECTIONS

CNS infection with *Toxoplasma gondii* occasionally occurs in HSCT recipients. Reactivation of latent toxoplasmic infection is a well-described entity in the immunocompromised host such as a patient with AIDS. The number of cases in HSCT does not exceed 50.[90–95] The incidence of reactivated toxoplasmosis in HSCT recipients has been calculated to be 2% of those who are seropositive prior to transplantation.

The most common presentations of toxoplasmosis in patients undergoing HSCT are encephalitis, pneumonitis, and myocarditis. Retinitis has also been reported. Almost all the cases occurred within the first 6 months after transplantation. Correct diagnoses may be difficult because spinal fluid examination and serologic test results are variable and may be atypical or inconclusive in immunocompromised hosts. Analysis using polymerase chain reaction (PCR) may be helpful but must be interpreted with caution as previously reported.[96] CT is a valid tool for detection and follow-up of some cases of cerebral toxoplasmosis, as shown in Figure 49–2. In some cases, stereotactic biopsy of a mass lesion may be necessary to make the definite diagnosis. This is rarely performed, however, because invasive procedures in HSCT recipients carry a high risk for complications. A combination of pyrimethamine and sulfadiazine is the standard treatment of toxoplasmosis. Myelosuppression with pyrimethamine remains a concern in these patients. Trimethoprim-sulphamethoxazole (TMP-SMX) is believed to protect against reactivation of toxoplasmoses in immunoincompetent patients such as patients with AIDS. Cases of reactivation have been described in patients undergoing HSCT and receiving TMP-SMX prophylaxis, however. It is possible that standard prophylaxis using 2 or 3 days of TMP-SMX per week may not provide adequate prophylaxis against *Toxoplasma*.

VIRAL INFECTIONS

Viral infections of the CNS are uncommon. They are usually due to cytomegalovirus (CMV), Epstein Barr virus, herpes simplex virus, varicella-zoster, and human herpesvirus type 6.

CMV can cause pneumonitis and gastrointestinal disease

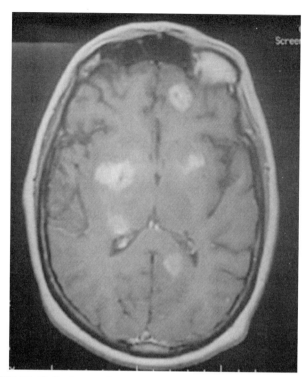

FIGURE 49–2. Computed tomograph of multiple central nervous system lesions of *Toxoplasma*.

in HSCT recipients. For unclear reasons, retinitis and encephalitis, which are common in the AIDS populations, are rare in HSCT recipients.[97–99] Patchell et al. reviewed the autopsy files of the Johns Hopkins Oncology Center from 1977 to 1982.[1] Systemic CMV infections were present in 28 of 780 patients. In seven patients, scattered microglial nodules and rod cells were found in gray and white matter. No cytomegalic or viral inclusions were present. Immunocytochemical stains for CMV were not performed. All seven patients had systemic CMV infections, and three of them had nonfocal encephalopathies that could not be explained by metabolic abnormalities. CMV cultures from brain showed no growth. Graus et al.[2] evaluated the neurologic complications in 425 patients who underwent HSCT. CNS infections occurred in nine patients, and in three of them CMV was the causative agent. In these three patients, there was severe systemic infection in multiple organs. All three died, and in two an autopsy was performed. The brain had microglial nodules and multiple areas of necrosis with hemorrhage and macrophage infiltrates in the cerebral hemispheres and brain stem.

After allogeneic HSCT, Epstein-Barr virus (EBV) infections may present with a wide range of clinical manifestations.[100, 101] A case of EBV meningoencephalitis has so far been reported in the literature.[101] The patient was successfully treated with ganciclovir. Herpesvirus type I reactivates in 80% of serologically positive recipients. Acyclovir is used routinely in these patients as prophylaxis to prevent viral shedding.[102] Despite the high incidence of reactivation, herpes encephalitis is rare. Patchell reported two cases of herpes simplex encephalitis.[101] Both patients had systemic infections that began less than 1 month after transplantation and persisted until death. The clinical manifestations were of a subacute nonfocal encephalopathy with progressive obtundation but no seizures. The diagnosis was confirmed before death in one patient by culture of the spinal fluid.

Varicella-zoster virus (VZV) infection is an issue in transplant recipients.[103, 104] VZV infection usually results from reactivation. The usual manifestation is in the form of dermatomal (localized) infection. Atkinson et al.[104] found that almost 50% of patients undergoing allogeneic transplantation for aplastic anemia or leukemia who survived at least 6 months experienced VZV infection. Clinical encephalitis developed in 4% of the HSCT recipients with active VZV infection. This study was done before the routine use of prophylactic acyclovir. The risk of VZV infection in the autologous transplant population is lower and depends on the underlying disease, with a risk of greater than 40% in patients with Hodgkin disease and 10–15% in solid tumors. Primary infection with this virus is rare but may be life threatening. This issue is more problematic in pediatric patients.

Human herpesvirus 6 (HHV-6) is a recently discovered herpesvirus that has been implicated as a pathogen in both normal and immunocompromised patients.[105] HHV-6 has been linked with exanthema subitum in the normal host. Most recently it has been associated with pneumonitis, encephalitis (Fig. 49–3), and marrow suppression in bone marrow and solid organ transplant recipients.[106–112] In some of the patients, HHV-6 has been successfully treated with antiviral medications, either ganciclovir or foscarnet. The diagnosis in the few cases reported has varied from visualization of the virus in pathology specimens to DNA detection in the spinal fluid in the absence of isolation of other pathogens. There are too few reported patients thus far to recognize a pattern of disease. HHV-6 activity has been studied in 15 allogeneic cases and in 11 autologous cases.[106] After transplantation, HHV-6 has been isolated from the peripheral blood mononuclear cells in almost 50% of the cases.

Adenovirus can cause infection of the lungs, liver, and kidneys in patients undergoing allogeneic transplantation. There is a single case of adenovirus meningoencephalitis in the literature.[113] Progressive multifocal leukoencephalopathy is extremely rare in this patient population but has been reported.[114] Viral infections are discussed in Chapters 36 (Prevention) and 43 (Treatment).

IMMUNE-MEDIATED NEUROMUSCULAR DISEASES

Immune-mediated neurologic complications of HSCT affect mainly the peripheral nervous system as opposed to the CNS. These complications include inflammatory demyelinating polyneuropathy, myasthenia gravis, and polymyositis. The clinical hallmark of all these three complications is lower motor neuron muscle weakness (muscle flaccidity, hypoactive deep tendon reflexes, and absence of extensor plantar reflex). Differential localization of the involved anatomic site usually needs further testing with electromyography, nerve conduction velocity, serologic testing for anticholinesterase antibody, and sometimes muscle biopsy.

DEMYELINATING DISEASES

The commonly accepted pathologic criteria for demyelinating disease are the destruction of myelin sheath of nerve fibers with relative sparing of neurons and axons. Such destruction is associated with perivascular mononuclear infiltrate followed by glial sclerosis. Diagnostic tests include slowing of nerve conduction by electromyography, elevated protein and immunoglobulin levels in the spinal fluid (oligoclonal bands, elevated IgG index) with or without pleocytosis, detection of cerebrospinal fluid myelin basic protein (CSF-MBP) by radioimmunoassay, complement-mediated antimyelin serum antibody, anti–T cells in CSF reactive to MBP, and antinerve antibody. Clinical features of demyelinating diseases are based on anatomic location of nerve fiber involvement.

Acute disseminated encephalitis usually follows infectious diseases. Cerebral demyelination after allogeneic transplantation has been described. Donor lymphocytes sensitized to CNS antigen are considered to be responsible for widespread cerebral demyelination.[115] Multiple sclerosis, on the other hand, is not a neurologic complication of HSCT. In contrast, HSCT is being used to treat a subset of patients with multiple sclerosis with a progressive clinical course.[116]

Acute inflammatory demyelinating polyneuropathy (Guillain-Barré syndrome) commonly follows acute viral syndrome and *Campylobacter jejuni* infection leading to paresthesias and rapid quadriplegia. Both humoral and cellular immune reactions against peripheral nerve antigen and MBP are defined. Acute inflammatory demyelinating polyneuropathy is described in allogeneic recipients with

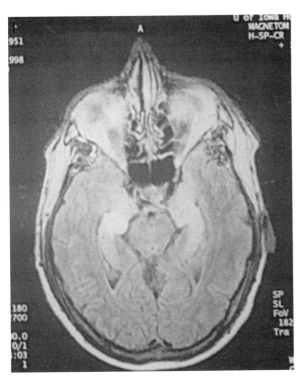

FIGURE 49–3. Magnetic resonance image of bilateral mesotemporal changes consistent with herpetic encephalitis.

or without any evidence of GVHD.[117] It usually occurs 2 to 3 months after allogeneic transplantation. Lymphocytes from patients with this disorder show mitogenic response after stimulation with crude peripheral myelin extract, whereas lymphocytes from donors and patients after recovery show no such reaction.[118] Early Guillain-Barré syndrome has been described within 1 month after autologous transplantation, supporting the hypothesis regarding cellular immune alteration in the pathogenesis of this complication.[119] Early onset of Guillain-Barré syndrome is also described in a patient with chronic myelogenous leukemia receiving donor buffy coat and interferon therapy for relapsed disease after allogeneic transplantation.[120, 121]

Chronic demyelinating polyneuropathy is an uncommon disorder that resembles Guillain-Barré but follows a more indolent and relapsing course. Nerve conduction is delayed along with elevated protein in the spinal fluid. Immunoglobulin deposits in peripheral nerves and the presence of anti-MBP suggest an immune origin with this disorder. Severe exacerbation of quiescent chronic inflammatory demyelinating polyneuropathy leading to quadriplegia and death has been reported during conditioning or immediately after HSCT.[122]

MYASTHENIA GRAVIS

Myasthenia gravis, a rare complication of transplantation, is a disease of unknown etiology in which muscle weakness is due to a disorder of the neuromuscular transmission. Frequent occurrence of this disease with thymoma, thymic hyperplasia, and other autoimmune diseases strongly suggests an underlying immune mechanism. Antiacetylcholine receptor antibody found in this condition not only interrupts postsynaptic signal transmission but causes complement-mediated destruction of postsynaptic membrane with loss of normal folds and receptor sites.

Few cases of myasthenia gravis have been reported in the setting of HSCT.[123–127] This disease manifestation mainly occurs in allogeneic HSCT recipients after discontinuation of immunosuppressive therapy for previously evident chronic GVHD.[126] Antibodies to acetylcholine receptor are present, as are the occasional antibodies to striated muscles. Myasthenia gravis usually responds satisfactorily to pyridostigmine treatment in addition to immunosuppressive therapy for chronic GVHD. Plasmapheresis may be temporarily required for respiratory failure. In several studies, serial peripheral blood and bone marrow studies of cytogenetics and red blood cell markers have shown evidence of donor cells only. No donor or family members had evidence of neurologic or muscular disease before or after transplantation. Other characteristic features of myasthenia gravis in HSCT recipients besides the demonstration of antiacetylcholine receptor antibody are the presence of chronic GVHD; absence of thymoma; increased frequency of human leukocyte antigens (HLA) CW1, CW7, and DR2 with no statistically significant association with HLA A2, B7, or B35; or donor-recipient sex mismatch.[127] Treatment of myasthenia in transplant recipients is similar to that of nonrecipients and includes intensive care management, immunosuppression, avoidance of drugs that may affect neuromuscular transmission, and the use of plasmapheresis

and intravenous immunoglobulin. Of interest, 11 of 54 patients without this disorder whose serum was examined after transplantation had low levels of antibodies against the acetylcholine receptor.[128] Furthermore, in one of these patients the concentration of antibodies increased over years before the disease became clinically apparent.

POLYMYOSITIS

Polymyositis has been described as a rare complication of patients undergoing HSCT. It is reported after both allogeneic and autologous HSCT. The disease is characterized by proximal muscle weakness and tenderness with elevation of muscle enzymes (creatine phosphokinase, aldolase). Electromyography shows characteristic myopathic changes. There are several reports of polymyositis in patients with chronic GVHD after allogeneic transplantation.[129] Chronic GVHD–related polymyositis responds well to prednisone and cyclosporin.[130, 131] There are some reported cases of polymyositis in patients undergoing autologous transplantation.[132]

VASCULAR COMPLICATIONS

Hemorrhagic complications are relatively rare in HSCT recipients because prophylactic platelet transfusion is performed if platelet number is under 10,000 or 20,000/mm³. These complications are more common in patients who experience platelet transfusion refractoriness, abnormal coagulation, and sepsis. Autologous transplantation is associated with a higher risk of CNS hemorrhagia. Graus et al. reviewed the neurologic complications of 425 (310 allogeneic and 115 autologous) patients who underwent transplantation.[2] Cerebral hemorrhage occurred in 16 patients (3.8%). Eleven of the 16 patients had subdural hematomas, which were more frequent in autologous (8%) than in allogeneic (0.6%) cases. This risk was related to platelet refractoriness and the diagnosis of acute myelogenous leukemia.[133]

Patients undergoing autologous transplantation for acute myelogenous leukemia experience a prolonged hematologic recovery. This delayed recovery results in a higher requirement for platelet transfusions and probably a higher risk of platelet refractoriness that favors the development of hemorrhagic complications. In an autopsy study of 109 patients undergoing allogeneic transplantation, subdural hematomas were present in 12% of the patients, but some were probably incidental findings without clinical relevance.[6] In the same series, 13% of recipients had subarachnoid bleedings and 5% intraparenchymal hematomas. In another study, the frequency of symptomatic subdural hematomas was 5% in HSCT recipients, with no difference between allogeneic and autologous recipients.[134]

Subdural hematomas can be overlooked early in their course, particularly in patients who are sedated or encephalopathic for metabolic reasons, because subdural hematomas may have no or mild lateralizing signs. CT is preferable to MRI in evaluating patients with possible CNS bleeds.[135] Treatment may be conservative or involve surgery and aggressive platelet support.[136, 137]

Ischemic stroke is infrequent in patients undergoing HSCT. Pathogenic mechanisms include hypercoagulability, chemotherapy-induced vasospasm, or chemotherapy-induced endothelial activation or damage. After autologous transplantation, temporary decreases of anticoagulants such as protein C and antithrombin C with a concomitant increase in fibrinogen have occurred.[138, 139] A report of an ischemic stroke attributed to reduced protein C level in an allogeneic transplant recipient has been published.[140] Increased levels of von Willebrand factor (as a marker for endothelial damage after HSCT) have been reported.[141] Cerebral infarction may also result from local thrombosis or an embolus from nonbacterial thrombotic endocarditis. An examination of all autopsies done at Johns Hopkins Oncology Center from 1972 to 1982 showed that nonbacterial thrombotic endocarditis occurred with a significantly higher frequency in HSCT recipients than the general autopsy population (7.7% vs. 1.9%).[142] With an increase in the number of transplantations being performed, it is possible that more cases of ischemic complications will be reported.

LEUKOENCEPHALOPATHY

Atkinson et al. first described leukoencephalopathy in marrow transplant recipients in 1977.[143] The combined application of CNS irradiation and intrathecal chemotherapy can result in irreversible brain damage. In a review of 415 patients receiving allogeneic transplants, Thompson et al. reported 7 patients with leukoencephalopathy.[144] They confirmed that the complication occurred exclusively in patients who had received cranial irradiation and/or intrathecal chemotherapy before conditioning and post-transplantation intrathecal methotrexate. The majority of patients with leukoencephalopathy have had acute lymphoblastic leukemia.[145] Thompson et al. also reported that the conditioning regimen by itself and post-transplantation methotrexate do not appear to increase the risk of this complication in patients who have not previously undergone CNS therapy or prophylaxis. These authors also suggested that there was no added benefit for the prevention of CNS relapse from the administration of more than four to five doses of post-transplantation intrathecal methotrexate and that more doses were associated with increased risk of leukoencephalopathy.

This complication may occur days to months after transplantation. The most common neurologic signs include dysarthria, ataxia, dysphasia, confusion, and decreased sensorium. The complication is not age-related, but it does occur more frequently in young patients. This is most likely related to the age distribution of acute lymphoblastic leukemia. Leukoencephalopathy is a degenerative process with no known effective therapy. CT of the brain and MRI are helpful diagnostic tools. Myelin basic protein is elevated in the spinal fluid during the early phase of the disorder.

NEUROLOGIC FINDINGS IN LONG-TERM SURVIVORS

The neurologic complications so far described usually occur during the immediate post-transplantation period. With more and more patients undergoing HSCT and being cured of their diseases, it is important to know if these patients are also at risk for long-term neurologic complications.

To our knowledge, only one report relates to long-term neurologic effects. Padovan et al. described the neurologic, neuropsychological, and neuroradiologic findings in 66 long-term marrow transplant survivors.[146] Fifty-nine patients had undergone allogeneic transplantation, whereas 7 had received autologous transplants. They underwent clinical examination, brief neuropsychological testing, and cranial MRI at 34 ± 26 months post transplantation. Neurologic examination results were abnormal in 64% of patients, and MRI results were abnormal in 65% (white matter lesions in 54% and atrophy in 11%). These findings were associated with the presence of chronic GVHD and with steroid and cyclosporine therapy. Neuropsychological impairment (cognitive deficits in 37%) was associated with long-term cyclosporine use and age. The authors concluded that the frequent neurologic abnormalities in long-term survivors of allogeneic transplantation are associated with chronic GVHD and with resulting immunosuppression. They also suggested the possibility of cerebral involvement in chronic GVHD.

In animal models, perivascular lymphocytes and donor-derived immune cells have been found in the CNS.[148, 149] The human neuropathologic data are controversial, however. A possible association with GVHD has been discussed for several histologic CNS changes such as multifocal cerebellar Purkinje and granular cell degeneration, necrotizing vasculitis, astrocytic gliosis, small foci of leukoencephlopathy, and lymphohistiocytic aggregates.[1, 5] In contrast, other series have found no autopsy-confirmed signs of central GVHD. The authors hypothesize a cerebral small vessel disease as consequence of GVHD leading to the long-term neurologic sequelae. We are likely to see more reports in the future dealing with this issue.

CONCLUSION

Neurologic complications are not considered among the most common causes of morbidity and mortality in patients undergoing HSCT. The complications can be caused by the toxicity of the chemotherapeutic agents, either directly on the CNS or indirectly through metabolic imbalance created by impairing functions of the renal, digestive, and /or other organ systems. They can also be caused by immunosuppressants used in treatment of GVHD/and/or infections of the CNS by bacterial, viral, fungal, or parasitic organisms, although the incidence of CNS infection after HSCT is low. Metabolic encephalopathy can be treated by reduction of exogenous nitrogen load. Withdrawal of immunosuppressants must be balanced against the severity of GVHD. Complications in the peripheral nervous system are usually induced by immunologic elements following allogeneic HSCT. Although the importance of neurologic complications appears to be minor immediately after HSCT, the late effects in long-term survivors remain relatively unknown. Additional studies are needed to clarify the effects of HSCT on long-term survivors.

REFERENCES

1. Patchell RA, White CL, Clark AW, et al: Neurologic complications of bone marrow transplantation. Neurology 35:300–306, 1985.
2. Graus F, Saiz A, Sierra J, et al: Neurologic complications of autologous and allogeneic bone marrow transplantation in patients with leukemia: a comparative study. Neurology 46:1004–1009, 1996.
3. Davis DG, Patchell RA: Neurologic complications of bone marrow transplantation. Neurol Clin 6:377–387, 1988.
4. Snider S, Bashir R, Bierman P: Neurologic complications after high dose chemotherapy and autologous bone marrow transplantation for Hodgkin's disease. Neurology 44:681–684, 1994.
5. Witznitzer M, Parker RJ, August CS, et al: Neurologic complications of bone marrow transplantation in childhood. Ann Neurol 16:569–576, 1984.
6. Mohrmann RL, Mah V, Vinters HV: Neuropathologic findings after bone marrow transplantation: an autopsy study. Hum Pathol 21:630–639, 1990.
7. Gallardo D, Ferra BC, Berlanga JJ, et al: Neurologic complications after allogeneic bone marrow transplant. Bone Marrow Transplant 18:1135–1139, 1996.
8. Guerrero A, Perez-Simon JA, Gutierrez N, et al: Neurological complications after autologous stem cell transplantation. Eur Neurol 41:48–50, 1999.
9. Mitchell RB, Wagner MD, Karp EJ, et al: Syndrome of idiopathic hyperammonemia after high-dose chemotherapy: review of nine cases. Am J Med 85:662–667, 1988.
10. Davies Sm, Szabo E, Wagner JE, et al: Idiopathic hyperammonemia: a frequently fatal complication of bone marrow transplantation. Bone Marrow Transplant 17:1119–1125, 1996.
11. del Rosario, Werlin SL, Lauer SJ: Hyperammonemic encephalopathy after chemotherapy: survival after treatment with sodium benzoate and sodium phenylacetate. J Clin Gastroenterol 25:682–684, 1997.
12. Bleggi-Torres LF, de Medeiros BC, Ogasawara VSA, et al: Iatrogenic Wernicke's encephalopathy in allogeneic bone marrow transplantation: a study of eight cases. Bone Marrow Transplant 20:391–395, 1997.
13. Matolino I, Caponetto A, Scime R, et al: Wernicke-like encephalopathy after autologous bone marrow transplantation. Haematologica 75:282–284, 1990.
14. Torres LFB, Ogassawara VSA, Pasquini R: Acute deficiency of thiamin in bone marrow transplanted patients. Neuropathol Appl Neurobiol 19:451, 1993.
15. Perry MC: Toxicity: ten years later. Semin Oncol 19:453–609, 1992.
16. Burger PC, Kamenar E, Schold SC, et al: Encephalomyelopathy following high-dose BCNU therapy. Cancer 48:1318–1327, 1981.
17. Jagannath S, Armitage JO, Dicke K, et al: Prognostic factors for response and survival after high-dose cyclophosphamide, carmustine, and etoposide with autologous bone marrow transplantation for relapsed Hodgkin's disease. J Clin Oncol 7:179–185, 1989.
18. De La Camara R, Tomas JF, Figuera A, et al: High dose busulfan and seizures. Bone Marrow Transplant 7:363–364, 1991.
19. Hartmann O, Banhamou E, Beaujean F, et al: High-dose busulfan and cyclophosphamide with autologous bone marrow transplantation support in advanced malignancies in children: a phase II study. J Clin Oncol 12:1804–1810, 1986.
20. Vassal G, Deroussent A, Hartmann O, et al: Dose dependent neurotoxicity of high-dose busulfan in children: a clinical and pharmacological study. Cancer Res 50:6203–6207, 1990.
21. Grigg AP, Shepherd JD, Phillips GL: Busulfan and phenytoin. Ann Intern Med 111:1049–1050, 1989.
22. Ghany AM, Tutschka PJ, McGhee RB, et al: Cyclosporin associated seizures in bone marrow recipients given busulfan and cyclophosphamide preparative regimen. Transplantation 52:310–315, 1991.
23. Vose JM: Dose-intensive ifosfamide for the treatment of non-Hodgkin's lymphoma. Semin Oncol 23(3 Suppl 6):33–37, 1996.
24. Elias A, Elder JP, Shea T, et al: High dose ifosfamide with mesna uroprotection: a phase I study. J Clin Oncol 8:170–178, 1990.
25. Pratt CB, Green AA, Horowitz ME, et al: Central nervous system toxicity following the treatment of pediatric patients with ifosfamide/mesna. J Clin Oncol 4:1253–1261, 1986.
26. Cerny T, Castiglione M, Brunner K, et al: Ifosfamide by continuous infusion to prevent encephalopathy. Lancet 335:175, 1990.
27. Goren MP, Wright RK, Pratt CB, et al: Dechloroethylation of ifosfamide and neurotoxicity. Lancet 2:1219–1220, 1986.
28. Kahan DB: Cyclosporin. N Engl J Med 321:1725–1738, 1987. Allen RD, Hunnisett AG, Morris PJ: Cyclosporin and magnesium. Lancet 1:1283–1284, 1985.
29. Joss DV, Barrett AJ, Kendra JR, et al: Hypertension and convulsions in children receiving cyclosporin [Letter] Lancet 1:906, 1982.
30. Lucey MR, Kolars JC, Merion RM, et al: Cyclosporin toxicity at therapeutic levels and cytochrome P-450 IIA. Lancet 335:11–15, 1990.
31. Famiglio L, Racusen L, Fivush B, et al: Central nervous system toxicity of cyclosporin in a rat model. Transplantation 48:316–321, 1989.
32. De Groen PC, Aksamt AJ, Rakela J, et al: Central nervous system toxicity after liver transplantation. N Engl J Med 317:861–866, 1987.
33. Zoja C, Furci L, Ghilardi F, et al: Cyclosporin-induced endothelial cell injury. Lab Invest 55:455–462, 1986.
34. Holler E, Kolb HJ, Hiller E, et al: Microangiopathy in patients with cyclosporin prophylaxis who developed acute graft versus host disease after HLA-identical bone marrow transplantation. Blood 73:2018–2024, 1989.
35. van Buren D, van Buren CT, Flechner SM, et al: De novo hemolytic uremic syndrome in renal transplant recipients immunosuppressed with cyclosporin. Surgery 95:54–62, 1985.
36. Kalhs P, Brugger S, Schawarzinger I, et al: Microangiopathy following allogeneic marrow transplantation: association with cyclosporin and methylprednisolone for graft versus host disease prophylaxis. Transplantation 60: 949–957, 1995.
37. Kunzerdof U, Brockmoller J, Jochimsens I, et al: Immunosuppressive properties of cyclosporin metabolites. Lancet 1:734–735, 1989.
38. Kunzerdof U, Brockmoller J, Jochimsen F, et al: Cyclosporin metabolites and central nervous system toxicity. Lancet 1:1223, 1988.
39. Trull AK, Tan KKC, Roberts NB, et al: Cyclosporin metabolites and neurotoxicity. Lancet 2:448, 1989.
40. O' Sullivan DP: Convulsions associated with cyclosporin A. Bone Marrow J 290:858, 1985.
41. Appleton RE, Farrell K, Teal P, et al: Complex partial status epilepticus associated with cyclosporin A therapy. J Neurosurg Psychiatry 52:1068–1071, 1989.
42. Reece DE, Frei-Lahr DA, Shepherd JD, et al: Neurologic complications in allogeneic bone marrow transplant patients receiving cyclosporin. Bone Marrow Transplant 8:393–401, 1991.
43. June H, Thompson B, Kennedy S, et al: Profound hypomagnesemia and renal magnesium wasting associated with the use of cyclosporin for marrow transplantation. Transplantation 39:620–624, 1985.
44. Deleted in proof.
45. Thompson C, June CH, Sullivan KH, Thomas DE: Association between cyclosporin neurotoxicity and hypomagnesaemia. Lancet 2:1116–1120, 1984.
46. Durrant S, Chipping PM, Palmer S, et al: Cyclosporin A, methylprednisolone, and convulsions [Letter] Lancet 2:829–830, 1982.
47. Moody H, Matz L, Hurst P: Vascular lesions as manifestations of cyclosporin nephrotoxicity [Letter]. Lancet 1:1221–1222, 1986.
48. Shulman H, Striker G, Deeg HJ, et al: Nephrotoxicity of cyclosporin A after allogeneic marrow transplantation. N Engl J Med 305:1392–1395, 1981.
49. Freeman DJ, Laupacis A, Keown PA, et al: Evaluation of cyclosporin-phenytoin interaction with observations on cyclosporin metabolites. Br J Clin Pharmacol 18:887–893, 1984.
50. Fischman MA, Hull D, Bartus SA, et al: Valproate for epilepsy in renal transplant recipients receiving cyclosporin. Transplantation 48:542, 1989.
51. Hillebrand G, Castro LA, Van Scheidt W, et al: Valproate for epilepsy in renal transplant patients receiving cyclosporin. Transplantation 43:915–916, 1987.
52. Memon M, deMagalhaes-Silverman M, Bloom EJ, et al: Reversible cyclosporine induced cortical blindness in allogeneic bone marrow transplant recipients. Bone Marrow Transplant 15:283–286, 1995.
53. Rubin AM, Kang H: Cerebral blindness and encephalopathy with cyclosporin A toxicity. Neurology 37:1072–1076, 1987.
54. Turwit CL, Denaro CP, Lake JR, et al: MR imaging of reversible cyclosporin A–induced neurotoxicity. Am J Neuroradiol 12:651–659, 1991.
55. Lind MJ, Mcwilliam L, Jip J, et al: Cyclosporin associated demyelination following allogeneic bone marrow transplantation. Hematol Oncol 7:49–52, 1989.
56. Berden JHM, Hoitsma AJ, Merx JL et al: Severe central nervous

system toxicity associated with cyclosporin. Lancet 1:219–220, 1985.

57. Fiorani L, Bandini G, D' Allessandro R, et al: Cyclosporin A neurotoxicity after allogeneic bone marrow transplantation. Bone Marrow Transplant 14:175–176, 1994.

58. Nash RA, Pineiro LA, Storb R, et al: FK506 in combination with methotrexate for prevention of graft-versus-host disease after marrow transplantation from matched unrelated donors. Blood 88:3634–3641, 1996.

59. Koehler MT, Howrie D, Mirro J, et al: FK506 (tacrolimus) in the treatment of steroid-resistant acute graft-versus-host disease in children undergoing bone marrow transplantation. Bone Marrow Transplant 15:895–899, 1995.

60. Spencer CM, Goa KL, Gillis JC: Tacrolimus: an update of its pharmacology and clinical efficacy in the management of organ transplantation. Drugs 54:925–975, 1997.

61. Thyagarajan GK, Cobanoglu A, Johnston W: FK506-induced fulminant leukoencephalopathy after single-lung transplantation. Ann Thorac Surg 64:1461–1464, 1997.

62. Hall RCW, Popkin MK, Stickney SK, et al: Presentation of the steroid psychosis. J Nerv Ment Dis 167:229–236, 1979.

63. Askari A, Vignos PJ, Moskowitz RW: Steroid myopathy in connective tissue disease. Am J Med 61:485–492, 1976.

64. Khaleeli AA, Edwards RHT, Gohil K, et al: Corticosteroid myopathy: a clinical and pathological study. Clin Endocrinol 18:155–166, 1983.

65. Guegan Y, Fardoun R, Launois B, et al: Spinal cord compression by extradural fat after prolonged corticosteroid therapy. J Neurosurg 56:267, 1982.

66. Rovelli A, Arrigo C, Nesi F, et al: The role of thalidomide in the treatment of refractory chronic graft-versus-host disease following bone marrow transplantation in children. Bone Marrow Transplant 21:577–581, 1998.

67. Forsyth CJ, Cremer PD, Torzillo P, et al: Thalidomide responsive chronic pulmonary GVHD. Bone Marrow Transplant 17:291–293, 1996.

68. Clemmensen DJ, Olsen PZ, Andersen KE: Thalidomide neurotoxicity. Arch Dermatol 120:338–341, 1984.

69. Fullerton PM, O' Sullivan DJ: Thalidomide neuropathy: a clinical electrophysiological, and histological follow-up study. J Neurol Neurosurg Psychiatry 31:543–551, 1968.

70. Snavely SR, Hodges GR: The neurotoxicity of antibacterial agents. Ann Intern Med 101:92–104, 1984.

71. Frytak S, Moertel CG, Childs DS: Neurologic toxicity associated with high-dose metronidazole therapy. Ann Intern Med 88: 361–362, 1978.

72. Eng RHK, Munsif AN, Yangco BG, et al: Seizure propensity with imipenem. Arch Intern Med 149:1881–1883, 1989.

73. Wade JC, Meyers JD: Neurologic symptoms associated with parenteral acyclovir treatment after marrow transplantation. Ann Intern Med 98:921–925, 1983.

74. Cohen SMZ, Minkove JA, Zevley JW, et al: Severe but reversible neurotoxicity from acyclovir. Ann Intern Med 100:920, 1984.

75. Davis CL, Springmeyer S, Gmerek BJ: Central nervous system side effects of gancyclovir. N Engl J Med 322:933–934, 1990.

76. Chrisp P, Clissold SP: Foscarnet: a review of its antiviral activity, pharmacokinetic properties and therapeutic use in immunocompromised patients with cytomegalovirus retinitis. Drugs 41:104–129, 1991.

77. Walter EA, Bowden RA: Infection in the bone marrow transplant recipient. Infect Dis Clin North Am 9:823–847, 1995.

78. Meyers JD, Atkinson K: Infection in bone marrow transplantation. Clin Haematol 12:791–811, 1983.

79. Ringden O, Lonnqvist B, Lundgren G, et al: Experience with a cooperative bone marrow transplantation program in Stockholm. Transplantation 33:500–504, 1982.

80. Winston DJ, Gale RP, Meyer DV: Infectious complications of human bone marrow transplantation. Medicine 58:1–31, 1979.

81. Lenarsky C: Immune recovery after bone marrow transplantation. Curr Opin Hematol 2:409–412, 1995.

82. D, Antonio D, DiBartolomeo P, Iacone A, et al: Meningitis due to penicillin-resistant *Streptococcus pneumoniae* in patients with chronic graft versus host disease. Bone Marrow Transplant 9:299–300, 1992.

83. Gubbins PO, Bowman JL, et al: Antifungal prophylaxis to prevent invasive mycoses among bone marrow transplantation recipients. Pharmacotherapy 18:549–564, 1998.

84. Khoury H, Adkins D, Miller G, et al: Resolution of invasive central nervous system aspergillosis in a transplant recipient. Bone Marrow Transplant 20:179–180, 1997.

85. Denning DW, Stevens DA: Antifungal and surgical treatment of invasive aspergillosis. Rev Infect Dis 20:1147–1201, 1990.

86. Gaziev D, Baronciani D, Galimberti M, et al: Mucormycosis after bone marrow transplantation: report of four cases of thalassemia and review of the literature. Bone Marrow Transplant 17:409–414, 1996.

87. Cutsem V, Boogaerts MA, Tricot G: Multiple brain abcesses caused by *Torulopsis glabrata* in an immunocompromised patient. Mykosen 29:306–308, 1986.

88. Guppy KH, Thomas K, Anderson D: Cerebral fungal infections in the immunocompromised host: a literature review and a new pathogen—*Chaetomum atrobrunneum*: a case report. Neurosurgery 43:1463–1469, 1998.

89. Verfaillie C, Weisdorf D, Haake R, et al: Candida infections in bone marrow transplant recipients. Bone Marrow Transplant 8:177–184, 1991.

90. Brinkman K, Debast S, Sauerwein R, et al: Toxoplasma retinitis/encephalitis 9 months after allogeneic bone marrow transplantation. Bone Marrow Transplant 21:635–636, 1998.

91. Slavin MA, Meyers JD, Remington JS, et al: *Toxoplasma gondii* infection in bone marrow transplant recipients: a 20 year experience. Bone Marrow Transplant 13:549–557, 1994.

92. Seong DC, Przepiorka D, Bruner JM, et al: Leptomeningeal toxoplasmosis after allogeneic marrow transplantation. Am J Clin Oncol 16:105–108, 1993.

93. Deroiun F, Gluckman E, Beauvais MB, et al: Toxoplasma infection after human allogeneic bone marrow transplantation. Bone Marrow Transplant 1:167–173, 1986.

94. Hirsch R, Burke BA, Kersey JH: Toxoplasmosis in BMT recipients. J Pediatr 105:426–428, 1984.

95. Lowenberg B, Gijn J, Prins E, et al: Fatal cerebral toxoplasmosis in a BMT recipient with leukemia. Transplantation 35:30–34, 1983.

96. Johnson JD, Butcher PD, Savva D, et al: Application of the polymerase chain reaction to the diagnosis of human toxoplasmosis. J Infect 26:147–158, 1993.

97. Cordonnier C, Feuilhade F, Vernant JP, et al: Cytomegalovirus encephalitis occurring after bone marrow transplantation. Scand J Haematol 31:248–252, 1983.

98. Dorfman LJ: Cytomegalovirus encephalitis in adults. Neurology 23:136–144, 1973.

99. Vinters HV, Kwok MK, Ho HW, et al: Cytomegalovirus in the nervous system of patients with acquired immune deficiency syndrome. Brain 112:245–268, 1989.

100. Dellemijn PLI, Brandenburg A, Niesters HGM, et al: Successful treatment with gancyclovir of presumed Epstein-Barr meningo-encephalitis following bone marrow transplant. Bone Marrow Transplant 16:311–312, 1995.

101. Oettle H, Wilborn F, Schmidt H, Siegert W: Treatment with gancyclovir and Ig for acute Epstein-Barr virus infection after allogeneic bone marrow transplantation. Blood 82:2257–2262, 1993.

102. Saral R, Burns WH, Laskin OL, et al: Acyclovir prophylaxis of herpes simplex virus infection. N Engl J Med 305:63–67, 1981.

103. Locksley RM, Flournoy N, Sullivan KM, et al: Infection with varicella zoster virus infection after marrow transplantation. J Infect Dis 152:1172–1181, 1985.

104. Atkinson K, Meyers JD, Storb R, et al: Varicella-zoster virus infection after bone marrow transplantation for aplastic anemia or leukemia. Transplantation 29:47–50, 1980.

105. Kimberlin DW: Human herpes virus 6 and 7: identification of newly recognized viral pathogens and their association with human disease. Pediatr Infect Dis J 17:59–67, 1998.

106. Kadakia MP, Rybka WB, Stewart JA, et al: Human herpes virus 6: infection and disease following autologous and allogeneic bone marrow transplantation. Blood 87:5341–5354, 1996.

107. Knox KK, Carrigan DR: Chronic myelosuppression associated with persistent bone marrow infection due to human herpes virus 6 in a bone marrow transplant recipient. Clin Infect Dis 22:174–175, 1996.

108. Yanagihara K, Tanaka-Taya K, Itagaki Y, et al: Human herpesvirus 6 meningoencephalitis with sequelae. Pediatr Infect Dis J 14:240–242, 1995.

109. Novoa LJ, Nagra RM, Nakawatase T, et al: Fulminant demyelinating encephalomyelitis associated with productive HHV-6 infection in an immunocompetent adult. J Med Virol 52:301–308, 1997.

110. Rieux C, Gautheret-Dejean A, Challine-Lehmann D, et al: Human herpes virus-6 meningoencephalitis in a recipient of an unrelated allogeneic bone marrow transplantation. Transplantation 65:1408–1411, 1998.
111. Mookerjee BP, Vogelsang G: Human herpes virus-6 encephalitis after bone marrow transplantation: successful treatment with gancyclovir. Bone Marrow Transplant 35:905–906, 1997.
112. Drobyski WR, Knox KK, Majewski D, et al: Brief report: fatal encephalitis due to variant B human herpesvirus-6 infection in a bone marrow transplant recipient. N Engl J Med 22:171–173, 1994.
113. Davis DG, Henslee J, Markesberry WR: Fatal adenovirus meningoencephalitis in a bone marrow transplant patient. Ann Neurol 23:385–389, 1988.
114. Przepiorka D, Jaeckle KA, Birdwell RR, et al: Successful treatment of progressive multifocal leukoencephalopathy with low-dose interleukin-2. Bone Marrow Transplant 20:983–987, 1997.
115. Kelly P, et al: Multifocal remitting-relapsing cerebral demyelination twenty years after allogeneic transplantation. J Neuropathol Exp Neurol 55:992, 1996.
116. McAlester LD, Betty PG, Rose J: Allogeneic bone marrow transplantation for chronic myelogenous leukemia in a patient with multiple sclerosis. Bone Marrow Transplant 19:395, 1997.
117. Wen PY, Alyea EP, Simon D, Herbest RS, et al: Guillain-Barré syndrome following allogeneic bone marrow transplantation. Neurology 49:1711, 1997.
118. Eliashiv S, Brenner T, Abramsky O, et al: Acute inflammatory polyneuropathy following bone marrow transplantation. Bone Marrow Transplant 8:315, 1991.
119. Mudad R, Hussain A, Peters WP: Guillain-Barré syndrome following autologous bone marrow transplantation. Am J Clin Oncol 18:167, 1995.
120. Johnson NT, Crawford SW, Sargur M: Acute acquired demyelinating polyneuropathy with respiratory failure following high dose systemic cytosine arabinoside and marrow transplantation. Bone Marrow Transplant 2:203, 1987.
121. Schwarzer A, et al: Guillain Barré syndrome—a possible side effect of buffy coat transfusion and IFN alpha therapy in relapsed CML after bone marrow transplantation. Ann Oncol 6:617, 1995.
122. Openshaw H, et al: Exacerbation of inflammatory demyelinating polyneuropathy after bone marrow transplantation. Bone Marrow Transplant 7:411, 1991.
123. Lefvert AK, Bolme P, Hammarstrom L, et al: Bone marrow grafting selectively induces the production of acetylcholine receptor antibodies, immunoglobulins bearing related idiotypes and anti-idiotype antibodies. Ann N Y Acad Sci 505:825, 1987.
124. Gray JM, Casademont J, Monforte, et al: Myasthenia gravis after allogeneic bone marrow transplantation: report of new case and pathogenic consideration. Bone Marrow Transplant 5:435, 1990.
125. Lefvert AK, Bjorkholm M: Antibodies against acetylcholine receptor in hematologic disorder: report of myasthenia gravis after bone marrow grafting. N Engl J Med 317:170, 1987.
126. Zaja F, Barillari G, Russo D: Myasthenia gravis after allogeneic bone marrow transplantation: a case report and a review of the literature. Acta Neurol Scand 96:256, 1997.
127. Mackey JR, Desai S, Larratt L, et al: Myasthenia gravis in association with allogeneic bone marrow transplantation: clinical observation, therapeutic implication and review of literature. Bone Marrow Transplant 19:939, 1997.
128. Smith CIE, Hammarstrom L, Levert AK: Bone marrow grafting induces acetylcholine receptor antibody formation. Lancet 1:978, 1985.
129. Parker PM, Penshaw H, Forman SJ: Myositis associated with graft versus host disease. Curr Opin Rheumatol 9:513, 1997.
130. Anderson BA, Young PV, Kean WF, et al: Polymyositis in chronic graft versus host disease. Arch Neurol 39:188, 1982.
131. Parker P, et al: Polymyositis as a manifestation of chronic graft versus host disease. Medicine 75:279, 1996.
132. Scmidley JW, Galloway P: Polymyosistis following autologous bone marrow transplantation in Hodgkin's disease. Neurology 40:1003, 1990.
133. Pomeranz S, Naparstek E, Ashkenasi E, et al: Intracranial haematomas following bone marrow transplantation. J Neurol 241:252–256, 1994.
134. Adams JA, Gordon AA, Jiang YZ, et al: Thrombocytopenia after bone marrow transplantation for leukemia: changes in megakaryocyte growth promoting activity. Br J Haematol 75:195–201, 1990.
135. Nakamura N, Akiyama H, Mishima K, et al: Subdural hematoma during allogeneic bone marrow transplantation for chronic myelogenous leukemia. Acta Haematol 88:163–164, 1992.
136. Bender MB, Christoff N: Nonsurgical treatment of subdural hematomas. Arch Neurol 31:73–79, 1974.
137. Croce MA, Dent DL, Menke PG, et al: Acute subdural hematoma: nonsurgical management of selected patients. J Trauma 36:820–827, 1994.
138. Kaufman PT, Joneds RB, Greenberg CS, et al: Autologous bone marrow transplantation and factor XII, factor VII, and protein C deficiencies. Cancer 66:515–521, 1990.
139. Gordon B, Haire W, Kessinger A, et al: High frequency of antithrombin 3 and protein C deficiency following autologous bone marrow transplantation and lymphoma. Bone Marrow Transplant 8:497–502, 1991.
140. Gordon BG, Saving KL, McCallister JAM, et al: Cerebral infarction associated with protein C deficiency following allogeneic bone marrow transplant. Bone Marrow Transplant 8:323–325, 1991.
141. Collins PW, Gutteridge CN, O'Driscoll A, et al: Von Willebrand factor as a marker of endothelial cell activation following BMT. Bone Marrow Transplant 10:499–506, 1992.
142. Patchell RA, White CL, Clark AW, et al: Nonbacterial thrombotic endocarditis in bone marrow transplant patients. Cancer 55:631–635, 1985.
143. Atkinson K, Clink H, Lawler S, et al: Encephalopathy following bone marrow transplantation. Eur J Cancer 13:623–625, 1977.
144. Thompson CB, Sanders JE, Flournoy N, et al: The risks of central nervous system relapse and leukoencephalopathy in patients receiving marrow. Blood 67:195–199, 1986.
145. Johnson Fl, Thomas ED, Clark BS, et al: A comparison of marrow transplantation with chemotherapy for children with acute lymphoblastic leukemia in second or subsequent remission. N Engl J Med 305:846–851, 1981.
146. Pavodan CS, Tarek AY, Schleuning M, et al: Neurological and neuroradiological findings in long-term survivors of allogeneic bone marrow transplantation. Ann Neurol 42:627–633, 1998.
147. Hickey WF, Kimura H: Graft-vs-host disease elicits expression of class I and class II histocompatibility antigens and the presence of scattered T lymphocytes in rat central nervous system. Science 239:1035–1038, 1988.
148. Unger ER, Sung JH, Manivel JC, et al: Male donor-derived cells in the brains of female sex-mismatched bone marrow transplant recipients: a Y-chromosome specific in situ hybridization study. J Neuropathol Exp Neurol 52:460–470, 1993.
149. Hoogerbrugge PM, Suzuki K, Poorhuis BJ, et al: Donor derived cells in the central nervous system of twitcher mice after bone marrow transplantation. Science 239:1035–1038, 1988.

CHAPTER FIFTY

Transfusion Support in Hematopoietic Stem Cell Transplantation

Ileana López-Plaza, M.D., and Darrell J. Triulzi, M.D.

The transfusion service plays an important supporting role in hematopoietic stem cell transplantation (HSCT) by providing blood components and guidance on optimal blood component therapy during the peritransplantation period. The number of blood components available for transfusion has increased, allowing for more-specific transfusion therapy. Blood component requirements depend on donor and/or recipient factors (i.e., human leukocyte antigen [HLA] match grade and ABO compatibility), the patient's pretransplantation conditioning regimen, the source of stem cells, use of growth factors, and post-transplantation immunosuppressive therapy), all of which influence hematologic engraftment and immune reconstitution. Table 50–1 summarizes the transfusion requirements in autologous and allogeneic HSCT at our institution. The shift toward peripheral blood progenitor cells (PBPC) has markedly decreased transfusion requirements.

The introduction of recombinant hematopoietic growth factors has substantially reduced transfusion requirements, largely by augmenting PBPC collections quantitatively and qualitatively. Granulocyte and granulocyte-macrophage stimulating factors enhance the peripheral mobilization of noncommitted and committed hematopoietic stem cells.[1–3] The transfusion of these products enriched for hematopoietic stem cells has significantly shortened the period of the neutropenia,[1–3] shortened the time to platelet engraftment, and decreased platelet transfusion requirements.[2–4] More recently, two thrombopoietic growth factors have been identified. Clinical studies have shown that treatment with recombinant human interleukin-11 can reduce the time to platelet recovery and the number of platelet transfusions after chemotherapy.[5] This growth factor is now approved and commercially available. The other thrombopoietic factor, thrombopoietin,[6] is in clinical trials to assess its impact on platelet engraftment and transfusion support. Erythropoietin is not routinely used in the HSCT patient population because of its marginal impact on red blood cell transfusions.[7–9]

PROPHYLACTIC PLATELET TRANSFUSIONS

Prophylactic platelet transfusion has been the standard of care for hematologic malignancy/chemotherapy-induced thrombocytopenia for several decades. This intervention, first used in acute leukemias, has decreased the incidence of fatal bleeding during therapy to less than or equal to 1% and currently is a widespread practice in oncology.[10] Multiple studies have been conducted to evaluate whether and when prophylactic platelet transfusion should be given. Because early studies observed that gross hemorrhage would rarely occur with platelet counts of greater than or equal to 20,000/mm^3,[11] later studies were able to show that the risk of bleeding significantly increased only when the thrombocytopenia reaches platelet counts of less than 10,000/mm^3.[12] It was also observed that an increased bleeding risk of 5000–20,000/mm^3 correlated with the presence of clinical factors such as fever, the clinical setting in which thrombocytopenia occurred, and the underlying disease.[13, 14] Although a platelet count of 20,000/mm^3 is still the most

TABLE 50–1. BLOOD USE IN STEM CELL TRANSPLANTATION*

DIAGNOSIS	N	TYPE	SOURCE	RED BLOOD CELLS (UNITS)	PLATELETS‡
Breast	40	Auto	PBPC	8 ± 4	5 ± 4
	14	Auto	Marrow	17 ± 17	17 ± 16
Lymphoma	40	Auto	PBPC	10 ± 10	11 ± 16
AML	17	Auto	Marrow†	65 ± 58	80 ± 76
	27	Allo	Marrow	28 ± 23	30 ± 25
CML	33	Allo	Marrow	33 ± 25	39 ± 35
ALL	15	Allo	Marrow	36 ± 33	55 ± 56
Other	15	Allo	PBPC	15 ± 12	16 ± 20

*Consecutive transplantations performed between July 1991 and December 1995. Includes transfusions leading up to and post-transplantation.
†Monoclonal antibody purged.
‡Transfusion episode, 1 unit/kg dose.
AML, CML, lymphoma, chronic lymphocytic leukemia, multiple myeloma, myelodysplastic syndrome, severe combined immunodeficiency.
Allo, allogeneic; Auto, autologous; AML, acute myelogenous leukemia; CML, chronic myelogenous leukemia; ALL, acute lymphoblastic leukemic; PBPC, peripheral blood progenitor cell.

often used trigger for prophylactic platelet transfusion, a National Institutes of Health consensus determined in 1986 that this number can be safely lowered in some patients with close clinical observation.[15] In our institution, a prophylactic platelet transfusion threshold of less than 10,000/mm^3 is used for otherwise clinically stable patients. For patients presenting with complications such as fever, sepsis, or other clinical conditions in which the risk of bleeding is augmented, the threshold is still 20,000/mm^3.

PLATELET REFRACTORINESS

Platelet refractoriness is defined as a poor platelet count increment (defined later) after a platelet transfusion. Refractoriness develops in approximately 50% of patients undergoing multiple transfusions.[16] Most commonly, clinical factors are responsible for the poor platelet transfusion response.[13, 17] Clinical factors such as fever, sepsis, HSCT, splenomegaly, bleeding, use of amphotericin, veno-occlusive disease, and disseminated intravascular coagulation are associated with decreased survival of transfused platelets. Immune refractoriness, in contrast with clinical refractoriness, is caused by allo- or autoantibodies with specificities to the HLA, ABO, or platelet-specific antigen systems. Prior to the widespread use of leukoreduction (white blood cell removal) of blood components by filtration in the early 1990s, immune refractoriness occurred in 25–50% of patients with leukemia and as many as 80% of those with aplastic anemia.[18]

The most frequent cause of platelet alloimmunization is the development of antibodies against class I major histocompatibility antigens (HLA). These anti-HLA antibodies cause platelet transfusion refractoriness and also fever/chill nonhemolytic transfusion reactions.[19] These antibodies may spontaneously decrease or disappear entirely in 30% of patients.[20] HLA alloimmunization can occur via natural courses (i.e., pregnancy) or via medical intervention (i.e., blood transfusion, bone marrow, or solid organ transplantation). The median time to the development of primary HLA alloimmunization is 4 weeks (3–26 weeks) from the first transfusion exposure.[21] Approximately 10% of patients present with refractoriness even to the initial platelet transfusion due to previous sensitization by transfusion or pregnancy.[22] The presence of antibodies against platelets does not necessarily cause refractoriness because only 30% of alloimmunized patients, mostly with multispecific HLA antibodies, are refractory to random platelet transfusions.[22] In contrast, when HLA antibodies are accompanied by platelet-specific antibodies, the likelihood of refractoriness is higher.[18]

Less frequently, alloimmunization is defined by antibodies to human platelet–specific antigens (HPA), ABO antigens, or the presence of autoantibodies. Kickler reported a 2% alloimmunization rate for HPA, this rate increasing to 9% in patients who also have HLA antibodies.[18] The antibodies with HPA specificity identified as causing refractoriness are mostly directed against epitopes that are expressed on glycoprotein IIb/IIIa (i.e., anti HPA-1a or P1A1).[23] ABO platelet incompatibility occurs when the recipient has isohemagglutinins against ABO antigens expressed on the transfused platelets (i.e., platelets from an A donor to an O

recipient). Platelet ABO incompatibility can cause up to a 46% reduction in platelet recovery.[24] Transient platelet autoantibodies may develop in 50% of HSCT recipients but are rarely associated with refractoriness.[22]

MANAGEMENT OF PLATELET IMMUNE REFRACTORINESS

When platelet refractoriness is suspected, platelet counts at 1 hour and 24 hours after transfusion should be obtained for two consecutive transfusion episodes. Results obtained at 1 hour generally distinguish clinical versus immune refractoriness, which is necessary for appropriate management.[25] Studies have shown that a 10-minute post-transfusion platelet count is as useful as the 60-minute count for evaluating platelet recovery.[26] To standardize the platelet transfusion response with respect to the recipient's size and dose of platelets transfused, a corrected count increment (CCI) (Fig. 50–1)[27] should be calculated. Characteristically, patients with clinical refractoriness demonstrate an adequate 1-hour CCI with a return to pretransfusion baseline level at 24 hours post transfusion (i.e., poor survival of transfused platelets). Immune refractoriness is typically associated with a poor 1-hour CCI due to rapid removal of transfused platelets by the reticuloendothelial system (i.e., poor recovery).

Once a patient is shown to have poor post-transfusion platelet recovery, laboratory data should be sought to document the presumptive diagnosis of immune-mediated refractoriness. An HLA antibody screen should be obtained as part of the evaluation. If the HLA antibody screen is negative, other antibody specificities (i.e., HPA, ABO) should be investigated. If ABO incompatibility has been identified in prior transfusions, ABO-compatible platelets should be used and the CCI evaluated.

If the HLA antibody screen is positive, several alternatives exist to provide "matched" platelets. The first is to provide platelets from donors who are matched at the class I HLA-A and -B loci with the recipient. Duquesnoy et al. designed a system to grade matches based on the degree of identity or cross-reactivity (Table 50–2).[28] Three fourths of patients treated with identical (grade A) four antigen-matched platelets respond to the transfusion. The polymorphism of the HLA system makes it difficult to provide grade A matches, however. By taking advantage of the cross-reactivity observed between the histocompatibility antigen groups, investigators have produced successful responses with transfused platelets expressing cross-reactive

---

Corrected Count Increment (CCI) Formula:

$$CCI = \frac{(\text{platelet count post} - \text{platelet count pre}) \times (BSA)}{\text{number of units transfused or number of platelet transfused } (10^{11} \text{ multiples})}$$

For 1 hour CCI, consider an adequate response:

1. If platelet units are used in denominator, CCI 4000-5000
2. If platelets number is used in denominator, CCI 7000-10000

FIGURE 50–1. Corrected count increment (CCI) formula. (Adapted from Vengeler-Tyler V: Technical Manual, 13th ed. Bethesda, MD, American Association of Blood Banks, 1999:456.)

TABLE 50–2. GRADING SYSTEM FOR HUMAN LEUKOCYTE ANTIGEN (HLA)-MATCHED PLATELETS

MATCH GRADE*	ANTIGEN MATCH DESCRIPTION
A	4 Antigens identical
B	2 or 3 antigens identical
	1 or 2 antigens unknown or cross-reactive
C	3 Antigens identical
	1 Antigen mismatched
D	≥ 2 Antigens mismatched

*HLA-A and -B loci only.

Adapted from Duquesnoy RJ, Filip DJ, Rodey GE, et al: Successful transfusion of platelets "mismatched" for HLA antigens to alloimmunized thrombocytopenic patients. Am J Hematol 2:219–226, 1977.

but not identical HLA (grade B matches).[28] Another alternative is to provide a "selective mismatch" (grade C or D matches) by using HLA types that lack the antigen against which the HLA antibodies are expressing specificity. Possible causes of poor responses to HLA-matched platelets include unidentified clinical factors, suboptimal matches, antibodies to other antigen systems (ABO, HPA), or antibodies induced through other mechanisms (autoantibodies, drug-induced, immune complexes). Because antibodies against the HPA system are rare and require specialized testing for identification,[23] HPA-negative platelets should be provided only when antibodies with specificity for the HPA system have been identified and the patient has not responded to HLA-matched platelets.

An alternative in the management of HLA alloimmunization consists of selecting platelets based on in vitro compatibility by testing the patient's serum against the potential donor platelets (platelet cross-match). Multiple studies have looked not only at the different cross-match methods[29, 30] but also at factors that can influence the transfusion response to cross-matched platelets.[31] Among the various techniques used for platelet cross-matches are the platelet immunofluorescence test,[29] complement-dependent cytotoxicity,[29] the radiolabeled antiglobulin test,[32] the solid phase red blood cell adherence assay,[31, 33, 34] and the enzyme-linked immunoassay (ELISA).[29] A positive cross-match has been shown to have a high predictive value of poor in vivo platelet recovery. Several investigators have reported that alloimmunized recipients can be successfully supported with platelet donors identified by platelet cross-matching.[24, 32, 33] The success of a platelet transfusion associated with a negative cross-match, however, depends on the patient's clinical factors.[31]

The management of clinical refractoriness to platelet transfusion depends on the clinical situation. Increasing the dose and/or frequency of transfusion is recommended until the underlying clinical problems have resolved. In our experience, HLA-matched products have not provided any additional benefit to patients with clinical refractoriness unless alloimmunization was also present.

Some alloimmunized patients do not achieved adequate increments with either HLA-matched or cross-matched platelets. Numerous strategies have been used to treat these patients with conflicting results, including plasmapheresis,[35] high-dose (400 mg/kg body weight for 5 days) intravenous gammaglobulin (IVIG),[36, 37] massive platelet trans-

fusion,[38] and *Staphylococcus* protein A column.[39] Aminocaproic acid appears to be useful in controlling bleeding in patients with thrombocytopenia due to bone marrow hypoplasia.[40–42] For this infrequent clinical occurrence, our recommendations for such a thrombocytopenic patient in the setting of life-threatening bleeding or undergoing a major invasive procedure is the following: Try to obtain an HLA-A or -B match if possible or initiate platelet transfusion support with 1.5–2 times the dose indicated for patient weight. Continue platelet transfusions support every 6–8 hours until bleeding is controlled. If more intensive platelet support is unsuccessful, IVIG (1 g/kg × 2 days) may be given when short-term control of bleeding is required because its effects are short lived.[37] If necessary, the correction of abnormalities in the other components of the coagulation system should be pursued. If not contraindicated, the patient should be started on an antifibrinolytic agent (i.e., ε-aminocaproic acid). The goal of this therapeutic approach is not solely to increase the platelet count but also to prevent, decrease, or stop the bleeding. When the etiology of bleeding is predominantly thrombocytopenia, these measures decrease the amount of bleeding in most cases.

PREVENTION OF ALLOIMMUNIZATION

Difficulty in adequately supporting the alloimmunized patient with platelet transfusion has provided the impetus for development of preventive strategies. The primary mechanism of transfusion-induced alloimmunization has been summarized elsewhere.[14, 43] Briefly, donor-derived antigen-presenting cells expressing class II histocompatibility antigens are considered necessary for the initiation of the primary immune response. Antigen-presenting cells process foreign antigen in a way recognizable to the recipient's T-helper cells. By extrapolation of the results obtained from studies with mice,[44] it was found that more than 10^7 donor leukocytes are needed for HLA alloimmunization. This information led to clinical studies to evaluate the effect of leukoreduction on the risk of alloimmunization. Early studies reported conflicting results due to the different methods used for leukoreduction and the variable use of leukoreduction for red blood cells and platelets. More recent studies have shown that alloimmunization can be delayed or avoided when cellular blood components are leukoreduced to a residual white blood cell (WBC) content of less than 5×10^6.[45] Current leukocyte reduction filters are capable of 3-log (99.9%) WBC removal, resulting in blood components with a residual WBC content less than 10^6/bag. The residual alloimmunization rate of 5–15% is most likely due to undetected previously alloimmunized patients and less frequently to filter failure.

Limiting donor exposure to alloantigens by transfusing single-donor platelets and ultraviolet irradiation (UV-B) of cellular blood components, which inactivates donor antigen-presenting cells, has been investigated. Despite promising preliminary animal and in vitro data, clinical studies have been discouraging.[46] A recently completed multi-institutional study (TRAP—trial to reduce alloimunization in platelets) completed in 1997 compared the rate of alloimmunization in patients with leukemia receiving pooled random platelets or a product designed to decrease the risk of alloimmunization (i.e., leukoreduced pooled random platelets, leukoreduced single-donor platelets, or UV-B irradiated platelets). Results from this study showed that the risk of alloimmunization to platelets is equally reduced by the use of leukoreduced pooled random platelets, leukoreduced single-donor platelets, or UV-B irradiated platelets.[47] Current practice in our institution for prevention of alloimmunization consists of pooled random platelets leukoreduced (filtered) in the laboratory. Platelets filtered at the bedside may not be as effective in reducing the risk of alloimmunization.[48] Single-donor platelets are reserved for patients needing HLA matches, providing directed donor platelets when requested, or as a supplement to the random platelet inventory.

TRANSFUSION-ASSOCIATED GRAFT-VERSUS-HOST DISEASE

Transfusion-associated graft-versus-host disease (TAGVHD) results from the passive transfer of donor immunocompetent T cells capable of engrafting and initiating an immune response against the recipient.[49–52] It is a rare transfusion complication, most often occurring in severely immunocompromised patients, but it also has been reported in immunocompetent patients.[53, 54] The recipient's inability to eliminate these donor lymphocytes may result from severe immunosuppression. HSCT recipients are presumed to be at risk for TAGVHD because they may experience graft-derived GVHD, even in the autologous setting.[52, 55–57]

Another potential setting for TAGVHD is when a patient receives a cellular blood component from a donor who is homozygous for a shared HLA haplotype (antigens) in the patient (Fig. 50–2). Under these circumstances, the patient may not be able to recognize the donor T cells as foreign. The donor T cells, however, can recognize the unshared HLA haplotype (antigens) in the recipient as foreign and can initiate an unopposed immune response. The transfusion of blood components such as HLA-matched platelets or blood components from biologic relatives create an increased risk for this complication.[58–61]

The TAGVHD syndrome is characterized by high fever and an erythematous skin rash occurring 3–30 days after transfusion of a nonirradiated cellular blood component.[62] Like transplant-associated GVHD, the gastrointestinal tract, liver, and skin are involved but to a more severe degree. The key feature that differentiates TAGVHD from transplant-associated GVHD is a profound pancytopenia caused by the donor T lymphocyte–derived destruction of the bone marrow. TAGVHD is typically refractory to all current therapies for GVHD and has an associated mortality rate of over 90%. The cellular blood components associated with this syndrome include red blood cells, platelets, granulocytes, hematopoietic stem cells, and liquid plasma. "Acellular" blood components such as fresh-frozen plasma, cryoprecipitate, and coagulation factor concentrates are not associated with TAGVHD.

Because no successful treatment is currently available, the best option is to prevent the syndrome. TAGVHD is prevented by gamma-irradiation of cellular blood components prior to transfusion for patients who are at risk. Blood irradiators typically use cesium-137 as a source of gamma-radiation, although a cobalt-60 source or a linear accelerator can also be used. The minimum recommended dose of gamma-radiation is 2500 cGy.[63–66] This dose results in a less than 5-log reduction in the T-cell proliferative (blastic) response.[63] At this level of irradiation, the function of the red blood cells,[67, 68] platelets,[69–71] or granulocytes[72] is not affected; however, the ability of red blood cells to tolerate storage is slightly decreased.[73]

All HSCT recipients are considered at risk for TAGVHD and should receive irradiated components. Outside of the transplant setting, irradiated components are recommended for patients with Hodgkin disease; however, it remains controversial whether irradiated components are required for all patients with leukemia or non-Hodgkin lymphoma. Patients with solid tumors do not appear to be at increased risk for TAGVHD unless they receive a bone marrow transplant. Regardless of the diagnosis or immune status, the component should be irradiated in any patient who receives directed donor blood from a blood relative or an HLA-matched component.[53, 54, 58–60, 74, 75]

TRANSFUSION-ASSOCIATED CYTOMEGALOVIRUS INFECTION

Cellular blood components (whole blood, red blood cells, platelets, leukocytes) may contain latently infected leukocytes capable of transmitting cytomegalovirus (CMV) to susceptible recipients. Noncellular blood components (fresh-frozen plasma, cryoprecipitate) do not transmit CMV but may passively transfer antibodies to CMV. Serologic assays are used to screen for the presence of antibodies against CMV in blood donors. Seroprevalence in donors ranges between 40% and 90% and increases with age.[76] Recipient seroconversion studies suggest that only 10% of seropositive donors are infectious.[77] CMV polymerase chain reaction (PCR) studies in seropositive donors have shown that only 8% are PCR-positive.[78] Risk factors for seroconversion include the number of units transfused[77] as well as the immunologic status of the host.[79] In addition, leukoreduction significantly reduces the risk of transmission by removing the potential source of the transmission.[77, 80]

Because of the high prevalence of seropositivity among

TAGVHD in an Immunocompetent Host

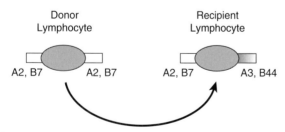

FIGURE 50–2. Transfusion-associated graft-versus-host disease (GVHD) in the immunocompetent host. Donor homozygosity for a shared human leukocyte antigen haplotype. The donor lymphocytes are not recognized as foreign by the recipient; however, the donor lymphocytes recognize the recipient A3, B44 antigens as foreign and may initiate a cellular immune response (GVHD).

donors, the availability of seronegative blood products is limited. Several studies looking at alternatives to CMV-negative products have demonstrated that leukoreduction using the current 3-log WBC removal filters can markedly reduce the risk of CMV transmission,[81–85] even converting PCR-positive units into PCR-negative units.[81] A large clinical study randomized 502 HSCT recipients (303 allogeneic, 3 syngeneic, 196 autologous) to receive either CMV-seronegative or filtered red blood cells and platelets.[85] Patients were then followed up for development of CMV infection between day 21 and day 100 post transplantation (primary end point). Five CMV infections occurred during this period, 2 of 249 in the seronegative and 3 of 247 in the filtered arm (P = NS). None of the patients in the seronegative arm but all three in the filtered arm had evidence of CMV disease (P = NS). A secondary analysis of all infections occurring between day 0 and 100 post transplantation found a higher probability of CMV disease in the filtered arm (2.4% vs. 0%, P = .03); however, this was less than the predefined acceptable rate of less than or equal to 5%. Overall, the probability of CMV infection was equivalent between the CMV-seronegative and the filtered blood components. The difference in disease rate between the two arms could not be explained by CMV pathobiology or study randomization. In addition, it is well known that development of CMV disease depends on recipient immune status rather than the type of exposure. Bowden et al. concluded that seronegative components and filtered components are equivalent in their risk of CMV transmission.[85] These data support the use of blood rendered CMV-safe by filtration as an alternative to seronegative blood. At our institution, CMV-safe (filtered) blood components are provided to CMV-negative autologous transplant recipients. CMV-negative recipients of allogeneic HSCT receive seronegative blood components when available and CMV-safe components when the latter are not available.

IMMUNOHEMATOLOGIC CONSEQUENCES OF ABO-MISMATCHED BONE MARROW TRANSPLANTS

Because ABO and HLA genes are inherited independently, providing the best HLA match during allogeneic HSCT results in recipient/donor ABO/Rh mismatching in up to 15–20% of recipients.[86] Although ABO mismatching may have hematologic consequences, ABO incompatibility does not affect engraftment of myeloid or megakaryocytic elements[87] or increase the risk of graft rejection[88] or GVHD.[89]

ABO compatibility between donor and recipient in allogeneic HSCT can be subdivided into four categories: ABO-identical, minor ABO incompatibility, major ABO incompatibility, and minor and major ABO incompatibility. Depending on the type of incompatibility, manipulation of the donor marrow or PBPC and/or alteration on component ABO selection may be required. The appropriate component selection during the post-transplantation period can minimize the consequences of ABO mismatching (Table 50–3). When blood components are selected, red blood cells should be compatible with both donor and recipient plasma. Plasma components should be compatible with both donor and recipient red blood cells. Transfusion of

incompatible plasma in cellular components (i.e., red blood cells, platelets) should be minimized. Appropriate component ABO selection can minimize the risk and/or severity of delayed hemolysis or delayed red blood cell engraftment in ABO-mismatched transplants.

MINOR ABO INCOMPATIBILITY

Minor ABO incompatibility occurs when donor plasma is incompatible with recipient erythrocytes (e.g., O to A, A to AB). Complications from this type of incompatibility may include acute or delayed hemolysis. Acute immune hemolysis can occur during bone marrow or PBPC infusion because of the presence of isohemagglutinins in the donor plasma. By removing the donor plasma from the graft prior to the infusion, acute hemolysis can be prevented.[87] ABO component selection is intended to minimize the transfusion of plasma incompatible with recipient red blood cells (see Table 50–3). Delayed immune hemolysis has occurred 1–3 weeks after transplantation and was due to the production of isohemagglutinins by the immunocompetent passenger donor lymphocytes infused with the bone marrow or PBPC.[90–96] The diagnosis is made by demonstrating a positive direct antiglobulin test result due to ABO antibodies with laboratory and/or clinical evidence of hemolysis. The diagnosis may be complicated when the patient has received components that contain incompatible plasma.

Detectable donor-derived isohemagglutinins are found in as many as 25%[87] to 57%[94] of patients receiving a bone marrow transplant, although hemolysis occurs in only 13–29%[87, 94] of these patients. Hemolysis is generally mild and can be adequately treated with transfusions. Delayed hemolysis after bone marrow transplantation in the setting of minor ABO incompatibility appears to be limited to situations in which cyclosporine,[90] FK 506,[93] and/or T-cell depletion[94] is used. Studies have suggested that the profound inhibition/depletion of T-cell regulatory function may facilitate unopposed B-cell proliferation with consequent antibody production.[90] Similarly, it has been shown that if other immunosuppressive agents that are cytotoxic to B cells are used in combination with T-cell depletion or T-cell-inhibitory agents, the delayed hemolysis does not occur.[93, 94] Although the frequency of this type of hemolysis in association with PBPC transplants is still unknown, the cases reported have involved severe hemolysis.[95, 96] The lymphocyte yield in a PBPC collection has been reported to be 10 times higher than in a bone marrow harvest.[97] The Heme/BMT Laboratory Research division at our institution has measured the B-cell content of 12 allogeneic PBPC collections with a mean of 17.9% per product and a calculated mean infusion dose of 1.03×10^8 B cells per kilogram of recipient's weight. Therefore, the pathogenesis of the severe hemolysis observed in these cases may be associated to the larger B-cell population passively infused at the time of the transplantation.

MAJOR ABO INCOMPATIBILITY

Major ABO incompatibility occurs when the donor erythrocytes are incompatible with recipient plasma (i.e., A to

TABLE 50–3. COMPONENT SELECTION IN ABO-INCOMPATIBLE STEM CELL TRANSPLANTATION

DONOR	RECIPIENT	RBC	WBC	PLASMA	PLATELETS (1ST CHOICE)	PLATELETS (2ND CHOICE)
A	A	A	A	A, AB	A, AB	B, O*
B	B	B	B	B, AB	B, AB	A, O*
O	O	O	O	O	O	A, B, AB
AB	AB	AB	AB	AB	AB	A, B, O*
Minor ABO Incompatibility						
O	A	O	O	A, AB	A, AB	B, O*
O	B	O	O	B, AB	B, AB	A, O*
A	AB	A	A	AB	AB	A, B, O*
B	AB	B	B	AB	AB	A, B, O*
O	AB	O	O	AB	AB	A, B, O*
Major ABO Incompatibility						
A	O	O	O	A, AB	A, AB	B, O*
B	O	O	O	B, AB	B, AB	A, O*
AB	O	O	O	AB	AB	A, B, O*
AB	A	A	A	AB	AB	A, B, O*
AB	B	B	B	AB	AB	A, B, O*
Major and Minor ABO Incompatibility						
A	B	O	O	AB	AB	A, B, O*
B	A	O	O	AB	AB	A, B, O*

*Concentrate second-choice platelets to remove incompatible plasma.

O, AB to A). Complications expected from this type of incompatibility may include acute or delayed hemolysis and delayed red blood cell engraftment. Incompatible red blood cells in the harvested bone marrow are sufficient to cause acute immune hemolysis when infused.[89] Several management options can be used to prevent this complication. Most frequently, the harvested marrow is processed prior to infusion to remove red blood cells.[86, 87, 98] Procedures for red blood cell depletion are discussed in Chapter 28. Alternatively, recipient isohemagglutinins can be depleted by intensive plasma exchange and/or in vivo antibody adsorption or by extracorporeal (ex vivo) immunoadsorption.[99–102] Both techniques have been used when the recipient isohemagglutinin titers are greater than or equal to 1:128.[103, 104] Studies have shown that a delay in erythroid engraftment (reticulocyte count < 1% for more than 40 days) occurs in 15% to 40% of recipients. Limited hemolysis at the time of red blood cell engraftment is associated with the persistence of recipient isohemagglutinins.[86, 105] Hemolysis occurs in 11% to 50% of patients and is associated with increased red blood cell transfusion requirements (20 U vs. 6 U in ABO-compatible HSCT).[86, 87] The diagnosis is made by demonstrating a positive direct antiglobulin test result due to ABO antibodies with laboratory and/or clinical evidence of hemolysis. Generally, no treatment is necessary except to transfuse with red blood cells compatible with recipient and donor isohemagglutinins.

ABO MAJOR AND MINOR MISMATCH

Recipients of a major and minor ABO incompatible marrow (i.e., A to B, B to A) are at risk for the hematologic complications of both types of incompatibility (i.e., hemolysis during infusion, hemolysis 7–10 days post transplantation, delayed red blood cell engraftment, and hemolysis when donor red blood cells engraft). The marrow

should be processed to remove both plasma and red blood cells. Component ABO selection is limited to O cells and AB plasma (see Table 50–3).

ALLOGENEIC HEMATOPOIETIC STEM CELL DONOR BLOOD COMPONENT REQUIREMENTS

The amount of allogeneic marrow harvested for transplantation depends on the patient's body weight. For most marrow donors, red blood cell requirements can be met by preharvest autologous blood donation. When both the recipient and the donor are CMV-seronegative, allogeneic transfusions should be with CMV-seronegative or filtered (CMV-safe) components. Donor allogeneic transfusions should be irradiated to avoid the theoretical risk of TAGVHD by the passive transfer of immunocompetent lymphocytes from a third person at the time of transplantation to the recipient.[106] Leukoreduction of cellular blood products for the donor is not routinely necessary unless filtered products are being used as a substitute for CMV-negative products. Hematopoietic stem cells harvested by PBPC collection rarely if ever require transfusion support. If transfusion support were needed, the guidelines already described for marrow donors would apply.

GRANULOCYTE TRANSFUSIONS

Because of the profound neutropenia that develops post transplantation, HSCT recipients are at risk for life-threatening bacterial and fungal infections. Results obtained from both controlled and uncontrolled studies of granulocyte transfusions have shown that there is a clinical benefit in a selected group of transplant recipients as summarized by Strauss[107] and McCullough.[108] These are patients with the following characteristics: absolute neutropenia (absolute neutrophil count <500/mm³), documented sepsis, unresponsiveness to at least 48 hours of adequate antibiotic therapy, and an expected bone marrow recovery.[107, 108] A daily therapeutic dose of greater than 1×10^{10} granulocytes is of critical importance for a beneficial clinical response.[107, 108] In the past, donors have been treated with corticosteroids prior to leukapheresis to increase the granulocyte yield per harvest with limited success (average yield, $1-2 \times 10^{10}$ WBC per collection). Clinical studies using granulocyte colony-stimulating factor (G-CSF) in volunteer donors have reported an increase in collection yields as much as six times (4×10^{10} granulocytes) over unprimed donors.[109] In addition to the higher mobilization achieved with G-CSF, the granulocytes collected after G-CSF stimulation have enhanced phagocytic and bactericidal activities.[110]

Granulocyte transfusions are frequently accompanied by mild to severe side effects. Mild reactions such as fever and chills can be controlled by treating the patient with antipyretics or short-acting steroids and meperidine. More severe reactions such as respiratory distress might require the discontinuation of the granulocyte transfusion therapy. Because of the synergistic effects on pulmonary function, simultaneous infusion of amphotericin and granulocytes should be avoided.[111] CMV infection and TAGVHD can be complications of a granulocyte infusion. Therefore, the component should be irradiated for all HSCT recipients. If the patient is CMV-seronegative, a CMV-seronegative component is indicated. The risk of alloimmunization is higher for recipients of granulocytes. Special considerations for granulocyte transfusions include the following: Never administer through a leukoreduction filter; transfuse as soon as possible after collection (ideally within 6 hours of collection); if HLA antibodies are present, the component should be HLA-matched; and donor/recipient ABO compatibility is required because of red blood cell contamination.

Our recommendation is to use granulocyte transfusion therapy primarily in neutropenic patients with severe progressive bacterial infection who are already receiving G-CSF and proper antibiotic therapy. In such cases, a minimum of 4 days of therapy is recommended. Clinical benefits of granulocyte transfusion for fungal sepsis are controversial for the neutropenic patient.[112]

CONCLUSION

Blood transfusion support remains a critical part of HSCT despite the availability of hematopoietic growth factors. Currently available growth factors for clinical use, such as granulocyte macrophage CSF (GM-CSF), G-CSF, IL-11, erythropoietin, and those under clinical investigation such as thrombopoietin shorten but do not eliminate the pancytopenia in this patient population.

Future consideration in blood transfusion support for HSCT will include alternatives such as the development of blood substitutes as well as ex vivo clonal expansion of the hematopoietic stem cells, which is discussed in detail in Chapter 32.[113] Blood substitutes currently under study include infusable platelet membrane[114] and chemically modified hemoglobin.[115] Ideally, by using ex vivo clonal expansion of the patient's own bone marrow or PBPC harvest, more differentiated hematopoietic cells could be obtained

for transfusion during the early post-transplantation period to reduce or eliminate the duration of pancytopenia.

REFERENCES

1. Siena S, Bregni M, Brando B, et al: Circulation of CD34+ hematopoietic stem cells in the peripheral blood of high-dose cyclophosphamide-treated patients: enhancement by intravenous recombinant human granulocyte-macrophage colony-stimulating factor. Blood 74:1905–1914, 1989.
2. Applebaum FR: Allogeneic marrow transplantation and the use of hematopoietic growth factors. Stem Cells 13:344–350, 1995.
3. Besinger WI, Weaver CH, Applebaum FR, et al: Transplantation of allogeneic peripheral blood stem cells mobilized by recombinant human granulocyte colony stimulating factor. Blood 85:1655–1658, 1995.
4. Sheridan WP, Begley CG, Juttner CA, et al: Effect of peripheral-blood progenitor cell mobilized by filgastrin (G-CSF) on platelet recovery after high dose chemotherapy. Lancet 339:640–644, 1992.
5. Isaacs C, Robert NJ, Bailey FA, et al: Randomized placebo-controlled study of recombinant human interleukin-11 to prevent chemotherapy-induced thrombocytopenia in patients with breast cancer receiving dose-intensive cyclophosphamide and doxorubicin. J Clin Oncol 15:3368–3377, 1997.
6. Metcalf D: Thrombopoietin—at last. Nature 369:519–520, 1994.
7. Beguin Y, Clemons JK, Oris R, Fillet G: Circulating erythropoietin levels after bone marrow transplantation: inappropriate response to anemia in allogeneic transplants. Blood 77:868–873, 1991.
8. Lazarus HM, Goodnough LT, Golswasser E, et al: Serum erythropoietin levels and blood component therapy after autologous bone marrow transplantation: implications for erythropoietin therapy in this setting. Bone Marrow Transplant 63:90–95, 1992.
9. Weinthal JA: The role of cytokines following bone marrow transplantation: indications and controversies. Bone Marrow Transplant 18(Suppl 3):S10–S14, 1996.
10. Baer MR, Bloomfield CD: Controversies in transfusion medicine: prophylactic platelet transfusion therapy: pro. Transfusion 266:377–380, 1992.
11. Gaydos LA, Freireich EJ, Mantel N: The quantitative relation between platelet count and hemorrhage in patients with acute leukemia. N Engl J Med 266:905–909, 1962.
12. Gmur J, Burger J, Schanz U, et al: Safety of stringent prophylactic platelet transfusion policy for patients with acute leukaemia. Lancet 338:1223–1226, 1991.
13. Bishop JF, McGrath K, Wolf MM, et al: Clinical factors influencing the efficacy of pooled platelet transfusion. Blood 71:383–387, 1988.
14. Slichter SJ: Platelet transfusion therapy. Hematol Oncol Clin North Am 4:291–311, 1991.
15. Platelet Transfusion Therapy Consensus Conference. JAMA 257:1777–1780, 1987.
16. Murphy MF, Waters AH: Platelet transfusions: the problem of refractoriness. Blood Rev 4:16–24, 1990.
17. McFarland JG, Anderson AJ, Slichter SJ: Factors influencing the transfusion response to HLA-selected apheresis donor platelets in patients refractory to random platelet concentrates. Br J Hematol 73:380–386, 1989.
18. Kickler TS: The challenge of platelet alloimmunization: management and prevention. Transfus Med Rev 4:8–18, 1990.
19. Stack G, Judge JV, Snyder EL: Febrile and non immune transfusion reactions. In Rossi EC, Simon TL, Moss GS, Gould SA (eds): Principles of Transfusion Medicine. Baltimore, Williams & Wilkins, 1996.
20. Lee EJ, Schiffer CA: Serial measurements of lymphocytotoxic antibody in alloimmunised patients. Blood 66:280a, 1985.
21. Dutcher JP, Schiffer CA, Aisner J, Wiernik PH: Alloimmunization following platelet transfusion: the absence of a dose-response relationship. Blood 57:395–398, 1981.
22. Murphy MF, Waters AH: Platelet transfusions: the problem of refractoriness. Blood Rev 4:16–24, 1990.
23. Kickler T, Kennedy SD, Braine HG: Alloimmunization to platelet-specific antigens on glycoproteins IIb/IIIa and Ib/IX in multiply transfused thrombocytopenic patients. Transfusion 30:622–625, 1990.
24. Heal JM, Blumberg N, Masel D: An evaluation of crossmatching, HLA, and ABO matching for platelet transfusions to refractory patients. Blood 70:23–30, 1987.

25. Daly PA, Schiffer CA, Aisner J, Wiernik PH: Platelet transfusion therapy: one-hour posttransfusion increments are valuable in predicting the need for HLA-matched preparations. JAMA 243:435–438, 1980.

26. O'Connell B, Lee EJ, Schiffer CA: The value of 10-minute posttransfusion platelet count. Transfusion 28:66–67, 1988.

27. Walters RH (ed): AABB Technical Manual, 11th ed. Bethesda, MD, American Association of Blood Banks, 1993.

28. Duquesnoy RJ, Filip DJ, Rodey GE, et al: Successful transfusion of platelets "mismatched" for HLA antigens to alloimmunized thrombocytopenic patients. Am J Hematol 2:219–226, 1977.

29. Freedman J, Gafni A, Garvey MB, Blanchette V: A cost-effectiveness evaluation of platelet crossmatching and HLA matching in the management of alloimmunized thrombocytopenic patients. Transfusion 29:201–207, 1989.

30. Kakaiya RM, Gudino MD, Miller WV, et al: Four crossmatch methods to select platelet donors. Transfusion 24:35–41, 1984.

31. Friedberg RC, Donnelly SF, Boyd JC, et al: Clinical and blood bank factors in the management of platelet refractoriness and alloimmunization. Blood 81:3428–3434, 1993.

32. Kickler TS, Ness PM, Braine HG: Platelet crossmatching: a direct approach to the selection of platelet transfusions for the alloimmunized thrombocytopenic patient. Am J Clin Pract 90:69–72, 1988.

33. O'Connell BA, Lee EJ, Rothko K, et al: Selection of histocompatible aphersis platelet donors by cross-matching random donor platelet concentrate. Blood 79:527–531, 1992.

34. Rachel JM, Sinor LT, Tawfik OW, et al: A solid-phase red cell adherence test for platelet cross-matching. Med Lab Sci 42:194–195, 1985.

35. Bensinger WI, Buckner CD, Clift RA, et al: Plasma exchange for platelet alloimmunisation. Transplantation 41:602–605, 1986.

36. Zeigler ZR, Shadduck RK, Rosenfeld CS, et al: Intravenous gamma globulin decreases platelet-associated IgG and improves transfusion responses in platelet refractory states. Am J Hematol 38:15–23, 1991.

37. Kickler T, Braine HG, Piantadosi S, et al: A randomized, placebo-controlled trial of intravenous gammaglobulin in alloimmunized thrombocytopenic patients. Blood 75:313–316, 1990.

38. Nagasawa T, Kim BK, Baldini MG: Temporary suppression of circulating antiplatelet alloantibodies by the massive transfusion of fresh, stored or lyophilized platelets. Transfusion 18:429–435, 1978.

39. Christie DJ, Howe RB, Lennon SS, Sauro SC: Treatment of refractoriness to platelet transfusion by protein A column therapy. Transfusion 33:234–242, 1993.

40. Gardner FH, Helmer RE: Aminocaproic acid: use in control of hemorrhage in patients with amegakaryocytic thrombocytopenia. JAMA 243:35–37, 1980.

41. Dean A, Tuffin P: Fibrinolytic inhibitors for cancer-associated bleeding problems. J Pain Symptom Management 13:20–24, 1997.

42. Shpilberg O, Blumenthal R, Safer O, et al: A controlled trial of tranexamic acid therapy for the reduction of bleeding during treatment of acute myeloid leukemia. Leuk Lymph 19:141–144, 1995.

43. Merryman HT: Transfusion-induced alloimmunization and immunosuppression and the effects of leukocyte depletion. Transfus Med Rev 3:180–193, 1989.

44. Blachjman MA, Bardossy L, Carmen RA, et al: An animal model of allogeneic donor platelet refractoriness: the effect of the time of leukodepletion. Blood 79:1371–1375, 1992.

45. Bordin JO, Heddle NM, Blajchman MA: Biologic effects of leukocytes present in transfused cellular blood products. Blood 84:1703–1721, 1994.

46. Andreu G, Boccaccio C, Klaren J, et al: The role of UV radiation in the prevention of human leukocyte antigen alloimmunization. Transfus Med Rev 6:212–224, 1992.

47. The Trial to Reduce Alloimmunization to Platelets Study Group: Leukocyte reduction and ultraviolet B irradiation of platelets to prevent alloimmunization and refractoriness to platelet transfusions. N Engl J Med 337:1861–1869, 1997.

48. Williamson LM, Wimperis JZ, Williamson P, et al: Bedside filtration of blood products in the prevention of HLA alloimmunization—a prospective randomized study. Blood 83:3028–3035, 1994.

49. Leitman SF: Posttransfusion graft-versus-host disease. In Smith DM, Silvergleid AJ (eds): Special Considerations in Transfusing the Immunocompromised Patient. Arlington, VA, American Association of Blood Banks, 1985.

50. Linden JV, Pisciotto PT: Transfusion-associated graft-versus-host disease and blood irradiation. Transfus Med Rev 6:116–123, 1992.

51. Anderson KC, Weinstein HJ: Transfusion-associated graft-versus-host disease. N Engl J Med 323:315–321, 1990.

52. Brubaker DB: Immunopathogenic mechanisms of posttransfusion graft-vs-host disease. Proc Soc Exp Biol Med 202:122–147, 1993.

53. Capon SM, DePond WD, Tyan DB, et al: Transfusion-associated graft-versus-host disease in an immunocompetent patient. Ann Intern Med 114:1025–1026, 1991.

54. Otsuka S, Kunieda K, Kitamura F, et al: The critical role of blood from HLA-homozygous donors in fatal transfusion-associated graft-versus-host disease in immunocompetent patients. Transfusion 31:260–264, 1991.

55. Rappeport JM, Mehm N, Reinherz EL, et al: Acute graft-vs-host disease in recipients of bone marrow transplants from identical twin donors. Lancet 2:717–720, 1979.

56. Gluckman E, Devergie A, Sohler J, Sauret JH: Graft-versus-host disease in recipients of syngeneic bone marrow. Lancet 8162:253–254, 1980.

57. Vogelsang GB, Jones RJ, Hess AD, et al: Induction of autologous graft-versus-host disease. Transplant Proc 21:2997–2998, 1989.

58. Wagner FF, Flegel WA: Transfusion-associated graft-versus-host disease: risk due to homozygous HLA haplotypes. Transfusion 35:284–291, 1995.

59. Petz LD, Calhoun L, Yam M, et al: Transfusion-associated graft-versus-host disease in immunocompetent patients: report of a fatal case associated with transfusion of blood from a second-degree relative, and a survey of predisposing factors. Transfusion 33:742–750, 1993.

60. Shivdasani RA, Haluska FG, Dock NL, et al: Brief report: graft-versus-host disease associated with transfusion of blood from unrelated HLA-homozygous donors. N Engl J Med 328:766–770, 1993.

61. McMillin KD, Johnson RL: HLA homozygosity and the risk of related-donor transfusion-associated graft-versus-host disease. Transfus Med Rev 7:37–41, 1993.

62. Vogelsang GB, Hess AD: Graft-versus-host disease: new directions for a persistent problem. Blood 84:2061–2067, 1994.

63. Pelszynski MM, Moroff G, Luban NLC, et al: Effect of γ irradiation of red blood cell units on T-cell inactivation as assessed by limiting dilution analysis: implications for preventing transfusion-associated graft-versus-host disease. Blood 83:1683–1689, 1994.

64. AABB Standards for Blood Banks and Transfusion Services: 1994–1995 Standards Committee of the American Association of Blood Banks, 17th ed. Bethesda, MD, American Association of Blood Banks, 1996.

65. Draft guidance for irradiation of blood products issued. AABB Blood Bank Week 10:1–2, 1993.

66. Rosen NR, Weidner JG, Boldt HD, Rosen DS: Prevention of transfusion-associated graft-versus-host disease: selection of an adequate dose of gamma radiation. Transfusion 33:125–127, 1993.

67. Moore GL, Ledford ME: Effects of 4000 rad irradiation on the in vitro storage properties of packed red cells. Transfusion 25:583–585, 1985.

68. Brugnara C, Churchill WH: Effect of irradiation on red cell cation content and transport. Transfusion 32:246–252, 1992.

69. Read EJ, Kodis C, Carter CS, Leitman SF: Viability of platelets following storage in the irradiated state: a pair controlled study. Transfusion 28:446–450, 1988.

70. Rock G, Adams A, Labow RS: The effects of irradiation on platelet function. Transfusion 28:451–455, 1988.

71. Moroff G, George VM, Siegl AM, Luban NLC: The influence of irradiation on stored platelets. Transfusion 26:453–456, 1986.

72. Valerius NH, Johansen KS, Nielsen OS, et al: Effect of in vitro X-irradiation on lymphocyte and granulocyte function. Scand J Haematol 27:9–18, 1981.

73. Davey RJ, McCoy NC, Yu M, et al: The effect of prestorage irradiation on posttransfusion red cell survival. Transfusion 32:525–528, 1992.

74. Grishaber JE, Birney SM, RG Strauss: Potential for transfusion-associated graft-versus-host disease due to apheresis platelets matched for HLA class I antigens. Transfusion 33:910–914, 1993.

75. Kanter MH: Transfusion-associated graft-versus-host disease: do transfusions from second-degree relatives pose a greater risk than those from first-degree relatives? Transfusion 32:323–327, 1992.

76. Tegtmeier G: Posttransfusion cytomegalovirus infections. Arch Pathol Lab Med 113:236–245, 1989.

77. Hillyer CD, Emmiens RK, Zago-Novaretti M, Berkman EM: Methods for the reduction of transfusion-transmitted cytomegalovirus infection: filtration versus the use of seronegative donor units. Transfusion 34:929–934, 1994.

78. Smith KL, Kulski JK, Cobain T, Dunstan RA: Detection of cytomegalovirus in blood donors by polymerase chain reaction. Transfusion 33:497–503, 1993.

79. Preiksaitis JK, Brown L, McKenzie M: The risk of cytomegalovirus infection in seronegative transfusion recipients not receiving exogenous immunosuppression. J Infect Dis 157:523–529, 1988.

80. Sayers MH, Anderson KC, Goodnough LT, et al: Reducing the risk for transfusion-transmitted cytomegalovirus infection. Ann Intern Med 116:55–62, 1992.

81. Smith KL, Cobain T, Dunstan RA: Removal of cytomegalovirus DNA from donor blood by filtration. Br J Haematol 83:640–642, 1993.

82. Bowden RA, Slichter SJ, Sayers MH, et al: Use of leukocyte-depleted platelets and cytomegalovirus-seronegative red blood cells for the prevention of primary cytomegalovirus infection after marrow transplant. Blood 78:246–250, 1991.

83. De Graan-Hentzen YCE, Gratama JW, Mudde GC, et al: Prevention of primary cytomegalovirus infection in patients with hematologic malignancies by intensive white cell depletion of blood products. Transfusion 29:757–760, 1989.

84. De Witte T, Schattenberg A, Van Dijk BA, et al: Prevention of primary cytomegalovirus infection after allogeneic bone marrow transplantation by using leukocyte-poor random blood products from cytomegalovirus-unscreened blood bank donors. Transplantation 50:964–968, 1990.

85. Bowden RA, Slichter SJ, Sayers M, et al: A comparison of filtered leukocyte-reduced and cytomegalovirus (CMV) seronegative blood products for the prevention of transfusion-associated CMV infection after marrow transplant. Blood 86:3598–3603, 1995.

86. Sniecinsky IJ, Petz LD, Oien L, Blume KG: Immunohematologic problems arising from ABO incompatible bone marrow transplantation. Transplant Proc 19:4609–4611, 1987.

87. Lasky LC, Warkenin PI, Kersey JH, et al: Hemotherapy in patients undergoing blood group incompatible bone marrow transplantation. Transfusion 23:277–285, 1983.

88. Hershko C, Gale RP, Ho W, Fitchen J: ABH antigens and bone marrow transplantation. Br J Haematol 44:65–73, 1980.

89. Buckner CD, Clift RA, Sanders JE, et al: ABO-incompatible marrow transplants. Transplantation 26:233–238, 1978.

90. Gajewski JL, Petz LD, Calhoun L, et al: Hemolysis of transfused group O red blood cells in minor ABO-incompatible unrelated-donor bone marrow transplants in patients receiving cyclosporine without posttransplant methotrexate. Blood 79:3076–3085, 1992.

91. Hows J, Beddow K, Gordon-Smith E, et al: Donor-derived red blood cell antibodies and immune hemolysis after allogeneic bone marrow transplantation. Blood 67:177–181, 1986.

92. Hazlehurst GRP, Brenner MK, Wimperis JZ, et al: Haemolysis after T-cell depleted bone marrow transplantation involving minor ABO incompatibility. Scand J Haematol 37:1–3, 1986.

93. Greeno EW, Perry EH, Ilstrup SJ, Weisdorf DJ: Exchange transfusion the hard way: massive hemolysis following transplantation of bone marrow with minor ABO incompatibility. Transfusion 36:71–74, 1996.

94. Robertson VM, Henslee PJ, Jennings CD, et al: Early appearance of anti-A isohemagglutinin after allogeneic, ABO minor incompatible, T cell depleted bone marrow transplant. Transplant Proc 29:4612, 1989.

95. Broketa G, Simpson JK, Hammert L, et al: Delayed hemolysis after minor ABO mismatched peripheral blood stem cell transplantation [Abstract]. Transfusion 37:37S, 1997.

96. Oziel-Taieb S, Faucher-Barbey C, Chabannon C, et al: Early and fatal immune haemolysis after so-called "minor" ABO-incompatible peripheral blood stem cell allotransplantation. Bone Marrow Transplant 19:1155–1156, 1997.

97. Weaver CH, Longin K, Buckner CD, Besinger W: Lymphocyte content in peripheral blood mononuclear cells collected after the administration of recombinant human granulocyte colony-stimulating factor. Bone Marrow Transplant 13:411–415, 1994.

98. Blacklock HA, Gilmore MJML, Prentice HG, et al: ABO-incompatible bone-marrow transplantation: removal of red blood cells from donor marrow avoiding recipient antibody depletion. Lancet 8307:1061–1064, 1982.

99. Tichelli A, Gratwohl A, Wenger R, et al: ABO-incompatible bone marrow transplantation: in vivo adsorption, an old forgotten method. Transplant Proc 19:4632–4637, 1987.

100. Bensinger WI, Buckner CD, Clift RA, et al: Comparison of techniques for dealing with major ABO-incompatible marrow transplants. Transplantation 19:4605–4608, 1987.

101. Anderson KC: The role of the blood bank in hematopoietic stem cell transplantation. Transfusion 32:272–285, 1992.

102. Petz LD: Bone marrow transplantation. In Petz LD, Swisher SN, Kleinman S, et al (eds): Clinical Practice of Transfusion Medicine, 3rd ed. New York, Churchill Livingstone, 1996.

103. Hows JM, Chipping PM, Palmer S, Gordon-Smith EC: Regeneration of peripheral blood cells following ABO incompatible allogeneic bone marrow transplantation for severe aplastic anemia. Br J Haematol 53:145–151, 1983.

104. Gmur JP, Burger J, Schaffner A, et al: Pure red cell aplasia of long duration complicating major ABO-incompatible bone marrow transplantation. Blood 75:290–295, 1990.

105. Braine HG, Sensenbrenner LL, Wright SK, et al: Bone marrow transplantation with major ABO blood group incompatibility using erythrocyte depletion of marrow prior to infusion. Blood 60:420–425, 1982.

106. Drobyski W, Thibodeau S, Truitt RL, et al: Third party mediated graft rejection and graft-versus-host disease after T-cell depleted bone marrow transplantation as demonstrated by hypervariable DNA probes and HLA-DR polymorphism. Blood 74:2285–2294, 1989.

107. Strauss RG: Granulocyte transfusion. In Rossi EC, Simon TL, Moss GS, Gould SA (eds): Principles of Transfusion Medicine, Baltimore, Williams & Wilkins, 1996.

108. McCullough J: Granulocyte transfusion. In Petz LD, Swisher SN, Kleinman S. et al (eds): Clinical Practice of Transfusion Medicine, 3rd ed. New York, Churchill Livingstone, 1996.

109. Bensinger WI, Price TH, Dale DC, et al: The effects of daily recombinant human granulocyte colony stimulating factor administration on normal granulocyte donors undergoing leukapheresis. Blood 81:1883–1887, 1993.

110. Roilides E, Walsh TJ, Pizzo PA, Rubin M: Granulocyte colony stimulating factor enhances the phagocytic and bactericidal activity of normal and defective human neutrophils. J Infect Dis 63:579, 1991.

111. Wright DG, Robichaud KJ, Pizzo PA, Deisscroth AB: Lethal pulmonary reaction associated with the combined use of amphotericin B and leukocyte transfusions. N Engl J Med 304:1185–1189, 1981.

112. Bhatia S, McCullough J, Perry EH, et al: Granulocyte transfusions: efficacy in treating fungal infections in neutropenic patients following bone marrow transplantation. Transfusion 34:226–232, 1994.

113. Cottler-Fox M, Klein HG: Transfusion support of hematology and oncology patients: the role of recombinant hematopoietic growth factors. Arch Pathol Lab Med 118:417–420, 1994.

114. Chao FC, Kim BK, Houranieh AM, et al: Infusable platelet membrane microvesicles: a potential transfusion substitute for platelets. Transfusion 36:536–542, 1996.

115. Ogden JE, Mac Donald SL: Haemoglobin-based red cell substitutes: current status. Vox Sang 69:302–308, 1995.

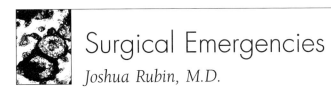

CHAPTER FIFTY-ONE

Surgical Emergencies

Joshua Rubin, M.D.

The treatment regimens for patients undergoing hematopoietic stem cell therapy (HSCT) predispose patients to a variety of gastrointestinal and intra-abdominal complications, some of which require operative intervention.[1–3] Caring for these patients is particularly challenging because the clinical presentation is often vague. The symptoms and signs of the underlying disease process may be obscured by narcotics, glucocorticoids, or altered mental status. The perioperative risk in these patients is significantly increased because of the profound immunosuppression associated with HSCT. Nevertheless, surgical intervention is often required when a potentially life-saving maneuver is indicated.

PATIENT EVALUATION

Surgeons are usually asked to assist in the evaluation of abdominal pain. This is a common symptom, which usually is a manifestation of nonsurgical disease, and the differential diagnosis in patients who are being treated with chemotherapy for hematologic malignancies is large. The salient task for the surgeon is to ensure that the patient does not have an ongoing problem that requires operative intervention. This evaluation has been eloquently described by others and will only be summarized here.[4]

The patient's history and review of systems can be helpful, particularly if the patient is suffering from a more common gastrointestinal disorder, such as cholecystitis, peptic ulcer disease, or diverticulitis. Patients with cholecystitis may have a documented history of gallstones and may have suffered episodes of postprandial colicky upper abdominal pain in the past. The new onset of unremitting, well-localized right upper quadrant abdominal pain suggests that the patient has acute cholecystitis.

Patients with a history of peptic ulcer disease are prone to reactivation during periods of significant stress. A history of increasingly severe dyspepsia in a patient with known peptic ulcer disease suggests that the patient has a recurrent ulcer. Many of these patients are also treated with steroids, which further raises suspicion of peptic ulcer disease. The clinical picture may be obscured by steroid-induced pancreatitis, which if uncomplicated is rarely a surgical disease.

Diverticulitis is most common in the elderly. It usually presents as increasingly severe lower abdominal discomfort, which initially may be crampy. A history of diverticulitis or diverticulosis may be obtained. High doses of chemotherapeutic agents or steroids can interfere with the body's ability to isolate a colon perforation, and it is our experience that diverticulitis runs a more fulminant course in these patients.

Surgeons are also called on to evaluate perirectal pain in immunocompromised patients. A history of diarrhea or constipation is common. It is not unusual for these patients to experience perianal irritation. The immunocompromised state predisposes patients to perianal sepsis in this setting. A history of constipation and the sudden development of perianal pain after passage of stool is typical for an anal fissure. The more indolent development of perirectal discomfort, exacerbated by bowel movement and associated with fever, is more suggestive of a perirectal abscess or perirectal cellulitis. Hemorrhoidal disease can be exacerbated by an alteration of bowel habits, which often accompanies chemotherapy, immunosuppression, and bed rest. A history of hemorrhoidal disease is significant in this respect and should prompt a close evaluation of the anorectum.

Abdominal pain, diarrhea, fever, abdominal tenderness, and distention may herald the development of a particularly serious lesion in patients who are profoundly neutropenic. Typhlitis, or neutropenic colitis, may occur in leukemic patients as early as 1 day after development of chemotherapy-induced neutropenia as a result of mucosal ulcers, which may lead to localized infection of the cecal wall. The clinical presentation varies from vague and nonspecific symptoms and signs, as noted above, to fulminant pancolitis with colonic bleeding, perforation, and/or necrosis. If the condition is recognized early, patients can usually be successfully treated with broad-spectrum antibiotics. Suggested regimens include drugs active against clostridial species, *Pseudomonas*, and anaerobes. Antidiarrhea medication should be avoided. Nasogastric tube decompression of the bowel should be instituted. Colon resection may be lifesaving for patients who manifest clinical deterioration or who develop clear-cut signs of a "surgical abdomen." These patients should be evaluated early on by surgeons for this reason.[5–8]

Gastrointestinal bleeding is usually due to peptic ulcer disease or graft-versus-host disease. A history of retching prior to the onset of hematemesis suggests that the patient experienced a Mallory-Weiss tear. A history of profound thrombocytopenia or coagulopathy raises the suspicion of a retroperitoneal bleed. In this case, patients complain not only of abdominal pain but also of flank or back discomfort. A history of trauma is often absent, although retroperitoneal bleeding has occurred after attempted femoral artery or vein cannulation. A history of splenomegaly suggests splenic rupture and bleeding into the abdominal cavity. In addition to abdominal pain, some patients may complain of left shoulder discomfort or the Kerr sign.

PHYSICAL EXAMINATION

The evaluation of immunocompromised patients who have abdominal pain requires meticulous inspection, auscultation, and palpation. Patients with peritonitis prefer to lie still and complain of increased pain as a result of any voluntary or involuntary movement. Close inspection of the eyes is important in order to determine whether or not the patient has jaundice. Although cholecystitis rarely presents with clinically significant jaundice, associated choledocholithiasis could cause sepsis and jaundice in patients with known gallstones. A right pleural effusion could be a manifestation of underlying liver disease. Hepatic abscesses can develop in immunocompromised patients with diverticulitis. Hepatic vein thrombosis may complicate the treatment of hematologic malignancy. The thrombosis may present with acute abdominal findings but is not a surgically reversible disease.

The abdominal examination is difficult to interpret in critically ill patients. Usually there is a paucity or absence of bowel sounds. Active bowel sounds are unusual in surgical diseases of the abdomen, although this sign is not specific enough to be reliable. If vomiting has been a significant component of the patient's clinical presentation, ventral and inguinal hernias should be sought. The presence of the Grey-Turner or Cullen sign suggests that the patient has a retroperitoneal bleed. Abdominal distention is a nonspecific finding in many of these patients. It can usually be attributed to ascites or intestinal distention due to an ileus. Occasionally it is the manifestation of mechanical bowel obstruction. Some chemotherapeutics, most commonly vincristine and vinblastine, can cause many of these signs.

Palpation of the abdomen should enable the examining physician to determine whether the patient has peritonitis and whether it is localized. Many nonsurgical conditions are associated with abdominal tenderness, such as intestinal distension, bladder distension, and passive congestion of the liver. Peritoneal irritation manifested by rebound tenderness, abdominal rigidity, and pain on movement, however, usually belies a more sinister intra-abdominal process. Diffuse peritonitis without any localizing signs is a surgical emergency in these patients.

Patients who complain of perianal pain should first be examined by an inspection of the perineum. Perirectal sepsis is usually accompanied by perineal cellulitis. This area becomes tender and may be indurated. Fluctuance is rare but suggests that the patient has a perirectal abscess.[9] Internal hemorrhoids may prolapse and become incarcerated. This leads to their strangulation and necrosis, which can also lead to local sepsis. Strangulated hemorrhoids are evident on physical examination. Anal fissures can be difficult to detect because of the pain associated with physical examination. Gently spreading the buttocks apart to inspect the anus often reveals a small mucosal injury at either end of the midline. Digital rectal examination should always be attempted in patients who will tolerate it. Pelvic fullness or unilateral tenderness suggests perirectal abscess.

LABORATORY EVALUATION

The laboratory evaluation of immunocompromised patients with abdominal pain should be guided by two considerations. Some laboratory abnormalities may provide insight into the etiology of abdominal pain. Of equal importance is the need to define abnormalities that should be corrected in the event the patient requires an operation.

The patient's white blood cell count is usually of little diagnostic help in this setting because most of these patients are neutropenic at the time they experience abdominal pain. The platelet count and coagulation profile, however, are important for the preoperative preparation of the patient. Patients with platelet counts of less than 30,000/mm^3 are prone to significant intraoperative and postoperative bleeding complications and should undergo preoperative platelet transfusion in order to maintain their platelet count above this level. Anemia should also be corrected, particularly in older patients with suspected or documented heart disease. Electrolyte abnormalities should be corrected as expeditiously as possible before general anesthesia is induced. Biliary tract disease may be accompanied by mild elevation of the liver function test results and bilirubin. Cholangitis is often associated with more-significant elevations of serum bilirubin and alkaline phosphatase. Profound elevations of hepatic transaminase are more suggestive of chemical or viral hepatitis (see Chapter 46), both of which are nonsurgically treated lesions. Amylase and lipase should be measured to rule out pancreatitis.[10]

Blood cultures sometimes can identify the source of infection. Patients with gram-negative or anaerobic bacteremia are likely to have an intestinal source of their abdominal pain. Urosepsis can be manifested as lower abdominal discomfort but does not require operative therapy.

RADIOGRAPHIC EVALUATION

The etiology of abdominal pain in immunocompromised patients often remains an enigma despite a thorough history and meticulous physical examination. Radiographs have become the most useful diagnostic studies, and chest radiography is an appropriate first diagnostic test for evaluating abdominal pain. Pneumonia sometimes presents as upper abdominal pain. The chest radiograph should be obtained with the patient upright so that free air underneath the diaphragm may be detected. The presence of free intra-abdominal air is the sine qua non of a perforated intra-abdominal viscus, and this finding should prompt urgent operative therapy.

Clinical impression can be useful in guiding the radiologic work-up. Patients with known gallstones, upper abdominal pain, and right upper quadrant tenderness may be evaluated with ultrasonography or a hepatoiminodiacetic acid (HIDA) scan. Ultrasound findings consistent with acute cholecystitis include pericholecystic fluid, thickening of the gallbladder wall, gallstones, and gas within the wall of the gallbladder in severe cases. These findings can be diagnostic in the appropriate clinical setting. Because it is less specific and may appear abnormal in a variety of clinical settings, a HIDA scan is less useful. It would be unusual to have either acute calculus or acute acalculus cholecystitis in the presence of a normal HIDA scan result.

Contrast studies of the gastrointestinal tract are rarely recommended, even though this organ is frequently damaged in the setting of immunocompromise. Rather, the most specific and sensitive survey of the abdominal cavity is a well-performed, contrast-enhanced computed tomograph. Although the barium used for computed tomography (CT) is very dilute, a water-soluble contrast medium should be requested if there is a possibility that the patient may require surgery. Findings on CT can reliably be used to diagnose appendicitis, diverticulitis, and neutropenic typhlitis.[11] The latter occasionally occurs in neutropenic patients and is thought to be due to breakdown of the normal mucosal defenses against the microflora of the colon. The disease can rapidly progress to full-thickness necrosis of the colon if not recognized early and treated appropriately. Broad-spectrum antibiotics directed against gram-negative and anaerobic bacteria are often successful in treating this disease. More-advanced cases or treatment failures require emergency colectomy.

Clostridium difficile colitis is a disease that is not unique to immunocompromised patients.[12] It is thought to develop as a result of changes in the colonic flora due to broad-spectrum antibiotics.[12] Most patients treated with HSCT either receive a course of prophylactic antibiotics or antibiotics for infectious complications. *Clostridium difficile* colitis, when recognized early and treated with metronidazole (Flagyl), often resolves. More-advanced cases lead to sepsis and ultimately death unless an emergent colectomy is performed. CT is useful in identifying *Clostridium difficile* colitis as a diagnostic possibility. Flexible sigmoidoscopy may be used to confirm the diagnosis by documenting pseudomembranes. Stool should be evaluated for *Clostridium difficile* toxin. Other colonic lesions that can present as right lower quadrant peritoneal findings include leukemic infiltration of the bowel wall and ischemic colitis. Findings on CT are nonspecific and have to be incorporated into the clinical evaluation of the patient. Colonoscopy can help to further distinguish these lesions.

CT can also identify splenomegaly, splenic rupture, and intraperitoneal bleeding. Retroperitoneal hematomas due to coagulapathy or thrombocytopenia can also be diagnosed by CT, which is a sensitive test for the demonstration of small amounts of free intra-abdominal air that might have been missed on plain chest radiograph or decubitus abdominal radiographs.[11] Evaluation of the pelvis by CT may demonstrate perirectal inflammation suggestive of a perirectal abscess. Profoundly neutropenic patients may not have a discreet abscess, obviating the need for surgical intervention.

TREATMENT

The goal in evaluating an immunocompromised patient with abdominal pain is to distinguish a lesion requiring surgical intervention from one that does not. Findings of free intra-abdominal air on radiograph or diffuse peritonitis on physical examination should prompt urgent operative intervention. Localized peritoneal signs due to diverticulitis, limited neutropenic colitis, or pseudomembranous colitis can be treated conservatively with antibiotics and close clinical observation. Deterioration in the patient's clinical condition should prompt urgent surgical intervention.

The greatest risks patients face perioperatively are bleeding, infection, and wound disruption. Chemotherapeutics and steroids may delay wound healing. Steroids also have an anti-inflammatory effect. Some of these patients are malnourished at the time of surgery, which further impairs their healing ability and predisposes to infection. This has implications for the conducting of an abdominal operation. We often fashion an intestinal stoma rather than re-establish intestinal continuity with an anastomosis in patients who require a bowel resection in order to avoid anastomotic leak. Intestinal continuity can be re-established at a later date if the patient survives the surgical disease and the underlying disease for which the HSCT was performed. Reliable closure of an abdominal wound is challenging for the same reasons. It is our practice to leave the skin open and to place retention sutures in patients whose surgery is contaminated by intra-abdominal infection.

These patients often have a coagulation disorder or are thrombocytopenic as a result of the conditioning regimen (see Chapter 41). This should be corrected preoperatively in order to minimize the risk of postoperative bleeding. Preoperative preparation of these patients should also include vigorous intravenous hydration in order to avoid intraoperative hypotension and oliguria, both of which predispose patients to postoperative renal failure or intraoperative cardiac events. Steroids should be administered in "stress" doses if the patient is or has recently been on steroids, because the stress response of the adrenal glands may be impaired in these patients.

Laparoscopy has become increasingly important in the evaluation and management of immunocompromised patients with abdominal pain.[13] Despite meticulous evaluation, the etiology of the patient's abdominal pain and even the need for surgical intervention may remain unclear. The laparoscopic survey can identify cholecystitis, bowel perforation, and ischemic or necrotic intestine. A laparoscopic approach can occasionally be used to treat the patient's surgical disease. Cholecystectomy is performed almost routinely by laparoscope, with less than 10% of cases requiring conversion to an open procedure. Previous intra-abdominal surgery and massive intestinal distention limit the usefulness of laparoscopy in this setting.

CONCLUSION

Abdominal pain is a frequent but nonspecific complaint in immunocompromised patients such as those who are undergoing hematopoietic stem cell transplantation. Careful evaluation is necessary in order to rule out a surgical intra-abdominal lesion. The history and physical examination often suggest a particular disease but usually are not diagnostic. The most useful studies are radiographic. In the absence of a presumptive diagnosis, abdominal and pelvic CT is the test of choice. CT often leads to a fairly limited differential diagnosis. In the absence of free intra-abdominal air or diffuse peritonitis, many of these lesions can be treated expectantly if they appear to be inflammatory on radiograph. A worsening clinical condition usually necessitates operative intervention. The radiographic evaluation of bleeding is often not only diagnostic but may be therapeutic. The mainstay of therapy is endoscopic. Finally, although exotic diseases occur with increased frequency in the immunocompromised patient, surgical lesions are most usual and must be considered in the evaluation of these patients.

REFERENCES

1. Downey RJ, Espat J, Hsu FI: Surgical problems in the critically ill oncologic patient. *In* Shoemaker WC, Ayres SM, Grenvik A, Holbrook PR (eds): Textbook of Critical Care, ed 4. Philadelphia, WB Saunders, 1999, pp 1769–1777.
2. Glenn J, Funkhouser WK, Schnieder PS: Acute illness necessitating urgent abdominal surgery in neutropenic cancer patients. Surgery 105:778–789, 1989.
3. Villor HV, Wareke JA, Peck MD, et al: Role of surgical treatment in the management of complications of the gastrointestinal tract in patients with leukemia. Surg Gynecol Obstet 165:217–222, 1987.
4. Silen W: Cope's Early Diagnosis of the Acute Abdomen, ed 20. New York, Oxford University Press, 2000.
5. Moir CR, Scudamore CH, Bonny WB: Typhlitis: Selective surgical management. Am J Surg 151:563–566, 1986.
6. Wade DS, Douglas HO: Neutropenic enterocolitis: Clinical diagnosis and treatment. Cancer 69:17–23, 1992.
7. Shaked A, Shinar E, Freund H: Neutropenic typhlitis: A plea for conservativism. Dis Colon Rectum 26:351–352, 1983.
8. Gandy W, Greenberg BR: Successful medical management of neutropenic enterocolitis. Cancer 51:1551–1555, 1983.
9. Nunes FA, Lucey MR: Gastrointestinal complications of immunosuppression. Gastroenterol Clin North Am 28:233–245, 1999.
10. Shore T, Bow E, Greenberg H, et al: Pancreatitis post-bone marow transplantation. Bone Marrow Transplant 17:1181–1184, 1996.
11. Horton KM, Corl FM, Fishman EK: CT of nonneoplastic diseases of the small bowel: Spectrum of disease. J Comput Assist Tomogr 23:417–428, 1999.
12. Gerding DN, Johnson S, Peterson LR, et al: *Clostridium difficile*-associated diarrhea and colitis. Infect Control Hosp Epidemiol 16:459–477, 1995.
13. Willsher PC, Sanabria JR, Gallinger S, et al: Early laparoscopic cholecystectomy for acute cholecystitis: A safe procedure. J Gastrointest Surg 3:50–53, 1999.

CHAPTER FIFTY-TWO

Late Graft Failure

Jian Chen, M.D., Ping Law, Ph.D., and Edward D. Ball, M.D.

Late or secondary graft failure is a serious complication of hematopoietic stem cell (HSC) transplantation (HSCT). It is presented as complete or partial recovery of hematopoiesis of donor origin followed by profound pancytopenia with a markedly hypocellular marrow in the absence of moderate to severe graft-versus-host disease (GVHD). Its causes are multifactorial. Table 52–1 is a summary of reported incidences of allogeneic and autologous late graft failure.

In allogeneic HSCT, secondary graft failure is more common in recipients of human leukocyte antigen (HLA)-nonidentical marrow and T cell–depleted marrow grafts. This is usually characterized by the disappearance of donor HSC in the circulation. The origin of circulating blood cells or the chimerism status can be examined either by a specific probe to sex chromosomes if the donor and recipient are sex-discordant or by individual-specific short-tandem-repeat and variable-number tandem-repeat assay. Chronic GVHD can inflict extensive damage to the host marrow microenvironment and lead to graft failure.

In autologous HSCT, the common causes include an inadequate number of HSC infused, damaged HSC due to prior chemotherapy or ex vivo manipulations (such as purging with pharmacologic agents), pre-existing abnormal HSC at an undetectable level by routine histologic examinations, and relapse of original malignancy. Secondary graft failure after autologous HSCT is usually presented as myelodysplastic syndrome with pancytopenia. The true incidence of secondary graft failure is difficult to access because some patients die in the post-transplantation period from a variety of causes before their grafts actually fail. Viral infections and some medications can also suppress the marrow function and cause graft failure. The causes and risk factors of late graft failure are summarized in Table 52–2.

ALLOGENEIC HSCT

HLA DISPARITY

The effect of HLA incompatibility on graft failure has been analyzed by several groups. In one report, the incidence of

TABLE 52–1. INCIDENCE OF LATE GRAFT FAILURE

INSTITUTION	NO.	INCIDENCE (%)	YEAR (REFERENCE)
Allogeneic HSCT Using HLA-Identical Related Donor			
FHCRC	50	10	1986 (1)
U. Perugia	171	14	1987 (2)
IBMTR	615	7.8	1989 (3)
FHCRC	930	0.4	1989 (4)
U. Minnesota	151	0.7	1994 (5)
U. Perugia	54	0	1999 (6)*
Allogeneic HSCT Using HLA-Identical Unrelated Donor			
NMDP	462	8	1993 (7)
U. Minnesota	20	15	1994 (5)
FHCRC	192	2.1	1998 (8)
Allogeneic HSCT Using HLA-Nonidentical Donor			
FHCRC	269	4.1	1989 (4)
U. Minnesota	20	25	1994 (5)
Hahnemann U.	25	0	1996 (9)†
U. Perugia	43	0	1998 (10)‡
Autologous HSCT			
Dana Farber Cancer Center	552	7.4	1999 (44)

*Transplantation-related mortality, 16.6%; 28 of 54 achieved long-term survival.
†Transplantation-related mortality, 36%.
‡Transplantation-related mortality, 40%; 12 of 43 patients survived with a median follow-up of 18 months.
FHCRC, Fred Hutchinson Cancer Research Center; HLA, human leukocyte antigen; IBMTR, International Bone Marrow Transplant Registry; NMDP, National Marrow Donor Program.

TABLE 52–2. COMMON CAUSES OF LATE GRAFT FAILURE

HLA incompatibility
T-cell depletion
Graft-versus-host disease
Inadequate number of hematopoietic stem cells
Infections: cytomegalovirus, Epstein-Barr virus, herpes simplex virus, parvovirus B19, hepatitis virus
Dysfunction of bone marrow stroma cells
Damage to hematopoietic stem cells by prior chemotherapy, irradiation, ex vivo purging

HLA, human leukocyte antigen.

secondary graft failure was 4.1% in patients who received HLA-nonidentical marrow compared with 0.4% in patients who received HLA-identical marrow from their siblings.[4] In another report, the incidence of secondary graft failure was 0.7%, 15%, and 25% for patients who received marrow from fully-matched related donors, serologically matched unrelated donors, and partially matched unrelated donors, respectively.[5] The results of unrelated donor transplantation have improved significantly, however. In 1998, a report from the Fred Hutchinson Cancer Research Center (FHCRC) reported only four cases of secondary graft failure in a series of 192 patients who underwent transplantation for chronic myelogenous leukemia using HLA-matched unrelated donors.[8] Several factors contributed to the low incidence of secondary graft failure, including the relative young age of the recipients, improved HLA-matching techniques, conditioning regimens containing total body irradiation (TBI), and prophylaxis against cytomegalovirus and fungal infections.

T-CELL DEPLETION

Depletion of T cells from donor marrow has been used to overcome the limited supply of HLA-identical related donors and HLA incompatibility. Despite the success in reducing the incidence and severity of acute GVHD, early experience with T cell–depleted marrow transplantation yielded a higher graft failure rate ranging from 20% to 50% before 1990.[11] This has declined significantly since then. An analysis of the National Marrow Donor Program (NMDP) data reported an 8% incidence of secondary graft failure in 462 patients. T-cell depletion was the only significant factor associated with secondary graft failure.[7] Several strategies have been successfully applied to overcome the higher incidence of graft failure associated with T-cell depletion, including a more-intensive conditioning regimen,[12] a larger dose of infused marrow cells,[10] and limited T-cell depletion.[13] Two groups of investigators from the United States and Italy reported no secondary graft failure in their experience of T cell–depleted bone marrow transplantation with an intensive conditioning regimen.[6, 10, 12] The transplantation-related mortality rate, however, was 24% in one report[6] and 40% in the other report.[10]

GRAFT-VERSUS-HOST DISEASE AND PROPHYLAXIS

Acute and chronic GVHD has been associated with secondary graft failure. In one analysis of 171 recipients of HLA-matched allogeneic bone marrow transplants, the rate of secondary graft failure was 14%. The presence of severe acute GVHD (grade II–IV) was the major risk factor.[2] Chronic GVHD can inflict extensive damage to bone marrow stromal cells and lead to secondary graft failure. Persistent pancytopenia is a common manifestation of chronic GVHD. On the other hand, the immunosuppressive agents to prevent and treat GVHD are associated with high incidence of opportunistic infections, especially cytomegalovirus infection, which is another common cause of secondary graft failure. Detailed discussions on GVHD can be found in Chapters 39 and 45.

AUTOLOGOUS HSCT

QUANTITY AND QUALITY OF HEMATOPOIETIC STEM CELLS

The source and the number of HSC are both important factors for late graft failure in autologous HSCT. Bentley et al. analyzed the effect of infused HSC dose by measuring colony-forming units—granulocyte macrophage (CFU-GM) as well as the source of HSC on late graft failure.[14] A total of 51 patients underwent autologous HSCT, and 24 of them received both autologous peripheral blood progenitor cells (PBPC) and bone marrow. Eleven patients had less than 1×10^5 CFU-GM/kg. Seven of them were PBPC recipients, and six of seven experienced late graft failure. In contrast, no late graft failure occurred in four patients who received low-dose autologous bone marrow. The low-dose PBPC recipients, however, had undergone significantly more prior chemotherapy, and a significantly higher proportion received TBI as part of the conditioning regimens. The authors concluded that low-dose CFU-GM, especially for PBPC, was an important cause of late graft failure. The number of HSC infused in autologous HSCT has been studied extensively.[15–17] An inadequate quantity of cells results in delayed engraftment, transfusion dependency, and an increased incidence of late graft failure.[18–20] Hematopoiesis after autologous HSCT is characterized by a prolonged and severe deficiency of erythroid and megakaryocyte progenitors in marrow, whereas peripheral white blood cells and marrow cellularity have recovered to relatively normal values shortly after transplantation. This persistent hematopoietic deficiency is the consequence of impaired HSC self-renewal and a marrow microenvironment too damaged to support hematopoiesis.

Previous cytotoxic therapy and irradiation can inflict damage to both HSC and the marrow microenvironment. The interruption of this complex cell-to-cell interaction is one of the important factors in late graft failure with autologous HSCT. In addition, ex vivo marrow purging by a variety of techniques may adversely effect the number and function of HSC. In one study of 14 autograft recipients in whom purging was performed by immunotoxin and 4-hydroperoxycyclophosphamide, engraftment failed in one patient and late graft failure developed in two.[21] A high incidence of relapse of the original malignancy is another common cause of late graft failure in autologous transplants.

MYELODYSPLASTIC SYNDROME

Secondary myelodysplastic syndrome (MDS) is a well-known complication of cytotoxic chemotherapy. An increased incidence of late graft failure presented as MDS has been reported after autologous HSCT.[22, 23] A retrospective study has addressed whether the HSC damage is caused by pretransplantation high-dose chemotherapy or is already present in pretransplantation hematopoietic precursors. The investigators studied pretransplantation marrow or PBPC samples from 12 patients by a sensitive fluorescence in situ hybridization method to detect abnormal cytogenetic markers. In 9 of 12 cases, the same cytogenetic abnormality observed at the time of MDS diagnosis was detected in pretransplantation specimens. The abnormal cell population consisted of 5–46% of pretransplantation HSC cells prior to high-dose chemotherapy. In 3 of 12 patients, the cytogenetic abnormalities found at the time of myelodysplasia diagnosis were not detected in their pretransplantation samples. These findings suggest that in many cases of post-transplantation MDS, the HSC damage may not be related to high-dose chemotherapy or the transplantation procedure itself.[24]

STROMAL DAMAGE

The role of the bone marrow micronenvironment in sustaining engraftment has not been clearly established. A complex interaction between infused HSC and marrow stromal cells takes place after transplantation. In allogeneic transplantation, the genetic disparity between donor and recipient can certainly compromise the functions of the marrow microenvironment. The intensive conditioning regimen or chemotherapy prior to transplantation can cause permanent damage to marrow stromal cells. Because marrow stromal cells retain their host origin after an intensive conditioning regimen, the donor-derived immune cells are capable of attacking and damaging these cells. A graft-versus-host stroma effect has been documented in patients who received HLA-nonidentical transplants.[25] The presence of alloreactive cytotoxic T lymphocytes capable of lysing host stromal cells has been shown in an in vitro experiment.[26] The deficiency of stromal cell function in patients with graft failure can be studied in long-term bone marrow culture. Results show decreased production of stimulatory growth factors such as granulocyte colony-stimulating factor (G-CSF) and increased production of inhibitory cytokines such as transforming growth factor β.[27] In addition, viral infections have been associated with stromal cell dysfunction and decreased hematopoietic growth factor production in vitro.[28–30]

INFECTION

Infection can cause late graft failure in both autologous and allogeneic HSCT. The effect can be particularly pronounced in T cell–depleted allogeneic marrow transplants. Acute parvovirus-B19 infection has been reported as the cause of graft failure by several investigators.[31–34] These patients presented with persistent severe anemia or sudden onset

of aplastic anemia, and they were usually treated with intravenous immunoglobulin after the diagnosis was made. One patient received second bone marrow transplantation from the same donor. Several cases of late graft failure caused by human herpesvirus-6 have been reported.[35, 36] Most of these patients received T cell–depleted marrow transplantation.

Some viruses may act directly on the HSC, whereas other viruses may act on marrow stromal cells. Experimental studies using long-term culture techniques have shown that marrow stromal cells are the targets of reproductive cytomegalovirus (CMV) and Epstein-Barr virus.[28, 29] The presence of CMV antigen in stromal cells has been associated with decreased production of G-CSF mRNA. In one animal model, the investigators demonstrated that CMV infection was not associated with significant loss of marrow HSC but with markedly reduced gene expression of stem cell factor, G-CSF, and IL-6.[30]

Viral hepatitis is a common complication after HSCT and has been associated with increased incidence of veno-occlusive disease. Although hepatitis has been associated with aplastic anemia independent of HSCT, it is uncommon as a cause of secondary graft failure. Only a small number of reports of acute hepatitis have been implicated in late graft failure. One case of non-A, non-B hepatitis was reported to be the cause of graft failure and required second marrow transplantation.[37] In 1997, Korn et al. reported from Germany that two patients with co-infection of hepatitis C and hepatitis G experienced late graft failure requiring second transplantation.[38] These data suggest that persistent hepatotropic viral infection may have significant effects on the marrow graft.

MANAGEMENT OF LATE GRAFT FAILURE

Once secondary graft failure is detected, possible causes should be carefully reviewed. Relapse of the original malignancy should first be eliminated as the cause of pancytopenia. Treatment options common to both allogeneic and autologous HSCT include discontinuation or gradual dose-reduction of marrow suppressive medications, effective treatment of identifiable infections, and judicious use of hematopoietic growth factors. G-CSF and granulocyte-macrophage CSF (GM-CSF) are the most commonly used growth factors after transplantation. A combination of growth factors has been shown to rescue graft failure, including G-CSF, GM-CSF, M-CSF, erythropoietin, and IL-1β.[39]

ALLOGENEIC HSCT

The chimerism status of circulating blood cells in recipients of allografts should be assessed by molecular techniques, such as sex-chromosome probes, short-tandem-repeat, and variable-number tandem-repeat. One should also consider the balance of the immune suppression necessary for controlling GVHD and the infection. Second HSCT should be considered in selected patients, such as those of young age, of good performance status, and with potentially curable underlying disease. The HSCT source of the second transplant can come from the same donor, a different donor, or autologous back-up collections if performed and if there is no recurrence of original malignacy.[39–44] No prospective study has addressed this issue, and the decision has to be made individually. The outcome of second transplantation for late graft failure appears to be better than for primary graft failure.[3] In one report, none of 19 patients who suffered primary graft failure survived for the long term, including 10 patients who had undergone second transplantation. Among 47 patients who experienced late graft failure, 27 received a second transplant and 16 of them survived for the long term.[3]

AUTOLOGOUS HSCT

Second HSCT should be considered in selected patients of young age and good performance status with potentially curable disease. The choice of HSC source is an HLA-identical sibling or, if such a person is not available, an HLA-matched unrelated donor or mismatched related donor. No prospective study has addressed this issue, and the decision has to be made individually. The outcome remains poor for patients who received an autograft and presented with myelodysplasia. In a 1999 report, 13 patients underwent second allogeneic HSCT for myelodysplasia after autologous transplantation. All of them died from transplant-related toxicity and relapse.[45]

CONCLUSION

Secondary graft failure is rare in HSCT. The common causes are HLA incompatibility, T-cell depletion, and GHVD in allogeneic transplants. For autografts, an inadequate number of HSC, a dysfunctional marrow microenvironment, recurrence of malignancy, extensive chemotherapy, and irradiation prior to transplantation are the major causes of late graft failure. Infections, especially viral infections, should be considered in the differential diagnosis of late graft failure. Second HSCT is the treatment of choice for eligible patients whenever a suitable donor is available.

REFERENCES

1. Anasetti C, Doney KC, Storb R, et al: Marrow transplantation for severe aplastic anemia: long-term outcome in fifty "untransfused" patients. Ann Intern Med 104:461, 1986.
2. Peralvo J, Bacigolupo A, Pittaluga PA, et al: Poor graft function associated with GVHD after allogeneic marrow transplantation. Bone Marrow Transplant 2:279, 1987.
3. Champlin RE, Horowitz MM, van Bekkum DW, et al: Graft failure following bone marrow transplantation for severe aplastic anemia; risk factors and treatment results. Blood 73:606, 1989.
4. Anasetti C, Amos D, Beatty PG, et al: Effect of HLA compatibility on engraftment of bone marrow transplants in patients with leukemia and lymphoma. N Engl J Med 320:197, 1989.
5. Davies SM, Ramsay NKC, Haake RJ, et al: Comparison of engraftment in recipients of matched sibling or unrelated donor marrow allografts. Bone Marrow Transplant 13:51, 1994.
6. Aversa F, Terenzi A, Carotti A, et al: Improved outcome with T-cell-depleted bone marrow transplantation for acute leukemia. J Clin Oncol 17:1545, 1999.
7. Kernan NA, Bartsch G, Ash RC, et al: Analysis of 462 transplantations from unrelated donors facilitated by the National Marrow Donor Program. N Engl J Med 328:593, 1993.
8. Hansen JA, Gooley TA, Martin PJ, et al: Bone marrow transplants from unrelated donors for patients with chronic myeloid leukemia. N Engl J Med 338:962, 1998.
9. Topolsky D, Crilley P, Styler MJ, et al: Unrelated donor bone marrow transplantation without T cell depletion using a chemotherapy only conditioning regimen: low incidence of failed engraftment and severe acute GVHD. Bone Marrow Transplant 17:549, 1996.
10. Aversa F, Tabilio A, Velardi A, et al: Treatment of high-risk acute leukemia with T-cell-depleted stem cells from related donors with one fully mismatched HLA haplotype. N Engl J Med 339:1186, 1998.
11. Champlin R: T-cell depletion to prevent GVHD after bone marrow transplantation. Hematol Oncol Clin North Am 4:687, 1990.
12. Papadopoulos EB, Carabasi MH, Castro-Malaspina, et al: T-cell-depleted allogeneic bone marrow transplantation as postremission therapy for acute myelogenous leukemia: freedom from relapse in the absence of GVHD. Blood 91:1083, 1998.
13. Drobyski WR, Ash RC, Casper JT, et al: Effect of T-cell depletion as GVHD prophylaxis on engraftment, relapse, and disease-free survival in unrelated marrow transplantation for CML. Blood 83:1980, 1994.
14. Bentley SA, Brecher ME, Powell E, et al: Long-term engraftment failure after marrow ablation and autologous hematopoietic reconstitution: differences between peripheral blood stem cell and bone marrow recipients. Bone Marrow Transplant 19:557, 1997.
15. To LB, Dyson PG, Juttner CA: Cell-dose effect in circulating stem cell autografting. Lancet 2:404, 1986.
16. Juttner CA, To LB, Ho JQK, et al: Early lymphohematopoietic recovery after autografting using peripheral blood stem cell in acute non-lymphoid leukemia. Transplant Proc 20:40, 1988.
17. Bender J, To JB, Williams S, et al: Defining a therapeutic dose of peripheral blood stem cells. J Hematother 1:329, 1992.
18. Kiss JE, Rybka WB, Winkelstein A, et al: Relationship of CD34+ cell dose to early and late hematopoiesis following autologous peripheral blood stem cell transplantation. Bone Marrow Transplant 19:303, 1997.
19. Weaver CH, Potz J, Redmond J, et al: Engraftment and outcomes of patients receiving myeloablative therapy followed by autologous peripheral blood stem cells with a low CD34+ cell content. Bone Marrow Transplant 19:1103, 1997.
20. Zimmerman TM, Lee WJ, Bender JG, et al: Quantitative CD34 analysis may be used to guide peripheral blood stem cell harvest. Bone Marrow Transplant 9:439, 1995.
21. Uckun FM, Kersey JH, Vallera DA, et al: Autologous bone marrow transplantation in high-risk remission T-lineage acute lymphoblastic leukemia using immunotoxins plus 4-hydroperoxycyclosphosphamide for marrow purging. Blood 76:1723, 1990.
22. Miller JS, Arthur DC, Craig EL, et al: Myelodysplastic syndromes after autologous bone marrow transplantation: an additional late complication of curative cancer therapy. Blood 83:3780, 1994.
23. Stone RM, Neuberg D, Soiffer R, et al: Myelodysplastic syndrome as a late complication following autologous bone marrow transplantation for non-Hodgkin's lymphoma. J Clin Oncol 12:2535, 1994.
24. Abruzzese B, Radford JE, Miller JS, et al: Detection of abnormal pretransplant clones in progenitor cells of patients who developed myelodysplasia after autologous transplantation. Blood 94:1814, 1999.
25. Torok-Storb R, Holmberg L: Role of marrow microenvironment in engraftment and maintenance of allogeneic hematopoietic stem cells. Bone Marrow Transplant 14(Suppl 4):571, 1994.
26. Torok-Storb B, Simmons PJ, Przepiorka D: Impairment of hemopoiesis in human allografts. Transplant Proc 19(Suppl 7):33, 1987.
27. Greenberger JS: Toxic effects on the hematopoietic microenvironment. Exp Hematol 19:1101, 1991.
28. Rothstein L, Pierce JH, Klassen V, et al: Amphotropic retrovirus vector transfer of the v-ras oncogene into human hematopoietic and stromal cells in continuous bone marrow culture. Blood 65:744, 1985.
29. Simmons P, Kaushansky K, Torok-Storb B: Mechanism of a CMV-mediated myelosuppression: perturbation of stromal cell function versus direct infection of myeloid cells. Proc Natl Acad Sci U S A 87:1386, 1990.
30. Mayer A, Podlech J, Kurz S, et al: Bone marrow failure by cytomegalovirus is associated with an in vivo deficiency in the expression of essential stromal hemapoietin genes. J Virol 71:4589, 1997.
31. Weiland HT, Salimans MMM, Fibre WE, et al: Prolonged human parvovirus B19 infection with severe anemia in a bone marrow transplant patient. Br J Haematol 71:300, 1989.

32. Azzi A, Fanci R, Ciappi S, et al: Human parvovirus B19 infection in bone marrow transplantation patients. Am J Hematol 44:207, 1993.

33. Solano C, Juan O, Gimeno C, et al: Engraftment failure associated with peripheral blood stem cell transplantation after B19 parvovirus infection. Blood 88:1515, 1996.

34. Itala M, Kotilainen P, Nikkari S, et al: Pure red cell aplasia caused by B19 parvovirus infection after autologous blood stem cell transplantation in a patient with chronic lymphocytic leukemia. Leukemia 11:171, 1997.

35. Drobyski WR, Dunne WM, Burd EM, et al: Human herpesvirus-6 infection in allogeneic bone marrow transplant recipients: evidence of a marrow-suppressive role for HHV-6 in vivo. J Infect Dis 167:73 5, 1993.

36. Rosenfeld CS, Rybka WB, Weinbaum D, et al: Late graft failure due to dual bone marrow infection with variants A and B of human herpesvirus-6. Exp Hematol 23:626, 1995.

37. Niki T, Nakao S, Ueda M, et al: Incomplete marrow recovery associated with hepatitis after syngeneic bone marrow transplant for aplastic anemia: successful treatment with second marrow transplantation without preconditioning. Br J Haematol 75:285, 1990.

38. Korn K, Schmidt B, Greil J, et al: Hepatitis G virus—association with graft failure after hematopoietic stem cell transplantation? Beitrage Infusionsther Transftisionsmed 31:16, 1997.

39. Yokota T, Tsuboi A, Okajima Y, et al: Treatment of graft failure after bone marrow transplantation. Leuk Res 18:875, 1994.

40. Mehta J, Powles R, Singhal S, et al: Outcome of autologous rescue after failed engraftment of allogeneic marrow. Bone Marrow Transplant 17:2 13, 1996.

41. Fouillard L, Deconinck E, Tiberghien P, et al: Prolonged remission and autologous recovery in two patients with CML after graft failure of allogeneic bone marrow transplantation. Bone Marrow Transplant 21:943, 1998.

42. Lipton JH, Messner H: The role of second bone marrow transplant using a different donor for relapsed leukemia or graft failure. Eur J Haematol 58:133, 1997.

43. Remberger M, Ringden O, Ljungman P, et al: Booster marrow or blood cells for graft failure after allogeneic bone marrow transplantation. Bone Marrow Transplant 22:73, 1998.

44. Grandage VL, Comish JM, Pamphilon DH, et al: Second allogeneic bone marrow transplants from unrelated donors for graft failure following initial unrelated donor bone marrow transplantation. Bone Marrow Transplant 21:687, 1998.

45. Friedberg JW, Neuberg D, Stone RM, et al: Outcome in patients with myelodysplastic syndrome after autologous bone marrow transplantation for non-Hodgkin's lymphoma. J Clin Oncol 17:3128, 1999.

CHAPTER FIFTY-THREE

Infection and Immunization

David J. Tweardy, M.D., and
Scott M. White, M.D.

The late postengraftment period (~6 months and later) following hematopoietic stem cell transplantation (HSCT) is characterized by a number of immune system defects relating to the continuing recovery and normalization of B- and T-lymphocyte functions. Chronic graft-versus-host disease (GVHD) and its treatment prolong the time for these functions to recover and superimpose additional disruptions of host defenses. Because of the nature of these defects in host immunity and their accentuation by chronic GVHD, patients undergoing HSCT are susceptible to specific infectious agents during this late period.

The recovery of normal immune system activity after both autologous HSCT (autoHSCT) and allogeneic HSCT (alloHSCT) begins with restoration of basic phagocytic and nonspecific cytotoxic defenses.[1] Normal serum levels of immunoglobulin IgM and IgG are achieved within 3–4 months after both types of HSCT.[1, 2] Inversion of the normal CD4+/CD8+ T-cell ratio occurs as lymphocyte populations recover from post-HSCT immunosuppressive regimens.[1, 2] Because of this aberrant T-cell development and interaction, B-cell development and subsequent Ig production in response to neoantigens are impaired until well into the late phase, recovering by 9–12 months after transplantation as the CD4/CD8 ratio normalizes.[1, 2] Secretory IgA production specifically may remain impaired for years after autoHSCT or alloHSCT.[1, 2] Eventually, long-term healthy survivors of HSCT experience essentially normal specific immune responses. After alloHSCT, however, this pattern of immune system recovery is frequently disrupted by chronic GVHD and its treatment.

GVHD is becoming increasingly understood as a complex interplay of alloreactive T lymphocytes, autoreactive T lymphocytes, and an inflammatory cytokine response promoting cytotoxic tissue damage.[3] As donor and recipient human leukocyte antigen (HLA) identity become increasingly disparate, GVHD occurs more frequently and with greater intensity. Relative HLA disparity has even been found by some investigators to be an independent risk factor for infections during the late period after HSCT.[4] T-cell depletion of donor marrow and immunosuppressive agents are used to reduce the incidence and severity of GVHD. For chronic GVHD, the measures taken to reduce its incidence and its treatment all act to disrupt T-cell development and therefore T cell–mediated immune functions, inducing greater delays in the recovery of a normal CD4+/CD8+ ratio, defective primary responses to neoantigens, failure of IgM to IgG class switching, and further reduction in secretory IgA production.[1, 5, 6] Active chronic

GVHD typically affects the skin, liver, and mouth, with other areas such as the eyes, sinuses, esophagus, lungs, vagina, and muscles less commonly involved.[5, 6] Because of the disruption of these dermal and mucosal membranes by chronic GVHD, along with impaired reticuloendothelial cell system function, afflicted patients have a much higher risk of infection compared with patients without chronic GVHD.[5] Discussions on acute and chronic GVHD can be found in Chapters 39, 45, and 54.

INFECTIONS

BACTERIAL INFECTIONS

Encapsulated Bacteria

Epidemiology

As patients undergoing HSCT survived 6 months and longer, it was noticed that their incidence of sinopulmonary pneumococcal infections was much greater than in the normal population (27% vs. 0.2% in the normal population).[7] In one report, 7 of 26 long-term survivors (>7 months post transplantation) experienced pneumococcal infections, of which 5 were associated with bacteremia. These patients had normal hematopoietic function and were not receiving immunosuppressive therapy. They were found to have a decreased serum opsonic activity for *Streptococcus pneumoniae* based on decreased levels of antipneumococcal IgG and or impaired complement activity. Later studies confirmed that pneumococcal disease was occurring more frequently in transplant recipients and identified defects in production of IgA and IgG₂, which persisted into the late period following both autoHSCT and alloHSCT, and contributed to the increased susceptibility to pneumococcal infections.[1, 8–11] Although some studies could not identify chronic GVHD as being specifically associated with an increased risk of pneumococcal infections, it does alter host mucosal barriers and influence reticuloendothelial cell functions, making patients functionally asplenic and therefore theoretically making afflicted patients even more susceptible to infection.[6, 7, 12, 13]

Although less frequent than pneumococcal infections, *Haemophilus influenzae* type B (HIB) infections also occur with increased frequency in patients undergoing HSCT over normal hosts.[14–16] Given the encapsulated nature of this organism, similar to pneumococci, the same risk factors apply regarding the predisposition of transplant recipients to infections with this agent. HIB tends to be the etiologic agent in patients receiving prophylactic penicillin to prevent pneumococcal infection who develop pneumonia.[15] *Neisseria meningitidis* is another encapsulated organism that is not as well studied because of its lower incidence relative to infections caused by *Streptococcus pneumoniae* and *H. influenzae*; however, patients undergoing HSCT are potentially more susceptible to this agent than normal hosts for the same reasons.

Treatment

The treatment of pneumococcal infections has changed since the mid-1980s because of the emergence of penicillin-resistant strains.[17] Most strains of pneumococci in the United States have minimum inhibitory concentrations (MIC) for penicillin of 0.05–0.1 μg/mL. Ten percent or more of clinical isolates are now found to be intermediate in resistance, with MIC in the range of 0.1–1.0 μg/mL. There are also a small number (~1%) of strains displaying high-level resistance to penicillin with MIC greater than 2.0 μg/mL.[18] This resistance is mediated by mutations in the penicillin-binding proteins of the pneumococcus.[19] In the case of high-level resistance, it is thought that the direct transfer of genetic material from another species is responsible because of other antimicrobial resistance genes also found in these high-level penicillin-resistant strains.[20] Increased MIC for second- and third-generation cephalosporins are also found in the penicillin-resistant pneumococcal isolates, which is not surprising because these drugs also work via penicillin-binding protein.[21, 22] No resistance to vancomycin has been identified thus far, and no studies of penicillin use for resistant pneumococcal infections in immunocompromised hosts have been reported.

The clinical implications of these newly emerging penicillin-resistant pneumococci were examined in immunocompetent patients with severe pneumonia. Patients infected with a penicillin-resistant pneumococcal strain had no increase in mortality compared with patients infected with penicillin-sensitive strains, even though both groups were treated with penicillin or ampicillin.[17] The findings may be explained by the fact that intravenous penicillin G, when given at 2–4 million units every 4–6 hours, provides serum and lung tissue concentrations well above the MIC of even high-level resistant strains. Cerebrospinal fluid levels of penicillin, however, would not be adequate even at maximum recommended dosages. Therefore, the recommendation for treatment of suspected pneumococcal disease in patients undergoing HSCT is to start with vancomycin and add a third-generation cephalosporin if meningeal disease is suspected because of variable penetration of vancomycin into cerebrospinal fluid. Once an isolate is obtained and is tested for penicillin sensitivity, antimicrobial coverage may then be adjusted.

Treatment of *Haemophilus influenzae* must account for the presence of β-lactamase production by many clinical isolates.[23, 24] Susceptibility to trimethoprim-sulfamethoxazole (TMP-SMX), second- and third-generation cephalosporins, ampicillin or amoxicillin plus a β-lactamase inhibitor, and fluoroquinolones provide many options for treatment of *Haemophilus* infections.[23, 25] For treatment of minor infections, such as mild sinusitis or otitis, oral TMP-SMX or a second-generation cephalosporin is adequate. For more severe disease, such as pneumonia or meningitis, the third-generation cephalosporins are the preferred agents, with fluoroquinolones being useful in these cases for patients allergic to cephalosporins.

Prevention and Vaccination

Because of the penicillin resistance found in *Haemophilus influenzae* and *Streptococcus pneumoniae*, TMP-SMX given two or three times weekly is presently the most appropriate choice for antibiotic prophylaxis, with penicillin or ampicillin being given daily to those patients unable to take TMP-SMX.[6] For patients without evidence of chronic GVHD, this prophylaxis may be discontinued 9–12 months after transplantation as production of IgG recovers. For those patients with chronic GVHD or on immunosupressive agents as treatment for chronic GVHD, however, such prophylaxis should continue until chronic GVHD resolves.

The utility of available vaccines has been examined for both *S. pneumoniae* and *H. influenzae*. The protective antibodies generated by these vaccines are against the polysaccharide capsules of the organisms. Typically, the titers of IgM and IgG to these organisms fall significantly after the HSCT conditioning regimen. The pneumococcal 14-valent and 23-valent polysaccharide vaccines have been studied in a variety of situations. In general, the immunogenicity of these pure polysaccharide vaccines is poor, even 2 years after both alloHSCT and autoHSCT.[12, 26, 28] Even when the donor is immunized with pneumococcal vaccine prior to transplantation and the recipient is vaccinated 18–24 months after transplantation, responses to most pneumococcal serotypes remain below normal. This is most likely because polysaccharides are not T cell–dependent antigens.[27, 28] B cells responding to T cell–independent antigens, as the designation indicates, do not generate a concomitant memory T-cell expansion and tend to have decreased B-cell expansion upon re-exposure to antigen. These B cells also produce only IgM and IgG_2 in response to these polysaccharide antigens, as opposed to B cells responding to T cell–dependent antigens, which produce a much broader variety of immunoglobulin types.[29] Interestingly, even though it is associated with impaired immunoglobulin class switching, the presence of chronic GVHD does not seem to further diminish the response to pneumococcal vaccination, perhaps because the antibody response to the pneumococcal vaccine fails to progress to the level at which chronic GVHD could even have an impact.[12, 26]

The general lack of efficacy of the polysaccharide pneumococcal vaccine is most unfortunate because the very patients who are most at risk for pneumococcal disease—those during the first 1–2 years after transplantation or those with chronic GVHD—are the poorest responders to pneumococcal vaccination. The meningococcal vaccine presently available is also a pure polysaccharide preparation and likely results in similar poor responses in this population. Even though these vaccines induce only limited antibody responses, some authors continue to recommend their routine use at 12 months post transplantation.[30] Newer protein conjugated pneumococcal vaccines are being examined for their ability to elicit a T cell–dependent response and therefore provide an improved initial response as well as a booster effect. The efficacy of these conjugate vaccines is being examined in infants and immunosuppressed adults with some encouraging results. More evaluation is required, however, before recommendations regarding their use can be made with confidence.[31–35]

For HIB, newer vaccines that conjugate HIB capsular polysaccharide to a protein, such as diphtheria or tetanus toxoid, have been found to be effective in infants and other populations who respond poorly to pure polysaccharide vaccines.[36–38] In patients undergoing HSCT, HIB protein conjugate vaccines appear to be much more effective than polysaccharide pneumococcal vaccines or older HIB capsular polysaccharide vaccines at producing significant antibody responses and have minimal side effects.[15, 28] In one study, patients undergoing alloHSCT were noted to react to the HIB conjugate vaccine as early as 4 months after transplantation.[15] In a later study, in which donors were also immunized with HIB conjugate vaccine, antibody production in response to vaccination was significantly increased as early as 3 months post transplantation, whereas patients whose donors were not immunized did not respond until 12–24 months after HSCT.[28] In either case, the response rate and antibody titer are much better in those receiving conjugate vaccine than in those receiving pure capsular polysaccharide vaccine. These study results and safety profile suggest that the HIB conjugate vaccine be given to patients undergoing autoHSCT and alloHSCT as early as 4–6 months after transplantation with two additional doses given at 12 and 18–24 months.

Other Bacterial Infections

Other bacterial infections that complicate the late period following HSCT typically relate to the presence of chronic GVHD and its attendant immunosuppressive therapy. Because of skin ulceration and fibrosis resulting from the scleroderma-like nature of chronic GVHD, cellulitis and skin abscesses account for up to 9% of the infections occurring during this period.[16] These are most commonly due to *Staphylococcus* or *Streptococcus* and should be treated with an antistaphylococcal penicillin or vancomycin along with local drainage if fluctuance is clinically evident. Chronic GVHD also produces a Sjögren-like sicca syndrome with decreased lacrimal and salivary secretions. This leaves patients at risk for bacterial conjunctivitis and keratitis, which can be due to a variety of agents, including *Staphylococcus, Streptococcus, Haemophilus, Chlamydia,* or *Pseudomonas.* Cultures of the conjunctiva or cornea should be obtained and topical therapy initiated. In the case of keratitis, immediate ophthalmologic evaluation is recommended because of the risk of corneal perforation. The administration of appropriate systemic antimicrobials should be based on Gram stain of the corneal scrapings and adjusted according to culture results.

VIRAL INFECTIONS

Varicella-Zoster Virus

Varicella-zoster virus (VZV) infections typically occur as single events of reactivation of latent virus in patients who were seropositive prior to transplantation, with both autologous and allogeneic transplant recipients being at risk.[39, 40] Disease occurs at a median of approximately 5 months after alloHSCT and 3 months after autoHSCT with a similar incidence of 25–40% in both groups. The majority of cases are noted within the first year.[39, 41] Typical VZV disease presents as dermatomal zoster, but in 16% of cases it initially presents as varicella. Asymptomatic seroconversion has also been documented.[42] Of those patients who initially present with dermatomal disease, up to 36% eventually experience dissemination if not treated, with a mortality rate of 10%.[39] More severe disease is associated with acute GVHD and onset within 7 months of transplantation.[6, 40] Prophylaxis for VZV reactivation extending from 6 months to 1 year after transplantation is recommended by some authors, with acyclovir, 200 mg orally four times daily, reported to be effective at reducing the rate of recurrence.[43] Other authors have found that VZV prophylaxis only delays the occurrence of VZV infection until prophylaxis is stopped and reduces the VZV-specific T-cell response because of reduced antigen exposure.[44]

Treatment for VZV infection using oral acyclovir is available, but the poor absorption of this drug and higher MICs required for activity against VZV make such therapy unreliable.[13] Newer oral agents with improved bioavailability and longer half-lives, such as brivudin, famciclovir, penciclovir, and valacyclovir, are in development or currently available, but their efficacy in immunosuppressed patients is still under evaluation. For single dermatome disease, oral therapy with any of the available agents is appropriate. When dissemination involves multiple dermatomes or with involvement of the nasocilliary branch of the trigeminal nerve, therapy with intravenous acyclovir at doses of 10–15 mg/kg every 8 hours is recommended.

Other Viral Infections

Beyond 6 months after HSCT, viral infections other than with VZV are rare.[6, 13, 16] Patients at this stage of recovery with chronic GVHD and/or on immunosuppressive therapy have been reported to experience severe infections with cytomegalovirus, adenovirus, or polyomavirus; others present with lymphoproliferative disease associated with Epstein-Barr virus; however, these are case reports.[13, 45, 46] Therapy for such infections is limited to supportive care, reduction in immunosuppressive therapy, and antivirals for cytomegalovirus disease. Immunization for specific viral diseases is discussed later.

FUNGAL INFECTIONS

Fungal infections other than oropharyngeal candidiasis in the late period following HSCT are unusual.[6, 16] Patients with chronic GVHD or on continued immunosuppressive therapy are at greater risk for fungal infections.[6, 13]

PROTOZOAN INFECTIONS

Six months or more after transplantation, protozoan infections, as with most viral and fungal pathogens, are uncommon in healthy transplant recipients.[6, 13] Agents such as *Pneumocystis carinii* or *Toxoplasma gondii* are only problematic for patients on immunosuppressive therapy for chronic GVHD.[47] Prophylaxis with trimethoprim-sulfamethoxazole given as one single-strength tablet three times weekly is reasonable in those patients at risk.

IMMUNIZATION OF HEMATOPOIETIC STEM CELL TRANSPLANT RECIPIENTS

TOXOIDS AND INACTIVATED-VIRUS VACCINES

It has been documented that after autoHSCT or alloHSCT, antibody titers to vaccines, including diphtheria, measles, mumps, polio, rubella, and tetanus, decrease over time.[48–53] The presence of chronic GVHD is associated with lower antibody titers to these agents as well as a poor response to revaccination.[1, 52] Inactivated virus vaccines such as the Salk polio vaccine and toxoid vaccines for diphtheria and tetanus have been shown to be safe and effective at restoring protective antibody levels as compared with those in normal vaccine recipients.

For diphtheria, immunization has been shown to be effective when a series of three doses of vaccine were given starting 2 years or more after alloHSCT.[48] Tetanus toxoid also stimulates an antibody response in patients undergoing alloHSCT, with response rates and antibody titers improved with a three-dose series relative to a single-dose regimen.[48, 50] Polio vaccination has been shown to be effective as early as 6 months after both autoHSCT and alloHSCT, though the recipients of allogeneic grafts had lower antibody titers at the end of the study.[52] Three doses of the trivalent inactivated polio vaccine appear to provide superior antibody titers to one- or two-dose regimens.[49]

Interestingly, one study that examined the antibody response to tetanus toxoid after HSCT identified normal antibody titers as early as 4 months post HSCT; however, the clonality of the response was markedly reduced.[54] This findings may result from decreased numbers of memory B cells found as patients continue to recover after HSCT, suggesting that although antibody titers in response to various vaccinations may appear normal, qualitatively these antibodies may not function as effectively. Recommendations for vaccination for diphtheria, tetanus, and polio based on the present data would be for immunization to begin at 12 months after transplantation, with two subsequent doses given over the following 12–18 months.

INFLUENZA A

Vaccination against influenza A viruses is recommended for all elderly or immunocompromised persons.[55] In the case of patients undergoing HSCT, this risk is greatest in the first 1–2 years after transplantation, when their immune response is weakest. A trial of immunization with a trivalent vaccine given to both autologous and allogeneic transplant recipients at 2–82 months after HSCT found that only 25% of patients responded to all three virus strains in the vaccine after a single dose.[56] When a second dose was given, the response rate increased by 4–10% for specific strains. None

of the patients who were less than 7 months beyond transplantation responded to the vaccine, even after the second dose. The response rate in the 7-months to 2-years post-HSCT group was 13% after the first dose, increasing from 21% to 29% after the second dose for specific strains. The group that was more than 2 years beyond HSCT responded at rates of 64–71% after the first dose, without significant improvement after the second dose.

Recommendations drawn from these results are to give amantadine or rimantadine prophylaxis to patients who are less than 2 years beyond HSCT and to vaccinate their household contacts. For patients who are more than 2 years beyond HSCT, immunization with a single dose of vaccine along with immunization of their household contacts is indicated.

LIVE ATTENUATED VIRUS VACCINES

Measles, Mumps, and Rubella

Measles, mumps, and rubella (MMR) vaccines are all live attenuated virus preparations, raising concern for their administration to potentially immunosuppressed persons. In one study, the loss of immunity to these agents after autoHSCT was examined: only 6–18% of patients became seronegative at 1 year after transplantation.[57] Some of these patients then received a live vaccine, none of whom developed significant side effects. Another study showed that the MMR vaccine was safe when given to patients undergoing alloHSCT without evidence of chronic GVHD and who did not receive any immunosuppressive agents.[53] Although seroconversion occurred in only about 70% of these patients, no serious side effects were noted. Even though herd immunity makes the risk of acquiring MMR quite low, it is still recommended that patients who are 2 or more years beyond transplantation, who lack evidence of chronic GVHD, and who are not receiving immunosuppressive agents should then receive the MMR vaccination along with confirmation of similar vaccination of household contacts.[43]

Varicella-Zoster Virus

The vaccine for the varicella-zoster virus (VZV) is a live attenuated virus preparation and shares the same risks as the MMR vaccine for administration to patients undergoing HSCT.[58] Because most patients who experience severe reactivation of VZV do so early after HSCT (<6–7 mo), its use is unsafe during the period when patients are at highest risk for severe disease. This fact, in addition to the availability of safe and effective pharmacologic therapy for VZV infections, makes the use of the VZV vaccine unwarranted in patients undergoing HSCT. For patients who are seronegative and exposed to VZV, especially those patients with chronic GVHD or who are receiving immunosuppressive agents, varicella-zoster immune globulin should be administered within 4 days after exposure as an attempt to abort clinical varicella infection.

INTRAVENOUS IMMUNOGLOBULIN

The use of intravenous immunoglobulin in patients undergoing HSCT has been examined for its effects on acute and chronic GVHD as well as on infectious complications at all stages of marrow engraftment.[59-61] In the late period after HSCT, no clear benefit has been identified; no decrease in the incidence of chronic GVHD or late infectious complications has been documented.[59, 60] At this time, the use of intravenous immunoglobulin beyond 3 months from transplantation for the purpose of reducing chronic GVHD and/ or the incidence of infection is not warranted.

CONCLUSION

Once transplant recipients have survived into the sixth month after transplantation, their risk of infection decreases significantly. After 2 years, their immunologic defenses are considered essentially normal except for decreased production of secretory IgA. Chronic GVHD and its treatment can seriously delay this recovery, inflicting persistent defects on both immunoglobulin production and cell-mediated immunity. The most common infectious complications during this final recovery stage after transplantation are sinopulmonary infections with encapsulated bacteria and reactivation of latent VZV. Through the use of prophylactic antimicrobials and advances in vaccine immunogenicity, the incidence of such complications can be reduced. Reimmunization for childhood illnesses and yearly influenza vaccination also play an important role in maintaining the health of bone marrow transplant recipients.

REFERENCES

1. Lum LG: The kinetics of immune reconstitution after human marrow transplantation. Blood 69(2):369–380, 1987.
2. Atkinson K: Reconstruction of the haemopoietic and immune systems after marrow transplantation. Bone Marrow Transplant 5, 1990.
3. Vogelsang GB, Hess AD: Graft-versus-host disease: new directions for a persistent problem. Blood 84(7):2061–2067, 1994.
4. Ochs L, et al: Late infections after allogeneic bone marrow transplantations: comparison of incidence in related and unrelated donor transplant recipients. Blood 86(10):3979–3986, 1995.
5. Siadak M, Sullivan KM: The management of chronic graft-versus-host disease. Blood Rev 8(3):154–160, 1994.
6. Sable CA, Donowitz GR: Infections in bone marrow transplant recipients. Clin Infect Dis 18(3):273–281, 1994.
7. Winston DJ, et al: Pneumococcal infections after human bone-marrow transplantation. Ann Intern Med 91(6):835–841, 1979.
8. Kiesel S, et al: B-cell proliferative and differentiative responses after autologous peripheral blood stem cell or bone marrow transplantation. Blood 72(2):672–678, 1988.
9. Aucouturier P, et al: Long lasting IgG subclass and antibacterial polysaccharide antibody deficiency after allogeneic bone marrow transplantation. Blood 70(3):779–785, 1987.
10. Sheridan JF, et al: Immunoglobulin G subclass deficiency and pneumococcal infection after allogeneic bone marrow transplantation. Blood 75(7):1583–1586, 1990.
11. Velardi A, et al: Acquisition of Ig isotype diversity after bone marrow transplantation in adults: a recapitulation of normal B cell ontogeny. J Immunol 141(3):815–820, 1988.
12. Lortan JE, et al: Class- and subclass-specific pneumococcal antibody levels and response to immunization after bone marrow transplantation. Clin Exp Immunol 88(3):519–529, 1992.
13. Wingard JR: Advances in the management of infectious complications after bone marrow transplantation [see comments]. Bone Marrow Transplant 6(6):371–383, 1990.
14. Cordonnier C, et al: Pulmonary complications occurring after allogeneic bone marrow transplantation: a study of 130 consecutive transplanted patients. Cancer 58(5):1047–1054, 1986.
15. Barra A, et al: Immunogenicity of Haemophilus influenzae type b

16. conjugate vaccine in allogeneic bone marrow recipients. J Infect Dis 166(5):1021–1028, 1992.
16. Atkinson K, et al: Analysis of late infections in 89 long-term survivors of bone marrow transplantation. Blood 53(4):720–731, 1979.
17. Pallares R, et al: Resistance to penicillin and cephalosporin and mortality from severe pneumococcal pneumonia in Barcelona, Spain [see comments]. N Engl J Med 333(8):474–480, 1995.
18. Appelbaum PC: Antimicrobial resistance in Streptococcus pneumoniae: an overview. Clin Infect Dis 15(1):77–83, 1992.
19. Markiewicz Z, Tomasz A: Variation in penicillin-binding protein patterns of penicillin-resistant clinical isolates of pneumococci. J Clin Microbiol 27(3):405–410, 1989.
20. Dowson CG, et al: Horizontal transfer of penicillin-binding protein genes in penicillin-resistant clinical isolates of Streptococcus pneumoniae. Proc Natl Acad Sci USA 86(22): 8842–8846, 1989.
21. Marchese A, et al: Susceptibility of Streptococcus pneumoniae strains isolated in Italy to penicillin and ten other antibiotics. J Antimicrob Chemother 36(5):833–837, 1995.
22. Chesney PJ, et al: Penicillin- and cephalosporin-resistant strains of Streptococcus pneumoniae causing sepsis and meningitis in children with sickle cell disease. J Pediatr 127(4):526–532, 1995.
23. Wollschlager CM, et al: Controlled, comparative study of ciprofloxacin versus ampicillin in treatment of bacterial respiratory tract infections. Am J Med 82(4A):164–168, 1987.
24. Scheifele DW, Fussell SJ: Frequency of ampicillin-resistant Haemophilus parainfluenzae in children. J Infect Dis 143(3):495–498, 1981.
25. Watanakunakorn C, Glotzbecker C: Comparative susceptibility of Haemophilus species to cefaclor, cefamandole, and five other cephalosporins and ampicillin, chloramphenicol, and tetracycline. Antimicrob Agents Chemother 15(6):836–838, 1979.
26. Guinan EC, et al: Polysaccharide conjugate vaccine responses in bone marrow transplant patients. Transplantation 57(5):677–684, 1994.
27. Giebink GS, et al: Titers of antibody to pneumococci in allogeneic bone marrow transplant recipients before and after vaccination with pneumococcal vaccine. J Infect Dis 154(4):590–596, 1986.
28. Molrine DC, et al: Donor immunization with Haemophilus influenzae type b (HIB)-conjugate vaccine in allogeneic bone marrow transplantation. Blood 87(7):3012–3018, 1996.
29. Yount WJ, et al: Studies on human antibodies: VI. Selective variations in subgroup composition and genetic markers. J Exp Med 127(3):633–646, 1968.
30. Ambrosino DM, Molrine DC: Critical appraisal of immunization strategies for prevention of infection in the compromised host. Hematol Oncol Clin North Am 7(5):1027–1050, 1993.
31. Ahmed F, et al: Effect of human immunodeficiency virus type 1 infection on the antibody response to a glycoprotein conjugate pneumococcal vaccine: results from a randomized trial. J Infect Dis 173(1):83–90, 1976.
32. Chan CY, et al: Pneumococcal conjugate vaccine primes for antibody responses to polysaccharide pneumococcal vaccine after treatment of Hodgkin's disease. J Infect Dis 173(1):256–258, 1996.
33. Kayhty H, et al: Pneumococcal polysaccharide-meningococcal outer membrane protein complex conjugate vaccine is immunogenic in infants and children. J Infect Dis 172(5):1273–1278, 1995.
34. Sarnaik S, et al: Studies on Pneumococcus vaccine alone or mixed with DTP and on Pneumococcus type 6B and Haemophilus influenzae type b capsular polysaccharide-tetanus toxoid conjugates in two- to five-year-old children with sickle cell anemia. Pediatr Infect Dis J 9(3):181–186, 1990.
35. Molrine DC, et al: Antibody responses to polysaccharide and polysaccharide-conjugate vaccines after treatment of Hodgkin disease. Ann Intern Med 123(11):828–834, 1995.
36. Weinberg GA, Granoff DM: Polysaccharide-protein conjugate vaccines for the prevention of Haemophilus influenzae type b disease. J Pediatr 113(4):621–631, 1988.
37. Anderson P, Insel RA: Prospects for overcoming maturational and genetic barriers to the human antibody response to the capsular polysaccharide of Haemophilus influenzae type b. Vaccine 6(2):188–191, 1988.
38. Robbins JB, Schneerson R: Polysaccharide-protein conjugates: a new generation of vaccines [see comments]. J Infect Dis 161(5):821–832, 1990.
39. Locksley RM, et al: Infection with varicella-zoster virus after marrow transplantation. J Infect Dis 152(6):1172–1181, 1985.
40. Han CS, et al: Varicella zoster infection after bone marrow transplanta-

tion: incidence, risk factors and complications. Bone Marrow Transplant 13(3):277–283, 1994.

41. Wacker P, et al: Varicella-zoster virus infections after autologous bone marrow transplantation in children. Bone Marrow Transplant 4(2):191–194, 1989.

42. Ljungman P, et al: Clinical and subclinical reactivations of varicella-zoster virus in immunocompromised patients. J Infect Dis 153(5):840–847, 1986.

43. Fielding AK: Prophylaxis against late infection following splenectomy and bone marrow transplant. Blood Rev 8(3):179–191, 1994.

44. Sempere A, et al: Long-term acyclovir prophylaxis for prevention of varicella zoster virus infection after autologous blood stem cell transplantation in patients with acute leukemia. Bone Marrow Transplant, 10(6):495–498, 1992.

45. Cervoni JP, et al: Exudative gastropathy associated with cytomegalovirus infection after allogenic bone marrow transplantation. Gastroenterol Clin Biol 18(8–9):775–778, 1994.

46. Zutter MM, et al: Epstein-Barr virus lymphoproliferation after bone marrow transplantation. Blood 72(2):520–529, 1988.

47. Sepkowitz KA: *Pneumocystis carinii* pneumonia in patients without AIDS. Clin Infect Dis 17(Suppl 2):S416–S422, 1993.

48. Li Volti S, et al: Immune status and immune response to diphtheria-tetanus and polio vaccines in allogeneic bone marrow-transplanted thalassemic patients. Bone Marrow Transplant 14(2):225–227, 1994.

49. Pauksen K, et al: Immunity to poliovirus and immunization with inactivated poliovirus vaccine after autologous bone marrow transplantation. Clin Infect Dis 18(4):547–552, 1994.

50. Ljungman P, et al: Response to tetanus toxoid immunization after allogeneic bone marrow transplantation. J Infect Dis 162(2):496–500, 1990.

51. Ljungman P, Duraj V, Magnius L: Response to immunization against polio after allogeneic marrow transplantation. Bone Marrow Transplant 7(2):89–93, 1991.

52. Engelhard D, et al: Immune response to polio vaccination in bone marrow transplant recipients. Bone Marrow Transplant 8(4):295–300, 1991.

53. Ljungman P, et al: Efficacy and safety of vaccination of marrow transplant recipients with a live attenuated measles, mumps, and rubella vaccine. J Infect Dis 159(4):610–615, 1989.

54. Gerritsen EJ, et al: Clonal dysregulation of the antibody response to tetanus-toxoid after bone marrow transplantation. Blood 84(12):4374–4382, 1994.

55. Anonymous: Prevention and control of influenza: recommendations of the Immunization Practices Advisory Committee (ACIP). MMWR Morbid Mortal Wkly Rep 39(RR-7):1–15, 1990.

56. Engelhard D, et al: Antibody response to a two-dose regimen of influenza vaccine in allogeneic T cell-depleted and autologous HSCT recipients. Bone Marrow Transplant 11(1):1–5, 1993.

57. Pauksen K, et al: Immunity to and immunization against measles, rubella and mumps in patients after autologous bone marrow transplantation. Bone Marrow Transplant 9, 1992.

58. Krause PR, Klinman DM: Efficacy, immunogenicity, safety, and use of live attenuated chickenpox vaccine. J Pediatr 127(4):518–525, 1995.

59. Guglielmo BJ, Wong-Beringer A, Linker CA: Immune globulin therapy in allogeneic bone marrow transplant: a critical review. Bone Marrow Transplant 13(5):499–510, 1994.

60. Sullivan KM: Immunomodulation in allogeneic marrow transplantation: use of intravenous immune globulin to suppress acute graft-versus-host disease. Clin Exp Immunol 104(Suppl 1):43–48, 1996.

61. Sullivan KM, et al: Immunomodulatory and antimicrobial efficacy of intravenous immunoglobulin in bone marrow transplantation. N Engl J Med 323(11):705–712, 1990.

CHAPTER FIFTY-FOUR

Chronic Graft-Versus-Host Disease

Deborah C. Marcellus, M.D., and Georgia B. Vogelsang, M.D.

Although the literature had long contained case reports of patients with chronic graft-versus-host disease (GVHD), the first thorough review on the subject was published by Sullivan et al. in 1981.[1] It described the manifestations of severe end-stage chronic GVHD and the initial experience of treating patients at Fred Hutchinson Cancer Research Center, Seattle. Many of their early observations continue to apply.

Chronic GVHD remains the most common late complication of allogeneic hematopoietic stem cell transplantation (HSCT). It continues to be a significant cause of morbidity and mortality. Although there have been significant improvements in the prevention and treatment of acute GVHD, these advances have not resulted in a decreased incidence of chronic GVHD. The persistence of this significant problem can probably be attributed to specific changes in clinical practice. First, allogeneic HSCT is being used in increasingly older persons and the risk of chronic GVHD is known to increase with age.[2, 3] The use of unrelated donors as well as related but not human leukocyte antigen (HLA)-identical donors is expanding. Both acute and chronic GVHD are significantly greater problems with these transplants compared with related sibling donor HSCT. The use of a new therapy, donor lymphocyte infusion, to treat relapsed disease after allogeneic transplantation has resulted in a substantial number of these patients experiencing chronic GVHD. Finally, there is a suggestion that patients receiving allogeneic peripheral blood progenitor cell transplants have a lower incidence of acute GVHD but that their incidence of chronic GVHD is as high or higher than that of comparable patients receiving marrow grafts. For these reasons, chronic GVHD must be considered one of the major problems still facing the field of blood and marrow transplantation.

PATHOGENESIS

Our understanding of the pathophysiology of chronic GVHD has lagged significantly behind our understanding of acute GVHD for a number of clinical and laboratory-related reasons. Clinical studies of patients with chronic GVHD are hampered by the fact that patients are frequently back in their local communities and thus at a distance from the transplant center by the time chronic GVHD develops. Early manifestations of the disease may be missed by physicians unfamiliar with the disease. The ability to clinically investigate the disease and the response to therapy may be impaired by the constraints of distance. Many assumptions about chronic GVHD have been influenced by how often patients are seen back at major transplant centers.

In addition, animal models of chronic GVHD exist but are expensive as well as time- and labor-intensive to establish. This has hampered both the investigation of basic immunobiology and the evaluation of therapy in animal models. Inoculation of T cells into allogeneic or congeneic, immunoincompetent mice or rats leads to GVHD-related changes such as diarrhea, skin lesions, severe wasting, and death within 1–3 weeks. This model is consistent with acute GVHD. Surviving animals might succumb later, usually 1–3 months after inoculation, with features consistent with chronic GVHD. The animals experience hepatosplenomegaly, immunodeficiency, and evidence of autoimmune phenomena before death. The symptoms of human chronic GVHD can be established in different ways, including performing HSCT across an isolated class I barrier or transplanting from parent to F1 (semiallogeneic HSCT).[4, 5] The model of cyclosporine-induced syngeneic GVHD reported by Hess et al. also results in a condition mimicking chronic GVHD.[6]

The ways in which these murine systems can be manipulated in order to alter the course and severity of GVHD do shed some light on potential factors that contribute to the development of GVHD. Variables such as the number and proportion of CD4+ versus CD8+ lymphocytes injected, the type and extent of recipient immunosuppression, the age of donors and recipients, and the presence or absence of tissue injury caused by chemotherapy, radiation, or infections result in different manifestations of GVHD.

The exact pathogenesis of chronic GVHD, however, remains unclear. In addition to donor-derived alloreactive T cells that are so important in acute GVHD, post-thymic CD4+ T cells are thought to play an important role in chronic GVHD.[7] The T-cell precursors may undergo aberrant "thymic education" after HSCT, which effectively makes them self-reactive or *autoreactive*. Additionally, the activation of different helper T-cell subsets (Th1 vs. Th2) may be responsible for distinct manifestations of acute and chronic GVHD.[4, 5, 8]

Investigators continue to try to delineate the role of alloreactivity versus autoreactivity in the pathogenesis of chronic GVHD. Alloreactivity to minor histocompatibility antigens is thought by some to explain chronic GVHD as a late phase of acute GVHD. The importance of autoreactivity, however, is suggested by clinical manifestations of chronic GVHD, which frequently mimic those of autoimmune diseases—the finding of autoantibodies in some patients with chronic GVHD and experimental data suggest the importance of thymic education in the pathogenesis of chronic GVHD. As new information becomes available about the pathogenesis of autoimmune disorders outside the setting of HSCT, the immunobiology of chronic GVHD may be further illuminated.

INCIDENCE

Chronic GVHD occurs in about one third of patients receiving HLA-identical sibling transplants, one half of patients undergoing HLA-nonidentical related HSCT, and about two thirds of those undergoing matched unrelated HSCT.[9] For patients receiving mismatched unrelated transplants, the incidence is even higher.

The diagnosis may be made early (occasionally >100 days post HSCT) and is rarely made later than 500 days post HSCT. The median day of diagnosis is 201 after HLA-identical sibling HSCT, 159 days after HLA nonidentical related HSCT, and 133 days after unrelated HSCT.[9]

RISK FACTORS

Several groups have looked at factors that predict chronic GVHD. HLA disparity is probably the most potent predictor of risk. Age of the recipient is also important. Among HLA-identical sibling transplant recipients, the risk of chronic GVHD rises from 13% in those less than 10 years of age to 46% in those over 20 years of age.[9] Another strong risk factor is prior acute GVHD.[2] The type of acute GVHD prophylaxis used may influence the risk of chronic GVHD. For example, patients receiving a vigorously lymphocyte-depleted marrow graft have a lower incidence of chronic GVHD.[2] This may be related to the lower incidence of acute GVHD in this setting.

Other proposed risk factors appear more controversial. Some consider the duration of cyclosporine prophylaxis to influence the development of chronic GVHD.[10-12] Transfusion of nonirradiated donor buffy coat or marrow boosts has been associated with an increased risk of chronic GVHD, whereas random red blood cell transfusions given shortly before HSCT have been reported to lead to decreased rates of chronic GVHD.[13, 14] The role of latent herpes infections, such as cytomegalovirus, in either the donor or the recipient has been implicated as an additional risk, but others have disputed this observation.[15, 16]

Loughran et al. reported a study looking at the value of day-100 screening in predicting chronic GVHD.[17] In 169 patients, screening tests were performed to determine whether chronic GVHD could be predicted. Seventeen clinical and laboratory factors were evaluated. Multivariate analysis was then performed and showed that finding GVHD on skin biopsy or oral mucosal biopsy, despite the lack of clinically evident GVHD or a history of acute GVHD, was a strong predictor for subsequent development of chronic GVHD. These features independently predicted a threefold relative risk of chronic GVHD.

Despite their predictive value, skin and oral mucosal biopsies are not routinely performed in the absence of clinically evident disease. No data suggest that treatment initiated in the absence of clinically evident disease is needed. Patients with a history of acute GVHD need to be closely monitored for the development of chronic disease.

Patients undergoing high-risk transplantation, such as those using unrelated or mismatched related donors, need to be frequently evaluated by those familiar with chronic GVHD.

CLASSIFICATION OR STAGING

Although a staging system has been developed and is widely accepted for acute GVHD, the same cannot be said for chronic GVHD. Chronic GVHD has been classified according to three basic models, which use the pattern of onset, extent of disease, or clinicohistologic features (Table 54-1).

Categorizing patients according to the onset of chronic GVHD in relation to acute GVHD, as described by Sullivan et al., is one of the most common approaches.[1] Three patterns of onset were identified—*de novo, quiescent*, and *progressive*. The least common onset is *de novo* chronic GVHD, in which patients have no antecedent acute GVHD. More commonly, chronic GVHD occurs in patients who have had documented acute disease. The onset of chronic GVHD is considered *quiescent* when the acute GVHD has completely resolved before chronic GVHD sets in. Patients whose disease evolves directly from acute GVHD have a *progressive* onset of chronic GVHD.

A fourth pattern of onset, *explosive* GVHD, was described by Vogelsang et al. in 1993.[18] This category describes a picture of multiorgan GVHD that shifts within days of presentation from erythroderma (i.e., like severe acute) to a diffuse lichenoid eruption. Patients have a mixed picture of acute organ GVHD involving the liver and/or gut and chronic GVHD of the mouth, eyes, and skin. As opposed to progressive chronic GVHD, many of these patients have had no prior acute GVHD. Some of these patients have had known chronic GVHD. The onset of explosive GVHD has been associated with abrupt cessation of immunosuppressive agents (usually due to noncompliance) or severe skin injury, such as occurs with sunburn or herpes zoster infections.

A second method of classifying chronic GVHD was also developed by investigators at Fred Hutchinson Cancer Research Center.[1] Patients are divided according to the extent of their disease and described as having either *limited* or *extensive* chronic GVHD. Localized skin involvement, with or without hepatic dysfunction, is considered limited disease. Extensive chronic GVHD is defined as either generalized skin involvement or localized skin involvement in association with eye involvement, oral involvement, hepatic dysfunction, and abnormal liver histology results (chronic progressive hepatitis, bridging necrosis, or cirrhosis) or involvement of any other target organ. Although this division of chronic GVHD is relatively simple, it has no utility in comparing patients undergoing treatment because patients with limited disease require little or no therapy.

Finally, patients may also be divided according to their primary clinical and histologic pattern. Thus, patients are described as having *lichenoid* or *sclerodermatous* disease. Although these are sometimes called *early* and *late* chronic GVHD, it is probably more meaningful to describe chronic GVHD in terms of the clinicopathologic manifestations. Although lichenoid disease usually occurs early and may evolve into the sclerodermatous form of the disease, li-

TABLE 54–1. CLASSIFICATION OF CHRONIC GVHD

MODEL	TYPE OF CHRONIC GVHD	CHARACTERISTICS
Pattern of onset	De novo	No antecedent acute GVHD
	Quiescent	Onset after complete resolution of acute GVHD
	Progressive	Direct evolution from acute GVHD
	Explosive	Acute and chronic GVHD features are concomitant at the time of onset and very aggressive
Extent of disease	Limited	Skin (localized) associated/none to mild liver involvement
	Extensive	Skin (generalized) and/or liver (severe), eye, mouth, or any other target organ involvement
Clinical/histologic pattern	Lichenoid	Maculopapular rash. Skin is thick and rough. Common oral and ocular involvement. Can evolve to scleroderma.
	Sclerodermatous	Thickening and tautness of the skin, usually patchy, occasional blisters and ulcers. Associated or isolated facial involvement causes severe limitation in the range of motion.

chenoid eruptions can occur very late in the course of the disease, particularly in patients with poorly controlled chronic GVHD.

CLINICAL AND HISTOLOGIC MANIFESTATIONS

The diagnosis of chronic GVHD is largely a clinical one, with confirmatory evidence being obtained histologically. The organ systems involved are described in the following paragraphs. Many of the clinical manifestations of chronic GVHD are similar to recognized autoimmune diseases that occur outside the transplant setting.[19] Infectious complications and, to a lesser extent, autoimmune phenomena contribute significantly to the clinical course of patients with chronic GVHD and are discussed separately.

SKIN

The most commonly involved organ in chronic GVHD is the skin.[20] Although an occasional patient has just oral, ocular, or hepatic disease, most patients have cutaneous manifestations. The majority of disease begins with raised, lichenoid papules. This eruption can occur anywhere and does not show the typical distribution of acute GVHD. Skin damaged either from acute GVHD, sun, or herpetic infection may be more susceptible to chronic GVHD. Clinically, the picture in lichenoid chronic GVHD does not differ significantly from other lichenoid skin eruptions such as lichen planus.[21, 22] Likewise, the sclerodermatous form of the disease clinically appears similar to systemic sclerosis.[23] Patients experience significant dermal sclerosis with hair loss and loss of sweat glands. Affected skin may become either hyperpigmented or hypopigmented. Patients with sclerotic disease have fragile skin that heals poorly, likely because of capillary and lymphatic damage. Rarely, patients experience blistering of their skin, which is a severe manifestation of sclerotic chronic GVHD.[24] Sclerotic skin involvement needs to be separated from deeper fascial involvement.

The histopathologic findings in the lichenoid skin lesions of chronic GVHD resemble those in idiopathic lichen planus. These include hyperkeratosis, acanthosis, dyskeratosis, and vacuolar alterations in the basal cell layer, together with monocytic and lymphocytic infiltrates in the papillary dermis. The intensity of inflammation in lichenoid chronic GVHD is less than that in idiopathic lichen planus. The lesions heal without dermal fibrosis or loss of elastic tissue. In contrast, the sclerodermoid form of chronic GVHD is associated with sclerosis and thickening of the reticular dermis, loss of distinction between the papillary and reticular dermis plus loss of rete pegs due to increased collagen deposition, and a mild perivascular lymphocytic infiltrate. Characteristically, the sweat glands are infiltrated with lymphocytes and melanophages. It has been reported that there is an initial increase in type III procollagen in the upper dermis, with a transition to type I procollagen in the later stages of disease.

MOUTH

Oral disease is also common.[25] Odynophagia (pain on swallowing) and xerostomia (dryness of the mouth) are frequent oral manifestations of chronic GVHD. In its earliest manifestations, patients may simply complain of dryness or food sensitivity and examination may reveal no more than mild erythema. As the disease progresses, however, a fine white reticular pattern or whitish plaques may appear on the buccal mucosa or tongue, mimicking oral lichen planus. These lichenoid changes may evolve to frank ulceration. Atrophy of the gums can occur, and this predisposes the patient to severe dental damage. Salivary glandular disease also contributes to the dryness, predisposing to dental disease. Furthermore, numerous dental caries may result from decreased secretions and deficiencies in local immunity. Secondary infections, particularly due to herpes simplex and *Candida*, are common. Changes in symptoms are frequently due to infection, and cultures should be obtained in any patient complaining of increased oral pain.

Salivary gland and mucosal involvement can be demonstrated by biopsy. The histopathologic features of lichenoid oral lesions are similar to those in the lichenoid form of cutaneous chronic GVHD. Fibrosing sialoadenitis, as seen in Sjögren sicca syndrome, may be demonstrated by biopsy of minor salivary glands.

EYES

Ocular disease is common in conjunction with oral disease. Photophobia, burning of the eyes, and dryness of the eyes are common symptoms in patients with extensive chronic GVHD.[26] The factors leading to dry eyes are not reversible. All patients with manifestations of chronic GVHD should be monitored with Schirmer tests because ocular damage may occur before symptoms are present. Conjunctival disease, with hyperemia progressing to pseudomembranes, is a severe manifestation of GVHD and has a very poor prognosis.[27] Left untreated, corneal damage may occur.

Lymphocytic infiltration, fibrosis, and destruction of lacrimal glands result in decreased tear production and chemosis plus corneal scarring and ulceration. These pathologic changes in the lacrimal apparatus resemble those in the sicca syndrome of Sjögren.

LIVER

Hepatic disease is also fairly common in chronic GVHD. Clinically, liver disease is associated with moderate elevations in alkaline phosphatase, bilirubin and, to a lesser extent, transaminases. Patients typically have few symptoms referable to their liver until their hepatic disease becomes severe. Portal hypertension, cirrhosis, and frank hepatic failure are rare.[28, 29]

Many of the findings are nonspecific; liver biopsy may be necessary to make the diagnosis. The portal triads have a dense, mixed infiltrate of lymphocytes, histiocytes, and often eosinophils and plasma cells. The infiltrate extends into the lobule with piecemeal hepatocellular involvement. The bile ducts usually show lymphocyte-associated necrosis of the epithelium and prominent periportal bile stasis. There is increased portal fibrosis, occasionally leading to micronodular cirrhosis. After long-standing active disease, the ducts in the portal triads may be decreased in number or absent.

RESPIRATORY TRACT

Some patients with chronic GVHD may have chronic sinopulmonary infections, cough, and bronchospasm. Although infiltration of submucosal glands with lymphocytes and plasma cells is common, these cellular infiltrates are not found in the bronchial and bronchiolar mucosa.

Obliterative bronchiolitis may also be associated with antecedent or concomitant chronic GVHD. This condition may be the result of any or all of the following factors: the underlying immune deficiency related to chronic GVHD and its treatment, the breakdown of the mucociliary defense system in the mainstem bronchi, and epithelial injury, as occurs in lymphocytic bronchiolitis. Bronchiolitis obliterans is considered a severe manifestation of chronic GVHD involving the lung.[30–32]

Unlike interstitial pneumonitis, which generally occurs during the first 100 days after transplantation, bronchiolitis obliterans occurs later on. Symptoms include progressive dyspnea, wheezing, and cough. Chest radiographs may be completely normal or they may show signs of hyperinflation, bleb formation, interstitial pneumatosis, pneumothorax, or pneumomediastinum. Studies of pulmonary function reveal a marked decrease in the forced expiratory volume in 1 second (FEV$_1$) compared with the forced vital capacity (FVC), decreased expiratory flow, reduced vital capacity, and increased residual lung volume. These findings are consistent with obstructive lung disease. In this setting, such disease may have either an acute or insidious onset.

Bronchiolitis obliterans carries a very poor prognosis, and no therapy has been shown to improve survival. In light of the prognostic importance of bronchiolitis obliterans, an adequate biopsy of lung tissue is required. Bronchiolitis obliterans must be distinguished histologically from bronchiolitis obliterans with organizing pneumonia because the latter condition does not carry the same grave prognosis as the former. In the absence of histologic confirmation of true bronchiolitis obliterans, reports of survival should be interpreted with caution.

Histopathologic findings in this late-onset obstructive airway disease are best detected in the terminal bronchioles. Open-lung biopsy is frequently required in order to obtain the tissue of interest. Lymphocytic and mononuclear cell infiltrates and hyperplasia of bronchiolar smooth muscle may be noted. Focal or transmural necrosis of bronchioles and bronchi is present. The most striking feature is the intraluminal accumulation of inflammatory cells and granulation tissue, which leads to partial or even complete occlusion of the bronchioles. Mucus plugging with atelectasis or emphysema of distal air spaces may be present. Hyperplasia of bronchial mucous glands and destruction of alveoli, as occur in chronic bronchitis and emphysema, are absent in cases of bronchiolitis obliterans. Although focal interstitial inflammatory reactions may occur, the intensity and extent of these changes are minimal. In contrast, such lesions are extensive in interstitial pneumonitis.

GASTROINTESTINAL TRACT

The gastrointestinal (GI) tract is rarely involved in chronic GVHD today. In the past, it occurred in untreated patients or as a sequela of severe acute GVHD affecting the gut. When involved, the symptoms include esophageal reflux, dysphagia, substernal pain, diarrhea, and weight loss. Abnormal motility, mucosal desquamation, and formation of webs or strictures may occur in the esophagus.[33] Bullous esophagitis has been described by Minocha et al.[34] Although mucosal or submucosal fibrosis is most common in the esophagus and very rare in the large intestine, it may occur anywhere along the upper GI tract. Mononuclear cell infiltrates as occur in the lamina propria may arise anywhere in the GI tract. The cellular infiltrates are associated with shortening of the villi and hyperplasia of the crypts of Lieberkühn, which is most evident in the small intestine. Even in the absence of histologically documented GI involvement, a wasting syndrome may develop.

MUSCULOSKELETAL

Myositis and myopathy have both been described in patients with chronic GVHD.[35, 36] Rarely, patients have myositis with tender muscles and elevated muscle enzymes. Parker et al. suggest that the clinical manifestations and treatment of myositis associated with chronic GVHD are similar to idiopathic or autoimmune myositis.[37] More commonly, limitation in function results from contractures or fasciitis. These possibilities should be considered in patients with limitations in strength or function. Patients frequently complain of muscle cramps, the exact etiology of which remains unclear.

As noted earlier, fascial involvement may be mistaken for thickening or sclerosis of the skin. When the overlying skin is soft and subtle but exhibits a peau d'orange characteristic, fascial involvement is the likely explanation. Janin et al., who originally reported this manifestation of chronic GVHD, used biopsies of deep tissue to document it.[38] Fascial involvement can be determined clinically in the presence of the findings already noted plus impaired range of motion. Patients may also have significant edema and myalgia. Patients with chronic GVHD should be monitored carefully for range of motion to look for this complication.

NEUROLOGIC

Neurologic conditions have been reported in patients with chronic GVHD, including peripheral neuropathy and myasthenia gravis.[39–41] Nerve biopsy and autoantibody studies may help in diagnosing these complications. No convincing evidence suggests direct central nervous system involvement with chronic GVHD, but the immunocompromised state of these patients puts them at risk for opportunistic infections such as toxoplasmosis, which neurologic symptoms might make apparent.

HEMATOPOIETIC SYSTEM

In many patients with chronic GVHD, peripheral blood counts are suppressed.[42, 43] It is not clear whether this is due to a direct effect on marrow stroma from the chronic GVHD or a specific autoimmune manifestation. Isolated neutropenia, anemia, or thrombocytopenia, as well as pancytopenia, may occur in patients with chronic GVHD. Investigators at Fred Hutchinson Cancer Research Center found thrombocytopenia to be a marker for severe chronic GVHD, whereas investigators at Johns Hopkins Oncology Center found that this was simply a reflection of progressive chronic GVHD.[44] Occasionally, patients have eosinophilia.

OTHER SYSTEMS

Women have been noted to have vaginitis and vaginal strictures that have been attributed to chronic GVHD.[45] These effects must be differentiated from those resulting from ovarian failure induced by the conditioning regimen.[46]

Kidney involvement by chronic GVHD has been reported in two patients,[47] but renal impairment is more commonly attributable to medications used in the treatment of GVHD than to a direct effect of the disease.

INFECTIOUS COMPLICATIONS

Patients with chronic GVHD must be considered profoundly immunocompromised. The basis for impaired immunity is multifactorial and includes disrupted mucosal barriers, thymic injury, functional asplenia, hypogammaglobulinemia, and qualitative T-cell and B-cell abnormalities.[48, 49] Increased susceptibility to infection is attributable to both features of the disease and its treatment. All patients should be carefully monitored for bacterial, viral, and fungal infections because infection is the leading cause of death among patients with chronic GVHD.

AUTOIMMUNE PHENOMENA

Many of the common features of chronic GVHD mimic autoimmune disorders. Essentially every autoimmune disorder has been reported in patients with chronic GVHD. This includes autoimmune cytopenia, myasthenia gravis, myositis, and vasculitis. Although these manifestations are frequently fascinating and may be very disabling to individual patients, they are simply a reflection of the disordered immune system in these patients.

PREVENTION

Because the occurrence of acute GVHD is a strong predictor of chronic GVHD, steps to reduce the incidence of acute GVHD have been evaluated to determine whether they also decrease chronic GVHD. For example, T-cell depletion of donor marrow has reduced the incidence of chronic GVHD by about 50%.[50] The effect is less pronounced with T-cell depletion of marrow from unrelated donors.[51] It will be of interest to see whether the use of molecular class I typing to identify and select unrelated donors will reduce the incidence of acute GVHD in this setting. Perhaps a more effective strategy for the prevention and treatment of acute GVHD will translate into a lower incidence of chronic GVHD. This is an area of active research around the world.

With the observation that weekly administration of intravenous immunoglobulin (IVIG) until day 90 post HSCT reduced the incidence and mortality of acute GVHD, Sullivan et al. conducted a randomized study to see whether continuation of IVIG administration would affect the incidence of chronic GVHD.[52, 53] No difference was observed among patients who received and those who did not receive IVIG monthly between days 90 and 360 post HSCT.

Other approaches have included prolonged administration of cyclosporine, transplantation of thymic tissue grafts, and administration of thymic factors. Extended cyclosporine administration has been reported to reduce the incidence of chronic GVHD,[10–12] whereas modulation of thymic function through tissue grafts or factor administration has not proven successful.[54, 55] Chao et al. reported results of a prospective, randomized, double-blind study comparing thalidomide with placebo as prophylaxis against chronic GVHD.[56] This group randomized 59 patients to receive either placebo or thalidomide (200 mg orally twice a day) starting on day 80 after allogeneic HSCT. Fifty-four patients were evaluable at the time of the first interim analysis, and the study was stopped at that time. Not only was there a higher incidence of chronic GVHD among the patients receiving thalidomide than among those receiving placebo ($P = .06$), but overall survival was significantly worse among those receiving thalidomide (P = .006). The authors concluded that the early use of thalidomide shifted the balance between GVHD and induction of tolerance, thus leading to the negative effects of thalidomide on incidence of chronic GVHD and overall survival.

EVALUATION

Once the diagnosis of chronic GVHD has been suspected clinically and confirmed histologically in one tissue, the extent of current involvement must be established. The initial evaluation should be comprehensive, looking at all organs or systems commonly involved in the disease, whether or not existing symptoms are referable to those organs. This initial evaluation can then be used as a baseline to assess progression of the disease or response to therapy. The elements of the initial and subsequent evaluations are shown in Table 54–2.

TREATMENT

The most successful treatment of patients with chronic GVHD results when a systematic approach to diagnosis,

management, and evaluation is undertaken by a multidisciplinary team whose members share an interest in this complex disorder. In addition to HSCT physicians and nurses, team members should include dermatologists, ophthalmologists, dieticians, physical and occupational therapists, and social workers. Pathologists with special expertise in the histologic features of GVHD are crucial. Because chronic GVHD can affect virtually any organ system, consultants in subspecialty areas such as dentistry, gastroenterology, neurology, and infectious diseases can be invaluable resources for the team.

Treatment of patients with chronic GVHD can be considered under two main categories, disease-halting therapy and supportive care. The first category includes therapy aimed at arresting disease progression. The second category deals with minimizing or preventing complications of the disease. A successful treatment approach addresses both categories of therapy.

DISEASE-HALTING THERAPY

The choice of therapy has evolved over time, but one of the first papers describing chronic GVHD also established

TABLE 54–2. EVALUATION OF THE PATIENT WITH CHRONIC GVHD

ORGAN SYSTEM	TESTS TO BE PERFORMED*	INDICATION
Skin	Biopsy	Papular rash, thickened skin, folliculitis, hyperpigmentation, severe dry skin to establish diagnosis
Mouth	Biopsy (buccal mucosa or salivary gland)	In absence of skin abnormality, affected buccal mucosa or salivary gland may be diagnostic
	Cultures	White plaques, ulcers may need to be cultured to rule out fungal/viral infection
Eyes	Schirmer test	All patients should have baseline ophthalmologic evaluation, including Schirmer test (positive result if tear production in 5 minutes is <5 mL) Evaluation of cornea prior to PUVA or etretinate
Liver	Bilirubin, aspartate aminotransferase, alanine aminotransferase, alkaline phosphatase	All patients at baseline
	Liver biopsy	For abnormal liver function test results, particularly when they occur in absence of skin/mouth when liver changes of chronic GVHD would require systemic therapy
Respiratory tract	Pulmonary function tests (forced vital capacity [FVC], forced expiratory volume in 1 second [FEV$_1$], diffusing capacity of the lungs for carbon monoxide [DL$_{CO}$])	All patients at baseline; repeat every 3–6 mo if chronic GVHD persists despite therapy or if patient becomes symptomatic.
	Helium lung volumes Transbronchial or open-lung biopsy to confirm	If FEV$_1$ and DL$_{CO}$ are significantly decreased.
GI tract	Endoscopy with biopsies and cultures	For patients with persistent nausea or dyspepsia.
	Colonoscopy with biopsies and cultures	For patients with diarrhea. Be sure to check for cytomegalovirus infection.
Musculoskeletal	Physical and occupational therapy assessment	All patients at baseline. Repeat serially to monitor response to therapy.
Immune system	Immunoglobulin levels	All patients at baseline. Repeat monthly if IgG less than 500 mg/dL and patient receiving supplemental intravenous immunoglobulin. Every 3–6 mo for other patients until off therapy for 6 mo.
Hematopoietic	Complete blood counts	All patients at baseline and at least monthly. Add reticulocyte count, haptoglobin, Coombs test, examination of peripheral smear if there is concern about hemolysis.
Other systems	Bone density studies	At baseline and every year for patients treated with steroids.
	Neurologic evaluation	In patients with signs or symptoms of peripheral neuropathy. MRI if concern regarding CNS side effects of cyclosporine/FK 506 or focal neurologic signs.
	Others	As indicated by symptoms

*In addition to clinical examination.
CNS, central nervous system; MRI, magnetic resonance imaging; PUVA, 8-methoxypsoralen plus ultraviolet A irradiation.

the need for therapy in most patients.[1] Fifty-two of 175 survivors of allogeneic transplantation experienced chronic GVHD. Five of these patients had limited chronic GVHD and received no therapy. They did well despite the lack of therapy. Today such patients might also be observed for progression and not immediately started on systemic therapy. On the other hand, among the 47 patients with extensive disease identified in this early report, 13 received no therapy and only two (18%) of the 13 survived. Mortality resulted from infection. Another 13 patients received therapy with drugs that today would be considered inadequate in terms of both nature and timing in the course of the disease. Three (23%) of these patients survived without significant disability. The final group of 21 were treated early in the course of their disease with a combination of prednisone and an alkylating agent. Seventy-six percent of these patients survived.

Basing their work on these findings, Sullivan et al. undertook a randomized double-blind study of prednisone and azathioprine versus prednisone plus placebo as early treatment of extensive chronic GVHD.[57] Patients with thrombocytopenia were defined as high risk and were not eligible for randomization because of concern about myelosuppression with azathioprine. These high-risk patients were treated with an equivalent dose of alternate-day prednisone. Results with 164 patients enrolled between 1980 and 1983 were reported (63 standard-risk patients in each of the two randomized groups and 38 high-risk, nonrandomized patients). The median duration of therapy was 2 years. All patients were treated with trimethoprim and sulfamethoxazole (TMP-SMX) prophylaxis. The nonrelapse mortality rate was 21% among randomized patients receiving prednisone alone and 40% in the randomized group receiving prednisone plus azathioprine (P = .003). The excess mortality among patients receiving combination therapy was attributed to infection. The overall survival rate was 61% in the prednisone arm and 47% in the combination therapy arm (P = .03). The 38 nonrandomized, high-risk patients treated concurrently with prednisone alone did worse than both standard-risk groups. These patients experienced a 58% nonrelapse mortality rate, resulting in 26% overall survival among the 38 patients with thrombocytopenia.

Subsequently, the same group studied the combination of alternate-day cyclosporine and prednisone in high-risk patients.[58] Among the 40 patients receiving initial treatment for high-risk disease, the actuarial survival rate was 52%. The cause of death was primarily related to infection and relapse of the primary disease.

Other approaches to initial therapy in high-risk patients have also been reported. A phase I–II trial of thalidomide for chronic GVHD resulted in a 48% 3-year survival rate among high-risk patients.[59] Again, infection was the major cause of death. Other groups have also tested thalidomide in chronic GVHD.[60, 61]

At this time, the mainstay of initial disease-halting therapy for chronic GVHD is immunosuppression. In patients with newly diagnosed extensive disease, a combination of cyclosporine and steroids is usual. Our group starts with daily prednisone at 1 mg/kg/day and daily cyclosporine at 10 mg/kg/day divided into two doses based on ideal or actual weight, whichever is less. After 2 weeks, provided the disease has comes under control, we begin tapering the steroids gradually (by 25% per week) such that patients

end up on 1 mg/kg of prednisone on alternate days. Once the steroid taper has been completed and patients are on 1 mg/kg of prednisone every other day without a flare in GVHD, we then taper the cyclosporine on the days when patients are getting their prednisone. On those days, cyclosporine is reduced by 25% per week. In this way, patients ultimately end up on alternate-day dosing such that the patient takes cyclosporine (10 mg/kg in two divided doses) on 1 day alternating with prednisone (1 mg/kg) the next day.

Given the chronic nature of the disease, response is usually evaluated after about 3 months on this final alternate-day dosing regimen. The 3-month time frame for evaluation of response to a given therapy is based on the observation that 90% of patients who are ultimately going to respond to that therapy show signs of some response by 3 months. If the disease has completely resolved, patients are gradually weaned off medication, with dose reductions made about every 2 weeks. Patients who are continuing to respond are kept on the same therapy and are re-evaluated in another 3 months. Once patients reach their maximal response, therapy is continued for another 3 months and then gradually weaned over 30–60 days. The drugs should not be discontinued abruptly or a flare may occur. For those who have not responded by the 3-month time point or in whom disease progresses during this period of observation, adjustments must be made.

Disease that is refractory to initial steroid therapy has been treated in a number of ways with variable success. Refractory cases were included in both the Fred Hutchinson Cancer Research Center study evaluating the combination of alternate-day cyclosporine and prednisone[58] and the Johns Hopkins Oncology Center study of thalidomide.[59] Sullivan's group reported a 67% survival rate among 21 patients receiving alternate-day cyclosporine and prednisone as salvage therapy. Vogelsang et al. saw a 78% survival rate in 23 refractory cases treated with thalidomide. Azathioprine is sometimes used in steroid-refractory cases but is probably better avoided because of its myelosuppressive effect.

The use of tacrolimus (FK506) in steroid-resistant cases has been reported by Tzakis et al.[62] Among 17 patients with extensive chronic GVHD after at least 2 months of first-line therapy had failed, persistent disease, or adverse reactions to first-line medication, six were judged to have incurred an unequivocally beneficial response. The authors described possible differential responsiveness in involved organs, with the best responses observed in skin and gut.

A retrospective review of 26 patients with refractory chronic GVHD treated with the steroid-sparing combination of mycophenolate mofetil and tacrolimus at Johns Hopkins Oncology Center was undertaken. The combination was well tolerated, and nearly half the patients experienced an objective response. Further studies are ongoing.

Particularly challenging are those patients with refractory sclerodermatous chronic GVHD. We reviewed the Johns Hopkins Oncology Center experience with etretinate, a synthetic retinoid, in 32 such patients.[63] This group was heterogeneous in many ways, but all had sclerodermatous GVHD that had failed to improve or was progressing on standard immunosuppressive therapy. The addition of etretinate to the treatment regimen led to clinical responses in 20 of the 32 patients. These results are considered encouraging, and further study is underway. In a similar vein, borrowing from the experience in treatment of non-GVHD dermatologic conditions, Lee et al. reported encouraging results using clofazimine.[64] This antimycobacterial drug has anti-inflammatory activity and has been used successfully in treating leprosy and chronic autoimmune skin disorders. Because of its effectiveness in other dermatologic diseases and the reports of in vitro studies, hydroxychloroquine (Plaquenol) is another agent of interest in chronic GVHD therapy.[65–67]

Patients with refractory disease may also benefit from the addition of nonpharmacologic approaches such as 8-methoxypsoralen plus ultraviolet A irradiation (PUVA). This approach was originally reported in 1985 by Hymes et al. and in 1986 by Atkinson et al.[68, 69] A review of 40 patients treated with PUVA at Johns Hopkins Oncology Center with either refractory disease (n = 35) or high-risk disease (n = 5) was undertaken.[70] Eleven patients had disease limited to the skin, and five obtained a complete response. Among 22 patients with systemic lichenoid disease, 11 complete skin responses and 6 partial skin responses were seen. Unfortunately, no systemic effects occurred in the patients with multiorgan disease. PUVA may be an effective therapy for cutaneous chronic GVHD. PUVA is currently being evaluated in combination with thalidomide and cyclosporine (found to be effective in an animal model). Rossetti et al. treated lymphocytes, ex vivo, with PUVA, then reinfused them into patients—good results were reported in five of eight patients treated.[71] Others have reported the use of low-dose total lymphoid irradiation. In a report of nine patients receiving 100 cGy of thoracoabdominal irradiation, six experienced significant improvements in their chronic GVHD.[72, 73]

Although virtually all patients with extensive disease require systemic therapy, patients with symptomatic disease limited to the oral cavity may benefit from topical steroids, thus sparing them the effects of systemic immunosuppression. We find that dexamethasone (Decadron) elixir (0.5 mg/5 mL) can be effective local therapy when the patient swishes 10 mL around the mouth for 2–3 minutes at least four times a day. Patients are instructed to spit this solution out rather than swallow it at the end of the swishing. Topical steroids such as fluocinonide (Lidex) have been tried. When local steroids alone fail to control the oral disease, we have tried cyclosporine swishes, again having the patient spit the solution out at the conclusion of a 2- to 3-minute swish. If the oral disease fails to resolve with topical therapy, a trial of oral PUVA or systemic immunosuppressive therapy may be warranted. Patients meeting the definition of limited disease at presentation generally do not require immediate initiation of systemic therapy, but such patients do require careful follow-up because their disease may progress to a more-extensive category.

SUPPORTIVE CARE

No less important than the disease-halting therapy just discussed are the measures taken for supportive care. Chronic GVHD is a cause of significant morbidity and mortality. Supportive-care measures aim to minimize both and, thus, improve both the quantity and the quality of life

for patients with chronic GVHD. The primary cause of death in patients with chronic GVHD is infection. Owing to their immunosuppressed state, all patients should receive antimicrobial prophylaxis. This is perhaps the most important factor in the care of these patients and should include *Pneumocystis carinii* prophylaxis (such as TMP-SMX) as well as prophylaxis against encapsulated organisms, including *Pneumococcus* (such as penicillin). Although the risk from *P. carinii* probably decreases once immunosuppressive anti-GVHD therapy is completed, we believe that poor splenic function persists. For this reason, our practice is to discontinue *P. carinii* prophylaxis 6 months after GVHD therapy is completed but to maintain patients on penicillin prophylaxis for life. Additionally, patients should receive antibiotic prophylaxis for dental and other invasive procedures, according to the "endocarditis" prophylaxis recommendations of the American Heart Association.

Topical antifungal prophylaxis with clotrimazole (Mycelex) troches or nystatin swishes should be used in all patients receiving local steroid therapy for oral GVHD. If thrush occurs despite this, systemic antifungal therapy is indicated. Acute episodes of herpetic infection should be treated with antiviral therapy. To avoid dissemination of dermatomal herpes zoster, we often initiate therapy with intravenous acyclovir rather than use one of the newer oral antiviral agents. Patients who were serologically positive to cytomegalovirus (CMV) coming into transplantation should undergo frequent surveillance cultures or testing for CMV antigenemia. Patients with documented CMV disease must be treated with ganciclovir and immunoglobulin infusion acutely and then maintained on ganciclovir prophylaxis while still on steroid therapy because there is a risk of reactivation of the disease.

Additional protection is afforded patients by supplemental IVIG if they have very low serum IgG levels. The goal of such therapy would be to keep the IgG level greater than 500 mg/dL. While still receiving immunosuppressive therapy, patients with chronic GVHD may or may not respond to vaccination. Vaccinations used in transplant populations should be delayed until 1 year after GVHD therapy has been completed and only given when there is no evidence of active disease. Antibody titers can be used to check response to inactivated vaccines that are typically given to patients after HSCT, such as inactivated polio, diphtheria, and tetanus toxoid. Polyvalent influenza, pneumococcal, and *Haemophilus influenzae B* immunization can also be given at that time. Live vaccines should not be given for at least 2 years after completion of therapy for chronic GVHD.

In addition to prophylaxis, having a high index of suspicion for and aggressively investigating potential infections is important in minimizing morbidity and mortality in chronic GVHD. Symptomatic management is also important in patients with chronic GVHD. Dry skin should be aggressively lubricated. Agents that are free of perfume and preservatives are best. Petroleum jelly offers excellent lubrication, but patients often complain about the messiness of this therapy. To get around this, we advise patients to apply petroleum jelly liberally before bedtime and to wear old night clothes. Trauma should be avoided because many of these patients have very frail skin that is prone to abrasion. Patients should avoid sunburn and should wear sunblock with at least a sunblock factor of 15. For those in whom sweat glands are affected, precautions must be taken to avoid getting overheated. Unfortunately, heat prostration and heat stroke may occur in patients who do not take precautions during extreme weather.

For patients with sicca syndrome, the use of preservative-free artificial tears at least every 4 hours during the day and preservative-free ointment at night is important. Careful ophthalmologic follow-up is needed to prevent long-term damage to the eyes. Artificial saliva may be used for the dry mouth. Topical analgesic products may be used, with caution, in patients with painful oral GVHD. Patients with dry mouths are at increased risk for dental caries, so close dental follow-up is essential.

Muscular aches and cramps are common complaints of unknown etiology. Electrolyte imbalances should be corrected with supplemental calcium, magnesium, and potassium. Quinine may be added. For cramps that persist and are disabling, we have tried dantrolene. This must be used cautiously with careful attention to side effects, which include muscle weakness, drowsiness, diarrhea, abnormal liver function test results, and sun sensitivity. It should not be used in patients being treated with PUVA.

Poor appetite is common in these patients, and malnutrition may result. The cause of the poor appetite is probably multifactorial and includes oral disease, dry mouth, altered taste, and side effects of drugs. Additionally, infections in the mouth or esophagus may contribute to poor oral intake. Nutritional assessment and monitoring is important to maintain the patient's well-being. Patients who are unable to maintain adequate caloric intake by mouth may need parental nutrition or enteral feeds through surgically placed tubes. Chronic GVHD may have a significant impact on growth and development in children.[74]

A thorough physical therapy evaluation and an individually designed program of activity can be invaluable in maintaining and increasing strength, range of motion, and mobility. For patients with the sclerodermatous variety of chronic GVHD, range-of-motion exercises may preserve joint mobility and decrease pain associated with joint contractures. Although detailed literature on its efficacy is lacking, our practice is to have all patients evaluated by a physical therapist familiar with the disease. Patients are given a personalized prescription for activity and exercise with their initial evaluation, and their progress is monitored about every 3 months. Occupational therapy can also be instrumental in maximizing functional capability in activities of daily living, employment opportunities, and sexual satisfaction. Support groups or individual therapy may benefit patients as they learn to cope with this chronic illness.

PROGNOSIS

Wingard et al. evaluated factors that predicted for poor outcome from chronic GVHD.[44] In 85 patients with chronic GVHD, baseline characteristics before therapy were examined to determine whether there were risk factors for death. In a multivariate proportional hazards analysis, three baseline factors emerged as independent predictors of death: progressive presentation of chronic GVHD, lichenoid changes on skin histology, and elevated serum bilirubin. Patients with one of these risk factors had a 70% chance of survival at 6 years, whereas patients with two or three of these risk factors had a survival chance of only 20%.

In a similar analysis of 143 patients treated with alternating-day cyclosporine and prednisone, Sullivan et al. identified progressive onset, advanced stage of malignancy, and thrombocytopenia as independent risk factors for death.[75] Patients with extensive, as compared with limited, disease experience higher mortality.

Mortality in chronic GVHD is largely attributable to infection. Death may also result from pulmonary failure due to bronchiolitis obliterans but is rarely due to other organ dysfunction. Death due to the autoimmune manifestations of the disease is uncommon.

CONCLUSION AND FUTURE DIRECTIONS

Chronic GVHD remains a major complication in allogeneic HSCT. The disease involves multiple organs and can be treated with various regimens of immunosuppressive medications. Supportive care is also important in ameliorating the effects of chronic GVHD. The current trend of increased utilization of peripheral blood progenitor cells with myeloablative and nonmyeloablative conditioning regimens may increase the incidence of chronic GVHD.

With an increasing number of patients undergoing allogeneic HSCT, particularly those involving donors other than HLA-identical siblings, the challenge of chronic GVHD will continue to be one faced by transplantation experts. Additional research is needed to better understand the pathogenesis of this entity so that new therapeutic approaches may be developed.

REFERENCES

1. Sullivan KM, Shulman H, Storb R, et al: Chronic graft versus host disease in 52 patients: adverse natural course and successful treatment with combination immunosuppression. Blood 57:267–276, 1981.
2. Atkinson K, Horowitz MM, Gale RP, et al: Risk factors for chronic graft-versus-host disease after HLA-identical sibling bone marrow transplantation. Blood 75:2459–2464, 1990.
3. Niederweiser D, Pepe M, Storb R, et al: Factors predicting chronic graft-versus-host disease after HLA-identical sibling bone marrow transplantation for aplastic anemia. Bone Marrow Transplant 4:151–156, 1989.
4. Allen RD, Staley TH, Sidman CL: Differential cytokine expression in acute and chronic murine graft-versus-host disease. Eur J Immunol 23:333–337, 1993.
5. de Wit D, van Mechelen M, Zanin C, et al: Preferential activation of Th2 cells in chronic graft-versus-host reaction. J Immunol 150:361–366, 1993.
6. Hess AD, Horwitz LR, Laulis MK: Cyclosporine-induced syngeneic graft-versus-host disease: recognition of self-MHC class II antigens in vivo. Transplant Proc 25:1218–1221, 1993.
7. Perreault C, Decary F, Brochu DA, et al: Minor histocompatibility antigens. Blood 76:1269–1280, 1990.
8. Ferrara JL, Krenger W: Graft-versus-host disease: the influence of type 1 and type 2 T cell cytokines. Transfus Med Rev 12:1–17, 1988.
9. Sullivan K, Agura E, Anasetti C: Chronic graft versus host disease in other late complications of bone marrow transplantation. Semin Hemtol 28:250–259, 1991.
10. Ruutu T, Volin L, Elonen E: Low incidence of severe acute and chronic graft-versus-host disease as a result of prolonged cyclosporine prophylaxis and early aggressive treatment with corticosteroids. Transplant Proc 20:491–493, 1988.

11. Lonnqvist B, Aschan J, Ljungman P, Ringden O: Long-term cyclosporin therapy may decrease then risk of chronic graft-versus-host disease. Br J Haematol 74:547–548, 1990.

12. Bacigalupo A, Maiolini A, Van Lint MT, et al: Cyclosporin A and graft versus host disease. Bone Marrow Transplant 6:341–344, 1990.

13. Bolger GB, Sullivan KM, Storb R, et al: Second marrow infusion for poor graft function after allogeneic marrow transplantation. Bone Marrow Transplant 1:21–30, 1986.

14. de Gast GC, Beatty PG, Amos A: Transfusions shortly before HLA-matched marrow transplantation for leukemia are associated with a decrease in chronic graft versus host disease. Bone Marrow Transplant 7:293–295, 1991.

15. Bostrom L, Ringden O, Jacobsen N, et al: European Multicenter Study of Chronic Graft Versus Host Disease—the role of cytomegalovirus serology in recipients and donors, acute graft-versus-host disease, and splenectomy. Transplantation 49:1100–1105, 1990.

16. Ljungman P, Niederweiser D, Pepe MS, et al: Cytomegalovirus infection after marrow transplantation for aplastic anemia. Bone Marrow Transplant 6:295–300, 1990.

17. Loughran TP Jr, Sullivan K, Morton T, et al: Value of day 100 screening studies for predicting the development of chronic graft versus host disease after allogeneic bone marrow transplantation. Blood 76:228–234, 1990.

18. Vogelsang GB, Altomonte V, Farmer E, et al: Explosive graft-versus-host disease [Abstract]. Blood 82(Suppl 1):422a, 1993.

19. Siadak M, Sullivan KM: The management of chronic graft-versus-host disease. Blood Rev 8:154–160, 1994.

20. Shulman HM, Sale GE, Lerner KG, et al: Chronic cutaneous graft-versus-host disease in man. Am J Pathol 91:545–570, 1978.

21. Saurat JH, Gluckman E, Bussel A, et al: The lichen planus-like eruption after bone marrow transplantation. Br J Dermatol 93:675–681, 1975.

22. Van Vloten WA, Scheffer E, Dooren LJ: Localized scleroderma-like lesions after bone marrow transplantation in man. Br J Dermatol 96:337–341, 1977.

23. Lawley TJ, Peck GL, Moutsopoulos HM, et al: Scleroderma, Sjögren-like syndrome, and chronic graft-versus-host disease. Ann Intern Med 87:707–709, 1977.

24. Hymes SR, Farmer ER, Burns WH, et al: Bullous sclerodermatous like changes in chronic graft-vs-host disease. Arch Dermatol 121:1189–1192, 1985.

25. Schubert MM, Sullivan KM, Morton TH, et al: Oral manifestations of chronic graft-versus-host disease. Arch Intern Med 144:1591–1595, 1984.

26. Johnson DA, Jabs DA: The ocular manifestations of graft-versus-host disease. Int Ophthalmol Clin 37:119–33, 1997.

27. Jabs DA, Wingard J, Green WR, et al: The eye in bone marrow transplantation: III. Conjunctival graft-versus-host disease. Arch Ophthalmol 107:1343–1348, 1989.

28. Yau JC, Zander AR, Srigley, et al: Chronic graft-versus-host disease complicated by micronodular cirrhosis and esophageal varices Transplantation 41:129–130, 1986.

29. Knapp AB, Crawford JM, Rappepart JM, Gollan JL: Cirrhosis as a consequence of graft-versus-host disease. Gastroenterology 92:513–519, 1987.

30. Holland HK, Wingard JR, Beschorner WE, et al: Bronchiolitis obliterans in bone marrow transplantation and its relationship to chronic graft-v-host disease and low serum IgG. Blood 72:621–627, 1988.

31. Clark JG, Crawford SW, Madtes DK, Sullivan KM: The clinical presentation and course of obstructive lung disease after allogeneic marrow transplantation. Ann Intern Med 111:368–376, 1989.

32. Crawford SW, Clark JG: Bronchiolitis associated with bone marrow transplantation. Clin Chest Med 14:741–749, 1993.

33. McDonald GB, Sullivan KM, Schuffler MD, et al: Esophageal abnormalities in chronic graft-versus-host disease in humans. Gastroenterology 80:914–921, 1981.

34. Minocha A, Mandanas RA, Kida M, Jazzar A: Bullous esophagitis due to chronic graft-versus-host disease. Am J Gastroenterol 92:529–530, 1997.

35. Reyes MG, Noronha P, Thomas W Jr, Heredia R: Myositis of chronic graft versus host disease. Neurology 33:1222–1224, 1983.

36. Urbano-Marquez A, Estruch R, Grau JM, et al: Inflammatory myopathy associated with chronic graft-versus-host disease. Neurology 36:1091–1093, 1986.

37. Parker PM, Openshaw H, Forman SJ: Myositis associated with graft-versus-host disease. Curr Opin Rheumatol 9:513–519, 1997.

38. Janin A, Socie G, Devergie A, et al: Fasciitis in chronic graft-versus-host disease—a clinicopathologic study of 14 cases. Ann Intern Med 120:993–998, 1994.

39. Greenspan A, Deeg HJ, Cottler-Fox M, et al: Incapacitating peripheral neuropathy as a manifestation of chronic graft-versus-host disease. Bone Marrow Transplant 5:349–351, 1990.

40. Smith CIE, Aarli JA, Biberfeld P, et al: Myasthenia gravis after bone-marrow transplantation. N Engl J Med 309:1565–1568, 1983.

41. Bolger GB, Sullivan KM, Spencer AM, et al: Myasthenia gravis after allogeneic bone marrow transplantation: relationship to chronic graft-versus-host disease. Neurology 36:1087–1091, 1986.

42. Hirabayashi N: Studies on graft versus host (GvH) reactions: I. Impairment of hematopoietic stroma in mice suffering from GvH disease. Exp Hematol 9:101–110, 1981.

43. Atkinson K, Norrie S, Chan P, et al: Hemopoietic progenitor cell function after HLA-identical sibling bone marrow transplantation: influence of chronic graft-versus-host disease. Int J Cell Cloning 4:203–220, 1986.

44. Wingard J, Piantadosi S, Vogelsang G, et al: Predictors of death from chronic graft versus host disease after bone marrow transplantation. Blood 74:1428–1435, 1989.

45. Corson SL, Sullivan K, Batzer F, et al: Gynecologic manifestations of chronic graft-versus-host disease. Obstet Gynecol 60:488–492, 1982.

46. Schubert MA, Sullivan KM, Schubert MM, et al: Gynecological abnormalities following allogeneic bone marrow transplantation. Bone Marrow Transplant 5:425–430, 1990.

47. Gomez-Garcia P, Herrera-Arroyo C, Torres-Gomez A, et al: Renal impairment in chronic graft-versus-host disease: a report of two cases. Bone Marrow Transplant 3:357–362, 1988.

48. Atkinson K, Farewell V, Storb R, et al: Analysis of the infections after human bone marrow transplantation: role of genotypic nonidentity between marrow donor and recipient and of nonspecific suppressor cells in patients with chronic graft-versus-host disease. Blood 60:714–720, 1982.

49. Lapp WS, Ghayur T, Mendes M, et al: The functional and histological basis for graft-versus-host-induced immunosuppression. Immunol Rev 88:107–133, 1985.

50. Marmont AM, Horowitz MM, Gale RP, et al: T-cell depletion of HLA-identical transplants in leukemia. Blood 78:2120–2130, 1991.

51. Ash RC, Casper JT, Chitambar CR, et al: Successful allogeneic transplantation of T-cell depleted bone marrow from closely HLA-matched unrelated donors. N Engl J Med 322:485–494, 1990.

52. Sullivan KM, Kopecky KJ, Jocom J, et al: Immunomodulatory and antimicrobial efficacy of intravenous immunoglobulin in bone marrow transplantation. N Engl J Med 323:705–712, 1990.

53. Sullivan KM, Mori M, Sanders J, et al: Late complications of allogeneic and autologous marrow transplantation. Bone Marrow Transplant 10(Suppl 1):127–134, 1992.

54. Atkinson K, Storb R. Ochs HD, et al: Thymus transplantation after allogeneic bone marrow graft to prevent chronic graft-versus-host disease in humans. Transplantation 33:168–173, 1982.

55. Witherspoon RP, Sullivan KM, Lum LG, et al: Use of thymic factors to augment immunologic recovery after bone marrow transplantation: brief report with 2 to 12 years' followup. Bone Marrow Transplant 3:425–435, 1988.

56. Chao NJ, Parker PM, Niland JC, et al: Paradoxical effect of thalidomide prophylaxis on chronic graft-vs-host disease. Biol Blood Marrow Transplant 2:86–92, 1996.

57. Sullivan KM, Witherspoon R, Storb R, et al: Prednisone and azathioprine compared with prednisone and placebo for treatment of chronic graft-v-host disease: prognostic influence of prolonged thrombocytopenia after allogeneic marrow transplantation. Blood 72:546–554, 1988.

58. Sullivan K, Witherspoon R, Storb A, et al: Alternating day cyclosporine and prednisone for treatment of high risk chronic graft versus host disease. Blood 72:555–561, 1988.

59. Vogelsang GB, Farmer ER, Hess AD, et al: Thalidomide for the treatment of chronic graft versus host disease. N Engl J Med 326:1055–1058, 1992.

60. Cole CH, Rogers PCJ, Pritchard S, et al: Thalidomide in the management of chronic graft-versus-host disease in children following bone marrow transplantation. Bone Marrow Transplant 14:937–942, 1994.

61. Parker PM, Chao N, Nademanee A, et al: Thalidomide as salvage therapy for chronic graft-versus-host disease. Blood 86:3604–3609, 1995.

62. Tzakis AG, Abu-Elmagd K, Fung JJ, et al: FK506 rescue in chronic graft-versus-host disease after bone marrow transplantation. Transplant Proc 23:3225–3227, 1991.

63. Marcellus DC, Altomonte VL, Farmer ER, et al: Etretinate therapy for refractory sclerodermatous chronic graft-versus-host disease. Blood 93:66–70, 1999.

64. Lee SJ, Wegner SA, McGarigle CJ, et al: Treatment of chronic graft-versus-host disease with clofazimine. Blood 89:2298–2302, 1997.

65. Schultz KR, Nelson D, Bader S: Synergy between lysosomotropic amines and cyclosporin A on human T cell responses to an exogenous protein antigen, tetanus toxoid. Bone Marrow Transplant 18:625–631, 1996.

66. Schultz KR, Bader S, Nelson D, Immune suppression by lysosomotropic amines and cyclosporin on T-cell responses to minor and major histocompatibility antigens: does synergy exist? Transplantation 64:1055–1065, 1997.

67. Schultz KR, Gilman AL: The lysosomotropic amines, chloroquine and hydroxychloroquine: a potentially novel therapy for graft-versus-host disease. Leukemia Lymph 24:201–210, 1997.

68. Hymes SR, Morison WL, Farmer ER, et al: Methoxsalen and ultraviolet A radiation in treatment of chronic cutaneous graft-versus-host reaction. Acad Dermatol 12:30–37, 1985.

69. Atkinson K, Weller P, Ryman W, Biggs J: PUVA therapy for drug resistant graft versus host disease. Bone Marrow Transplant 1:227–236, 1986.

70. Vogelsang GB, Wolff D, Altomonte V, et al: Treatment of graft-versus-host disease with ultraviolet irradiation and psoralen (PUVA). Bone Marrow Transplant 17:1061–1067, 1996.

71. Rossetti F, Dall'Amico R, Crovetti G, et al: Extracorporeal photochemotherapy for the treatment of graft-versus-host disease. Bone Marrow Transplant 18(Suppl 2):175–181, 1996.

72. Socie G, Devergie A, Cosset J, et al: Low dose total lymphoid irradiation for extensive, drug resistant chronic graft versus host disease. Transplantation 49:657–658, 1990.

73. Bullorsky EO, Shanley CM, Stemmelin GR, et al: Total lymphoid irradiation for treatment of drug resistant chronic GVHD. Bone Marrow Transplant 11:75–76, 1993.

74. Sanders JE: Effects of chronic graft-vs-host disease on growth and development. *In* Burakoff SJ, Deeg HJ, Ferrara J, Atkinson K (eds): Graft-vs-host disease: immunology, pathophysiology, and treatment. New York, Marcel Dekker, 1990, pp. 665–680.

75. Sullivan KM, Mori M, Witherspoon R, et al: Alternating-day cyclosporine and prednisone (CSP/PRED) treatment of chronic graft-vs-host disease(GVHD): predictors of survival [Abstract]. Blood 76(Suppl 1):568a, 1990.

Endocrine and Metabolic Complications

Stephen J. Winters, M.D., and Mushtaq Syed, M.D.

Endocrine dysfunction is common among hematopoietic stem cell transplantation (HSCT) patients. The acute illness of transplantation as well as the alkalating agents, irradiation, and glucocorticoids in high doses used to treat these patients have pronounced effects on the function of most endocrine glands. The major complications are electrolyte and mineral disturbances, poor growth in children, hypothyroidism, and reproductive failure in adults. Certain abnormalities occur during conditioning, whereas other complications may take many years to develop and require lifelong follow-up.

MINERAL AND ELECTROLYTE DISORDERS

HYPOKALEMIA

Hypokalemia occurs with decreased oral intake, redistribution of potassium between the extracellular and intracellular compartments, or loss of potassium through the kidney, gastrointestinal tract, or skin. Patients who are unable to eat require potassium supplementation parenterally to meet the normal daily potassium requirement of approximately 0.35–0.5 mEq/kg/day. Medications that are nephrotoxic and produce potassium wasting include amphotericin B, cyclosporine, and aminoglycosides. Various chemotherapeutic agents, especially ifosfamide and cisplatin, also contribute to hypokalemia in patients undergoing HSCT. Total parenteral nutrition (TPN) may result in hypokalemia because the glucose and amino acids infused intravenously stimulate insulin release. Hyperinsulinemia redistributes extracellular potassium into the intracellular space, thereby lowering the serum potassium without actually depleting the total body stores.[1] Glycosuria also increases loss of potassium in the urine. Potassium is readily replaced parenterally in intravenous fluids or in TPN solution. Potassium depletion secondary to hypomagnesemia is usually refractory to treatment until magnesium deficiency is corrected, however.[2]

HYPOMAGNESEMIA

Magnesium balance is maintained by consuming approximately 5 mg/kg/day of elemental magnesium in the diet. With starvation or impaired intestinal absorption, urinary magnesium excretion declines to negligible values. Patients undergoing HSCT experience magnesium deficiency most often because of inappropriate urinary loss of magnesium due to cyclosporine, cisplatin, ifosfamide, vinblastine, bleomycin, and various aminoglycosides.[3] Other causes of renal magnesium wasting include diabetes mellitus, hypercalcemia, diuretics, renal failure, and the use of TPN.

Approximately half of patients in intensive care units are magnesium depleted, and these patients experience increased morbidity and mortality.[4] Symptoms attributable to hypomagnesemia occur when the plasma level declines below 1.2 mEq/L, which may occur abruptly. Myoclonus, weakness, muscular fasciculations, athetosis, or tetany suggests hypomagnesemia. If hypokalemia or hypocalcemia develops secondary to magnesium deficiency, the amount of magnesium deficit is usually in excess of 250–300 mEq.[5] Patients undergoing HSCT should be carefully monitored for magnesium deficiency, and adequate supplementation should be provided either separately or in the TPN solution.

HYPOPHOSPHATEMIA

Phosphorus is abundant in the diet, and its intestinal absorption is thought to proceed by passive diffusion. Normal phosphorus balance is maintained by precise renal excretion, which, like that for magnesium, declines as the oral intake falls. Serum phosphate is maintained at normal levels at the expense of loss of intracellular stores. In patients with acidosis, there is a net shift of phosphate ions from the intracellular to the extracellular space, which increases renal clearance. When the acidosis is corrected, hypophosphatemia may occur.[6] Hypophosphatemia is relatively common in transplant recipients, especially those with respiratory alkalosis or receiving TPN. Hypophosphatemia results in erythrocyte dysfunction with impaired oxygen delivery. Muscular weakness, cardiac dysfunction, and respiratory failure are the major complications of hypophosphatemia. They occur if the serum phosphate level falls below 1.0 mg/dL.[7]

Mild hypophosphatemia (>2 mg/dL) resulting from a temporary interruption of the diet does not require treatment. When patients are able to take oral fluids, skim milk, which is rich in calcium and phosphate, is suggested. If the phosphate level falls to less than 1 mg/dL, intravenous treatment is necessary. Neutral potassium phosphate (80% K_2HPO_4 and 20% KH_2PO_4), at a dose of 1–2 mmol/kg over 24 hours, is administered with careful monitoring of the serum calcium, phosphate, magnesium, and potassium level because overzealous treatment can decrease the plasma level of these electrolytes and cause calcium precipitation in soft tissues including blood vessels.

HYPERCALCEMIA AND HYPOCALCEMIA

Hypercalcemia is a common complication of many malignant disorders. The mechanisms through which hypercalcemia occurs in cancer patients include local osteolytic hypercalcemia, humoral hypercalcemia due principally to the production of parathyroid hormone-related protein, increased production of 1,25-dihydroxyvitamin D, and paraneoplastic secretion of parathyroid hormone (reviewed in references 8 and 9). Dehydration during conditioning chemotherapy may unmask hypercalcemia by lowering urinary calcium excretion. Immobilization contributes to hypercalcemia in adolescents among whom bone turnover rates are increased. 13-Cis-retinoic acid has been used in the treatment and prevention of several malignancies including neuroblastoma and may produce hypercalcemia as a side effect.[10]

Hyperparathyroidism may occur as a long-term complication of neck irradiation.[11] The usual biochemical findings are hypercalcemia, hypophosphatemia, and an elevated plasma parathyroid hormone level. Parathyroid adenomas are the predominant cause of hypercalcemia in patients with radiation exposure as well as in nonirradiated patients. Most of the patients had received low-dose radiation for benign conditions such as acne and tonsillar enlargement. The applicability of these findings to HSCT recipients is unknown.

Hypocalcemia is common in patients with hypomagnesemia and is corrected with magnesium replenishment. Hypocalcemia in cancer patients has also been attributed to increased uptake of calcium into bone in a few cases. Hypoparathyroidism has been reported as a long-term sequel of ^{131}I treatment for thyroid disease and could occur after use of other radiation modalities.

HYPERNATREMIA AND HYPONATREMIA

Leukemic infiltration of the hypothalamic-pituitary region may produce diabetes insipidus characterized by the excretion of large amounts of dilute urine and by polydipsia. Dehydration results in hypernatremia. There is one report of a patient whose diabetes insipidus resolved after bone marrow transplantation (BMT), presumably because treatment eradicated central nervous system disease.[12] Renal resistance to vasopressin (nephrogenic diabetes insipidus) may occur in patients with multiple myeloma or lymphoma or during treatment with cisplatin, amphotericin B, or foscarnet.

Hyponatremia is a relatively common metabolic abnormality in cancer patients. In one series,[13] 3 of 43 children with lymphoid malignancies who received methyl-CCNU, high-dose cyclophosphamide, and autologous peripheral blood progenitor cells experienced severe hyponatremia (<125 mEq/L). Because cyclophosphamide metabolites produce hemorrhagic cystitis, large volumes of fluid are given parenterally with the drug and patients are encour-

aged to drink fluids. Cancers, especially small cell lung cancer, may produce vasopressin (antidiuretic hormone) leading to water retention.[14] Central nervous system disease may produce hyponatremia by resetting the osmostat. Vinca alkaloids and cyclophosphamide are believed to stimulate the inappropriate secretion of vasopressin. The production of atrial natriuretic peptide by tumors may lead to renal salt loss.[15] Finally, vomiting contributes to fluid and electrolyte losses. Therefore, careful monitoring of the serum electrolytes is essential during conditioning for HSCT.

PARENTERAL NUTRITION

The anorexia, nausea, vomiting, diarrhea, and mucositis that occur in bone marrow transplant recipients as side effects of cytotoxic drugs and radiotherapy substantially reduce the oral intake of nutrients. One approach to overcome the nutritional deficit is to supply nutrients parenterally. TPN, therefore, is considered to be standard therapy in HSCT recipients by some investigators. The data on the effectiveness of TPN in relation to the outcome of HSCT are incomplete, however. Very few randomized controlled trials are available concerning HSCT.

In one trial, 137 patients were randomly assigned to receive TPN together with oral feeding or 5% dextrose in water intravenously plus oral feeding beginning 1 week before and for 4 weeks after transplantation. Because of low calorie intake, 61% of the control group were given intravenous nutrition support prior to discharge. The incidence of bacterial infection in the TPN groups was higher than in the control group, but the median day of discharge was similar for both groups. Interestingly, patients who received TPN were less likely to experience relapse and had longer survival than those who received 5% dextrose.[16] Szeluga et al.[17] on the other hand, using the results of a similar although smaller trial, concluded that TPN was not clearly superior to individualized enteral feeding and recommended that TPN be used judiciously. In the latter series, TPN was associated with more days of diuretic use, frequent hyperglycemia, and more catheter-related complications, but hypomagnesemia occurred less often than in patients on the enteral feeding program. TPN was found to be more effective in preserving the body cell mass calculated by isotope dilution methods, but the cost of therapy was 2.3 times the cost of the individualized oral feeding program. No significant differences were found between the two groups in terms of hematologic recovery, graft-versus-host disease, length of hospitalization, or long-term survival. In a third study, patients with solid tumors were randomized to receive TPN or partial parenteral nutrition and continuous tube feedings. Both modalities were found to be equally effective.[18]

At present, the indications for TPN in patients undergoing HSCT are loosely defined. If parenteral nutrition is initiated, patients must be constantly evaluated for under- and over-hydration, and plasma levels of magnesium, potassium, calcium, and phosphate must be carefully monitored because rapid anabolic responses may cause redistribution of these elements from the extracellular to the intracellular compartments.[19]

THE THYROID

Thyroid dysfunction is a relatively common endocrine complication of HSCT. Abnormalities in thyroid function can result from the pre-existing condition or disease; the stress of the preconditioning regimen; the consequences of irradiation of the thyroid, hypothalamus, and pituitary; and finally, post-transplantation sequelae such as graft-versus-host disease.

The various thyroid abnormalities observed depend on the temporal relationship to HSCT. During the preconditioning stage, thyroid function test results may be abnormal because of nonthyroidal illness (low T_3 or euthyroid sick syndrome). The thyroid is generally unaffected by chemotherapy but is relatively sensitive to radiation exposure. Many types of delayed thyroid dysfunction have been described after irradiation and HSCT. By far the most common is mild thyroid failure (borderline hypothyroidism). Primary and secondary hypothyroidism, thyroid neoplasms, hyperthyroidism, and autoimmune thyroiditis may also occur. Recombinant interferon-α, which is widely used to treat malignant disease, may stimulate autoimmune disease, most notably thyroid disease.

NONTHYROIDAL ILLNESS

Patients undergoing preconditioning regimens for HSCT are stressed, febrile, and inactive, and they eat poorly. The changes in thyroid indices are not unique but instead occur in most patients who are seriously ill.[20] The most characteristic laboratory findings are low plasma T_3 and thyroid-stimulating hormone (TSH) levels. Plasma T_4 levels are in the low-normal range or are reduced, and free T_4 levels are usually normal but may be low or high.[21] Abnormal thyroid function test results return to normal with recovery from illness. TSH levels may slightly exceed the normal range for a few weeks and then return to normal. This pattern of changes in thyroid function test results over time is illustrated in Figure 55–1. Reverse T_3 levels may be elevated in nonthyroidal illness but do not reliably distinguish between the hypothyroid sick and the euthyroid sick patient.[22]

The mechanisms for these changes are only partly understood. T_4 is a relatively weak hormone, and it is converted to T_3 in target tissues to achieve full bioactivity. During illness, the conversion of T_4 to T_3 is suppressed because of decreased activity of the deiodinases in peripheral tissues such as the liver and kidney. Altered cell uptake of T_4 may also lead to decreased T_3 production. Substances, including the drugs diphenylhydantoin and furosemide, bilirubin, and fatty acids—which are believed to inhibit the binding of T_4 to thyroid-binding globulin—may increase the percentage of free hormone concentration and enhance the clearance of T_4. The low TSH level also contributes to reduced T_4 concentrations. Cytokines[24] and glucocorticoids[25] suppress the hypothalamic production of thyroid-releasing hormone, which in turn decreases TSH production. TSH glycosylation is also altered, producing molecules that appear to have reduced biologic activity.[26] These thyroidal modifications during nonthyroidal illness teleologically may represent the energy or calorie conservation of the starving or hibernating animal. Finally, treating the thyroid abnormalities in nonthyroidal illness with thyroid hormones has not been shown to improve clinical outcomes.[27]

PRIMARY HYPOTHYROIDISM

Hypothyroidism is common after irradiation, either incidental or therapeutic, of the thyroid gland.[28–31] The most common finding after HSCT is borderline hypothyroidism characterized by an elevated TSH but normal T_4 level, but overt hypothyroidism (low T_4 level) may also occur.[32] In one longitudinal study, 13 of 27 children with leukemia treated with cyclophosphamide and single-fraction total body irradiation experienced borderline (n = 10) or overt (n = 3) hypothyroidism during 7 years of follow-up.[33] The likelihood of hypothyroidism is higher with single-dose than with fractionated irradiation. In one study, thyroid dysfunction occurred in 73% of patients receiving single-fraction radiation, whereas only 25% of patients undergoing fractionated irradiation experienced thyroid dysfunction.[34] In a second study of 13 patients with chronic myelogenous leukemia, no cases of hypothyroidism occurred 3–25 months (median, 14 months) after fractionated irradiation with 10.2 Gy in six doses.[35] Hyperfractionated irradiation was associated with a 15% prevalence of hypothyroidism at 11–88 months (mean, 49 months).[36] Chemotherapy further increases the risk of hypothyroidism in children receiving craniospinal irradiation for brain tumors,[29] although the applicability of this finding to HSCT is unproved.

Overt hypothyroidism is treated with thyroxin. Patients with subclinical hypothyroidism are also generally treated with thyroxin to suppress stimulation of the thyroid by TSH because such stimulation predisposes to goiter and may increase the risk of cancer in the irradiated thyroid.[37] The presence of elevated plasma cholesterol levels, fatigue, and depression are additional reasons for treating these patients.

SECONDARY HYPOTHYROIDISM

Secondary hypothyroidism represents a low serum thyroxin level due to inadequate thyrotropin (TSH) stimulation. Thyrotropin deficiency occurs after HSCT because of radiation damage to the hypothalamus or pituitary. Radiation-

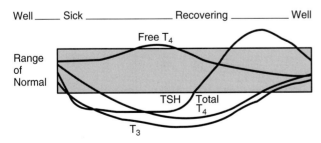

FIGURE 55–1. Time course of changes in total and free thyroxin (T4), triiodothyronine (T3), and thyrotropin (TSH) in patients before, during, and after recovery from acute illness such as that brought on by bone marrow transplantation.

induced hypothalamic-pituitary damage is dose-dependent,[28] and 50 Gy is believed to be a threshold dose for hypothyroidism.[38] In a study of 32 Japanese children who underwent conditioning irradiation before BMT, no children had overt hypothyroidism at 1 year, but 8 children had a subnormal or delayed TSH response to stimulation of thyroid-releasing hormone.[39] In patients given supplemental cranial irradiation prior to BMT, both secondary and primary hypothyroidism may occur and the elevated TSH level characteristic of primary hypothyroidism may be blunted. Therefore, thyroxin as well as TSH levels should be monitored.

HYPERTHYROIDISM

Hyperthyroidism occasionally occurs after thyroid irradiation. The mechanism is variable, ranging from injury to Graves disease. Again, most of the information originates from the literature on therapeutic irradiation of the thyroid for malignancies such non-Hodgkin lymphoma,[40, 41] whereas there are only a few case reports of hyperthyroidism after BMT.[42–44]

Subacute thyroiditis, a spontaneously remitting inflammatory disorder of the thyroid characterized by fever and a tender goiter in which both hyperthyroidism and hypothyroidism may develop, has occurred after HSCT, where it has been attributed to radiation damage or to viral infection. Graves disease results from the production of immunoglobulins that activate TSH receptors. Several cases of Graves disease have been reported after allogeneic BMT in which recipients may have acquired clones of programmed lymphocytes from the donor.[43]

Hyperthyroidism due to thyroiditis can be differentiated from Graves disease by measuring the radioactive iodine uptake by the thyroid gland. The radioactive iodine uptake is usually high in Graves disease but low in hyperthyroidism due to thyroiditis. The presence of immunoglobulins that bind to the TSH receptor support the diagnosis of Graves disease. Treatment options for hyperthyroidism are the thyroid hormone synthesis inhibitors propylthiouracil and methimazole, radioactive iodine ablation, and thyroidectomy. Beta-blockers are used to control symptoms.

THYROID NEOPLASMS

The incidence of thyroid neoplams is increased in populations exposed to radiation. These cancers are usually well differentiated, indolent, and rarely fatal. The risk for cancer increases linearly with doses of 6.5–1500 cGy, but higher doses tend to destroy the glandular tissue, so the risk of cancer actually declines.[45] The peak incidence of thyroid tumors is between 5 and 30 years after exposure, but it has been reported as late as 50 years.[46] Several cases of differentiated thyroid cancer after BMT have been reported,[47] but surveillance studies suggest that thyroid cancer is rare after BMT.[48]

All patients who receive head and neck or total body irradiation should be followed at least yearly with a careful thyroid examination. Detection of a new thyroid nodule, cyst, or surface irregularity should raise the suspicion of

malignancy, and fine-needle aspiration biopsy and cytologic examination of the specimen should be performed.

THYROID AND INTERFERON-α

Recombinant interferon-α is used to treat patients with hepatitis, solid tumors, chronic myelogenous leukemia, hairy cell leukemia, essential thrombocythemia, and multiple myeloma, some of whom may undergo HSCT. Patients treated with interferon-α may experience autoimmune thyroid disease with hypothyroidism or, less commonly, hyperthyroidism.[49] Prevalence rates varying from 5% to 20% have been reported in different populations, perhaps because interferon-α unmasks or activates pre-existing autoimmune thyroid disease. Serum antibodies to thyroglobulin and to thyroid peroxidase (antimicrosomal antibodies) are usually present in high titer, with suppressed T_4 and increased TSH levels. In cases of hyperthyroidism, the TSH level is suppressed while T_4 and/or T_3 levels are elevated. TSH receptor antibodies may be present. Thyroid dysfunction associated with interferon-α is often reversible but may persist after therapy is discontinued.[50] Therefore, a conservative approach is indicated. Interferon-α and irradiation may have an additive effect to cause hypothyroidism.

GROWTH AND DEVELOPMENT

Growth retardation and delayed pubertal development are common among children after HSCT. Growth is influenced by multiple factors including multigenic predisposition, nutrition, psychophysiologic stress, and hormones such as growth hormone (GH) and insulin-like growth factor-1 (IGF-1; somatomedin), thyroid hormone, glucocorticoids, and sex steroids. The major factors thought to contribute to reduced growth in children after HSCT are listed in Table 55–1.

During the phase of acute illness and chemotherapy, patients are febrile, are physically inactive, eat poorly, may be treated with glucocorticoids, and do not grow normally. Part of this immediate growth arrest results from a suppression of hepatic production of IGF-1, a mediator of the growth-promoting actions of GH.[51] Plasma GH levels are normal or increased, however.[52] The reduced circulating levels of IGF-1 are instead due to GH resistance, which is thought to relate to dietary protein deficiency and decreased insulin production. There is evidence for resistance to the growth-promoting actions of IGF-1 as well. Thyroid hormone production, which is important in bone maturation, is also reduced in acute illness (see above). When

TABLE 55–1. FACTORS CONTRIBUTING TO DECREASED GROWTH AFTER BMT

Acute illness
Central nervous system irradiation
Delayed sexual development
Glucocorticoid treatment for graft-vs-host disease
Hypothyroidism
Radiation of the epiphyseal growth plates

chemotherapy is completed, IGF-1 and thyroxin levels normalize.[53]

Recovery of endocrine function subsequent to acute illness may be associated with a compensatory increase in growth velocity know as "catch-up growth." For example, in children with acute lymphoblastic leukemia who received multidrug chemotherapy and intrathecal methotrexate but did not undergo HSCT, growth velocity was significantly less than normal 1 year after diagnosis and rebounded to exceed normal values between years 2 and 4 so that their absolute height 5 years after treatment was normal.[54] Similarly, final height was not adversely affected by BMT with cyclophosphamide conditioning in children with aplastic anemia[55] or in children with leukemia treated with BMT after busulfan, cyclophosphamide, and L-PAM treatment.[56]

Conditioning regimens that include irradiation to the central nervous system can produce a loss of height potential, however. For example, among 72 children with acute leukemia, the height 4 years after BMT with total body irradiation (TBI) conditioning was 2 SD below the mean in 25%.[57] In the large series from Fred Hutchinson Cancer Research Center with longer follow-up, all patients were more than 2 SD below the mean height,[58] whereas the outcome in a more recent study was more favorable, with a final height of 2 SD below the mean in only 1 of 25 children treated with TBI.[55] The variable outcomes in these reports may relate to total radiation dose, dose rate, duration of treatment, underlying and complicating illness, and type of chemotherapy, among other factors. Several studies have shown that the growth disturbance after single-dose TBI is more severe than with fractionated treatment.[34, 58, 59] As shown by Giorgiani et al.[56] (Fig. 55–2) as well as by others,[55, 57] prophylactic cranial irradiation results in poorer growth than TBI alone. Moreover, the radiation effect is dose-dependent in that central nervous system prophylaxis with 24 Gy resulted in lower final height than with 18 Gy.[60] In one uncontrolled study,[61] growth after single-dose total lymphoid irradiation (7.5 Gy) was close to normal at 3 years. Children younger than age 5 years at the time of HSCT may experience greater height loss than older children.

The major cause of growth failure after cranial irradiation is believed to be GH deficiency due to damage to the hypothalamus and pituitary. Although GH secretion is most readily impaired among the pituitary hormones, the precise nature of the defect is uncertain.[62] Children with brain tumors who receive high doses of radiation are likely to become GH deficient,[63] whereas GH secretion in patients receiving the smaller doses of radiation used in conditioning for HSCT is variable.

At present, there is no single definitive test for the accurate diagnosis of GH deficiency, so multiple tests are usually used. Provocative tests examine peak GH levels after arginine infusion, insulin-induced hypoglycemia, L-dopa, or clonidine administration. Many normally growing children have abnormal responses ("growth without growth-hormone syndrome"), and poorly growing children may demonstrate normal responses to these tests. Evaluation of spontaneous GH secretory patterns in blood samples drawn every 20 minutes for 12–24 hours with analysis using newer two-site GH assays may be a more-sensitive

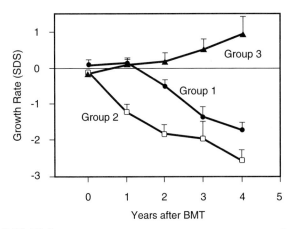

FIGURE 55–2. Effects of different conditioning regimens on growth in children with various malignancies treated by bone marrow transplantation (BMT). The data represent the mean (± SEM) growth rate standard deviation score (SDS) before and after BMT in three groups of children who received autologous or allogeneic bone marrow transplants. The SD score (or Z-score) represents the difference between the individual value and the normal mean in standard deviations. The children were 0.5–12 years old (median 7 years) at the time of BMT. Group 1 consists of 37 children who received total body irradiation and cytotoxic drugs. Group 2 represents 17 children who received additional prophylactic cranial radiation (18 Gy in 12 fractions). Group 3 consisted of 22 children conditioned with busulfan and cyclophosphamide with or without L-PAM. (Data from Giorgiani G, Bozzola M, Locateli F, et al: Role of busulfan and total body irradiation on growth of prepubertal children receiving bone marrow transplantation and results of treatment with recombinant human growth hormone. Blood 86:825, 1995.)

and specific approach but is very expensive. Plasma levels of IGF-1 and IGF-binding protein 3 are low in most patients with GH deficiency, although overlap with normal values also occurs.[64] The inadequate correlation between GH testing and growth may also reflect the contribution of factors other than GH to growth.

Through an endocrine-independent mechanism, spinal irradiation—for example, to children with medulloblastoma—damages the growth plates and nourishing blood vessels, limiting spinal growth and predisposing to scoliosis.[65] Spinal growth can be followed by measuring the sitting height. Disproportionate growth is more pronounced when irradiation is applied to young children, but it may not be evident until puberty.

Glucocorticoid treatment for graft-versus-host disease also suppresses growth through complex mechanisms.[66] Sanders et al.[58] reported that growth velocity was decreased in those children with graft-versus-host disease receiving glucocorticoid therapy compared to those not receiving it but that catch-up growth occurred after glucocorticoid treatment was discontinued. Although little data are available from patients undergoing HSCT, GH secretion is reduced in other patient groups receiving long-term high-dose prednisone treatment. Experimental studies indicate that glucocorticoids also decrease GH receptor binding and uncouple GH from its signal transduction pathways.[67] Plasma levels of IGF-1 and IGF BP-3 in prednisone-treated children are within the normal range, however.[68] Glucocorticoids also effect growing tissues directly by decreasing collagen synthesis and chondrocyte mitosis. Glucocorticoids reduce sex-hormone production by decreasing gonadotropin secretion, which suppresses growth further. Alternate-day glucocorticoid therapy reduces, but does not eliminate, growth suppression.[69] In addition, glucocorticoids decrease muscle mass, increase fat mass, and predispose to osteoporosis.

Defining the presence of GH deficiency is important because short stature due to GH deficiency can be treated with recombinant GH replacement. GH treatment of patients undergoing BMT has been reported to increase height velocity for 1–3 years,[56, 57] but the effect is substantially less than in patients with idiopathic GH deficiency, probably because the short stature after BMT is multifactoral in etiology. Long-term studies are needed to determine the ultimate benefit of GH treatment and to define those children undergoing HSCT who are likely to respond favorably. Because many children treated with HSCT grow to a final height that is within the normal range for the population, the decision to treat with GH requires clinical experience and careful longitudinal testing as well as an awareness of potential treatment side effects. GH treatment is also very expensive. GH and IGF-1 stimulate cell lines to proliferate, and the incidence of gastrointestinal tumors may be increased in patients with GH-producing pituitary adenomas (acromegaly). The report of a slightly increased incidence of leukemia in GH-treated children was not confirmed, however, and there is presently no evidence that GH replacement therapy increases cancer recurrence rates.[70]

PUBERTAL DEVELOPMENT

Puberty is the activation of hypothalamic-pituitary-gonadal function, which occurs at the age of 10–15 years. Although genetically determined, the onset and progression of puberty are often delayed by chronic illness. Stress, weight loss, and nutritional deficiency are thought to contribute to this delay in pubertal development. Puberty often occurs normally in children conditioned with cyclophosphamide alone, although a detailed longitudinal study has not been performed. Girls age 9–12 with leukemia who received TBI (10–13.2 Gy) as well as high-dose cyclophosphamide may enter into puberty, but ovarian failure usually occurs once they reach their mid-teens.[71, 72] Pubertal boys with Hodgkin disease treated with alkylating agents experience Leydig cell as well as seminiferous tubule damage, and gynecomastia may occur.[73] Luteinizing hormone levels are often elevated, indicating Leydig cell dysfunction, in boys after BMT with TBI and cyclophosphamide conditioning.[22] Treatment of testicular relapse of acute lymphoblastic leukemia with testicular radiation damages Leydig cells as well as seminiferous tubules.[74] High doses of central nervous system radiation may also impair gonadal function by damaging the hypothalamus and pituitary.[38] There are also a few reports of precocious puberty in young children treated with cranial irradiation before BMT and TBI, and a tendency for accelerated puberty, including menarche, among girls younger than age 7 years at BMT has been described, although the comparison of pubertal timing was with a historical control population.[60]

Puberty is associated with a sudden acceleration of the growth velocity that is known as the adolescent growth spurt. During this time, GH secretion increases substantially.[75] As shown in Figure 55–3, growth curves for chil-

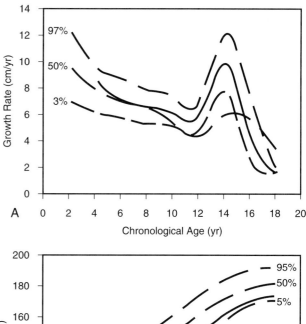

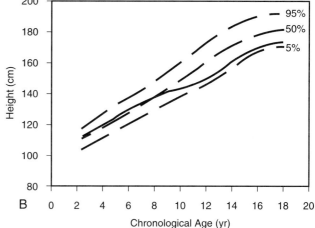

FIGURE 55–3. Effects of illness and pubertal delay on growth rate in cm/yr (*A*) and height in cm (*B*). In *A*, the values represent the variation in height velocity from the 3rd to 97th percentile versus age in years in normal boys. The *solid line* represents the growth rate of a boy in whom acute lymphoblastic leukemia developed at age 8. His growth rate declined immediately. With successful treatment growth resumed, but his pubertal growth spurt was delayed and prolonged. *B*, A plot of chronologic age versus height reveals that as a young boy he had been growing at the 50th percentile for height but that he crossed growth lines during his illness; his final height of 164 cm placed him instead at about the 10th percentile. (The normative data are adapted from Tanner JM, Whitehouse RH: Clinical longitudinal standards for height, weight, height velocity, weight velocity, and stages of puberty. Arch Dis Child 51:170–179, 1976.)

dren undergoing BMT reveal that height loss occurs in the prepubertal period but is more pronounced during puberty. This attenuation of the adolescent growth spurt may reflect the additive effects of GH and sex hormone deficiencies. Inasmuch as circulating estrogens increase GH secretion, impaired gonadal steroid production after TBI contributes to reduced adolescent growth. In addition, low-dose cranial irradiation impairs GH production and blunts the pubertal growth spurt.[76] The impact of sex steroid deficiency on growth is observed in children with thalassemia, in whom transfusional hemochromatosis leads to pronounced hypogonadism but only marginal GH deficiency.[77] In these children, the growth rate fell off after BMT in teenagers but remained stable, at slightly reduced pretreatment values, in those below age 7 years.[78] Accordingly, teenagers who have undergone HSCT with TBI should be evaluated yearly for the need for sex steroid replacement. If women are having regular monthly menstrual periods, their gonadal axis is almost certainly normal. In men, the plasma level of testosterone is recommended for screening.

REPRODUCTIVE SYSTEM

Chemotherapy and irradiation to the pelvis have pronounced adverse effects on the reproductive system that substantially influence the quality of life for persons undergoing HSCT. The disturbance is both immediate and long-term. Damage to the hypothalamic-pituitary unit as well as to the gonads may produce a complex diagnostic and therapeutic condition. Sex, age, pubertal status, disease state, treatment regimen, and dose all influence the prognosis for reproductive failure.

MALES

Chemotherapeutic drugs accelerate programmed cell death (apoptosis) not only in tumor cells but in proliferating normal tissues such as testicular germinal epithelium.[79] Among the anticancer drugs, alkylating agents, in particular nitrogen mustard and cyclophosphamide, deplete germ cells in a dose-dependent fashion. Treatment with cyclophosphamide at a dose of 50–100 mg daily for 2 months may produce oligospermia, and the high-dose pulses of cyclophosphamide used in HSCT produce azoospermia in most men within a few months.[80, 81] Animal toxicology studies indicate that busulfan and procarbazine are also gonadotoxic.

The addition of radiation therapy to chemotherapy further damages the testes. The cytotoxic effects of radiation are thought to be due to the ionization of water, which generates free radicals, which damage DNA. Dose/injury curves of ionizing radiation on testicular tissue reveal transient oligospermia at doses of 10–30 cGy and irreversible azoospermia with doses of 200 cGy.[82]

Differentiating spermatogonia, the male gamete stem cell, is the most susceptible germ cell to damage by radiation and chemotherapy. Damage to the DNA of spermatogonia results in loss of all germ cells from the testes. The histologic term for this condition is the *Sertoli-cell-only syndrome* or *germinal aplasia*.[83] Figure 55–4 compares the testicular biopsy photo from a patient with germinal aplasia to a normal testicular biopsy photo. The diameter of the seminiferous tubules is reduced, germ cells are absent, and electron microscopy reveals that Sertoli cells are abnormal. On the other hand, Leydig cells, found in clusters in the loose intertubular connective tissue, are structurally normal. Damage may be focal, however, so a portion of the seminiferous tubules may contain germ cells at various states of maturation arrest. Because the seminiferous tubules account for about 85% of the cross-sectional area of the testis, extensive damage to the germinal epithelium results in a decrease in testis size.

The biochemical marker of impaired spermatogenesis is a rise in circulating follicle-stimulating hormone (FSH) levels. It is now well established that a decrease in inhibin secretion by Sertoli cells is responsible for the rise in FSH.[84]

Elevated FSH levels are observed within a few months of HSCT.[84] This delay does not necessarily indicate a lag in testicular damage; rather, the acute illness of HSCT suppresses hypothalamic-pituitary function,[86] masking the gonadotropin response to testicular failure. Leydig cell dysfunction may also occur after HSCT, resulting in a rise in plasma LH levels, and occasionally circulating testosterone concentrations decrease. When the brain is treated with large doses of irradiation, gonadotropin insufficiency may occur,[38] further lowering testosterone production, and clinical androgen deficiency may occur. Prolactin levels may also increase slightly.[80]

Less information is available on the long-term effects of conditioning therapy administered to children. Sanders et al.[58] noted that sperm counts were normal in six of eight boys treated before puberty with BMT and 200 mg/kg of cyclophosphamide conditioning. On the other hand, germ cell failure is to be expected when prepubertal males are treated with TBI together with alkylating agents.[86] Supplemental testicular radiation (18–24 Gy) for acute lymphoblastic leukemia invariably leads to testosterone deficiency as well as seminiferous tubular damage.[58, 87] Mackie et al.[86] reported that 89% of boys with Hodgkin disease treated with chlorambucil, vinblastine, procarbazine, and prednisone (ChlVPP) between ages 8 and 15 years had elevated plasma FSH levels when re-examined 2.5–11 years later, although less gonadal toxicity has been observed when drugs other than alkylating agents have been used to treat leukemia.[87]

Testicular dysfunction occurs among men with malignant disease even before conditioning chemotherapy is begun. For example, semen analysis results were abnormal in one of three young adult men with Hodgkin disease at diagnosis.[88] The most frequent abnormality is a reduction in sperm motility and morphology.[89] In men with Hodgkin disease, fever and advanced disease appear to be predictive of testicular dysfunction.[90] Men should be advised that a temporary decrease in libido and a decline in sexual performance are common during and immediately after treatment.

Sperm production generally resumes in about 10% of men 2–5 years after treatment, but the sperm density is low and sperm quality is poor.[89, 91] Rarely, men have fathered children after HSCT.[92] Unfortunately, there is no currently available treatment that protects the testes from the effects of cancer chemotherapeutic drugs and radiation. Pretreatment with testosterone, medroxyprogesterone acetate, or gonadotropin-releasing hormone analogues to suppress spermatogenesis prior to chemotherapy has been ineffective.[93] Therefore, sperm banking has been used to preserve fertility in male cancer patients before beginning chemotherapy. The poor-quality semen in cancer patients, however, even prior to treatment, cryopreserves poorly[94] so that subsequent artificial insemination was often unsuccessful. For example, only 3 of 11 couples conceived after intrauterine insemination of cryopreserved sperm in one series reported in 1987.[95]

More recent assisted reproductive methods, such as in vitro fertilization and intracytoplasmic sperm injection (ICSI), have allowed for pregnancies even with low-quality semen.[96] With ICSI, a single sperm cell is injected into the ooplasm, and the fertilized egg is incubated in vitro fol-

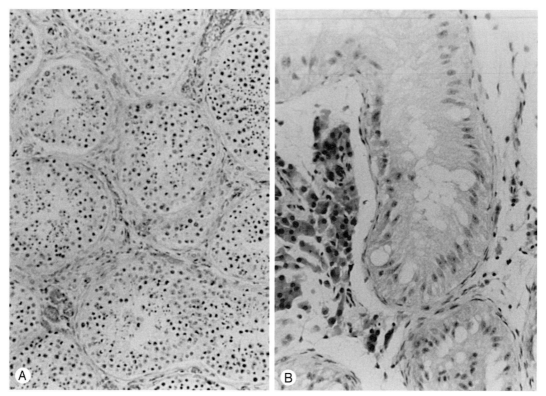

FIGURE 55–4. *A*, Biopsy of a normal adult testis (×50). Seminiferous tubules have a diameter of 150–300 μm. There is an organized arrangement of germ cells. Sertoli cells extend from the basment membrane to the tubular lumen and are recognizable by their prominent nucleoli. Between the seminiferous tubules is loose connective tissue containing single and clusters of Leydig cells. *B*, Testicular biopsy from an azoospermic man that reveals germinal aplasia (×64). A seminiferous tubule is shown longitudinally (*right*) and in cross-section (*left*). The seminiferous tubules contain only Sertoli cells. The darkly stained cluster of cells are Leydig cells, which appear more prominent than in *A* partly because the tubules are collapsed.

lowed by embryo transfer to the uterus if fertilization is successful.[97] There is a potential genetic risk of using sperm from cancer patients for ICSI. With this qualification, cryopreservation of sperm should be considered for all men prior to HSCT whose ejaculates contain sperm. In vitro fertilization can be performed after HSCT with poorly motile sperm, and ICSI can be effective even if the ejaculate contains only nonmotile sperm. Testosterone replacement using intramuscular testosterone esters or transdermal testerone preparations is indicated if testosterone deficiency is documented.

FEMALES

Amenorrhea is nearly uniform after HSCT.[98] Stress, infection, and immunotherapy in the immediate post-transplantation period suppress cyclic gonadotropin secretion, leading to anovulation. Within a few months gonadotropin levels rise, often to values that exceed the normal range, in most women who have received high-dose chemotherapy with or without irradiation.[99] Menopausal symptoms may occur. This change may indicate ovarian failure, or it may be transient, and instead reflect recovery of hypothalamic-pituitary-gonadal function. In fact, menses often resume in women treated with chemotherapy alone. For example, in the Fred Hutchinson Cancer Center study of women with aplastic anemia treated by BMT, menses resumed within 18 months in approximately 50% of young adult women.[98] Chemotherapy appears to accelerate the menopause, how-

ever, and resumption of menses is much less common among women treated beyond age 26 years.[98, 100]

TBI greatly reduces ovarian function compared with chemotherapy alone. It has been estimated that a dose of 4 Gy causes the death of 50% of oocytes.[101] Sanders et al.[98] found that women with leukemia who received TBI as well as high-dose cyclophosphamide were 7–9 times more likely to experience permanent ovarian failure than were women with aplastic anemia treated with cyclophosphamide alone. Elevated plasma LH and FSH and reduced estradiol levels were present 1 year after BMT in nearly all women who received combination therapy. Fractionated TBI has also produced uniform ovarian failure.[102] A few women experience return of menstruation a few years after BMT. As with cyclophosphamide alone, older age at treatment increases the risk of permanent ovarian failure after radiotherapy.[103] Women receiving more than 10 Gy also appear more likely to experience permanent ovarian failure than those receiving smaller doses of TBI.

The long-term pituitary-ovarian consequences of HSCT in girls appear to be similar to those of adult women. Among 32 girls ages 9–15 years with Hodgkin disease who received ChlVPP but no radiotherapy below the diaphragm, 53% experienced elevated gonadotropin levels 2–11 years later, but 9 women had conceived.[86] The dose dependency of the cyclophosphamide effect is applicable to prepubertal girls, with predictable ovarian failure occurring at doses of 500 mg/kg but no apparent impact of doses less than 200 mg/kg.[98] TBI is associated with nearly uniform ovarian failure in teenage girls as in adults.[98] There is a suggestion that fewer children experience gonadal failure if TBI is fractionated rather than delivered as a single dose.[34] HSCT with busulfan/cyclophosphamide conditioning was associated with elevated plasma FSH levels in 80% of prepubertal girls with thalassemia re-evaluated after 1–5 years.[77] Interestingly, the boys in the same study had persistent gonadotropin deficiency, suggesting a sex difference in iron deposition in the hypothalamus-pituitary.

Many pregnancies have been reported in women after HSCT for aplastic anemia (Table 55–2). A comprehensive analysis of the experience at Fred Hutchinson Cancer Research Center reveals a pregnancy rate of at least 25% in this group, unadjusted for women not wishing to conceive.[104] Pregnancy is not without risk in these women, however. Cytopenia may occur because the damaged bone marrow cannot respond to the demands of pregnancy and aplastic anemia has relapsed.[105] Pregnancy termination may be necessary. By contrast, pregnancy is rare among women who have received TBI, and when pregnancies have occurred, the dose of TBI has been less than 12.5 Gy.[104, 106, 107]

Moreover, very few women who received TBI after age 25 years have become pregnant.[106] Pregnancy after busulfan/cyclophosphamide conditioning appears to be just as unlikely as with TBI.[56] No consistent pre-, peri-, or postpartum complications have been described, although the risk for late abortion may be increased,[104] perhaps because of radiation-induced uterine dysfunction. The incidence of preterm low-birth-weight babies may also rise. There is a theoretical risk for hemolysis in the offspring of the polytransfused patient owing to the presence of antibodies to fetal blood group antigens.[100] There is no evidence, however, that pregnancy predisposes to cancer relapse or that the prevalence of congenital malformations is increased.[104, 108]

Unfortunately, there is no readily available approach to protect the ovary from the damage caused by radiation and high-dose chemotherapy. However, ovarian tissue cryopreservation and autotransplantation are promising recent developments. Medical treatment to suppress pituitary-ovarian function using gonadal steroids or gonadotropin-releasing analogues has been attempted as in men but was also unsuccessful. Therefore, pretreatment oocyte retrieval and embryo cryopreservation can be considered.[109] A second approach is the use of donor oocytes.[110] Estrogen-progestin replacement therapy is recommended within months of HSCT because of troubling menopausal symptoms such as hot flashes, irritability, insomnia, and dyspareunia and the increased long-term risk for osteoporosis

and coronary artery disease. Patient education is important because there is frequent anxiety about sterility, femininity, and appearance after HSCT.

PITUITARY-ADRENAL FUNCTION

Hypothalamic-pituitary-adrenal function is usually normal after HSCT conditioning regimens. Spontaneous adrenocorticotropic hormone (ACTH) and cortisol secretion were normal in 20 children with acute lymphoblastic leukemia who were studied 3.6–10 years after chemotherapy and fractional (18–24 Gy) cranial irradiation.[111] The same investigators found that the cortisol response to insulin-provoked hypoglycemia was normal in 29 and equivocal in 2 children 0.5–8 years after BMT.[72]

Primary adrenal failure presents with nausea, vomiting, and hypotension. Although the adrenal glands are resistant to radiation damage and the effects of chemotherapy, profound bleeding into both adrenals may produce acute adrenal failure in the setting of sepsis and coagulopathy. Laboratory clues to this diagnosis include hyponatremia and hyperkalemia, an unexplained decline in the hematocrit, azotemia, and acidosis. If the diagnosis is suspected, plasma cortisol and ACTH levels should be drawn and the patient should be treated immediately with high doses of hydrocortisone. Computed tomography generally reveals bilateral enlargement of the adrenal glands.[112]

The use of glucocorticoids for 1–2 weeks is unlikely to be associated with significant side effects. Although suppression of ACTH secretion can be demonstrated, recovery of function is rapid. With prolonged therapy, on the other hand, as for graft-versus-host disease, recovery is delayed and it is not possible to accurately predict the time course of recovery of function. In general, pharmacologic doses of glucocorticoids can be reduced rapidly to 7.5–10 mg of prednisone daily in divided doses if the underlying disorder does not relapse. Thereafter, slow tapering is necessary. The cortisol response 60 minutes after synthetic ACTH administration is often measured to monitor recovery. A normal response is a plasma cortisol level above 18 μg/dL. Persistence of suppression should be suspected for 12 months after discontinuation of glucocorticoid treatment, however, so that 200–300 mg of hydrocortisone should be administered over 24 hours in the event of surgery or other severe stress.

TABLE 55–2. PREGNANCY AFTER BONE MARROW TRANSPLANTATION*

DIAGNOSIS	TREATMENT	NO. OF PATIENTS	RESUMED MENSES	PREGNANT
Aplastic anemia				
Giorgiani et al.[56]	Cy 50 mg/kg/day ×4	103	56 (54%)	28
Marky et al.[52]	Cy 200 mg/kg/day ×4	6	4 (66%)	3
Leukemia				
Giorgiani et al.[56]	Cy + TBI	532	53 (10%)	13
Marky et al.[52]	"	14	0	0
Katz et al.[54]	"	10	0	0
Giorgiani et al.[56]	Cy + BU	73	1 (1.4%)	0

*Additional single case reports have also been published.
Cy, cyclosporine; BU, busulfan; TBI, total body irradiation.

METABOLIC COMPLICATIONS

DIABETES MELLITUS

Few patients with diabetes mellitus have been reported to have undergone HSCT. From the limited information available, diabetics appear to be at high risk for immediate complications, including infection and renal insufficiency.[113] There is no information about the impact of HSCT on the long-term complications of diabetes, such as retinopathy and nephropathy. Because of poor oral intake, fever, a catabolic state, and the propensity for dehydration, the insulin-dependent diabetic in the acute conditioning period should probably be managed with a controlled intravenous infusion of regular insulin and dextrose.[114] Treatment options for patients with non-insulin-dependent diabetes mellitus are more variable, and therapy should be individualized.

Secondary diabetes due to hemochromatosis may develop in patients with aplastic anemia or thalassemia. Glucose intolerance may improve in these patients after HSCT in part because of a decrease in the need for transfusion. On the other hand, glucose tolerance may worsen temporarily in diabetics and nondiabetics during conditioning because of the stress of illness and glucocorticoid therapy. There is no evidence, however, that HSCT predisposes to the delayed development of diabetes mellitus.[115] Adoptive transfer of polyendocrine failure including diabetes mellitus occurred in a patient whose HLA-identical sister donor experienced hypothyroidism 9 years later[116] and in a woman whose donor was an HLA-identical brother who likewise experienced insulin-dependent diabetes.

OBESITY

Obesity was diagnosed in nearly 50% of childhood survivors of HSCT for acute lymphoblastic leukemia.[60] Potential etiologic factors for obesity in these patients include GH and sex hormone deficiency, treatment with glucocorticoids, and physical inactivity. Fat mass is increased and muscle mass is decreased in untreated GH deficiency.[117] GH lowers the activity of lipoprotein lipase, the main enzymatic regulator of triglyceride uptake, and thereby reduces the volume of mature adiposites. Because increased visceral fat in GH-deficient adults is inversely correlated with high-density lipoprotein cholesterol levels and with increased risk of atherosclerotic disease, HSCT survivors may be at increased risk for coronary and peripheral vascular disease as they grow older. Recombinant GH therapy improves muscle mass, strength, and endurance in young adults with hypopituitarism. The cost is substantial, however, and the indications for GH replacement in adults remain controversial.

OSTEOPOROSIS

Osteoporosis is another delayed metabolic complication of HSCT. Potential etiologic factors include GH and sex hormone deficiency and glucocorticoid therapy. GH and sex steroids are important in the development of peak bone mass, which occurs between puberty and young adulthood.

Bone mineral density in adults with childhood-onset GH deficiency[118] or delayed puberty[119] of various causes is reduced, and the results are likely to be applicable to children and adolescents treated with HSCT. Glucocorticoids decrease bone mass by direct suppression of bone formation and by impairing calcium absorption, resulting in secondary hyperparathyroidism.

Glucocorticoids also decrease GH and sex hormone production. As occurs in most patients treated with glucocorticoids in high doses, bone density declines rapidly during treatment for graft-versus-host disease.[120] In a study of young adult survivors of childhood acute lymphoblastic leukemia treated according to a variety of protocols, including HSCT in five patients, bone mineral density in patients with GH deficiency was significantly lower than in patients who were not GH deficient, and treatment with GH prevented osteopenia.[121] Further studies are needed to identify effective preventive therapy. For the present, adult survivors of HSCT should be monitored for osteopenia using dual energy x-ray absorptiometry, and they should be treated if osteopenia is detected.

REFERENCES

1. Tulikorua I, Liewendahl K, Taskinen MR, et al: Effect of parenteral nutrition on the blood levels of insulin, glucagon, growth hormone, thyroid hormones and cortisol in catabolic patients. Acta Chir Scan 148:315, 1982.
2. Blachley JD, Hill JB: Renal and electrolyte disturbances associated with cisplatin. Ann Intern Med 95:628, 1981.
3. Jones DP, Chesney RW: Renal toxicity of cancer chemotherapeutic agents in children: ifosfamide and cisplatin. Curr Opin Pediatr 7:208, 1995.
4. Olerich MA, Rude K: Should we supplement Mg in critically ill patients? New Horizons 2:186, 1994.
5. Rude R: Magnesium metabolism and deficiency. Endocrinol Metab Clin North Am 22:377, 1993.
6. Knochel JP: The pathophysiology and clinical characteristics of severe hypophosphatemia. Arch Intern Med 137:203, 1977.
7. Newman JH, Neff TA, Ziporin P: Acute respiratory failure associated with hypophosphatemia. N Engl J Med 296:1101, 1977.
8. Grill V, Martin TJ: Parathyroid hormone-related protein as a cause of hypercalcemia in malignancy. In Bilezikian JP, Marcus R, Levine MA (eds): The Parathyroids: Basic and Clinical Concepts. New York, Raven Press, p 1994, 295.
9. Black KS, Mundy GR: Other causes of hypercalcemia: local and ectopic secretion syndromes. In Bilezikian JP, Marcus R, Levine MA (eds): The Parathyroids: Basic and Clinical Concepts. New York, Raven Press, 1994, p 341.
10. Villablanca JG, Khan AA, Avramis VI, et al: Hypercalcemia: a dose-limiting toxicity associated with 13-cis retinoic acid. Am J Pediatr Hematol Oncol 15:410, 1993.
11. Cohen J, Gierlowski TC, Schneider AB: A prospective study of hyperthyroidism in individuals exposed to radiation in childhood. JAMA 264:581, 1990.
12. Pagano L, Voso MT, Sica S: Recovery from diabetes insipidus associated with AML after a BMT conditioning regimen including busulfan. Bone Marrow Transplant 11:175, 1993.
13. Abe T, Takaue Y, Okamoto Y, et al: Syndrome of inappropriate antidiuretic hormone secretion (SIADH) in children undergoing high-dose chemotherapy and autologous peripheral blood stem cell transplantation. Pediatr Hematol Oncol 12:363, 1995.
14. Comis RL, Miller M, Ginsberg SJ: Abnormalities in water metabolism in small cell anaplastic lung cancer. Cancer 45:2414, 1980.
15. Campling BG, Sarda IR, Baer KA, et al: Secretion of atrial natriuretic peptide and vasopressin by small cell lung cancer. Cancer 75:2442, 1995.
16. Weisdorf SA, Lysne J, Wind D, et al: Positive effect of prophylactic TPN on long term outcome of BMT. Transplantation 43:833, 1987.
17. Szeluga DJ, Stuart RK, Brookmeyer R, et al: Nutritional support of bone marrow transplant recipient. Cancer Res 47:3309, 1987.

18. Mulder POM, Bouman JG, Gietema JA, et al: Hyperalimentation in autologous bone marrow transplant for solid tumors. Cancer 64:2045, 1989.

19. Knochel JP: Complications of total parenteral nutrition. Kidney Int 27:489–496, 1984.

20. Vexiau P, Perez-Castiglioni P, Socie G, et al: The "euthyroid sick syndrome": incidence, risk factors, and prognostic value soon after allogeneic bone marrow transplantation. Br J Haematol 85:778, 1993.

21. Hershman JM, Eriksin E, Kaufman N, et al: Thyroid function tests in patients undergoing bone marrow transplantation. Bone Marrow Transplant 6:49, 1990.

22. Burmeister LA: Reverse T3 does not reliably differentiate hypothyroid sick syndrome from euthyroid sick syndrome. Thyroid 5:434, 1995.

23. Chopra IJ, Tien-Shang H, Hurd RE, et al: A competitive ligand binding assay for measurement of thyroid homone-binding inhibitor in serum and tissues. J Clin Endocrinol Metab 58:619, 1984.

24. Pang X-P, et al: Impairment of hypothalamic-pituitary function in rats treated with human tumor necrois factor alpha (cachectin). Endocrinology 125:76, 1989.

25. Brabant G, Brabant A, Ranft U, et al: Circadian and pulsatile thyrotropin secretion in euthyroid men under influence of thyroid hormone and glucocorticoid administration. J Clin Endocrinol Metab 65:83, 1987.

26. Weintraub BD, Stannard BS, Magner JA, et al: Glycosylation and post translational processing of thyroid stimulating hormone: clinical implications. Rec Prog Horm Res 41:577, 1985.

27. Brent GA, Hershman JM: Thyroxine therapy in adults with severe non-thyroidal illness and low serum thyroxine concentration. J Clin Endocrinol Metab 63:1, 1986.

28. Littley MD, Shalet SM, Beardwell CG, et al: Radiation induced hypopituitarism is dose-dependant. Clin Endocrinol 31:363, 1989.

29. Ogilvy-Stuart AL, Shalet SM, Gattamaneni HR: Thyroid function after treatment of brain tumors in children. J Pediatr 119:733, 1991.

30. Bruning P, Bonfrer J, DeJongBakker M, et al: Primary hypothyroidism in breast cancer patients with irradiated supraclavicular nodes. Br J Cancer 51:659, 1985.

31. Grande C: Hypothyroidism following radiotherapy for head neck cancer: multivariate analysis of risk factors. Radiother Oncol 25:31, 1992.

32. Sklar CA, Kim TH, Ramsay NKC: Thyroid dysfunction among long-term survivors of bone marrow transplantation. Am J Med 73:688, 1982.

33. Borgstrom B: Thyroid function in children after allogeneic bone marrow transplantation. Bone Marrow Transplant 13:59, 1994.

34. Thomas BC, Stanhope R, Plowman PN, et al: Endocrine function following single fraction and fractionated TBI for bone marrow transplantation in childhood. Acta Endocrinol 128:508, 1993.

35. Lio S, Ariese W, Papa G, et al: Thyroid and pituitary function following allogeneic bone marrow transplantation. Arch Intern Med 148:1066, 1988.

36. Boulad F, Fromley M, Black P, et al: Thyroid dysfunction following bone marrow transplantation using hyperfractionated radiation. Bone Marrow Transplant 15:71, 1995.

37. Hancock SL, McDougall IR, Constine LS, et al: Thyroid abnormalities after therapeutic external radiation. Int J Radiat Oncol Biol Phys 31:1165, 1995.

38. Constine LS, Woolf PD, Cann D, et al: Hypothalamic-pituitary dysfunction after radiation for brain tumors. N Engl J Med 328:87, 1993.

39. Kubota C, Shinohara O, Hinohara T, et al: Changes in hypothalamic-pituitary function following bone marrow transplantation in children. Acta Paediatr Japon 36:37, 1994.

40. Hancock SL, Cox RS, McDougall IR: Thyroid disease after treatment of Hodgkin's disease. N Engl J Med 325:599, 1991.

41. Wasnich RD, Grumet FC, Payne RO, et al: Graves' ophthalmopathy following external neck irradiation for non-thyroidal neoplastic disease. J Clin Endocrinol Metab 37:703, 1973.

42. Constine LS, Donaldson SS, McDougall IR, et al: Radiation therapy for Hodgkin's disease followed by hypothyroidism and then Grave's hyperthyroidism. Clin Nucl Med 7:69, 1982.

43. Ichihashi T, Yoshida H, Kiyoi H, et al: Development of hyperthyroidism in donor and recipient after allogeneic bone marrow transplantation. Bone Marrow Transplant 10:397, 1992.

44. Aldouri MA, Ruggier R, Epstein O, et al: Adoptive transfer of hyperthyroidism and autoimmune thyroiditis following allogeneic

bone marrow transplantation for chronic myelogenous leukemia. Br J Haematol 74:118, 1990.

45. Ron E, Lubin JH, Shore RE, et al: Thyroid cancer after exposure to external radiation: a pooled analysis of seven studies. Radiat Res 141:259, 1995.

46. Greenspan FS: Radiation exposure and thyroid cancer. JAMA 237:2089, 1977.

47. Uderzo C, van Lint MT, Rovelli A, et al: Papillary thyroid carcinoma after total body irradiation. Arch Dis Child 71:256, 1994.

48. Kolb HJ, Guenther W, Duell T, et al: Cancer after bone marrow transplantation: IBMTR and EMBT/EULEP Study Group on Late Effects. Bone Marrow Transplant 1:135, 1992.

49. Nagayama Y, Ohta K, Tsuruta M: Exacerbation of thyroid autoimmunity by interferon alpha treatment in patients with chronic viral hepatitis: our studies and review of the literature. Endocrinol J 41:565, 1994.

50. Chen F-Q, Okamura K, Sato K: Reversible primary hypothyroidism with blocking or stimulating type TSH binding inhibitor immunoglobulin following recombinant interferon-α therapy in patients with pre-existing thyroid disorders. Clin Endocrinol 45:207, 1996.

51. Jones JI, Clemmons DR: Insulin-like growth factors and their binding proteins: biological actions. Endocrinol Rev 16:3, 1995.

52. Marky I, Mellander L, Lannery B, et al: A longitudinal study of growth and growth hormone secretion in children during treatment for acute lymphoblastic leukemia. Med Pediatr Oncol 19:258, 1991.

53. Nivot S, Benelli C, Clot JP: Nonparallel changes of growth hormone (GH) and insulin growth factor-1, insulin-like growth factor binding protein-3, and growth hormone binding protein, after cranial spinal irradiation and chemotherapy. J Clin Endocrinol Metab 78:597, 1994.

54. Katz JA, Chambers B, Everhart C, et al: Linear growth in children with acute lymphoblastic leukemia treated without cranial irradiation. J Pediatr 118:575, 1991.

55. Cohen A, Rovelli A, Van-Lint MT: Final height of patients who underwent bone marrow transplantation during childhood. Arch Dis Child 74:737, 1996.

56. Giorgiani G, Bozzola M, Locateli F, et al: Role of busulfan and total body irradiation on growth of prepubertal children receiving bone marrow transplantation and results of treatment with recombinant human growth hormone. Blood 86:825, 1995.

57. Huma Z, Boulad F, Black F, et al: Growth in children after bone marrow transplantation for acute leukemia. Blood 86:819, 1995.

58. Sanders JE and the Seattle Marrow Transplant Team: The impact of marrow transplant preparative regimens on subsequent growth and development. Semin Hematol 28:244, 1991.

59. Brauner R, Rappaport R, Prevot C, et al: A prospective study of the development of growth hormone deficiency in children given cranial irradiation, and its relation to statural growth. J Clin Endocrinol Metab 68:346, 1989.

60. Davies HA, Didcock E, Didi M, et al: Growth, puberty and obesity after treatment for leukemia. Acta Pediatr Suppl 411:45, 1995.

61. Bushhouse S, Ramsay NK, Pescovitz OH, et al: Growth in children following irradiation for bone marrow transplant. Am J Pediatr Hematol Oncol 11:134, 1989.

62. Littley MD, Shalet SM, Beardwell CG, et al: Hypopituitarism following external radiotherapy for pituitary tumors in adults. Q J Med 262:145, 1989.

63. Brauner R, Fontura M, Zucker JM, et al: Growth and growth hormone secretion after bone marrow transplantation. Arch Dis Child 68:458, 1993.

64. Cianfarani S, Boemi S, Spagnoli A, et al: Is IGF binding protein-3 assessment helpful for the diagnosis of GH deficiency? Clin Endocrinol 43:43, 1995.

65. Oberfield SE, Allen JC, Pollack JC, et al: Long-term endocrine sequelae after treatment of medulloblastoma: prospective study of growth and thyroid function. J Pediatr 108:219, 1986.

66. Allen DB: Growth suppression by glucocorticoid therapy. Endocrinol Metab Clin North Am 25:699, 1996.

67. Gabrielsson BG, Carmignac DF, Flavell DM, et al: Steroid regulation of growth hormone (GH) receptor and GH-binding protein messenger ribonucleic acids in the rat. Endocrinology 136:209, 1995.

68. Hokken-Koelega ACS, Stijnen T, de Muinck Keizer-Schrama SMPF, et al: Drop in SLS levels of growth hormone, insulin-like growth factor I (IGF-1) and II, IGF-binding protein-1 and -3, and cortisol in prednisone-treated children with growth retardation after renal transplantation. J Clin Endocrinol Metab 77:932, 1993.

69. Reimer LH, Morris HG, Ellis EE: Growth of asthmatic children

during treatment with alternate day steroids. J Allergy Clin Immunol 55:224, 1975.

70. Oglivy-Stuart AL: Safety of growth hormone after treatment of a childhood malignancy. Horm Res 44(Suppl 3):73, 1995.

71. Giri N, Davis EA, Vowels MR: Long term complications following bone marrow transplantation in children. J Pediatr Child Health 29:201, 1993.

72. Oglivy-Stuart AL, Clark DJ, Wallace WHB, et al: Endocrine deficit after fractionated total body irradiation. Arch Dis Child 67:1107, 1992.

73. Sherins RJ, Olweny CLM, Ziegler JL: Gynecomastia and gonadal dysfunction in adolescent boys treated with combination chemotherapy for Hodgkin's disease. N Engl J Med 299:12, 1978.

74. Blatt J, Poplack DG, Sherins RJ: Testicular function in boys after chemotherapy for acute lymphoblastic leukemia. N Engl J Med 304:1121, 1981.

75. Martha PM, Gorman KM, Blizzard RM, et al: Endogenous growth hormone secretion and clearance rates in normal boys, as determined by deconvolution analysis: relationship to age, pubertal status, and body mass. J Clin Endocrinol Metab 74:336, 1992.

76. Crowne EC, Moore C, Wallace MHB, et al: A novel variant of growth hormone insufficiency following low dose cranial irradiation. J Clin Endocrinol 22:375, 1992.

77. De Sanctis V, Galimberti M, Lucarelli G, et al: Gonadal function after allogenic bone marrow transplantatin for thalassaemia. Arch Dis Child 66:517, 1991.

78. De Simone M, Olioso P, Di Bartolomeo P, et al: Growth and endocrine function following bone marrow transplantation for thalassemia. Bone Marrow Transplant 15:227, 1995.

79. Allan DJ, Harmon BV, Kerr JFR: Cell death in spermatogenesis. *In* Potten CS (ed): Perspectives on Mammalian Cell Death. London, Oxford University Press, 1987, p 229.

80. Chapman RM, Rees LH, Sutcliffe SB, et al: Cyclical combination chemotherapy and gonadal function. Lancet 8111:285, 1979.

81. Chatterjee R, Mils W, Katz M, et al: Germ cell failure and Leydig cell insufficiency in post-pubertal males after autologous bone marrow transplantation with BEAM for lymphoma. Bone Marrow Transplant 13:519, 1994.

82. Clifton DDK, Bremner WJ: The effect of testicular x-irradiation on spermatogenesis in man: a comparison with the mouse. J Androl 4:387, 1983.

83. Sherins RJ, DeVita VT: Effect of drug treatment for lymphoma on male reproductive capacity. Ann Intern Med 79:216, 1973.

84. Wallace EM, Groome NP, Riley SC, et al: Effects of chemotherapy-induced testicular damage on inhibin, gonadotropin and testosterone secretion: a prospective, longitudinal study. J Clin Endocrinol Metab 82:3111, 1997.

85. Spratt DI, Cox P, Orav J, et al: Reproductive axis suppression in acute illness is related to disease severity. J Clin Endocrinol Metab 76:1548, 1993.

86. Mackie EJ, Radford M, Shalet SM: Gonadal function following chemotherapy for childhood Hodgkin's disease. Med Pediatr Oncol 27:74, 1996.

87. Blatt J, Sherins RJ, Niebrugge D, et al: Leydig cell function following treatment for testicular replase of acute lymphoblastic leukemia. J Clin Oncol 3:1227, 1985.

88. Marmor D, Elefant E, Dauchez C: Semen analysis in Hodgkin's disease before the onset of treatment. Cancer 57:1986, 1986.

89. Viviani S: Testicular dysfunction in Hodgkin's disease before and after treatment. Eur J Cancer 27:1389, 1991.

90. Vigersky RA, Chapman RM, Berenberg J, et al: Testicular dysfunction in untreated Hodgkin's disease. Am J Med 73:482, 1982.

91. Chapman RM, Sutcliffe SB, Malpas JS: Male gonadal dysfunction in Hodgkin's disease: a prospective study. JAMA 245:1323, 1981.

92. Pakkala S, Lukka M, Helminen P, et al: Paternity after bone marrow transplantation following conditioning with total body irradiation. Bone Marrow Transplant 13:489, 1994.

93. Morris ID, Shalet SM: Endocrine-mediated protection from cytotoxic-induced testicular damage. J Endocrinol 120:7, 1989.

94. Agarwal A, Shekarriz M, Sidhu RK, et al: Value of clinical diagnosis in predicting the quality of cryopreserved sperm from cancer patients. J Urol 155:934, 1996.

95. Redman JR, Bajorunas DR, Goldstein MC, et al: Semen cryopreservation and artificial insemination for Hodgkin's disease. J Clin Oncol 5:233, 1987.

96. Sanger WG, Olson JH, Sherman JK, et al: Semen cryobanking for men with cancer—criteria change. Fertil Steril 60:1024, 1992.

97. Payne D, Flaherty SP, Jeffrey R, et al: Successful treatment of severe male factor infertility in 100 consecutive cycles using intracytoplasmic sperm injection. Hum Reprod 9:2051, 1994.

98. Sanders JE, Buckner CD, Amos D, et al: Ovarian function following marrow transplantation for aplastic anemia or leukemia. J Clin Oncol 6:813, 1988.

99. Chatterjee R, Mills W, Katz M: Prospective study of pituitary-gonadal function to evaluate short-term effects of ablative chemotherapy of total body irradiation with autologous or allogeneic marrow transplantation in post-menarchal female patients. Bone Marrow Transplant 13:511, 1994.

100. Hinterberger-Fischer M, Kier P, Kalhs P, et al: Fertility, pregnancies and offspring complications after bone marrow transplantation. Bone Marrow Transplant 7:5, 1991.

101. Wallace WHB, Shalet SM, Hendry JH, et al: Ovarian failure following abdominal irradiation in childhood: the radiosensitivity of the human oocyte. Br J Radiol 62:995, 1989.

102. Littley MD, Shalet SM, Morgenstern GR, Deakin DP: Endocrine and reproductive function following fractionated total body irradiation in adults. Q J Med 78:265, 1991.

103. Lushbaugh GC, Casarett GW: The effects of gonadal irradiation in clinical radiation therapy: a review. Cancer 37:1111, 1976.

104. Sanders JE, Hawley J, Levy W, et al: Pregnancies following high-dose cyclophosphamide with or without high-dose busulfan or total-body irradiation and bone marrow transplantation. Blood 87:3045, 1996.

105. Pajor A, Kelemen E, Szakacs Z, et al: Pregnancy in idiopathic aplastic anemia (report of 10 patients). Eur J Obstet Gynecol Reprod Biol 45:19, 1992.

106. Lipton JH, Derzko C, Fyles G, et al: Pregnancy after BMT: three case reports. Bone Marrow Transplant 11:415, 1993.

107. Maruta A, Matsuzaki M, Miyashta H, et al: Successful pregnancy after allogeneic bone marrow transplantation following conditioning with total body irradiation. Bone Marrow Transplant 15:637, 1995.

108. Kawamura S, Suzuki Y, Tamai Y, et al: Pregnancy outcome among long-term survivors with acute leukemia. Int J Hematol 62:157, 1995.

109. Winkel CA, Fossum GT: Current reproductive technology: considerations for the oncologist. Oncology 7:40, 1993.

110. Lydic ML, Liu JH, Rebar RW, et al: Success of donor oocyte in in vitro fertilization—embryo transfer in recipients with and without premature ovarian failure. Fertil Steril 65:98, 1996.

111. Crowne EC, Wallace WHB, Gibson S, et al: Adrenocorticotrophin and cortisol secretion in children after low dose cranial irradiation. Clin Endocrinol 39:297, 1993.

112. Rao RH: Bilateral massive adrenal hemorrhage. Med Clin North Am 79:107, 1995.

113. Schouten HC, Maragos D, Vose J, et al: Diabetes mellitus or an impaired glucose tolerance as a potential complicating factor in patients treated with high-dose therapy and autologous bone marrow transplantation. Bone Marrow Transplant 6:333, 1990.

114. Gavin LA: Perioperative management of the diabetic patient. Endocrinol Metab Clin North Am 21:457, 1992.

115. Lorini R, Cortona L, Scaramuzza A, et al: Hyperinsulinemia in 34 children and adolescents after bone marrow transplantation. Hormone Res 41:63, 1994.

116. Vialettes B, Maranichi D, San Marco MP, et al: Autoimmune polyendocrine failure type 1 (insulin-dependent) diabetes mellitus and hypothyroidism after allogeneic bone marrow transplantation in a patient with lymphoblastic leukemia. Diabetologia 36:541, 1993.

117. Jorgensen JOL, Muller J, Moller J, et al: Adult growth hormone deficiency. Hormone Res 42:235, 1994.

118. Kaufman J-M, Taelman P, Vermeulen A, et al: Bone mineral status in growth hormone–deficient males with isolated and multiple pituitary deficiencies of childhood onset. J Clin Endocrinol Metab 74:118, 1992.

119. Finkelstein JS, Klibanski A, Neer RM, et al: Osteoporosis in men with idiopathic hypogonadotropic hypogonadism. Ann Intern Med 106:354, 1987.

120. Stern IM, Chestnut CH, Bruemmer B, et al: Bone density loss during treatment of chronic GVHD. Bone Marrow Transplant 17:395, 1996.

121. Nusey SS, Hyer SL, Brada M, et al: Bone mineralization after treatment of growth hormone deficiency in survivors of childhood malignancy. Acta Paediatr Suppl 399:9, 1994.

CHAPTER FIFTY-SIX

Relapse After Hematopoietic Stem Cell Transplantation: Mechanisms and Treatment

Sergio A. Giralt, M.D., and Richard E. Champlin, M.D.

Disease relapse after hematopoietic stem cell transplantation (HSCT) remains the most important cause of treatment failure for this procedure.[1–4] Because of the increase in the number of autologous and allogeneic transplant procedures performed during earlier phases of the disease and the unchanging relapse rates, the number of patients presenting with their initial relapse after transplantation will increase.[1, 5, 6] These patients will more than likely be young, have a good performance status, and demand therapy with curative intent. Therefore, searches for novel and potentially curative strategies for patients experiencing relapse after transplantation need to be explored.

MECHANISMS OF RELAPSE

Intuitively, the most common cause of disease recurrence after autologous or allogeneic HSCT is residual disease resistant to the conditioning. For allogeneic transplantation, however, other mechanisms of disease recurrence exist.

ORIGIN OF DISEASE RELAPSE

After successful allogeneic HSCT, hematopoiesis and immunity are reconstituted from donor-derived cells. Leukemia relapses generally occur in recipient-derived cells. Donor-cell leukemia is a rare but well-documented phenomenon. Most cases of donor-cell leukemia occur late after HSCT and have been associated with total body irradiation. The mechanisms postulated for leukemic transformation of donor cells include radiation-facilitated viral leukemogenesis, persistence of the leukemogenic stimulus with de novo leukemic transformation, or transfer of oncogenic genetic material from host-derived leukemic cells to normal donor HSC.[7–10]

Recipients of autologous transplants for lymphoma or solid tumors usually experience relapse at the sites of prior disease, suggesting that the major source of recurrent disease is the residual disease left in the body after the preparative regimen. Gene-marking experiments have documented that cells in the infused HSC product also contribute to relapse in chronic myelogenous leukemia (CML), acute myelogenous leukemia (AML), and neuroblastoma.[11, 12]

MECHANISMS OF RESISTANCE TO THE CONDITIONING REGIMEN

Resistance to chemoradiotherapy is due to a variety of mechanisms, such as intrinsic resistance of the leukemic progenitor cell, immune phenotype, kinetic resistance, enhanced DNA repair, and excessive leukemic cell burden.[13, 14] Mechanisms of resistance to alkylating agents include: genetic instability, glutathione synthesis, enhanced DNA repair, kinetic resistance, and others.[15, 16]

GRAFT-VS.-LEUKEMIA EFFECT

The response to donor lymphocyte infusions in patients who experience relapse after allogeneic transplantation is the most conclusive evidence for the existence of an immune-mediated effect that prevents disease recurrence after allogeneic transplantation (the graft vs. leukemia effect [GVL]).[17–27] Additional discussions about GVL can be found later in this chapter and in Chapters 4 and 31.

The cell populations that mediate the GVL effect are unknown. In humans, donor-derived cytotoxic T lymphocytes with antileukemic activity without normal host tissue reactivity can be isolated in vitro, but cells with dual reactivity also exist.[28–30] Both CD4+ and CD8+ cytotoxic clones have been reported, suggesting that antigens presented in the context of major histocompatibility complex class I and class II loci are involved.[26, 28–30] Lymphokine-activated killer (LAK) cells and natural killer (NK) cells have also been reported to mediate GVL effects in vivo and in vitro.[31] Cytokines also may play a role in the GVL phenomenon. Both CD4+ and CD8+ cells secrete interleukin-2 (IL-2), IL-3, granulocyte macrophage colony-stimulating factor (GM-CSF), interferon-γ, tumor necrosis factor (TNF), and other cytokines when activated. These cytokines could potentially mediate a direct or indirect cytotoxic effect.[32–34]

LEUKEMIA TOLERANCE

Patients with acute or chronic GVHD still experience relapse. This indicates that leukemic clones can overcome the GVL effect. This phenomenon of immune escape may be due to change in the leukemic phenotype with loss of expression of antigens essential for immune recognition.[25]

Tumor tolerance has been described in animal models and may be associated with the production of transforming growth factor β or other inhibitory cytokines.[35, 36] The existence of inhibitory cytokines would explain the presence of in vitro alloreactive cells in the setting of clinical tolerance.[37]

NATURAL HISTORY OF RELAPSE AFTER TRANSPLANTATION

LEUKEMIA

The survival of patients who experience relapse after HSCT depends on the specific leukemia diagnosis, stage of disease, interval from transplantation to recurrence, patient performance status, type of initial transplant, and salvage therapy. Patients with acute leukemia who experience relapse after allogeneic HSCT and receive no further treatment have a median survival time of 3–4 months, with no long-term survivors.[38–40]

Complete remission is the major prognostic factor for survival. The median survival duration for patients who achieve a complete remission is 8 months (those with AML) and 14 months (those with acute lymphoblastic leukemia [ALL]). Survival in patients not achieving a complete remission is comparable to that of patients receiving supportive care alone. In most series, the duration of post-transplantation remission emerges as the most important prognostic factor for complete remission and survival.[38, 39]

Patients with CML who experience relapse after allogeneic HSCT have a different natural history, depending on the status of their disease at the time of relapse. For patients with isolated cytogenetic relapses, median survival is greater than 6 years, compared with 3 years for those whose disease relapses into a clinical chronic phase.[41] Spontaneous cytogenetic remissions have been reported in up to 20% of patients receiving non—T-cell–depleted allografts with cytogenetic relapses; in contrast, with recipients of T cell–depleted allografts, disease progression seems to be the rule.[42, 43] Patients who experience relapse into a more-advanced phase have a median survival duration of less than 6 months, with poor response to interferon or conventional chemotherapy.[41]

Granulocytic sarcoma as a sole manifestation of relapse is uncommon after allogeneic transplantation. In a retrospective review, 26 of 5824 patients were identified with these sarcomas. All of these patients had received allografts for AML, myelodysplastic syndromes (MDS), or CML. The granulocytic sarcomas appeared between 4 and 56 months post transplantation (median, 13 months), presenting as single or multiple lesions on the trunk, limbs, or breasts. The risk of progression to overt leukemia and death was related primarily to the stage of the disease at the time of transplantations, with no long-term survivors among patients receiving transplants beyond first remission. Eight patients were alive and free of disease between 15 and 132 months after a variety of treatments, ranging from involved-field radiation to second allogeneic transplantation.[44] Other sites of extramedullary relapses, such as central nervous system and testicular relapses, are more frequent. These can occur in up to 20% of allograft recipients for AML and 6–30% of patients with ALL. Most occur concurrently with marrow relapse.[38, 39]

MYELOMA

High-dose chemotherapy with autologous HSC support is rapidly becoming an integral part of the primary therapy of patients with multiple myeloma. This therapeutic modality has been shown to increase complete remission rates and improve disease-free survival and overall survival; even so, the disease appears to relapse invariably, which remains the most important cause of treatment failure.[45, 46]

In a study of 94 patients experiencing relapse after high-dose chemotherapy and autologous HSCT, the presalvage level of β$_2$-microglobulin and the post-transplantation remission time emerged as the most important predictors for response to salvage therapy. The overall survival rate for patients with a β$_2$-microglobulin level of 2.5 mg/L or less or a post-transplantation remission of greater than 12 months was 80% at 2 years, in contrast with 38% for patients with higher β$_2$-microglobulin or shorter remission duration after transplantation. Although patients who received a second autologous transplant as part of salvage therapy experienced a higher complete remission rate than patients receiving conventional chemotherapy, salvage transplantation did not emerge as a prognostic factor for overall survival in a multivariant analysis.[47]

The natural history of relapse after allografts for myeloma has not been well defined.[48, 49] The median survival of patients who do not experience remission after allogeneic transplantation is less than 12 months, with a 3-year survival rate of approximately 12%. Studies defining the utility of post-transplantation chemotherapy, cytokines, and second transplantation are needed to determine the impact of these therapies on survival in this setting.

LYMPHOMA

Autologous transplantation is being used more frequently as part of the initial therapy or as salvage therapy for a variety of lymphomas.[50] Relapses post transplantation occur in 30–70% of the patients, depending on the status of the disease at the time of transplantation, disease histology, chemosensitivity, and other pretransplantation prognostic factors.[50–53]

Vose et al., at the University of Nebraska Medical Center, reviewed the outcomes of 169 patients who had progressive disease after autologous transplantation for either Hodgkin disease or non-Hodgkin lymphoma. The median survival for the 95 patients with Hodgkin disease was 10.5 months from the time of relapse. These patients received a variety of salvage therapies. The achievement of a complete remission any time prior to transplantation or with HSCT was the most important prognostic factor for survival after relapse post transplantation.[51] The median survival after progression for patients with non-Hodgkin lymphoma was 3 months, with duration of remission after transplantation being the most important prognostic factor for survival.

For patients who experienced relapse longer than 12 months post transplantation, median survival was greater than 36 months versus 6 months for patients with a shorter remission duration. Salvage therapy was varied and did not predict for survival in this series of patients.[54]

BREAST CANCER

Relapse after high-dose chemotherapy for breast cancer occurs primarily in the sites of prior disease.[55, 56] The natural history of these patients has not been well documented in the literature. As with other malignancies, one would expect that survival after progression would be short and determined primarily by the disease status at the time of transplantation, disease stage at transplantation, number and sites of metastatic disease, and response to salvage therapy.

With the increasing use of high-dose chemotherapy as intensification for patients with high-risk stage 2 and 3 disease, many patients will manifest their first recurrence after a high-dose chemotherapy program. Understanding the natural history of this disease will be essential in making treatment decisions for both patients and physicians.

TREATMENT OF RELAPSE AFTER HSCT

RELAPSES AFTER ALLOGENEIC TRANSPLANTATION

Patients experiencing relapse after allogeneic HSCT are usually in a chimeric state in which the recurrent leukemia is of recipient origin, but the residual normal hematopoietic and immune systems remain donor in origin. Strategies to induce remission should therefore not only consider conventional antineoplastic chemotherapy but also novel therapeutic approaches that exploit this unique chimeric situation. Such strategies may employ selective stimulation of donor-derived hematopoiesis or augmentation of the GVL reaction through either cytokines or cellular therapy.[26]

Leukemia
Cyclosporine Withdrawal

Cyclosporin withdrawal has been reported to induce complete remissions in patients with CML, AML, and ALL. All patients reported having experienced GVHD, and most had received an allograft that was not T-cell depleted, suggesting that an immune-mediated mechanism was involved in the reinduction of remission.[57-59] A retrospective analysis from the Fred Hutchinson Cancer Research Center suggests that patients with CML and two consecutive abnormal cytogenetic test results benefitted from cyclosporin discontinuation without exacerbation of GVHD.[60]

Conventional Chemotherapy and Radiotherapy

Chemotherapy with conventional antileukemic agents can prolong survival and improve quality of life in patients obtaining a complete remission. Patients with AML can be successfully treated with a combination of cytosine arabinoside and anthracyclines, whereas patients with ALL have responded to combination therapy with vinca alkaloids, steroids, and anthracyclines.[38-40, 61, 62] Patients with central nervous system, testicular, or symptomatic extramedullary disease may receive localized radiation therapy. Isolated extramedullary relapses precede overt marrow relapses in most cases, and further therapy may be warranted for long-term disease control.[38, 39, 44, 61-65]

Cytokine Therapy

Granulocyte colony-stimulating factor (filgrastim, G-CSF) can induce cytogenetic and hematologic remissions in patients with leukemia who experience relapse after allogeneic HSCT.[66] In a recent follow-up of the initial experience, 7 of 23 patients responded. All responding patients have subsequently experienced relapse a median of 12 months after G-CSF therapy (range, 3–20 months). The responding patients had lower numbers of peripheral blood and bone marrow blasts than the nonresponding patients. This novel approach to therapy requires further evaluation to determine the mechanism of response and utility of this strategy. G-CSF therapy and withdrawal of immunosuppression constitute our initial therapeutic approach to patients experiencing early acute leukemia relapse (cytogenetic relapse or hematologic relapse without peripheral blood blasts).[67]

Interferon-α (IFN-α) has direct activity against leukemic cells and may enhance a GVL effect by up-regulating MHC antigen expression and stimulating T-lymphocyte and NK-cell activity.[68] IFN-α has been reported to reinduce remissions in selected patients with recurrent CML after allogeneic HSCT.[41, 68-70] IFN-α therapy increases the cytogenetic response rate for patients experiencing relapse after HSCT from 2% to 22% and delays disease progression. IFN-α therapy emerges as an independent prognostic factor for survival in patients with CML relapse after allogeneic HSCT, although the survival benefit seems to be lost after 6 years.[41]

IL-2 is in theory an ideal agent for the treatment of relapse post HSCT. IL-2 has modest single activity against acute leukemia, is a potent immune stimulant, and is probably involved in the GVL effect.[71-73] Unfortunately, the experience with IL-2 in the setting of post-HSCT relapse has been limited and shows conflicting results.[74-76]

In a pilot trial, we have explored the combination of IFN-α and low-dose IL-2 for patients with acute or chronic leukemia experiencing relapse after allogeneic HSCT. One of five patients with acute leukemia responded, but this patient died from fungal pneumonia. Three patients experienced exacerbation of acute GVHD, and four patients required dose reduction.[74] Other investigators have reported good responses to combination cytokine therapy with donor lymphocyte infusion, but further studies of these approaches are needed.[75-77]

Second Allogeneic Transplants

Second transplants have been successful in selected patients who experience relapse after allogeneic HSCT (Table 56–1). The treatment-related mortality rate is between 30% and 40%, with approximately 20% of the patients becoming long-term survivors.[78-87] Early relapse post transplantation,

TABLE 56–1. RESULTS OF SECOND TRANSPLANTS FOR RELAPSE AFTER ALLOGENEIC TRANSPLANTATION

REFERENCE	DIAGNOSIS/NO.	RELAPSE RATE (%)	100-DAY TRM (%)	POSITIVE PROGNOSTIC FACTORS	DFS AT 4 YEARS
80	Leukemia/25	60	50	>12 mo from BMT1	17%
81	Leukemia/77	70	36	AGVHD, age <10 yr, CML	14%
82	Leukemia/42	NS	NS	CML, >6 mo from BMT1	12%
83	Leukemia/23	24	42	CML, >6 mo from BMT1	29%
84	Leukemia/87 Other/3	69	47	>18 mo from BMT1 CGVHD during BMT2	11%
85	Leukemia/114	65	40	>6 mo from BMT1 PS >80, age <26 yr, CML	21%

BMT1, bone marrow transplant #1; BMT2, bone marrow transplant #2; TRM, transplant-related mortality; DFS, disease-free survival; CML, chronic myelogenous leukemia; CGVHD, chronic graft-versus-host disease; AGVHD, acute graft-versus-host disease; NS, not stated; PS, performance status.

older age, poor performance status, and prior toxicity from the initial transplant are poor prognostic factors for a second conventional transplant. Alternative therapies should be offered to these patients.[26]

For patients with more than one possible donor, no data support the use of an alternative HLA-compatible donor as a means to achieve a greater GVL effect. For patients experiencing relapse after syngeneic HSCT, an allogeneic transplant could be considered if an HLA-compatible donor is available. Allogeneic peripheral blood progenitor cells have been successfully used to support salvage high-dose regimens, but whether the enhanced hematologic recovery and the large lymphocyte dose infused will decrease treatment-related mortality and relapse is not known.[88–90]

Donor Lymphocyte Infusion

The antileukemic effects of donor peripheral blood lymphocytes has been confirmed by multiple investigators.[17–23, 76, 91] Results from the largest reported series suggest that patients with CML that recurs as an isolated cytogenetic relapse or in chronic phase respond better to this treatment than do patients with more-advanced disease or acute leukemia. Patients with CML who receive donor lymphocytes after relapse experience a median survival of more than 30 months as opposed to less than 1 year for patients with acute leukemia, of whom only a handful of patients obtain long-term disease control.[23, 91] Prognostic factors for response and complications have been identified from two large registry trials (Table 56–2).[23, 91]

The effector cells responsible for the antileukemic effect of donor lymphocyte infusion (DLI) have not been identified. Selective T-cell depletion of donor lymphocytes may help dissect the roles that different lymphocyte subsets play in the antileukemic effect. CD8-depleted DLI induced complete hematologic and cytogenetic remissions in seven of seven patients in either cytogenetic or chronic-phase relapse of CML after allogeneic HSCT and in one of three patients in an accelerated phase. Two patients in this series experienced acute GVHD, and two cases of chronic GVHD occurred. This preliminary observation suggests that CD8-depleted donor lymphocytes are as effective as unmanipulated DLI and that CD8+ cells are not essential for the GVL effect in CML.[92]

The optimum lymphocyte dose for treatment of relapse post transplantation has not been identified. Mackinnon et al. reported that doses of less than 1×10^7 CD3+ cells/kg do not regularly induce remissions in patients with CML in hematologic relapse, but lower doses may be effective in less-advanced phases of the disease.[93, 94]

GVHD and pancytopenia secondary to marrow aplasia have been important causes of treatment failure in most published series of DLI. These complications account for most of the 20% rate of treatment-related mortality.[23, 24, 91] Aplasia post lymphocyte infusion appears to be related to the degree of residual donor hematopoiesis at the time of DLI, occurring less frequently in patients who undergo DLI with less-advanced disease (cytogenetic relapse vs. hematologic relapse).[20] GVHD has been reported to occur in up to 80% of patients receiving DLI.[23, 24, 91]

Patients with acute leukemia experiencing relapse after allogeneic HSCT have a lower response rate and a shorter remission duration after DLI than do patients with CML. The biologic basis for this difference in response rates is not understood but could depend on expression of costimulatory molecules or inadequate numbers of class I and II antigen expression. The fact that acute leukemias generally have a faster doubling time than CML does not explain the difference in response rates because DLI after chemotherapy has not been shown to be dramatically more effective than DLI alone. The contribution of concomitant chemotherapy or other maneuvers is uncertain. Chemotherapy is probably beneficial in patients with rapid proliferating disease, in whom disease control is needed to give time for the DLI to exert its effect.[23, 91, 95] Most investigators have administered conventional salvage therapy prior to DLI containing anthracyclines, cytosine arabinoside, vinca alkaloids, or steroids, but it seems more appropriate to use new agents with different mechanism of actions in this setting. It is possible that infusion of donor CD34+ cells (obtained by G-CSF mobilization or from the donor bone marrow) could facilitate recovery after salvage chemotherapy for these patients, but this has not been shown to prevent pancytopenia or aplasia after lymphocyte infusions.[95, 96]

Myeloma

DLI has been reported to be effective in treating myeloma relapses after allogeneic HSCT.[91, 97–99] Preliminary results

TABLE 56–2. PREDICTORS FOR RESPONSE AND COMPLICATIONS AFTER DONOR LYMPHOCYTE INFUSIONS

SERIES	DISEASE/RESPONSES	FAVORABLE PREDICTORS FOR RESPONSE	PREDICTORS FOR GVHD	PREDICTORS FOR APLASIA
Kolb et al., 1995[23]	CML 54/75	Chronic phase at HSCT T cell–depleted HSCT Non-transformed relapse GVHD after DLI Cytopenia after DLI GVHD after HSCT not a predictor	T-cell depletion Interferon	T-cell depletion Hematologic relapse
	Acute leukemia 6/33	Diagnosis AML	None identified	None identified
Collins et al., 1995[91]	CML 34/57	Lymphocyte dose $<5 \times 10^8$/kg Sex: male to female Time to DLI <2 years Chronic phase at DLI	Not stated	Not stated
	Acute leukemia 12/61	None identified	Not stated	Not stated

CML, chronic myelogenous leukemia; DLI, donor lymphocyte infusion; AML, acute myelogenous leukemia; GVHD, graft-versus-host disease.

from Dana-Farber Cancer Institute also suggest that the graft-versus-myeloma effect does not require CD8+ cells.[98] Other salvage strategies, such as interferon, conventional chemotherapy, and second transplants, have been attempted with variable degrees of success.[100]

Lymphoma

A graft-versus-lymphoma effect has also been shown to exist in lymphoma as documented by disease regression with withdrawal of immunosuppression, appearance of GVHD, and DLI.[91, 101–103] Treatment of lymphoma relapse post allogeneic transplantation remains controversial, however. Treatment options vary from observation alone (in the case of low bulk low-grade lymphoma) to second transplants (in the case of lymphoblastic lymphoma).[101–104] As with other diseases, treatment needs to be individualized and depends on the extent of the disease, the remission duration after transplantation, performance status, and histologic subtype. These patients should preferentially be treated on investigational protocols involving immune modulation or novel treatment strategies.

RELAPSE AFTER AUTOLOGOUS TRANSPLANTATION

Leukemia

A fraction of leukemia patients experiencing relapse after autologous transplantation respond to salvage therapy and achieve long-term disease control with a second autograft or an allogeneic transplant.[41, 105–107] Use of allogeneic transplantation in this setting has the theoretical advantage of exploiting a GVL effect. Use of alternative donors, such as partially mismatched related donors and unrelated donors, has been attempted successfully in small numbers of pa-

tients with acute leukemia experiencing relapse after autologous transplantation who did not have an HLA-compatible sibling.[108] Allogeneic HSCT after autologous transplantation is associated with a high risk of early mortality but can produce long-term remissions and should be studied further.[104–107] Patients unwilling or unable to undergo second transplantation can still obtain benefits from conventional-dose chemotherapy or radiotherapy in terms of survival and quality of life and therefore should be considered for therapy.

Lymphoma and Myeloma

Patients with lymphoid malignancies who experience relapse after autologous transplantation generally respond to conventional-dose salvage therapy if the initial HSCT was early in the course of the disease and the post-transplantation remission was greater than 12 months.[47, 54] Salvage strategies usually consist of combination chemotherapy with or without involved-field radiation. The role of a second course of high-dose chemotherapy with autologous or allogeneic HSC support has not been well established but has been reported to induce long-term remission in selected patients.[104–106]

Breast Cancer

No established therapy exists for patients experiencing relapse after autologous transplantation for breast cancer. As with other tumors, further responses to chemotherapy can be expected in patients with low tumor bulk at the time of relapse, minimal prior therapy, and long post-transplantation remission. These patients should be considered for further therapy with agents proven to be effective in the metastatic setting, such as anthracyclines and the new taxane derivatives, or with investigational protocols exploring novel therapeutic strategies such as allogeneic HSCT. Patients with hormone-responsive tumors can be treated with a variety of hormonal manipulation, but the response to these agents in the setting of post-transplantation relapse has not been well established.

SUMMARY AND THERAPEUTIC RECOMMENDATIONS

Until recently, relapses after transplantation were generally considered incurable and treatment was mainly palliative. Experience with second transplants showed that a small fraction of these patients could achieve long-term disease control, although at the expense of high treatment-related mortality. With novel immune-modulatory strategies, such as DLI and cytokine manipulation, a new therapeutic avenue has become available. Unfortunately, only patients with CML regularly respond to immune modulation with either interferon or DLI. Better approaches need to be developed for patients with acute leukemia and patients who experience relapse after autologous transplantation. Table 56–3 summarizes the most commonly available therapeutic options for patients experiencing relapse after transplantation.

With the exception of the case with CML, there is no well-established therapy for patients experiencing relapse after allogeneic or autologous transplantation.[26] Even in CML, controversies exist with regard to what cases should be treated (i.e., molecular relapse vs. cytogenetic relapse vs. hematologic relapse) and whether initial therapy should be interferon, DLI, or both.[26]

Treatment of patients with CML whose only evidence of relapse is a positive polymerase chain reaction test for the bcr/abl rearrangement should not be routinely recommended.[109] The risk of cytogenetic and hematologic progression in these patients has not been well established.[110–115] Mackinnon et al. reported that in patients given T cell–depleted allografts, two or more positive test results predict for a high likelihood of cytogenetic and hematologic progression and that therapeutic intervention should thus be considered.[110] In general, initial therapy should involve interferon or DLI in all patients experiencing cytogenetic and hematologic relapse in chronic phase with or without clonal evolution.[26] Patients experiencing relapse in more-advanced phases of the disease should be considered for more-aggressive therapy involving chemotherapy and second allogeneic transplantation.

Patients with acute leukemia or lymphoma who experience relapse after allogeneic transplantation should be considered for investigational protocols exploring immune modulation with cytokines or DLI, if possible. Patients refusing investigational therapy should receive further chemotherapy or radiotherapy if warranted by the clinical circumstances. Young patients with good performance status and no history of major complications with the first transplantation should be considered for a second marrow or peripheral blood progenitor cell transplant, followed by some form of investigational therapy to prevent relapse.

TABLE 56–3. THERAPEUTIC STRATEGIES FOR PATIENTS RELAPSING POST TRANSPLANTATION

STRATEGY	RESPONSE RATES	TOXICITY	COMMENTS
Chemotherapy	40–60% for remission >1 yr <20% for remissions <1 yr	10–40% reinduction deaths	Reduce tumor burden Palliation Data available for leukemia, lymphoma, myeloma; little data for breast cancer Few long-term survivors
Radiotherapy	Local control	Local toxicity Can trigger GVHD	Treatment of isolated extramedullary relapse (central nervous system, testicles)
Cytokines			
Interferon	10–30% cytogenetif remissions for early relapses	Myelosuppression Fatigue	Delays disease progression Some long-term remissions Effective mainly in CML
Filgrastim	10–20% in patients with indolent relapses	Bone pain Disease progression	Limited experience; well tolerated; no long-term survivors
Interleukin-2	Responses in acute leukemia with donor lymphocytes	GVHD Capillary leak	Limited experience, may be valuable adjuvant to donor lymphocytes
Cyclosporine withdrawal	Unknown	GVHD	Initial approach for most patients experiencing relapse
Donor lymphocytes	CML 60–80% CR AML 20% CR ALL 20% CR Lymphoma: case reports Myeloma: case reports	GVHD Aplasia 20% death in remission	Most effective strategy for reinduction of remission in CML; main goals in the future are to make donor lymphocyte infusion safer in CML and more effective in acute leukemia
Second allografts	10–20% disease-free survival	50–70% treatment-related mortality	Limited to patients with donors and good performance status
Second autografts	Unknown, but positive preliminary experience in myeloma and lymphoma	10–20% mortality	Limited by stem cell quality; may become more useful if enough cells collected routinely prior to initial transplantation
New agents or strategies	Unknown		Interesting new strategies *New agents:* decitabine, radioimmunotherapy *Relapse prevention:* linomide, cytokine stimulation of donor lymphocytes

ALL, acute lymphocytic leukemia; AML, acute myelogenous leukemia; CML, chronic myelogenous leukemia; GVHD, graft-versus-host disease.

Patients experiencing relapse after an autograft should also be considered for salvage therapy using a risk-oriented approach. Patients with chemosensitive disease and long remission durations after initial transplantation can be considered for a second high-dose intensification with either autologous or allogeneic HSC support, although the benefit of this type of therapy has not been well defined in this setting.

All patients experiencing relapse after transplantation should be encouraged to participate in current ongoing clinical trials exploring new drugs or immune-modulating agents or that compare treatment strategies. Many patients are unwilling or unable to receive further therapy. Ensuring the best quality of life for these patients requires the utmost diligence. Rapid attention to symptom management, appropriate supportive care, palliative chemotherapy or radiotherapy when indicated, and timely referral to hospice agencies should ensure a comfortable and less painful death for these patients.

CONCLUSION

New therapeutic avenues are now available for patients experiencing relapse after transplantation with a variety of malignant disorders. Interferon and DLI have rapidly become the standard treatments for relapse of CML after HSCT. The optimal cell dose and timing of DLI remain to be determined. For other diseases, further study into the cause of relapse and continued investigation of novel treatment strategies for post-transplantation relapse will aid in developing the most effective therapy, which needs to include prophylaxis, early intervention, and risk determination.

REFERENCES

1. Bortin M, Horowitz M, Rimm A: Increasing utilization of allogeneic bone marrow transplantation: results of the 1988–1990 survey. Ann Intern Med 116:505, 1992.
2. Champlin R, McGlave P: Allogeneic bone marrow transplantation for chronic myelogenous leukemia. In Forman S, Blume K, Thomas E (eds): Bone Marrow Transplantation. Boston, Blackwell Scientific, 1994, pp 595–606.
3. Long G, Blume K: Allogeneic bone marrow transplantation for acute myeloid leukemia. In Forman S, Blume K, Thomas E (eds): Bone Marrow Transplantation. Boston, Blackwell Scientific, 1994, pp 607–618.
4. Chao N, Forman S: Allogeneic bone marrow transplantation for acute lymphoblastic leukemia. In Forman S, Blume K, Thomas E (eds): Bone Marrow Transplantation. Boston, Blackwell Scientific, 1994, pp 618–628.
5. Bortin M, Horowitz M, Gale R, et al: Changing trends in allogeneic bone marrow transplantation for leukemia in the 1980s. JAMA 268:607, 1992.
6. Aurer I, Gale RP: Are new conditioning regimens for transplants in acute myelogenous leukemia better? Bone Marrow Transplant 7:255–261, 1991.
7. Goh K, Klemperer M: In vivo leukemic transformation: cytogenetic evidence of in vivo leukemic transformation of engrafted marrow cells. Am J Hematol 2:283, 1990.
8. Elfenbein G, Brogaonkar D, Bias W, et al: Cytogenetic evidence for recurrence of acute myelogenous leukemia after allogeneic bone marrow transplantation in donor hematopoietic cells. Blood 52:627, 1987.
9. Fialkow P, Thomas E, Bryant J, Neiman P: Leukemic transformation of engrafted human marrow cells in vivo. Lancet 1:251, 1971.
10. Newburger P, Latt S, Pesando J, et al: Leukemia relapse in donor cells after allogeneic bone marrow transplantation. N Engl J Med 304:712, 1981.
11. Deisseroth AB, Zu Z, Claxton D, et al: Genetic marking shows that Ph+ cells present in autologous transplant of chronic myelogenous leukemia contribute to relapse after autologous bone marrow in CML. Blood 83:3068, 1994.
12. Brenner MK, Rill DR, Mour RC, et al: Gene marking to trace origin of relapse after autologous bone marrow transplantation. Lancet 341:85, 1993.
13. Tubiami M: The causes of clinical radioresistance. In Stell G, Adams G, Peckham M (eds): The Biological Basis of Radiotherapy. New York, Elsevier, 1983, pp 13–20.
14. Uckun F, Ramsay N, Waddick K, et al: In vitro and in vivo radiation resistance associated with CD3 surface antigen expression in T-lineage acute lymphoblastic leukemia. Blood 78:2945, 1991.
15. Dalton W: Drug resistance: modulation in the laboratory and the clinic. Semin Oncol 20:64, 1993.
16. Hilton J: Role of aldehyde dehydrogenase in cyclophosphamide resistant L1210 leukemia. Cancer Res 44:5156, 1984.
17. Kolb H, Mittermuller J, Clemm C, et al: Donor leukocyte transfusions for treatment of recurrent chronic myelogenous leukemia in marrow transplant patients. Blood 76:2462, 1990.
18. Porter D, Roth M, McGarigle C, et al: Induction of graft-versus-host disease as immunotherapy for relapsed chronic myeloid leukemia. N Engl J Med 330:100, 1994.
19. Drobyski W, Keever C, Roth M, et al: Salvage immunotherapy using donor leukocyte infusions as treatment for relapsed chronic myelogenous leukemia after allogeneic bone marrow transplantation: efficacy and toxicity of a defined T-cell dose. Blood 82:2310, 1993.
20. van Rhee F, Lin F, Cullis J, et al: Relapse of chronic myeloid leukemia after allogeneic bone marrow transplant: the case for giving donor leukocyte transfusions before the onset of hematologic relapse. Blood 83:3377, 1994.
21. Bar B, Schattenberg A, Mensink E, et al: Donor leukocyte infusions for chronic myelogenous leukemia after allogeneic bone marrow transplantation. J Clin Oncol 11:513, 1993.
22. Hertenstein B, Wiesneth M, Novotny J, et al: Interferon-α and donor buffy coat transfusions for treatment of relapsed chronic myeloid leukemia after allogeneic bone marrow transplantation. Transplantation 56:1114, 1993.
23. Kolb H, Schattenberg A, Goldman J, et al: Graft-versus-leukemia effect of donor lymphocyte transfusions in marrow grafted patients. Blood 86:2041, 1996.
24. Antin J: Graft-versus-leukemia: no longer an epiphenomenon. Blood 82:2273, 1993.
25. Barrett J, Malkovska V: The graft-versus-leukemia effect. Curr Opin Oncol 8:89, 1996.
26. Giralt S, Champlin RE: Leukemia relapse after allogeneic bone marrow transplantation: a review. Blood 84:3603, 1994.
27. Theobald M: Allorecognition and graft-versus-host disease. Bone Marrow Transplant 15:489, 1995.
28. Sosman J, Oettel K, Smith S, et al: Specific recognition of human leukemic cells by allogeneic T cells: II. Evidence for HLA-D restricted determinants on leukemic cells that are cross reactive with determinants present on unrelated non leukemic cells. Blood 75:2005, 1990.
29. van Lochem E, de Gast B, Goulmy E: In vitro separation of host specific graft-versus-host disease and graft-versus-leukemia cytotoxic T-cell activities. Bone Marrow Transplant 10:181, 1992.
30. Faber L, Van-Luxemburg-Heijs S, Willemze R, Falkenburg F: Generation of leukemia reactive cytotoxic T-lymphocyte clones from the HLA-identical bone marrow donor of a patient with leukemia. J Exp Med 176:1283, 1992.
31. Hausch M, Gazzola M, Small T, et al: Anti leukemia potential of interleukin-2 activated natural killer cells after bone marrow transplantation for chronic myelogenous leukemia. Blood 75:2250, 1990.
32. Ferrara J, Deeg H: Graft-versus-host disease. N Engl J Med 324:667, 1991.
33. Fong T, Mosmann T: Alloreactive murine CD8+ T-cell clones secrete the Th1 pattern of cytokines. J Immunol 144:1744, 1990.
34. Kelso A: Frequency analysis of lymphokine secreting CD4+ and CD8+ T-cells activated in a graft versus host reaction. J Immunol 144:1744, 1990.

35. Rakhmilevich AL, North RJ, Dye FS: Presence of CD4+ T-suppressor cells in mice rendered unresponsive to tumor antigens by intravenous injection of irradiated tumor cells. Int J Cancer 55:338, 1993.

36. Bergman L, Schui DK, Brieger J, et al: Inhibition of lymphokine-activated killer cells in acute myeloblastic leukemia is mediated by transforming growth factor-beta 1. Exp Hematol 23:1574, 1995.

37. Araten DJ, Lawton D, Ferrara J, et al: In vitro alloreactivity against host antigens in an adult HLA-mismatched bone marrow recipient despite in vivo host tolerance. Transplantation 55:76, 1993.

38. Frassoni F, Barrett J, Granena A, et al: Relapse after allogeneic bone marrow transplantation for acute leukemia: a survey of the EBMTR of 117 cases. Br J Hematol 70:317, 1988.

39. Mortimer J, Binder M, Schulman S, et al: Relapse of acute leukemia after marrow transplantation: natural history and results of subsequent therapy. J Clin Oncol 7:50, 1989.

40. Mehta J, Powles R, Treleaven J, et al: Outcome of acute leukemia relapsing after bone marrow transplantation: utility of second transplants and immunotherapy. Bone Marrow Transplant 19:709–719, 1997.

41. Arcese W, Goldman J, Arcangelo E, et al: Outcome of patients who relapse after allogeneic bone marrow transplantation for chronic myeloid leukemia. Blood 82:3211, 1993.

42. Arthur C, Apperley J, Guo A, et al: Cytogenetic events after bone marrow transplantation for chronic myeloid leukemia in chronic phase. Blood 71:1179, 1988.

43. Hughes T, Economou K, Mackinnon S, et al: Slow evolution of chronic myeloid leukemia relapsing after bone marrow transplantation with T-cell depleted donor marrow. Br J Hematol 73:462, 1989.

44. Bákássy A, Hermans J, Gorin NC, Gratwohl A: Granulocytic sarcoma after allogeneic bone marrow transplantation: a retrospective European multicenter survey. Bone Marrow Transplant 17:801, 1996.

45. Vesole DH, Tricot G, Jagannath S, et al: Autotransplants in multiple myeloma: what have we learned? Blood 88:838, 1996.

46. Attal M, Harousseau JL, Stoppa AM, et al: A prospective, randomized trial of autologous bone marrow transplantation and chemotherapy in multiple myeloma: Intergroupe Francais de Myelome. N Engl J Med 335:91, 1996.

47. Tricot G, Jagannath S, Vesole DH, et al: Relapse of multiple myeloma after autologous transplantation: survival after salvage therapy. Bone Marrow Transplant 16:7, 1996.

48. Gahrton G, Tura S, Ljungman P, et al: Prognostic factors in allogeneic bone marrow transplantation for multiple myeloma. J Clin Oncol 13:1312, 1995.

49. Barlogie B, Anderson K, Berenson J, et al: Transplants for multiple myeloma. Bone Marrow Transplant 15(Suppl 1):S234, 1995.

50. Armitage J: Bone marrow transplantation. N Engl J Med 330:827, 1994.

51. Vose J, Armitage J, Bierman P, et al: Salvage therapy for relapsed or refractory non-Hodgkins lymphoma utilizing autologous bone marrow transplantation. Am J Med 87:285, 1989.

52. van Besien K, Tabocoff J, Rodriguez M, et al: High-dose chemotherapy with BEAC regimen and autologous bone marrow transplantation for intermediate grade and immunoblastic lymphoma: durable complete remissions, but a high rate of regimen-related toxicity. Bone Marrow Transplant 15:549, 1995.

53. van Besien K, Mehra R, Giralt S, et al: Allogeneic bone marrow transplantation for poor prognosis lymphoma: response, toxicity, and survival depend on disease histology. Am J Med 100:299, 1990.

54. Vose J, Bierman PJ, Anderson JR, et al: Progressive disease after high-dose therapy and autologous transplantation for lymphoid malignancy: clinical course and patient follow up. Blood 80:2142, 1992.

55. Peters WP, Shpall EJ, Jones RB, et al: High dose combination alkylating agents with bone marrow support as initial treatment for metastatic breast cancer. J Clin Oncol 6:1368, 1988.

56. Dunphy FR, Spitzer G, Buzdar AU, et al: Treatment of estrogen receptor-negative or hormonally refractory breast cancer with double high-dose chemotherapy intensification and bone marrow support. J Clin Oncol 8:1207, 1990.

57. Odom L, Githers J, Morse H, et al: Remission of relapsed leukemia during a graft-versus-host reaction: a graft-versus-leukemia reaction in man? Lancet 2:537, 1978.

58. Higano C, Brixey M, Bryant E, et al: Durable complete remission of acute nonlymphocytic leukemia associated with discontinuation of immunosuppression following relapse after allogeneic bone marrow transplantation: a case report of a probable graft-versus-leukemia effect. Transplantation 50:175, 1990.

59. Collins R, Rogers Z, Bennett M, et al: Hematologic relapse of chronic myelogenous leukemia following allogeneic bone marrow transplantation: apparent graft-versus-leukemia effect following abrupt discontinuation of immunosuppression. Bone Marrow Transplant 10:391, 1992.

60. Flowers M, Clift R, Schoch G, et al: Discontinuation of cyclosporine to induce a graft-versus-leukemia effect in patients with cytogenetic relapse after allogeneic bone marrow transplantation for chronic myelogenous leukemia. Blood 84: (Suppl 1): 540a, 1994.

61. Bostrom B, Woods W, Nesbit M, et al: Successful reinduction of patients with acute lymphoblastic leukemia who relapse following bone marrow transplantation. J Clin Oncol 5:376, 1987.

62. Barrett A, Tew C, Joshi R: How should acute lymphoblastic leukemia relapse after bone-marrow transplantation be treated? Lancet 1:1188, 1985.

63. Chak L, Sapozink M, Cox R: Extramedullary lesions in non-lymphocytic leukemia results of radiation therapy. Int J Radiat Oncol Biol Phys 9:1173, 1983.

64. Bowman W, Aur R, Hustu H, Rivera G: Isolated testicular relapse in acute lymphocytic leukemia of childhood: categories and influence on survival. J Clin Oncol 2:924, 1984.

65. Singhal S, Powles R, Treleaven J, et al: Central nervous system relapse after bone marrow transplantation for acute leukemia in first remission. Bone Marrow Transplant 17:637, 1996.

66. Giralt S, Escudier S, Kantarjian H, et al: Treatment with filgrastim for relapse of leukemia and myelodysplasia after allogeneic bone marrow transplantation: preliminary observations. N Engl J Med 329:357, 1993.

67. Giralt S, Hester J, Talpaz M, et al: Cytokine therapy for patients relapsing after allogeneic bone marrow transplantation. J Cell Biochem Suppl 18B:88a, 1994.

68. Baron S, Tyring S, Fleischmann W, et al: The interferons: mechanism of action and clinical applications. JAMA 266:1375, 1991.

69. Arcese W, Mauro F, Alimena G, et al: Interferon therapy for Ph positive CML patients relapsing after T-cell depleted allogeneic bone marrow transplantation. Bone Marrow Transplant 5:309, 1991.

70. Higano C, Raskind W, Singer J: Use of α-interferon for the treatment of relapse of chronic myelogenous leukemia in chronic phase after allogeneic bone marrow transplantation. Blood 80:1437, 1992.

71. Rosenberg S, Grimm E, McGrogan M, et al: Biological activity of recombinant human interleukin-2. Science 223:1412, 1984.

72. Maraninchi D, Blaise D, Viens P, et al: High dose recombinant interleukin-2 and acute myeloid leukemias in relapse. Blood 78:218, 1991.

73. Foa R, Meloni G, Tosti S, et al: Treatment of acute myelogenous leukemia patients with recombinant interleukin-2: a pilot study. Br J Haematol 77:491, 1991.

74. Giralt S, O'Brien S, Talpaz M, et al: Alpha interferon and interleukin-2 as treatment for leukemia relapse after allogeneic bone marrow transplantation. Cytokines Mol Ther 1:115, 1995.

75. Mehta J, Powles R, Singhal S, et al: Cytokine-mediated immunotherapy with or without donor leukocytes for poor-risk acute myeloid leukemia relapsing after allogeneic bone marrow transplantation. Bone Marrow Transplant 16:133, 1995.

76. Slavin S, Naperstek E, Nagler A, et al: Allogeneic cell therapy for relapsed leukemia after bone marrow transplantation with donor peripheral blood lymphocytes. Exp Hematol 23:1553, 1995.

77. Slavin S, Naparstek E, Nagler A, et al: Allogeneic cell therapy with donor peripheral blood cells and recombinant human interleukin-2 to treat leukemia relapse after allogeneic bone marrow transplantation. Blood 87:2195, 1996.

78. Wright S, Thomas E, Buckner C, et al: Experience with second marrow transplants. Exp Hematol 4:221, 1976.

79. Champlin R, Ho W, Lenarsky C, et al: successful second bone marrow transplantation for AML or ALL. Transplant Proc 17:496, 1985.

80. Sanders J, Buckner C, Clift R, et al: Second marrow transplants in patients with leukemia who relapse after allogeneic marrow transplantation. Bone Marrow Transplant 3:11, 1988.

81. Radich J, Sanders J, Buckner C, et al: Second allogeneic marrow transplantation for patients with recurrent leukemia after initial transplant with total body irradiation containing regimens. J Clin Oncol 11:304, 1993.

82. Stern L, Landan M, Feig S, Gajewski J: Outcome of second bone marrow transplants. Blood 80:334a, 1992.

83. Wagner J, Vogelsang G, Zehnbauer B, et al: Relapse of leukemia after bone marrow transplantation: effect of second myeloablative therapy. Bone Marrow Transplant 9:205, 1992.

84. Barrett A, Locatelli F, Treleaven J, et al: Second transplants for leukemic relapse after bone marrow transplantation: high early mortality but favorable effect of chronic GVHD on continued remission. Br J Haematol 78:561, 1991.

85. Mrsic M, Horowitz M, Atkinson K, et al: Second HLA-identical sibling transplants for leukemia recurrence. Bone Marrow Transplant 9:269, 1992.

86. Blume K, Forman S: High dose busulfan/etoposide as a preparatory regimen for second bone marrow transplants in hematologic malignancies. Blut 55:49, 1987.

87. Atkinson K, Biggs J, Concannon A, et al: Second marrow transplants for recurrence of hematological malignancy. Bone Marrow Transplant 1:159, 1986.

88. Nemunaitis J, Albo V, Zeigler Z, et al: Reduction of allogeneic transplant morbidity by combining peripheral blood and bone marrow progenitor cells. Leuk Lymphoma 10:405, 1993.

89. Russell N, Hunter A, Rogers S, et al: Peripheral blood stem cells as an alternative to marrow for allogeneic transplantation. Lancet 341:1482, 1993.

90. Körbling M, Przepiorka D, Engel H, et al: Allogeneic blood stem cell transplantation for refractory leukemia and lymphoma: potential advantage of blood over marrow allografts. Blood 85:159, 1995.

91. Collins R, Shpilberg O, Drobyski W, et al: Donor leukocyte infusions for post bone marrow transplant relapse-retrospective cohort analysis of 141 cases. Blood 86(Suppl 1):563a, 1995.

92. Giralt S, Hester J, Huh Y, et al: CD8-depleted donor lymphocyte infusion as treatment for relapsed chronic myelogenous leukemia after allogeneic bone marrow transplantation. Blood 86:4337, 1995.

93. Mackinnon S, Papadopoulos E, Carabasi M, et al: Adoptive immunotherapy evaluating escalating doses of donor leukocytes for relapse of chronic myeloid leukemia following bone marrow transplantation: separation of graft-versus-leukemia responses from graft-versus-host disease. Blood 86:1261, 1995.

94. Mackinnon S, Papadopoulos E, Carabasi M, et al: Adoptive immunotherapy using donor leukocytes following bone marrow transplantation for chronic myeloid leukemia: is T-cell dose important in determining biologic response? Bone Marrow Transplant 15:591, 1995.

95. Szer J, Grigg A, Phillips G, Sheridan W: Donor leucocyte infusions after chemotherapy for patients relapsing with acute leukemia following allogeneic BMT. Bone Marrow Transplant 11:109, 1993.

96. Flowers MED, Sullivan KM, Martin P, et al: G-CSF stimulated donor peripheral blood infusions as immunotherapy in patients with hematologic malignancies relapsing after allogeneic transplantation. Blood 86:564a, 1995.

97. Verdonck LF, Lokhorst HM, Dekker AW, et al: Graft-versus-myeloma effect in two cases. Lancet 347:800, 1996.

98. Alyea E, Soiffer R, Murray C, et al: Adoptive immunotherapy following allogeneic bone marrow transplantation (BMT) with donor lymphocytes depleted of CD8+ T-cells: Blood 86(Suppl 1):293a, 1995.

99. Tricot G, Vesole D, Jagannath S, et al: Graft-versus-myeloma effect: proof of principle. Blood 87:1196, 1996.

100. Hunault M, Rio B, Zittoun R, et al: Pattern of relapse and treatment of multiple myeloma after high dose therapy. Blood 86(Suppl 1):835a, 1995.

101. Van Besien KW, de Lima M, Giralt SA, et al: Management of lymphoma recurrence after allogeneic transplantation: the relevance of the graft-versus-lymphoma effect. Bone Marrow Transplant 19:977–982, 1997.

102. van Besien K, Khouri I, Giralt S, et al: Allogeneic bone marrow transplantation for refractory and recurrent low grade lymphoma: the case for aggressive management. J Clin Oncol 13:1096, 1995.

103. van Besien K, Mehra R, Giralt S, et al: Allogeneic bone marrow transplantation for poor prognosis lymphoma: response, toxicity, and survival depend on disease histology. Am J Med 100:299, 1990.

104. de Lima M, van Besien KW, Giralt SA, et al: Bone marrow transplantation after failure of autologous transplant for non-Hodgkin's lymphoma. Bone Marrow Transplant 19:121–127, 1997.

105. Schouten HC, Armitage JO, Klassen LW, et al: Allogeneic bone marrow transplantation in patients with lymphoma relapsing after autologous transplantation. Bone Marrow Transplant 4:119, 1989.

106. Tsai T, Goodman S, Schiller G, et al: Allogeneic bone marrow transplantation for relapse after autologous bone marrow transplantation in lymphomas and acute leukemia. Blood 86:969a, 1995.

107. Schwella N, Schwerdtfeger R, Konig V, et al: Allogeneic bone marrow transplantation for recurrence of leukemia after autologous bone marrow transplantation. Transplantation 57:1263, 1994.

108. Godder K, Pat A, Abhyarkar S, et al: Partially mismatched related donor transplants as salvage therapy for patients with refractory leukemia who relapse post bone marrow transplantation. Bone Marrow Transplant 17:49, 1996.

109. Giralt SA, Kolb HJ: Donor lymphocyte infusions. Curr Opin Oncol 8:96, 1996.

110. Mackinnon S, Barnett L, Heller G: Polymerase chain reaction is highly predictive of relapse in patients following T cell–depleted allogeneic bone marrow transplantation for chronic myeloid leukemia. Bone Marrow Transplant 17:643, 1996.

111. Lee M, Khouri I, Champlin R, et al: Detection of minimal residual disease by polymerase chain reaction of bcr/abl transcripts in chronic myelogenous leukaemia following allogeneic bone marrow transplantation. Br J Haematol 82:708, 1992.

112. Roth MS, Antin JH, Ash R, et al: Prognostic significance of Philadelphia chromosome–positive cells detected by the polymerase chain reaction after allogeneic bone marrow transplant for chronic myelogenous leukemia. Blood 79:276, 1992.

113. Radich JP, Gehly G, Gooley T, et al: Polymerase chain reaction detection of the BCR-ABL fusion transcript after allogeneic marrow transplantation for chronic myeloid leukemia: results and implications in 346 patients. Blood 85:2632, 1995.

114. Delage R, Soiffer RJ, Dear K, Ritz J: Clinical significance of bcr-abl gene rearrangement detected by polymerase chain reaction after allogeneic bone marrow transplantation in chronic myelogenous leukemia. Blood 78:2759, 1991.

115. Cross NCP, Feng L, Chase A, et al: Competitive polymerase chain reaction to estimate the number of BCR-ABL transcripts in chronic myeloid leukemia patients after bone marrow transplantation. Blood 82:1929, 1993.

CHAPTER FIFTY-SEVEN

Myelodysplasia and Second Malignancies

Peter R. Holman, M.B., B.Ch.

The development of a second malignancy after high-dose therapy (HDT) is a devastating event after cure of a primary malignancy. In many cases, this is a terminal event. This chapter focuses on factors contributing to the development of second malignancy and the spectrum of malignant disorders encountered in this situation. Treatment considerations are also considered.

The occurrence of second malignancy after conventional chemotherapy and radiation is well established. In particular, alkylating agents,[1-4] radiation therapy alone or in combination with chemotherapy,[4-7] and epipodophyllotoxins[8-13] have been implicated as causative agents. In addition, primary malignancy and splenectomy are reported to predispose to the development of second malignancy.[14-16]

Most patients undergoing HDT have previously been exposed to one or more leukemogenic agents before transplantation, complicating the interpretation of studies examining the incidence of second malignancy. Other factors implicated include allogeneic hematopoietic stem cell transplantation (alloHSCT), T-cell depletion, and immunosuppression for prophylaxis or treatment of graft-versus-host disease (GVHD) (Table 57–1). Three main categories of second malignancy can be identified. The first includes myelodysplastic syndromes and acute myelogenous leukemia. These occur rarely after alloHSCT but account for significant mortality after autologous HSCT (autoHSCT). The second category is solid cancers, and the third includes post-transplantation lymphoproliferative disorders (Table 57–2).

MYELODYSPLASIA/ACUTE MYELOGENOUS LEUKEMIA AFTER HIGH-DOSE THERAPY

INCIDENCE

Many studies have examined the incidence of myelodysplastic syndromes/acute myelogenous leukemia (MDS/

AML) in patients receiving conventional chemotherapy.[7, 17-20] The incidence after Hodgkin disease has been most studied (Table 57–3). The Stanford group reported on 1507 patients treated for Hodgkin disease.[18] Ninety-eight secondary cancers developed including 28 cases of leukemia (1.9%). The risk of leukemia was significantly increased in all treatment groups but highest in patients receiving chemotherapy, with a more than 100-fold increased risk over the expected incidence. The cumulative risk at 9 years was 3.3%. All cases occurred within the group receiving mechlorethamine, vincristine, procarbazine, and prednisone (MOPP). No cases occurred in the small number of patients receiving doxorubicin, bleomycin, vinblastine, and dacarbazine (ABVD), procarbazine, melphalan, and vinblastine (PAVe), or vinblastine, bleomycin, and methotrexate (VBM). No cases occurred after 9 years of follow-up, similar to findings previously reported from the National Cancer Institute.[21] The NSABP reported an increased incidence of leukemia after adjuvant chemotherapy and radiotherapy in breast cancer patients.[22] More-recent reports have confirmed these data. In a cohort study involving 82,700 women with breast cancer, the relative risk was 2.4, 10, and 17.4 for radiation alone, alkylating agents alone, and radiation with chemotherapy, respectively.[23]

MDS/AML occurs only rarely after alloHSCT.[24] MDS/AML after autoHSCT, however, is not infrequent (Table 57–4). The causative role of HDT remains difficult to establish because patients have generally received standard induction therapy, maybe radiation, and often one or more salvage regimens prior to transplantation. Interpretation of studies is further complicated by difficulty in the diagnosis of MDS after HDT. Dysplastic features affecting one or more lineages are common after standard chemotherapy in addition to HDT. Most studies examining the incidence of MDS/AML post transplantation have therefore excluded patients with only morphologic evidence of dysplasia. Interpretation of cytogenetic abnormalities post transplantation is impossible in the absence of pretransplantation cytogenetics, and abnormal cytogenetics have been reported

TABLE 57–1. FACTORS IMPLICATED IN THE DEVELOPMENT OF SECOND MALIGNANCIES

Pretransplantation chemotherapy
Pretransplantation radiation
Allogeneic transplant
T-cell depletion
Post-transplantation immunosuppression

TABLE 57–2. SPECTRUM OF MALIGNANCIES OCCURRING AFTER HIGH-DOSE THERAPY

Myelodysplastic syndrome and acute leukemia
Solid cancers
Post-transplantation lymphoproliferative disorder

TABLE 57–3. RELATIVE RISK OF SECOND MALIGNANCY AFTER THERAPY FOR HODGKIN DISEASE

SITE OR TYPE	OBSERVED CASES	EXPECTED CASES	RELATIVE RISK (OBSERVED/EXPECTED)	95% CONFIDENCE INTERVAL
All cancers	342	99.1	3.5	3.1–3.8
Leukemia	75	2.3	32.4	25.5–40.6
Acute nonlymphocytic leukemia	68	1.0	70.8	55.0–89.8
Non-Hodgkin lymphoma	49	2.6	18.6	13.8–24.6
Solid tumors	219	92.4	2.4	2.1–2.7
Lung	77	18.5	4.2	3.3–5.2
Mouth and pharynx	6	0.8	7.6	2.8–16.5
Stomach	11	5.1	2.1	1.1–3.8
Colon	20	6.9	2.9	1.8–4.5
Rectum	5	4.0	1.3	0.4–2.9
Bone	4	0.3	12.2	3.3–31.4
Connective tissue	5	0.7	7.0	2.3–16.3
Melanoma	9	2.1	4.2	1.9–8.0
Female breast	42	16.9	2.5	1.8–3.4
Bladder	7	4.0	1.8	0.7–3.6
Thyroid	3	0.6	4.7	1.0–13.7
All solid tumors except lung cancer	142	73.9	1.9	1.6–2.3

Adapted from van Leeuwen FE: Second cancers. In DeVita VT, Hellman S, Rosenberg SA (eds): Cancer: Principles and Practice of Oncology. Philadelphia, Lippincott-Raven, 1997, pp 2773–2796.

post transplantation in the absence of any other evidence of MDS/AML.[25]

In the Minnesota study of 206 patients undergoing transplantation for Hodgkin disease (HD) or non-Hodgkin lymphoma, 9 experienced MDS/AML at a median of 34 months post transplantation. Of the 9 patients, 2 were excluded from the incidence analysis because they had received further therapy for relapsed disease post transplantation. The cumulative actuarial risk at 5 years was 14.5% ± 14.7%, similar for both HD and NHL. All 9 patients had normal pretransplantation morphology, and of 3 examined all had normal cytogenetics.[26] Updated results from this group showed an estimated cumulative probability of experiencing MDS/AML of 13.5% ± 4.8% at 6 years.[27]

In the Dana Farber Cancer Institute (DFCI) study of 262 patients undergoing autoHSCT for NHL, the preparative regimen was cyclophosphamide/total body irradiation and patients had received a variety of pretransplantation regimens. With a median follow-up of 31 months, 20 patients experienced MDS/AML for an overall crude incidence of 7.6%. The actuarial risk at 6 years was 18% (CI ± 9%). The median time to the development of MDS was 31 months after HDT and 69 months from the initial treatment of the NHL.[28] In a recent update from the DFCI of patients followed up after autoHSCT for diffuse, aggressive NHL,

the actuarial incidence of MDS was 19.8%. Forty-one cases occurred among 552 patients who underwent transplant. All patients received a conditioning regimen of cyclophosphamide and TBI. Thirty patients had received more than one previous regimen. Following diagnosis of MDS, the median survival was 9.4 months.[29]

Of 511 patients reported from the Omaha group undergoing autoSCT for HD or NHL, 12 patients experienced MDS/AML at a median of 44 months post-HDT and 68 months since initial diagnosis. The cumulative incidence at 5 years was 4%, increasing to 10% at 7 years. For patients alive at 5 years, the probability of developing MDS/AML was 11% for HD and 12% for NHL. Among patients with NHL, MDS/AML only occurred in the group receiving total body irradiation.[30]

A University of Chicago study described seven cases of MDS/AML after autoHSCT or autologous bone marrow transplantation in 649 patients.[31] This included one case of acute lymphoid leukemia developing after treatment for breast cancer. The disease-specific incidences for the development of MDS/AML were 0.3% for breast cancer, 6.3% for HD, and 1% for NHL. The City of Hope reported on the cumulative probability of clonal cytogenetic abnormalities after HDT. Of 275 patients at risk, the incidence was 9% at 8 years. Pretransplantation cytogenetics were normal

TABLE 57–4. INCIDENCE OF MYELODYSPLASTIC SYNDROMES/ACUTE MYELOGENOUS LEUKEMIA AFTER HIGH-DOSE THERAPY AND AUTOLOGOUS STEM CELL THERAPY

SERIES	NO. OF PATIENTS	PRIMARY DISEASE	INCIDENCE (%)	ACTUARIAL INCIDENCE
University of Minnesota[26]	206	NHL/HD	9 (4)	15.2% ± 18 for HD at 5 yr 14% ± 14.7 for NHL at 5 yr
DFCI[28]	262	NHL	20 (7.6)	18% ± 9 at 6 yr
University of Nebraska[30]	511	NHL/HD	12 (2.3)	11% for HD at 5 yr 12% for NHL at 5 yr
City of Hope[25]	275	NHL/HD	10 (4)	6.4% at 2 yr
Duke University[32]	864	Breast cancer	5 (0.58)	1.6% at 4 yr

HD, Hodgkin disease; NHL, non-Hodgkin lymphoma.

in the 10 patients experiencing abnormalities post transplantation. Abnormalities were noted a median of 3.9 years after induction therapy and 1.4 years after HDT. Five patients had associated morphologic abnormalities, two with frank AML and three with MDS.[25]

MDS/AML has been reported after autoHSCT for breast cancer. The Duke study retrospectively examined 864 patients. Normal cytogenetics were observed in all patients before transplantation. Five patients experienced MDS/AML for a crude cumulative incidence of 0.58% and a 4-year probability of 1.6%. The time to development of MDS/AML was 26–71 months after initial diagnosis and 2–41 months after HDT.[32] This incidence was similar to that previously reported by the NSABP after conventional chemotherapy[22] and supports a primary causative role for pretransplantation therapy rather than the preparative regimen.

PRESENTATION

As noted earlier the diagnosis of MDS post transplantation may be complicated by changes attributable to previous therapy. Cytopenias may persist after partial recovery from HDT, and morphologic evidence of dysplasia is common in this setting. Of nine patients experiencing MDS/AML in the Minnesota study, five had delayed or persistent cytopenias post transplantation. Four had normal engraftment with later development of cytopenias, and all nine had dysplastic features in at least one lineage after transplantation. At diagnosis of MDS/AML, the median hemoglobin was 8.8 g/dL, median WBC $2.8 \times 10^3/mm^3$, and median platelet count $56 \times 10^3/mm^3$. Peripheral blood blasts were not elevated. Morphologic abnormalities were common, including dysgranulopoiesis, hyposegmented neutrophils, and hypogranular cytoplasm. Bone marrow abnormalities were common, with a median myeloblast count of 3.2% (range, 0.8–14.7%). Other features included erythroid hyperplasia with dyserythropoiesis, megaloblastic changes, nuclear karyorrhexis, and coarse basophilic stippling. Of eight patients examined, three had 10–20% ringed sideroblasts, eight had mild to moderate dysgranulopoiesis, and three had increased eosinophils ranging from 5.2% to 13%. Six patients had atypical megakaryocytes with increased nuclear-to-cytoplasmic ratio and hyposegmented nuclei.[26]

Abnormal cytogenetics, involving chromosomal breakpoints characteristically involved in de novo and therapy-related MDS/AML have been reported post transplantation without other hematologic evidence of MDS/AML. Of the 20 patients experiencing MDS/AML in the Dana Farber series, 12 of 15 analyzed had cytogenetic abnormalities. Monosomy 7 or 7q− was apparent in 10 patients, and 5q− was detected in 4. Combined 5 and 7 abnormalities were detected in two patients. Interestingly, cytogenetics were abnormal in 50% of patients analyzed post transplantation without morphologic evidence of MDS/AML.[28]

After excluding patients with typical therapy-related cytogenetic findings, the City of Hope group described 10 of 275 patients experienced clonal cytogenetic abnormalities after autoHSCT for HD or NHL.[25] Dysplasia in all three cell lines in addition to the cytogenetic findings was required for a definitive diagnosis of MDS. All had normal morphology prior to transplantation. Cytogenetic abnormalities developed a mean of 3.9 years after initial induction chemotherapy and 1.4 years post transplantation. In four cases, abnormalities of chromosomes 5 or 7 were detected and in three cases the abnormalities were those usually ascribed to the use of topoisomerase II inhibitors. Two patients had a combination of both abnormalities. These abnormalities were similar to those reported in therapy-related MDS after conventional chemotherapy.[33–35] In a study of 62 patients with AML followed post transplantation, 7 had abnormal cytogenetics. At a median follow-up of 30 months, only 1 had other features suggestive of MDS.[36]

In the City of Hope study, of 10 patients with clonal cytogenetic abnormalities, frank AML and MDS occurred in 2 and 3 patients, respectively. Five patients had no clinical or morphologic abnormalities.[25] Of these 10 patients with normal pretransplantation cytogenetics, the morphology of 9 was correlated with karyotype and survival. Four patients had an aggressive course with short survival and had significantly more trilineage dysplasia prior to transplantation suggesting that the stem cell damage was primarily due to pretransplantation therapy.[37] In the breast cancer cohort from Duke University, all patients experiencing MDS post transplantation had normal pretransplantation cytogenetics.[32]

The necessity of obtaining routine pretransplantation cytogenetic evaluation has been addressed by City of Hope investigators. Of approximately 170 patients, pretransplantation cytogenetic evaluation was obtained in half. Four with abnormal cytogenetics were excluded from transplantation. No cases of MDS/AML occurred in the remainder of the tested group who proceeded to transplantation. Three cases, however, occurred in the group with unknown cytogenetics prior to transplantation.[38]

A recommendation for routine pretransplantation cytogenetic study should be based on the ability to identify subgroups of patients with a reasonable likelihood of cytogenetic abnormalities predicting progression of stem cell damage. Newer molecular techniques or fluorescent in situ hybridization may allow improved identification of such persons who may not benefit from transplantation. High-risk patients include those with extensive prior exposure to alkylating agents or epipodophyllotoxins. Cytogenetic testing should be performed in such cases. Morphology does not appear to correlate with cytogenetic findings, and the significance of certain chromosomal abnormalities after chemotherapy or transplantation remains unknown.

ETIOLOGY OF MDS/AML AFTER TRANSPLANTATION

A number of factors may contribute to the development of MDS/AML after autoHSCT (Table 57–5). The interval to development of MDS/AML post transplantation supports a primary role for pretransplantation therapy rather than the conditioning regimen. After conventional chemotherapy, the median time to onset is 4–7 years.[34, 39–41] The interval following HDT and MDS/AML is significantly shorter. Timing from initial pretransplantation therapy, however, is similar for patients not receiving transplants.

An Arkansas study examined two groups of patients undergoing tandem transplantation for multiple myeloma.

TABLE 57–5. VARIABLES POSSIBLY AFFECTING DEVELOPMENT OF MDS/AML AFTER TRANSPLANTATION

Primary malignancy
Pretransplantation chemotherapy or radiotherapy
Time interval between previous chemotherapy and high-dose therapy
Pelvic irradiation
Lower platelet count
Peripheral blood stem cell source
Preparative regimen
Age >35 years
Changes in bone marrow microenvironment
Decreased immune surveillance
Post allogeneic transplantation methotrexate use
Increased endogenous secretion of myeloid growth factors
Transfer of genetic material from residual abnormal cells to donor cells

The median duration of pretransplantation therapy in the two groups was 7.6 months and 24 months. All seven MDS/AML cases occurred in the latter group.[42]

The contribution of additional risk factors for development of MDS/AML post transplantation is difficult to ascertain because of the small numbers in most studies. In the Dana Farber study, patients receiving pelvic irradiation and those with a longer interval between initial diagnosis and HDT had a significantly higher incidence of MDS/AML on univariate analysis. On multivariate analysis, a pretransplantation platelet count of less than $152 \times 10^3/mm^3$ was a significant risk factor.[28] The lower platelet count may reflect previously unidentified stem cell damage, but cytogenetics were not routinely performed prior to transplantation. In the Minnesota study, a higher incidence was noted in patients receiving peripheral blood rather than marrow stem cells and in patients older than 35 years.[27]

Malignant transformation of endogenous hematopoietic stem cells surviving and receiving damage from the preparative regimen is another possible contributing factor. These effects have been examined, but because of many confounding variables, the precise role remains unclear.[42–45] Similarly, despite the well-established link between radiation exposure and subsequent malignancy, the role of radiation-containing preparative regimens remains unknown.[46, 47] More likely, however, is the reinfusion of previously damaged stem cells because some patients never regain normal hematopoiesis.[26] Other possible factors are changes in the bone marrow stromal microenvironment, decreased immune surveillance, and increased endogenous secretion of myeloid growth factors in the setting of post-transplantation leukopenia.[48, 49]

ETIOLOGY OF MDS/AML IN THE ALLOGENEIC TRANSPLANTATION SETTING

The majority of MDS/AML cases after alloHSCT reflects relapse rather than second malignancy. Malignant transformation of the donor cells has been described by many investigators, however.[50–56] Most reports describe donor cell leukemia occurring relatively early, often within the first 36 months following transplantation. The incidence is difficult to establish because of the small numbers reported and the differing methods used to determine the cell of origin of the relapse. These methods have varying degrees of sensitivity. Restriction fragment length polymorphism analysis has limited sensitivity, whereas cytogenetic analysis is limited by the ability to detect only cells in metaphase. Cytogenetics may detect residual normal host cells rather than the donor-derived malignant clone. Variable number tandem repeat analysis has also been used to assign the cell of origin.[57]

Witherspoon et al.[58] reported a patient with AML probably occurring in the donor cells 6 years after a human leukocyte antigen (HLA) identical sibling transplant for probable acute lymphoblastic leukemia. Leukemia may also result from previous genotoxic therapy in the donor. Fluorescent in situ hybridization demonstrated donor cell origin in AML occurring post transplantation for Ph[1]-positive chronic myelogenous leukemia. The donor had previously received chemotherapy for malignant melanoma.[56] The donor, however, showed no hematologic changes, suggesting a role for additional recipient extrinsic factors with transforming effects on the infused stem cells. Possibilities include abnormal stimuli from the marrow microenvironment or direct transfer of genetic material from residual malignant cells to donor cells. Abnormal activation resulting from antigenic stimulation may also play a role. Direct damage by post transplantation methotrexate or impaired immune surveillance post transplantation has also been implicated.[58] In addition, inadvertent transplantation of leukemia from an affected donor has also been described.[59]

TREATMENT OF POST-TRANSPLANTATION MDS/AML

The treatment of MDS remains unsatisfactory. Most patients experience poor outcomes, with a median survival of 4–6 months. Eighty percent of cases are refractory to current treatments. Options similar to those in the nontransplant setting include no treatment, transfusion support, growth factors, differentiating agents, and low- or conventional-dose chemotherapy. Biologic response modifiers may also have a role. All these approaches have been reported in de novo MDS with limited success. The study of amifostine, an agent shown to protect cells from chemotherapy or radiation-induced stress, continues in clinical trials. Decreased transfusion requirements were noted in a phase I/II trial.[60] Further evaluation continues to define this drug's role in MDS. 5-Azacytidine, a differentiating agent, has been reported to result in improved survival, more-frequent hematologic responses, and delayed progression to AML in a randomized trial.[61]

Chemotherapy agents, including low-dose cytarabine, etoposide, hydroxyurea, and more recently topotecan either alone or in combination with cytarabine, have also been studied in MDS. Encouraging results have been reported for the latter combination.[62] Immunosuppressive agents, including antithymocyte globulin and cyclosporin A, have produced promising results.[63, 64] Autologous and allogeneic transplants have been applied to both de novo MDS/AML and therapy-related MDS/AML.[65–72] A study of 46 patients undergoing allogeneic or syngeneic transplantation for the treatment of therapy-related or MDS-related AML reported a 5-year actuarial disease-free survival rate of 24.4%. The cumulative incidences of relapse and nonrelapse mortality were 31.3% and 44.3%, respectively. Therapy-related AML resulted in a higher relapse rate and lower disease-free survival than de novo leukemia.[73]

In the allogeneic HSCT setting, nonrelapse mortality has been high, and studies examining the use of peripheral blood stem cells are under way. Studies of allogeneic HSCT specifically for MDS/AML after autologous transplantation have not been performed. Many patients will be precluded from an allogeneic HSCT as a result of age, general medical condition, or lack of a suitable donor. Nonmyeloablative transplant approaches deserve consideration in this setting. The ability to restore polyclonal hematopoiesis after induction chemotherapy is well established.[74] Collection of normal stem cells after cytotoxic chemotherapy has also been demonstrated. AutoHSCT has also been investigated.[75–77] To date, no long-term follow-up is available, although nonrelapse mortality should be significantly lower than in the allogeneic setting.

SOLID MALIGNANCY AFTER TRANSPLANTATION

Patients who have undergone HDT are at increased risk for solid malignancy.[24, 27, 78–81] This is best characterized in the allogeneic transplant setting. Etiologic factors include the occurrence of the primary malignancy, chemotherapy or irradiation prior to transplantation, the preparative regimen, and treatment given after the development of GVHD.[24, 43, 45, 81–85] Numerous studies, both animal and human, have established the contribution of radiation to the development of malignancy. Survivors of Hiroshima and Nagasaki had a markedly increased risk of hematologic malignancy,[46, 47] and the increased risk of malignancy after irradiation for lymphoma is well established.[18] Chronic GVHD appears to increase the risk of epithelial malignancy.

INCIDENCE

A number of reports have described the incidence of solid malignancy occurring after transplantation.[24, 27, 79, 86] More recently, a large multicenter study incorporating 19,229 patients from the International Bone Marrow Transplant Registry (IBMTR) and the Fred Hutchinson Cancer Research Center detailed the incidence and risk factors for solid cancers after allogeneic or syngeneic transplantation. Patients underwent HSCT at 235 centers between 1964 and 1992. Allogeneic HSCT accounted for 97.2% of the cases, and 3200 patients survived 5 or more years. Eighty solid cancers occurred during the follow-up period, yielding a relative risk of 8.3. At 5 and 10 years, respectively, the cumulative incidence was 0.7% (95% CI, 0.4–0.9) and 2.2% (95% CI, 1.5–3.0) and continued to increase, reaching 6.7% (95% CI, 3.7–9.6) at 15 years.

The spectrum of malignancy included buccal mucosa and salivary gland cancers, bone and connective tissue and brain and other central nervous system tumors, and invasive melanomas. Two cases of malignant fibrous histiocytoma involving the liver occurred. An increase in the more-common breast, gastrointestinal, pulmonary, and genitourinary tumors was not apparent. The highest incidence of

solid malignancy occurred in children aged less than 10 years at the time of transplantation. Tumors in this group included brain and thyroid malignancy and were most common among patients receiving cranial irradiation prior to transplantation. The observed incidence was 36.6 times higher than expected. In patients older than 30, the risk approached that in the general population. Risk factors for solid malignancy post HSCT included previous limited-field irradiation, increasing doses of total body irradiation, and the presence of chronic GVHD. Limited-field irradiation was associated with a marked increase in the risk of buccal cavity malignancy. In patients receiving fractionated total body irradiation, a dose-response relationship was noted. Chronic GVHD was associated with an increased incidence of squamous cell carcinoma of the buccal cavity and skin, particularly in patients on immunosuppressive therapy for 2 or more years. Medications including anti-thymocyte globulin (ATG) for the treatment or prevention of acute GVHD had no effect on the incidence in this series.[78] In an earlier Seattle series, an increased risk of solid cancers was associated with the use of ATG. There was a 6.69 times higher age-adjusted incidence of all secondary cancers.[24]

In a study by Lowsky et al., 557 adult patients undergoing allogeneic related, unrelated, or syngeneic HSCT were reviewed for the incidence of secondary malignancy. Most patients underwent HSCT for hematologic malignancy. Of 10 cancers developing in 9 patients, 8 were solid cancers. The age-adjusted incidence was 4.2 times higher than in the general population. A higher incidence was detected after the use of total body irradiation and acute GVHD grade II or higher. Again, chronic GVHD was a risk factor for epithelial cancers.[81]

POST-TRANSPLANTATION LYMPHOPROLIFERATIVE DISORDERS

PATHOPHYSIOLOGY

Much has been written regarding post-transplantation lymphoproliferative disorders (PTLD) in solid organ transplant recipients. There is less information regarding the disease post SCT. Most cases occur in the setting of T-cell dysfunction and Epstein-Barr virus (EBV) infection.[87] EBV-negative PTLD occurring in solid organ recipients has been reported.[88] By adulthood, 95% of the population is EBV-positive. The virus persists in a latent form in B lymphocytes and certain epithelial cells. Initial infection in children is usually asymptomatic, but 50% of adolescents and adults may experience a mononucleosis syndrome.

EBV infection of B lymphocytes is associated with the expression of nine proteins required for transformation. These include six EBV-determined proteins, nuclear antigens (EBNA) 1–6. In addition, three membrane-spanning determinants are detectable. All except EBNA-1 can effectively elicit a cytotoxic T-cell CTL response. It is postulated that on initial infection of resting B lymphocytes, expression of all these proteins may result in transformation (reviewed in 89). A powerful CTL response may follow, with resultant elimination of transformed cells. Some infected B cells, however, assume the resting state, with down-regulation of all transforming proteins except EBNA-1. A state of equilibrium between EBV-infected B cells and host surveillance results. On reactivation, a CTL response restores the latent state in normal persons.

In the setting of congenital or acquired immunodeficiency, reactivation may occur without an appropriate immune response to control the proliferation. Post-SCT EBV cellular immunity is diminished but tends to recover by 6 months.[90, 91] It is during this window of EBV immunosuppression that conditions permissible for the development of PTLD exist. Without the cellular immune response, the initial polyclonal EBV-associated lymphoproliferation fails to regress and oligoclonal and monoclonal proliferations may develop. High levels of EBV DNA have been demonstrated to correlate with the subsequent development of PTLD.[92–94]

INCIDENCE

In solid organ recipients, there is a variable incidence ranging up to approximately 10% in heart-lung transplant recipients.[95] Following allogeneic HSCT, the incidence varies from 0.6% to 1.6%. A higher incidence occurs with T-cell depletion (TCD), unrelated transplants, and greater degrees of immunosuppression for acute GVHD. PTLD has also been reported following autologous HSCT.[96] Of 506 allogeneic HSCT from the University of Minnesota, there were 8 (1.6%) cases of PTLD. The incidence was 24% in 25 patients receiving mismatched TCD HSCT and only 0.2% in 424 patients receiving matched non-TCD HSCT.[97] Of 2475 allogeneic HSCT reported from Fred Hutchinson Cancer Research Center, 15 cases occurred for an incidence of 0.6%. An increased incidence was noted in patients receiving TCD transplants (3.1%) and in patients receiving an anti-CD3 monoclonal antibody for treatment of acute GVHD.[98] Of 462 unrelated transplant recipients from the National Marrow Donor Program (NMDP), 5% receiving TCD marrow experienced PTLD as opposed to 1% in patients receiving non-TCD HSCT.[99] A combined analysis of data from the IBMTR and the Fred Hutchinson Cancer Research Center described 78 cases of PTLD occurring in more than 18,000 allogeneic bone marrow transplants. Sixty-four cases occurred less than 1 year from transplant, and the cumulative incidence was 1.0% ± 0.3% at 10 years. The maximal risk occurred in the first 5 months following transplant. Significant risk factors for early-onset PTLD included a mismatched or unrelated donor, selective T-cell depletion (as opposed to combined B and T cell depletion), and the use of ATG or an anti-CD3 monoclonal antibody for prophylaxis or treatment of aGVHD. Extensive chronic GVHD was the only risk factor associated with the later-onset PTLD.[100]

In 1997, Orazi and colleagues described 10 cases among 245 allogeneic HSCT recipients.[101] All occurred in the 110 patients receiving TCD HSCT. The incidence ranged from 16% among unrelated patients to 2% among related HSCT. Other series have reported detection rates of 1–2%, with most cases occurring in the setting of TCD.[102, 103] In 1998, the Vancouver group described PTLD in 8 of 428 allogeneic HSCT. Six followed unrelated HSCT. In multivariate analysis, significant risk factors were TCD (relative risk [RR]

30.5), anti-T-cell therapy (RR, 12.7), and acute GVHD grades 3–4 (RR, 7.7).[104] A recent article reported on the incidence of Hodgkin disease following allogeneic BMT. Eight cases were observed among a cohort of more than 18,000 patients. Two of these cases were HIV positive. The absolute excess risk was calculated at 1.6 cases per 10,000 person-years at risk. Interestingly, although the number of cases was small, no correlation was noted between the development of Hodgkin disease and T-cell depletion, HLA mismatch, or the use of unrelated donors.[105]

CLINICAL FEATURES

PTLD occurrs a median of 3–5 months post HSCT.[101, 106] Common presenting features include fever, lymphadenopathy, hepatitis, abdominal pain, rash, central nervous system symptoms, and hepatosplenomegaly (Table 57–6). Organ involvement at diagnosis commonly included lymph nodes, liver, or spleen with one-third having kidney, lung, or bone marrow involvement. Single-organ involvement occurs in 25%[101, 106] (Table 57–7). Most patients present with disseminated involvement. PTLD may be an incidental finding at autopsy. The disease tends to be aggressive, with a high associated mortality.[97, 98, 101, 106, 107]

PATHOLOGY

The features of PTLD after solid organ transplantation has been well characterized[101] (reviewed in reference 108). The initial classification was proposed by Frizzera et al.[109, 110] More recently, three distinct entities were grouped together as the post-transplantation lymphoproliferative disorders.[111] Plasmacytic hyperplasia most commonly arose in the oropharynx or lymph nodes. Most cases are polyclonal. Polymorphic B-cell hyperplasia (PBCH) or polymorphic B-cell lymphoma (PBCL) occurs in lymph nodes or extranodal sites, and most cases are monoclonal. Immunoblastic lym-

TABLE 57–6. SYMPTOMS AND SIGNS IN 32 CASES OF POST-TRANSPLANTATION LYMPHOPROLIFERATIVE DISORDERS

SYMPTOM/SIGN	PERCENT
Fever	68
Lymphadenopathy	47
Hepatitis	37.5
Abdominal pain	31.3
Anorexia	25
Lethargy	19
Central nervous system symptoms	16
Respiratory symptoms	16
Hepatomegaly	16
Splenomegaly	12.5
Pharyngitis	12.5
Thrombocytopenia	12.5
Renal disease	6.3
Weight loss	6.3
Dysphagia, laryngeal ulceration, diarrhea	3

Data from Cohen JI: Epstein-Barr virus lymphoproliferative disease associated with acquired immunodeficiency. Medicine 70(2):137–160, 1991.

TABLE 57–7. ORGAN DISTRIBUTION IN 32 CASES OF POST-TRANSPLANTATION LYMPHOPROLIFERATIVE DISORDERS

ORGAN INVOLVED	PERCENT	ORGAN INVOLVED	PERCENT
Lymph nodes	81	Uterus	6
Liver	50	Lacrimal gland	6
Spleen	50	Salivary gland	6
Kidney	41	Gallbladder	6
Lung	37.5	Conjunctiva	3
Bone marrow	31	Esophagus	3
Small intestine	16	Bladder	3
Large intestine	16	Prostate	3
Heart	12.5	Pancreas	3
Central nervous system	12.5	Tongue	3
Peripheral blood	9	Nasopharynx	3
Adrenal	9	Retroperitoneum	3
Thymus	9	Parathyroid	3
Stomach	6	Appendix	3
Ovary	6	Thyroid	3

Data from Cohen JI: Epstein-Barr virus lymphoproliferative disease associated with acquired immunodeficiency. Medicine 70(2):137–160, 1991.

phoma or multiple myeloma is widely disseminated and monoclonal.

In 1997, the Society for Hematopathology Workshop reviewed 20 cases of PTLD. Most cases followed solid organ transplantation. Five distinct entities were identified. They included (1) early lesions, (2) polymorphic PTLD, (3) monomorphic PTLD, B-cell lymphomas, and T-cell lymphomas, (4) plasmacytoma-like lesions, and (5) T-cell-rich large B-cell lymphoma/Hodgkin disease–like lesions.[112] An updated classification has been proposed with the recent World Health Organization Classification of Neoplastic Diseases of the Hematopoietic and Lymphoid Tissues (Table 57–8).[113]

Differing morphologic patterns were described in the post-HSCT series reported by Orazi and colleagues.[101] Polymorphic or monomorphic cell infiltrates were detected. The polymorphic infiltrates were either PBCH or PBCL.

TABLE 57–8. CATEGORIES OF POST TRANSPLANT LYMPHOPROLIFERATIVE DISORDERS

Early lesions
  Reactive plasmacytic hyperplasia
  Infectious mononucleosis-like
PTLD, polymorphic
  Polyclonal (rare)
  Monoclonal
PTLD, monomorphic
  B-cell lymphomas
    Diffuse large B-cell lymphoma (immunoblastic, centroblastic, anaplastic)
    Burkitt/Burkitt-like lymphoma
    Plasma cell myeloma
  T-cell lymphomas
    Peripheral T-cell lymphoma, not otherwise categorized
    Other types (hepatosplenic, γ-δ, T/NK)
Other types, rare
  Hodgkin disease–like lesions (associated with methotrexate therapy)
  Plasmacytoma-like lesions

Adapted from Harris NL, Jaffe ES, Diebold J, et al: World Health Organization Classification of Neoplastic Diseases of the Hematopoietic and Lymphoid Tissues: report of the Clinical Advisory Committee Meeting—Airlie House, Virginia, November 1997. J Clin Oncol 17:3835–3849, 1999.

The monomorphic infiltrate was malignant lymphoma-immunoblastic. The three cases of malignant lymphoma-immonoblastic examined were monoclonal, whereas in seven cases of PBCL only four were monoclonal. All cases were CD20-positive. Fifty percent expressed varying levels of p53 protein. Two patterns of growth were noted in the Vancouver series. Diffuse large B-cell lymphoma occurred in five, and PBCH was observed in three cases. All eight were EBV-positive, and seven were monoclonal. No correlation between morphology, EBV positivity, and clonality clinical behavior was noted.[104]

Most cases occurring post HSCT are of donor origin.[97, 98, 106] Of 32 cases reviewed by Cohen, 6 were of recipient origin, 15 were monoclonal, 7 were polyclonal, and 9 had both polyclonal and monoclonal lesions present.[106] In solid organ donor transplants, most cases are of recipient origin.[114] Initially, polyclonal proliferations are usual. Ultimately, oligoclonal and monoclonal proliferations may develop. After solid organ transplantation, polyclonal proliferations are usual.[111, 114–118] Numerous distinct monoclonal proliferations occurring simultaneously have been described.[119]

THERAPY

Because certain risk factors for PTLD are inherent to transplantation the development of strategies to identify patients who may benefit from prophylactic or early treatment measures is important. The early identification of EBV-associated lymphoproliferation using the outgrowth of transformed B lymphocytes ex vivo and the detection of EBV DNA by a polymerase chain reaction (PCR) method was associated with EBV-associated lymphoproliferation prior to the onset of clinical disease.[93] PCR and an end-point dilution technique were used to demonstrate markedly elevated levels of EBV DNA in four of five patients with PTLD at or before clinical diagnosis. EBV DNA levels fell dramatically with effective therapy.[120] Improved techniques for selective TCD may also reduce the incidence of PTLD. Counterflow elutriation depletes B cells in addition to T cells and may reduce the EBV load with a resultant decrease in PTLD.[121]

Therapeutic options used include combination chemotherapy[122] and withdrawal of immunosuppressive drugs.[102, 123, 124] Combination chemotherapy has been used with little success in the SCT setting. The combination of post-transplantation immunosuppression and chemotherapy results in increased mortality,[122] but combination chemotherapy has been successfully used after solid organ transplantation.[125, 126]

High-dose acyclovir and ganciclovir have been used.[97, 98, 127] Interferon-α and donor lymphocyte infusions have also been used.[101, 128–130] The Memorial Sloan-Kettering Cancer Center reported five patients with PTLD after TCD allogeneic HSCT receiving one to three transfusions of donor lymphocytes from their EBV-seropositive donors. All responded with no evidence of lymphoma, but two died from respiratory failure. Of those surviving, two experienced cutaneous grade II acute GVHD and all three experienced mild chronic GVHD.[129]

A 1998 report from St. Jude Children's Research Hospital described the administration of gene marked cytotoxic T cells to 39 high-risk patients after TCD matched unrelated or mismatched related HSCT.[130] EBV-specific T-cell lines were generated by culture with autologous irradiated lymphoblastoid cells. In six patients experiencing high EBV DNA levels post transplantation, levels fell by 3–5 logs within 2–3 weeks of cytotoxic T-lymphocyte infusion. No patients experienced PTLD. Of 61 control patients, 7 with increasing EBV DNA levels post transplantation progressed to PTLD, for an incidence of 11.5%. No toxicity was directly attributed to the donor lymphocyte infusion, although chronic GVHD worsened in 1 patient. Gene marked T cells were present in regenerated EBV-specific T-cell lines for up to 38 months.

CONCLUSION

Second malignancy after HSCT is a major and increasing problem. Three separate groups of malignancy can be identified to occur during well-defined time periods post transplantation. Early post transplantation, the risk is highest for PTLD. These are EBV-associated lymphoproliferations occurring in the setting of immunosuppression. They primarily occur in the allogeneic HSCT setting and are associated with TCD and the use of agents to prevent or treat GVHD. Treatment is initially aimed at reduction in immunosuppression. Recent studies using adoptive immunotherapy have proven promising. Chemotherapy is usually poorly tolerated in this population.

Patients are subsequently most at risk for MDS/AML. This complication occurs almost exclusively in the autologous HSCT setting and appears to be primarily related to the pretransplantation therapy rather than to the preparative regimen or other transplant factors. The precise contribution of the latter factors remains to be defined. The risk of MDS/AML appears to disappear by 9 years post transplantation. In contrast with these two disorders, the incidence of solid malignancy continues to rise over time post HSCT. The occurrence of a second malignancy post HSCT can account for significant morbidity and mortality

in a patient who is cured of primary malignancy. There is an increasing tendency in certain diseases toward earlier HSCT, resulting in reduced exposure to mutagenic agents, which may result in a decreased incidence of second malignancy. Also, improved methods of TCD and a better understanding of lymphocyte subsets should also allow for immune manipulation without an increased incidence of malignancy. Until better understanding leads to prevention of these disorders, patients need to be made aware of the risks of second malignancy prior to HSCT.

REFERENCES

1. Lerner HJ: Acute myelogenous leukemia in patients receiving chlorambucil as long-term adjuvant chemotherapy for stage II breast cancer. Cancer Treat Rep 62(8):1135–1138, 1978.
2. Berk PD, Goldberg JD, Silverstein MN, et al: Increased incidence of acute leukemia in polycythemia vera associated with chlorambucil therapy. N Engl J Med 304(8):441–447, 1981.
3. Tucker MA, Meadows AT, Boice JD Jr, et al: Leukemia after therapy with alkylating agents for childhood cancer. J Natl Cancer Inst 78(3):459–464, 1987.
4. Sont JK, van Stiphout WA, Noordijk EM, et al: Increased risk of second cancers in managing Hodgkins disease: the 20-year Leiden experience. Ann Hematol 65(5):213–218, 1992.
5. Travis LB, Curtis RE, Boice JD Jr, et al: Second cancers following non-Hodgkin's lymphoma. Cancer 67(7):2002–2009, 1991.
6. Abrahamsen JF, Andersen A, Hannisdal E, et al: Second malignancies after treatment of Hodgkin's disease: the influence of treatment, follow-up time, and age [see comments]. J Clin Oncol 11(2):255–261, 1993.
7. Boivin JF, Hutchison GB, Zauber AG, et al: Incidence of second cancers in patients treated for Hodgkin's disease [see comments]. J Natl Cancer Inst 87(10):732–741, 1995.
8. Pedersen-Bjergaard J, Philip P, Larsen SO, et al: Therapy-related myelodysplasia and acute myeloid leukemia: cytogenetic characteristics of 115 consecutive cases and risk in seven cohorts of patients treated intensively for malignant diseases in the Copenhagen series. Leukemia 7(12):1975–1986, 1993.
9. Pedersen-Bjergaard J, Daugaard G, Hansen SW, et al: Increased risk of myelodysplasia and leukaemia after etoposide, cisplatin, and bleomycin for germ-cell tumours [see comments]. Lancet 338(8763):359–363, 1991.
10. Whitlock JA, Greer JP, Lukens JN: Epipodophyllotoxin-related leukemia: identification of a new subset of secondary leukemia. Cancer 68(3):600–604, 1991.
11. Thirman MJ, Larson RA: Therapy-related myeloid leukemia. Hematol Oncol Clin North Am 10(2):293–320, 1996.
12. Yagita M, Ieki Y, Onishi R, et al: Therapy-related leukemia and myelodysplasia following oral administration of etoposide for recurrent breast cancer. Int J Oncol 13(1):91–96, 1998.
13. Smith MA, Rubinstein L, Anderson JR, et al: Secondary leukemia or myelodysplastic syndrome after treatment with epipodophyllotoxins. J Clin Oncol 17(2):569–577, 1999.
14. van Leeuwen FE, Somers R, Taal BG, et al: Increased risk of lung cancer, non-Hodgkin's lymphoma, and leukemia following Hodgkin's disease. J Clin Oncol 7(8):1046–1058, 1989.
15. Chung CT, Bogart JA, Adams JF, et al: Increased risk of breast cancer in splenectomized patients undergoing radiation therapy for Hodgkin's disease. Int J Radiat Oncol Biol Phys 37(2):405–409, 1997.
16. Dietrich PY, Henry-Amar M, Cosset JM, et al: Second primary cancers in patients continuously disease-free from Hodgkin's disease: a protective role for the spleen? Blood 84(4):1209–1215, 1994.
17. Travis LB, Curtis RE, Glimelius B, et al: Second cancers among long-term survivors of non-Hodgkin's lymphoma. J Natl Cancer Inst 85(23):1932–1937, 1993.
18. Tucker MA, Coleman CN, Cox RS, et al: Risk of second cancers after treatment for Hodgkin's disease. N Engl J Med 318(2):76–81, 1988.
19. van Leeuwen FE, Klokman WJ, Hagenbeek A, et al: Second cancer risk following Hodgkin's disease: a 20-year follow-up study. J Clin Oncol 12(2):312–325, 1994.
20. Swerdlow AJ, Douglas AJ, Hudson GV, et al: Risk of second primary

cancers after Hodgkin's disease by type of treatment: analysis of 2846 patients in the British National Lymphoma Investigation. BMJ 304(6835):1137–1143, 1992.

21. Blayney DW, Longo DL, Young RC, et al: Decreasing risk of leukemia with prolonged follow-up after chemotherapy and radiotherapy for Hodgkin's disease. N Engl J Med 316(12):710–714, 1987.

22. Fisher B, Rockette H, Fisher ER, et al: Leukemia in breast cancer patients following adjuvant chemotherapy or postoperative radiation: the NSABP experience. J Clin Oncol 3(12):1640–1658, 1985.

23. Curtis RE, Boice JD Jr, Stovall M, et al: Risk of leukemia after chemotherapy and radiation treatment for breast cancer [see comments]. N Engl J Med 326(26):1745–1751, 1992.

24. Witherspoon RP, Fisher LD, Schoch G, et al: Secondary cancers after bone marrow transplantation for leukemia or aplastic anemia [see comments]. N Engl J Med 321(12):784–789, 1989.

25. Traweek ST, Slovak ML, Nademanee AP, et al: Clonal karyotypic hematopoietic cell abnormalities occurring after autologous bone marrow transplantation for Hodgkin's disease and non-Hodgkin's lymphoma. Blood 84(3):957–963, 1994.

26. Miller JS, Arthur DC, Litz CE, et al: Myelodysplastic syndrome after autologous bone marrow transplantation: an additional late complication of curative cancer therapy [see comments]. Blood 83(12):3780–3786, 1994.

27. Bhatia S, Ramsay NK, Steinbuch M, et al: Malignant neoplasms following bone marrow transplantation. Blood 87(9):3633–3639, 1996.

28. Stone RM, Neuberg D, Soiffer R, et al: Myelodysplastic syndrome as a late complication following autologous bone marrow transplantation for non-Hodgkin's lymphoma. J Clin Oncol 12(12):2535–2542, 1994.

29. Friedberg JW, Neuberg D, Stone RM, et al: Outcome in patients with myelodysplastic syndrome after autologous bone marrow transplantation for non-Hodgkin's lymphoma. J Clin Oncol 17:3128–3135, 1999.

30. Darrington DL, Vose JM, Anderson JR, et al: Incidence and characterization of secondary myelodysplastic syndrome and acute myelogenous leukemia following high-dose chemoradiotherapy and autologous stem-cell transplantation for lymphoid malignancies. J Clin Oncol 12(12):2527–2534, 1994.

31. Sobecks RM, Le Beau MM, Anastasi J, Williams SF: Myelodysplasia and acute leukemia following high-dose chemotherapy and autologous bone marrow or peripheral blood stem cell transplantation. Bone Marrow Transplant 23(11):1161–1165, 1999.

32. Laughlin MJ, McGaughey DS, Crews JR, et al: Secondary myelodysplasia and acute leukemia in breast cancer patients after autologous bone marrow transplant. J Clin Oncol 16(3):1008–1012, 1998.

33. Kantarjian HM, Keating MJ, Walters RS, et al: Therapy-related leukemia and myelodysplastic syndrome: clinical, cytogenetic, and prognostic features. J Clin Oncol 4(12):1748–1757, 1986.

34. Le Beau MM, Albain KS, Larson RA, et al: Clinical and cytogenetic correlations in 63 patients with therapy-related myelodysplastic syndromes and acute nonlymphocytic leukemia: further evidence for characteristic abnormalities of chromosomes no. 5 and 7. J Clin Oncol 4(3):325–345, 1986.

35. Rowley JD, Golomb HM, Vardiman JW: Nonrandom chromosome abnormalities in acute leukemia and dysmyelopoietic syndromes in patients with previously treated malignant disease. Blood 58(4):759–767, 1981.

36. Imrie KR, Dubae I, Prince HM, et al: New clonal karyotypic abnormalities acquired following autologous bone marrow transplantation for acute myeloid leukemia do not appear to confer an adverse prognosis. Bone Marrow Transplant 21(4):395–399, 1998.

37. Wilson CS, Traweek ST, Slovak ML, et al: Myelodysplastic syndrome occurring after autologous bone marrow transplantation for lymphoma: morphologic features. Am J Clin Pathol 108(4):369–377, 1997.

38. Chao NJ, Nademanee AP, Long GD, et al: Importance of bone marrow cytogenetic evaluation before autologous bone marrow transplantation for Hodgkin's disease. J Clin Oncol 9(9):1575–1579, 1991.

39. Kantarjian HM, Keating MJ: Therapy-related leukemia and myelodysplastic syndrome. Semin Oncol 14(4):435–443, 1987.

40. Pedersen-Bjergaard J, Ersbll J, Srensen HM, et al: Risk of acute nonlymphocytic leukemia and preleukemia in patients treated with cyclophosphamide for non-Hodgkin's lymphomas: comparison with results obtained in patients treated for Hodgkin's disease and ovarian carcinoma with other alkylating agents. Ann Intern Med 103(2):195–200, 1985.

41. Coleman CN, Williams CJ, Flint A, et al: Hematologic neoplasia in patients treated for Hodgkin's disease. N Engl J Med 297(23):1249–1252, 1977.

42. Govindarajan R, Jagannath S, Flick JT, et al: Preceding standard therapy is the likely cause of MDS after autotransplants for multiple myeloma. Br J Haematol 95(2):349–353, 1996.

43. Deeg HJ, Witherspoon RP: Risk factors for the development of secondary malignancies after marrow transplantation. Hematol Oncol Clin North Am 7(2):417–429, 1993.

44. Deeg HJ, Storb R, Thomas ED: Bone marrow transplantation: a review of delayed complications. Br J Haematol 57(2):185–208, 1984.

45. Kolb HJ, Bender-Geotze C: Late complications after allogeneic bone marrow transplantation for leukaemia. Bone Marrow Transplant 6(2):61–72, 1990.

46. Finch SC: The study of atomic bomb survivors in Japan. Am J Med 66(6):899–901, 1979.

47. Preston D: Cancer risks and biomarker studies in the atomic bomb survivors. Stem Cells Dayt 13(Suppl 1):40–48, 1995.

48. Kawano Y, Takaue Y, Saito S, et al: Granulocyte colony-stimulating factor CSF, macrophage-CSF, granulocyte-macrophage CSF, interleukin-3, and interleukin-6 levels in sera from children undergoing blood stem cell autografts. Blood 81(3):856–860, 1993.

49. Cairo MS, Suen Y, Sender L, et al: Circulating granulocyte colony-stimulating factor G-CSF levels after allogeneic and autologous bone marrow transplantation: endogenous G-CSF production correlates with myeloid engraftment [see comments]. Blood 79(7):1869–1873, 1992.

50. Newburger PE, Latt SA, Pesando JM, et al: Leukemia relapse in donor cells after allogeneic bone-marrow transplantation. N Engl J Med 304(12):712–714, 1981.

51. Fialkow PJ, Thomas ED, Bryant JI, Neiman PE: Leukaemic transformation of engrafted human marrow cells in vivo. Lancet 1(7693):251–255, 1971.

52. Boyd CN, Ramberg RC, Thomas ED: The incidence of recurrence of leukemia in donor cells after allogeneic bone marrow transplantation. Leukemia Res 6(6):833–837, 1982.

53. Thomas ED, Bryant JI, Buckner CD, et al: Leukemic transformation of engrafted human marrow. Transplant Proc 4(4):567–570, 1972.

54. Thomas ED, Bryant JI, Buckner CD, et al: Leukaemic transformation of engrafted human marrow cells in vivo. Lancet 1(7764):1310–1313, 1972.

55. Browne PV, Lawler M, Humphries P, McCann SR: Donor-cell leukemia after bone marrow transplantation for severe aplastic anemia. N Engl J Med 325(10):710–713, 1991.

56. Lowsky R, Fyles G, Minden M, et al: Detection of donor cell derived acute myelogenous leukaemia in a patient transplanted for chronic myelogenous leukaemia using fluorescence in situ hybridization. Br J Haematol 93(1):163–165, 1996.

57. Cransac M, Boiron JM, Merel P, et al: Burkitt-type acute lymphoblastic leukemia in donor cells after allogeneic bone marrow transplantation for acute nonlymphoblastic leukemia. Transplantation 56(1):120–123, 1993.

58. Witherspoon RP, Schubach W, Neiman P: Donor cell leukemia developing six years after marrow grafting for acute leukemia. Blood 65(5):1172–1174, 1985.

59. Niederwieser DW, Appelbaum FR, Gastl G, et al: Inadvertent transmission of a donor's acute myeloid leukemia in bone marrow transplantation for chronic myelocytic leukemia. N Engl J Med 322(25):1794–1796, 1990.

60. List AF, Brasfield F, Heaton R, et al: Stimulation of hematopoiesis by amifostine in patients with myelodysplastic syndrome. Blood 90(9):3364–3369, 1997.

61. Silverman LR, Demakos EP, Peterson B, et al: A randomized controlled trial of subcutaneous azacitidine (aza-c) in patients with the myelodysplastic syndrome (MDS): a study of the Cancer and Leukemia Group B (CALGB). Proc Am Soc Clin Oncol 17:14a, 1998.

62. Beran M, Kantarjian H, Keating M, et al: Results of combination chemotherapy with topotecan and high-dose cytosine arabinoside (ara-C) in previously untreated patients with high-risk myelodysplastic syndrome (MDS) and chronic myelomonocytic leukemia (CMML). Blood 90(Suppl 1):583a, 1997.

63. Jonasova A, Neuwirtova R, Cermak J, et al: Promising cyclosporine A therapy for myelodysplastic syndrome. Leukemia Res 21(Suppl):842, 1997.

64. Molldrem JJ, Caples M, Mavroudis D, et al: Antithymocyte globulin for patients with myelodysplastic syndrome. Br J Haematol 99(3):699–705, 1997.

65. Anderson JE, Appelbaum FR, Fisher LD, et al: Allogeneic bone marrow transplantation for 93 patients with myelodysplastic syndrome. Blood 82(2):677–681, 1993.

66. de Witte T, Suciu S, Peetermans M, et al: Intensive chemotherapy for poor prognosis myelodysplasia MDS and secondary acute myeloid leukemia sAML following MDS of more than 6 months' duration: a pilot study by the Leukemia Cooperative Group of the European Organisation for Research and Treatment in Cancer EORTC-LCG. Leukemia 9(11):1805–1811, 1995.

67. Longmore G, Guinan EC, Weinstein HJ: Bone marrow transplantation for myelodysplasia and secondary acute nonlymphoblastic leukemia. J Clin Oncol 8(10):1707–1714, 1990.

68. De Witte T, Zwaan F, Hermans J, et al: Allogeneic bone marrow transplantation for secondary leukaemia and myelodysplastic syndrome: a survey by the Leukaemia Working Party of the European Bone Marrow Transplantation Group EBMTG [see comments]. Br J Haematol 74(2):151–155, 1990.

69. Bandini G, Rosti G, Calori E: Allogeneic bone marrow transplantation for secondary leukaemia and myelodysplastic syndrome [letter; comment]. Br J Haematol 75(3):442–444, 1990.

70. Sutton L, Leblond V, Le Maignan C, et al: Bone marrow transplantation for myelodysplastic syndrome and secondary leukemia: outcome of 86 patients. Bone Marrow Transplant 7(Suppl 2):39, 1991.

71. O'Donnell MR, Long GD, Parker PM, et al: Busulfan/cyclophosphamide as conditioning regimen for allogeneic bone marrow transplantation for myelodysplasia. J Clin Oncol 13(12):2973–2979, 1995.

72. Ballen KK, Gilliland DG, Guinan EC, et al: Bone marrow transplantation for therapy-related myelodysplasia: comparison with primary myelodysplasia. Bone Marrow Transplant 20(9):737–743, 1997.

73. Anderson JE, Gooley TA, Schoch G, et al: Stem cell transplantation for secondary acute myeloid leukemia: evaluation of transplantation as initial therapy or following induction chemotherapy. Blood 89(7):2578–2585, 1997.

74. Delforge M, Demuynck H, Vandenberghe P, et al: Polyclonal primitive hematopoietic progenitors can be detected in mobilized peripheral blood from patients with high-risk myelodysplastic syndromes. Blood 86(10):3660–3667, 1995.

75. Demuynck H, Delforge M, Verhoef GE, et al: Feasibility of peripheral blood progenitor cell harvest and transplantation in patients with poor-risk myelodysplastic syndromes. Br J Haematol 92(2):351–359, 1996.

76. Verhoef GE, Demuynck H, Delforge M, et al: Autologous peripheral blood progenitor cell transplantation in patients with high-risk myelodysplastic syndromes. Pathol Biol 45(8):651–655, 1997.

77. Wattel E, Solary E, Caillot D, et al: Autologous bone marrow (ABMT) or peripheral blood stem cell (ABSCT) transplantation after intensive chemotherapy in myelodysplastic syndromes (MDS). Leuk Res 21(Suppl 1):S52, 1997.

78. Curtis RE, Rowlings PA, Deeg HJ, et al: Solid cancers after bone marrow transplantation [see comments]. N Engl J Med 336(13):897–904, 1997.

79. Deeg HJ, Sociae G, Schoch G, et al: Malignancies after marrow transplantation for aplastic anemia and fanconi anemia: a joint Seattle and Paris analysis of results in 700 patients. Blood 87(1):386–392, 1996.

80. Witherspoon RP, Deeg HJ, Storb R: Secondary malignancies after marrow transplantation for leukemia or aplastic anemia. Transplant Sci 4(1):33–41, 1994.

81. Lowsky R, Lipton J, Fyles G, et al: Secondary malignancies after bone marrow transplantation in adults. J Clin Oncol 12(10):2187–2192, 1994.

82. Bender-Geotze C: Late effects of allogeneic bone marrow transplantation in children. Pediatrician 18(1):71–75, 1991.

83. Kolb HJ, Guenther W, Duell T, et al: Cancer after bone marrow transplantation. IBMTR and EBMT/EULEP Study Group on Late Effects. Bone Marrow Transplant 10(Suppl 1):135–138, 1992.

84. Witherspoon RP, Storb R, Pepe M, et al: Cumulative incidence of secondary solid malignant tumors in aplastic anemia patients given marrow grafts after conditioning with chemotherapy alone [letter; comment]. Blood 79(1):289–291, 1992.

85. Deeg HJ, Sanders J, Martin P, et al: Secondary malignancies after marrow transplantation. Exp Hematol 12(8):660–666, 1984.

86. Sociae G, Henry-Amar M, Bacigalupo A, et al: Malignant tumors occurring after treatment of aplastic anemia: European Bone Marrow Transplantation—Severe Aplastic Anaemia Working Party. N Engl J Med 329(16):1152–1157, 1993.

87. Locker J, Nalesnik M: Molecular genetic analysis of lymphoid tumors arising after organ transplantation. Am J Pathol 135(6):977–987, 1989.

88. Leblond V, Davi F, Charlotte F, et al: Posttransplant lymphoproliferative disorders not associated with Epstein-Barr virus: a distinct entity? J Clin Oncol 16(6):2052–2059, 1998.

89. Klein G: Epstein-Barr virus strategy in normal and neoplastic B cells. Cell 77(6):791–793, 1994.

90. Lucas KG, Pollok KE, Emanuel DJ: Post-transplant EBV induced lymphoproliferative disorders. Leukemia Lymphoma 25(1–2):1–8, 1997.

91. Crawford DH, Mulholland N, Iliescu V, et al: Epstein-Barr virus infection and immunity in bone marrow transplant recipients. Transplantation 42(1):50–54, 1986.

92. Riddler SA, Breinig MC, McKnight JL: Increased levels of circulating Epstein-Barr virus EBV-infected lymphocytes and decreased EBV nuclear antigen antibody responses are associated with the development of posttransplant lymphoproliferative disease in solid-organ transplant recipients. Blood 84(3):972–984, 1994.

93. Rooney CM, Loftin SK, Holladay MS, et al: Early identification of Epstein-Barr virus–associated post-transplantation lymphoproliferative disease. Br J Haematol 89(1):98–103, 1995.

94. Savoie A, Perpaete C, Carpentier L, et al: Direct correlation between the load of Epstein-Barr virus–infected lymphocytes in the peripheral blood of pediatric transplant patients and risk of lymphoproliferative disease. Blood 83(9):2715–2722, 1994.

95. Randhawa PS, Yousem SA, Paradis IL, et al: The clinical spectrum, pathology, and clonal analysis of Epstein-Barr virus–associated lymphoproliferative disorders in heart-lung transplant recipients. Am J Clin Pathol 92(2):177–185, 1989.

96. Shepherd JD, Gascoyne RD, Barnett MJ, et al: Polyclonal Epstein-Barr virus–associated lymphoproliferative disorder following autografting for chronic myeloid leukemia. Bone Marrow Transplant 15(4):639–641, 1995.

97. Shapiro RS, McClain K, Frizzera G, et al: Epstein-Barr virus associated B cell lymphoproliferative disorders following bone marrow transplantation. Blood 71(5):1234–1243, 1988.

98. Zutter MM, Martin PJ, Sale GE, et al: Epstein-Barr virus lymphoproliferation after bone marrow transplantation. Blood 72(2):520–529, 1988.

99. Kernan NA, Bartsch G, Ash RC, et al: Analysis of 462 transplantations from unrelated donors facilitated by the National Marrow Donor Program [see comments]. N Engl J Med 328(9):593–602, 1993.

100 Curtis RE, Travis LB, Rowlings PA, et al: Risk of lymphoproliferative disorders after bone marrow transplantation: a multi-institutional study. Blood 94:2208–2216, 1999.

101. Orazi A, Hromas RA, Neiman RS, et al: Posttransplantation lymphoproliferative disorders in bone marrow transplant recipients are aggressive diseases with a high incidence of adverse histologic and immunobiologic features. Am J Clin Pathol 107(4):419–429, 1997.

102. Nalesnik MA, Jaffe R, Starzl TE, et al: The pathology of posttransplant lymphoproliferative disorders occurring in the setting of cyclosporine A-prednisone immunosuppression. Am J Pathol 133(1):173–192, 1988.

103. Simon M, Bartram CR, Friedrich W, et al: Fatal B-cell lymphoproliferative syndrome in allogeneic marrow graft recipients: a clinical, immunobiological and pathological study. Virchows Arch B Cell Pathol Mol Pathol 60(5):307–319, 1991.

104. Micallef I, Chhanabhai M, Gascoyne R, et al: Lymphoproliferative disorders following allogeneic bone marrow transplantation: the Vancouver experience. Bone Marrow Transplant 22(10):981–987, 1998.

105. Rowlings PA, Curtis RE, Passweg JR, et al: Increased incidence of Hodgkin's disease after allogeneic bone marrow transplantation. J Clin Oncol 17:3122–3127, 1999.

106. Cohen JI: Epstein-Barr virus lymphoproliferative disease associated with acquired immunodeficiency. Medicine 70(2):137–160, 1991.

107. Martin PJ, Shulman HM, Schubach WH, et al: Fatal Epstein-Barr virus–associated proliferation of donor B cells after treatment of acute graft-versus-host disease with a murine anti-T-cell antibody. Ann Intern Med 101(3):310–315, 1984.
108. Nalesnik M: Clinicopathologic features of posttransplant lymphoproliferative disorders. Ann Transplant 2(4):33–40, 1997.
109. Frizzera G: Atypical lymphoproliferative disorders. *In* Knowles DM (ed): Neoplastic Hematopathology. Baltimore, Williams & Wilkins, 1992.
110. Frizzera G, Hanto DW, Gajl-Peczalska KJ, et al: Polymorphic diffuse B-cell hyperplasias and lymphomas in renal transplant recipients. Cancer Res 41(11 Pt 1):4262–4279, 1981.
111. Knowles DM, Cesarman E, Chadburn A, et al: Correlative morphologic and molecular genetic analysis demonstrates three distinct categories of posttransplantation lymphoproliferative disorders. Blood 85(2):552–565, 1995.
112. Harris NL, Ferry JA, Swerdlow SH: Posttransplant lymphoproliferative disorders: summary of Society for Hematopathology Workshop. Semin Diagn Pathol 14(1):8–14, 1997.
113. Harris NL, Jaffe ES, Diebold J, et al: World Health Organization Classification of Neoplastic Diseases of the Hematopoietic and Lymphoid Tissues: report of the Clinical Advisory Committee Meeting—Airlie House, Virginia, November 1997. J Clin Oncol 17:3835–3849, 1999.
114. Chadburn A, Suciu-Foca N, Cesarman E, et al: Post-transplantation lymphoproliferative disorders arising in solid organ transplant recipients are usually of recipient origin. Am J Pathol 147(6):1862–1870, 1995.
115. Seiden MV, Sklar J: Molecular genetic analysis of post-transplant lymphoproliferative disorders. Hematol Oncol Clin North Am 7(2):447–465, 1993.
116. O'Reilly RJ, Lacerda JF, Lucas KG, et al: Adoptive cell therapy with donor lymphocytes for EBV-associated lymphomas developing after allogeneic marrow transplants. Import Adv Oncol 149–166, 1996.
117. Cleary ML, Nalesnik MA, Shearer WT, Sklar J: Clonal analysis of transplant-associated lymphoproliferations based on the structure of the genomic termini of the Epstein-Barr virus. Blood 72(1):349–352, 1988.
118. Kaplan MA, Ferry JA, Harris NL, Jacobson JO: Clonal analysis of posttransplant lymphoproliferative disorders, using both episomal Epstein-Barr virus and immunoglobulin genes as markers. Am J Clin Pathol 101(5):590–596, 1994.
119. Chadburn A, Cesarman E, Liu YF, et al: Molecular genetic analysis demonstrates that multiple posttransplantation lymphoproliferative disorders occurring in one anatomic site in a single patient represent distinct primary lymphoid neoplasms. Cancer 75(11):2747–2756, 1995.
120. Kenagy DN, Schlesinger Y, Weck K, et al: Epstein-Barr virus DNA in peripheral blood leukocytes of patients with posttransplant lymphoproliferative disease. Transplantation 60(6):547–554, 1995.
121. Gross TG, Hinrichs SH, Davis JR, et al: Depletion of EBV-infected cells in donor marrow by counterflow elutriation. Exp Hematol 26(5):395–399, 1998.
122. Nalesnik MA, Makowka L, Starzl TE: The diagnosis and treatment of posttransplant lymphoproliferative disorders. Curr Probl Surg 25(6):367–472, 1988.
123. Starzl TE, Nalesnik MA, Porter KA, et al: Reversibility of lymphomas and lymphoproliferative lesions developing under cyclosporin-steroid therapy. Lancet 1(8377):583–587, 1984.
124. Hanto DW, Frizzera G, Gajl-Peczalska KJ, Simmons RL: Epstein-Barr virus, immunodeficiency, and B cell lymphoproliferation. Transplantation 39(5):461–472, 1985.
125. Swinnen LJ: Durable remission after aggressive chemotherapy for post-cardiac transplant lymphoproliferation. Leuk Lymphoma 28(1–2):89–101, 1997.
126. Garrett TJ, Chadburn A, Barr ML, et al: Posttransplantation lymphoproliferative disorders treated with cyclophosphamide-doxorubicin-vincristine-prednisone chemotherapy. Cancer 72(9):2782–2785, 1993.
127. Skinner J, Finlay JL, Sondel PM, Trigg ME: Infectious complications in pediatric patients undergoing transplantation with T lymphocyte-depleted bone marrow. Pediatr Infect Dis 5(3):319–324, 1986.
128. Hromas R, Cornetta K, Srour E, et al: Donor leukocyte infusion as therapy of life-threatening adenoviral infections after T-cell–depleted bone marrow transplantation [letter]. Blood 84(5):1689–1690, 1994.
129. Papadopoulos EB, Ladanyi M, Emanuel D, et al: Infusions of donor leukocytes to treat Epstein-Barr virus–associated lymphoproliferative disorders after allogeneic bone marrow transplantation [see comments]. N Engl J Med 330(17):1185–1191, 1994.
130. Rooney CM, Smith CA, Ng CY, et al: Infusion of cytotoxic T cells for the prevention and treatment of Epstein-Barr virus–induced lymphoma in allogeneic transplant recipients. Blood 92(5):1549–1555, 1998.
131. van Leeuwen FE: Second cancers. *In* De Vita VT, Hellman S, Rosenberg SA (eds): Cancer: Principles and Practice of Oncology. Philadelphia, Lippincott-Raven, 1997, pp 2773–2796.

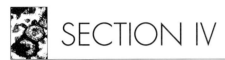

SECTION IV

Post-transplant Therapy

Conventional Biologic Therapy

CHAPTER FIFTY-EIGHT

Biologic Therapy After Hematopoietic Stem Cell Transplantation

Hans-Georg Klingemann, M.D., Ph.D.

RATIONALE FOR THE USE OF BIOLOGIC THERAPY AFTER TRANSPLANTATION

THE "CYTOKINE RELEASE SYNDROME" DURING GRAFT-VS.-HOST DISEASE AND ITS POTENTIAL CONTRIBUTION TO A GRAFT-VS.-TUMOR EFFECT

When the disease-free survival (DFS) data of patients undergoing syngeneic, autologous, T cell–depleted allogeneic hematopoietic stem cell (HSC) transplantation (HSCT) are compared with those after unmanipulated allogeneic HSCT, it becomes evident that transplantation of unmanipulated allogeneic HSC preparations have the lowest recurrence rate.[1–3] Moreover, the presence of either acute or chronic graft-vs.-host disease (GVHD) can further reduce the recurrence rate. Immunologically competent T lymphocytes transplanted with the allograft can induce a graft-vs.-tumor (GVT) effect that seems to be particularly effective if only minimal disease remains. Likewise, the infusion of donor T cells has been shown to induce remissions after allogeneic HSCT particularly in patients who have recurrent disease after transplantation for chronic myelogenous leukemia.[4]

A GVT reaction is often associated with the clinical manifestation of GVHD, and the separation of the effector mechanisms of these two immunologic entities has been impossible thus far. It is possible that shared epitopes are recognized by alloreactive T cells and that this makes it difficult to separate the two mechanisms. Because an allogeneic immune response does not occur after autologous transplantation owing to the lack of alloantigen differences, the post-transplantation relapse rate after autologous HSCT is at best similar to what occurs after syngeneic HSCT. Hence, immunotherapeutic maneuvers are increasingly considered in autologous transplant recipients to achieve a GVT-like effect and overcome tumor tolerance.

Although an allo-immune response and GVHD are initiated by clonally expanding T cells that recognize differences of either major histocompatibility complex (MHC) or minor (non-MHC) antigens on host target cells, secondary reactions during such a reaction involve the release of cytokines such as interleukins (IL), interferons (IFN), and tumor necrosis factor (TNF), all of which have immune-enhancing functions or direct antitumor effects. The release of cytokines during GVHD has been compared with a "cytokine storm," and these secondary cytokines can further support the generation and activation of cytolytic cells such as natural killer (NK) cells, monocytes/macrophages, and neutrophils, all of which can have antitumor effects. In addition, TNF-α and nitric oxide are released from these cells and may also contribute to the GVT effect. Collectively, these observations form the basis for the use of cytokines, particularly after autologous transplantation but also after allografting to enhance GVT effects in high-risk malignancy.

CYTOKINE TREATMENT OF HEMATOLOGIC MALIGNANCY CAN BE EFFECTIVE

Although the work by Rosenberg et al.[5] showed that even patients with chemotherapy-resistant malignancy can achieve a remission with IL-2 treatment, the side effects of high doses of IL-2 were significant. Also, because of the advanced nature of those cancers, only a minority of patients achieved complete remission. For these reasons, treatment of advanced cancer with IL-2 has largely been abandoned. Rather, treatment with biologic therapy is likely to be more effective if only minimal malignant disease remains after primary therapy. In several studies, biologics were given to patients with hematologic malignancy after initial treatment with conventional-dose chemotherapy. The results from those studies have provided the rationale for their use after HSCT.

In patients with multiple myeloma, IFN-α can induce occasional tumor responses in untreated as well as chemotherapy-resistant patients. When IFN-α was given as maintenance treatment after conventional chemotherapy, overall survival was superior in the IFN group and some patients experienced objective responses.[6, 7] A randomized multicenter trial of the Nordic Myeloma Study Group confirmed that progression-free survival was superior when IFN-α was added to melphalan/prednisone for initial and maintenance therapy.[8] Similar results were obtained in a randomized trial of the National Cancer Institute of Canada.[9] IFN is also known to induce cytogenetic remissions in a subpopulation of patients with chronic myelogenous leukemia. It has also been shown to prolong progression-free survival in patients with lymphoma after they had been given conventional chemotherapy.[10]

IL-2 can induce tumor regression in some patients with advanced hematologic disease such as myeloma or acute myelogenous leukemia.[11, 11] Some of these patients responded, particularly those in whom the marrow was not completely replaced by leukemic blasts. Likewise, a meta-analysis of single-center observations in patients with ma-

TABLE 58–1. APPROACHES OF USING IMMUNE MODULATING MOLECULES AFTER HSCT

Clinically Tested
- Infusion of donor-derived T-cells ("buffy coat") or donor lymphocytic infusions (Chapters 30, 31, 56)
- Induction of autologous graft-vs.-host disease with cyclosporine and interferon
- Administration of cytokines (IL-2, IFN)
- Culture of autograft in cytokines
- Infusion of IL-2 activated NK cells (Chapter 31)

Experimental Stage
- Tumor immunization with cytokine transfected tumor cells
- Infusion of tumor-antigen specific T-cells
- Dendritic cells, engineered to present tumor antigens

IL-2, interleukin-2; IFN, interferon; NK, natural killer.

lignant lymphoma receiving either IL-2 alone or in combination with adoptively transferred lymphokine-activated killer (LAK) cells allows for the conclusion that IL-2 has some activity, particularly against follicular and diffuse non-Hodgkin lymphoma, and may also have some activity in Hodgkin disease.[15]

Collectively, these data suggest that the cytokines IFN and IL-2 (which are the only cytokines currently approved for clinical use) can induce favorable responses in a subset of patients with hematologic malignancy and that their administration after autologous or allogeneic HSCT could be beneficial by controlling residual disease post transplantation. Importantly, immunotherapy is considered "non-cross-reactive" with chemotherapy or radiation administered in preparation for transplantation. Malignant cells resistant to chemotherapy and radiation can still respond to immunotherapy.[16] It is also known that IL-2-responsive lymphocytes and NK cells recover early after autologous and allogeneic HSCT and provide the "substrate" for immune-active cytokines.

Various approaches of using immune modulating molecules and activated cells are summarized in Table 58–1.

INTERFERON AFTER STEM CELL TRANSPLANTATION

Both IFN-α and IFN-γ have been given together with cyclosporin early after autologous transplantation to induce autologous GVHD. When IFN-α and IFN-γ were compared, the addition of IFN-γ to cyclosporin seemed to provide some antitumor effect in patients undergoing HSCT for lymphoma, an observation that needs to be confirmed in a randomized trial. In those studies, IFN had no serious adverse effects, although the treatment duration was limited (3 weeks) and the dose was relatively low. The dose and possibly the timing of IFN seem to be crucial: IFN-α, when started the day after HSC infusion and combined with cyclosporine, was found to cause significant nausea, vomiting, fatigue, fever, and even respiratory distress, particularly at doses exceeding 1×10^6 U/m²/day.[17] Side effects of IFN administration are summarized in Table 58–2.

Three noncontrolled studies have suggested a prolonged progression-free survival in patients with multiple myeloma when IFN-α was part of the management after autologous

HSCT.[18–20] No randomized trial has been conducted that could confirm whether there is any benefit in giving IFN-α to these patients.

In 1996, the group at Fred Hutchinson Cancer Research Center published results from a randomized study in children after allogeneic HSCT for acute lymphocytic leukemia who were given natural leukocyte IFN for a limited time after transplantation to prevent cytomegalovirus pneumonia.[21] Although this particular complication could not be prevented by IFN treatment, analysis of the data revealed that the relapse rate was significantly lower in patients who had been assigned to the IFN group. Surprisingly, no follow-up studies were conducted, although the same group had an activated IFN-α protocol. The side effects related to IFN-α, especially when it is given early after transplantation, made the compliance rate low, causing discontinuation of IFN-α therapy in a majority of patients.

A phase I/II study in which 11 allograft and 3 autograft recipients were given escalating doses of recombinant IFN-α confirmed this initial observation. The dose of recombinant IFN-α in that study[22] could not be escalated beyond 0.5×10^6 U/m² when given daily to patients within the first 100 days after grafting. Marrow depression, nausea, vomiting, and failure to thrive posed significant obstacles. In 2 of 11 allogeneic recipients, IFN-α triggered acute GVHD, which was easily controlled with prednisone. Although almost all patients in that study underwent HSCT for a disease that had poor prognostic features, the relapse-free survival rate continued to be 50% at 7 years, suggesting that IFN-α may indeed have an antitumor effect.

IFN-α treatment for patients with chronic myelogenous leukemia who experience relapse after unmanipulated or T lymphocyte–depleted allogeneic HSCT can occasionally re-induce hematologic and/or cytogenetic remissions.[23] Because buffy coat infusions have been shown to be effective in inducing remission in these patients, however, IFN-α is no longer given. It is unclear whether "pretreatment" with IFN-α prior to administering buffy coat would increase the response rate further. IFN-α is also administered to patients

TABLE 58–2. SIDE EFFECTS OF CYTOKINE TREATMENT IN HSCT RECIPIENTS

Interferon
- Marrow suppression
- Nausea, vomiting, lack of appetite
- Induction of acute graft-vs.-host disease
- Graft rejection

Interleukin-2
Low/intermediate doses:
- Fever
- Fatigue, nausea, vomiting
- Rash
- Skin nodules after subcutaneous injection
- Myalgia
- Fluid retention
- Increased incidence of bacterial infections[57]
- Autoimmune hemolytic anemia[13]
- Autoimmune thyroiditis[58]
- Cholecystitis with thickening of the gallbladder wall[59]

High doses (all of the above plus):
- Anemia/thrombocytopenia
- Hypotension due to left ventricular dysfunction
- Fluid retention and pulmonary edema

after autologous HSCT for chronic myelogenous leukemia,[24] and some patients convert to a Ph+ chromosome–negative state. The overall benefit of such a strategy is unclear.

INTERLEUKIN-2 AFTER STEM CELL TRANSPLANTATION

Initial studies by Blaise et al.[25] and Higuchi et al.[26] in patients with acute leukemia were aimed at obtaining feasibility and safety data for IL-2* when administered after autologous HSCT. In both studies, the cytokine was given after neutrophil and platelet engraftment had occurred. In the trial by Blaise et al.,[25] IL-2 was administered to patients as a constant infusion for 6 days at a dose of 6×10^6 IU/m²/day beginning at a median of 79 days post grafting. All 10 patients had undergone autologous HSCT for advanced disease and hence had received increased doses of chemotherapy prior to grafting. A rash occured in all patients, and three patients experienced a drop in blood pressure under 85 mm Hg (systolic) that did not respond to albumin infusions. Some temporary suppression of marrow function occurred, but all side effects were fully and quickly reversible after IL-2 was discontinued.

The treatment schedule for IL-2 in the study by Higuchi et al.[26] was different, consisting of an induction treatment during which escalating doses of IL-2 were given ($0.9–13.5 \times 10^6$ IU/m²/day for 5 days) followed by a nonescalating maintenance dose of 1.6×10^6 IU/m²/day for 10 days. At the maximum tolerated dose of 9×10^6 IU/m²/day, hypotension and thrombocytopenia occurred, which were fully reversible after stopping the cytokine. In addition, high temperature, nausea, diarrhea, and a rash occurred in most patients who received 9×10^6 IU/m²/day. Side effects of administrating low and high doses of IL-2 are summarized in Table 58–2.

Patient data from this phase I study obtained in patients with acute myelogenous leukemia and non-Hodgkin lymphoma have matured, and results are encouraging. Patients with acute myelogenous leukemia had disease that was subjected to transplantation beyond the first complete remission, and the disease-free survival for this group continued to be around 50%. Likewise, patients with non-Hodgkin lymphoma seemed to have benefited from IL-2 treatment, and this is currently being tested in a multicenter randomized trial by the Southwest Oncology Group.

In contrast with those two trials in which IL-2 was given to autograft recipients after they had experienced sufficient engraftment, Weisdorf et al.[27] administered IL-2 by continuous infusion for the first 3 weeks beginning on day +1. All 14 patients were suffering from acute lymphoblastic leukemia and the HSCT was performed in remission (CR1: one patient; CR2: eight patients; CR3–4: five patients). The dose of IL-2 was escalated, with groups of patients receiving 1.3, 3, and 6×10^6 IU/m²/day.

The side effects of IL-2 in this trial were significant. Only 10 of 14 patients completed the 3-week treatment as planned. In addition, two patients experienced progressive

interstitial pulmonary edema and died 7 and 15 days later, respectively. Severe organ toxicity was most common at the highest dose level of IL-2 and generally developed during the second or third week of IL-2 treatment. The investigators believe that the course of two additional patients who ultimately died was complicated by IL-2 toxicity. There was no negative effect of IL-2 on marrow engraftment. Relapse of leukemia occurred in 9 of 10 patients, suggesting that the IL-2 had no obvious antileukemic effect when given according to this schedule.[27] This observation is supported by results from a randomized multicenter trial from France that also concluded that IL-2 had no significant impact on relapse prevention after autografting for acute lymphoblastic leukemia.[28]

It is possible that the radiation (patients received 125 cGy $\times$ 11 fractions over 4 days) given as part of the conditioning regimen contributed to the severe side effects that occurred with IL-2 in the study by Weisdorf et al. This is supported by observations in patients receiving IL-2 for the first week after autologous transplantation for acute myelogenous leukemia in whom radiation was not part of the conditioning regimen.[29] The side effects in that study of 24 patients were much less, and all but one patient finished the planned treatment with IL-2 of 7 days. The preparation of IL-2 (in this case natural), the dose of IL-2 (lower), and the duration (7 vs. 21 days), however, were different from those in the study by Weisdorf et al., and it is possible that this accounted for the lower incidence of side effects. Another side effect of IL-2 that deserves attention is its ability to reduce neutrophil chemotaxis, which can lead to an increased risk of bacterial infection during IL-2 treatment.

Although animal studies have suggested that the combination of pentoxifylline and ciprofloxacin could prevent some of the IL-2–related side effects, this could not be confirmed; in fact, most patients experienced side effects related to pentoxifylline.[30]

IL-2 has also been given after allogeneic HSCT. In animal models, IL-2 has been reported to induce a GVT effect and to either trigger or protect against GVHD, depending on the mouse model, the timing of IL-2 administration, and the dose.[31] A "protective" effect of IL-2 could not be confirmed in a clinical study, however.[32]

A patient who experienced relapse after allogeneic T cell–depleted HSCT was treated with IL-2 at a dose of 3×10^6 IU/m² given daily as a continuous infusion for two cycles of 5 days each.[33] Although the patient died of *Aspergillus* pneumonia, no leukemia was found on autopsy and, importantly, no GVHD had developed. In a dose-finding study, IL-2 was administered to 17 children who received HLA-matched sibling transplants beyond CR1 and in whom no active GVHD had developed after discontinuation of immunosuppressive medication.[34] IL-2 was given according to the same schedule that was established for autologous transplants by the Fred Hutchinson Cancer Research Center. Usual side effects (fever, nausea, weight gain, rash) occurred during the induction phase, and the maximum tolerated dose of IL-2 was one third of the dose for autologous recipients (3×10^6 IU/m²). De novo acute GVHD developed in 2 of 16 patients and resolved without additional therapy. In 5 of 16 patients, however, extensive chronic GVHD developed, especially in those patients who

---

*Biologic activity of IL-2 preparation: Cetus/Chiron (Proleukin): 1 unit = 6 IU; Roche: 1 unit = 3 IU.

had received the higher dose of IL-2 for induction. In contrast, no acute GVHD occurred when IL-2 was administered at low doses ($2–6 \times 10^5$ IU/m²/day) for 3 months by continuous infusion to patients who had undergone T cell–depleted allogeneic HSCT. Although the incidence of relapse seemed to be less when compared with historical controls, it is impossible to draw conclusions from these noncontrolled studies as to the efficacy of IL-2.

Both IL-2 and IFN are given either concurrently or sequentially at some centers to patients who have experienced post-transplantation relapse and may even have experienced failure of reinduction treatment with buffy coat or lymphocyte infusions from the donor. Patients who do not respond to cell-mediated immunotherapy, however, only rarely show a durable response after administration of biologics.[35]

EX VIVO CULTURE OF STEM CELL PREPARATIONS IN IMMUNE-ACTIVE CYTOKINES

When marrow or peripheral blood progenitor cells (PBPC) are incubated with IL-2, leukemia cells are purged. Animals who have received transplants with such purged marrow experienced superior disease free survival compared with those who were given untreated marrow.[36] NK cells activated by IL-2 (LAK cells) are responsible for the purging effect. Malignant cells are still susceptible to NK cell–mediated lysis, even when they have become resistant to chemotherapy.[16] Studies in mice have suggested that a short ex vivo incubation of marrow with IL-2 followed by IL-2 injections immediately post transplantation resulted in better survival than when only IL-2-activated marrow was given.[37] The rationale of this approach is to maintain the cytotoxic activity of autologous HSC preparations after infusion.

Based on those observations, a clinical trial was initiated that used an 8-day ex vivo incubation of marrow and subsequently of PBPC with IL-2 followed by 1 week of daily injections of IL-2.[29] Preclinical data confirmed that NK cells could be fully activated by IL-2 during the 8-day culture period and, most importantly, that the hematopoietic progenitor function was not compromised under these conditions.[38] It was also observed that IL-2-cultured cells produce cytokines such as TNF-α and IFN-γ, which could contribute to an ex vivo purging effect.[39]

A dose-escalation study confirmed that IL-2 at doses up to 0.5×10^6 IU/m²/day was tolerated early after transplantation, although almost all patients experienced fever, fatigue, and in some cases a rash. Engraftment in the first cohort of 10 patients, who received IL-2-cultured marrow, was delayed. Subsequently, patients received IL-2-cultured bone marrow together with PBPC, and engraftment occurred in a timely fashion. Currently, patients are given IL-2-cultured PBPC preparations obtained from one leukapheresis.

Other centers are using a shorter incubation of HSC preparations (24–48 hours) together with high concentrations of IL-2 in the culture medium (5000 IU/mL). This approach is currently being tested for autologous transplants in patients with acute myelogenous or lymphoblastic leukemia in CR2,[16] non-Hodgkin lymphoma, and breast cancer.[40] Because all of these studies are uncontrolled, it will be difficult to conclude whether this culture procedure in IL-2 offers any benefit to patients.

Instead of culturing marrow/PBPC in IL-2 ex vivo, the cytokine has been administered to patients shortly before marrow or PBPC harvesting in an attempt to harvest activated cytotoxic cells with the graft.[41] Although this is tolerated by patients, more data are needed to decide whether it decreases posttransplantation relapse.

TREATMENT WITH NONSPECIFIC (NATURAL KILLER) AND SPECIFIC (T-CELL) ANTITUMOR CELLS

LAK cells can be generated from patients early after autologous transplantation. Infusion of these cells after high-dose chemotherapy and autografting is feasible with no adverse effects on engraftment.[42] Preliminary results from LAK cell infusions have suggested that there may be a decrease in the post-transplantation recurrence rate in patients with lymphoma.[43] The collection of LAK cells early after transplantation, however, has not been without problems: The leukapheresis can induce significant thrombocytopenia and the IL-2 can cause significant side effects. Cell lines with LAK cell–like activity have been shown to have remarkable antitumor effects in cell culture and animal experiments.[44] These cells, which can be expanded ex vivo, have a much higher cytotoxic activity against a broader spectrum of malignant target cells than autologous LAK cells. In particular, the NK-92 cell line holds promise for ex vivo purging and in vivo treatment because the cells are highly cytolytic against various malignant targets and have been shown to be able to eliminate human leukemia in severe combined immunodeficient (SCID) mice.[45]

Specific cytotoxic T lymphocytes directed against tumor-specific antigens can be generated ex vivo. Autologous T cells can be generated against malignant target cells.[46, 47] Because auologous tumor cells are usually poor antigen-presenting cells, may express Fas ligand (FasL), or produce suppressor factor for T cells, it could be more useful to use allogeneic (HLA-matched) T cells. This can be achieved either by immunizing the donor prior to transplantation or by using allogeneic T cells for ex vivo expansion.[48, 49] The latter approach has been shown to generate effective cytotoxic lymphocytes against cytomegalovirus and Epstein-Barr virus.

ANTIBODY-DIRECTED THERAPY AFTER TRANSPLANTATION

Serotherapy with monoclonal antibodies directed against tumor-specific surface molecules is an interesting treatment modality to overcome residual disease, but thus far the clinical results have been somewhat disappointing. Although antibodies can bind to the tumor antigen, they often lack the ability to activate cytotoxic mechanisms sufficiently to kill the tumor cells. Further, antigen-antibody complexes may be shed from the tumor surface, or circulating antigen may prevent the binding of the antibody to the tumor surface. Various cytotoxic entities, such as radioisotopes, toxins, or drugs, have been linked to the antibody.

Currently undergoing clinical evaluation are the anti-CD19 or anti-CD20 antibodies, which recognize B cells, for the post-transplantation treatment of patients with B-cell non-Hodgkin lymphoma.[50] Studies with an anti-CD15 monoclonal antibody are ongoing in myeloid leukemia.[51]

As commonly occurs with murine antibodies, antimouse antibodies can develop that neutralize the antibody. This will likely become less of a problem with the use of "humanized" antibodies that can be engineered to contain human constant regions and variable framework portions. Bifunctional antibodies are also at the stage of clinical exploitation. These antibodies can simultaneously recognize a tumor-cell-specific antigen and antigens on immune cells (i.e., CD3 or CD56).

NEW EXPERIMENTAL APPROACHES

Although a number of different cytokines and chemokines have been cloned, few have been tested thus far in patients. Particularly IL-12 can effectively generate LAK cells from lymphocytes of patients early after autologous or allogeneic transplantation.[52] It can also augment the purging of leukemia from PBPC collections when cocultured with IL-2.[53] Unfortunately, most of the cytokines, although effective in cell culture studies and animal experiments, will likely have unacceptable side effects in patients. This result has led to approaches that make use of targeted, site-specific cytokine release. One group of obvious carriers for cytokines are hematopoietic progenitor cells or marrow fibroblasts that are expected to "home" to the marrow after infusion, a site at which residual disease would remain.[54]

Most tumor cells are poor antigen-presenting cells and are incapable of inducing a cytotoxic T-cell response. This can be due to incomplete HLA expression or lack of expression of costimulatory molecules, such as B7.1/B7.2 and/or adhesion molecules, which are essential to provide the second activating signal to T cells after T-cell receptor engagement. Cytokine treatment (especially with IL-2) may circumvent these requirements and activate T cells directly. Further, certain cytokines are known to induce expression or up-regulation of adhesion molecules, allowing for better conjugate formation between effector and target cells.[55]

More recently, the use of dendritic cells as tumor antigen-presenting cells has developed into a new area of immunotherapy that could become particularly useful after HSCT. Initial reports from patients with B-cell lymphoma are encouraging.[56] Dendritic cells, which can easily be cultured and expanded from marrow or blood, can be engineered to present a tumor peptide on their surface. They can also be generated directly from malignant stem cells.[47] Certain cytokines are currently exploited with respect to augmenting either antigen presentation (e.g., granulocyte-macrophage colony-stimulating factor, GM-CSF) or specific lymphocyte proliferation (e.g., IL-2). Lastly, gene therapy–based approaches are being considered. Although some have shown antitumor effects in animal models, results in patients are not yet conclusive. The ex vivo transfer of cytokines or costimulatory surface antigen (e.g., B7) can

induce a systemic antitumor effect when the transfected malignant cells (after they have been irradiated) are returned to the animal.

The field of immunotherapy will continue to develop rapidly in coming years, and it is likely that it will assume an important role together with radiotherapy and chemotherapy in the treatment of malignant disease with allogeneic or autologous stem cell transplantation.

CONCLUSION

Therapy after autologous HSCT is needed to reduce the high relapse rate. Administration of new or higher doses of chemotherapeutic agents is limited by prior therapy and the conditioning regimen already given to the patient. Use of immune modulating cytokines or other drugs represents an attractive alternative. Dosing schedule and safety for molecules such as IFN, IL-2, and cyclosporine had been defined by various Phase I/II clinical trials, and the results showed that acceptable toxicity to patients could be achieved. For administration of IL-2 immediately after HSCT, some of the toxicity might be related to the use of total body irradiation in the conditioning regimen. Preliminary results on clinical outcome demonstrated that the therapy could reduce the relapse rate and improve disease-free survival. The timing is ripe for multi-center Phase III clinical trials to confirm the activity of the cytokines.

Phase I/II clinical trials using antibody directed against tumor makers after HSCT have just been initiated. Preliminary results were not as encouraging as those using cytokines or biologic response modifiers. Since the immunity of the patient is compromised and will take time for recovery, the antibodies may have to be conjugated with cytotoxic entities such as radioisotopes, toxins, and drugs to be effective. Additional Phase I/II trials are needed in this application. Trials testing therapeutic modalities combining immune modulating cytokines to activated T cells and/or dendritic cells are just beginning. Preliminary results on safety and toxicity are encouraging, but clinical outcomes are not yet available.

REFERENCES

1. Weiden PL, Flournoy N, Thomas ED, et al: Antileukemic effect of graft-versus-host disease in human recipients of allogeneic-marrow grafts. N Engl J Med 300:1068, 1979.
2. Gale RP, Horowitz MM, Ash RC, et al: Identical-twin bone marrow transplants for leukemia. Ann Intern Med 120:646, 1994.
3. Horowitz MM, Gale RP, Sondel PM, et al: Graft-versus-leukemia reactions after bone marrow transplantation. Blood 75:555, 1990.
4. Kolb HJ, Schattenberg A, Goldman JM, et al: Graft-versus-leukemia effect of donor lymphocyte transfusions in marrow grafted patients. Blood 86:2041, 1995.
5. Rosenberg SA, Lotze MT, Yang JC, et al: Prospective randomized trial of high-dose interleukin-2 alone or in conjunction with lymphokine-activated killer cells for the treatment of patients with advanced cancer. J Natl Cancer Inst 85:622, 1993.
6. Ludwig H, Cohen AM, Polliack A, et al: Interferon-alpha for induction and maintenance in multiple myeloma: results of two multicenter randomized trials and summary of other studies. Ann Oncol 6:467, 1995.
7. Westin J, Rodjer S, Turesson I, et al: Interferon alpha-2b versus no maintenance therapy during the plateau phase in multiple myeloma: a randomized study. Br J Haematol 89:561, 1995.

8. The Nordic Myeloma Study Group: Interferon-a2b added to melphalan-prednisone for initial and maintenance therapy in multiple myeloma. Ann Intern Med 124:212, 1996.

9. Browman GP, Bergsagel D, Sicheri D, et al: Randomized trial of interferon maintenance in multiple myeloma: a study of the National Cancer Institute of Canada Clinical Trials Group. J Clin Oncol 13:2354, 1995.

10. Smalley RV, Andersen JW, Hawkins MJ, et al: Interferon alfa combined with cytotoxic chemotherapy for patients with non-Hodgkin's lymphoma. N Engl J Med 327:1336, 1992.

11. Peest D, Leo R, Bloche S, et al: Low-dose recombinant interleukin-2 therapy in advanced multiple myeloma. Br J Haematol 89:328, 1995.

12. Maraninchi D, Blaise D, Viens P, et al: High-dose recombinant interleukin-2 and acute myeloid leukemias in relapse. Blood 78:2182, 1991.

13. Meloni G, Foa R, Vignetti M, et al: Interleukin-2 may induce prolonged remissions in advanced acute myelogenous leukemia. Blood 84:2158, 1994.

14. Foa R: Interleukin 2 in the management of acute leukaemia. Br J Haematol 92:1, 1996.

15. Gisselbrecht C, Maraninchi D, Pico JL, et al: Interleukin-2 treatment in lymphoma: a phase II multicenter study. Blood 83:2081, 1994.

16. Margolin KA, Wright C, Forman SJ: Autologous bone marrow purging by in situ IL-2 activation of endogenous killer cells. Leukemia 11:723–728, 1997.

17. Ratanatharathorn V, Uberti J, Karanes C, et al: Phase I study of alpha-interferon augmentation of cyclosporine-induced graft vs host disease in recipients of autologous bone marrow transplantation. Bone Marrow Transplant 13:625, 1994.

18. Powles R, Raje N, Cunningham D, et al: Maintenance therapy for remission in myeloma with intron A following high-dose melphalan and either an autologous bone marrow transplantation or peripheral stem cell rescue. Stem Cells 13(Suppl 2):114, 1995.

19. Attal M, Huguet F, Schlaifer D, et al: Maintenance treatment with recombinent alpha interferon after autologous bone marrow transplantation for aggressive myeloma in first remission after conventional induction chemotherapy. Bone Marrow Transplant 8:125, 1991.

20. Harousseau J, Attal M, Divine M, et al: Autologous stem cell transplantation after first remission induction treatment in multiple myeloma: a report of the French Registry on autologous transplantation in multiple myeloma. Blood 85:3077, 1995.

21. Meyers JD, Flournoy N, Sanders JE, et al: Prophylactic use of human leukocyte interferon after allogeneic marrow transplantation. Ann Intern Med 107:809, 1987.

22. Klingemann H-G, Grigg AP, Wilkie-Boyd K, et al: Treatment with recombinant interferon (lal-2b) early after bone marrow transplantation in patients at high risk for relapse. Blood 78:3306, 1991.

23. Higano CS, Raskind WH, Singer JW: Use of lal interferon for the treatment of relapse of chronic myelogenous leukemia in chronic phase after allogeneic bone marrow transplantation. Blood 80:1437, 1992.

24. Barnett MJ, Eaves CJ, Phillips GL, et al: Autografting with cultured marrow in chronic myeloid leukemia: results of a pilot study. Blood 84:724, 1994.

25. Blaise D, Olive D, Stoppa AM, et al: Hematologic and immunologic effects of the systemic administration of recombinant interleukin-2 after autologous bone marrow transplantation. Blood 76:1092, 1990.

26. Higuchi CM, Thompson JA, Petersen FB, et al: Toxicity and immunomodulatory effects of interleukin-2 after autologous bone marrow transplantation for hematologic malignancies. Blood 77:2561, 1991.

27. Weisdorf DJ, Anderson PM, Blazar BR, et al: Interleukin-2 immediately after autologous bone marrow transplantation for acute lymphoblastic leukemia—a phase I study. Transplantation 55:61, 1993.

28. Attal M, Blaise D, Marit G, et al: Consolidation treatment of adult acute lymphoblastic leukemia: a prospective, randomized trial comparing allogeneic versus autologous bone marrow transplantation and testing the impact of recombinant interleukin-2 after autologous bone marrow transplantation. Blood 86:1619, 1995.

29. Klingemann H-G, Eaves CJ, Barnett MJ, et al: Transplantation of patients with high risk acute myeloid leukemia in first remission with autologous marrow cultured in interleukin-2 followed by interleukin-2 administration. Bone Marrow Transplant 14:389, 1994.

30. Thompson JA, Bianco JA, Benyunes MC, et al: Phase Ib trial of pentoxifylline and ciprofloxacin in patients treated with interleukin-

31. Sykes M, Romick ML, Hoyles KA, Sachs DH: In vivo administration of interleukin-2 plus T cell–depleted syngeneic marrow prevents graft-vs-host disease mortality and permits alloengraftment. J Exp Med 171:645, 1990.

32. Przepiorka D, Ippoliti C, Koberda J, et al: Interleukin-2 for prevention of graft-versus-host disease after haploidentical marrow transplantation. Bone Marrow Transplant 58:858, 1994.

33. Verdonck LF, van Heugten HG, Giltay J, Franks CR: Amplification of the graft-versus-leukemia effect in man by interleukin-2. Transplantation 51:1120, 1991.

34. Robinson N, Sanders JE, Benyunes MC, et al: Phase I trial of interleukin-2 after unmodified HLA-matched sibling bone marrow transplantation for children with acute leukemia. Blood 87:1249, 1996.

35. Mehta J, Powles R, Singhal S, et al: Induction of graft-versus-host disease as immunotherapy of leukemia relapsing after allografting: single-center experience of 28 adults. Blood 88(Suppl 1):260a, 1996.

36. Long GS, Hiserodt JC, Harnaha JB, Cramer DV: Lymphokine-activated killer cell purging of leukemia cells from bone marrow prior to syngeneic transplantation. Transplantation 46:433, 1988.

37. Charak BS, Brynes RK, Groshen S, et al: Bone marrow transplantation with interleukin-2-activated bone marrow followed by interleukin-2 therapy for acute myeloid leukemia in mice. Blood 76:2187, 1990.

38. Klingemann H-G, Deal H, Reid D, Eaves CJ: Design and validation of a clinically applicable culture procedure for the generation of interleukin-2 activated natural killer cells in human bone marrow autografts. Exp Hematol 21:1263, 1993.

39. Klingemann H-G, Neerunjun J, Schwulera U, Ziltener HJ: Culture of normal and leukemia bone marrow in interleukin-2: analysis of cell activation, cell proliferation, and cytokine production. Leukemia 7:1389, 1993.

40. Meehan KR, Verma UN, Arun Kilic B, et al: Survival following interleukin-2 (IL-2) activated autologous PBSC transplantation and post transplant IL-2 therapy in women with breast cancer. Blood 88(Suppl 1):127a, 1996.

41. Messina C, Zambello R, Rossetti F, et al: Interleukin-2 before and/or after autologous bone marrow transplantation for pediatric acute leukemia patients. Bone Marrow Transplant 17:729, 1996.

42. Lister J, Donnenberg AD, deMagalhaes-Silverman M, et al: Autologous peripheral blood stem cell transplantation and adoptive immunotherapy with activated natural killer cells in the immediate post-transplant period. Clin Cancer Res 1:607, 1995.

43. Benyunes MC, Higuchi C, York A, et al: Immunotherapy with interleukin 2 with or without lymphokine activated killer cells after autologous bone marrow transplantation for malignant lymphoma: a feasibility trial. Bone Marrow Transplant 16:283, 1995.

44. Gong J, Maki G, Klingemann H-G: Characterization of a human cell line (NK-92) with phenotypical and functional characteristics of activated natural killer cells. Leukemia 8:652, 1994.

45. Klingemann H-G, Wong E, Maki G: A cytotoxic NK-cell line (NK-92) for ex vivo purging of leukemia from blood. Biol Blood Marrow Transplant 2:68, 1996.

46. Faber LM, van Luxemburg-Heijs SAP, Rijnbeek M, et al: Minor histocompatibility antigen-specific, leukemia-reactive cytotoxic T cell clones can be generated in vitro without in vivo priming using chronic myeloid leukemia cells as stimulators in the presence of α-interferon. Biol Blood Marrow Transplant 2:31, 1996.

47. Choudhury A, Gajewski JL, Liang JC, et al: Use of leukemia dendritic cells for the generation of antileukemic cellular cytotoxicity against philadelphia chromosome-positive chronic myelogenous leukemia. Blood 89:1133, 1997.

48. Kwak LW, Taub DD, Duffey PL, et al: Transfer of myeloma idiotype-specific immunity from an actively immunised marrow donor. Lancet 345:1016, 1995.

49. Heslop HE, Ng CYC, Li C, et al: Long-term restoration of immunity against Epstein-Barr virus infection by adoptive transfer of gene-modified virus-specific T lymphocytes. Nature Med 2:551, 1996.

50. Grossbard M, Press O, Appelbaum F, et al: Monoclonal antibody-based therapies of leukemia and lymphoma. Blood 80:863, 1992.

51. Ball ED, Selvaggi K, Hurd D, et al: A phase I clinical trial of serotherapy in patients with acute myeloid leukemia with an IgM monoclonal antibody to CD15. Clin Cancer Res 1:965, 1995.

52. Lindgren CG, Thompson JA, Robinson N, et al: Interleukin-12 induces cytolytic activity in lymphocytes from recipients of autologous and allogeneic stem cell transplants. Bone Marrow Transplant 19:867, 1987.
53. Wong EK, Eaves C, Klingemann H-G: Comparison of natural killer activity of human bone marrow and blood cells in cultures containing IL-2, IL-7 and IL-12. Bone Marrow Transplant 18:63, 1996.
54. Kühr T, Dougherty GJ, Klingemann H-G: Transfer of the tumor necrosis factor 1al gene into hematopoietic progenitor cells as a model for site-specific cytokine delivery after marrow transplantation. Blood 84:2966, 1994.
55. Maki G, Kristal G, Dougherty G, et al: Induction of sensitivity to NK-mediated cytotoxicity by TNF-α treatment: possible role of ICAM-3 and CD44. Leukemia 12:1565, 1998.

56. Hsu FJ, Benike C, Fagnoni F, et al: Vaccination of patients with B-cell lymphoma using autologous antigen-pulsed dendritic cells. Nature Med 2:51, 1996.
57. Blaise D, Stoppa AM, Viens P, et al: Intensive immunotherapy with recombinant IL2 after autologous bone marrow transplantation is associated with a high incidence of bacterial infections. Bone Marrow Transplant 10:193, 1992.
58. Caligiuri MA, Murray C, Soiffer RJ, et al: Extended continuous infusion low dose recombinant interleukin-2 in advanced cancer: prolonged immunomodulation without significant toxicity. J Clin Oncol 9:2110, 1991.
59. Powell FC, Spooner KM, Shawker TH, et al: Symptomatic interleukin-2 induced cholecystopathy in patients with HIV infection. Am J Roentgenol 163:117, 1994.

CHAPTER FIFTY-NINE

Post-Transplant Cytotoxic Therapy

Margarida de Magalhães-Silverman, M.D.

Hematopoietic stem cell transplantation (HSCT) is widely used in the treatment of acquired or genetic, neoplastic or non-neoplastic disorders.[1] The curative effect of allogeneic HSCT has been ascribed to high-dose chemotherapy with or without radiation and the antitumor effect of the graft.[2, 3] The considerable mortality and morbidity, together with the need for a human leukocyte antigen (HLA)-compatible donor, limit the application of allogeneic transplants to a small portion of younger patients (≤50 years old). Autologous HSCT has been widely used to treat patients with leukemia, lymphoma, myeloma, and certain solid tumors. The transplant-related mortality and morbidity associated with autografting is much lower than that associated with allografting. The success of autologous HSCT, however, is limited by a high incidence of relapses. This is attributed to residual malignant cells, which survive the conditioning regimen, and/or tumor cells, which may have been infused with the graft.

Thus, strategies to improve outcomes of patients receiving high-dose therapy and autologous HSCT must be designed to enhance antitumor effects. Such strategies may include more dose-intensive chemotherapy regimens, the use of more-effective induction regimens, induction of an autologous graft-versus-tumor effect, and post-transplantation therapies. This chapter reviews the use of post-transplantation cytotoxic chemotherapy. Special attention focuses on metastatic breast cancer.

BREAST CANCER

Breast cancer is the most frequently diagnosed cancer in American women and the second most common cause of death.[4] Although approximately 80% of patients with breast cancer present with disease limited to the breast and/or axilla, almost half of these patients eventually experience metastatic disease and succumb to it. Therefore, better therapies for patients with high-risk primary and advanced breast cancer are needed. The role of high-dose chemotherapy and autologous HSC support as treatment for breast cancer remains controversial (see Chapter 10). The rationale for autotransplants in breast cancer is based on the dose-response relationship between many chemotherapy agents and breast cancer. Most studies of high-dose chemotherapy have been uncontrolled phase I and II trials.[5-7] Until recently, only several small phase III trials[8-10] had

appeared in the literature, but in general these trials were too small or the follow-ups were too short to draw firm conclusions. Preliminary data from four trials were presented at the 1999 American Society of Clinical Oncology meeting.[11-14] Although it is still unclear whether benefit can be derived from high-dose chemotherapy with HSC support when applied in addition to conventional chemotherapy, the relatively low disease-free survival rate demanded that investigations into new approaches be conducted.

Tallman et al.[15] reported on a series of patients with metastatic breast cancer treated with an Adriamycin-based induction regimen, high-dose chemotherapy consisting of cyclophosphamide and thiotepa with autologous HSC rescue, and finally post-transplantation 5-fluorouracil and cisplatin. The goal of post-transplantation cytotoxic therapy was the eradication of a small number of malignant cells that might have been unknowingly reinfused with the autograft. Patients were eligible to receive post-transplantation chemotherapy if they achieved either complete response or partial response, or had stable disease after high-dose therapy and adequate hematopoietic reserve, defined as a platelet count of at least 50,000/mm³ and an absolute neutrophil count (ANC) of 1,000/mm³. The therapy was to begin no earlier than 60 days after transplantation or when the platelet count and ANC count met the given criteria.

Four cycles delivered every 3–4 weeks were planned. A total of 48 patients were enrolled in the study. Thirty-three patients (69%) received at least one cycle of therapy. Fifteen patients (31%) were able to receive all four planned cycles. Fifteen patients (31%) did not receive post-transplantation chemotherapy because of either early death (two patients) or progressive disease. Toxicities of the chemotherapy were quite limited among the 33 patients receiving at least one cycle. Ten patients (33%) experienced myelosuppression. No reason was stated for why 18 patients received only one cycle of therapy instead of the planned four.

The overall survival rate for patients receiving all four cycles was reported to be 40% (95% CI, 11–74%), compared with 20% for patients not receiving post-transplantation chemotherapy. The event-free survival and overall survival among the patients receiving four cycles of post-transplantation therapy was better than those for patients not receiving such treatment. The authors, however, cautioned that the results should be interpreted carefully. It is possible that the patients eligible to receive the post-transplantation therapy were those with the least amount of disease at transplantation. Alternatively, these patients might have had the more chemosensitive disease. Because this was not a prospective randomized trial, it is possible that these patients would have done as well without the post-transplantation therapy.

In another trial,[16] 21 patients with metastatic breast cancer were treated with cyclophosphamide followed by HSC collection. Notably, the trial design did not include induction chemotherapy to determine chemoresponsiveness. All patients received the STAMP V (cyclophosphamide, thiotepa, carboplatin) regimen followed by HSC support. Upon recovery from hematopoietic and gastrointestinal toxicities, three cycles of doxorubicin at 60 mg/m² were planned. Fifty-five of the 63 cycles of post-transplantation therapy were delivered. All but one patient received post-transplantation chemotherapy. The median time from HSCT to the first cycle was 38 days. After STAMP V, 13 patients (62%) experienced a complete or partial response. The response rate increased to 81% after post-transplantation chemotherapy. The authors concluded that post-transplantation administration of doxorubicin was feasible.

In a subsequent study,[17] the same investigators attempted to deliver three cycles of doxorubicin and taxol after STAMP V and HSCT for metastatic breast cancer. The authors assumed that the high relapse rate after autografting reflected the survival of resistant cancer cells among heterogeneous clones in the original tumor and that post-transplantation therapy with non–cross-resistant agents would eliminate additional clones. Twenty-four patients were treated with high-dose cyclophosphamide and etoposide followed by HSC collection. Patients then proceeded to receive STAMP V with HSC support. All patients, irrespective of response, were eligible to receive three cycles of post-transplantation doxorubicin at 50 mg/m² and Taxol at 150 mg/m². A total of 69 (87% of planned) cycles of post-transplantation therapy was delivered. The median time from transplantation to the first cycle was 38 days. Because the possibility of progressive decline of marrow reserve with the use of chemotherapy immediately after transplantation was a major concern, autograft stability was examined 6 months after transplantation, with all patients demonstrating a normal platelet and leukocyte count. With this strategy, the overall response rate was 66%.

In another study concerning metastatic breast cancer, Rahman et al.[18] tested the feasibility of administering multiple cycles of escalating doses of paclitaxel after HSCT. The fear of irreversibly damaging the newly engrafted HSC with post-transplantation chemotherapy was alleviated by transducing the marrow progenitor cells with the multidrug-resistant (MDR-1) gene. The transduced cells were shown to exhibit preferential resistance to paclitaxel in preclinical laboratory studies.[19, 20]

In the trial, autologous CD34+ cells from patients with metastatic breast cancer were exposed to a replication-incompetent retroviral vector carrying MDR-1 complementary DNA and then reinfused after high-dose chemotherapy. The hypothesis was that transduced autologous HSC would be less sensitive to paclitaxel and, by giving paclitaxel immediately after transplantation, it is possible that the tumor cells damaged by high-dose chemotherapy would

be more sensitive to paclitaxel in the immediately post-transplantation period.

Ten patients were enrolled. The marrow cells of three patients contained vector MDR-1–positive cells only at the time of the first course of post-transplantation paclitaxel, indicating that the MDR-1 vector–modified cells had only short-term engrafting potential. Most of the courses of paclitaxel were therefore delivered in the absence of detectable MDR-1 transduced cells. A total of 83 courses of paclitaxel was administered starting at a median of 30 days from transplantation. The median dose of paclitaxel was 225 mg/m².

All patients except one tolerated the post-transplantation cytotoxic therapy well without excessive toxicity. No delayed toxicity or bone-marrow failure was noted in these patients at a median follow-up of 2 years after transplantation, and no myelodysplasia was reported. Three patients who had achieved less than a complete response to high-dose chemotherapy were converted to complete response during post-transplantation paclitaxel therapy. The investigators concluded that paclitaxel could be safely administered after transplantation and that post-transplantation therapy could further improve the response of patients with metastatic breast cancer.

These studies suggest that post-transplantation chemotherapy can be safely delivered. Patients tolerated well the additional chemotherapy, which did not appear to irreversibly damage the newly engrafted HSC. The choice of drugs and timing of administration would likely depend on the induction chemotherapy and conditioning regimens. Large phase I/II clinical trials may address this issue. Whether the use of post-transplantation cytotoxic chemotherapy is of value remains to be investigated. This question can only be answered by randomized controlled trials. In view of the controversy and the disappointing success rates of a single course of high-dose therapy with autologous HSCT for metastatic breast cancer, this disease would be a highly appropriate target for the study of post-transplantation cytotoxic therapy.

OTHER MALIGNANCY

Bregni et al.[21] reported on seven patients with stage III ovarian cancer who achieved a partial response or progression after high-dose chemotherapy supported by autologous peripheral blood progenitor cells (PBPC). Patients received epirubicin (50–80 mg/m²) and paclitaxel (175 mg/m²). A median of seven cycles was delivered, and the time between cycles was 21 days. In only one case, treatment was delayed by 1 week. At the end of post-transplantation therapy, two patients were in pathologic complete remission. The authors concluded that in patients with ovarian cancer who do not achieve a pathologic complete remission after transplantation, conventional-dose post-transplantation therapy is feasible, and in some cases additional responses might be achieved.

A randomized study[22] showed that high-dose chemotherapy with autologous HSC rescue improves both disease-free and overall survival in previously untreated patients with multiple myeloma compared with conventional chemotherapy. A study by the Southwest Oncology Group[23] comparing high-dose therapy and autologous transplantation with conventional chemotherapy confirmed those results. A majority of patients experienced relapse, however. In an attempt to decrease the relapse rate, several approaches were investigated, including tandem autotransplants and post-transplantation vaccination using anti-idiotype or dendritic cells.

Several investigators are exploring post-transplantation cytotoxic therapy. A combination of dexamethasone pulsing with 4 days' continuous infusion of cyclophosphamide, etoposide, and cisplatin (DCEP) has been found to be an effective therapy after HSCT.[24] This post-transplantation regimen has been evaluated in a trial for high-risk myeloma patients. Preliminary results in 48 patients (Barlogie B: Personal communication) demonstrated superior event-free survival and overall survival compared with similar patients not given DCEP. Other investigators are exploring the alternation of DCEP with a combination of dexamethasone, paclitaxel, and cisplatin in the same patient population.

Bassan et al.[25] reported on a trial in newly diagnosed adult acute lymphoblastic leukemia (ALL) using an idarubicin-containing regimen for induction followed by consolidation with unpurged autologous bone marrow supported with high-dose therapy. Additional post-transplantation chemotherapy consisted of vincristine, cyclophosphamide, teniposide, and cytarabine given for 12 weeks and low-dose maintenance for 6 months. Ninety-six patients were enrolled in this trial, and 74 patients received post-transplantation therapy. A total of 273 cycles were delivered. Toxicity was minimal. The 5-year disease-free survival rate with this approach was 31%. Post-transplantation cytotoxic therapy was delivered with the goal of eliminating acute leukemia cells infused with the autograft. The authors concluded that post-transplantation therapy could be safely delivered but its place in the treatment of patients with ALL in first remission remains ill-defined.

In another study, Powles et al.[26] evaluated the use of maintenance chemotherapy after autografting for ALL. Fifty consecutive patients in first remission received melphalan and total body irradiation followed by autologous HSC (marrow or PBPC) transplantation. After hematologic recovery, 6-mercaptopurine and methotrexate were administered for 2 years. No graft failure resulted from the post-transplantation cytotoxic therapy. The 5-year overall survival rate was 56.2%, and the relapse rate was 30.6%. When results were compared with results in patients receiving chemotherapy alone, the investigators concluded that the administration of maintenance chemotherapy after autografting might reduce relapse in adult ALL. A randomized study is necessary to evaluate the role of that form of post-transplantation therapy, however.

CONCLUSION

Relapse after autologous HSCT remains a major cause of treatment failure. Preliminary studies using post-transplantation cytotoxic therapy indicate that this form of treatment is feasible within a short time after HSCT and is associated with acceptable toxicity. Several questions remain unanswered: Whether this form of therapy can im-

prove the overall cure rate of HSCT, the optimal timing, and the most-effective drug with respect to different diseases and prior treatment regimens. The role of post-transplantation cytotoxic therapy in tumor eradication can only be determined by well-designed phase III clinical trials.

REFERENCES

1. de Magalhaes-Silverman M, Donnenberg AD, Pincus SM, Ball ED: Bone marrow transplantation: a review. Cell Transplant 2:75–98, 1993.
2. Horowitz, MM, Gale RP, Sondel PM, et al: Graft-versus-leukemia reactions after bone marrow transplantation. Blood 75:555–562, 1990.
3. Weiden PL, Sullivan KM, Flournoy N, et al: Antileukemic effect of chronic graft-versus-disease: contribution to improved survival after allogeneic marrow transplantation. N Engl J Med 304:1529–1533, 1981.
4. Landis SH, Murray T, Bolden S, et al: Cancer statistics, 1998. CA Cancer J Clin 48:6–29, 1998.
5. Peters WP: Autologous bone marrow transplantation for breast cancer. Curr Opin Oncol 4:279–282, 1992.
6. Antman KH, Rowlings PA, Vaughn WP, et al: High-dose chemotherapy with autologous hematopoietic stem cell support for breast cancer in North America. J Clin Oncol 15:1870–1879, 1997.
7. Lazarus HM: Hematopoietic progenitor cell transplantation in breast cancer: current status and future directions. Cancer Invest 16:102–126, 1998.
8. Bezwoda WR, Seymour L, Dansey RD: High-dose chemotherapy with hematopoietic rescue as primary treatment for metastatic breast cancer: a randomized trial. J Clin Oncol 13:2483–2489, 1995.
9. Rutqvist LE: Randomized adjuvant breast cancer trials in Sweden. Cancer 74(Suppl 3):1135–1138, 1994.
10. Rodenhuis S, Richel DJ, Van der Wall E: Randomized trial of high-dose chemotherapy and haematopoietic progenitor cell support in operable breast cancer with extensive axillary lymph-node involvement. Lancet 352(9127):515–521, 1998.
11. Stadtmauer E, O'Neal A, Goldstein L, et al: Phase III randomized trial of high-dose chemotherapy and stem cell support shows no difference in overall survival or severe toxicity compared to maintenance chemotherapy with cyclophosphamide, methotrexate and 5-fluorouracil (CMF) for women with metastatic breast cancer who are responding to conventional induction chemotherapy: the "Philadelphia" Intergroup Study (PBT-1) [Abstract 1]. Proc ASCO 18, 1999.
12. Peters W, Rosner G, Vredenburgh J, et al: A prospective randomized comparison of two doses of combination alkylating agents (AA) as consolidation after CAF in high-risk primary breast cancer involving ten or more axillary lymph nodes (LN): preliminary results of CALGB 9082/SWOG 9114/NCIC MA-13 [Abstract 2]. Proc ASCO 18, 1999.
13. The Scandinavian Breast Cancer Study Group 9401: Results from a Randomized Adjuvant Breast Cancer Study with high dose chemotherapy with CTCb supported by autologous bone marrow stem cells versus dose escalated and tailored FEC therapy [Abstract 3]. Proc ASCO 18, 1999.
14. Bezwoda WR: Randomized controlled trial of high dose chemotherapy (HD-CNVp) versus standard dose (CAF) chemotherapy for high risk surgically treated primary breast cancer [Abstract 4]. Proc ASCO 18, 1999.
15. Tallman MS, Rademaker AW, Jahnke L, et al: High-dose chemotherapy, autologous bone marrow or stem cell transplantation and post-transplant consolidation chemotherapy in patients with advanced breast cancer. Bone Marrow Transplant 20:721–729, 1997.
16. de Magalhães-Silverman M, Bloom E, Lembersky B, et al: High-dose chemotherapy and autologous stem cell support followed by post-transplantation doxorubicin as initial therapy for metastatic breast cancer. Clin Cancer Res 3:193–197, 1997.
17. de Magalhaes-Silverman M, Hammert L, Lembersky B, et al: High-dose chemotherapy and autologous stem cell support followed by post-transplant doxorubicin and Taxol as initial therapy for metastatic breast cancer: hematopoietic tolerance and efficacy. Bone Marrow Transplant 21:1207–1211, 1998.
18. Rahman Z, Kavanagh J, Champlin R, et al: Chemotherapy immedi-

ately following autologous stem-cell transplantation in patients with advanced breast cancer. Clin Cancer Res 4:2717–2721, 1998.

19. Hanania E, Giles R, Claxton D, et al: Post-transplant frequency of genetically modified cells using retroviral-mediated multiple drug resistance (MDR-1) stromal transduction protocol in breast and ovarian cancers [Abstract 2363]. Proc Am Assoc Cancer Res 37, 1996.

20. Hanania E, Fu S, Zu Z, et al: Chemotherapy resistance to taxol in clonogenic progenitor cells following transduction of CD34 selected marrow and peripheral blood cells with a retrovirus that contains the MDR-1 chemotherapy resistance gene. Gene Ther 2:285–294, 1995.

21. Bregni M, Marzola M, Di Nicola M, et al: Full-dose conventional chemotherapy is feasible and effective after tandem high-dose treatments supported by mobilized blood autografting [Abstract 342]. Proc ASCO 17, 1998.

22. Attal M, Harrousseau J, Stoppa A, et al: A prospective, randomized trial of autologous bone marrow transplantation and chemotherapy in multiple myeloma. N Engl J Med 335:91–97, 1996.

23. Barlogie B, Jagannath SW, Desikan KR, et al: Total therapy with tandem transplants for newly diagnosed multiple myeloma. Blood 93:55–65, 1999.

24. Munshi N, Desikan KR, Jagannath S, et al: Dexamethasone, cyclophosphamide, etoposide, and cis-platinum (DCEP), an effective regimen for relapse after high-dose chemotherapy and autologous transplantation (AT) [Abstract 586a]. Blood 88, 1996.

25. Bassan R, Lerede T, Di Bona E, et al: Induction-consolidation with an idarubicin-containing regimen, unpurged marrow autograft, and postgraft chemotherapy in adult acute lymphoblastic leukemia. Br J Haematol 104:755–762, 1999.

26. Powles R, Mehta J, Singhal S, et al: Autologous bone marrow or peripheral blood stem cell transplantation followed by maintenance chemotherapy for adult acute lymphoblastic leukemia in first remission: 50 cases from a single center. Bone Marrow Transplant 16:241–247, 1995.

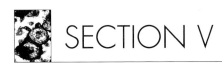

SECTION V

Associated Issues

Psychosocial Considerations

CHAPTER SIXTY

Psychosocial Considerations: A Family Approach to Patient Care

Joyce Herschl, M.S.W.

Hematopoietic stem cell transplantation (HSCT) has been improved by numerous technological advances.[1-4] In spite of the advances, HSCT continues to be associated with a high risk of physical and psychosocial morbidity along with a significant risk of mortality.[3] HSCT is a rigorous medical and psychological experience that often results in psychosocial distress that permeates the entire family unit,[5, 6] and alters the emotional balance of even previously well-adjusted patients and families.[7]

This chapter addresses the often complex psychosocial aspects of the transplantation experience. An adult patient's care can be measurably improved when the patient/family unit is understood as an interdependent system with the needs of the patient, donor, and family being addressed.[8] The concept of family in this discussion includes both traditional and nontraditional relationships.

BIOPSYCHOSOCIAL STAGES OF TRANSPLANTATION

The stages of transplantation were first delineated by Brown and Kelly.[9] The stages encompass the entire spectrum of the transplantation experience: (1) the decision, (2) evaluation and care planning, (3) immunosuppression and isolation, (4) transplantation, (5) graft rejection or "take," (6) Graft-versus-host disease (GVHD), (7) discharge, and (8) adaptation.[9] Haberman similarly identified six phases of HSCT: (1) making the decision, (2) preadmission, (3) conditioning, (4) immunosuppression, (5) transplantation, and (6) discharge to outpatient status.[2] With each stage/phase, congruent psychosocial markers are identified, emphasizing that the psychological responses are not indicative of rigid patterns.[2, 9] The process, in fact, is often nonlinear, with transient responses that may overlap.[2] Common to both models is the concomitance of medical and psychosocial factors. Acknowledging both approaches, this chapter chronicles three phases of the biopsychosocial experience: (1) evaluation and preparation for transplantation, (2) the transplantation process, and (3) transition to ambulatory care and recovery (Table 60–1).

EVALUATION AND PREPARATION FOR TRANSPLANTATION

The process begins with determining eligibility and the patient's decision to proceed with transplantation. It is important to recognize that family members often play a crucial role in the decision-making process.[10] Consequently, inclusion of the family in the evaluation for HSCT reinforces the utmost importance of family in the plan of treatment.

A multidisciplinary team approach is most effective in the evaluation of candidates for HSCT. A model for such an approach is illustrated in Figure 60–1. The team includes HSCT physicians, protocol coordinators, nurse practitioners, a utilization review/case manager, a clinical social worker, a financial analyst, and a patient care coordinator. Each plays a significant role, working synergistically together to complete a medical, physical, and psychosocial evaluation.[11]

With a goal of establishing protocol eligibility, a medical history, physical examination, blood work, and bone marrow biopsies are routinely performed. Then begins the process of informed consent, discussed later in greater detail, with the candid explanation of the risks and benefits of HSCT.[2, 9] Patients and families come to the intake evaluation with wide variations in their baseline knowledge of HSCT. This can range from sophisticated data acquired from the National Cancer Institute or professional journals to personalized accounts obtained from magazines, the Internet, and/or other patients. It is important to evaluate their cognitive understanding in order to rectify myths and/or incorrect information.

The evaluation process is designed to provide optimal information, including clarification of previously held ideas, in order to increase the knowledge base and facilitate the decision-making of the patient and family. Andrykowski suggests that the provision of information by the HSCT physician may actually have a minimal impact on the patient's decision.[3] Most patients make their decision in favor of HSCT before coming to the transplant center because of their hope for a cure.[2, 9] Only a small portion of patients who meet the selection criteria for HSCT decline the procedure.[3, 12] Patients are also strongly influenced by the recommendation of their referring physician, who often states much-higher rates for survival with HSCT.[2, 13] This is in contrast to the more-realistic statistics and in-depth information offered by the HSCT physician.[2] The discordant information at times leads to feelings of disbelief, anger, and/or resentment directed toward the referring physician. The resulting cognitive dissonance seldom affects the patient's decision to undergo HSCT, but may affect the professional relationship with the referring physician.

TABLE 60–1. BIOPSYCHOSOCIAL STAGES OF BLOOD AND MARROW TRANSPLANTATION

CHRONOLOGY OF STAGES	PSYCHOSOCIAL CONSIDERATIONS
1. Evaluation and preparation for transplantation	Process of informed consent
	Hope for a cure
	Risks and benefits
	Financial and insurance concerns
	Rigorous testing—waiting for results
	Organization of personal affairs
	Advanced directives
	Vocational/educational disruption
	Tension and anxiety
	Anxious anticipation
2. The transplantation process	Geographic dislocation
	Family disruption
	Role reversal
	Isolation
	Toxic conditioning regimen
	Noxious side effects
	Dependence
	Regression
	Pervasive uncertainty
	Pain and despair
	Complications
	Family stress
	Engraftment
3. Transition to ambulatory care and recovery	Renewed hope
	Caregiver stress
	Separation anxiety
	Re-entry into family life
	Altered body image
	Chronic symptoms
	Cognitive impairment
	Rigorous follow-up regimen
	Role changes
	Sexual reconnection
	Catastrophic financial constraints
	Vocational/educational re-entry
	Renormalization
	Adaptation

Adapted from Brown H, Kelly M: Stages of bone marrow transplantation: a psychiatric perspective. Psychosom Med 38(6):439–446, 1976; and Haberman M: Psychosocial aspects of bone marrow transplantation. Semin Oncol Nurs 4(2):55–59, 1988.

After the provision of medical information and the comprehensive assessment for HSCT, the entire team meets to present and discuss each HSCT candidate. The treatment plan, which may or may not include a recommendation for HSCT, is agreed on by the team and subsequently presented to patient and family by the physician. Again, the emphasis is on inclusion of the family. Most centers will not deny HSCT as a treatment option solely because of psychological and/or psychosocial factors.[1, 5, 14] Instead, candidates are usually excluded from HSCT as the result of disease status alone.[13] Moreover, if an acceptable candidate presents with premorbid psychological and/or behavioral problems, it becomes imperative to develop a psychotherapeutic treatment plan, which may include psychopharmacologic agents, to effectively care for the patient.[1, 15]

INFORMED CONSENT

As stated, discussion of the risks and benefits of HSCT in the evaluation process initiates the process of informed consent. The process is typically one of extreme anxiety for patient and family. Consent forms are both explicit and terrifying. The risks, such as drug toxicities, veno-occlusive disease, and graft rejection—to name a few—are often incomprehensible. Patients subsequently tend to selectively absorb the information presented by the physician, redefining the biomedical data to make them more acceptable to themselves.[16] This phenomenon, which usually leads to unrealistic optimism, is indicative of a defense mechanism used in the face of stress and adversity.[3] Overly optimistic expectations, however, have been correlated with poor postoperative adjustment in renal transplant studies.[17] It is therefore essential for the physician to provide a realistic assessment of the potential outcome without compromising healthy amounts of denial.[3, 9, 17]

In spite of information and data that may seem equivocal to the patient and family, a decision to undergo HSCT becomes a calculated gamble based on one's personal philosophy of life.[2, 16, 18] At the foundation of the decision is the knowledge that HSCT can "cure or kill."[16] Patients and families typically latch on to the possibility of "cure" and are therefore willing to take the risk. Patients tend to focus on more tangible concerns, such as hair loss, rather than address the more emotionally charged issues of morbidity and mortality.[9] This is typically a coping strategy used by the patient to diffuse and minimize the inherent vulnerability of undergoing transplantation.[14]

PSYCHOEDUCATIONAL MODEL

A psychoeducational model for teaching is proposed to promote a sense of mastery for each patient and family prior to admission. Education, support, and reinforcement should be provided by all members of the transplant team. This should include a tour of the transplant unit and the ambulatory care clinic and a step-by-step explanation of what to expect during treatment and after discharge from the hospital. This is a dynamic process that should include on-site visits and informational sessions along with ongoing telephone contacts. An exploration of available resources should also be included, with patients and families being made aware of peer support programs, self-image programs, behavioral medicine, support groups, psychosexual counseling, reproductive counseling (including sperm banking), and other support services. A certain amount of bonding takes place between patient/family and the HSCT team during this period of preparation. The resulting sense of intimacy in the professional relationship can be maximized to promote trust and encourage patient/family participation in the plan of treatment.[1, 15]

PSYCHOSOCIAL ASSESSMENT

Critical to the evaluation process for HSCT is a psychosocial assessment of patient and family completed by a clinical social worker.[10, 19] Included in the assessment interview is preparatory information about what to expect during the transplantation process.[16] A patient may be interviewed separately or with his or her family. Generally, the latter promotes a more insightful assessment of the support system, roles, communication patterns, and family dynamics.

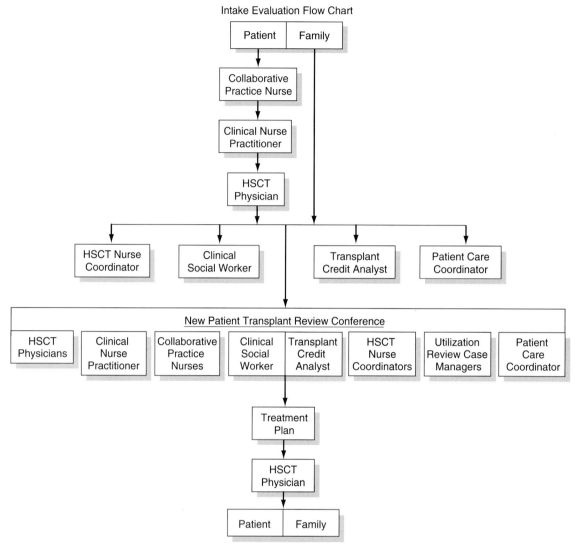

FIGURE 60–1. Hematopoietic stem cell transplant (HSCT) team approach to the evaluation of the potential transplant candidate.

The intrinsic goal of an assessment is to develop a better understanding of the patient as an individual[9] and how he or she functions within the family system. A clinician can then more effectively predict the patient's ability to tolerate the often formidable process of transplantation.[1] Additionally, insight to the family's capacity to maintain its equilibrium throughout the patient's treatment can also be assessed.[10]

Quantitatively, a psychosocial assessment should include a significant amount of concrete data, such as demographics, insurance coverage, medical history, employment/income status, education, and use of resources. Qualitatively, the psychological component of the assessment should most importantly include (1) prior psychiatric history, (2) quality of family and social support, and (3) prior history of coping.[5] Finally, a comprehensive evaluation should include other salient information such as quality of affect, meaning and impact of illness, roles and responsibilities, proneness to anxiety, strengths and weaknesses, mental status, functional ability, cultural and spiritual needs, and repertoire of coping strategies.[1, 5, 15, 17, 19, 20] The domain of coping, in particular, may range from denial to mastery. How a patient

has coped with previous stressful life events is usually an indicator of how he or she will cope with transplantation.

The HSCT experience permeates the entire family unit; consequently, an assessment of the family system is an essential part of the screening process. Because the family is traditionally the mainstay of support, the family unit needs to remain functional and strong.[8] Regardless of how functional they may appear at the onset, families will undoubtedly be affected by the stressors of the procedure.[7, 10, 19] More specifically, the emotional impact may lead to problems in communication, role performances, and disruption of the patient's care. In general, families have inherent weaknesses that can lead to dysfunction when triggered by a serious life event such as a health crisis.[8] The stressors of transplantation can also exacerbate dysfunction that had previously been dormant.[8] Crucial to the assessment is the determination of how the family system operated before the health crisis and what changes to expect with the recommendation for HSCT.[9]

Given the current paradigm shift to ambulatory care in HSCT, a caregiver evaluation becomes a key component of the psychosocial assessment as far more caregiving responsibilities are being placed on family members.[21] A caregiver, whether family member or friend, should be a responsible adult who is available 24 hours per day to assist the patient as needed. Some patients, out of necessity, choose to have more than one caregiver share the responsibility. To ensure continuity, however, it is advisable to limit the caregiver selection to no more than two persons. Designated caregivers must then be assessed for the capacity to monitor the patient's condition, manage the side effects of treatment, monitor medications, and provide therapy in the home or temporary lodging.[22] A caregiver assessment can be accomplished through an interview and/or a specifically designed questionnaire. In particular, a caregiver's willingness and ability to perform the role need to be evaluated. Caregivers should then be reassured that in-depth instruction and ongoing educational reinforcement will be provided by the HSCT team.

In allogeneic transplantation, the social worker needs to assess the donor's psychological stability, his or her attitude toward being a donor, the existence of any family pressures, and the premorbid history of the donor/recipient relationship.[1, 6] Although there are few physiologic consequences of donating marrow, intense emotions can surface if the recipient experiences GVHD or dies.[17] Consequently, it is important for the donor to be an active participant in the evaluation process when education is provided regarding the inherent complications of HSCT and the related emotional responses.[6, 17] In particular, donors should be counseled with regard to the fantasy of "rescue" often experienced by marrow donors, the potential for graft failure or GVHD, and the possibility of recipient death.

Lastly, psychometric testing used in concert with a screening interview is effective as a predictive tool in the evaluation process.[23] Standardized testing may be used to measure family functioning, roles, social support, self-esteem, coping, mood, distress, life satisfaction, and psychiatric morbidity, all key elements of a comprehensive screening evaluation.[24] The subsequent measurement of psychosocial variables systematically identifies psychological, psychosocial, and/or behavioral problems early on and therefore facilitates prevention and intervention.[23, 25]

Many standardized instruments can be used in conjunction with a clinical interview. Measurement through screening tools, however, should be standard with psychosocial oncology.[24] Secondary to usefulness in the initial evaluation, psychosocial variables measured before transplantation may be used in quality-of-life studies post discharge. The Brief Symptom Inventory (BSI) is advocated as an effective screening tool that can quickly identify high-risk patients.[10, 24] A short version of Symptom Checklist–90–Revised (SCL-90-R), the BSI consists of 53 items that have been validated in large samples of psychiatric patients as well as normative samples.[26] More specifically, the BSI measures psychological symptoms of distress.[26] Given the prevalence of high distress during all phases of transplantation, vulnerable patients may be identified early on through the BSI. The subsequent psychological profile can then be used in planning intervention while also establishing a database for research studies.[27]

FINANCIAL/INSURANCE ISSUES

Financial/insurance concerns are critical to the decision-making process for most patients and families. Financial issues are often overwhelming to patients and families at a time when they are most distraught and vulnerable. Consequently, these issues must be addressed up front and included in the screening process. Meeting with the financial analyst, who is employed by the hospital to evaluate insurance coverage and is part of the HSCT team, helps to identify any specific gaps in coverage.[19] Related and/or ongoing financial/insurance concerns can be further addressed with the social worker. The following examples illustrate potential difficulties related to finances and insurance. First, third-party payers may still consider HSCT for certain diseases as experimental therapy and thus deny coverage.[28] Second, donor expenses in allogeneic HSCT are not always covered by the donor's or the recipient's insurance plans.[28] Third, insurance coverage may be approved for HSCT but with a significant copayment for the patient (i.e. 20–30%) or with a limited yearly or lifetime maximum of insurance benefits. Finally, in addition to gaps in insurance coverage, families are also confronted with the extraordinary expense of having to relocate to the geographic area of the transplant center, including housing, transportation, meals, long-distance phone calls, and child care, to name a few. These additional expenses come at a time when the family income has often been significantly reduced. It has been my experience that some patients who do not want to become a burden to their families choose not to undergo HSCT when financial indebtedness is likely.

Financial concerns need to be candidly discussed to help patients and families in mobilizing any available resources.[19] Although resources are scarce in the present economy, the social worker can make referrals to assist the patient and family with transplant-related expenses, such as medications, supplies, durable medical equipment, temporary lodging, transportation, and meals. Referrals can also be made to programs specifically designed to assist with formal fund raising, payment for human leukocyte antigen (HLA) testing, and other extraordinary expenses. Such resource utilization encompasses internal (hospital-sponsored) programs, community agencies, and national organizations.

PATIENT SEQUELAE

Once the physician and the transplant candidate agree to proceed with HSCT, the patient begins what may seem like an endless process of testing, procedures, consultations, and waiting.[16] This phase is typically filled with tension and anxiety.[9, 19] In addition, because of the pervasive fear of disease progression during this waiting period, a sense of urgency may prevail.[9, 16] It is also common for patients to have "second thoughts" about their decision to undergo HSCT, but most proceed with the treatment.[12]

Preparing for admission requires a great deal of organization and planning at a time when the patient is often overwhelmed by the emotional aspects of the treatment. For example, there are arrangements to prepare for absence from work, school, and/or home. Child care is a major issue when the patient is a young parent. As discussed, financial and insurance matters must be addressed, along with the burdensome process of applying for disability benefits and/or supplemental income.[19] Patients should also explore the feasibility of having their insurance plan switched to the Consolidated Omnibus Budget Reconciliation Act (COBRA) to ensure coverage while disabled.

In organizing their personal affairs, patients should be encouraged to make advanced-directive decisions in the form of a living will or durable power of attorney. This may be a highly sensitive issue for physicians and patients because the introduction of the subject alone may be perceived as taking away hope. The HSCT team can be instrumental in facilitating a discussion of advanced directives by emphasizing the natural aspects of making decisions about all phases of one's life, including death. Such decisions made in advance of HSCT tend to bring peace of mind to the patient and the family.

FAMILY SEQUELAE

Families face multiple challenges as they embark on the journey of transplantation. Their concerns may be especially heightened if the procedure is still considered experimental or has a relatively high risk of mortality.[1] Family lifestyle, in general, becomes fragmented and requires reorganization to accommodate the needs of the patient.[1, 5] Some families find it difficult or even impossible to adapt to the stressors of treatment.[8] Consequently, this may lead to disturbed family interactions prior to admission and throughout the transplantation course.[8] Adjustment difficulties need to be identified early on by the social worker in order to plan and initiate psychotherapeutic intervention.

Complicating the transplant experience is the possibility that a spouse may feel ambivalent or angry because he or she does not agree with the patient's decision to undergo HSCT.[6] A spouse may also feel trapped or overwhelmed by the increased responsibility and role changes.[5] Moreover, the inherent stress of having to relocate to a distant city can be considerable.[1, 10] As previously stated, the financial implications of relocation can be far-reaching, with long-term effects on the economic stability of the family.

Children of patients undergoing HSCT often become the "hidden" members of the family if not permitted or encouraged to become part of the transplantation experience.[29] It has only been within recent years that the needs of children of cancer patients have been recognized.[30] In studies that have addressed the impact of cancer on children in the family, it has been noted that most children yearn for the lost parenting of both parents and feel resentment about being ignored.[29] Children of a parent with cancer often retrospectively describe the experience as having been profoundly stressful, leaving permanent scars.[29] Based on such knowledge, consultation, social work, and/or psychology consultations should be offered to assist parents in helping their children cope and adapt to the health crisis.

Lastly, the interruption of employment and/or education can be a painful experience for the patient and the family. Options should be discussed, such as taking a medical leave and/or applying for disability benefits, in order to decrease the level of anxiety. For family members who wish to spend additional time with the patient, information should be offered regarding the Family and Medical Leave Act, which entitles a patient and/or family member to take a 12-week leave of absence from work without the threat of job loss.

THE TRANSPLANTATION PROCESS

Length of stay (LOS) in the hospital, in an era of increased cost containment, is changing dramatically. Care is being shifted to lower-cost units, such as ambulatory care, "hospitel," and/or care at home with a designated caregiver. Consequently, the LOS for many patients undergoing HSCT has declined, particularly for those undergoing peripheral blood progenitor cell transplantation.[22] In fact, it had not been unusual, prior to this paradigm shift, for transplant recipients to be hospitalized for 8–10 weeks, whereas the current LOS may be as short as 1 week.[18] In spite of decreased LOS, hospitalization can be physically and emotionally stressful, placing great demands on the coping abilities of the patient, family, and staff.[1, 14, 31] The stress begins with the patient entering an isolation unit that can vary from laminar air flow chambers to less stringent reverse isolation units.[18]

ISOLATION

When rigid isolation is required, patients tend to feel secluded at a time when they are most in need of physical and emotional support.[1, 2, 9] In addition, entering an isolation unit is a graphic reminder of the seriousness of the disease and treatment, often taking away, at least temporarily, the use of denial in coping. In response, some patients regret their decision to undergo HSCT. Others appear apathetic. Spouses, who may have been opposed to the patient's decision, may appear angry or distant.[5, 6] In spite of the prodigious amount of information and education provided about what to expect during HSCT, most patients arrive ill prepared, as previously mentioned, because of selective listening.[2] Consequently, the HSCT team physicians, nurses, and social worker should continue to provide detailed information throughout all phases of the process of transplantation in spite of the thought that the information may be repetitive or redundant.

CONDITIONING REGIMEN

There are a variety of considerations for adjustment and coping throughout this phase of treatment. For example, psychological stability during immunosuppression, according to Holland, appears to be directly related to the quality of individual nursing care.[32] Quality nursing usually depends on a dedicated staff of HSCT nurses who have received extensive training in the process of transplantation and the subsequent psychosocial implications. Loss of control is also a major issue during the conditioning regimen secondary to the noxious side effects such as nausea, vomiting, and diarrhea.[7, 9, 17] Furthermore, patients tend to become preoccupied with bodily concerns along with a heightened awareness of sensations and functions.[15] Moreover, many feel defenseless and lose their sense of dignity during this intense period of distress.[9]

Another perspective suggests that adaptive coping may depend on the patient's internal locus of control, a belief that physical and psychological distress can be affected by positive coping strategies such as prayer, hope, and diversion.[31] Also, steady support from family and/or significant others is critical to effective coping.[15] Families, however, often feel ineffective and helpless while discounting "just being there" as an important aspect of support.

Families with a previous history of dysfunction may become more chaotic and disruptive during this early phase of treatment.[8, 10] Because maladaptive coping responses and behavior often escalate as the treatment progresses, family-oriented treatment strategies are recommended.[8] Families whose systems were dysfunctional prior to the health crisis are in fact the most in need of help.[8] Social work intervention with families having a difficult time coping is imperative to patient management. Patients do not do well when stressed by negative family interactions.

BLOOD AND MARROW TRANSPLANTATION

The actual process of infusing marrow or peripheral blood progenitor cells during this next phase of treatment has been described by many as undramatic and/or anticlimactic.[1, 9, 17] The procedure itself is unremarkable, with cells infused in the same manner as a blood transfusion. Although the process is simplistic compared with the arduous conditioning regimen, the experience can be profoundly emotional and therefore highly dramatic for patient and family.[2] The emotionality is related to the existential significance of the procedure. More specifically, the infused HSC are symbolic of renewed life. Patients may use hope-maintaining strategies, a means of managing the impact of threat while sustaining hope, and subsequently describe the actual transplantation as a commencement celebration.

Ironically, the day of transplantation may also denote discharge from an acute care setting for some patients.[22] The feelings associated with early discharge, such as fear, anxiety, and apprehension, may confound the exhilarated feeling of having just received potentially life-saving cells. Staff members can be most efficacious if they validate the affective aspects of the day of transplantation. This response helps patients and families with intense feelings that often go unspoken.

WAITING FOR ENGRAFTMENT

The passage of time wherein the patient and family are waiting for signs of engraftment is often physically and psychologically intolerable.[31] The interval after transplantation is characteristically dominated by the noxious side effects of neurotoxic drug regimens, infections, antibiotic therapy, sleep deprivation, and pain.[11, 17] Consequently, a sense of helplessness prevails for patient and family during this unpredictable period of time.[17] The stress may in fact lead to psychiatric symptoms.[33] Futterman and Wellisch, however, report that the stress and pressure of HSCT do not always correlate with the patient's clinical status.[6] For example, fear, anxiety, and expectations can in fact create

stress when the patient is actually doing well.[6] Consequently, patients and family members alike should be encouraged by the staff to express these pent-up emotions. This may be accomplished through individual counseling and/or addressed in a support group setting.

PATIENT SEQUELAE

Anxiety, grief, regression, ambivalence, and neuropsychiatric disregulation of the brain (or central nervous system) are described as inherent reactions to the process of transplantation.[5] The responses are essentially normal reactions of persons placed in abnormally stressful situations.[6] Problems in adaptation often arise as the result of an imbalance between the demands of treatment and the coping abilities of patients and families.[15] Successful adaptation may then be contingent on the patient's ability to give up at least some degree of autonomy and control in order to allow the staff to provide care.[1] At the same time, dependence can lead to an increased sense of helplessness and regressive behavior.[15] Nearly all patients, regardless of developmental stage, regress while undergoing HSCT, particularly while awaiting engraftment.[5, 6] Even so, the spectrum of regression as a defense mechanism can range from functional (a minimal response), to infantile (a severe, autistic-like response).[5, 6] Additionally, there is greater evidence of regression in patients who are the most sick. Regressive behavior tends to resolve when patients begin to show signs of engraftment.[5, 6]

Pain and discomfort associated with the toxic conditioning regimen for HSCT are also significant issues during the wait for engraftment. Patients can experience a variety of side effects, such as oral mucositis, stomatitis, vomiting, diarrhea, and hemorrhagic cystitis, in addition to the effects of bacterial and fungal infections. Higher levels of anxiety and distress during this difficult period may be associated with the magnitude of pain.[31] More specifically, common emotions associated with pain are feelings of depression, despair, powerlessness, fear, and indignity.[34] The subsequent management of pain as a phenomenon of sensory, affective, and cognitive components can be enhanced by assessing the patient's perception of pain and use of coping strategies.[31] In order to treat pain associated with HSCT, increased attention must be paid to the roles of emotion and cognition in conjunction with the sensory report.[31] Therefore, care of the patient experiencing pain, by physician and nurse alike, must include careful listening and communicating, educating, and being open to compromise.[34] Supportive interventions include increasing the patient's control over pain relief and teaching pain-coping strategies.[24]

The strains of complications, symptoms, procedures, and the usual "ups and downs" of the transplantation process demand strategy for and discipline in coping.[15] Consequently, patients who present with premorbid psychological problems may face even greater distress during the wait for engraftment. Pre-existing problems combined with the normal emotional difficulties experienced during this phase warrant close monitoring by staff. The responses may vary but can include anxiety, depression, withdrawal, hostility, anger, noncompliance, apathy, paranoia, acting-out behavior, and/or suicidality.[1, 14] Unless the emotional conflict has a negative effect on the patient's treatment, Neuser et al. recommend not intervening with any pre-existing psychiatric disorders.[15] Instead, intervention should be focused on maximizing strengths and abilities in order to maintain psychological functioning.[1, 15]

FAMILY SEQUELAE

Stress-induced behavioral and psychological responses of patients often incite further stress in families. Nonetheless adversity and crisis are inherent to family systems and therefore an integral part of living.[8] In fact, disturbed family interactions in previously well-functioning families are not uncommon during this troubling phase of treatment. For example, a spouse or child may feel guilty because he or she resents having to assume increased responsibilities at home.[8] These uncomfortable feelings, which often go unspoken, may lead to tension or conflict in the patient/family relationship. Family members, however, regardless of behavior or style, continue to be the most significant factors in the patient's ability to cope. High family cohesion and enmeshment, although bothersome to staff, may result in better psychosocial adjustment.[35] Conversely, low family cohesion and disengagement undoubtedly have a negative impact on the patient.[35] Consequently, because family constitutes the patient's primary source of moral support, efforts should be focused on helping families remain functional and strong.[8] Hill recommends examining the adequacy of family members' role performances, family flexibility, and the meaning of the health crisis to the family.[36]

In addressing such issues, family conferences with the HSCT primary care team can be effective in assessing family strengths and weaknesses. Problem areas can be better delineated during a family conference, and support can be elicited in setting goals for patient management.[19] A subsequent contract can be developed with patient and family to reach these goals. This type of intervention reinforces the family's understanding of being essential to patient recovery.

Patient and family support groups are also an effective way to reduce stress through communication and catharsis.[37] The concept of patient/family-oriented groups, rather than exclusive patient or family groups, is a fundamental shift in thinking.[5] Family focus in the group setting is another means of reinforcing the importance of family support and cohesion. Although time consuming for staff, the group setting is an optimal method of providing encouragement, education, and a forum for mutual sharing. The group, facilitated by a social worker and or nurse, can help to establish bonds between patients and families on the unit.[38, 37] Groups are characteristically cross-generational and open-ended, with the common denominator being the transplantation experience. Offering group meetings consistently serves to fill the gap of unmet psychosocial needs. For instance, participation in a support group reinforces that one is not alone in his or her battle with cancer. Consequently, the healing aspect of group support may be more beneficial than individual counseling.[5] Verbal endorsement of the group by HSCT nurses and physicians helps to validate the importance of group support and education.[38]

TRANSITION TO AMBULATORY CARE AND RECOVERY

With clinical signs of engraftment, the acute level of psychosocial stress for patient and family usually begins to subside and is replaced initially with feelings of joy and renewed hope.[1] At the same time, the elation is often tempered with the realization that adjustment and adaptation to life outside the hospital can be traumatic.[11] Although viewed as a milestone on the road to recovery, being discharged from an acute care setting can be both energizing and anxiety provoking.[39] For example, feelings of ambivalence appear to prevail as patients look forward to being in their own environment while mourning the loss of staff support and the availability of life-sustaining technology at their bedside.[1, 2, 9, 11, 40]

Successful transition to the ambulatory care setting requires extensive preparation and education from the staff.[39] Once again, family members should be included when discharge instructions are given. This will give them firsthand knowledge of the "DOs and DON'Ts" while reinforcing the importance of their roles in caregiving. Patients and family members should be encouraged to articulate their expectations and concerns so that appropriate modifications can be suggested.[40] Formal caregiver educational programs can be effective when initiated prior to discharge.

PATIENT SEQUELAE

Most patients have unrealistic expectations for recovery after discharge from the hospital.[19] More specifically, in spite of education during the pretransplantation phase and at the time of discharge, patients are often ill-prepared for the diligent follow-up regimen, possible postdischarge complications, chronic symptoms, and potential readmissions to the hospital.[11, 19] Patients for the most part want to be treated as normally as possible when they return to their home environment. Re-entering normal activities, however, can be a difficult process.

First, patients often remain physically weak, lethargic, and anorexic, becoming easily fatigued with the normal activities of daily living.[11] Moreover, they are disappointed that total recovery from HSCT is not guaranteed or that recovery will take longer than anticipated.[1] Additionally, the patient's lifestyle, at home or in temporary lodging, is subject to restrictions in diet, activity, and social interaction.[15]

Second, as patients re-enter the world outside the hospital, they may also experience the emotional impact of an altered body image secondary to alopecia and facial and body changes. The normalcy of such an emotional response should be addressed by the staff in order to prevent feelings of low self-esteem and isolative behavior.

Third, roles and responsibilities, which had been placed on hold during hospitalization, come to the forefront as the patient returns to family life.[9] The ability to resume these roles with ease is unlikely during the early phase of recovery. Furthermore, self-worth is often threatened by the patient's ongoing dependence on others.[15] Conversely, some patients are unwilling to give up the "sick role" and the subsequent relinquishment of special attention.[17]

Fourth, adaptation may also be hampered by changes in cognitive performance secondary to the neurotoxicity of conditioning regimens.[4, 41] Cognitive impairment may be manifested in slowed reaction time, poor concentration, reduced attention span, and poor problem solving.[41] Common deficits may also include psychomotor impairment, impaired perceptive motor tasks, and deficits in abstract thinking.[11] Education is imperative to prepare patients for any possible cognitive changes.

Finally, changes in sexual functioning may also be a major issue for patients and their partners, but the concerns are often not articulated or sought out by the health care team. Sexual dysfunction can be the result of one or more factors: fear of infection, decreased desire, low stamina, infertility, low self-esteem, generalized anger, changes in body image, endocrine toxicity, and depression.[1, 3, 4, 42] The impact of early menopause is also significant for young women and may lead to negative sexual self-esteem. In response to such issues, assessment and psychosexual counseling should be made available on a routine basis to address and validate these concerns. Additionally, reproductive counseling should also be made available for young patients faced with infertility to inform them of medically assisted reproduction technology.[43]

Emotional and psychological distress generally varies from patient to patient after discharge.[11] More specifically, factors that can affect the patient's psychological well-being are personality type, locus of control, pre-existing psychological problems, coping style, and social support.[11] In the first few months after HSCT, patients may experience post-transplantation anxiety disorders, similar to post-traumatic stress disorders, and depressive symptoms.[5, 44] Anxiety and depression can be potentiated by a multiplicity of factors, including familial stresses, economic constraints, clinical status, functional limitations, and role changes.[45] Fear of relapse also remains paramount to all patients.[1] Most patients continue to worry about relapse on a daily basis months or years after transplantation. They become particularly anxious when facing yearly follow-up examinations or scans. Their anxiety should be acknowledged as normal and assuaged by education and reassurance from staff.

The recovery process from a sick role to a healthy role tends to be lengthy, sometimes extending far beyond any evidence of symptoms. Consequently, patients may benefit from the HSCT team's ongoing interest in their well-being. This may be demonstrated through periodic phone calls, correspondence, the availability of a post-transplantation support group, and planned reunions of all patients and families.

FAMILY SEQUELAE

Little is known about the behavior and/or psychological experiences of family members after the patient is discharged from the hospital.[14] This deficit in studies is unfortunate in an era when far more caregiving responsibilities are being placed on family members.[21] In fact, family disruption is almost inevitable because of ongoing stresses and lifestyle changes.[1, 10] For example, marital/family conflict may result from altered role relationships, especially if family members are reticent to give up roles they were forced to assume when the patient was hospitalized.[4, 10, 17] Pre-existing marital conflict may also be exacerbated when the patient returns home.[1] Such conflict may in turn lead to flight, separation, or divorce. Additionally, as previously addressed, sexual reconnection may also be encumbered by feelings of anxiety, loss of desirability or self-esteem, or fear of infection.[5]

Anger is not uncommon during re-entry into home and family. For example, a patient may express anger toward the healthy spouse for being healthy, and the spouse may respond negatively to the ill partner for being ill.[46] Children may also seem less affectionate and attentive to the returning parent (patient) because of the length of separation, perceived feelings of rejection, fear of parental death, and/or prolonged lack of physical contact.[17] Feelings of anger are often replaced by guilt feelings during this complex period of transition and caregiving.

Little is also known about the short- or long-term sequelae associated with marrow donation.[14] Although studies have been limited, donors report minimal psychological distress and little change in the donor-recipient relationship after transplantation.[14] Death of the recipient may have a profound emotional impact on the donor, however.

In addition to the emotional impact of the transplantation experience, families often have to deal with ongoing catastrophic financial and insurance issues. They may be devastated by decreased family income, loss of savings, and a potential loss of earning power due to employment problems.[10] Family adaptation generally warrants closer attention in future studies. Family, marital, and psychosexual counseling should be provided within the institution, or through professional referrals, to enhance the recovery process.

QUALITY OF LIFE

In recent years, research efforts to evaluate the long-term effects of HSCT have increased. Measurements have included at least four general domains: social, physical, spiritual, and psychological.[45, 47] The concept of quality of life (QOL), in general and specific to HSCT, however, remains complex with diverse dimensions.[48]

Studies have shown a considerable variation in post-HSCT QOL.[3, 4, 41, 48–51] In general, survivors of HSCT experience the most difficulty with vocational activity, sexual activity, and vigorous physical activity.[3, 50, 52] QOL deficits and psychosocial distress are strongly linked to physical morbidity after transplantation.[49] The type of transplant, allogeneic or autologous, has not significantly affected QOL in recipients.[49] Although long-term treatment-related side effects are less traumatic in autologous transplantation, findings in the current literature are inconclusive.[48] Increased age at time of HSCT, however, has been associated with a greater decline in physical and psychosocial status.[3, 50] Although Murphy et al. report a high prevalence for depressive illness after HSCT, especially in females,[53] a majority of patients return to an acceptable QOL, with self-esteem playing a major predictive role in outcome.[49–51, 53] Being a survivor, in itself, reinforces the will to live, with patients redefining their perceptions of normality.[48]

CONCLUSION

HSCT is an aggressive and laborious therapeutic modality. In spite of technological advances and the subsequent hope for a cure, the treatment is inherently affected by a myriad of stress-producing factors. Although most long-term survivors return to a reasonable QOL, patients and families are often faced with chronic psychosocial distress.[45, 49, 50, 54]

Viewing the family as a system postulates that a change in any single element leads to a change in the system as a whole.[8] Transplantation, therefore, affects the family, but the family can also affect the transplantation process.[21] An emotionally healthy family, supported by the HSTC team, can buffer against the problems of treatment and recovery.[35]

A longitudinal psychoeducational approach is recommended to plan interventions for patient and family from the initial evaluation, throughout the course of HSCT, and during the extended period of readaptation to normal existence.[11] Increased educational efforts should be undertaken by all members of the transplantation team to prepare both patients and families for the inherent problems associated with transplantation. Most importantly, the HSCT team should encourage and support patients and families as proactive participants in the treatment plan.

REFERENCES

1. Lesko LM: Handbook of Psychooncology: Psychological Care of the Patient with Cancer. New York, Oxford University Press, 1989.
2. Haberman M: Psychosocial aspects of bone marrow transplantation. Semin Oncol Nurs 4(1):55–59, 1988.
3. Andrykowski M, et al: Returning to normal following bone marrow transplantation: outcomes, expectations and informed consent. Bone Marrow Transplant 15:573–581, 1995.
4. Wolcott D, Fawzy F, Wellisch D: Psychiatric aspects of bone marrow transplantation: a review and current issues. Psychiatric Med 41(3):299–317, 1987.
5. Wellisch D, Wolcott D: Psychological Issues in Bone Marrow Transplantation. Oxford, Blackwell Scientific, 1994.
6. Futterman A, Wellisch D: Psychodynamic themes of bone marrow transplantation: when I become thou. Hematol Oncol Clin North Am 4:699–709, 1990.
7. Paternaude A, Szymanski L, Rappaport J: Psychological costs of bone marrow transplantation in children. J Orthopsychiatry 49(3):409–422, 1979.
8. Parry J, Young A: The family as a system in hospital-based social work. Health Soc Work 3(2):55–70, 1978.
9. Brown H, Kelly M: Stages of bone marrow transplantation: a psychiatric perspective. Psychosom Med 38(6):439–446, 1976.
10. Zabora J, Smith E, Baker F, et al: The family: the other side of bone marrow transplantation. J Psychosoc Oncol 10(1):35–46, 1992.
11. Pot Mees C: Re-Adaptation to Normal Existence: Support of the Patient and Family. London, Churchill Livingstone, 1992.
12. Paternaude A, Rappaport J: Collaboration between hematologists and mental health professionals on a bone marrow transplant team. J Psychosoc Oncol 2(3–4):81–92, 1984.
13. Chauvenet A, Smith N: Referral of pediatric oncology patients for marrow transplantation and the process of informed consent. Med Pediatr Oncol 16:40–44, 1988.
14. Andrykowski M: Psychosocial factors in bone marrow transplantation: a review and recommendations for research. Bone Marrow Transplant 13:357–375, 1994.
15. Neuser J, et al: Principles of supportive psychological care for patients undergoing bone marrow transplantation. Hematol Blood Transfus 33:583–586, 1990.
16. Haberman M: The meaning of cancer therapy: bone marrow transplantation as an exemplar of therapy. Semin Oncol Nurs 11(1):23–31, 1995.
17. Folsom T, Popkin M: Current and future perspectives on psychiatric involvement in bone marrow transplantation. Psychiatric Med 4(3):319–329, 1987.
18. Rappaport B: Evolution of consultation-liaison services in bone marrow transplantation. Gen Hosp Psychiatry 10:346–351, 1988.
19. Kennedy V: The role of social work in bone marrow transplantation. J Psychosoc Oncol 11(1):103–116, 1993.
20. Futterman A, Willisch D, Bond G, Carr C: The psychosocial levels systems: a new rating scale to identify and assess emotional difficulties during bone marrow transplantation. Psychosomatics 32(2):117–186, 1991.
21. Spiegel D: Commentary. J Psychosoc Oncol 13(112):115–121, 1995.
22. Cavanaugh C: Outpatient autologous bone marrow transplantation: a new frontier. Qual Life Nurs Chall 3(2):25–29, 1994.
23. Grassi L, Rosti G, Albertazzi L, Marangolo M: Psychological stress symptoms before and after autologous bone marrow transplantation in patients with solid tumors. Bone Marrow Transplant 17:843–847, 1996.
24. Gotay C, Stern J: Assessment of psychological functioning in cancer patients. J Psychosoc Oncol 13(1/2):123–160, 1995.
25. Watson M: Screening for psychological morbidity in cancer patients. Cancer J 2:195–196, 1988.
26. Derogatis L, Melisaratos N: The brief symptom inventory: an introductory report. Psychol Med 13:595–605, 1983.
27. Zabora J, Smith E, Baker F, et al: An efficient method of psychosocial screening of cancer patients. Psychosomatics 31(2):192–196, 1990.
28. Rosenthal D: Oncology Social Work. Atlanta, American Cancer Society, 1993.
29. Rait D, Lederberg M: Family of the cancer patient. In Handbook of Psycho-oncology. New York, Oxford University Press, 1989, pp 585–597.
30. Hermann J: Oncology Social Work, A Clinician's Guide. Atlanta, American Cancer Society, 1993.
31. Gaston-Johansson F, Franco T, Zimmerman L: Pain and psychological distress in patients undergoing autologous bone marrow transplantation. Oncol Nurs Forum 19(1):41–48, 1992.
32. Holland JEA: Psychological response of patients with acute leukemia to germ free environments. Cancer 40:871–879, 1977.
33. Kaehler S, Goodwin J, Young L: Bone marrow transplantation: mastering the experience despite psychological risk factors. Psychosomatics 30(3):337–341, 1989.
34. Ferrell B, Johnston Taylor E, Sattler G, et al: Searching for the meaning of pain. Cancer Pract 1(3):185–193, 1993.
35. Fobair P, Zabora J: Family functioning as a resource variable in psychosocial cancer research: issues and measures. J Psychosoc Oncol 13(1/2):97–114, 1995.
36. Hill R: Genetic features of families under stress. Social Casework 42:139–151, 1958.
37. Cella D, Yellen S: Cancer support groups, the state of the art. Cancer Pract 1(1):56–61, 1993.
38. Paternaude A, Levinger L, Baker K: Group meeting for parents and spouses of bone marrow transplant patients. Social Work Health Care 12(1):51–65, 1987.
39. Chielens D, Herrick E: Recipients of bone marrow transplants: making a smooth transition to an ambulatory care setting. Oncol Nurs Forum 17(6):857–862, 1990.
40. Freund B, Siegel K: Problems in transition following bone marrow transplantation: psychosocial aspects. Am J Orthopsychiatry 56(2):244–252, 1986.
41. Andrykowski M, Altmaier E, Barnett R, et al: Cognitive dysfunction in adult survivors of allogeneic marrow transplantation: relationship to dose of total body irradiation. Bone Marrow Transplant 6:269–276, 1990.
42. Baruch J, Benjamin S, Treleaven J, et al: male sexual function following bone marrow transplantation. Bone Marrow Transplant 7(2):52, 1991.

43. Sanders J: Effects of bone marrow transplantation on reproductive function. *In* Green DM, D'Angio G (eds): Late Effects of Treatment for Childhood Cancer. New York, Wiley-Liss, 1992.

44. Heiney S, Neuberg R, Myers D, Bergman L: The aftermath of bone marrow transplant for parents of pediatric patients: a post-traumatic stress disorder. Oncol Nurs Forum 21(5):843–847, 1994.

45. Molassiotis A, vanden Akker O, Milligan D, et al: Quality of life survivors of marrow transplantation: comparison with a matched group receiving maintenance chemotherapy. Bone Marrow Transplant 17:249–258, 1996.

46. Stearns N: Celebrating life, lessons learned from a bone marrow transplant reunion. Cancer Pract 1(1):42–48, 1993.

47. Ferrell BEA: Quality of life in breast cancer. Cancer Pract 4(6):331–340, 1996.

48. Prieto J, et al: Physical and psychosocial functioning of 117 survivors of bone marrow transplantation. Bone Marrow Transplant 17:1133–1142, 1996.

49. Chao N, Tierney D, Bloom J, et al: Dynamic assessment of quality of life after autologous bone marrow transplantation. Blood 3:825–830, 1992.

50. Baker F, Wingard J, Curbow B, et al: Quality of life of bone marrow transplant long-term survivors. Bone Marrow Transplant 13:589–595, 1994.

51. Bush N, Haberman M, Donaldson G, Sullivan K: Quality of life of 125 adults surviving 6–18 years after bone marrow transplantation. Soc Sci Med 4:479–490, 1995.

52. Altmaier E, Gingrich R, Fyke M: Two year adjustment of bone marrow transplant survivors. Bone Marrow Transplant 7:311–316, 1991.

53. Murphy K, Jenkins P, Whittaker J: Psychosocial morbidity and survival in adult bone marrow transplant recipients—a follow-up study. Bone Marrow Transplant 18:199–201, 1996.

54. Whedon M, Ferrell B: Quality of life in adult bone marrow transplant patients: beyond the first year. Semin Oncol Nurs 10(1):42–57, 1994.

CHAPTER SIXTY-ONE

Specialized Nursing

Jennifer K. Simpson, M.S.N., Ph.D.

Hematopoietic stem cell (HSC) transplantation (HSCT) is an accepted treatment modality for both malignant and nonmalignant disorders. Despite advances in treatment, approximately 40% of patients require hemodynamic and/or electrocardiographic monitoring, ventilatory support, and hemodialysis during transplantation.[1] Because the scope of care can range from minimal care to intensive care management, the HSCT nurse must continually integrate advanced knowledge and skills to promote quality patient care.[2] This chapter reviews the complications associated with HSCT and the nursing intervention required in the recovery of the bone marrow transplant recipient.

PRETRANSPLANTATION CONDITIONING

Conditioning is considered to be bifunctional: immunosuppression and the removal of any remaining malignant cells. The type and duration of the conditioning regimen varies with the patient's disease state and treatment history. Nursing care during the conditioning phase is focused on symptom management. The HSCT nurse obtains a baseline assessment on admission. This includes the patient's height, weight, and vital signs (including postural blood pressure) and an assessment of the skin, cardiopulmonary system, and gastrointestinal system.

Nursing assessment of previous nausea and vomiting patterns and effective regimens used prior to admission can provide useful information when one is trying to prevent nausea and vomiting associated with the conditioning regimen. Nausea and vomiting, expected side effects of conditioning regimens, are controlled with various antiemetic regimens. Anticipatory nausea and vomiting may be minimized via relaxation techniques and sedation. The patient is encouraged to eat small, frequent meals consisting of bland, carbohydrate-rich foods to maintain oral intake with minimal nausea and vomiting. Eating and drinking should be stopped if oral intake persistently results in emesis. During the conditioning regimen, it is important to stress that persistent emesis may lead to further complications such as a Mallory-Weiss tear; therefore, it may be necessary to maintain nothing-by-mouth (NPO) status for a period of time.

Oral mucositis is directly related to the cytotoxic effects of the conditioning regimen and is a common cause of treatment-related pain.[3] Preventive measures include systematic oral care using chlorhexidine (Peridex) or saline rinses. The frequency and comprehensiveness of the nurses' oral assessments should be increased immediately after the HSC infusion, when mucositis is most prevalent.[3] Early detection of mucosal breakdown and prompt treatment for pain with topical and systemic analgesics are priority nursing care interventions. Oral mucositis may interfere with the patient's ability to swallow secretions. A suction catheter at the bedside is useful for the removal of secretions. The thrombocytopenic patient during the peak of oral mucositis must be cautioned to use the suction carefully because oral bleeding may occur if the mucosa is further traumatized.

Maintaining fluid and electrolyte balance is important during the conditioning phase. Aggressive hydration and the possibility of the cyclophosphamide-induced syndrome of inappropriate antidiuretic hormone secretion can place a patient at risk for fluid overload.[4] Nursing intervention involves daily monitoring of weight, intake/output, evidence of peripheral edema, and assessment of cardiopulmonary status.

Conditioning regimens that use cyclophosphamide include preventative measures to protect against hemorrhagic cystitis. These preventive measures include vigorous hydration, placement of a Foley catheter for bladder irrigation, and forced diuresis. Mercaptohethane sodium sulfonate (Mesna), a uroprotectant, may be used alone or in conjunction with bladder irrigation. Nursing care includes close monitoring of the patient's urine by Hemetest to evaluate for evidence of bleeding.

TRANSPLANTATION

Cryopreserved autologous HSC are brought to the patient's room in a dry-shipper and are thawed individually in a temperature-controlled water bath. The cells, once thawed, are pulled into a 50-mL syringe and are administered by intravenous push through the central venous catheter (CVC) by the physician, physician assistant, nurse practitioner, or other specially prepared personnel. Alternatively, thawed cells may be infused by gravity or pumps. Nursing responsibilities include educating the patient regarding possible side effects experienced during cell infusion, administration of antiemetics and premedications, and emotional support of the patient.

The HSCT nurse is responsible for placing the patient on a cardiac monitor and frequent monitoring of vital signs. Possible causes for adverse reactions during autologous transplantation include infusion of large graft volumes, damaged cells, products of cell lysis, and dimethylsulfoxide. Side effects associated with the infusion of autologous HSC include facial flushing, nausea and vomiting, abdominal cramping, diarrhea, dyspnea and chest tightness, headache, fever, bradycardia (defined as heart rate <60 beats per minute), and hypertension (defined as an increase in systolic blood pressure of 30 mm Hg or an increase in diastolic blood pressure of 25 mm Hg).[5]

Allogeneic bone marrow or peripheral blood progenitor cells are taken directly from the donor to the processing laboratory. Once processing is completed, the allogeneic cells are delivered to the in-patient unit, where the nurse directly infuses the cells via gravity into the patient's CVC. Side effects are those that would occur with a packed red blood cell or platelet transfusion and should be treated accordingly.

POST-TRANSPLANTATION COMPLICATIONS

POTENTIAL FOR INFECTION

For approximately 2–5 weeks after HSCT, patients experience severe immunosuppression.[8] Prevention of infection is a complex challenge for the nurse.[9] The patient's defenses are compromised by chemotherapeutic damage to the oral/gastrointestinal mucosa, profound neutropenia, and the presence of indwelling CVC. In addition, the routine use of prophylactic antibiotics can potentiate the overgrowth of opportunistic pathogens.[10] Nursing care is focused on infection prevention and early identification of infection in the immediate post-transplantation period.

Although the patient is neutropenic, signs of infection may be minimal or atypical. Often, persistent fever is the only sign. It is an important routine that the HSCT nurse monitor vital signs every 4 hours, with special attention to changes in the patient's baseline assessment. Evidence of potential infection includes fever, chills, tachycardia, tachypnea, hypotension, mental status changes, change in urinary patterns, change in the character of breath sounds, and erythema or tenderness at the CVC site. If any of these symptoms occur, the nurse can anticipate the need for blood cultures, urine culture, chest radiograph, and administration of additional antibiotics.

Measures to prevent infection should be initiated on admission to the hospital. The HSCT nurse educates the patient and family members regarding the importance of preventing infection by the use of protective isolation. These methods include the use of high-efficiency particulate air filtration, thorough handwashing, and masking to cover the mouth and nose when the patient is neutropenic. Instructing the patient on the importance of frequent, thorough mouth care; daily hygiene via showering; and the use of antimicrobial soap is essential. Patients are also instructed to follow an antimicrobial diet, which prohibits intake of fresh fruit, vegetables, and spices. The HSCT nurse performs CVC care per the institutional policy and procedure and assesses the line site for evidence of infection. Measures to promote optimal pulmonary toilet include instruction on coughing and deep breathing exercises, use

of an incentive spirometer, and encouraging physical activity.[7]

In the outpatient setting, instructions depend on the type of transplant the patient has received. Patients who continue to be neutropenic should be instructed to wear a mask when entering the hospital. Once the patient is in the examination room, the mask can be removed. For both the inpatient and outpatient setting, it is important for the HSCT nurse to instruct patients to avoid infectious persons and crowded places. Of particular concern are people who have varicella/herpes zoster. The nurse must emphasize the importance of prompt notification should contact occur because the patient may receive varicella zoster immunoglobulin if exposure has occurred within 72 hours. People who have had live vaccinations within the past 4 weeks should be avoided. This usually includes infants and toddlers receiving routine oral polio and measles-mumps-rubella vaccinations.

POTENTIAL FOR BLEEDING

Marrow aplasia is a direct result of the conditioning regimen. Thrombocytopenia, which can be severe, places patients at great risk for hemorrhage. The HSCT nurse must continually assess the patient for petechiae, ecchymosis, oral bleeding, epistaxis, hematuria, positive stool guaiac, or vaginal bleeding. Onset of headache, blurred vision, disorientation, seizures, or pupillary changes may indicate an intracranial bleed. The patient must be instructed about protective measures. These include the use of an electric razor and the avoidance of rectal suppositories, subcutaneous/intramuscular injections, finger/toenail cutting, forceful nose blowing, strenuous exercise, and lifting objects weighing more than 10 pounds. In addition, menses suppression via medroxyprogesterone acetate may be used for menstruating females. If epistaxis occurs, the patient should be placed in a sitting position with 90-degree elevation (high Fowler position). Ice packs and possibly nasal packing may also be used.[7]

Historically, the threshold for platelet transfusions has been set at 20,000/mm³ based on studies of leukemic patients in the 1960s, when aspirin and nonsteroidal anti-inflammatory drugs were widely used. More-recent studies have shown that the level for prophylactic platelet transfusion can be safely lowered in asymptomatic patients if platelet inhibitors are avoided and patients are carefully evaluated for signs of bleeding. This approach lowers the risk of transfusion-related adverse reaction, disease, and health care costs.[11]

All red blood cell and platelet products should be irradiated and filtered (leukocyte-depleted). The cytomegalovirus (CMV) status of a blood product depends on the status of the recipient. Leukocyte-depleted products carry a low risk of CMV transmission (CMV-safe).[12] If CMV-negative products are unavailable, CMV-safe products may be used for the CMV-negative recipient. Advantages of leukocyte-reduced blood products include reduced risk of alloimmunization, CMV infection, and immunologic refractoriness to random donor platelets.

GASTROINTESTINAL COMPLICATIONS

Nausea and vomiting are side effects of the conditioning regimen, organ damage secondary to the conditioning regimen, and the various medications used for supportive care. They can also occur secondary to complications such as graft-versus-host-disease (GVHD) and infections. HSCT nurses play an important role in managing nausea and vomiting. It is imperative to assess the nature, duration, timing, and intensity of each occurrence. Although several antiemetics are available, no one antiemetic has been found to be completely effective. Assessment of the patient's previous experience with nausea and vomiting, including previous use of antiemetics and their effectiveness, is helpful in determining an antiemetic regimen.

Nursing measures that may be useful include instructing the patient to eat small, frequent meals consisting of bland foods; eliminating noxious odors; applying cool compresses to the forehead; administering antiemetics; and administering pain medication if there is concurrent mucositis/stomatitis. Dietary interventions that have been anecdotally helpful include serving cool meals, allowing carbonated drinks to become "flat," and using clear-liquid diets. Relaxation techniques, including the use of tapes, music, and deep breathing, may also be beneficial. Liquid-diet supplementation may be used as well as total parenteral nutrition. Comprehensive evaluation and intervention by a clinical dietitian may enhance management.[7]

Diarrhea is frequently a problem in the HSCT recipient and is often multifactorial. Toxicity from conditioning regimens, GVHD, infection, and underlying bowel conditions is a possible cause of diarrhea. Stool cultures to rule out an infectious etiology should be evaluated prior to initiation of antidiarrheal medication. Colonoscopy with biopsies and cultures is necessary to identify GVHD and infection not found in stool culture. If infection or GVHD is the cause, treatment of the underlying disorder should stop the diarrhea. Hypermotility secondary to the conditioning regimen can be slowed through the use of antidiarrheal medication and nursing management. Instructing the patient to avoid foods that increase bowel motility (caffeinated beverages, lactose-containing beverages) may be useful. Strict assessment and care of the perianal area is important to prevent skin breakdown. Daily sitz baths and the use of topical creams and anti-inflammatory agents provide comfort to irritated skin.[7] It is important to closely monitor the amount of stool, total intake and output, vital signs, laboratory values, and patient's clinical status for evidence of dehydration.

SKIN INTEGRITY

An intact integument is the primary barrier to infection. Meticulous care is essential to prevent breakdown. The HSCT nurse instructs the patient on the importance of daily hygiene with an antimicrobial soap and the use of hypoallergenic emollients to maintain skin integrity. Careful attention to central line sites and areas that have been subjected to invasive procedures is important. Denuded areas secondary to adhesive dressings often occur around central line sites and are a potential source of infection as well as a source of pain. The use of antimicrobial ointments at the denuded areas and alternating the size and position of the dressing to prevent further breakdown can be helpful. The administration of pain medication prior to the dressing change may alleviate discomfort.

GRAFT-VERSUS-HOST DISEASE

Acute graft-versus-host disease (aGVHD) typically appears 10–40 days after HSCT. Incidence ranges from 20% to 80%, depending on the degree of histocompatibility, number of T cells in the graft, patient's age, and prophylactic regimen used. aGVHD may affect the skin, gastrointestinal tract, and/or liver. The presenting sign of skin GVHD is an erythematous maculopapular rash on the face, neck, palms, and soles. This may be associated with a tingling or burning sensation.[13]

Nursing care is centered on early recognition of these signs and symptoms and prompt reporting to the physician or nurse practitioner. The HSCT nurse must instruct the patient about meticulous skin care, with special attention to areas of desquamation. The use of bath oils and hypoallergenic lotion may help to decrease pruritus. The addition of corticosteroids to the prophylactic regimen for treatment of aGVHD and assessment of the patient's response are critical to the treatment course. Nursing care should also include prevention of injury to the skin through the use of specialized air flow beds, frequent turning and positioning of the patient, and maintaining nutritional support.[10] If skin bullae and desquamation occur, particular attention to insensible fluid loss and superinfection is critical.

Symptoms of gastrointestinal GVHD can include diarrhea with or without nausea and vomiting, abdominal pain, and/or ileus. Nursing management includes monitoring the amount, consistency, and characteristics of the diarrhea; guaiac testing of stool; monitoring the perirectal area for evidence of breakdown; and promoting meticulous hygiene. Assessment of fluid and electrolyte status through strict measurement of intake/output, daily weights, evaluation of serum laboratory values, and patient clinical status are imperative.

The HSCT nurse is responsible for administering electrolyte replacement, antiemetics, and analgesics as ordered. The use of platelet transfusions for support is also likely, with high volumes of stool output due to blood loss secondary to eroded mucosa from aGVHD of the gut.[10] Liver aGVHD is associated with an elevation of serum bilirubin alone or combined with increased serum activity of transaminases and possible prolongation of prothrombin time/partial prothrombin time. Nursing management includes monitoring the liver enzymes, coagulation studies, and degree of jaundice. Maintaining nutritional status through liquid supplementation or total parenteral nutrition is important while treatment for aGVHD is underway.[10]

VENO-OCCLUSIVE DISEASE

Veno-occlusive disease (VOD) of the liver is a life-threatening complication related to the conditioning regimen. The frequency varies greatly in reported series, from 1% to 54%.[14] Risk factors vary considerably. Elevated transaminases and a prior history of hepatitis C, however, have been identified as the most important risk factors. In allogeneic HSCT, the use of busulfan, methotrexate, and especially the combination of the two is associated with an increased risk of VOD. Extensive damage to structures in the centrilobular region (zone 3) of the liver is characteristic of the clinical syndrome of VOD.

Early injury occurs as subintimal edema with centrilobular congestion and hepatocyte degeneration. Fibrin deposition and accumulation of cell debris occurs in the vessel lumen secondary to microthrombus formation. The result is obstruction of venous blood flow through the liver.[15] A liver biopsy is often precluded because the syndrome is common in the presence of profound thrombocytopenia, generally within the first 21 days after transplantation.

Diagnosis of VOD is based on clinical criteria, which involves bilirubin greater than 2 mg/dL together with two of the following: hepatomegaly, weight gain greater than 2% of baseline, or ascites.[16]

Nursing management includes a baseline knowledge of the natural progression of VOD. Generally, insidious weight gain and jaundice precede abdominal pain, ascites, or encephalopathy.[17] Strict measurement of intake and output, daily weights, and monitoring of vital signs including postural blood pressure is important. Affected patients often experience fluid retention—thus, an adequate assessment of their fluid status is essential for treatment. Colloids, crystalloids, and packed red blood cells are generally administered if the patient is hypovolemic. If the patient is euvolemic or hypervolemic, fluid restrictions are often used. The intent is to maintain intravascular volume while minimizing capillary leak.[1] Administration of pain medication may also be necessary but should be undertaken cautiously because oversedation may occur in the setting of hepatic dysfunction.

Despite severe thrombocytopenia, heparin and tissue-plasminogen activator must be administered, predisposing the patient to bleeding. A vasodilator medication may also be used. Continuous assessment for evidence of bleeding is essential, as is the administration of blood products to prevent bleeding. Uncontrolled VOD often progresses to multiorgan failure and subsequent death.

RENAL COMPLICATIONS

Renal impairment in the HSC recipient is common in the setting of multiorgan failure. The most common type of renal insufficiency is prerenal failure.[18] Prerenal failure is a result of inadequate glomerular filtration secondary to diminished renal blood flow. Reasons for decreased renal blood flow are several: hypovolemia secondary to dehydration, capillary leak syndrome as a consequence of VOD, impaired blood flow secondary to sepsis, congestive heart failure, and vasoconstriction of renal arteries secondary to medications such as amphotericin B, cyclosporine, tacrolimus, acyclovir, and aminoglycosides.[17]

Treatment is aimed at correcting intravascular depletion through blood products and intravenous hydration, dose reduction of nephrotoxic medications, and correcting electrolyte imbalances.[19]

Acute tubular necrosis is the most common cause of intrarenal failure[20] and is often the result of administration of nephrotoxic medications that cause damage to the tubular cells. Hemodialysis is often required until tubular cells become functional. Nursing care includes close monitoring of the patient's weight, intake/output, urine studies, medication levels, and vital signs, including postural blood pressure and ongoing respiratory assessment.[17]

PULMONARY COMPLICATIONS

Pulmonary complications in the HSCT recipient, including infection, interstitial pneumonitis, and diffuse alveolar hemorrhage, carry significant morbidity and mortality. Predisposing factors include prior lung damage, immunosuppression, and profound neutropenia, which allows for the growth of opportunistic organisms.[17] Nursing management centers on prevention through ongoing pulmonary assessment, incentive spirometry, and good pulmonary toilet. Changes in the patient's respiratory rate/effort, abnormal breath sounds on lung assessment, and possibly changes in the patient's neurologic and/or mental status can signal hypoxia.[7] A pulse oximetry reading, a chest radiograph, and possibly an arterial blood gas measurement are conducted to further assess the patient's respiratory status. Nursing measures to improve oxygenation include placing the patient in high Fowler position, administration of oxygen via Venti mask, bronchodilators, anxiolytics, and diuretics as ordered. If the patient has thick oral secretions or increased sputum production, airway humidification, frequent turning and positioning, and the use of an oral suction device may alleviate discomfort.[7]

NEUROLOGIC COMPLICATIONS

Neurologic complications in HSCT recipients can occur at any stage of transplantation. Central nervous system complications that have been observed include leukoencephalopathy, drug-induced neurotoxicity, infections, hemorrhage, recurrence of malignancy, and metabolic encephalopathy.[21] Of these central nervous system complications, metabolic encephalopathy is the most common in this patient population.[13]

Continuous assessment of the HSCT recipient's mentation is key to early identification of subtle neurologic changes. Abnormal serum laboratory values and knowledge regarding their neurologic impact is useful in anticipating orders for electrolyte replacement. With changes in a patient's mentation comes an increased risk of injury. The HSCT nurse needs to maintain a safe environment through the use of raised bed rails, placing the call bell within reach, maintaining the bed in low position, using restraints, and assessing the need for constant supervision.[7] Frequent orientation to time, place, and person may ease patient anxiety. Fear of permanent damage may increase the anxiety of the patient as well as the family members. Constant reassurance and emotional support from the nurse is essential.[17]

PSYCHOLOGICAL COMPLICATIONS

Fear, anxiety, depression, and nervousness constitute the emotional response to the HSCT process.[22] On admission, many HSCT recipients generally face a hospital stay of at least 3 weeks. Many techniques and types of isolation are used to prevent nosocomial infections.[6] Special filtration systems to protect the patient during profound neutropenia often require the patient to remain in the hospital room until peripheral WBC count recovers. Social isolation secondary to protective isolation can have significant effects on a patient's psychological state, often leading to feelings of confinement and increased anxiety. The HSCT nurse should assess the patient and family for social support from friends and neighbors who may be helpful during the patient's hospitalization. Alternative modes of communication with family members and friends via phone calls, letters, and audio and video tapes may be explored. The nurse can remind family members of the importance of interaction with the patient to aid recovery.[7]

HSCT nurses can explore ways to decrease anxiety through relaxation techniques, support groups, consultation with the HSCT clinical or oncology social worker and hospital clergy, mild sedatives, or the use of psychology and psychiatry services. Reminding patients that routine complications are indeed routine can reassure them that their course is normal.[22] HSCT nurses can lessen anxiety regarding diagnostic tests by providing information about the sequence and timing of those tests.[23] Patients in critical condition pose a challenge for the bedside nurse. Through constant contact with patient and family members, the nurse often becomes the patient advocate. It is a challenge to balance the hope for a cure with the possibility of death.[23] Encouraging patients and their family members to verbalize their concerns and questions decreases the possibility of miscommunication and provides emotional support.

ROLE OF PHYSICIAN ASSISTANT OR ADVANCED PRACTICE NURSE

Traditionally, the physician assistant (PA) and nurse practitioner (NP) roles have been in primary care. Several subspecialties have developed, including HSCT. The PA or NP role provides an important service in both the inpatient and the outpatient setting. In both settings, the PA and/or NP work collaboratively with physicians to organize and deliver care to patients undergoing HSCT. The PA or NP performs physical examinations and assesses patients for side effects, toxicity, and disease response. Laboratory and diagnostic tests are ordered and interpreted as indicated. Diagnostic procedures, including bone marrow aspirate and biopsy, skin biopsy, and lumbar puncture, are performed by the PA or NP, who plays an active role in education of the patient and family regarding the recovery process, prevention and treatment of complications, and strategy for self-care.[24]

As the time for discharge approaches, coordination between the inpatient and outpatient staff, homecare services, and social work is crucial in facilitating a smooth transition from inpatient to outpatient status. This coordination is helpful in maintaining communication among all disciplines because HSC recipients require extensive outpatient care and are frequently readmitted with transplant-related complications.

CONCLUSION

HSCT provides a challenging environment of continued learning for specialized nurses. The intense physiologic and psychological stressors that affect the patient and family can be reduced significantly through the HSCT nurse's consistent and high-quality care. Integration of the nurse into the HSCT team compliments delivery of care and improves the patient's experience.[25]

REFERENCES

1. O'Quin T, Moravec C: The critically ill bone marrow transplant patient. Semin Oncol 4(1):25–30, 1988.
2. Ezzone S, Camp-Sorrell D (eds): Oncology Nursing Society Manual for Bone Marrow Transplant Nursing: Recommendations for Practice and Education. Pittsburgh, Oncology Nursing Press, 1994.
3. McGuire DB, Altomonte V, Peterson DE, et al: Patterns of mucositis and pain in patients receiving preparative chemotherapy and bone marrow transplantation. Oncol Nurs Forum 20(10):1493–1502, 1993.
4. DeFronzo RA, Braine H, Colvin M, et al: Water intoxication in man after cyclophosphamide therapy. Ann Intern Med 78:861–869, 1973.
5. Davis JM, Rowley SD, Braine HG, et al: Clinical toxicity of cryopreserved bone marrow graft infusion. Blood 75(3):781–786, 1990.
6. Zerbe MB, Parkerson SG, Spitzer T: Laminar air flow versus reverse isolation: nurses' assessments of moods, behaviors, and activity levels in patients receiving bone marrow transplants. Oncol Nurs Forum 21(3):565–568, 1994.
7. Ballard B, Caudell KA, Meriney D, et al: Nursing care plans for the hospitalized bone marrow transplant patient. In Whedon MB (ed): Bone Marrow Transplantation. Boston, Jones and Bartlett, 1991.
8. Richard-Smith A, Buh S: Reducing central line infections in bone marrow transplant patients. Nurs Clin North Am 30(1):45–52, 1995.
9. Storto Poe S, Larson E, NcGuire D, Krumm S: A national survey of infection prevention practices on bone marrow transplantation units. Oncol Nurs Forum 21(10):1687–1694, 1994.
10. Wujcik D, Ballard B, Camp-Sorrell D: Selected complications of allogeneic bone marrow transplantation. Semin Oncol Nurs 10(1):28–41, 1994.
11. Beutler E: Platelet transfusion, the 20,000 microL trigger. Blood 82(2):682–683, 1993.
12. Bowden RA, Slichter SJ, Sayers M, et al: A comparison of filtered leukocyte-reduced and cytomegalovirus (CMV) seronegative blood products for the prevention of transfusion-associated CMV infection after marrow transplant. Blood 86(9):3599–3603, 1995.
13. Ball ED, Bloom EJ, Donnenberg AD, et al: Bone marrow transplantation. In Ayers SM, Grenvik A, Holbrook PR, Shoemaker WC (eds): Textbook of Critical Care, 3rd ed. Philadelphia, WB Saunders, 1995.
14. Bearman SI: The syndrome of hepatic veno-occlusive disease after marrow transplantation. Blood 85(11):3005–3020, 1995.
15. Blostein MD, Paltiel OB, Thibault A, Rybka WB: A comparison of clinical criteria for the diagnosis of veno-occlusive disease of the liver after bone marrow transplantation. Bone Marrow Transplant 10(5):439–443, 1992.
16. Jones RJ, Lee KSK, Beschorner WE, et al: Veno-occlusive disease of the liver following bone marrow transplantation. Transplantation 44(6):778–783, 1987.
17. Wujcik D, Downs S: Bone marrow transplantation. Crit Care Nurs Clin North Am 4(1):149–166, 1992.
18. Zager RA, O'Quigley J, Zager BK, et al: Acute renal failure following bone marrow transplantation: a retrospective study of 272 patients. Am J Kidney Dis 13(3):210–216, 1989.
19. Klingemann HG: Kidneys and urinary tract. In Deeg HJ, Klingemann HG, Phillips GL (eds): A Guide to Bone Marrow Transplantation, 2nd ed. New York, Springer-Verlag, 1992.
20. Ballard B: Renal and hepatic complications. In Whedon MB (ed): Bone Marrow Transplantation. Boston, Jones and Bartlett, 1991.
21. Klingemann HG: Central nervous system. In Deeg HJ, Klingemann HG, Phillips GL (eds): A Guide to Bone Marrow Transplantation, 2nd ed. New York, Springer-Verlag, 1992.
22. Winters G, Miller C, Maracich L, et al: Provisional practice: the nature of psychosocial bone marrow transplant nursing. Oncol Nurs Forum 21(7):1147–1154, 1994.
23. Haberman MR: Psychosocial aspects of bone marrow transplantation. Semin Oncol Nurs 4(1):55–59, 1988.
24. Galassi A, Wheeler V: Advanced practice nursing: history and future trends. In Hubbard SM, Greene PE, Knobf T (eds): Oncology Nursing. Philadelphia, JB Lippincott, 1994.
25. Simpson JK: A day in the life of a bone marrow transplant nurse practitioner. Newsletter of the NP Special Interest Group, Oncology Nursing Society 7(3):1, 1996.

CHAPTER SIXTY-TWO

Coordination and Data Collection

Jennifer K. Simpson, M.S.N., Ph.D., and
Mary R. Burgunder, B.S.N.

A hematopoietic stem cell (HSC) transplantation (HSCT) program is a referral-based system that requires a structural component that facilitates the acquisition of patients and their introduction into the system.[1] The required evaluation and pretesting of a potential HSCT recipient is extensive and requires a systematic approach to ensure consistency. Most of the scheduled pretests are required to determine eligibility for investigational protocols and/or satisfy regulatory agency or third-party payor requirements. Adherence to the specific requirements of a transplant protocol is essential in order to maintain accuracy and validity of the data collected. This chapter reviews the procedures encountered by transplant recipients during the initial and referral period, pretesting, and data collection. The role and responsibilities of the HSCT coordinator and oncology registrar are reviewed.

In 1994, the Foundation for the Accreditation of Hematopoietic Cell Therapy (FAHCT) was established as the result of a merge in standards between the International Society for Hematotherapy and Graft Engineering (IS-HAGE) and the American Society for Blood and Marrow Transplantation (ASBMT). The primary goal of FAHCT is to promote quality practice in HSCT. Currently, FAHCT certification is voluntary and requires inspection and accreditation of HSCT facilities and procedures. To be accredited, centers must meet all criteria detailed in the FAHCT standards.[2]

ROLE OF THE HSCT COORDINATOR AND NURSING TEAM

FAHCT standards require that a minimum of 10 transplantations be performed in the year preceding an institution's application for accreditation, and further require programs to employ one or more designated staff members to provide efficient pretransplantation patient evaluation, and to coordinate treatment, post-transplantation follow-up and care.[2] A nurse coordinator is necessary to ensure protocol compliance and consistency. The size and complexity of an institution's HSCT program, as defined by the volume and types of transplantations performed annually, determine the number of coordinators needed. Programs performing more than 10 transplantations per year should have a full-time HSCT nurse coordinator.

The role of the coordinator varies by institution and may be program-based, clinically focused, research-based, or a combination of these components. Working titles may include Program Coordinator, Clinical Research Coordinator, Case Manager, or Clinical Coordinator. Programs performing transplants from unrelated donors may need a National Marrow Donor Program (NMDP) Coordinator. Many centers have a registered nurse in the role of coordinator. The registered nurse may have a diploma of nursing, an associate's degree, a baccalaureate of nursing (BSN), or a master's degree. The educational requirements may vary by institution and level of experience.

FAHCT accreditation requires HSCT program nurses and nurse supervisors to be formally trained and experienced in the management of patients receiving HSCT. Public and professional resources available for the education and practice of BMT nurses follow:

Manual for Bone Marrow Transplant Nursing: Recommendations for Practice and Education. Available through the Oncology Nursing Society (telephone number: 412/921–7373)

Bone Marrow Transplantation and Peripheral Blood Stem Cell Transplantation, Research Report. National Institutes of Health, National Cancer Institute, 1994

BMT Newsletter (for patients and families) (telephone number: 708/831-1913)

Leukemia Society of America (telephone number: 800/955-4572)

American Cancer Society (telephone number: 800/227-2345)

An essential component of the coordinator role is communication. The coordinator is the link between patient and physician and is responsible for communicating the treatment plan to the team. The coordinator maintains and ensures the continuity of care through all three phases of treatment—pretransplantation, intratransplantation, and post-transplantation.

The coordinator and nursing team may be responsible for a specific patient population (i.e., autologous peripheral blood progenitor cell transplants for lymphoma patients or allogeneic HSCT). The research coordinator may be assigned specific research studies and coordinate the patients enrolled in such studies. These duties include reviewing eligibility criteria and ensuring protocol compliance.

The coordinator's role may also include some responsibility for the clinical management of patients. For example, patients may call the coordinator with clinical issues such as central venous catheter problems or symptom management. Although most centers have an outpatient staff to manage the clinical care of the patient, the coordinator's role is still important in overseeing the patient's complete treatment course.

The coordinator role as a case manager has evolved in the modern era of managed care. Case management components of the role may include obtaining insurance approval, monitoring length of stay and resource utilization, and developing clinical pathway or care guidelines.

The NMDP requires a coordinator to perform unrelated donor searches, donor recruitment, and procurement. The NMDP coordinator may also be responsible for submitting data required by the Registry, or this may be performed by an oncology registrar.

The role of the coordinator is usually defined by the physician team and the institution. The role needs to fit the job categories available in the institution but also meet the needs of the transplant physician team as well as the patient. At many HSCT centers, a single person combines these roles. A center performing more than 100 transplantations per year may have two or three coordinators whose roles incorporate some or all of the responsibilities mentioned. Some coordinators also may have data management responsibilities, although centers performing more than 20 transplantations per year should have one full-time data management staff. This is discussed later in the chapter.

PHASES OF CARE

INITIAL (REFERRAL) PHASE

Referrals are usually made by the patient's primary care physician or hematologist/oncologist. Most centers have a dedicated intake telephone number to receive referrals. This may be in the physician's office, outpatient clinic, or coordinator's office with specially trained and/or assigned staff. The intake coordinator collects information regarding the patient's medical history, demographics, and insurance coverage. A clinical pathway may be initiated (Table 62–1). The amount of information required may vary by institution. For an example of a BMT referral sheet, see Figure 62–1.

After the information is reviewed by an HSCT physician, the patient is scheduled for an evaluation appointment. The evaluation may vary in length from one to several days. The purpose of the evaluation is to assess the patient's suitability for transplantation and to plan the timing of the transplantation. It is also the time for the patient and family to gain information regarding the procedure.[3] Detailed discussion of the evaluation process is described in Chapter 20.

The HSCT physician reviews all the patient's previous medical treatment. The physician or physician extender (certified registered nurse practitioner or physician assistant) performs a history and physical examination. The physician then presents the patient with the proposed treatment or research protocol and the potential acute and chronic complications that may occur during or after transplantation. This discussion begins the process of informed consent. The physician may discuss prognosis for long-term disease-free survival and answers any questions the patient or family may have. (If allogeneic HSCT is considered, the procedure for donor evaluation and harvesting is discussed with the patient and donor.) After the discussion with the HSCT physician and coordinator, the patient and family meet with the rest of the HSCT team. This may include a social worker, nutritionist, and financial analyst and a tour of the in-patient unit.

The coordinator discusses the proposed treatment plan and/or research protocol, provides education regarding the pretransplantation evaluation and timeline of testing, and answers any additional questions from the patient and family. A HSCT patient handbook is often provided at this point. The consent form is provided and thoroughly reviewed with the patient. The patient is encouraged to ask questions and may be required to sign a consent form prior to the initiation of pretesting. If there will be a search for an unrelated donor, the NMDP coordinator discusses the process and timeline.

The social worker performs a psychosocial assessment, reviewing the patient's coping skills and support mechanisms. The social worker provides the patient with information and resources for support services and programs available to the patient and family. A review of housing needs and facilities, if needed, also is conducted.

Even prior to and during the evaluation phase, the patient's insurance coverage and benefits have been under review. This is generally conducted by representatives from the institution's financial and contract departments. Prescription, outpatient, inpatient, and home health coverage are discussed with the patient and family. The process of obtaining financial clearance to proceed with HSCT is initiated at this time.

If a donor has not already been identified, human leukocyte antigen (HLA) typing may be needed after the initial consultation. The coordinator may arrange for typing the patient and siblings. If there is any difficulty in determining the HLA typing, the parents may need to be typed. Should no suitable family donor be found, a matched unrelated donor search may be initiated by the NMDP coordinator.

At the HSCT patient care conference, generally held each week, the physician and/or coordinator presents each patient currently undergoing evaluation and seeks input from the team regarding the patient's eligibility for transplantation, including clinical criteria, psychosocial status, and the patent's insurance coverage. The team decides how to proceed, and the coordinator communicates this decision to the patient and family. The transplant physician communicates the plan for the patient's care to the referring physician(s).

PRETRANSPLANTATION WORK-UP PHASE

The HSCT coordinator bases the pre-transplant work-up on the patient's disease, type of transplantation and treatment, and/or research protocol. The goal of the pretransplantation evaluation is to ensure that the patient meets the

TABLE 62–1. UNIVERSITY OF PITTSBURGH CANCER INSTITUTE (PCI)
CLINICAL PATHWAY BONE MARROW TRANSPLANT EVALUATION

COLLABORATIVE CARE PLAN	DATE: REFERRAL	DATE: EVALUATION DAY 1
1. Consults	Referred to HSCT program Received by HSCT coordinator *Actions and notifications:* a) Records requested from referring physician b) Physician/clinical director notified c) HSCT coordinator obtains patient demographics and financial information d) Potential donor information obtained, if appropriate e) Donor insurance verification obtained, if appropriate f) Patient contacted within 24 hours of referral g) Attending HSCT physician assigned h) Insurance verified by credit analyst *Notified of scheduled intake:* a) Clinical social work b) HSCT coordinator c) PCI outpatient services d) Orders sent to PCI OPS for laboratory testing e) HSCT unit f) HSCT attending physician	a) Multidisciplinary review of patient by 　Attending physician 　Nurse practitioner 　Clinical social worker 　HSCT nurse 　Credit analyst 　HSCT coordinator b) Payor medical clearance initiated by case manager
Initials:		
2. Tests		a) Complete blood count, differential, electrolytes, blood urea nitrogen, creatinine b) Mg, Ca, phosphorus, bilirubin c) Uric acid, lactate dehydrogenase, aspartate and alanine aminotransferase, alkaline phosphatase d) Cytomegalovirus e) Herpes simplex virus, herpes zoster virus f) Epstein-Barr virus, if potential allogeneic HSCT g) Hepatitis A, B, C h) Anti-HIV I/II i) Unilateral bone marrow aspiration and biopsy j) Cytogenetics if disease appropriate k) HLA typing, if potential allogeneic HSCT l) Serologic typing m) Molecular typing
Initials:		
3. Treatments		
Initials:		
4. Medications		
Initials:		
5. Nutrition		
Initials:		
6. Activity/safety		
Initials:		
7. Assessment Initials:		a) History and physical examination by physician b) Physical assessment by CRNP/physician c) Assignment of transplant type d) Donor search initiated, if allogeneic HSCT
8. Discharge planning		
Initials:		
9. Psychological/Social Initials:		a) Outpatient psychosocial assessment interview
10. Patient education Patient/significant other to understand:	a) Intake date and time b) Overview of intake process	a) Treatment options as identified by physician b) Overview of HSCT process c) Patient responsibilities d) Pretesting requirements prior to transplant e) Financial clearance process f) Orientation to inpatient hospitalization and outpatient follow-up

CRNP, certified registered nurse practitioner; OPS, outpatient services.

Date: _____

Patient Name: _____ Social Security Number: _____

Date of Birth: _____ Sex:_____ Race: _____

Address: _____

_____

Telephone: _____

Referring Doctor: _____

Address: _____

_____

Telephone: _____

Diagnosis: _____

Date of Diagnosis: _____

Disease State: _____

Stage: _____

HLA typing: _____

Siblings: _____

Course of Therapy:

_____

Complications/infections:

_____

_____

FIGURE 62–1. Hematopoietic stem cell transplantation referral information sheet.

transplant/protocol criteria and is sufficiently healthy to undergo high-dose chemotherapy and/or radiation therapy.

The referring physician may be requested to perform some or all of the pretransplantation testing. Pretesting by the referring physician is generally more convenient for patients, who may be required to travel long distances to transplant centers. Some centers require that all testing be performed at the transplant center; patients are asked to bring previous radiographic test results with them for comparison. Some patients may be required to stay at or near the transplant center for up to 1 week to complete the evaluation process.

Cardiac function is assessed by electrocardiography and multigated angiography. Respiratory function is evaluated by pulmonary function testing and chest radiography. Baseline laboratory values consisting of electrolytes, blood urea nitrogen, and creatinine are used to assess renal function. A creatinine clearance test may be required if an abnormality is identified[3] or if such a test is a protocol requirement.

Patients should be assessed for previous fungal, protozoan, viral, and bacterial infections. If an infection is identified, treatment may be required before proceeding to transplantation. Patients are required to undergo a dental evaluation, including cleaning and Panorex films. Because the oral cavity may be a source of infection, all dental work must be completed prior to transplantation.

Restaging of the disease is often required, and patients may undergo computed tomography (CT), bone marrow aspirate and biopsy, and lumbar puncture. Baseline laboratory studies to evaluate hematologic, immunologic, renal, and liver function are required within 30 days of transplantation.[3] Blood typing and antibody screening are required to ensure that the patient receives appropriate blood and platelet support. A complete list of tests that may be required during the pretransplantation work-up phase follows:

History and Physical Examination
Cardiac EKG, Multigated angiography with ejection fraction (if exposure to high doses of anthracycline or cardiac symptoms are present)
Pulmonary Chest radiograph, pulmonary function tests with diffusion capacity if there is question of respiratory compromise or infection
Neurologic Lumbar puncture, if indicated
Dental Clearing and evaluation for potential sources of infection or abscess
Renal Biochemistry profiles, assessment of glomerular filtration rate
Hematologic Complete blood count, differential, platelets, and retic count; bone marrow biopsy and aspirate, if indicated; blood group typing and antibody screen
Immunologic/Infectious Disease Human immunodeficiency virus (HIV), herpes zoster and simplex, cytomegalovirus, toxoplasmosis, Epstein-Barr virus, hepatitis A, B, and C, human T-cell lymphotropic virus, syphilis
Ophthalmologic Examination for cataracts, Schirmer test (if HSCT is allogeneic)

TRANSPLANTATION PHASE

Immediately prior to proceeding with transplantation, the physician re-reviews HSCT procedures and process with the patient and patient's family. The coordinator double-checks the chemotherapy orders to ensure protocol consistency and correct doses. These may be preprinted orders that are protocol specific. Many institutions have a one-page treatment matrix that can be individualized by the coordinator for the patient and/or protocol. The coordinator monitors the patients' course to ensure protocol compliance.

POST-TRANSPLANTATION PHASE

The HSCT physician and coordinator continue to follow the patient at the specific time intervals outlined in the treatment protocol. Follow-up may include quality-of-life assessment and restaging to determine disease response. Routine follow-up may be conducted in the outpatient setting. Table 62–2 is an example for follow-up care with allogeneic HSCT, and Table 62–3 is a typical follow-up schema for breast cancer patients after autologous transplantation using peripheral blood progenitor cells.

DONOR EVALUATION

Donor valuation should be performed at the transplant center. This may be done along with the patient evaluation or separately. The coordinator provides the donor with the appropriate consent. The donor also undergoes a medical history, physical examination, and assessment of cardiac, respiratory, and renal functions.[3] If a marrow harvest is planned, the donor is assessed for suitability to undergo general anesthesia. If peripheral blood progenitor cells are

to be collected, the donor is evaluated for peripheral venous access. This initial assessment may be performed by the apheresis staff. If peripheral venous access is inadequate, a surgical consultation may be initiated for a temporary apheresis catheter. A list of tests that may be performed for the donor evaluation follows:

History and physical examination
Chest radiograph
Electrocardiogram
Urinalysis
Viral titers: HIV, herpes simplex and zoster, cytomegalovirus, toxoplasmosis, Epstein-Barr virus, hepatitis A, B, and C
Biochemistry profile, complete blood count, differential, platelets
ABO, Rh typing
Venous access evaluation

If peripheral blood progenitor cells are mobilized with a cytokine, the donor's prescription coverage is evaluated. The cytokine may be covered by either the donor's or the patient's insurance. This step should be evaluated early in the planning process in order to minimize potential costs to the donor. After the completion of donor testing, the patient is cleared to proceed with transplantation.

DATA COLLECTION AND EVALUATION

HSCT is an accepted treatment modality for many diseases. Although many technologic advancements have been made, continuing research is needed to improve pretransplantation conditioning regimens, immunosuppression, and post-transplantation management, including infection and graft-versus-host disease.[4]

Patients are often enrolled in several research protocols, and the results are reported to varying HSCT registries, cancer clinical trials, cooperative groups, and/or (for industry-sponsored trials) pharmaceutical companies. Following is a listing of cooperative groups and registries:

Cooperative Groups
ECOG Eastern Cooperative Oncology Group
SWOG South West Oncology Group
CALGB Cancer and Leukemia Group B
CCG Childrens Cancer Group
POG Pediatric Oncology Group
Registries
IBMTR International Bone Marrow Transplant Registry
ABMTR Autologous Blood and Marrow Transplant Registry
EBMTR European Bone Marrow Transplant Registry
NMDP National Marrow Donor Program

Often the information is duplicated among varying cooperative groups, registries, and pharmaceutical groups and can be labor intensive. When the number of transplantations exceeds 20 per year, a full-time data manager is necessary to assist in collection of data for reporting to various agencies.[5]

Several computer software packages are now available for data management. One in particular, *StemSoft,* offers a variety of programs specific to HSCT for data management, reporting, or analysis. *BMTbase 095-Reports* incorporates all

TABLE 62-2. ALLOGENEIC HSCT FOLLOW-UP SCHEMA

EVERY VISIT	WEEKLY	DAY +28	DAY +90–100	4 MONTHS	5 MONTHS	6 MONTHS	9 MONTHS	1 YEAR
Complete blood count, differential, platelets	Cytomegalovirus cultures: Blood Urine Throat	Bone marrow sample	Chest radiograph	Clinic visit	Clinic visit	Clinic visit	Clinic visit	Clinic visit
SMAC-7, liver function tests	Albumin and total protein		Pulmonary function tests with diffusion capacity of lungs w/carbon monoxide	Laboratory work from weekly and every visit	Laboratory work from weekly and every visit	Lactate dehydrogenase/ follicle-stimulating hormone level	Computed tomography, if applicable	Bone marrow sample
						Testosterone (M), estrogen (F) Thyroid screen		Quantitative immunoglobulin levels Cytomegalovirus cultures if recently on immunosuppression
Lactate dehydrogenase	Reticulocyte count		Opthalmic examination			Quantitative immunoglobulin levels		Vaccines: Mitogen battery Tetanus Diphtheria Pneumovax *Haemophilus* flu Seasonal flus if b/w March and October
FK-506 level Cyclosporine level (C-mono)			Bone marrow sample Skin biopsy					
History and physical			Red blood cell phenotype					
			VNTR Computed tomography, if applicable Remove central line if no longer needed					
Ongoing: Intravenous immunoglobulin day +35, 58, 77, 97						Cytomegalovirus cultures		Pulmonary function tests with diffusion capacity of lungs w/carbon monoxide
Consults: as needed Transfusions: as needed						Bone marrow sample		Computed tomography, if applicable Ophthalmic exam
IV antibiotics: as needed						Computed tomography, if applicable Gynecologic evaluation Pulmonary function tests with diffusion capacity of lungs w/carbon monoxide		Electrocardiography Measles, mumps, rubella titer
								Purified protein derivative

TABLE 62–3. AUTOLOGOUS PERIPHERAL BLOOD PROGENITOR CELL TRANSPLANTATION BREAST CANCER FOLLOW-UP SCHEMA

EVERY VISIT	WEEKLY TILL DAY +30	DAY +30	3 MONTHS
History and physical	History and physical	Complete blood count, differential, platelets	Clinic visit
Complete blood count, differential, platelets	Complete blood count, differential, platelets	Na, K, glucose, Cl	Computed tomography, if applicable
NA, K, glucose, Cl	NA, K, glucose, Cl	Blood urea nitrogen, creatinine	Remove central line if no longer needed
Blood urea nitrogen, creatinine	Blood urea nitrogen, creatinine	Ca, CO_2, Mg	Complete blood count, differential, platelets
Ca, CO_2, Mg	Ca, CO_2, Mg	Aspartate aminotransferase, alanine aminotransferase, alkaline phosphatase	Na, K, glucose, Cl
Aspartate aminotransferase, alanine aminotransferase, alkaline phosphatase	Aspartate aminotransferase, alanine aminotransferase, alkaline phosphatase	LDH, total bilirubin	Blood urea nitrogen, creatinine
Lactate dehydrogenase (LDH), total bilirubin	LDH, total bilirubin	Uric acid	Ca, CO_2, Mg
Uric acid	Uric acid	Multigated angiogram	Aspartate aminotransferase, alanine aminotransferase, alkaline phosphatase
			LDH, total bilirubin
		Within 2 wk of absolute neutrophil count > 1500 mm^3 or PLT $> 100,000$/mm^3	Uric acid
		Electrocardiographic performance status 0 or 1	
		Gastrointestinal toxicity 0 or 1	
		Bilirubin < 2 mg/dL	
		Ejection fraction $> 40\%$ by multigated angiogram:	
		BEGIN	
		Doxorubicin 50 mg/m^2	
		Paclitaxel 150 mg/m^2	
		Granulocyte colony-stimulating factor 5 μm/kg	
		Day 3–12 after chemotherapy	
Ongoing: Pamidronate monthly, if needed Consults as needed Transfusions as needed			

of the necessary information required for the IBMTR 095 series reports. Through *BMTtransfer,* all 095 reports can be submitted to the IBMTR/ABMTR electronically. The *BMTstats* package enables the user to perform univariate, cross-tabulation, and survival analyses. These software packages can streamline the reporting process and in turn make statistical analysis more efficient.

Data collection and reporting may be the responsibility of one or more persons, and the credentials for each position vary among institutions. One approach is to have an oncology registrar and a HSCT coordinator. The oncology registrar is not required to have a postsecondary education but must have a minimum of 2 years of experience related to health care or education. The oncology registrar works with the physicians, nurses, and other allied health professionals to coordinate data collection for patients on clinical trials and reports to the clinical director of protocol implementation. Responsibilities include obtaining patient records; laboratory, radiology, and pathology reports; and other important information required to complete the case report forms. The registrar also assists HSCT coordinators in data retrieval, including prospective and retrospective data. Case report forms are monitored for quality assurance. Protocol activities and other pertinent information are distributed to the appropriate personnel by the oncology registrar.

Because the amount of data can be excessive, one option is to limit data collection to the transplant admission. Data

6 MONTHS	9 MONTHS	1 YEAR	EVERY 6 MONTHS
Clinic visit	Clinic visit	Clinic visit	Clinic visit
Complete blood count, differential, platelets	Complete blood count, differential, platelets	Bone scan, if applicable	Computed tomography, if applicable
Na, K, glucose, Cl	Na, K, glucose, Cl	Computed tomography	Bone scan, if applicable
Blood urea nitrogen, creatinine	Blood urea nitrogen, creatinine	Vaccines:	Complete blood count, differential, platelets
		Mitogen battery	
		Tetanus	
		Diphtheria	
		Pneumovax	
		Haemophilus influenzae flu	
		Seasonal flu vaccines between	
		March and October	
Ca, CO$_2$, Mg	Ca, CO$_2$, Mg	Measles, mumps, rubella titer	Na, K, glucose, Cl
Aspartate aminotransferase, alanine aminotransferase, alkaline phosphatase	Aspartate aminotransferase, alanine aminotransferase, alkaline phosphatase	Purified protein derivative	Blood urea nitrogen, creatinine
LDH, total bilirubin	LDH, total bilirubin	Complete blood count, differential, platelets	Ca, CO$_2$, Mg
Uric acid	Uric acid	Na, K, glucose, Cl	Aspartate aminotransferase, alanine aminotransferase, alkaline phosphatase
Bone scan, if applicable	Computed tomography	Blood urea nitrogen, creatinine	LDH, total bilirubin
Computed tomography		Ca, CO$_2$, Mg	Uric acid
		Aspartate aminotransferase, alanine aminotransferase, alkaline phosphatase	
		LDH, total bilirubin	
		Uric acid	

would be reviewed at 30 and 100 days after transplantation with the physician or nurse practitioner to review adverse events and toxicity. This method ensures compliance with FAHCT standards regarding adverse-event reporting and total quality management. If an adverse event occurs, the HSCT coordinator is responsible for reporting the event as specified in the protocol. On average, one registrar is required for every 50 transplant patients per year.

Another approach is to employ a protocol nurse. Qualifications generally include a baccalaureate degree in nursing (BSN) and several years of clinical experience, preferably in the area of hematology/oncology and HSCT. The protocol nurse is responsible for making sure patients adhere to the protocol and comply with all necessary testing. This person also is responsible for all data collection, adverse-event reporting, and site visits. In this model, the HSCT coordinator focuses on coordinating the patient through the various aspects of pretesting and clearance.

Randomized clinical trials are often used to evaluate new treatments; however, the number of patients, cost, time, and effort required for evaluation are often not feasible in the HSCT setting. For this reason, single-center series with treatment of consecutive patients is the most common type of HSCT study.[4] An observational database is now being used to analyze many questions previously answered by randomized clinical trials or single-center studies.[6] It is easier for centers to participate in an observational database because a commitment to a common protocol is not necessary, only the agreement to report comprehensive patient information. Several databases, including IBMTR, ABMTR North America, and EBMTR, are available.

IBMTR contains information on both allogeneic and autologous transplants. This database is an important resource consisting of over 200 transplant teams worldwide. These centers voluntarily contribute data on allogeneic and syngeneic transplants.[6] The database includes information on 40–50% of all allogeneic HSCT since 1968. Data is longitudinal, with a yearly follow-up for all survivors. The initial report form is due 100 days after transplantation, 1 year after transplantation, and every year thereafter. The ability to detect meaningful changes in outcome and the precision with which they can be detected is increased because the participation of many centers provides a representation of the general transplant population. An IBMTR advisory committee oversees the research priorities, collection and quality of data submitted, design and conduct of scientific studies, and approval of all manuscripts before publication. The committee is composed of more than 50 experts in HSCT as well as allied health fields.[6] Many of the other registries are modeled after the IBMTR.

The NMDP is an international registry created in 1986 to identify volunteer unrelated donors for marrow transplants to patients with leukemia, aplastic anemia, lymphomas, and other life-threatening diseases. Baseline data are collected before admission, then again at 100, 180, and 365 days and yearly thereafter. In addition, information regarding infection, engraftment, graft-versus-host disease, and veno-occlusive disease is required at 30, 60, 100, 180, and 365 days and then yearly thereafter.

CONCLUSION

Regardless of the size of the program or division of HSCT team roles and responsibilities, coordination and data management are essential for a viable HSCT program. Collaboration between these entities ensures protocol compliance and allows for accurate and consistent data collection. This information is not only integral to the individual center but may significantly contribute to the care of patients undergoing HSCT worldwide.

REFERENCES

1. Malmberg C, Wilson MW: Pretransplant care. *In* Buchsel P, Whedon MB (eds): Bone Marrow Transplantation: Administrative and Clinical Strategies. Boston, Jones & Bartlett, 1995.
2. Foundation for the Accreditation of Hematopoietic Cell Therapy: Standards for Hematopoietic Progenitor Cell Collection, Processing and Transplantation, 1st ed. Omaha, FAHCT, 1996.
3. Smith C: The role of the transplant co-ordinator. *In* Treleaven J, Barrett J (eds): Bone Marrow Transplantation in Practice. New York, Churchill Livingstone, 1992.
4. Horowitz M, Bortin M: The role of registries in evaluating the results of bone marrow transplantation. *In* Treleaven J, Barrett J (eds): Bone Marrow Transplantation in Practice. New York, Churchill Livingstone, 1992.
5. Mangan KF, Klumpp TR, Rosenfeld CS, Shadduck RK: Bone marrow transplantation. *In* Makowka L (ed): The Handbook of Transplantation Management. Austin, TX, RG Landes, 1991.
6. Sobocinski KA, Horowitz MM, Rimm AA, et al: The international bone marrow transplant registry. *In* Atkinson K (ed): Clinical Bone Marrow Transplantation. New York, Cambridge University Press, 1994.

Biostatistics

CHAPTER SIXTY-THREE

Biostatistics

John W. Wilson, Ph.D., and Haesook T. Kim, Ph.D.

Biostatistics is a discipline devoted to studying ways data can be used to address scientific (including clinical) questions. So defined, it is a broad field that includes the design of scientific studies, the quality assurance, storage, and manipulation of data gathered from such studies, and data analysis and presentation. Clearly, it is impossible to address all these issues in detail in this chapter. We have therefore chosen to discuss the aspects of biostatistics we think are the most likely to be useful in the field of hematopoietic stem cell transplantation (HSCT).

Specifically, the first part of this chapter focuses on statistical aspects of therapy development, especially phase I, II, and III clinical trials. The second portion of the chapter presents common methods of data presentation and summarization. Next, we present some of the most commonly used methods of hypothesis testing for continuous, categorical, and censored (i.e., survival) data. Finally, we briefly describe the basic ideas of Bayesian statistical analysis, which has received increasing attention in recent years in the clinical community. For further information on these and additional biostatistical topics, we refer the reader to other sources.[1–7]

Throughout this chapter, we assume that the reader has undertaken previous study of biostatistics, including summary measures commonly calculated from samples (e.g., sample mean and median, variance and standard deviation) and the basic notions of confidence intervals and hypothesis testing. Whenever there was a choice between "technical" references (from a mathematical statistics point of view) and references readable by physicians, we have attempted to provide the latter. More technical references, if desired, may be found within the references provided at the end of this chapter.

DEVELOPMENT OF NEW THERAPIES

The development of a new therapy typically passes through well-recognized phases. Phase I involves selection of a version of the therapy (e.g., dose) to be pursued for further clinical evaluation. In phase II investigations, preliminary evidence of therapeutic value is sought. Many therapies are abandoned at the completion of phase II because they do not appear sufficiently promising to warrant further investigation. If, at the completion of phase II, the therapy is considered promising, it may be compared with another (usually standard) therapy in phase III. The "winner" of the phase III comparison may be adopted as standard practice

in clinical care. Because of the different purposes of phase I, II, and III studies, they are usually carried out in different groups of patients and using different experimental designs. Each phase is now described in detail.

PHASE I

At the completion of a phase I clinical trial, a potential therapeutic procedure should be refined sufficiently to allow initial testing for efficacy. In many cases, this stage of therapy development involves the selection of a dose of a therapeutic agent. In some cases, however, phase I studies involve confirming that a selected procedure can be carried out without undue toxicity to the target patient population. This situation might arise if a small change is made in therapy and the change is judged sufficiently minor to not warrant a full-scale dose-finding investigation. For example, a substitution might be made of tacrolimus for cyclosporin A in a regimen of prophylaxis for acute graft-versus-host disease (GVHD). Because of the growing clinical experience with tacrolimus as an immunosuppressive drug, it may be thought that a dose can be selected without a dose-ranging study. In this case, the phase I study might involve confirming that the selected regimen could be used without undue toxicity.

A major component of many phase I clinical trials is the selection of the therapeutic agent's dose. Usually, an implicit assumption is that the higher the dose, the greater the likelihood of therapeutic benefit. Naturally, higher doses are often associated with increased toxicity, and an important goal of these studies is to discover the maximum dose that can be administered without unacceptable toxicity to the patient. This dose is called the *maximum tolerated dose,* or MTD, and is usually identified by means of a "dose-escalation" design. Toxicities that prohibit the administration of a therapy above a given dose are called *dose-limiting toxicities,* or DLT (usually grade 3 and higher).

In these phase I trials, it is usually assumed that any relationship between dose and toxicity does not vary by disease. Accordingly, the patients enrolled may have a variety of diseases. In addition, because the therapy being studied is experimental and may provide no benefit, patients are usually enrolled in these trials only after any therapies with known benefit have been tried.

Dose-finding studies commonly begin with the selection of a sequence of doses to be studied. Often, this sequence takes the form of a "modified Fibonacci sequence" with increases of 100%, 67%, 50%, 40%, and 33% from the previous dose.[6] The lowest dose is chosen to be unlikely to cause severe toxicity and may be that dose with a 10% probability of mortality in animal studies of the agent(s) being studied. In general, patients are enrolled at the lowest dose and, if the toxicity is considered acceptable in these patients, further patients are enrolled at higher doses. Patients are enrolled in successively higher doses until the patients at one dose experience unacceptable levels of toxicity. The dose below this one is identified as the MTD.

Although many study designs have been used for the identification of MTD, one has emerged as the most common in practice. This design proceeds along these lines[8]: Three patients are enrolled at the lowest dose. If DLT is observed in none of these patients, an additional three patients are enrolled at the next higher dose. If two or three patients experience DLT, this dose is considered unacceptable and dose escalation ceases. If, however, one patient exhibits DLT, an additional three patients are enrolled at the same dose. If one of the total of six patients experiences DLT, additional patients are enrolled at the next higher dose. If two or more of these six patients experience DLT, dose escalation ceases. The MTD is that dose below which two or more of six patients experience DLT.

Fields et al. employed a similar design to choose a dose of etoposide phosphate to administer in bone marrow transplantation protocols.[9] After evaluating previous experience with this drug, they identified doses of 250, 500, 750, 1000, 1200, 1400, and 1600 $mg/m^2/day$ infused over a 2-hour period. After escalating doses in the manner described, they found that toxicities (mucositis and fatigue) were excessive at the 1200 mg/m^2 dose. The investigators then extended the standard dose-escalation scheme by enrolling additional patients at doses of 1200, 1400, and 1600 mg/m^2, this time administered over a 4-hour period. They found that a dose of 1400 mg/m^2 was tolerated but that mucositis and fatigue were excessive at the 1600 mg/m^2 dose. The investigators concluded that 1000 mg/m^2 could be administered safely over a period of 2 hours and that 1400 mg/m^2 could be administered safely over 4 hours.

Although this decision procedure is commonly used in phase I clinical trials, it has drawbacks. First, several patients must be enrolled at the lowest dose levels. If it is true that higher doses are necessary for therapeutic benefit, these patients have little or no chance of benefiting from the treatment they receive. In addition, the decision process used at arriving at the MTD does not account for individual patient characteristics. For these and other reasons, alternative designs have been proposed for this stage of therapy development.

O'Quigley et al. proposed a design called the *continual reassessment method*.[10] This procedure incorporates an investigator's pretrial expectations of the probability of DLT (P_{DLT}) associated with each dose. First, the investigator decides on a target P_{DLT} that represents the maximum toxicity probability the MTD should have. As the study proceeds, one patient per dose is enrolled, not necessarily beginning with the lowest dose, and the estimated P_{DLT} for each dose is updated according to that patient's toxicity experience. The next dose is chosen as the dose whose estimated P_{DLT} is just below (or closest to) the target probability. After a specified number of patients are enrolled, say

20, the MTD is chosen as that dose whose estimated P_{DLT} is just below the target probability.

Although promising as a method for identifying the MTD while minimizing the number of patients on low doses, this method carries a risk of serious toxicity to patients before much experience with the therapy is gathered. Therefore, modifications have been suggested to minimize the chance of such toxicity. For example, Goodman et al. recommended that one to three patients be enrolled per dose, that the first dose administered be the lowest, and that dose changes be by, at most, one dose level.[11] Under simulated conditions, they found that these modifications reduced the risk of highly toxic treatment while preserving the original intent of minimizing the number of patients treated on very low doses.

Simon et al. proposed and evaluated three new designs aimed at addressing the shortcomings of the standard design.[8] In one design, dose escalation begins at the lowest dose, escalating through successive doses with one patient per dose until either the first DLT or the second grade 2 toxicity is observed. At that point, the "standard" decision process based on three or six patients per dose is instituted. Two additional designs were proposed in which doses were escalated two levels at a time. In one of these designs, escalation proceeds until the first DLT or second grade 2 toxicity is observed in the first course of treatment. In the second design, escalation proceeds until these landmarks are observed in any course of treatment. Under a variety of simulated conditions, these designs reduced the number of patients enrolled (and therefore the amount of time) before the MTD was identified. In addition, fewer patients were treated at the lowest doses.

Other investigators have approached the challenges of designing phase I trials by incorporating patient-specific information in the dose selection process. Mick and Ratain designed and evaluated a procedure for predicting leukopenia in individual patients using a linear model based on pretreatment white blood cell (WBC) count and dose.[12] In a simulation study, they found that the proposed procedure identified a "true" MTD more consistently than did the "standard" phase I design and led to treatment of fewer patients with subtherapeutic doses.

Piantadosi and Liu found that modifying the continual reassessment method to incorporate both dose and pharmacokinetic measurements (specifically, area under curve [AUC]) to predict toxicity improved estimates of MTD.[13] Babb et al. proposed a different method of minimizing the number of patients treated at low dose levels.[14] Called *escalation with overdose control,* or EWOC, this procedure is designed to approach the MTD as rapidly as possible, subject to the constraint that the predicted proportion of patients receiving an overdose does not exceed a specified value. These authors are currently investigating an extension of this procedure that will allow investigators to incorporate individual patient information to improve the choice of each patient's dose.[14]

PHASE II

At the close of a phase I trial, clinical investigators should have settled on a regimen that can be further studied for evidence of efficacy in phase II. If evidence of such efficacy is not found, the regimen is either abandoned or modified before trying again in another phase II trial. Many proposed clinical treatments are abandoned after the completion of a phase II trial because there is no evidence that they warrant further study.

In contrast with phase I trials, phase II trials are designed around the idea of obtaining a preliminary estimate of the efficacy rate of the new treatment. Therefore, the trial is carried out in a group of patients for whom the therapy is most likely to be useful (e.g., in patients with the target disease). In addition, the patients in phase II trials are often at an earlier disease stage than are patients of phase I trials. In some cases, the phase II regimen may be the first treatment these patients receive for their disease.

In the field of HSCT, it is not uncommon for phase II studies to take one of two different forms. The first is a long-term follow-up study in which patients are treated and followed for a specific outcome, such as disease-free survival (DFS) or overall survival (OS). The second study type, often of shorter duration, is one in which a prescribed number of patients are observed for evidence of objective response after treatment, such as tumor shrinkage or lack of evidence of disease. Each study type is described in more detail.

It occasionally happens that a treatment is used directly in clinical practice after it is finalized during the first phase of development. This may happen when the disease in question has no known cure or when there are several regimens used by different treatment centers with none having a clear advantage over the others. The outcome of interest may be short-term objective response (e.g., tumor shrinkage or lack of evidence of disease) but is often OS or DFS at, say, 3 or 5 years after treatment. These studies may not be designed using formal statistical design principles but may instead entail accumulating data on the outcome of treatment over time. As the study progresses, OS or DFS rates may be estimated, and there may be efforts to identify particular groups of patients who especially benefit from treatment.

As an example of this type of phase II trial, Selvaggi et al. summarized patient survival after autologous HSCT using marrow treated with monoclonal antibodies sensitive to leukemia cell surface markers.[15] The patients in this cohort were treated between August 1984 and April 1992. Among patients receiving transplants in CR2, CR3, or R1, they found that the 3-year DFS rate was estimated to be 21% when patients were conditioned with cyclophosphamide and total body irradiation. The corresponding DFS rate estimate among patients conditioned with busulfan and cyclophosphamide was 48%. Because this treatment was considered successful for this group of patients, the investigators have continued to use it at their institutions.

The second phase II design stems from the need to choose a treatment that has a short-term response rate of at least a given level and to reject a treatment that has a low response rate. For example, consider a prophylactic regimen administered after allogeneic HSCT to reduce the incidence of stage 2–4 acute GVHD. Such a treatment might be considered desirable if 80% or more of patients who underwent transplantation were GVHD-free 90 days post HSCT, but the treatment might be considered undesirable if 60% or fewer patients were GVHD-free during the same interval. In the former case, investigators would likely identify the new treatment as promising with a high probability. In the latter, investigators would likely reject the treatment with high probability.

One specific study design that would accomplish this goal would be the following: Treat 36 patients with the new regimen and observe them for GVHD in the first 90 days. If 25 or fewer patients are GVHD-free in the first 90 days, reject the treatment as being unpromising. On the other hand, if 26 or more patients survive GVHD-free, conclude that the treatment is promising enough to warrant further study. Standard calculations based on the binomial probability distribution show that the regimen would be rejected with 90% probability if the "true" probability of surviving GVHD-free until 90 days were 60% or less. On the other hand, the regimen would be rejected with only 10% probability if the probability of GVHD survival were 80% or more.

The key parameters for designing this type of phase II study are as follows:

p_0 The probability of response (i.e., response incidence rate) below which the therapy would not be considered useful

p_1 The probability of response (response incidence rate) above which continued use of the therapy would be highly desirable

α The probability of concluding that a therapy is useful when its probability of response is less than p_0 (i.e., "type I error")

β The probability of concluding that a therapy is not useful when its response probability is p_1 or greater (i.e., "type II error")

The choices for parameters p_0 and p_1 are determined by the current state of treatment for the disease and outcome under study. Typically, the difference between them is 20% or 15%. The larger the difference between these parameters, the smaller the number of patients that can be enrolled to meet the study's objectives. Conversely, decreasing the difference below 15% or choosing very small values for α and β may lead to sample sizes that are too high to be practical. Values commonly selected for α and β are 20%, 10%, and 5%, although any low value is permissible. If the consequences of rejecting a useful therapy when it is in fact valuable are more serious than those of continuing to use a poor therapy, investigators might consider setting β lower than α.

Although this design is useful as an illustration of phase II design principles, it is seldom used because of an ethical dilemma it poses: A large number of patients (e.g., 35–45) may be treated with a poor therapy before it is discarded. Therefore, "two-stage" designs have been proposed that allow investigators to evaluate the results after a smaller number of patients have been enrolled and, if the design appears not to be promising, to terminate the study early.

Perhaps the most widely used phase II design of this type is that proposed by Simon.[16] In the first stage of this design, n_1 patients are enrolled and the study is terminated and the therapy rejected if r_1 or fewer responses occur. If the study continues to the second stage, an additional n_2 patients are enrolled for a total study sample size of n patients. The therapy is rejected if r or fewer patients respond. The specific values for n_1, r_1, n, and r are chosen using the binomial probability distribution to satisfy all four of these design parameters.

As with the "single-stage" design, many designs satisfy a given set of parameters. In addition to the total sample size required, a criterion commonly used to choose among designs is the expected or average number of patients to be enrolled in the study of when the true response probability is p_0 or less, which is denoted $EN(p_0)$. Because of the ethical constraint to place as few patients as possible on an ineffective regimen, this quantity should be as low as possible (or nearly so) for any design employed. It usually happens that the design giving the minimum overall sample size is not that design for which $EN(p_0)$ is minimized. Accordingly, Simon listed designs for sets of design parameters that satisfied either the minimum total sample size ("minimax" designs) or the minimum $EN(p_0)$ ("optimal" designs). Tables giving phase II designs using Simon's approach are available in the references.[16, 17]

For the acute GVHD example given earlier, a two-stage study might be carried out as follows[16]: We would set $p_0 = 60\%$, $p_1 = 80\%$, $\alpha = 10\%$, and $\beta = 10\%$. The "optimal" design would require that 11 patients be enrolled initially, with study termination occurring if 6 or fewer patients are GVHD-free at 90 days. If 7 or more patients are GVHD-free, an additional 27 patients would be enrolled for a total of 38. Of these 38, the therapy will be rejected if 26 or fewer patients are GVHD-free. If 27 or more patients are GVHD-free, the therapy will be recommended for further study.

The "minimax" design has slightly different enrollments and rejection rules at both stages and enrolls a maximum of 35 patients. The expected numbers of patients enrolled when the true "success" rate is 60% are 25.4 and 28.5 for the optimal and minimax designs, respectively. On average, therefore, the optimal design will subject about three fewer patients to an ineffective regimen.

The design chosen, however, also depends on the philosophy of the investigators carrying out the study and the availability of patients. If, for instance, the particular disease under study is a rare one, the minimax design may be chosen because the accrual time for additional patients may be too long to wait. If patient accrual is not particularly slow, the "optimal" design may be chosen because of the low expected number of patients treated on an ineffective regimen.

Although the Simon-type designs are commonly used, they do not meet the needs of all diseases, outcomes, and investigators. Accordingly, modifications and extensions of this scheme have been proposed to meet specific needs. Ensign et al. proposed three-stage designs that allowed early rejection of a therapy after an initial string of failures (i.e., failures in the initial 5–10 patients).[18] Chen extended three-stage designs to more-general early restriction criteria and noted that these three-stage designs could lower the expected number of patients treated under an ineffective regimen and could be especially useful when patient accrual is expected to be slow.[19]

A therapy may be rejected early if there is early evidence that it is not promising. It is also reasonable to ask whether a therapy could be accepted early if there were early evidence of promise. In fact, early termination because of positive results is not routinely practiced at many centers.[20, 21] There

is not necessarily an ethical imperative to stop a study early if a therapy appears to be working. In this case, continued treatment with the therapy is desirable from the patient's point of view and enables more information about the therapy to be gathered. If, however, there is already a standard therapy for a given disease and the possibility exists of immediately beginning phase III research, it may be desirable to terminate a phase II trial early to take advantage of this possibility. Fleming therefore proposed an approach to phase II trials in which patients would be enrolled in two or three stages with rules for early termination at the end of each accrual stage.[22] These rules would allow early therapy rejection if the observed response rate was too low and early therapy acceptance if there was sufficient evidence for efficacy.

Multicenter phase II studies are relatively common and may require special consideration in study design. Suppose enough patients have been enrolled to satisfy either the first or second stage of enrollment in a two-stage design. It may well happen that additional patients have already been promised treatment with the experimental regimen. Because investigators are often reluctant not to enroll these patients, the exact sample sizes target for a particular design may not be achieved. Green and Dahlberg therefore proposed designs in which an initial hypothesis test of H_0: $p = p_1$ is carried out after the first stage of accrual.[20] That is, the study is terminated early if a low number of responses in the first stage would lead to a conclusion that $p < p_1$ with a probability of 2%, where p is the true response rate. If the study continues to the second stage, a second hypothesis test is carried out when the final sample size is reached, this time of H_0: $p = p_0$. If this test is *not* rejected using an α of 5.5% (i.e., if not enough patients respond in the entire study population), the therapy is rejected. Otherwise, the therapy may be considered for further study.

Clearly, this procedure may be carried out with a variety of sample sizes at each stage and has the flexibility required when target sample sizes are not exactly achieved. Green and Dahlberg found that this approach worked reasonably well under a variety of target enrollments, p_0, and p_1.[20] Chen and Ng extended the idea of flexible designs by assuming that, given a target first-stage accrual of n_1, any of eight sample sizes surrounding this target is equally likely.[21] Likewise, given a target final accrual of n, any of eight surrounding accruals is equally likely. Rejection rules r_1 and r are chosen for each attained sample size by criteria similar to those in the optimal and minimax Simon designs except that expected and maximal sample sizes are averaged over the $8 \times 8 = 64$ possible sample-size combinations.

As an example of how this approach works, consider the hypothetical phase II design described earlier in which it was desired to reject a therapy if the GVHD-free survival rate was no more than 60% and to recommend a therapy if this rate was at least 80%. According to the approach of Chen and Ng, one would still target 18 patients for initial accrual. The rejection rule, r_1, would be 6 if 15 or 16 patients were actually enrolled, 7 if 17, 18, or 19 patients were enrolled, 8 if 20 patients were enrolled, or 9 if 21 or 22 patients were enrolled. If the study continued to the second stage, an additional 28 patients would be targeted for accrual for a final target sample size of 28 plus the first stage's attained sample size. The final rejection rule, r, would be 21 if 44 or 45 patients were enrolled, 22 if 46 or 47 patients were enrolled, 23 if 48 or 49 were enrolled, or 24 if 50 or 51 were enrolled. Tables and further discussion of flexible optimal and minimax designs are presented in Chen and Ng's paper.[21]

Although phase II trials are nominally designed to provide an initial estimate of a therapy's efficacy, an important feature may be to gather toxicity information. The second purpose is especially important if the therapy in question does not lend itself to the traditional phase I dose-escalation framework. In this case, it may be desirable to combine the phase I and II purposes in a single study. Even if phase I studies have been carried out, the MTD selected may carry a higher risk of toxicity than was identified in an initial small sample of patients.

To account for these considerations, Conaway and Petronis[23, 24] and Bryant and Day[25] proposed group-sequential designs in which a therapy may be rejected because of either excessive toxicity or lack of efficacy. In addition to the parameters listed earlier for the design of phase II designs, these methods require the specification of a toxicity rate above which the therapy would be unacceptable as well as a toxicity rate below which the therapy would be acceptable.

Conaway and Petronis[23] and Bryant and Day[25] discuss and present phase II designs in which these probabilities are fixed. Conaway and Petronis extend the discussion to the case in which there may be a trade-off between response rates and toxicity.[24] For example, investigators may be willing to tolerate slightly more toxicity in a therapy that seems to be particularly efficacious. On the other hand, less toxicity may be tolerated in return for a lower response rate.

Additional references and discussion of phase II designs may be found in the review by Mariani and Marubini.[26]

PHASE III

At the close of phase II clinical trials, many therapies have not shown sufficient promise to warrant further development. At this point, the therapy might be modified in an effort to make it more efficacious or might be abandoned in favor of another treatment that investigators think shows more promise. A therapy that is judged successful at the completion of phase II studies may be adopted as medical practice if there is no standard therapy in place for a particular disease. If, on the other hand, there is a standard therapy, it is reasonable to ask whether the new therapy performs as well as the standard therapy or perhaps even better.

To aid in this decision, phase III trials are carried out to compare two or more therapies with respect to their effects on outcomes of interest. We discuss phase III trials as if they were comparing two treatments. The general principles extend to comparisons of any number of treatment groups. Several works discuss design principles for comparative studies in detail.[2, 4–6, 27–29] Because of limited space, only two issues related to phase III study design are discussed here—the method of treatment assignment and the choice of sample size.

Mechanism of Treatment Assignment

There are several methods of assigning treatments to patients in a comparative trial. For example, one might assign patients to treatments using a systematic scheme such as assigning even-numbered patients to treatment 1 and odd-numbered patients to treatment 2.

Systematic schemes have disadvantages, however.[2] Perhaps the most important is that it allows investigators to predict in advance which patients will receive which treatment, making it possible to manipulate patient enrollment according to the bias of the investigators. Although ethical investigators would not so manipulate a study to achieve desired results, it is possible that such bias might arise subconsciously. In any case, employment of a systematic treatment assignment procedure would reduce the credibility of the trial's results. The same criticism might be applied to treatment assignment schemes in which the investigators assigned treatments haphazardly, hoping to avoid biasing treatment assignment in that fashion. As with systematic schemes, subconscious investigator bias might come into play and this method of treatment assignment should be avoided.

The most widely accepted way of assigning patients to treatments in a comparative clinical trial is randomization, in which a formal random or pseudorandom mechanism is brought into play for the purpose of treatment assignment. Most often, treatments are assigned using computer-generated pseudorandom numbers. For example, a computer might routinely generate numbers between 0 and 1 as each patient is enrolled. The patient might be assigned to treatment 1 if the number generated is between 0 and 0.5 and to treatment 2 otherwise.

Randomization is often "blocked," meaning that the randomization scheme is restricted so that patients on the treatment arms would be balanced as of every four, six, or eight patients, say. This restriction minimizes the possibility that the sample sizes in the treatment groups would be significantly out of balance at the time of data analysis, a situation that would somewhat reduce the statistical power of the comparison.

There are several advantages to randomized treatment assignment.[2] First, the choice of treatment assignment is removed from the investigator so that the biases mentioned in connection with systematic and haphazard assignment are avoided. A second advantage is that, under the right circumstances, the randomization process may be used to keep the investigator and/or patient blinded to the assignment actually made. For example, in a study of a drug versus placebo, impartial pharmacy personnel can provide a patient's treatment in an unlabeled fashion so that neither the investigator nor the patient knows whether drug or placebo is being administered. Clearly, blinding will not be possible when the treatment is obvious by nature (e.g., surgery) or when the investigator is the attending physician administering the treatment. Nonetheless, blinding is an important tool for reducing potential biases and should be applied when possible. Third, randomization may aid in the balance of prognostic factors, known and unknown, among treatment groups, particularly in large trials with many patients. For example, it would be undesirable to compare 5-year DFS in two treatment groups if one group consisted primarily of patients with a poor prognosis and the other group consisted of patients with a good prognosis. It can be shown (e.g., using the binomial probability distribution) that extreme imbalance with respect to prognostic factors is unlikely in large studies when randomization is properly used to assign patients to treatments. Finally, in principle, randomization makes it possible to carry out formal statistical tests of group differences using a minimum of assumptions. As is discussed later in the chapter, the standard statistical tools used to carry out such tests all require assumptions for their valid application. Randomization may be used to reduce the number of assumptions required in carrying out these tests by making use of so-called randomization tests.[30, 31] These tests generate a reference distribution for test statistics that is based on the randomization process itself rather than assumptions about the shape of the underlying distribution of observations.

Randomization may be carried out nearly as easily as other methods of assignment and carries significant advantages over other methods. There is therefore no good reason not to use this approach in practice whenever possible.

CHOICE OF SAMPLE SIZE

One major feature in the design of any clinical trial is the choice of a sample size: How many patients should be enrolled? The means by which this decision is made depend on the purpose of the study and the study design. In most phase I and II studies, the sample size is determined as outlined previously in this chapter. Sample-size choice is discussed here for the cases when the purpose of a study is (1) to estimate a quantity with a specified level of precision and (2) to compare two or more groups with respect to a specified outcome.

If the goal of a study is primarily to estimate a given quantity, the sample size should be chosen to yield an estimate with acceptable precision so that it will be deemed trustworthy by the investigators and the clinical community. For example, suppose the purpose of the study is to estimate the proportion of patients that will experience engraftment after a certain treatment. Assuming that all patients are followed to engraftment (i.e., there are no deaths prior to engraftment), it is customary to estimate this proportion as the proportion of patients experiencing engraftment and to report this proportion with a 95% confidence interval[3]:

$$p \pm 1.96 \times \sqrt{\frac{p\,(1-p)}{n}}$$

where p is the proportion of patients experiencing engraftment, n is the number of patients treated, and

$$\sqrt{\frac{p\,(1-p)}{n}}$$

is the estimated standard error of p. In planning the study, the investigator may specify that the confidence interval should be no wider than a specified quantity, say W. Furthermore, he or she may think that the proportion is likely to be close to p_0. Then the projected confidence interval width can be expressed as

$$W = 2 \times 1.96 \times \sqrt{\frac{p_0(1-p_0)}{n}}$$

This expression can then be solved for n to give

$$n = \left[\frac{3.92}{W}\right]^2 \times p_0 \times (1-p_0)$$

For example, if an investigator thought that the observed proportion was likely to be close to 0.9 and wished to estimate the proportion with a total confidence interval width of 0.2, he or she would enroll

$$n = \left[\frac{3.92}{0.2}\right]^2 \times 0.9 \times (0.1) = 34.6$$

or 35 patients. In practice, the investigator would probably consider different combinations of target proportions and interval widths to be sure that the study would achieve the desired goal under circumstances other than those anticipated. A similar strategy could be followed to choose a number of patients if the outcome were a continuous variable rather than a proportion. That is, an expression for n could be obtained by rearranging an expression for the confidence interval width. The resulting expression for n could then be evaluated under likely experimental conditions.

It is in the arena of hypothesis testing that sample-size choice has received the most attention.[3, 28, 29] The basic procedure is as follows. A study question is phrased as a "null hypothesis," usually the hypothesis that there is no difference in the outcomes of two treatment groups. The opposing, or "alternative," hypothesis states that the outcomes will in fact differ in a specified way.

For example, suppose two regimens are to be compared to see whether one leads to shorter engraftment times. The null hypothesis would be that there is no difference in engraftment times of patients receiving the two regimens. The alternative hypothesis might be that the newer regimen, on average, decreases the engraftment time or that it changes the engraftment time in an unspecified fashion. The former case is called a "one-sided" alternative because it specifies the direction in which the difference is expected to be observed. The latter case, because it is not stated in a directional fashion, is called a "two-sided" alternative. It is common practice to test the null hypothesis and, if it is found inconsistent with the data, to conclude that the alternative hypothesis is true. Technically, a failure to reject the null hypothesis is exactly that: This failure is not considered proof that the null hypothesis is true, only that the data provide insufficient evidence to reject it.

For diverse study designs, the same major considerations come into play to influence the number of patients needed to test a hypothesis. These considerations are as follows:

1. α, the "false-positive" rate or type I error rate. This quantity is defined as the probability that the null hypothesis will be rejected when it is in fact true.

2. β, the "false negative" rate or type II error rate. This quantity is the probability that the null hypothesis will not be rejected when in fact the alternative hypothesis is true. The power of a test is defined as $1 - β$, the probability of rejecting the null hypothesis when the alternative is true.

3. δ, the level it is desired to detect with high probability. For example in designing the earlier-described study of engraftment, the investigators may wish to detect an improvement in engraftment time of 1 day with the new regimen.

4. σ, the level of variability inherent in the population from which the observations are assumed to be drawn. Frequently, this is expressed as the standard deviation of the population probability model underlying the observations.

With particular designs, additional information may be brought to bear on the problem of choosing a sample size. For example, in comparing the DFS of patients undergoing two different treatments, it may be necessary to consider the rates at which patients will be enrolled into the study and at which patients will be lost to follow-up.[32]

If there are no prior data on which to base an estimate of variability, it is often possible to combine (3) and (4) as δ/σ, the difference to be detected in units of standard deviation.

Further information about sample size calculations using all four considerations may be found in the references.[1–7, 27–29]

DATA SUMMARIZATION AND PRESENTATION

Addressing research questions using the data generated by clinical studies requires utilizing those data in a variety of ways. For example, although the chief aim of phase I studies is to find a therapeutic dose that will be used for further research, analysis usually does not stop when the MTD is defined. At the very least, investigators tabulate such factors as patient demographics, disease type and stage, and observed toxicities. In addition, pharmacokinetic information may be summarized to enhance the understanding of rates of absorption and bioavailability. Similarly, analysis of a phase II project does not stop with a simple determination of whether to continue to phase III research. Phase III and other comparative studies make use of a wealth of data to understand any group differences observed.

Once a clinical study has been completed, the major features of several types of data potentially need to be communicated in abstracts, manuscripts, or oral presentations. The most effective way to communicate these features varies according to the type of presentation and the type of data. In this discussion, we present several methods of summarizing data that we find useful in this field. The methods are organized around the type of data to be summarized—categorical, continuous, and censored (i.e., survival).

CATEGORICAL DATA

Categorical variables have a finite set of possible values for an observation and include nominal variables (e.g., school:

TABLE 63–1. FREQUENCY AND PERCENTAGE OF DEATH OR RELAPSE BY GENDER

GENDER	DEATH OR RELAPSE	FREQUENCY	%
Male	Yes	26	79
	No	7	21
	All	33	100
Female	Yes	18	60
	No	12	40
	All	30	100

A, B, C) and ordinal variables (e.g., drug response: poor, fair, good, excellent). Dichotomous variables are a special class of categorical variables with two categories (e.g., gender: male or female). The most basic summary for categorical variables is a simple listing of the categories and their frequencies. For example, among the patients undergoing autologous HSCT in the study of Selvaggi et al., there were 33 male patients and 30 female patients.[15] Of these 63 patients, 26 male and 18 female patients died or had experienced relapse as of October 1993. To summarize this information, we simply list the frequencies and corresponding percentages (Table 63–1).

A graphic representation of this frequency listing is a bar chart (Fig. 63–1). It shows that the male patients have a higher rate of death or relapse after HSCT than the female patients.

CONTINUOUS DATA

Continuous variables can take on any numeric value within a given range of numbers. Examples of this type of variable are body mass index and age. In practice, measurements of such variables are made discontinuous by limitations of measurement. Age, for example, may be measured at the level of years, months, days, hours, and so on but cannot be measured exactly by any instrument. The distinction between age and a bona fide categorical variable is that the "categories" of age are determined by units of measurement rather than by any quality intrinsic to the variable itself.

In describing continuous data, it is common to present (1) some measure of central tendency or "location," (2) a measure of the variability in the data, (3) the shape of the

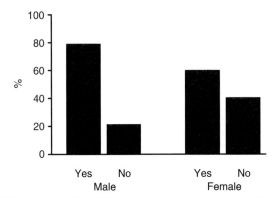

FIGURE 63–1. Bar chart of percentage of death or relapse after hematopoietic stem cell therapy by gender.

distribution of sample values, and (4) relationships among variables.

The most common measures of location are the sample mean and median. As is well known, the sample mean is calculated as

$$\bar{x} = \frac{\sum_{i=1}^{n} x_i}{n}$$

where x_i is a specific value in the sample, n is the number of values in the sample, and the symbol Σ is the standard notation for summation. If the number of sample values is odd, the median is the midpoint of the values when arranged from smallest to largest. If the sample size is even, then the median is the average of the two central observations (again ranked from smallest to largest). For example, if a sample consisted of the five observations 1, 3, 5, 7, and 10, the mean would be the average value (5.2) and the median would be the central value (5). In contrast, if there were four observations consisting of 1, 3, 5, and 7, the mean would be 4 and the median would be the average of 3 and 5 (or 4).

The variability (or "spread") of sample observations may be represented using any of several measures. The most common is the sample variance, calculated as

$$s^2 = \frac{\sum_{i=1}^{n} (x_i - \bar{x})^2}{n - 1}$$

where $\bar{x}$ is the sample mean and the other notations are as just described for the sample mean. The sample standard deviation, another common measure of variability, is simply the square root of the sample variance. An additional measure of data spread is the interquartile range, the difference between the 75th and 25th percentiles of the data. In general, the percentiles of a data set are slightly more complicated to calculate, and the reader is referred to the references for further details.

The shape of the distribution of sample values may be presented in several ways. One way is to divide a continuous variable such as age into intervals and present a table of counts of observations in each interval (Table 63–2).

Histograms may also be used to present the shape of a sample distribution. Figure 63–2 is a histogram of ages at HSCT.

Other useful methods of representing shape are the stem-and-leaf display and the box-and-whisker plot. A stem-and-leaf plot resembles a histogram except that it displays the actual measurements themselves. The "stem" is formed

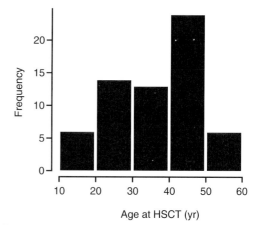

FIGURE 63–2. Histogram of age at time of transplantation.

from the initial one or more digits of the value and is displayed on the left side; the "leaf" is formed from remaining digit(s) and displayed on the right side of the plot. In Figure 63–3, for example, the age *11* is represented as a *1* in the stem column and a *1* in the leaf column. Other values are treated similarly.

A box-and-whisker plot is a diagram that depicts a five-number summary of a set of data values. The five quantities presented are the minimum value ("min" in Fig. 63–4), the 25th percentile ("Q1"), the median or 50th percentile ("Q2"), the 75th percentile ("Q3"), and the maximum ("max"). Figure 63–4 is a box-and-whisker plot of the age data.

Relationships among continuous variables are perhaps best summarized in bivariate scatterplots, in which each patient's values for two variables are plotted simultaneously. Features may be added to add additional information. For example, Figure 63–5 shows a scatterplot of body mass index (BMI, given in kg/m²) versus age at HSCT, with different symbols for men and women. If the relationship between BMI and age were different for men and women, the different relationships would be highlighted by the different symbols.

Numeric summaries of the degree of relationship between two variables are commonly provided by Pearson and Spearman correlation coefficients, which range between −1 (for perfectly negative associations) and +1 (for perfectly positive associations). The Pearson measure is designed to express the degree of *straight-line* relationship between two variables. The P values obtained for a test of the null hypothesis that the coefficient is zero depend on the bivariate normality of the observations. Therefore, tests based on the the Pearson coefficient are parametric procedures. In contrast, the Spearman coefficient is a procedure

TABLE 63–2. FREQUENCY BY AGE AT TIME OF TRANSPLANTATION

GROUP INTERVAL (AGE AT TRANSPLANTATION)	FREQUENCY	PERCENTAGE	CUMULATIVE FREQUENCY	CUMULATIVE PERCENTAGE
10 19	6	9.3	6	9.5
20–29	14	22.2	20	31.7
30–39	13	20.6	33	52.4
40–49	24	38.1	57	90.5
50–59	6	9.5	63	100.0

Stem	Leaf
1	1
1	68889
2	01334
2	556777788
3	02224
3	55666688
4	000012223344444
4	666778899
5	02244
5	7

FIGURE 63–3. Stem-and-leaf plot of age at time of transplantation.

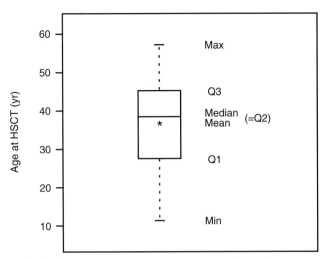

FIGURE 63–4. Box-and-whisker plot of age at time of transplantation (*denotes the mean).

that measures the degree of *monotonic* relationship (i.e., steadily increasing or decreasing but not necessarily linear). Because it makes use of the ranks of the observations, it is a nonparametric procedure and is not dependent on a particular distribution (e.g., the bivariate normal distribution) for the calculation of *P* values.

CENSORED DATA

It is common in research related to HSCT to summarize patient survival in a "survival curve" of patient survival versus time after HSCT. For example, Figure 63–6 shows estimated DFS after autologous HSCT from Selvaggi et al.[15] From such a plot, survival at any time point of interest may be read from the plot (or from a tabular listing that summarizes the plot's key points). In the rare event that all patients are followed until a follow-up time of interest (e.g., 1 year), the estimated survival at any time point is simply the proportion of patients surviving until that time.

In the much more common situation that patients are not all followed for the entire time period, survival is usually estimated using the Kaplan-Meier approach (e.g., see Collett[39]). The Kaplan-Meier procedure, although accounting for the fact that some patients are not followed for the entire time period, estimates what the complete survival curve would look like if all patients could be observed for the complete time interval.

Useful discussions of these and other approaches to data summarization may be found in the references.[1, 3, 7]

STATISTICAL METHODS FOR GROUP COMPARISONS

Group comparisons are an important part of scientific research. Often, scientific studies are designed so that two or more groups are assigned to different treatments, and comparisons of these groups with respect to an outcome of interest can shed light on scientific questions. The statistical

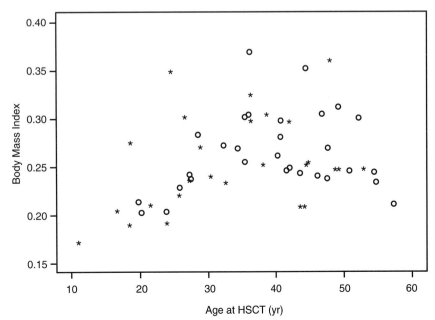

FIGURE 63–5. Bivariate scatterplot of body mass index versus age at time of transplantation (o, males; *, females).

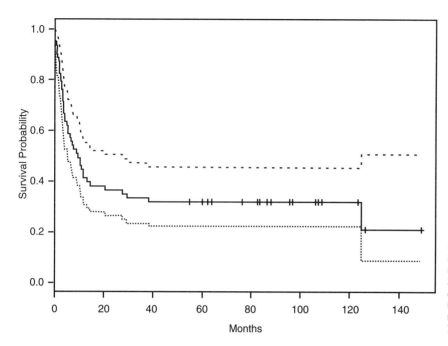

FIGURE 63–6. Kaplan-Meier survival curve and a 95% confidence interval for disease-free survival after hematopoietic stem cell therapy. (Data from Selvaggi KJ, Wilson JW, Mills LE, et al: Improved outcome for high-risk acute myeloid leukemia patients using autologous bone marrow transplantation and monoclonal antibody–purged marrow. Blood 83:1698–1705, 1994.)

procedures by which groups are compared vary according to the number of groups compared, the type of outcome studied, and whether adjustment for potential confounding variables is necessary. In the paragraphs that follow, we review standard statistical methods for carrying out group comparisons for three types of data—categorical data, continuous data, and survival data. As in the section describing methods of data presentation, the last type of data is treated separately from other continuous outcomes because of the special requirements imposed by the censorship of observations.

CATEGORICAL DATA

The simplest method of comparing categorical outcome variables in two groups is probably the chi-squared test. For example, Zittoun et al. recently compared OS and DFS in patients with acute myelogenous leukemia undergoing autologous or allogeneic HSCT and intensive chemotherapy.[33] Among the 126 patients randomized to receive intensive chemotherapy, the ages were as follows: 45 were 25 years old or younger, 71 were 26–45 years old, and 10 were 46 years old or older. The numbers of patients randomized to autologous HSCT were 42, 77, and 9, respectively. These data are summarized in Table 63–3. Rather than giving the formulas by which a chi-square test can be

carried out (and which may be found in references 1, 3, and 7), we simply note that the test proceeds by comparing the observed results to those expected if the null hypothesis of no group difference is true. The greater the discrepancy between observed and hypothesized values, the greater the evidence that the null hypothesis is false.

A similar test, Fisher's exact test, may also be used to test for group differences and is commonly used when cell counts or overall sample sizes are small. Although it is usually presented in introductory texts as a test for 2 × 2 tables, extensions for larger tables may be found, for example, in the SAS, Stata, and StatXact statistical software packages.[34–36] In this case, the chi-square and Fisher's exact tests yield P values of .825 and .850, respectively. There is no evidence to suggest that the age distributions were different in the two treatment groups.

It frequently happens that categorical variables are coded (or may be coded) into two categories (e.g., dead or alive, experienced or did not experience GVHD). If such a variable is the outcome or dependent variable of an analysis, it may be modeled as a function of independent or predictor variables using logistic regression.[37, 38]

To simplify the age comparison discussed earlier, suppose the ages were categorized into two groups, one with ages less than or equal to 45 years and the other with ages greater than or equal to 46 years. To see whether the two treatment groups differed with respect to age, it would be possible to treat age as the dependent variable in logistic regression analysis with a binary (0/1) variable indicating group membership as a predictor variable. The statistical significance of any association between the age and treatment groups would be assessed by testing the hypothesis that the regression coefficient associated with the predictor variable (treatment group) is 0. In this example, we would concur with the previous conclusion that there is no difference in age by treatment groups (P = .626). It is clear that if, as in this case, the outcome and predictor variables are binary, a 2 × 2 table analysis may be carried out using

TABLE 63–3. NUMBERS OF PATIENTS UNDERGOING CHEMOTHERAPY AND AUTOLOGOUS HSCT IN EACH AGE GROUP

	≤25 YR	26–45 YR	≥46 YR
HSCT	42	77	9
Chemotherapy	45	71	10
Total	87	148	19

logistic regression rather than a chi-square or Fisher's exact test. The value of logistic regression is that it can incorporate predictive information from more than one variable at a time. These joint predictors may be categorical or continuous predictor variables or combinations of the two types.

MULTIVARIABLE ANALYSIS IN REGRESSION

Predictor variables can be considered one at a time ("univariate" analysis) or in combination to adjust for confounder variables or to consider the effects of two or more predictors in concert (multivariable analysis). (The latter type of analysis is often incorrectly called *multivariate* analysis.) These considerations hold for logistic regression and, in addition, for the other types of regression addressed later in this section. Following Collett,[39] we distinguish two situations in which multivariable regression is used. In the first, we have several variables and are interested in seeing which are related to the outcome of interest. In the second case, we have one or two variables of primary interest and we are interested in including additional variables that may influence the size, direction, and precision of the treatment effect.

An important concept in multivariable analysis is interaction. Two variables are said to interact in their prediction of the outcome if the association between one variable and the outcome depends on the value of the second. For example, Selvaggi et al.[15] found a relationship between DFS and time in CR1 for patients undergoing transplantation in CR2 and CR3. The effect, however, was much stronger among patients who received busulfan and cyclophosphamide as a conditioning regimen than among patients whose conditioning regimen was cyclophosphamide and total body irradiation.

In the first case, it is common to use some kind of "stepwise" algorithm to add variables to a model.[37–39] That is, predictors are added to the model one at a time until all variables making a "significant" contribution in predicting the outcome have been added. One common algorithm is a "forward stepwise" approach, in which variables are added to the model one at a time with an opportunity for variables already added to drop out of the model if newly added variables make their information redundant. Typically, variables are first assessed in a univariate fashion for association with the outcome variable. The variable with the closest association is then added.

At the second stage, the remaining variables are assessed for their relationships to the outcome variable and the variable with the strongest association is entered into the model, along with a model term for the interaction with the first variable, if necessary. Further stages proceed along the same lines until variables not in the model show no significant association with the outcome and model-building ceases.

In the second case, there are one or two variables of primary interest, often treatment variables, and it is primarily their association with the outcome we seek.[37–39] It is often possible, however, that additional variables will modify an apparent association between treatment and outcome (i.e., provide an interaction). Therefore, it is customary to build a model using the secondary variables first (i.e., not including the primary interest variable) using an algorithm such as the stepwise algorithm described earlier. Then the variables of primary interest are allowed to enter the model along with any interactions that might be important.

It is unfortunately common that models are built using statistical criteria exclusively (using, for example, P values or the Akaike information criterion). Wherever possible, subject-matter criteria should be incorporated into the model-building process. It may be, for example, that including certain variables in the model together is not sensible. In other cases, certain variables may be known to influence outcome even though they don't show "statistical significance." In such cases, it may be advisable to include such terms in the model regardless of their lack of association in one's data set.

Another example of a binary outcome variable is engraftment within a certain time period after HSCT. Such an outcome would be suitable for contingency table analysis or logistic regression provided that all patients were observed for the entire time period and could be coded either "Yes" or "No" with respect to their engraftment. (If patients are not observable for engraftment during the entire time period—e.g., because of early death by infection—time-to-event models such as those listed later are appropriate.)

de Magalhaes-Silverman et al. studied factors influencing engraftment of peripheral blood progenitor cells (PBPC) in 38 patients with metastatic breast cancer undergoing PBPC transplantation.[40] Potential predictor variables for platelet engraftment were mobilization chemotherapy (cyclophosphamide and granulocyte colony-stimulating factor [G-CSF] vs. cyclophosphamide, VP-16, and G-CSF), the number of CD34 + cells infused, and the dose of G-CSF after PBPC infusion (5 μg/kg vs. 10 μg/kg). All patients who underwent infusion experienced platelet engraftment (20,000/mm^3) within 28 days. For the purpose of illustration, platelet engraftment can be coded as a binary variable (8–9 days vs. 10–28 days). When each predictor was considered alone, only the number of infused CD34 + cells showed a statistically significant relationship to platelet engraftment ($P = .005$). Mobilization chemotherapy and G-CSF dose, however, did not show such a relationship ($P = .178$ and $.840$, respectively).

Next, the number of infused CD34 + cells was included in the regression model together with each of the remaining predictors in turn. With CD34 + cells included in the model, neither mobilization chemotherapy nor G-CSF dose contributed additional predictive information ($P = .875$ and $.610$, respectively).

The interpretation and use of logistic regression, as is true of any statistical procedure, require caution. First, logistic regression is based on assumptions that are necessary for its validity and utility. In particular, any logistic regression model fit to a data set should be assessed for goodness of fit: Any conclusions drawn on the basis of a statistical model that does not fit the data to which it is applied are suspect. Therefore, any logistic regression analysis (in fact, any statistical analysis at all) should be accompanied by tests of model assumptions, including goodness of fit.

Second, the test results and confidence intervals obtained from most implementations of logistic regression are based on large-sample approximations to normal and chi-square probability distributions. For this reason, logistic regression analysis carried out on small samples should be interpreted with caution. Statistical software has become available to carry out logistic regression with small samples and without these large-sample approximations.[41]

An additional fact to keep in mind is that predictor variables may affect response variables in concert with other predictors (i.e., "interaction"). Finally, we emphasize that follow-up outcomes such as engraftment, acute and chronic GVHD, relapse, and death should be considered outcomes for logistic regression only if each patient is observed for the same amount of time after HSCT. If patients die or are otherwise lost to follow-up before an outcome can be observed, a time-to-event analysis such as the Cox regression and Kaplan-Meier procedures (described later) should be applied.

The use of logistic regression models in medical research is clearly described in books by Hosmer and Lemeshow[38] and Collett.[37]

CONTINUOUS OUTCOMES

Study variables may be continuous rather than discrete or categorical. Age, height, weight, numbers of cells harvested or transplanted, and time from transplantation to engraftment, death, or relapse are all variables that can be analyzed using statistical methods for continuous data.

Group comparisons of continuous data are geared toward testing the null hypothesis that means (or medians) of continuous outcomes are identical in different groups of patients. A common assumption is that the shape of the distribution, whatever it may be, is the same in all groups compared.[1, 3, 7] When one wishes to compare two groups with respect to a continuous variable whose distribution is unknown or probably not normal or bell-shaped, the most common procedure is a Wilcoxon rank sum test. Briefly, observations are ranked over both groups to be compared, and the ranks of one group are summed. If the first group is sampled from a population whose median is lower than the population from which the second group is sampled, the ranks in the first group will tend to be lower than those from the second and the rank sum will tend to be lower. The null hypothesis is rejected when the chosen group's rank sum is too low or high, indicating that the group samples probably are from different populations.

The same rationale underlies the Kruskal-Wallis test, which is a generalization of the rank sum test for three or more samples. Summaries of such distribution-free statistical methods (so called because they do not assume specific underlying probability distributions) can be found in the references.[1, 3, 7, 43] In the special case in which the data appear to represent a normal distribution or the observations can be transformed to appear normally distributed (e.g., by replacing each data value by its logarithm), groups may be compared using a t-test (two groups) or analysis of variance (ANOVA, three or more groups). These tests are described in most standard textbooks of statistical methods. As was the case for categorical variables, it is possible to use regression to address questions about interesting variables provided that the residuals (deviations of observed from fitted/predicted values) from such models are approxi-

mately normally distributed. Ordinary linear regression can be used to test whether two, three, or more groups are different by including variables representing the groups in the regression model. The value of regression over t-tests and ANOVA is that regression is capable of assessing multiple predictors' joint effects in predicting outcome. As in the case of logistic regression, the joint predictors may be categorical, continuous, or a combination of both types.

In addition to time to engraftment, de Magalhaes-Silverman et al. studied collection efficiency, defined as the total number of CD34+ cells collected divided by the number of aphereses required to obtain them.[40] Of interest was whether any of several predictor variables was associated with high collection efficiency. The predictors were mobilization chemotherapy (cyclophosphamide and G-CSF vs. cyclophosphamide, VP-16, and G-CSF), previous chemotherapy or radiation therapy, presence of marrow disease, and time from previous chemotherapy to mobilization. When the logarithm of collection efficiency was the outcome (dependent) variable in an ordinary linear regression model, none of the potential predictor variables was found to have a significant association.

Linear regression analysis is described in most introductory statistics textbooks.[1, 3, 7] In addition, there are readable introductions to regression analysis that assume some familiarity with basic statistical methods.[43, 44]

If the assumption of normality is not met by a particular set of data, nonparametric methods can be used to carry out regression analysis. One version of nonparametric regression analysis, generalized additive models, is described in the work of Hastie and Tibshirani.[45]

TIME-TO-EVENT ANALYSIS

In studies of HSCT, it is common to judge a procedure's success by considering follow-up events such as engraftment, GVHD incidence, OS, and DFS. Although the outcomes themselves are categorical (e.g., engraftment: yes/no; death: yes/no), it is customary to analyze not the yes/no outcome itself but rather the time to event.

This practice exists for two reasons. The first is that more information is gained by considering time to event than the binary outcome. Suppose that two groups are being compared for DFS at 3 years. At that time, assuming all patients have actually been observed for the entire time period, it would be possible to assign each patient's status as (1) dead or alive with relapse or (2) alive and disease-free. A group comparison such as a chi-squared test could be carried out. If the proportions of patients alive and disease-free did not differ substantially, one would probably conclude that there was no difference between the groups. But suppose that in one group, most relapses came early and that in the other group most relapses came later. The comparison of proportions would totally miss this fact, whereas a comparison based on times to death or relapse could pick up the fact that the post-HSCT experience was different in the two groups.

The second reason for considering the times to events is that most follow-up studies are carried out in such a way that patients are not observed for an event of interest for the entire time period of interest. A study examining the survival experience of patients after HSCT will include not only patients followed for a long period of time but also patients who underwent transplantation relatively recently and therefore were followed for a shorter period of time. For example, Selvaggi et al. reported follow-up results from 63 patients undergoing autologous HSCT.[15] Patients in this report received transplants between August 1984 and April 1992. Follow-up was summarized as of October 1993. Therefore, estimates of 3-year OS and DFS had to account for the fact that not every patient was followed for 3 years before the report was written. Time-to-event analysis, when properly carried out, accounts for the fact that some patients are not observed for the full follow-up period (i.e., that they are "censored").

When all patients can be observed for a time period of interest, it is customary to compare groups using a nonparametric test such as the Wilcoxon rank sum test (or Kruskal-Wallis test when there are three or more groups) to compare times to the events of interest.[3] Usually, however, there are censored observations and thus standard tests for continuous data are not applicable.

In this case, one standard procedure for carrying out group comparisons is the log rank test, which accounts for the fact that some observations are censored.[3, 39] A brief rationale for using this test to compare two groups is as follows. Suppose the event times (e.g., death times) from both groups occur at t_1, t_2, ..., t_j. Just prior to each time, there will be n_{11}, n_{12}, ..., n_{1j} patients at risk of death from the first group and n_{21}, n_{22}, ..., n_{2j} patients at risk for death from the second group. At each death time, it is possible to summarize the observed death(s) in each group and compare them to the numbers expected if the risk of death is the same for both groups. This information is combined over all time points to create an overall test of the equality of two overall survival curves. What makes this test suitable in the presence of censored observations is that patients are considered "at risk" only if they have survived event-free until the event in question.

For example, a patient who is followed for 90 days after transplantation (i.e., is censored at 90 days) would contribute information to the test at all time points until 90 days after transplantation. This patient, however, would not contribute information to the test at death times later than 90 days after transplantation. This test can be extended with a similar rationale to comparisons of more than two groups.[39]

As with categorical and continuous data, it is usually desirable to carry out group comparisons in the presence of one or more additional predictor variables. In the realm of survival analysis, this is usually done not by modeling the outcome itself or even the time to event but by modeling the hazard ratio. Although the term *hazard* has a precise mathematical definition, it can be described as follows when the event of interest is death[39]:

The *hazard function* is the probability that an individual dies at time t, conditional on he or she having survived to that time. The hazard function therefore represents the instantaneous death rate for an individual surviving to time t.

The hazard is therefore in some sense a measure of the risk of an event through time and may vary with time. For example, a surgical procedure may carry with it a risk of high perioperative mortality followed by a period of lower and relatively constant risk of death. The hazard of death would then be high immediately after the procedure and lower (and perhaps relatively stable) subsequently.

The most common procedure in the literature of HSCT for comparing the event-free survival of two or more groups is proportional hazards regression (or Cox regression).[46] In this approach, the actual hazard functions of the groups are left unspecified. It is assumed, however, that the ratio of the hazards of any two groups compared will be constant through time. The hazards themselves need not remain constant (as in the case of the perioperative mortality mentioned earlier). The ratio itself, however, is assumed to remain constant (at least in the "basic" form of proportional hazards regression). In proportional hazards regression, the natural logarithm (base e) of this constant ratio is what is modeled using a regression equation:

$$\ln\left(\frac{\lambda_1}{\lambda_0}\right) = \beta_1 X_1 + \beta_2 X_2 + \ldots + \beta_p X_p$$

where "ln" represents the natural logarithm; λ_1/λ_0 is the ratio of the hazards in the two groups being compared; X_1, X_2, etc. are the predictor variables of interest, and β_1, β_2, etc. are the usual regression coefficients associated with each predictor. As with other regression techniques, the statistical significance of a predictor is assessed by testing the null hypothesis that the corresponding regression coefficient is equal to zero. The information necessary for carrying out these tests is provided automatically in most statistical packages that include proportional hazards regression.

For example, Harousseau et al. studied CR, OS, and DFS in 517 adult patients with acute myelogenous leukemia who received intensive chemotherapy, allogeneic HSCT, or autologous HSCT.[47] As initial therapy, patients were randomized to receive either IV idarubicin or IV rubidazone. The 4-year OS rate in these patients was estimated at 40.5%, with no significant difference between the treatment groups. In a univariate analysis, French-American-British (FAB) classification (M2–M3 vs. others, $P < .0001$), initial WBC count ($< 30,000/mm^3$ vs. $\geq 30,000/mm^3$, $P < .001$), and karyotype (favorable, normal and intermediate, unfavorable, and missing, $P = .018$) were all significant predictors of OS. When variables were added to the proportional hazards model in a stepwise fashion, WBC count ($P = .004$) and FAB classification ($P = .004$) remained significant. In other words, karyotype was no longer considered predictive of OS when information about WBC count and FAB classification was accounted for. Treatment group was not predictive of OS either in univariate fashion or when FAB classification and WBC count were accounted for.

BAYESIAN STATISTICAL METHODS

In all of the data analytic situations described so far, we have assumed that some constant true parameter underlies the response of patients to treatment. Sample means, for example, were assumed to estimate true means of the populations from which the patients were drawn. Regression parameters calculated from a sample of patients are assumed to estimate unknown but constant parameters that would describe the true population of patients if all patients could be observed. We refer to such population parameters generically using the Greek letter θ.

In Bayesian statistics, parameters are assumed to be randomly varying quantities rather than constants and the goal of Bayesian analysis is to make probability statements about those parameters.[48] The interpretation of results in the Bayesian and non-Bayesian schools is therefore quite different. For example, in classic (or non-Bayesian) statistics, it is appropriate to speak of a 95% confidence interval (b_l, b_u, or "lower bound," "upper bound") by saying "the probability that the random interval (b_l, b_u) includes the true parameter θ is 95%." A Bayesian statistician refers to a 95% "credible" or "credibility" interval, saying "the probability that θ lies between b_l and b_u is 95%." In the non-Bayesian school of biostatistics, instructors take pains to point out that it is the lower and upper bounds that vary, not the parameter. In the Bayesian school, however, it is proper to speak of the parameter itself as varying according to probabilistic laws. Hypothesis tests may also be interpreted differently in the two schools. Whereas a classic statistician interprets the results of hypothesis tests in a "Yes/No" fashion (reject or fail to reject the null hypothesis), a Bayesian statistician could properly speak of the probability that the null hypothesis is correct.

The Bayesian approach incorporates a feature that the non-Bayesian approach does not, namely a "prior" probability distribution, $\pi(\theta)$, according to which the unknown parameter θ is assumed to vary *before data are collected*. The prior distribution may be based on the results of previous studies, in which several estimates of the parameter of interest were obtained. It may also be based on an investigator's degree of belief that the parameter of interest takes on certain values. The data x are considered to be generated according to a probability distribution $f(x|\theta)$, the probability density of "x given θ" or "x depending on θ."

Once the data are collected, they are considered given or fixed, and the task of a Bayesian statistician is to make inferences about θ based on the given data. The prior distribution, probability distribution of x given θ, and data values themselves are combined to create a posterior probability distribution of θ, $f(\theta|x)$. The distribution is called *posterior* because, unlike the prior distribution, it is derived after the data have been collected. The relationships among these entities is described as follows:

$$f(\theta|\underline{x}) = \frac{f(\underline{x}|\theta) \times \pi(\theta)}{\int f(\underline{x}|\theta) \times \pi(\theta) d\theta}$$

where "×" refers to multiplication and "$f \ldots d\theta$" refers to integration.

The controversial nature of Bayesian methods stems from acceptance of the validity of the prior distribution.[48] Some statisticians believe that the prior distribution is an appropriate way to summarize pre-experiment information and belief about the parameter of interest. To these statisticians, this distribution is a probability distribution like any other and can be validly manipulated according to the standard laws of probability. Other statisticians believe that in most situations the parameter θ is fixed and is not to be thought of as a random quantity. Furthermore, it would be possible for different investigators starting with different prior distributions for θ to arrive at different conclusions about likely values of θ, regardless of the data collected. These statisticians believe that the only time such a prior should be applied in a statistical problem is when there is substantial experience in the form of previous experiments in which θ has been estimated.

Most statisticians would agree that when a prior distribution is valid for a certain experiment, Bayesian methods are an appropriate way to analyze data.[48] Controversy, however, remains about how often such methods may validly be applied. Breslow[49] and Piantadosi[6] give recent perspectives on the use of Bayesian methods, particularly in clinical studies.

REFERENCES

1. Armitage P, Berry R: Statistical Methods in Medical Research. Oxford, UK, Blackwell, 1994.
2. Cox DR: The Planning of Experiments. New York, John Wiley and Sons, 1958.
3. Fisher L, van Belle G: Biostatistics: A Methodology for the Health Sciences. New York, John Wiley and Sons, 1993.
4. Fleiss JL: The Design and Analysis of Clinical Experiments. New York, John Wiley and Sons, 1986.
5. Meinert CL: Clinical Trials: Design, Conduct, and Analysis. New York, Oxford University Press, 1986.
6. Piantadosi S: Clinical Trials: A Methodologic Perspective. New York, John Wiley and Sons, 1997.
7. Rosner B: Fundamentals of Biostatistics. Belmont, CA, Duxbury Press, 1995.
8. Simon R, Freidlin B, Rubinstein L, et al: Accelerated titration designs for phase I clinical trials in oncology. J Natl Cancer Inst 89:1138–1147, 1997.
9. Fields SZ, Budman DR, Young RR, et al: Phase I study of high-dose etoposide phosphate in man. Bone Marrow Transplant 18:851–856, 1996.
10. O'Quigley J, Pepe M, Fisher L: Continual reassessment method: a practical design for phase I clinical trials in cancer. Biometrics 56:33–48, 1990.
11. Goodman SN, Azhurak ML, Piantadosi S: Some practical improvements in the continual reassessment method for phase I studies. Stat Med 14:1149–1161, 1995.
12. Mick R, Ratain MJ: Model-guided determination of maximum tolerated dose in phase I clinical trials: evidence for increased precision. J Natl Cancer Inst 85:217–223, 1993.
13. Piantadosi S, Liu G: Improved designs for dose escalation studies using pharmacokinetic measurements. Stat Med 15:1605–1618, 1996.
14. Babb J, Rogatko A, Zacks S: Cancer phase I clinical trials: efficient dose escalation with overdose control. Stat Med 17:1103–1120, 1998.
15. Selvaggi KJ, Wilson JW, Mills LE, et al: Improved outcome for high-risk acute myeloid leukemia patients using autologous bone marrow transplantation and monoclonal antibody-purged marrow. Blood 83:1698–1705, 1994.
16. Simon R: Optimal two-stage designs for phase II clinical trials. Control Clin Trials 10:1–10, 1989.
17. Simon R: Design and conduct of clinical trials. *In* DeVita VT, Hellman S, Rosenberg SA (eds): Cancer: Principles and Practices of Oncology. Philadelphia, JB Lippincott, 1993, pp 418–440.
18. Ensign LG, Gehan EA, Kamen DS, et al: An optimal three-stage design for phase II clinical trials. Stat Med 13:1727–1736, 1994.
19. Chen TT: Optimal three-stage designs for phase II cancer clinical trials. Stat Med 16:2701–2711, 1997.
20. Green SJ, Dahlberg S: Planned versus attained design in phase II clinical trials. Stat Med 11:853–862, 1992.
21. Chen TT, Ng T-H: Optimal flexible designs in phase II clinical trials. Stat Med 17:2301–2312, 1998.

22. Fleming TR: One-sample multiple testing procedure for phase II clinical trials. Biometrics 38:143–151, 1982.

23. Conaway MR, Petronis GR: Bivariate sequential designs for phase II trials. Biometrics 51:656–664, 1995.

24. Conaway MR, Petronis GR: Designs for phase II trials allowing for a trade-off between response and toxicity. Biometrics 52:1375–1386, 1996.

25. Bryant JL, Day RS: Incorporating toxicity considerations into the design of two-stage phase II clinical trials. Biometrics 51:1372–1383, 1995.

26. Mariani L, Marubini E: Design and analysis of phase II cancer trials: a review of statistical methods and guidelines for medical researchers. Int Stat Rev 64:61–88, 1996.

27. Peto R, Pike MC, Armitage P, et al: Design and analysis of randomized clinical trials requiring prolonged observation on each patient: I. Introduction and design. Br J Cancer 34:585–612, 1976.

28. Peto R, Pike MC, Armitage P, et al: Design and analysis of randomized clinical trials requiring prolonged observation on each patient: II. Analysis and examples. Br J Cancer 35:1–39, 1977.

29. Anderson S, Auquier A, Hauck WW, et al: Statistical Methods for Comparative Studies. New York, John Wiley and Sons, 1980.

30. Manly BFJ: Randomization, Bootstrap, and Monte Carlo Methods in Biology. New York, Chapman and Hall, 1997.

31. Edgington ES: Randomization Tests. New York, Marcel Dekker, 1995.

32. Lachin J, Foulkes MA: Evaluation of sample size and power for analyses of survival with allowances for nonuniform patient entry, losses to follow-up, noncompliance, and stratification. Biometrics 42:507–516, 1986.

33. Zittoun RA, Mandelli F, Willemze R, et al: Autologous or allogeneic bone marrow transplantation compared with intensive chemotherapy in acute myelogenous leukemia. N Engl J Med 332:217–223, 1995.

34. SAS Statistical Software, SAS Institute, Cary, NC.

35. Stata Statistical Software, Stata Corporation, College Station, TX.

36. StatXact Statistical Software, CYTEL Software Corporation, Cambridge, MA.

37. Collett D: Modelling Binary Data. London, Chapman-Hall, 1991.

38. Hosmer DW, Lemeshow S: Applied Logistic Regression. New York, John Wiley and Sons, 1989.

39. Collett D: Modelling Survival Data in Medical Research. London, Chapman-Hall, 1994.

40. de Magalhaes-Silverman M, Donnenberg AD, Lister J, et al: Factors influencing mobilization and engraftment in patients with metastatic breast cancer undergoing peripheral blood stem cell transplantation. J Hematother 8:167–172, 1999.

41. LogXact Statistical Software, CYTEL Software Corporation, Cambridge, MA.

42. Hollander M, Wolfe DA: Nonparametric Statistical Methods. New York, John Wiley and Sons, 1993.

43. Kleinbaum DG, Kupper LL: Applied Regression Analysis and Other Multivariable Methods. Scituate, MA, Duxbury Press, 1978.

44. Myers RH: Classical and Modern Regression with Applications. Belmont, CA, Duxbury Press, 1990.

45. Hastie T, Tibshirani R: Generalized Additive Models. London, Chapman and Hall, 1990.

46. Niland JC, Gebhardt JA, Lee J, Forman SJ: Study design, statistical analyses, and results reporting in the bone marrow transplantation literature. Biol Blood Marrow Transplant 1:47–53, 1995.

47. Harousseau J-L, Cahn J-Y, Pignon B, et al: Comparison of autologous bone marrow transplantation and intensive chemotherapy as postremission therapy in adult acute myeloid leukemia. Blood 90:2978–2986, 1997.

48. DeGroot MH: Probability and Statistics. Reading, MA, Addison-Wesley, 1986.

49. Breslow NE: Biostatistics and Bayes. Stat Sci 5:269–298, 1990.

The Economics of Hematopoietic Stem Cell Transplantation

CHAPTER SIXTY-FOUR

Economics

*Thomas J. Smith, M.D., Bruce E. Hillner, M.D., and
Saul A. Yanovich, M.D.*

THE RISING COST OF CANCER TREATMENT

The cost of cancer treatment increased from $35 billion (United States) in 1990[1] to $40 billion in 1994[2] to $50 billion in 1996[3] and now accounts for 5% of all health care expenses. The International Bone Marrow Transplant Registry (IBMTR) estimates that 17,000 allogeneic and over 30,000 autologous transplants were performed in 1999 worldwide. At a conservative estimate of $50,000 per autologous and $150,000 per allogeneic procedure, this amounts to a total cost of over $4 billion. At a time when health care resources are expected to decrease in coming years,[4, 5] the high individual cost of autologous and allogeneic hematopoietic stem cell transplantation (HSCT) has made it a lightning rod for health care economics. In general, data on such critically important aspects of HSCT as quality of life and cost-effectiveness have been roundly ignored, representing only 3–4% of published articles.[6] This chapter analyzes the available data on the economics of HSCT by cost, effectiveness, and cost-effectiveness, as well as strategies for improving cost-effectiveness, and cost implications for universal coverage.

COST OF HSCT

The HSCT financial data has been sketchy for many reasons.

HSCT has become proprietary, and even not-for-profit institutions are loath to release their full data because they are in an increasingly competitive market. It is anticipated that actual cost data will become more difficult to obtain as more insurers move to a capitated payment method. That is, if an institution is paid $60,000 to perform an HSCT procedure regardless of the resources used, there is less incentive for the hospital and providers to carefully study all the components except to ensure a reasonable return on investment. Most providers have been willing to accept $60,000 as a capitated case rate for autologous HSCT, depending on what is covered. There have been no reported cost data of matched unrelated HSCT experience with a case rate. Some of the anticipated problems include a longer period of acute care (up to 100 days) and more outliers (those with prolonged hospital stays and increased expense).

Table 64–1 lists some reported costs of HSCT for autologous, allogeneic matched and mismatched settings. These data are difficult to interpret unless details are specified for exactly what is covered in the HSCT; for instance, cost of catheters, hematopoietic growth factor priming, apheresis, and follow-up care could all be considered part of the HSCT "package" but are variably included. In the United States, the data of Bennett et al. included pre-high-dose chemotherapy (HDCT) and follow-up care but excluded those who died[7] (whose care often costs more because they die in the intensive care unit). Smith et al. reported full cost on all patients but only for the actual HSCT period.[8] In the reported studies, follow-up care costs have not varied much between types of care, generally less than 10% of the total.

Comparison by country is nearly impossible because of different patterns of care, cost structure, and pricing strategy; results from one country can at best be used as a guide to another. Randomized comparative trials, however, can illustrate differences in treatment.

Cost has been reported in more detail for alternative stem cell procedures—i.e., autologous bone marrow transplantation (BMT) vs. peripheral blood progenitor cell transplantation (PBPCT) (Table 64–2). Schmitz et al. showed that PBPCT saved an average of 6 hospital days and had better clinical effectiveness with less need for transfusion and fewer serious infections.[9] Smith et al. showed that expenditure was 23% less for PBPCT over autologous BMT, providing evidence that therapy with a better clinical outcome also had a better economic outcome (see Table 64–2).[8] Most of the savings were attributable to the period after HDCT because of shorter hospital stay, and the cost of filgrastim-mobilization of stem cells was more than offset by savings in hospitalization (Table 64–3). Hartmann et al. performed a similar study and found that PBPCT had significantly lower costs than autologous BMT, with equal short-term clinical efficiency.[10] Uyl-de Groot et al. showed that, compared with historical controls, patients who underwent PBPCT mobilized by filgrastim had a 30% lower expenditure than patients undergoing autologous BMT.[11] Lawless reported that charges to Blue Cross of Western Pennsylvania dropped by more than 50% when autologous BMT was replaced by PBPCT,[12] but actual cost or charges are not given and some of the change could be due to experience, hematopoietic growth factors, or the completeness of accounting.

Greater experience with the procedure might improve clinical outcome measures and lower the cost of the procedure. Experience may be as critically important to HSCT as it is for other aspects of medicine. For standard oncology

TABLE 64-1. REPORTED COST OF HEMATOPOIETIC STEM CELL TRANSPLANTATION

TYPE OF TRANSPLANT	FINANCIAL DATA, YEAR (ALL IN U.S. $)	COMMENT	REFERENCE
Autologous			
Auto BMT and PBPCT Hodgkin disease NHL	Cost, mean, 1991 $55,000–$74,000	Cost of hospitalization only before routine use of CSF, includes only survivors (underestimates costs, because those who die cost more)	Bennett et al., 1995[7]
Auto BMT and PBPCT Hodgkin disease NHL	Cost, mean, 1995 PBPBT $45,792 Auto BMT $59,214	Includes only HDCT phase, no follow-up care	Smith et al., 1997[8]
Auto BMT ± GM-CSF, lymphoma, and leukemia	Charges, 1994 OP $9,500 IP $54,100 Total $70,300	RCT of GM-CSF vs. none	Luce et al., 1994[54]
Auto BMT, AML	Cost, 1992 $74,098 for 2 years	Full 2-year costs	Dufoir et al., 1992[55]
Auto BMT, myeloma	Cost, 1992 $29,951	Very sketchy details on accounting	Henon et al., 1995[56]
Auto BMT, lymphomas	Cost, 1992 $34,445	Pre-HSCT and HSCT costs only; part of randomized study of CHOP vs auto BMT. Total average cost higher by $37,500	Uyl-de Groot et al., 1995[23]
Auto BMT, lymphomas, and solid tumors	Cost, 1992 $30,592–$32,443	No change if CSF used	Uyl-de Groot et al., 1994[11]
Allogeneic, Matched Related Donor			
AML 1st CR	Cost, 1992 $73,960 for 2 years	No more costly than auto HSCT, $74,098 for 2 years	Dufoir et al., 1992[55]
AML 1st CR	Cost, 1992 $242,000 for 5 years compared to $170,080 for standard	Includes all expenditures, but also mandatory ICU stay for transplant groups. Entire cost difference in first 6 months.	Welch and Larson, 1989[57]
AML 1st CR	Cost, 1992 $77,343	Compared with $86,423 for controls	Barr et al., 1996[36]
AML 2nd CR	Cost, 1992 $84,500	Compared with $43,500 for controls	Barr et al., 1996[36]
Allogeneic, Matched Unrelated Donor			
	No data available		

AML, acute myelogenous leukemia; auto BMT, autologous bone marrow transplantation; auto HSCT, autologous hematopoietic stem cell transplantation; CHOP, cyclophosphamide, doxorubicin, vincristine, prednisone; CR, complete response; CSF, colony-stimulating factor; GM-CSF, granulocyte-macrophage colony-stimulating factor; HDCT, high-dose chemotherapy; ICU, intensive care unit; IP, inpatient; NHL, non-Hodgkin lymphoma; OP, outpatient; PBPCT, peripheral blood progenitor cell transplantation; RCT, randomized clinical trial.

care, breast cancer treatment by specialist teams is associated with an absolute mortality rate reduction of 5%,[13, 14] gynecologic oncologists have improved outcomes over non-gynecologic surgeons in ovarian cancer treatment,[15] and specialized cancer centers have better results in the treatment of testicular cancer.[16]

No published data contradict these claims of specialist superiority, but there are also no randomized clinical trials of specialist versus generalist care in treatment. Bennett et al.[7] reported that toxic death rates decreased from 20–33% to 5%, and the cost of care diminished 8% per year for all patients undergoing HSCT at the University of Nebraska

TABLE 64-2. COMPARISON OF COST: PBPCT VERSUS AUTO BMT

STUDY	PBPCT, MEAN	ABMT	COMMENTS
Smith et al. (U.S., Europe, 1994)[58]	$45,792 −23%	$59,314	Costs, 1995 randomized controlled trial of filgrastim-mobilized PBPCT vs. auto BMT.
Uyl-de Groot et al. (Netherlands, 1994)[11]	$21,809 −30%	$32,443	Costs, 1992 historic cohorts; CSF used in both; $30,592 if auto BMT used without CSF
Bennett et al. (U.S., 1991)[7]	$69,870 if TBI not used; $102,560 if TBI used	$73,360 if TBI not used; $85,520 if TBI used	Costs, median, 1987–91 historic cohorts; only medians from 4-year period reported; CSF not routinely used; nonsurvivors excluded, making reported costs lower than true means.
Hartmann et al. (France, 1994)[10]	$21,688 −17%	$26,136	Costs, 1995 randomized controlled auto BMT as PBPCT; costs of HSCT alone

auto BMT, autologous bone marrow transplantation; CSF, colony-stimulating factor; HSCT, hematopoietic stem cell transplantation; PBPCT, peripheral blood progenitor cell transplantation; TBI, total body irradiation.

TABLE 64–3. SAVINGS FROM PBPCT ARE DUE TO EARLIER HOSPITAL DISCHARGE

CATEGORY	PBPCT COSTS ($)	AUTO BMT COSTS ($)
Autograft collection	5,760	8,531
High-dose chemotherapy, BEAM	10,019	10,030
Post-BEAM hospitalization	30,013	40,752
Total	45,792	59,314
Difference	−23%	

autoBMT, autologous bone marrow transplantation; BEAM, carmustine, etoposide, cytosine arabinoside, melphalan; PBPCT, peripheral blood progenitor cell transplantation.

Modified from Smith TJ, Hillner BE, Schmitz N, et al: Economic analysis of a randomized clinical trial to compare filgrastim-mobilized PBPC transplantation and autologous BMT in patients with Hodgkin's and non-Hodgkin's lymphoma. J Clin Oncol 15:5–10, 1997.

from 1987 to 1991. The average hospitalization cost and length of stay diminished markedly although the daily cost stayed nearly the same, suggesting that patients were hospitalized for a shorter period of time but experienced more-intensive resource use during their hospitalization. The University of Nebraska experience was that expenditure was approximately the same for autologous BMT vs. PBPCT during that time; data after 1991 have not been reported. Similar results were reported from the Medical College of Virginia.[17]

EFFECTIVENESS OF STEM CELL TRANSPLANTATION COMPARED WITH OTHER TREATMENTS

A first principle for cost-effectiveness analysis is that the effectiveness be established. The effectiveness of HDCT compared with standard treatment is a major area of concern to those interested in cost-effectiveness as well as clinical medicine. The standard for efficacy has been a randomized phase III clinical trial (with the assumption that effectiveness in the community will follow given similar types of patient, although there is only one oncology study that supports the assumption).[18] Table 64–4 shows a representative sampling of how phase II evidence has translated into phase III evidence when available. In general, the trend is for highly effective therapy in phase II trials to be translated into some observed benefit in phase III trials, but there are exceptions.

LYMPHOMA AND HODGKIN DISEASE

At least one randomized clinical trial has established HSCT as more effective than standard treatment in recurrent Hodgkin disease,[19] recurrent non-Hodgkin lymphoma (NHL),[20] and high-risk NHL.[21, 22] Phase II apparent benefit has not translated into phase III benefit in standard-risk NHL in first remission. No better disease-free survival (DFS) and overall survival (OS) is seen, except possibly for those patients at highest risk for recurrence[22] and "slow responders" to chemotherapy, in which patients experience no better and possibly worse outcomes.[23]

BREAST CANCER

Phase II HDCT trials for metastatic breast cancer have typically shown better clinical outcomes than historical controls.[24] There has, however, been a strong selection bias toward younger patients (which may or may not influence prognosis), healthier patients, and higher socioeconomic status (which gives better prognosis in other diseases) in clinical trials.[25, 26] In addition, more intense pre-HSCT staging may preclude up to 20–25% of patients who would have experienced recurrence earlier, leading to better results than with historical controls.[27] The first published random-

TABLE 64–4. AVAILABLE DATA OF EFFICACY IN SOLID TUMORS AND LYMPHOMA FOR HIGH-DOSE CHEMOTHERAPY AND STEM CELL TRANSPLANTATION

DISEASE	PHASE III RANDOMIZED CLINICAL TRIAL DATA	PHASE II CLINICAL TRIAL DATA
Breast Stage II	The largest RCT showed no difference in DFS or OS, even for those who achieved complete response; the smaller trial has significant methodologic problems	Multiple small series showing possible prolongation of DFS and OS
Breast Stage IV[24, 30]	Two small series showing no change in DFS or OS; one large RCT showing no change in DFS or OS; if there is any effect, it must be small; OS doubled from 10.4 to 20.8 months in one small trial	Multiple small series showing possible prolongation of DFS and OS, possible survival "tail"
Hodgkin disease, recurrent[59]	Small difference in DFS, but not OS favoring HDCT	Multiple small series showing possible prolongation of DFS and OS
Lymphoma, first remission[22]	464 patients; no difference in DFS or OS. Benefit in patients at higher risk (P = 0.09)	Multiple small series showing possible prolongation of DFS and OS
Lymphoma, slow responding[59]	Equivalent DSF and OS	Multiple small series showing possible prolongation of DFS and OS
Lymphoma recurrent[20]	Better OS at 5 years, 53% vs 32%, P = 0.035	Multiple small series showing possible prolongation of DFS and OS
Lymphoma, high risk[21]	Better OS at 7 years, 76% vs 46%	Multiple small series showing possible prolongation of DFS and OS

DFS, disease free survival; OS, overall survival; HDC, high dose chemotherapy; RCT, randomized clinical trial; CHOP, cyclophosphamide, doxorubicin, vincristine, prednisone.

ized clinical trial shows better survival in the HDCT group but has been criticized for poorer survival of the control arm.[28] Some authorities have argued that because the response and survival of the control arm was so poor, and the much higher number of responders in the HDCT arm then received tamoxifen, the results should not be interpreted as conclusive.[29] Current results of the largest randomized clinical trial show no difference in survival between standard and high-dose chemotherapy, even for those who achieved complete response.[30]

The use of HSCT in the adjuvant treatment of breast cancer shows early DFS and OS advantages in phase II single-institution historical controls.[31] Two randomized controlled trials of standard vs. standard followed by high-dose chemotherapy plus HSCT have shown *no* DFS or OS benefit.[32, 33] Both trials were powered to prove or disprove a 30% DFS benefit seen in the phase II trials but did not rule out a smaller benefit. The largest randomized clinical trial of HSCT in the adjuvant setting shows no DFS or OS benefit, but results are only preliminary.[34]

The rapid growth of HSCT for patients with breast cancer and its high cost to society has occurred before proof of its efficacy. Of great concern to health service researchers is that proof of effectiveness may be less important to rapid dissemination of HSCT procedures than fear of litigation, adverse public relations, or loss of market share by not performing HSCT.[35] This has made evaluation of effectiveness problematic as less than 1% of patients with breast cancer undergoing SCT enter phase III randomized clinical trials.

LEUKEMIAS

In contrast, the effectiveness of allogeneic transplantation for acute and chronic leukemia is not questioned. Allogeneic HSCT is accepted as a preferred therapy for chronic myelogenous leukemia. In acute leukemia, better DFS and OS are complicated by higher mortality rates in the transplant arm, usually leading to small differences in OS that vary by disease.[36] These issues are covered extensively in Chapters 2, 3, 4, and 9.

COST-EFFECTIVENESS OF STANDARD TREATMENT COMPARED WITH HSCT

The available data on cost and cost-effectiveness of HSCT are shown in Table 64–5. Using reasonable assumptions about the efficacy of the procedure, Hillner et al. estimated that HSCT for metastatic breast cancer compared with standard treatment would add about 6 months of survival, although at a cost of $116,000 per additional year of life (LY) gained.[37] Through careful attention to costs and being further down the learning curve, the cost-effectiveness can drop to about $70,000/LY.[17] The unstated but generally accepted threshold for cost-effectiveness has been about $50,000/LY associated with renal dialysis,[38] or the proposed standards for use in the evaluation of new technologies (if <$20,000/LY, accept; at $20,000–100,000/LY, examine on a case-by-case basis; >$100,000/LY, reject).[39] This standard

from the Canadian experience in which government expenditure is the sole source of revenue; this situation of socialized medicine is profoundly different from the context of the United States, in which patients may be willing to assume greater financial burden and risk.[40] The trial of Bezwoda et al. in metastatic breast cancer, which showed prolonged OS, has not been subjected to an economic analysis.[28]

Adjuvant HSCT for stage 2 high-risk cancer compared with standard treatment with CAF (cyclophosphamide, doxorubicin, and 5-flurouracil) would have a cost-effectiveness of about $50,000/LY.[41] This estimate is similar to the $43,000/LY obtained by Peters et al. using results from a Duke University phase II trial.[42] Both these results depend on several factors, including (1) that the results in selected phase II patients can be replicated in phase III and subsequent community settings and (2) the care is provided by experienced teams with similar outpatient facilities, low costs, and low toxicity.

Allogeneic HSCT for acute leukemia in second remission has cost-effectiveness ratios within the standard accepted benchmark of $50,000/LY, according to several studies listed in Table 64–5. Of note, the alternative (nontransplant) strategies to HSCT generally cost as much with worse outcomes. Autologous HSCT may prove to be more cost-effective if comparable long-term outcomes can be demonstrated in a randomized clinical trial.

Autologous HSCT for patients with relapsed NHL appears to have a cost-effectiveness ratio well under accepted limits. Messori et al. use the clinical data from a multicenter European study (Parma study) and the economic data reported by Uyl-de Groot to model the cost-effectiveness of HSCT.[43] The Parma study showed a doubling of overall survival and an average survival benefit of about 3 years per patient. The cost-effectiveness of autologous HSCT compared with standard therapy was $9,229/LY (95% CI $5,390–24,012), making it one of the most cost-effective interventions in modern health care. Although this model used separate data sets, the magnitude of the clinical benefit makes the cost-effectiveness data appear to be quite sound.

STRATEGY TO IMPROVE COST EFFECTIVENESS

Table 64–6 outlines strategies to perform HSCT in a cost-effective manner. Chief among these would be withholding HSCT outside of a well-designed clinical trial until efficacy has been established. This approach, however, may not be possible in the United States if preliminary evidence is positive.[35, 40] Our desire for rapid dissemination of technology (such as magnetic resonance imaging or coronary artery bypass grafting), knowledge of poor results with conventional therapy, and a willingness of informed patients to assume risks make such hesitation difficult.

Other published operational changes that have been proven to reduce expenditure without lowering the quality of care include (1) use of outpatient facilities for chemotherapy[44] and total body radiation,[45] (2) use of glutamine-containing total parental nutrition for patients undergoing HSCT with expected long inpatient stays,[46] and (3) outpa-

TABLE 64–5. AVAILABLE COST AND COST-EFFECTIVENESS DATA FOR STEM CELL TRANSPLANTATION, COMPARED WITH STANDARD CARE

DISEASE	TYPE OF EVIDENCE	COST		RESULTS	COMMENTS
		Std	HSCT		
Autologous					
Breast cancer metastatic[33]	Phase II	$36,100	$89,700	$116,000/LY	Used reasonable conservative estimate of effect for HSCT, similar to that observed in subsequent randomized clinical trials[24]
Breast cancer adjuvant[41, 42]	Phase II	$36,600	$107,200	$43,000–50,000/LY	Used Duke data for HSCT, best available data for standard treatment. All treatments include chest wall radiation.
Multiple myeloma[56]	Phase II			Standard $/LY cannot be calculated from the data given. Authors report $3,848–50,232/QALY.	Major methodologic problems. Compares historical cohorts of 12 patients treated with HDCT to patients treated with conventional therapy, but patients are dissimilar in age, comorbidity, and refusal to participate. Utility values based on physician estimate of disability using instrument that has not been validated. Unable to calculate standard cost-effectiveness measures or standard cost-utility measures.
Lymphoma, slow responders[23]	Phase III	$3,118	$34,445	Auto BMT group more expensive and patients had 0.14 fewer LYs and 0.22 fewer QALYs than CHOP group.	Well-designed randomized clinical trial, careful accounting, validated instrument for utility assessment.
Hodgkin disease[60]	Phase II	$16,300	$76,500	Auto SCT in 2nd relapse gave best survival at $26,200/LY.	Decision-analysis study
Allogeneic					
AML in 2nd CR[36]	Comparative trial based on donor availability	$51,800	$100,600	1.67 LYs added; $29,200/LY	Used local Ontario data for costs and efficacy; extensive sensitivity analyses bear out conclusions (1992 Canadian $)
ALL in 1st CR[36]	Phase III	$102,800	$92,000	0.37 LYs added; −$29,200/LY, or cost-saving	Used local Ontario data for costs and efficacy; extensive sensitivity analyses bear out conclusions
AML[53]	Matched cohorts	$170,080 5 years	$242,500 5 years	OS 21% vs. 40%	Improved OS offsets higher cost

ALL, acute lymphoblastic leukemia; AML, acute myelogenous leukemia; auto BMT, autologous bone marrow transplantation; auto SCT, autologous stem cell transplantation; CHOP, cyclophosphamide, doxorubicin, vincristine, prednisone; HDCT, high-dose chemotherapy; HSCT, hematopoietic stem cell transplantation; LY, life years; OS, overall survival; QALY, quality-adjusted life years.

tient bone marrow harvesting, if bone marrow is used.[47] Coordinated outpatient care reduces length of stay and costs remarkably,[48] but this strategy does require a caretaker friend or relative and adequate accommodation close to the HSCT facility (Table 64–7).

The concentration of some payers on low-cost regimens may be counterproductive to both clinical results and clinical research. The major problem in solid tumors is still disease relapse; more-toxic conditioning regimens that have increased short-term cost and toxicity may provide better long-term survival. There are no phase III data showing superiority of one conditioning regimen over another in any disease. A major concern is the proliferation of HSCT centers that administer only modestly elevated doses of chemotherapy, which may not even require HSC support.

The rapid proliferation of allogeneic mobilized a PBPC as a graft instead of bone marrow raises an additional set of problems. While cost may be lower, graft vs. host disease (GVHD) may be more prevalent, severe, or long-lasting

(Table 64–8).[49] Practitioners are urged to use caution in adopting this strategy until longer-term results are known.

IMPACT OF HSCT ON DISEASE PALLIATION AND QUALITY OF LIFE

There have been no published data on the palliation of symptoms by HSCT. In other diseases, tumor response does not correlate with quality or quantity of life, and antitumor response by itself does not justify treatment.[50] In the few studies reported, the quality of life of patients with breast cancer compares favorably after HSCT to that of patients treated with conventional therapy, but a significant number of patients (30%) experienced psychosocial problems.[51, 52] In the only reported study of patients with lymphoma, quality of life rapidly returned to 90% or more in both standard and HSCT groups.[23]

TABLE 64–6. WAYS TO USE HIGH-DOSE CHEMOTHERAPY RATIONALLY AND AT LEAST COST

- Enroll patients in national, randomized clinical trials (RCT) preferentially comparing standard and hematopoietic stem cell transplantation (HSCT) rather than in local trials.
- Do not perform transplantation off clinical trial unless the benefit is clearly established. Small phase II trials that purport to show benefit should not be valued more than a well-designed negative RCT.
- Once superiority of HSCT is shown in RCT, work to make it standard at your institution and community. This may mean transfer of care from a nontransplant physician to a transplant physician.
- Reduce costs, even if it means lower reimbursement. If two drug regimens have the same efficacy, use the less expensive. Use critical/clinical pathways and practice guidelines, and coordinate inpatient and outpatient services.
- Monitor costs and quality of life in clinical trials with the same accuracy as disease-free survival.
- Perform only clinical trials with sufficient subjects to answer a definite significant question.
- Restrict the use of HSCT to centers with sufficient volume, proven safety, and low cost.

COST IMPLICATIONS FOR UNIVERSAL COVERAGE OF HSCT

The large individual expense of HSCT requires careful balance of the needs of society against those of individuals. Uyl-de Groot et al. estimated that universal coverage of autologous HSCT for the Netherlands would cost an additional $4.9 to 6.7 million for patients with NHL and $2.2 million for patients with acute myelogenous leukemia.[53] Within the fixed budget of a health care system, those resources would be better spent in effective HSCT treatment of recurrent NHL and first-line treatment of high-risk NHL rather than for treatment of slow-responding or first-remission standard-risk NHL. The reference groups (those who need the money for other uses) could range from members of a health care plan, the neighborhood raising funds for an indigent patient, or an entire country. Some patients are willing to assume some or all of the additional financial burden themselves.

Barr et al. performed a "quick and dirty" analysis of allogeneic HSCT and its financial impact on the Province of Ontario in Canada.[36] This instructive analysis showed that the costs of HSCT may have been overestimated in the literature and that for some conditions, such as acute lymphoblastic leukemia in first remission, HSCT may reduce expenditure as well as be more effective. Even when

TABLE 64–7. REDUCING COSTS WITH COORDINATED OUTPATIENT CARE

	TYPE OF STAY		
	IP	Short Stay IP	OP
LOS (days)	17.3	8.2	2.7
Cost ($, 1996)	39,700	36,200	29,400

LOS, length of stay; IP, inpatient; OP, outpatient.
From Meisenberg, BR, Ferran K, Hollenbach K, et al: Reduced charges and costs associated with outpatient autologous stem cell transplantation. Bone Marrow Transplant 21:927–932, 1998.

TABLE 64–8. REDUCING COSTS OF ALLO BMT WITH G-CSF PRIMING OF PBPCT

	PBSCT (n = 21)	BMT (n = 13)
100 day OS, %	83	69; $P = 0.56$
Grade II–IV acute GVHD, %	57	46; $P = 0.20$
LOS, days	17	22
Total for IP, $	51,000	65,000
Total, $	77,000	96,000; $P<0.01$

OS, overall survival; GVHD, graft vs. host disease; IP, inpatient; PBPCT, peripheral blood progenitor cell transplant; BMT, bone marrow transplant.
Modified from Bennett C, Waters T, Stinson T, et al: Valuing clinical strategies early in development: a cost analysis of allogeneic peripheral blood stem cell transplantation. Bone Marrow Transplant 24:555–560, 1999.

HSCT was more expensive, the cost-effectiveness ratio was well within what society could be expected to bear.[38] The value of this analysis is to point out that alternative, non-HSCT therapy is often just as expensive with worse outcome.

The cost-effectiveness of HSCT can be put in some societal context by a comparison of cost-effectiveness ratios (Table 64–9).[38] In general, if a therapy is effective, its cost-effectiveness is within general accepted bounds of $50,000/LY. If not, as in HSCT for patients with metastatic breast cancer, the proponents of treatment have three choices: (1) improve the efficacy, (2) decrease the cost, or (3) not

TABLE 64–9. EFFICACY AND COST-EFFECTIVENESS OF CANCER TREATMENT

CANCER INTERVENTION	BENEFIT	COST/LY ($US 1992)
Auto BMT for all relapsed Hodgkin disease	8.2 yr	421,000
Auto BMT for limited metastatic breast cancer	6.0 mo	115,800
Chemotherapy vs. allo BMT for ANLL, 5-yr horizon	OS 21 vs. 48%	84,700
Chemotherapy for ANLL compared with no therapy	NA	80,300
Auto BMT for limited metastatic breast cancer current costs	6.0 mo	70,000
Auto BMT for stage II breast cancer	↑ DFS at 3 yr	50,000
Societal Benchmark, Dialysis		50,000
Auto BMT for Hodgkin disease, second relapse only	10.3 yr	26,200
Acute myeloid leukemia in 2nd CR	1.67 yr	24,550
Chemotherapy vs. allo BMT for ANLL, lifetime horizon	OS 21% vs. 48%	12,500
Autologous HSCT for relapsed NHL	OS 53% vs. 32% at 5 yr	9,229
Acute lymphoid leukemia in 2nd CR	0.37 yr	−24,550 (cost-saving)

allo BMT, allogeneic bone marrow transplantation; ANLL, acute nonlymphocytic leukemia; auto BMT, autologous bone marrow transplantation; CR, complete remission; DFS, disease-free survival; HDCT, high-dose chemotherapy; HSCT, hematopoietic stem cell transplantation; LY, life years; NHL, non-Hodgkin lymphoma; OS, overall survival.
Modified from Smith TJ, Hillner BE, Desch CE: Efficacy and cost-effectiveness of cancer treatment: rational allocation of resources based on decision analysis. J Natl Cancer Inst 85:1460–1474, 1993.

perform the procedure despite lack of other good treatment options. This last choice has been anathema to oncologists in the United States but one that will become increasingly common if resource allocation is based on efficacy.

CONCLUSION

The high initial cost of HSCT makes attention to outcome measures, including total disease expenditure, imperative regardless of the type of health care finance plan. In general, HSCT for leukemias and recurrent or high-risk lymphomas has acceptable cost and cost-effectiveness ratios because standard treatment is also very costly and the improved survival with HSCT can offset the higher initial cost. For other solid tumors, especially breast cancer, currently available data suggest that HSCT in the adjuvant setting meets accepted cost-effectiveness ratios. It is important to remember that cost-effectiveness ratios can be improved by both more effective therapy and reduced expenditure. Both are worthy goals and are just as important as improved clinical results.

REFERENCES

1. Brown ML: The national economic burden of cancer. J Natl Cancer Inst 82:1811–1814, 1990.
2. Brown ML, Hodgson TA, Rice DP: Economic impact of cancer in the U.S. In Schottenfeld D, Fraumeni J (eds): Cancer, Epidemiology, and Prevention. Oxford, Oxford University Press; 1996.
3. Rundle RL: Salick pioneers selling cancer care to HMOs. The Wall Street Journal Monday, August 12:B1–B2, 1996.
4. Callahan D: Controlling the costs of health care for the elderly—fair means and foul. N Engl J Med 335:744–746, 1996.
5. Levinsky NG: The purpose of advance medical planning—autonomy for patients or limitation of care? N Engl J Med 335:741–743, 1996.
6. Niland J, Gebhardt JA, Lee J, Forman SJ: Study design, statistical analyses, and results reporting in the bone marrow transplantation literature. Biol Blood Marrow Transplant 1:47–53, 1995.
7. Bennett CL, Armitage JL, Armitage GO, et al: Costs of care and outcomes for high-dose therapy and autologous transplantation for lymphoid malignancies: results from the University of Nebraska, 1987 through 1991. J Clin Oncol 13:969–973, 1995.
8. Smith TJ, Hillner BE, Schmitz N, et al: Economic analysis of a randomized clinical trial to compare filgrastim-mobilized peripheral blood progenitor cell transplantation and autologous bone marrow transplantation in patients with Hodgkin and non-Hodgkin lymphoma. J Clin Oncol 15:5–10, 1997.
9. Schmitz N, Linch DC, Dreger P, et al: Randomised trial of filgrastim-mobilised peripheral blood progenitor cell transplantation versus autologous bone-marrow transplantation in lymphoma patients. Lancet 347:353–357, 1996.
10. Hartmann O, Le Corroller A, Blaise D, et al: Peripheral blood stem cell and bone marrow transplantation for solid tumors and lymphomas: hematologic recovery and costs. Ann Intern Med 126:600–607, 1997.
11. Uyl-de Groot CA, Richel DJ, Rutten FF: Peripheral blood progenitor cell transplantation mobilised by r-metHuG-CSF (filgrastim); a less costly alternative to autologous bone marrow transplantation. Eur J Cancer 30A:1631–1635, 1994.
12. Lawless GD: Cost-effectiveness of autologous bone marrow transplantation. Am J Health Syst Pharm 52:S11–S14, 1995.
13. Gillis CR, Hole DJ: Survival outcome of care by specialist surgeons in breast cancer: a study of 3786 patients in the west of Scotland. BMJ 312:145–148, 1996.
14. Sainsbury R, Haward R, Rider L, et al: Influence of clinician workload and patterns of treatment on survival from breast cancer. Lancet 345:1265–1270, 1995.
15. Nguyen HN, Averette HE, Hoskins W, et al: National survey of ovarian carcinoma, Part V: the impact of physician's specialty on patient's survival. Cancer 72:3663–3670, 1993.
16. Feuer EJ, Frey CM, Brawley OW, et al: After a treatment breakthrough: a comparison of trial and population-based data for advanced testicular cancer. J Clin Oncol 12:368–377, 1994.
17. Smith TJ, Buonaiuto DA, Hillner BE, et al: The learning curve for cost of autologous bone marrow transplantation (ABMT) for breast cancer (Bca). Proc Am Soc Clin Oncol 12:54a, 1993.
18. Olivotto IA, Bajdik CD, Plenderleith IH, et al: Adjuvant systemic therapy and survival after breast cancer. N Engl J Med 330:805–810, 1994.
19. Linch DC, Winfield D, Goldstone AH, et al: Dose intensification with autologous bone-marrow transplantation in relapsed and resistant Hodgkin's disease: results of BNLI randomised trial. Lancet 341:1051–1054, 1993.
20. Philip T, Guglielmi C, Hagenbeek A, et al: Autologous bone marrow transplantation as compared with salvage chemotherapy in relapses of chemotherapy-sensitive non-Hodgkin's lymphoma. N Engl J Med 333:1540–1545, 1995.
21. Gianni AM, Bregni M, Brambilla C, et al: High-dose chemotherapy and autologous bone marrow transplantation compared with MA-COP-B in aggressive B-cell lymphoma. N Engl J Med 336:1290–1297, 1997.
22. Haioun C, Lepage E, Gisselbrecht C, et al: Comparison of autologous bone marrow transplantation with sequential chemotherapy for intermediate-grade and high-grade non-Hodgkin's lymphoma in first complete remission: a study of 464 patients. Groupe d'Etude des Lymphomes de l'Adulte. J Clin Oncol 12:2543–2551, 1994.
23. Uyl-de Groot CA, Hagenbeck A, Verdonck LF, et al: Cost-effectiveness of ABMT in comparison with CHOP chemotherapy in patients with intermediate- and high-grade malignant non-Hodgkin's lymphoma (NHL). Bone Marrow Transplant 16:463–470, 1995.
24. Antman K, Corringham R, de Vries E, et al: Dose intensive therapy in breast cancer. Bone Marrow Transplant 10:67–73, 1994.
25. Cella DF: The economics of cancer survival. Contemp Oncol 2:55–62, 1992.
26. Cella DF, Orav EJ, Kornblith AB, et al: Socioeconomic status and cancer survival. J Clin Oncol 9:1500–1509, 1991.
27. Crump M, Goss PE, Prince M, Girouard C: Outcome of extensive evaluation before adjuvant therapy in women with breast cancer and 10 or more positive axillary lymph nodes. J Clin Oncol 14:66–69, 1996.
28. Bezwoda WR, Seymour L, Dansey RD: High-dose chemotherapy with hematopoietic rescue as primary treatment for metastatic breast cancer: a randomized trial. J Clin Oncol 13:2483–2489, 1995.
29. Dose intensity and survival in metastatic breast cancer. Clin Onc Alert 10:89–91, 1995.
30. Stadtmauer EA, O'Neill A, Goldstein LJ, et al: Conventional-dose chemotherapy compared with high-dose chemotherapy plus autologous hematopoietic stem-cell transplantation for metastatic breast cancer. New Engl J Med 342:1069–1076, 2000.
31. Goldhirsch A, Wood WC, Senn H, et al: Meeting highlights: International Consensus Panel on the treatment of primary breast cancer. JNCI 87:1441–1445, 1995.
32. Rodenhuis S, Richel DJ, van der Wall E, et al: Randomised trial of high-dose chemotherapy and haemopoietic progenitor-cell support in operable breast cancer with extensive axillary lymph-node involvement. Lancet 352:515–521, 1998.
33. Hortobagyi GN, Buzdar AU, Theriault RL, et al: Randomized trial of high-dose chemotherapy and blood cell autografts for high-risk primary breast carcinoma. J Natl Cancer Inst 92:225–233, 2000.
34. Peters WP, Rosner G, Vredenburgh J, et al: A prospective, randomized comparison of two doses of combination alkylating agents (AA) as consolidation after CAF in high-risk primary breast cancer involving ten or more axillary lymph nodes (LN): Preliminary results of CALGB 9082/SWOG 9114/NCIC MA-13. Proceedings of ASCO, 1999, p 3A.
35. U.S. General Accounting Office: Health insurance: coverage of autologous bone marrow transplantation for breast cancer. B-260550:1329–1355, 1996.
36. Barr R, Furlong W, Henwood J, et al: Economic evaluation of allogeneic bone marrow transplantation: a rudimentary model to generate estimates for the timely formulation of clinical policy. J Clin Oncol 14:1413–1420, 1996.
37. Hillner BE, Smith TJ, Desch CE: Efficacy and cost-effectiveness of autologous bone marrow transplantation in metastatic breast cancer: estimates using decision-analysis while awaiting clinical trial results. JAMA 267:2055–2061, 1992.

38. Smith TJ, Hillner BE, Desch CE: Efficacy and cost-effectiveness of cancer treatment: rational allocation of resources based on decision analysis. J Natl Cancer Inst 85:1460–1474, 1993.

39. Laupacis A, Feeny D, Detsky AS, Tugwell PX: How attractive does a new technology have to be to warrant adoption and utilization? Tentative guidelines for using clinical and economic evaluation. Can Med Assoc J 146:473–481, 1992.

40. Smith TJ: A piece of my mind. Which hat do I wear? JAMA 270:1657–1659, 1993.

41. Smith TJ, Hillner BE: Decision analysis: a practical example. Oncology Suppl 37–45, 1995.

42. Peters WP, Ross M, Vredenburgh JJ, et al: High dose chemotherapy and autologous bone marrow support as consolidation after standard-dose adjuvant therapy for high-risk primary breast cancer. J Clin Oncol 11:1132–1143, 1993.

43. Messori A, Bonistalli L, Costantini M, Alterini R: Cost-effectiveness of autologous bone marrow transplantation in patients with relapsed non-Hodgkin's lymphoma. Bone Marrow Transplant 19:275–281, 1997.

44. Peters WP, Ross M, Vredenburgh JJ, et al: The use of intensive clinic support to permit outpatient autologous bone marrow transplantation for breast cancer. Semin Oncol 21:25–31, 1994.

45. Algara M, Valls A, Vivancos P, Granena A: Outpatient total body irradiation for bone marrow transplantation. Bone Marrow Transplant 14:381–382, 1994.

46. MacBurney M, Young LS, Ziegler TR, Wilmore DW: A cost-evaluation of glutamine-supplemented parenteral nutrition in adult bone marrow transplant patients. J Am Diet Assoc 94:1263–1266, 1994.

47. Brandwein JM, Callum J, Rubinger M, et al: An evaluation of outpatient bone marrow harvesting. J Clin Oncol 7:648–650, 1989.

48. Meisenberg BR, Ferran K, Hollenbach K, et al: Reduced charges and costs associated with outpatient autologous stem cell transplantation. Bone Marrow Transplant 21:927–932, 1998.

49. Bennett C, Waters T, Stinson T, et al: Valuing clinical strategies early in development: A cost analysis of allogeneic peripheral blood stem cell transplantation. Bone Marrow Transplant 24:555–560, 1999.

50. American Society of Clinical Oncology Outcomes Working Group (core members): Outcomes of cancer treatment for technology assessment and cancer treatment guidelines. J Clin Oncol 14:671–679, 1995.

51. Hann DM, Jacobsen PB, Martin SC, et al: Quality of life following bone marrow transplantation for breast cancer: a comparative study. Bone Marrow Transplant 19:257–264, 1997.

52. McQuellon RP, Craven B, Russell GB, et al: Quality of life in breast cancer patients before and after autologous bone marrow transplantation. Bone Marrow Transplant 18:579–584, 1997.

53. Uyl-de Groot CA, Okhuijsen SY, Hagenbeek A, et al: Costs of introducing autologous BMT in the treatment of lymphoma and acute leukemia in the Netherlands. Bone Marrow Transplant 15:605–610, 1995.

54. Luce BR, Singer JW, Weschler JM, et al: Recombinant human granulocyte-macrophage colony-stimulating factor after autologous bone marrow transplantation for lymphoid cancer. Pharmacol Econ 6:42–48, 1994.

55. Dufoir T, Saux MC, Terraza B, et al: Comparative cost of allogeneic or autologous bone marrow transplantation and chemotherapy in patients with acute myeloid leukaemia in first remission. Bone Marrow Transplant 10:323–329, 1992.

56. Henon P, Donatini B, Eisenmann JC, et al: Comparative survival, quality of life and cost-effectiveness of intensive therapy with autologous blood cell transplantation or conventional chemotherapy in multiple myeloma. Bone Marrow Transplant 16:19–25, 1995.

57. Welch HG, Larson EB: Cost-effectiveness of bone marrow transplantation in acute nonlymphocytic leukemia. N Engl J Med 321:807–812, 1989.

58. Smith TJ, Desch CE, Hillner BE: Ways to reduce the cost of oncology care without compromising the quality. Cancer Invest 12:257–265, 1994.

59. Verdonck LF, van Putten WL, Hagenbeek A, et al: Comparison of CHOP chemotherapy with autologous bone marrow transplantation for slowly responding patients with aggressive non-Hodgkin's lymphoma. N Engl J Med 332:1045–1051, 1995.

60. Desch CE, Lasala MR, Smith TJ, Hillner BE: The optimal timing of autologous bone marrow transplantation in Hodgkin's disease patients after a chemotherapy relapse. J Clin Oncol 10:200–209, 1992.

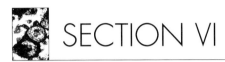

SECTION VI

Regulatory Issues

CHAPTER SIXTY-FIVE

Regulation of Hematopoietic Stem Cell Therapy

Adrian P. Gee, M.I.Biol., Ph.D.

Potential transmission of infectious agents has been a major force behind the development of regulations for the blood banking industry. In recent years, the discovery of the human immunodeficiency virus prompted the radical revision of these regulations and implementation of the product manufacturing approach known as current good manufacturing practice (cGMP).[1] The rapid growth in hematopoietic stem cell (HSC) transplantation (HSCT) in the therapy of refractory cancer, marrow failure syndromes, myelodysplasia, and inherited disorders has attracted the attention of the regulatory agencies in the United States, who have indicated that they intend to regulate the field. This chapter reviews relevant existing legislation and possible approaches to the development of specific new regulations.

LEVELS OF OVERSIGHT

VOLUNTARY STANDARDS

Oversight of any medical discipline or treatment may occur at a number of levels. In the case of HSC therapy, professional organizations, such as the Foundation for the Accreditation of Hematopoietic Cell Therapy (FAHCT)[2] and the American Association of Blood Banks (AABB), have published voluntary standards covering the collection, processing, and storage of these cells. In the case of FAHCT, the standards also encompass minimal guidelines for clinical transplantation programs. These standards do not have the power of law, but facilities that are not in compliance (as determined by on-site inspection) may be denied accreditation. Recent litigation in New Jersey[3] has nonetheless established that organizations that set voluntary standards may be held liable if they are thought to have been negligent in establishing appropriate standards based on currently available medical and scientific knowledge.

STATE REGULATIONS

Legally enforceable regulations have been established at the state level by New York and New Jersey. The New York regulations first went into effect in December 1988 and cover HSC derived from all sources (although more detailed regulations specific to placental and umbilical cord blood cells have recently been developed).[4] They detail general requirements, HSC collection services, donor qualifications, sterilization of instruments, collection and handling of HSC, HSC storage services, required records, quality assurance and safety requirements, compliance, and licensure.[5] Facilities in the state that collect and/or store HSC must be licensed and are subject to inspection by the State Department of Health.

The New Jersey regulations deal primarily with the requirement for a certificate of need for new HSC transplant programs (N.J.A.C. 8:33 Q-3/Q-2) but also indicate the intent to regulate cell collection, processing, and banking under the certificate of need when agreement is reached on specific standards. Other states, including Florida and California, are contemplating regulating the field or have particular legislation relating to the qualifications of staff involved in HSC collection and processing.

FEDERAL REGULATIONS

The primary responsibility for regulation, however, rests at the federal level, with the Food and Drug Administration (FDA). Within this complex body, the task falls mainly to the Center for Biologics Evaluation and Research (CBER), which is in turn composed of a number of offices and divisions. The mission of CBER is to "protect and enhance the public health through the regulation of biological and related products including blood vaccines and biological therapeutics according to statutory authorities."

Although specific details of which component of CBER covers which aspect of HSC collection and processing have yet to be resolved, it appears that this will be delegated according to the degree of manipulation of the cells (see later). Gene-modified, ex vivo expanded and extensively manipulated cells will fall under the Office of Therapeutics Research and Review, whereas placental/umbilical cord blood and minimally manipulated cells will be the responsibility of the Division of Blood Applications in the Office of Blood Research and Review. This situation, however, is still somewhat uncertain, and those seeking regulatory information on a particular cell source or specific manipulation are strongly advised to contact CBER directly. In addition to reviewing and developing a regulatory approach, the center also has the responsibility of enforcing the statutes through its Office of Compliance.

In developing regulations for a field, the FDA generally reviews existing legislation to see if and how it may apply to that field. This was the strategy adopted by CBER in seeking to regulate HSC therapy. Surprisingly, relevant laws considerably predated the therapy, with the first appearing at the turn of the century.

APPLICATION OF EXISTING LEGISLATION TO HSC THERAPY

Although the regulation of biologic products in the United States dates from the Biologics Control Act of 1902, blood and blood components were officially defined as biologic products under the United States Public Health Service Act of 1912. Under this Act, biologic products include "any virus, therapeutic serum, toxin, vaccine, blood, blood component or derivative . . . applicable to the prevention, treatment or cure of diseases or injuries of man."

Of particular importance to the present efforts to regulate the field is the Food, Drug and Cosmetic Act of 1938, which was enacted in response to the death of more than 100 people who had taken a toxic preparation of sulfanilamide. The Act established the cGMP for drug products for administration to humans or animals. In simple terms, this means that such products must be safe. The legislation was amended in 1962 in response to the thalidomide tragedy to state that prescription and nonprescription drug products must be *effective* and safe. This terminology underpins the current philosophy of regulation by the FDA and has given birth to a system for product preparation and testing to ensure both safety and efficacy. Blood banks and cell processing facilities are regarded as product manufacturers and are expected to comply with cGMP, and they are held to the same standards as drug and device manufacturers. In 1972, the FDA was officially given jurisdiction over the approval of human biologic products, therapeutics, and blood banking diagnostics. This was extended in 1976 to cover medical devices and in vitro diagnostics.

The first piece of legislation that officially addressed HSCT was the Transplant Amendment Act of 1990, under which the National Marrow Donor Program (NMDP) was established to set up a voluntary national bone marrow registry for matched unrelated donors. The NMDP was given the responsibility and authority to recruit donors, establish standards for quality, provide information on transplantation and support for studies, and ensure confidentiality of records. This legislation was developed in response to the dramatic growth in the number and types of HSCT beyond the use of traditional human leukocyte antigen–matched sibling donors. The NMDP publishes its own standards, which apply exclusively to HSC from unrelated donors. This was paralleled by increasing use of ex vivo manipulation of HSC in the form of depletion T cells from allogeneic grafts and tumor cells from autologous grafts. Further developments involving the insertion of genes into progenitor cells, ex vivo expansion of HSC, and the use of peripheral, placental, and umbilical cord blood-derived HSC have prompted regulatory agencies to propose regulations that specifically cover HSC therapy, which was included under the broader umbrella of "somatic cell therapy."

SOMATIC CELL THERAPY

In an attempt to clarify and provide guidance on how the FDA would apply its regulatory approach to somatic or gene therapy, the agency published "Application of Current Statutory Authorities to Human Somatic Cell Therapy Products and Gene Therapy Products" in the October 14, 1993 edition of the *Federal Register*. This document defined somatic cell therapy as "the prevention, treatment, cure, diagnosis or mitigation of disease or injuries in humans by the administration of autologous, allogeneic or xenogeneic cells that have been manipulated or altered ex vivo." Central to this definition is the use of the word *manipulated*, which is described as "ex vivo propagation, expansion, selection or pharmacological treatment of cells, or other alteration of their biological characteristics."

Under these combined definitions it would appear that the only HSC that would be subject to licensure as final products when used for somatic cell therapy would be autologous or allogeneic bone marrow transplants using activated or expanded bone marrow cells, and autologous or allogeneic somatic cells that have been genetically manipulated. Other cell types, now increasingly used in transplant-related immunotherapy, would also be subject to licensure. These included lymphocytes that were activated and expanded ex vivo (e.g., lymphokine-activated killer cells, tumor-infiltrating lymphocytes, and antigen-specific lymphocytes).

Excluded from approval prior to marketing were "minimally manipulated or purged bone marrow transplants"—a category that, again, is critically dependent on the definition of "minimal manipulation." In this case, the term was not defined more rigorously but examples of minimally manipulated products were given. These included autologous bone marrow transplants employing either "ex vivo tumor purging with an approved reagent," or "bone marrow enriched for stem cells by immunoadherence." Allogeneic marrow transplantation employing "ex vivo T cell purging with a monoclonal antibody approved for such purging" would also fall under minimal manipulation.

These proposals essentially left untouched the majority of commonly used graft processing and engineering procedures, with the exception of gene therapy and ex vivo expansion. It appeared that a relatively light regulatory hand was to guide the field and that the weight of that hand may be determined by the extent to which HSC were manipulated ex vivo. Within 2 years, this situation changed dramatically.

MANIPULATION REDEFINED

At a National Heart, Lung and Blood Institute (NHLBI)-sponsored workshop on stem cell processing held at the National Institutes of Health (NIH) in February 1995, Dr. Katherine Zoon, the Director of CBER, was invited to review the FDA's approach to the regulation of HSC. Her presentation radically redefined the term *minimal manipulation* with the result that many previously excluded categories of HSC transplants would now require regulatory approval.

In her introduction, Dr. Zoon indicated that this reevaluation was prompted by a number of factors. These included the emergence of new investigational sources of HSC and new technology for their purification, together with a lack of accepted specific standards and confusion in the interpretation of minimal manipulation as defined in the somatic cell therapy document of 1993. Elaborating on these issues, she detailed the agency's concerns. In the case of new sources of HSC, these related to how these cells were collected (including the use of closed systems and the logistics of collection); whether there were differences between HSC obtained from different sources; how many HSC were required for engraftment; what type of "genetic information" should be required for allogeneic transplantation; and the effects of long-term storage on HSC.

The use of new technology to purify HSC prompted questions on the effects of ancillary products on both the donor and the cells. These ancillary products may be intended to act on the donor (e.g., agents used for HSC mobilization and not approved for that indication) or require incorporation into the cells (e.g., anticoagulants and media infused with the graft). Other ancillary products may be intended to act on the cells and would include apheresis machines, separation devices, and collection and storage containers. The Agency was also concerned about the effects of manipulation on HSC engraftment and even the ultimate benefit of HSC support to the patient.

The lack of specific standards with respect to donor screening; HSC collection, processing, characterization, and storage; and the extent to which cells could be manipulated without rendering them a somatic cell product were also cited as factors that had prompted the reassessment of the regulatory strategy. The proposal was to redefine manipulated products as those "obtained after one or more procedures have been performed to intentionally purge or enrich the starting material of a subset(s) of nucleated cells." Conversely, minimally manipulated products would be those that "had not been subjected to a procedure(s) that selectively removes, enriches, expands or functionally alters specific nucleated cell populations (with the exception of neutrophils)." This drastically restricted procedures that would be considered to be minimal manipulation. This list no longer included tumor and T-cell purging and positive selection of CD34+ cells but was restricted to centrifugation, density gradient separation, erythrocyte lysis, addition of cryopreservation medium, transfer to storage containers, and storage in a liquid or frozen state.

A variety of regulatory mechanisms could be used to implement this strategy. These include obtaining an investigational new drug (IND) exemption to generate data that would be used to obtain product license approval. In order to manufacture the product, the facility would require both the product license approval and an establishment license approval, which demonstrates that the facility is in compliance with cGMP and has programs in place for process validation and quality management.

Alternatively, the 510(k) mechanism could be used, in which data generated under an investigational device exemption lead to premarket approval of the device. Additionally, facilities may be required to register with the Agency as blood establishments. Registration permits facilities to manufacture components for transfusion and further manufacture and, under specified conditions, to ship products across state lines or out of the country. These options were soon to be exercised in a draft proposal for the regulation of cord blood hematopoietic progenitor cell products.

PROPOSED REGULATION OF CORD BLOOD HEMATOPOIETIC STEM CELLS

On December 13, 1995, CBER and the NHLBI cosponsored a meeting at the NIH on "Cord Blood Stem Cells: Discussion of Procedures for Collection and Storage" at which it circulated a draft proposal concerning "the Regulation of Placental/Umbilical Cord Blood Stem Cell Products Intended for Transplantation or Further Manufacturing into Injectable Products."[6] The Agency had always indicated that it regarded cord blood HSC as a somewhat special case, and this was reflected in the proposal. It stated that, *regardless of the extent of manipulation*, cord blood HSC products intended for use in the prevention, treatment, cure, diagnosis, or mitigation of disease in humans would be subject to IND regulations during clinical development and, as final products, would be subject to licensure. The proposal also stated that "establishments collecting cord blood stem cells should consider the concepts found in blood regulations (21 Code of Federal Regulations [CFR] Parts 606 and 640) and relevant FDA recommendations to blood establishments." The proposal was published in the *Federal Register* in February 1996.[6]

This draft excited considerable comment from academic and community hospitals, professional organizations, and the cord blood banking companies. The latter believed that they could not remain commercially viable if they were required to function under IND regulations and lobbied Congress to adopt different legislation.

PROPOSED REGULATION OF PERIPHERAL BLOOD PROGENITOR CELLS

Following the same pattern used to launch draft regulations for cord blood transplantation, CBER held a meeting on February 22–23, 1996 to discuss peripheral blood progenitor cell (PBPC) transplantation, at which they circulated their "Draft Document Concerning the Regulation of Peripheral Blood Hematopoietic Stem Cell Products Intended for Transplantation or Further Manufacturing into Injectable Products." This more closely followed the regulatory strategy proposed by Dr. Zoon in 1995 in that it was partly based on the degree to which the cells were manipulated ex vivo. Nonmanipulated or minimally manipulated cells, as defined by the 1995 proposal, would not require an IND exemption, but if the product was intended for interstate commerce, licensure of the product and the establishment would be required.

Interestingly, there has been some discussion as to whether a patient who experienced engraftment and who is returning home from an out-of-state transplant center at which his or her cells had been collected, stored, and infused would constitute interstate commerce. The Agency also indicated that manufacturers of PBPC would be required to register as blood establishments, must operate under cGMP, and would be subject to FDA inspection. The proposal stated that nonmanipulated PBPC can be licensed when they meet product specifications and standards for collection, processing, and storage and that these standards were currently under development by the Agency. Because of the likelihood of interstate commerce, manufacturers of allogeneic PBPC should obtain product and establishment licenses.

Procedures that resulted in manipulated HSC would include centrifugal elutriation, negative or positive cell selection by monoclonal antibody–based technology, and cells expanded ex vivo using cytokines. Manipulated PBPC would be subject to IND regulations and, as final biologic products, would be subject to licensure. Ancillary products used in the manufacture of PBPC may be regulated as medical devices (e.g., apheresis machines, purging and selection equipment, and collection and storage containers) or as drugs or biologic products (e.g., investigational agents administered to HSC donors for mobilization—unlicensed cytokines, anticoagulants added to the collection container and infused with the product, and storage media and cryoprotectants).

The development of potentially different regulatory strategies for HSC derived from a variety of sources, combined with the increasing use of non–HSC–based cellular therapies and transplants, prompted the Agency to re-evaluate its approached in 1997. This was aimed at developing a single regulatory program for all human cellular and tissue-based products. Previously regulation had been on a case-by-case basis, with the result that some tissues were regulated as medical devices (under §201 of the federal Food, Drug and Cosmetic Act), for example, heart valve allografts and umbilical cord vein grafts, whereas others were considered to be biologic products (under §351 of the Public Health Service Act), for example, some genetically manipulated cells and somatic cell therapy products.

In announcing its new approach, the FDA said that it sought to achieve several goals, primary among them being "the improved protection of the public health without the imposition of unnecessary restrictions on research, development, or the availability of new products." These proposals were published in early 1997 in two documents, "Reinventing the Regulation of Human Tissue" and "A Proposed Approach to the Regulation of Cellular and Tissue-Based Products".[7] The major change was to regulate according to the degree of potential risk associated with the particular product. It was thought that this would allow the Agency to manage its resources more effectively and would result in a more consistent approach.

The Proposed Approach document details the criteria that will be used to evaluate risk: the potential to transmit communicable disease; the manufacturing controls that are used during handling to prevent contamination and maintain viability and function; the clinical safety and efficacy of the products; the type of labeling that is required for proper use of the products and the kind of promotion that would be permissible; and, finally, how the Agency should monitor and communicate with the practitioners of HSCT. It is important to emphasize that this proposal deals with a wide variety of types of cells and tissues, but it specifically mentions HSC derived from peripheral and placental and/or umbilical cord blood. It excludes minimally manipulated bone marrow, as this falls under the purview of the Health Resources Service Administration. Based upon this strategy, minimally processed tissues that are transplanted from one person to another for their normal structural functions would be subject only to infectious disease screening and testing and to meeting requirements for good handling procedures but would not require FDA premarket review or marketing approval. These would, however, be required for cells and tissues that are processed extensively, combined with noncellular components, labeled and promoted for purposes other than their normal function, or have a systemic effect. The proposed system for relating the degree of regulation to potential risk is summarized in Table 65–1. Because ex vivo manipulation is considered to be a risk factor, the differentiation between extensive and minimal manipulation remains central to this regulatory strategy. In the proposal, minimal manipulation does not alter the biologic characteristics of the cells or their function or integrity. Selection procedures, such as enrichment of stem cells, could be considered to be minimal manipulation.

TABLE 65–1. PROPOSED RELATIONSHIP BETWEEN POTENTIAL RISK FACTORS AND DEGREE OF REGULATION FOR PERIPHERAL AND PLACENTAL/UMBILICAL CORD BLOOD HEMATOPOIETIC PROGENITOR CELLS

TRANSPLANT TYPE	PROPOSED ACTION	FDA SUBMISSION
Risk Factor: Disease Transmission		
Allogeneic	Follow cGTP Require disease screening	None
Risk Factor: Processing		
Autologous or family member and minimal manipulation	Follow cGTP	None
Unrelated or manipulated	Follow cGTP	IND/IDE–PMA/BLA (comply with future standards)
Risk Factor: Clinical Safety		
Unrelated *or* 1. Manipulated 2. Non-normal function 3. Combined with noncellular component	Collect safety and/or efficacy data	IND/IDE–PMA/BLA effectiveness criteria based on biologics (includes PBPC)
Risk Factor: Labeling and Registration		
All tissue except autologous tissue transplanted in a single surgical procedure	Clear, accurate, non-misleading labeling Notify FDA	Depending on product, FDA submission may be required Registration and listing required

cGTP, current good tissue practices; IND, investigational new drug; IDE, investigational device exemption; PMA, pre-market approval; BLA, biologics license application; PBPC, peripheral blood progenitor cells; FDA, Food and Drug Administration.

More-than-minimal manipulation would involve processing that altered the biologic characteristics, function, and integrity of the cells and would include genetic modification and ex vivo expansion in culture. These procedures would be subject to IND/investigational device exemption (IDE) and the pre-market approval (PMA) mechanisms of regulations. The Agency also proposed to establish a Tissue Reference Group to help in the classification of particular types of manipulation.

For the first time, the Agency also mentioned the development of current good tissue practices that would be applied to this area in addition to GMP requirements applicable to drugs and devices. It also indicates that the Agency would need to assess the state of the industry (as it did not know its full size and scope), so that it could be regulated effectively. They would, therefore, require facilities to register. Centers that prepare cells and tissues that would be subject to the proposed regulations described above (i.e., manipulated, prepared for non-homologous use, combined with noncellular components, or having a systemic effect, except in the case of autologous use or transplantation into a first-degree relative) would be required to register with the FDA and list the products that are manufactured. Registration was subsequently discussed more extensively in the proposed rule Establishment Registration and Listing for Manufacturers of Human Cellular and Tissue-Based Products, published in the Federal Register on May 14, 1998.[8]

In March 1998, CBER updated its guidance on somatic and gene therapy products.[9] This provided more specific information on the development and characterization of cell populations for therapeutic administration, including sections on collection, cell culture, development of master and working cell banks, producer cells, and materials that are used during manufacture. Release criteria are also discussed and cover identity, potency, viability, sterility, purity, and safety testing. The guidance additionally contains specific sections on the production, characterization, and release testing of vectors for gene therapy. Importantly, information is provided on the types of preclinical evaluation that should be performed on cellular and gene therapy products.

In 2000, the field of cellular and gene therapy was shaken by the death of a patient in the United States who had received direct injection of an adenoviral vector. This prompted widespread review of regulatory strategies, visits by the FDA to centers conducting gene therapy trials, congressional hearings, and a general re-evaluation of how such studies should be designed, approved, and monitored. The fallout from this is likely to have an impact on the final design of the regulatory approach.

CURRENT GOOD MANUFACTURING PRACTICES

A recurring theme throughout the regulatory proposals is that cell collection and processing facilities will be required to follow cGMP. As described earlier, this is a system that originated in the Food, Drug and Cosmetic Act and that has been implemented and enforced in the blood banking industry. cGMP were established by the FDA to ensure that products are manufactured under a controlled, auditable process.

TABLE 65–2. CURRENT GOOD MANUFACTURING PRACTICES—21 CFR PART 606, SUBPART B: PERSONNEL REQUIREMENTS

Employees must be adequate in number, training, education, and experience.
Capabilities must be commensurate with assigned tasks.
Unauthorized personnel to be excluded from area.
Qualified director represents center to CBER.
Director is responsible for employee discipline, performance, and training in SOP and cGMP.
Director must understand scientific principles and techniques.

CBER, Center for Biologics Evaluation and Research; cGMP, Current Good Manufacturing Practices; SOP, standard operating procedure.

In the area of HSC, this would translate to the use of a system of values by which cells are processed to produce a safe finished product that effectively meets a medical need. The major composite elements are documentation, validation, facilities, equipment, personnel, training, management of standard operating procedures (SOP) and errors, labeling, auditing, and process control. The regulations as they primarily pertain to manufacturers of blood and blood products are detailed in Parts 606 and 640 of Title 21 of the Code of Federal Regulations (CFR), whereas Part 607 describes establishment registration and product listing. Additional regulations are found in Parts within the 200 series, including cGMP for manufacturers of drugs (Part 210) and finished pharmaceuticals (Part 211). Blood establishments are required to comply with the provisions of both the 600 and 200 Series because these are regarded as complementary and the more-specific regulation takes precedence only when there is a conflict.

The following summary of the major components of Part 606 is intended to provide an idea of how cGMP are structured. This Part of the (CFR) is divided into seven subparts that cover (A) general provisions, (B) organization and personnel (Table 65–2), (C) plant and facilities (Table 65–3), (D) equipment (Tables 65–4 and 65–5), (F—subpart E is reserved) production and process controls (Table 65–6), (G) finished product control (Table 65–7), (H) laboratory controls (Table 65–8), and (I) records and reports (Table 65–9). The general provisions section provides definitions of terminology. The major components of

TABLE 65–3. CURRENT GOOD MANUFACTURING PRACTICES—21 CFR PART 606, SUBPART C: PLANT AND FACILITIES

Adequate space for all procedures, including
  Donor examination
  Blood withdrawal with minimal exposure risk
  Blood and component storage during testing
  Finished product storage quarantine, handling, disposal of unsuitable products
  Orderly collection, processing, testing, and storage
  Performance of leukapheresis
  Packaging, labeling, and finishing operations
Maintained in clean orderly manner and of size and construction to facilitate cleaning, maintenance, and operation
Adequate space for procedures performed
Adequate lighting, ventilation, and screening of open windows and doors
Adequate bathroom facilities and drains
Safe and sanitary disposal of trash, blood, and components

TABLE 65–4. CURRENT GOOD MANUFACTURING PRACTICES—21 CFR PART 606, SUBPART D: EQUIPMENT

Maintained in clean orderly manner and located to facilitate cleaning and maintenance
Regularly scheduled standardization and cleaning as prescribed in standard operating procedures
Sterilizers must achieve defined operating parameters

TABLE 65–6. CURRENT GOOD MANUFACTURING PRACTICES—21 CFR PART 606, SUBPART F: PRODUCTION AND PROCESS CONTROLS

There shall be written, easily accessible standard operation procedures for all steps, including
 Donor suitability criteria
 Methods for donor screening and normal test ranges
 Solutions and methods to ensure sterile collection
 Methods to relate product to the donor
 Collection procedures
 Method(s) for component preparation
 All tests on blood and components
 Pretransfusion testing (crossmatch, etc.)
 Investigation of adverse reactions
 Storage methods and methods for temperature control
 Length of expiration
 Criteria for reissue of returned blood
 Methods to relate component from donor to disposition
 Labeling procedures and precautions to avoid mix-ups
 Procedures for leukapheresis and plasma salvage
 Record review before release or distribution

the subparts are briefly summarized in Tables 65–2 through 65–9 and reveal several major themes that permeate cGMP.

One of the most important of these is documentation to (1) facilitate tracking of each stage of the process from collection of the cells to their final disposition and (2) provide records of the history and current status of the facility, equipment and personnel, and details of how each product was prepared, including associated reagents and supplies. The use and management of SOP is probably the most important feature of documentation. It is recognized that deviations from SOP may occur, but these must be documented. All SOP must be approved by the quality control unit (see later).

A second major theme is quality management, which was traditionally associated with industrial manufacturing but is now a high priority in most institutions and has become a growth industry for consultants. Traditional quality inspection/assurance involved sampling and evaluating the quality of the finished product using predetermined criteria, identifying the nature and source of problems, and then implementing changes in production to correct those problems. The newer model is that of prevention, in which the manufacturing process is strictly controlled and designed to prevent problems from resulting in the final release of defective products. As discussed by Zuck,[10] this newer model is particularly appropriate for cell preparation facilities, where there is usually no control over the quality of the "raw materials" and it may not be possible to test each lot—the graft that is processed.

The aim of cGMP is to provide a system for control of the manufacturing process. Under cGMP (Title 21 CFR Part 211.22) there must be a quality-control unit with the responsibility to approve or reject all components of the

process and all procedures and specifications. The unit also has the authority to review production records to ensure that no errors have occurred and to fully investigate any errors that do occur. These responsibilities and the procedures for quality control must be in writing, and "such written procedures shall be followed." The quality-control unit should be independent in that it should not be composed of personnel without the direct daily responsibility of performing the procedures under review, although the unit should be knowledgeable about the work performed. In smaller facilities, this model may not be possible; under these circumstances, quality review should be performed at defined intervals, not immediately after completion of the procedure. CBER has published quality-assurance guidelines for blood establishments, many components of which would be applicable for HSC collection and processing facilities.[11]

The most frequently voiced concern from those involved in HSC collection, processing, and transplantation relates to cGMP: the design and construction of facilities. The research origins of most graft processing procedures have frequently resulted in clinical processing being performed in basic research laboratories rather than in purpose-de-

TABLE 65–5. CURRENT GOOD MANUFACTURING PRACTICES—21 CFR PART 606, SUBPART D: SUPPLIES AND REAGENTS

Store in safe, sanitary, and orderly manner
Surfaces in contact with blood must be sterile, pyrogen-free, and nonreactive
Containers must be observed for damage and contamination before and after filling
If there is no expiration date, oldest lots must be used first
Use according to manufacturer's instructions
Wherever possible, use sterile disposable items
There must be written procedures for receipt, identification, storage, handling, sampling, testing, etc.
Storage should prevent contamination and should be off floor
Record lot numbers and test lots (sampling techniques are described)
Identify acceptable lots and use oldest first

TABLE 65–7. CURRENT GOOD MANUFACTURING PRACTICES—21 CFR PART 606, SUBPART G: FINISHED PRODUCT CONTROLS

 Labeling
  Separate area to avoid mix-ups
  Labeling controls
   Hold and proof labels on receipt
   Store in way to prevent mix-ups
   Destroy obsolete labels
   Use checks during labeling
   Must be clear and legible
  Container labels must follow Guidelines for Uniform Labeling of Blood and Blood Components
  Instruction circular providing adequate directions for use must be available for distribution if product is intended for transfusion

TABLE 65–8. CURRENT GOOD MANUFACTURING PRACTICES—21 CFR PART 606, SUBPART H: LABORATORY CONTROLS

Establish standards specifications and test to ensure safety, purity, potency, and effectiveness
Provision to monitor test reliability, accuracy, precision, and performance
Adequately identify and test samples to relate them to the unit being tested or the recipient
Compatibility testing

signed facilities. This space is often inadequate and poorly designed for these procedures. At the other end of the spectrum, commercial organizations are spending large amounts of money to construct state-of-the-art cell processing centers that meet or exceed the cGMP followed by pharmaceutical manufacturers. If these standards were applied to most hospital or university-based cell processing facilities, they would have to close permanently because it is unlikely that the resources would be available to bring them into compliance.

The ultimate solution to this problem lies in compromise between the two extremes. This can be reached by considering the cost/benefit/risk ratios for the procedure that is being performed and the ability of a facility to comply with other aspects of cGMP as they relate to adequate space. There is a long history of successful routine HSC processing under non-cGMP conditions, but much can be learned by applying the cGMP philosophy (e.g., quality control, documentation, process control) in this environment without rebuilding every facility. In the case of extensive or prolonged ex vivo manipulation and culture, the necessity of specialized facilities should be examined case by case. When new facilities are being planned, it is wise to anticipate that extensive cell manipulation will become a routine component of many HSC therapies.

As indicated above, the FDA has voiced its intention to

TABLE 65–9. CURRENT GOOD MANUFACTURING PRACTICES—21 CFR PART 606, SUBPART I: RECORDS AND REPORTS

Must be maintained concurrently with each step during collection, processing, testing, storage, and distribution
Include
• Identity of person performing work
• Test results and interpretation
• Product expiration dates
• Complete history of work performed
• Lot numbers of supplies and reagents
• Donor records (described in detail)
• Information on storage and distribution
• Compatibility testing
• Transfusion reaction reports and complaints
• General information, to include:
   Sterilization records of supplies and reagents
   Responsible personnel
   Errors and accidents
   Maintenance records for equipment and facilities
   Details of supplies and reagents
   Disposition of rejected supplies and reagents
   Use of donor number for tracking
   Record retention
   Identification of unsuitable donors from records

develop a system of current good tissue practices (cGTP). These have not been finalized at the time of writing, but they will presumably cover the areas not adequately addressed by cGMP regulations covering drugs, devices, and blood-banking establishments. The Agency has stated that compliance with cGMP will remain a requirement where appropriate, even when cGTP is enforced.

PRODUCT VERSUS PROCESS

The components of cGMP described earlier were originally developed for drug manufacturers to ensure the safety and purity of the final product. The philosophy has more recently been extended to blood establishments, which necessitated the development of specific regulations (Parts 606 and 640 Title 21 CFR), many of which could be applied to HSC collection, processing, and storage.

There are, however, important differences between HSC "products" and blood components. In many cases, within limits, blood components can be used generically to support a variety of patients, and the patient's life rarely depends on a particular unit of a defined component. The reverse is true for HSC grafts, in which even unmanipulated HSC are designated for use by a particular individual. Criteria that would be mandatory for the acceptance of a blood component (e.g., sterility, negative screen for all infectious disease testing) may have to be waived for certain HSC grafts because of the unique nature of the product. In addition, present knowledge makes it almost impossible to define product specifications for these grafts.

Our primary criterion is that the cells should restore hematopoiesis and immune function in the recipient. For certain types of transplants, other parameters, such as T-cell content, extent of removal of tumor cells, and cellular composition of ex vivo expanded populations, may also be of great significance. It is, however, fair to say that there is no general consensus on which specific parameters should be measured and even how they should be measured. There is also little agreement on the value of numbers obtained from in vitro assays as to their value in predicting clinical outcome. Our greatest level of comfort in characterizing grafts comes from transplants for which we have the largest amount of clinical data (e.g., HLA-matched sibling donors, nonmanipulated autologous grafts), from which criteria such as nucleated cell doses of 1×10^8/kg recipient body weight have originated. Even here, however, these numbers are recognized to be targets rather than absolute requirements because engraftment is rapid and stable after patients receive much smaller cell doses, and vice versa.

As we progress to more-extensive types of graft manipulation, the characterization of the "product" becomes even more difficult because this therapy is in early evolution. The regulatory pressure, however, is greatest at this end of the continuum (Fig. 65–1). The challenge to the investigator and the regulatory agencies is to develop a system that does not freeze a new therapy at a suboptimal point in its development but allows it to evolve and improve as experience is gained. This mechanism must also ensure that (1) protocols are designed to protect the patient and generate useful data to evaluate safety and efficacy and (2) that

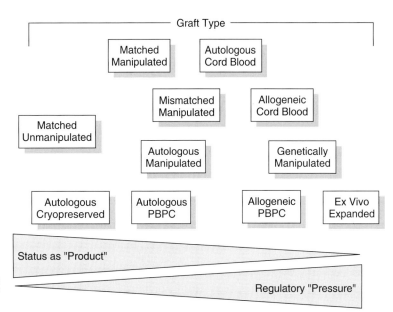

FIGURE 65–1. The opposing forces of regulatory pressure and status of hematopoietic stem cell grafts as "products." PBPC, peripheral blood progenitor cell.

grafts are collected, manipulated, and administered under conditions that meet the appropriate components of cGMP.

IMPLEMENTATION OF cGMP IN AN EXISTING FACILITY

Implementation of cGMP into HSC therapy is underway in North America, but the specific requirements for this field are still under development. There is, therefore, no recipe book approach that can be used to bring a facility into compliance, although Zuck has indicated how cGMP may be applied to cord blood banking.[12] Rather, until the regulatory strategy is clarified, the major components of the cGMP process need to be identified, implemented, tracked, and improved on an ongoing basis within any facility.

For collection and processing that is performed in a blood bank or regional blood center, the cGMP approach should already be in place and can be implemented for HSC collection and processing more easily. For laboratory and many hospital-based facilities, the concept of cGMP is entirely new and may seem to be overwhelming at first glance. As described earlier, however, the philosophy is based on a number of key elements that can be readily incorporated into the daily operation of most facilities.

First and foremost is training to ensure familiarity with cGMP. As defined in the regulations, this is the responsibility of the facility director. An understanding of the process is central to its successful application. In mixed research/clinical facilities, it is extremely important that the entire staff understands the basic principles so that the apparently inflexible approach of the clinical laboratory staff and the somewhat more liberal approach of most research staffs can coexist. A number of organizations, both commercial and professional, offer courses in cGMP; alternatively, staff members can visit facilities in which the system is already in place.

A major hurdle for most new facilities is documentation. The preparation of such components as SOP, flow sheets,

maintenance logs, and equipment files can be daunting. Most facilities that have gone through this process are sympathetic and are usually more than willing to share their forms, records, and files with others. In addition, computer templates for preparing SOP are available from the National Committee on Clinical Laboratory Standards. A basic SOP should include a title page (to include such items as protocol name, version, and effective dates), the purpose of the procedure, the scope of the procedure (the principle and the circumstances under which it is to be used), the materials and reagents required, a detailed description of the procedure, safety considerations, expected end-points, the responsibilities of the staff members involved, literature references, completed sample flow charts, signature pages for authors and staff, and a recorded history of revisions.

A flow chart for each product type, from collection to distribution, is of great value because it allows the identification of critical control points (i.e., the major steps in the procedure). These in turn can be used as "anchors" for the development of the quality management plan and the SOP. SOP should be sufficiently detailed to allow a trained staff member to perform the procedure but not so detailed that deviations must be routinely documented to cover inherent variability in the process due, for example, to the heterogeneity of the starting material.

Once the paper and electronic tracking system is in place, equal attention must be paid to ensure that it is used, maintained, reviewed, and updated as required. CBER has published guidelines for the validation of computer systems in blood establishments, which should also apply in large part to HSC collection and processing facilities.[13] As procedures evolve, or if specific changes have to be made during a procedure, these must be documented and approved. Annual review of manuals is mandatory.

Implementation of quality management systems is a requirement,[11] and in most larger centers there will be an institution-wide program that can be used by the HSC facility. In the traditional clinical testing laboratory, proficiency testing, either through an external agency (such as the College of American Pathologists) or by parallel testing of unknown samples with an approved facility, is a prerequisite to going "on-line." For cell processing facilities, there is no similar formal proficiency testing program, and it is not feasible to split grafts between centers for this purpose. Again, the best solution is to train personnel in an established facility and perform the first clinical procedures under the supervision of staff members from the established facility. Results from the clinical procedure should be reviewed regularly for consistency and to establish retrospective validation (i.e., the expected performance characteristics and range of results for the procedure). This would normally be carried out prospectively for most procedures, but this is impossible for most clinical-scale graft manipulation techniques. For in vitro testing procedures, prospective validation and parallel testing can be easily performed before the test is used clinically. In parallel, a formal training and competency testing program, with the associated documentation, should be established for the staff.

A system must be developed for the management of errors. Error reporting should be encouraged as part of the continuous quality-improvement process, and procedures should be changed to ensure error resolution and prevention. In parallel, facilities should develop a written audit program to search for unrecognized errors and ensure ongoing compliance.

For guidance regarding specific regulatory requirements, centers are advised to contact CBER directly. At this time, questions regarding procedures that involve ex vivo manipulation, cell expansion, and/or gene therapy should be directed to the Office of Therapeutics Research and Review. Inquiries regarding minimal manipulation and cord blood transplantation should be referred to the Division of Blood Applications of the Office of Blood Research and Review. Centers that are involved in collection of peripheral blood progenitor cells should contact the FDA to determine whether they should apply for establishment registration. The Agency is currently inspecting facilities involved in HSC collection and processing.

VOLUNTARY STANDARDS, INSPECTION, AND ACCREDITATION

In the mid-1990s, in the absence of specific governmental regulations, a number of organizations developed standards for HSC facilities and provided voluntary inspection and accreditation for their members. The most specific and comprehensive are those published by the FAHCT,[2] which cover collection, processing, manipulation, storage, and clinical transplantation. This document has now been adopted with minimal modifications by the Canadian and Mexican bone marrow transplant organizations and by ISHAGE-Europe and the European Group for Blood and Marrow Transplantation and their parallel inspection and accreditation arm—JACIE (the Joint Accreditation Committee of ISHAGE-Europe).

In March 2000, FAHCT and NetCord (the European pan-national cord blood transplant cooperative) published a draft first edition of Standards for Cord Blood Collection, Processing, Testing, Banking, Selection, and Release, to address the more specific requirements of placental and/or umbilical cord blood HSCT.

The AABB had previously included some standards for HSC in section Q of its Standards for Blood Bank and Transfusion Services. These included infectious disease testing, nucleated cell dose, labeling, record-keeping, and infusion. In 1996 they published a stand-alone standards document that covered HSC collection and processing but did not address clinical transplantation.[14] There were a number of meetings between FAHCT and the AABB to harmonize the two documents, with the result that they were remarkably consistent in their requirements. In 1998, the AABB released a draft second edition of their standards in a format based on the ISO 9000 approach to quality systems. The ISO (International Standards Organization) system and its various subsystems (ISO9001/2/3) is a quality-assurance system that is applicable to most processes that involve design, development, production, installation, servicing, final inspection, and testing. It provides a more generic approach in which the center establishes and validates the required processes to comply with the standard, rather than these being specifically defined by the standard itself.

These documents will undoubtedly have been forwarded to the FDA, who in January 1998 had requested submission of proposed standards for unrelated allogeneic peripheral and placental and/or umbilical cord blood hematopoietic stem/progenitor cell products. The Agency indicated that it also wished to receive supporting clinical and laboratory data, such as criteria for the acceptance of a unit of HSC. This could include numbers of CD34 + cells. The deadline for the submission of this information was Jan. 20, 2000.

CONCLUSION

There is no doubt that regulation of hematopoietic cell therapy, and cellular therapies in general, is imminent in the United States, and that other countries are not far behind. The development of a regulatory strategy has been complex, initially being based primarily on the use of genetic manipulation or extensive ex vivo manipulation. This subsequently was modified, based on the increasing use of HSC derived from other sources and the need to evaluate the safety and efficacy of new procedures and devices for cell manipulation. In an attempt to develop a more consistent approach, the FDA has now indicated that it will adopt a unified strategy for all types of cellular and genetic therapies, based upon the potential degree of risk posed to the potential recipient and the donor. The final regulations have yet to be published; however, there are several recurring themes that are likely to be central to the final rules. These include the use of cGMP (and the proposed cGTP) by facilities collecting, manipulating, and storing HSC; the registration of facilities performing these procedures; and more rigorous regulation of procedures that include extensive manipulation of the cells. Recent developments have placed gene therapy protocols under increased governmental scrutiny, and it is possible that this scrutiny will have an impact on the eventual regulatory approach. The challenge will be to develop a system that assures that patients are offered safe and potentially effective therapies while recognizing that the field is still in an early stage of development and will require flexibility to evolve.

REFERENCES

1. Menitove JE: Controversies in transfusion medicine: the recent emphasis on good manufacturing practices and the pharmaceutical manufacturing approach damages blood banking and transfusion medicine as medical care activities. Transfusion 33:439–442, 1995.
2. Standards for Hematopoietic Progenitor Cell Collection, Processing and Transplantation, 1st ed. Omaha, NE, Foundation for the Accreditation of Hematopoietic Cell Therapy, 1996.
3. American Association of Blood Banks outraged by court decision in HIV case. Random Harvest News Section. J Hematother 5:688–689, 1996.
4. New York State Department of Health: Stem Cell Banks. Subpart 58-5 of Title 10 (health) of the official compilation of codes, rules and regulations of the State of New York. New York State Register, October 2, 1991.
5. Ciavarella D, Linden JV: The regulation of hematopoietic stem cell collection and storage: the New York State approach. J Hematother 1:201–214, 1992.
6. Draft document concerning the regulation of placental/umbilical cord blood stem cell products intended for transplantation or further manufacturing into injectable products. Federal Register, February 26, 1996.
7. Proposed Approach to Regulation of Cellular and Tissue-Based Products: Availability and Public Meeting. Fed Regist 62:9721–9722, 1997.
8. Establishment Registration and Listing for Manufacturers of Human Cellular and Tissue-Based Products. Fed Regist 63:26744–26755, 1998.
9. Guidance for Human Somatic Cell Therapy and Gene Therapy: Guidance for Industry. Bethesda, MD, Center for Biologics Evaluation and Research, March 1998.
10. Zuck T: Current good manufacturing practices. Transfusion 35:955–966, 1995.
11. Quality Assurance Guidelines for Blood Establishments. Bethesda, MD, Center for Biologics Evaluation and Research, 1992.
12. Zuck T: The applicability of cGMP to cord blood banking. J Hematother 5:135–137, 1996.
13. Validation of computer systems in blood establishments. Bethesda, MD, Center for Biologics Evaluation and Research, 1993.
14. Standards for Hematopoietic Progenitor Cells. Bethesda, MD, American Association of Blood Banks, 1996.

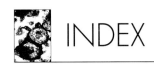

INDEX

Note: Page numbers in *italics* indicate figures; those followed by t indicate tables.

International Prognostic Scoring System (IPSS), for myelodysplastic syndrome, 52–54, 53t, 54t, 55
International Society of Hematotherapy and Graft Engineering (ISHAGE), stem cell quantification guidelines of, 300–302
Interstitial infiltrates, 571t
Interstitial pneumonia, and veno-occlusive disease of liver, 544
  cytomegalovirus, 516
  idiopathic, 563–564
  in acute myelogenous leukemia, 18
  in aplastic anemia, 8
Intestinal stoma, 601
Intracellular ice formation, in cryopreservation, 314–315, 315
Intracytoplasmic sperm injection (ICSI), 631–632
Intravenous immunoglobulin (IVIG), for adenoviruses, 421
  for bacterial infection, 430
  for chronic GVHD, 611–612, 618, 621
  for cytomegalovirus, 416
    interstitial pneumonia due to, 516
  for immunodeficiency disorders, 163
  for thrombocytopenia, 591
Invasive pulmonary aspergillosis, 568–569
Investigational new drug (IND) exemption, 724
IPS (idiopathic pneumonia syndrome), 563–564
IPSS (International Prognostic Scoring System), for myelodysplastic syndrome, 52–54, 53t, 54t, 55
Iron overload, in thalassemia, 186, 187
Irradiation. See Radiation therapy; Total body irradiation (TBI).
Ischemic stroke, 585
ISHAGE (International Society of Hematotherapy and Graft Engineering), stem cell quantification guidelines of, 300–302
Isolation, for bacterial infection, 430
  psychological effects of, 676, 686–687
Isotope controls, for rare-event analysis, 302–303
Itraconazole, for aspergillosis, 515, 569
  for fungal infection prophylaxis, 439–440, 440t
  with allogeneic transplantation, 447
  with autologous transplantation, 446
IVIG. See Intravenous immunoglobulin (IVIG).

J
Jaundice, evaluation of, 600
  in hepatic GVHD, 548–549
  in veno-occlusive disease of liver, 545, 545t

K
Kaplan-Meier survival curve, 705, 706
Keratan sulfate, in Morquio syndrome, 173
Keratinocytes, necrotic, in GVHD, 533, 533
Keratitis, with chronic GVHD, 610
Kerley lines, 571t
Kerr sign, 599
Kidneys. See Renal entries.
Klebsiella, pneumonia due to, 566
  posttransplant infection with, 511
Kostmann syndrome, 156t, 160
Kruskal-Wallis test, 708
Kurtzke Extended Status Disability Scale, 205–206, 206t

L
Laboratory controls, current good manufacturing practices for, 728t
Laboratory evaluation, of abdominal pain, 600
Laboratory testing, of umbilical cord blood, 293, 294t
LAD (leukocyte adhesion deficiency), 156t, 158
LAI (lupus activity index), 209
LAK (lymphokine-activated killer) cells, immunomodulation after transplantation with, 357, 662–663
  in graft-versus-leukemia effect, 637
Laminar airflow (LAF), for fungal infections, 438
Lamivudine, for hepatitis B virus, 420
Laparoscopy, 601
Large bowel crypts, in GVHD, 534, 534–535
Late graft failure. See Graft failure, late (secondary).
Lectin, for GVHD, 459, 459t
  with mismatched related bone marrow transplantation, 461, 461t
Length of stay (LOS), 676
Leukapheresis, donor recruitment for, 292
  donor tolerance to, 278
  in Gaucher disease, 197, 201
  large-volume, 280–281
  PBPC collection via, 279–281
Leukemia, acute lymphoblastic. See Acute lymphoblastic leukemia (ALL).
  acute myelogenous. See Acute myelogenous leukemia (AML).
  chronic lymphocytic, 95–98, 97, 97, 98
  chronic myelogenous. See Chronic myelogenous leukemia (CML).
  chronic myelomonocytic, 49, 50t, 51, 52
  conditioning regimen for, 408
  cost-effectiveness of HSCT for, 715, 716t
  efficacy of HSCT for, 715
  relapse of, 638, 639–640, 640t, 641, 641t
Leukemia tolerance, 637–638
Leukocyte adhesion deficiency (LAD), 156t, 158
Leukocyte count, and graft failure, 526–527
Leukocyte infusion, donor. See Donor lymphocyte infusion (DLI).
Leukocyte-depleted blood products, 684
Leukocytosis, due to G-CSF, 276–277
Leukodystrophy(ies), 170t, 174–180
  aspartylglucosaminuria as, 179
  fucosidosis as, 179
  Gaucher disease as, 178
  globoid cell, HSCT for, 176–177
    in utero transplantation for, 221
  GM₂ gangliosidoses as, 179–180
  mannosidosis as, 178–179
  metachromatic, 177–178
  mucolipidosis II (I-cell disease) as, 180
  Niemann-Pick disease as, 179
  Sandhoff disease as, 179–180
  Tay-Sachs disease as, 179–180
  Wolman disease as, 180
  X-linked adreno-, 174
    cerebral, 174–176
Leukoencephalopathy, 585
Leydig cell dysfunction, 630, 631
LH (luteinizing hormone), in males, 631
Lichenoid GVHD, 615–616, 616t
Linear regression analysis, 708
Linkage disequilibrium, 238
Lipofuscinosis, neuronal ceroid, 170t
Lipogranulomatosis, Farber, 170t
Lipomatosis, epidural, due to steroids, 580
Live attenuated virus vaccines, 611
Live/dead cell discrimination, absolute CD34+ cell counting using, 304

Liver. See also Hepatic entries; Hepatitis.
  pretransplantation evaluation of, 229
Liver biopsy, for veno-occlusive disease of liver, 546, 558
Liver disease, 541–553
  bacterial, 551t, 552
  cholangitis lenta as, 551t, 552
  drug-induced, 551t, 552–553
  fungal, 551t, 552
  in GVHD, acute, 548–551
    clinical manifestations of, 532, 548–549, 558
    histopathology of, 533–534, 534, 549–550, 550, 558
    mechanism of damage for, 550–551
    prognosis and treatment for, 551, 558–559
  chronic, 559, 617, 619t
  mycobacterial, 552
  veno-occlusive, 541–548
    clinical features of, 544–546, 545t
    coagulation system in, 543
    cytokines in, 543
    defined, 541
    diagnostic studies of, 546
    histopathology of, 541–542, 542
    incidence of, 544–545
    likelihood of subsequent complications with, 492t, 493
    morphologic changes in, 542–543
    nursing care for, 685–686
    onset of, 545
    outcome of, 545–546
    pathophysiology of, 542
    platelet transfusions and, 493, 494t
    prediction of, 546–547
    prophylaxis for, 547
    protein C and antithrombin III and, 493, 493, 494t, 495t
    risk factors for, 543–544
    treatment of, 547–548
  viral, 551–552, 551t
Liver transplantation, aplastic anemia after, 10
  for veno-occlusive disease of liver, 548
Liver/spleen scintigraphy, of veno-occlusive disease of liver, 546
Log rank test, 709
Logistic regression analysis, 706–707
  multivariable, 707–708
Long-term bone marrow culture (LTBMC). See Ex vivo stem cell expansion.
Long-term bone marrow culture (LTBMC) assay, 355
Long-term culture initiating cell (LTC-IC) assay, 355
Long-term follow-up study, in phase II clinical trials, 699
LOS (length of stay), 676
Loyola regimen, for ovarian carcinoma, 398, 399
Lung(s). See also Pulmonary entries.
  biopsy of, 572
  normal defense mechanisms of, 566
  pretransplantation evaluation of, 228
Lupus activity index (LAI), 209
Lupus erythematosus, systemic, 207–209, 210, 210t
  animal models of, 204t
  autologous HSCT for, 207–209, 210, 210t, 212t
Luteinizing hormone (LH), in males, 631
Lymphoblastic leukemia, acute. See Acute lymphoblastic leukemia (ALL).
Lymphoblastic lymphoma, 78

ISBN 0-443-07622-7

90038

9 780443 076220